THE ENCYCLOPEDIA OF AMERICAN CITIES

THE
ENCYCLOPEDIA
OF
AMERICAN
CITIES

BY THE EDITORIAL STAFF OF
UNIBOOK, INC

ORY MAZAR NERGAL
EDITOR IN CHIEF

E.P. DUTTON
NEW YORK

First published in 1980 by E. P. Dutton, a Division of Elsevier-Dutton
Publishing Company, Inc., New York

Copyright © 1980 by Unibook, Inc.
2323 South Voss Road, Houston, Texas 77052
(713) 977-2950
All rights reserved. Printed in U.S.A.

For information contact: E.P. Dutton, 2 Park Avenue, New York, N.Y. 10016

Library of Congress Catalog Card Number: 80-66112
ISBN: 0-525-93133-3

Published simultaneously in Canada
by Clarke, Irwin & Company Lmited,
Toronto and Vancouver
10 9 8 7 6 5 4 3 2 1

First Edition

TABLE OF CONTENTS

TABLE OF CONTENTS (Continued)

APPENDIXES

FOREWORD

While the American countryside was always the source, the base and the root of our economy, it was the American city that became the hub of progress, the setting for the great strides of achievement that is the great American contribution to human civilization.

Always the scene of electrified action, the American City is a place of restless dynamism, industrious drive and continuous change. City life is an interlocking network of activity. Indeed, it is the complexity of the workings of a large city, and the need to know about each major facet of it, that created the demand for a major comprehensive reference book to provide detailed information about the makeup of our cities. THE ENCYCLOPEDIA OF AMERICAN CITIES was created to fill that need.

The ENCYCLOPEDIA is a compendium of facts designed to serve the needs of the scholar, the student, the researcher, the businessman and the traveler, as well as the general reader. Individual sections are devoted to each of the 166 cities in the United States with populations of 100,000 or more. In addition to basic information describing a city's location and environs, such statistical facts and figures as those relating to population growth or decline, ethnic distribution, climatic conditions, economic development and banking activities are included.

A special section is devoted to the topography of the individual areas, embracing such components as soil, mountains, lakes, rivers, bayous, oceans and other characteristics of the terrain of each city. Flora and fauna comprise another independent section, in which plants and animals found in each area are listed. A transportation section consists of pertinent information concerning freeways, railroads, airports, airlines and bus lines. Radio stations as well as television broadcasting facilities are meticulously listed along with their national affiliations and the types of programs they feature. Newspapers and journals are described by name and frequency of publication.

The pulse of any city best appears in its history. Full sections are devoted to each city's origins, development and government as well as landmarks and sightseeing spots. Other sections include significant information on each city's most widely recognized hotels and motels, hospitals and clinics, universities, colleges and libraries, sporting events and teams. Sections on entertainment and cultural activities contain repertoires of annual events as well as descriptions of major festivals, museums, galleries, theaters, symphonies and operas, and dance and ballet performances. Such recreational facilities as resorts, golf courses, skating rinks, ski areas, tennis courts and parks are also portrayed.

To outline the distinctive features that contribute to the unique character of each city, maps as well as photographs are included. In addition, the work is fully and extensively indexed according to such various criteria as geographical features, population, size, zip code, area code and national legislative representatives.

A remarkable collection of information, THE ENCYCLOPEDIA OF AMERICAN CITIES will be revised and updated periodically in response to changes in the urban centers of the nation, which together constitute the heartbeat of our American civilization.

AKRON
OHIO

CITY LOCATION-SIZE-EXTENT. Akron, the seat of Summit Co., encompasses 58 sq. mi., 35 mi. S of Cleveland at 40°55' N lat. and 81°31' W long. The second largest city in NE OH, Akron is 40 mi. S of Lake Erie. Its met. area extends into surrounding Portage, Medina, Wayne and Stark counties. The Cuyahoga and the Tuscarawas rivers form parts of the city's N and S borders.

TOPOGRAPHY. The terrain of Akron, which is located in the Appalachian plateau region, is characterized by substantial hills and deep valleys, with rolling to flat areas in-between. There is at least one major hill in every quadrant of the city, whose name means "high place" in Greek. Its elev. ranges from 760' to 1200', with a mean of 1080'. Within the met. area are Summit and Nesmith lakes, parts of the OH and Erie canals and Portage Lakes which are five mi S of the city.

CLIMATE. Akron's climate is considerably influenced by Lake Erie, which tempers cold air masses moving into the area and also causes brief but heavy snow squalls during the winter. Spring generally arrives late in Akron, and summers are moderately warm and humid. There is a considerable amount of morning fog in the fall. Monthly mean temps. range from 26.7°F in Jan. to 72.3°F in July; the annual mean temp. is 49.7°F. The annual avg. rainfall of 36.38" is distributed throughout the year. Most of the 48.2" of snowfall occurs from Dec. to Mar. The RH ranges from 53% to 87%. The growing

season avgs. 166 days. Akron lies in the ESTZ and observes DST.

FLORA AND FAUNA. Animals native to Akron include the opossum, deer and raccoon. Common birds are the cardinal, robin, flickers, blue jay, thrasher and woodpecker. Frogs, turtles and snakes, including the venomous rattlesnake and the N copperhead, inhabit the area. Typical trees are the maple, oak, poplar, birch and dogwood. Flowering plants include the trillum and daisy.

POPULATION. According to the US census, the pop. of Akron in 1970 was 275,425. In 1978, it was estimated to have decreased to 245,000.

ETHNIC GROUPS. In 1978, the ethnic distribution of Akron was estimated to be 82.2% Caucasian, 17.3% Black and 0.7% Hispanic. (A percentage of the Hispanic total is included in the Caucasian total.)

TRANSPORTATION. Interstate hwys. 71, 76, 77, 80, 271 and 277, US hwy. 224 and state rts 5, 8, 18, 91, 93, 162 and 241 pass through Akron. The city is also served by four *railroads*, the Chessie System (B&O), ConRail, Akron & Barberton Belt and the Akron, Canton & Youngstown, a division of Norfolk & Western. *Airlines* serving the Akron-Canton Regional and Akron-Fulton Municipal airports are: US Air and UA. *Bus lines* are the Met. Regional Transit Authority, Trailways and Greyhound.

COMMUNICATIONS. Communications, broadcasting and print media serving Akron are: *AM radio stations* WHLO 640 (Indep., Contemp.); WSLR 1350 (ABC/E, C&W) and WAKR 1590 (Group Owned, News, Talk); *FM radio stations* WAUP 88.1 (ABC/I, Jazz, Spec. Ethnic); WAPS 89.1 (Indep., Educ.); WKDD 96.5 (Indep., AOR) and WAEZ 97.5; *television stations* WAKR, Ch. 23 (ABC) and WEAO, Ch. 49 (Educ.); *press*: one major newspaper is published in the city, the *Beacon Journal*, issued evenings and Sun. mornings. The *Cleveland Plain Dealer*, published daily and Sun., is widely distributed in Akron. *The Reporter* is a black weekly. Other publications serving the area include *Amateur Baseball News*, *Tire Review*, *Automotive Chain Store*, *Brake and Front End*, *Jobber/Retailer* and *Modern Tire Dealer*.

HISTORY. Akron was founded as a village in 1825 by Gen. Perkins and others, who expected the OH Canal to pass through the area. After the canal was opened to

A redeveloped area of the old Ohio Canal in central Akron, Ohio

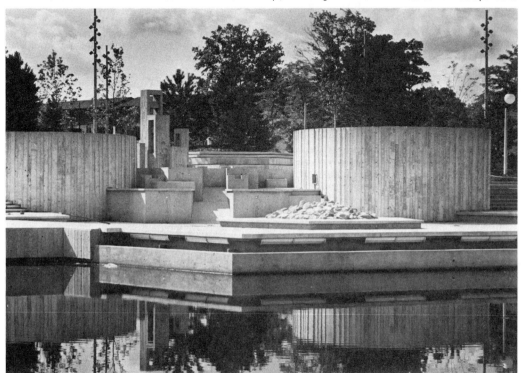

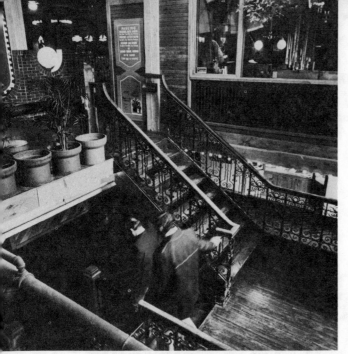

Interior view of Quaker Square, Akron, Ohio

traffic in 1827, Akron boomed, and was incorporated as a town in 1836. Plants which manufactured a variety of products were located on or near the canal. In 1863, German merchant Ferdinand Schumacher established a cereal mill in the city, founding what became a thriving cereal manufacturing industry. In 1865, Akron received a city charter. When B.F. Goodrich established a rubber factory in the city in 1870, it marked the beginning of a rubber trade that would eventually lead to Akron's prominence as "Rubber Capital of the World". By the end of the 1800s, Akron had become famous as a producer of farm machinery and clay products. The city grew steadily in the 1900s—its pop. soared from 69,000 to 209,000 between 1910 and 1920 —and eventually became the fifth largest city in OH.

GOVERNMENT. Akron has a strong mayor-council form of govt. The mayor, elected to a four-year term, is not a member of the council, which consists of 13 members. Ten councillors are elected by ward to two-year terms, while three are elected at large to four-year terms.

ECONOMY AND INDUSTRY. Akron is world headquarters for four intl. corps. with annual sales of more than one billion dollars. Rubber, plastics and chemicals are the predominant products. The city is the center of the nation's trucking industry. Non-electrical machinery, research and salt-mining are other significant parts of the city's industrial base. Recently, provision of services has increased, while production of goods has decreased. Avg. income per capita in 1978 was $4,802. The labor force totaled 115,000, while unemployment was 5.5% in 1978.

BANKING. There are five commercial banks and eight savings and loan assns. in Akron. In 1978, total deposits for the five banks headquartered in the city were $1,890,416,000 and the total assets were $2,282,744,000. Among the banks serving the city are BancOhio Natl., First Natl., Centran, Firestone and Goodyear.

HOSPITALS. There are four hospitals in Akron, Akron Gen. Medical Center, Akron City Gen., St. Thomas Gen. and Akron Children's Hosp. Portage Path Comm. Mental Health Center and Edwin Shaw Hosp., a treatment center for alcoholism, offer specialized medical treatment. The city fire dept. provides paramedic ambulance service.

EDUCATION. The U of Akron, a state-supported institution, offers engineering and liberal arts courses, as well as advanced programs in rubber and polymer chemistry. Established in 1870 as Buchtel Col., the U became the Municipal U of Akron in 1913 and achieved state-U status in 1967. Full-time undergrad. enrollment was approx. 23,000 in 1978, with more than 3,200 full-time grad. students. Other colleges and research institutions include NE OH University's Col. of Medicine (NEOUCOM)— established by both the U of Akron and nearby Kent State U in 1973 to prepare physicians oriented to the practice of primary care and family medicine at the comm. level—Hammel-Actual Business Col. and the McKim Technical Institute. Within a 40 mi. radius of the city, there are 24 colleges and universities. There are 46 elementary, 10 jr. and nine sr. high schools; 21 parochial schools—three of them high schools—as well as two private elementary and two private high schools. Libs. include the Akron-Summit Co. Public—over 100 years old—with 10 city and seven co. branches, the Akron Summit Co. Law and the U of Akron Bierce Lib. and Learning Resource Center.

ENTERTAINMENT. Intl. festivals, with street dances, ethnic food and entertainment, are held annually in Akron on May 30, July 4 and Labor Day. The annual All-American Soap Box Derby (Aug.), The Firestone Tournament of Champions—the largest stop on the pro bowlers' tour—are also held in the city. Akron, the "World Capital of Golf", is the site of the annual World Series of Golf, the fifth major tournament event, held at the Firestone Country Club. The 1960, 1966 and 1975 PGA Golf Tournaments were also held in the city. Akron is the home of the Professional Bowlers Assn. and the Natl. Headquarters of Amateur Baseball. The Cavaliers of the NBA and the Force Indoor Soccer Team of the NASL play at the 22,000-seat Coliseum located nearby in Summit Co. Other sports events are held at the Rubber Bowl of the U of Akron. The U's Zips participate in 13 intercollegiate sports.

ACCOMMODATIONS. There are several hotels and motels in Akron, including the Hilton, Holiday and Ramada inns and Travelodge.

FACILITIES. The 7,400-acre Akron met. park system includes 73 city parks, featuring a children's zoo and several swimming pools. Cuyahoga Valley Natl. Recreation Area, located on the edge of the city, extends for almost 30 mi. and encompasses the Cuyahoga River and parts of the old OH Canal. Swimming, hiking, water skiing, fishing and boating facilities are available on the 75 mi. of shoreline of the Portage Lakes chain S of the city. The 23-acre Lee R. Jackson Field of the U of Akron provides football and soccer fields, softball and baseball diamonds, an all-weather track, tennis courts and basketball courts.

CULTURAL ACTIVITIES. The Edwin J. Thomas Performing Arts Center on the campus of the U of Akron is the home of the Kenley Players, a theatrical group, and the Akron Symphony Orchestra. The OH Ballet, Tuesday Musical Club and Children's Concert Society, as well as other

Akron, Ohio

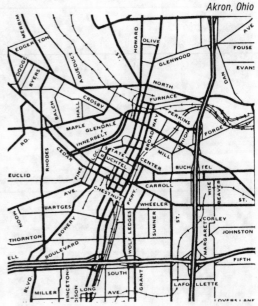

groups, also perform here. The Weathervane and Coach House theaters feature local dramatic performances. The 1835 Perkins Mansion built by Col. Simon Perkins, son of Akron's founder, houses a museum of old firearms and toys. Galleries in the city include the Akron Art Institute and Davis Art Gallery, located on the U of Akron Campus. The Cleveland Symphony Orchestra performs at the Blossom Music Center, eight mi. N of Akron, every summer.

LANDMARKS AND SIGHTSEEING SPOTS. The 1929 Akron Civic Theater, restored by the Comm. Hall Foundation and listed on the Natl. Register of Historic Places, houses a huge Wurlitzer theater organ and still presents films as well as other events. Also located in the city is the Stan Hywet Hall and Gardens, a 75-room English Tudor Revival mansion, built from 1911 to 1915 by Frank Seiberling, founder of Seiberling and Goodyear rubber companies. The grounds, open for tours—as are 28 art and antique-filled rooms of the house—contain a formal Japanese garden. Quaker Sq. in downtown Akron is a former Quaker Oats mill complex which has been converted into specialty shops, restaurants and the Railways of America Museum, which houses the largest model train display in the world. A unique Akron architectural landmark is the Goodyear Air Dock, the world's largest building without interior supports, which creates its own atmospheric changes. The 1825 Jonathan Hale Homestead, located eight mi. NW of the city, is an example of preserved "Western Reserve Style" architecture. Seven rooms are open for tours, as is a reconstructed pioneer village across the street. The home of abolitionist Tom Brown has also been preserved nearby.

ALBANY
NEW YORK

CITY LOCATION-SIZE-EXTENT. Albany, the capital of the state and seat of Albany Co., is located in E central NY on the W bank of the Hudson River, eight mi. S of the junction of the Mohawk and Hudson rivers. The city encompasses 21.5 sq. mi., 130 mi. N of NYC at 42°45' N lat. and 73°48' W long. The greater met. area includes Schenectady and Troy, and extends throughout Albany Co. and into Rensselaer Co. to the E, Schenectady and Saratoga counties to the N and Montgomery Co. to the W.

TOPOGRAPHY. Albany is located in the Hudson-Mohawk lowland region. Situated in the Hudson River Valley, its terrain consists of fertile plains surrounded by highlands. Gently rolling terrain extends W from the river to abruptly-rising land formations of the Appalachian Ridge. To the E, the terrain is more rugged, gradually rising to a range of hills 12 mi. E of Albany. The elev. ranges from 18' to 300'.

CLIMATE. The climate of Albany is continental, modified somewhat by the influence of the Atlantic Ocean. The avg. annual temp. of 48°F ranges from a Jan. mean of 22.9°F to a July mean of 72.4°F. The avg. annual rainfall of 36.55" is distributed evenly throughout the year, while most of the avg. annual snowfall of 66.4" occurs from Dec. through Mar. The RH ranges from 46% to 88%. The avg. growing season is 160 days. Albany lies in the ESTZ and observes DST.

FLORA AND FAUNA. Animals native to Albany include the raccoon, rabbit and beaver. Common birds are the loon, thrush, thrasher, woodpecker and wren. Spring peepers, slimy salamanders and milk snakes, as well as the venomous timber rattlesnake and copperhead, are found in the area. Typical trees include the maple, basswood and European buckthorn. Common flowers are the violet, chicory, day lily and buttercup.

POPULATION. According to the US census, the pop. of Albany in 1970

was 115,781. In 1978, it was estimated that it had decreased to approx. 107,000.

ETHNIC GROUPS. In 1978, the ethnic distribution of Albany was approx. 87.5% Caucasian, 12.2% Black and .3% other.

TRANSPORTATION. The NY State Thruway, Adirondack Northway, interstate hwys. 90, 87, 287 and 787, and US hwys. 20 and 9 provide major motor access to Albany. *Railroads* serving the city are ConRail, DL & Hudson, Albany Port District and AMTRAK. *Airlines* serving Albany Co. Airport are AA, US Air, BN, EA and various commuter lines. *Bus lines* serving the city include the local Capital District Transportation Authority, and Arrow, Bonanza, Greyhound, Trailways, Mt. View, Village and Yankee Trails. The city is a major inland seaport, accessible to ocean vessels via the 32' deep Hudson River channel. In 1978, the Port of Albany handled approx. 1,448,000 tons of cargo from ships of 19 countries.

COMMUNICATIONS. Communications, broadcasting and print media originating in Albany are: *AM radio stations* WROW 590; WGY 810; WTRY 980; WQBK 1300; WHAZ 1330; WABY 1400 (MBS, Mod. Ctry.); WOKO 1460 (ARC/I, Mod. Ctry.) and WPTR 1540 (CBS, Familiar Mus.); *FM radio stations* WVCR 88.5 (NPR, Var.); WAMC 90.3; WCDB 90.9 (Indep., Progsv.); WRPI 91.5; WFLY 92.3; WROW 95.5 (CBS, Familiar Mus.); WGFM 99.6; WWOM 100.9 (Indep., AOR); WHRL 103.1 (Indep., Btfl. Mus.); WQBK 104; WHSH 106.5 (Indep., Btfl. Mus.) and WGNA 107.7 (Indep., C&W); *television stations* WRGB, Ch. 6 (NBC); WTEN, Ch. 10 (ABC); WAST, Ch. 13 (CBS) and WMHT, Ch. 17 (PBS), *press:* two major dailies serve the city, the *Knickerbocker News*, published evenings except Sun., and *Albany Times-Union*, published mornings and Sun.; other publications include the *Rotterdam Reporter*, *Albany Student Press*, the

Nelson A. Rockefeller Empire State Plaza, Albany, New York

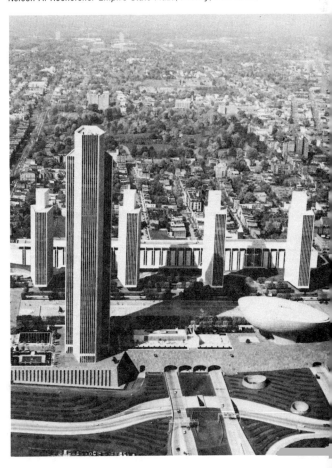

Evangelist, Capital District Business Review and the *Conservationist.*

HISTORY. The site of present-day Albany, the oldest continuous settlement of the 13 colonies, was originally inhabited by native Americans of the Iroquois Nation. Explorer Henry Hudson of the Dutch W India Co. arrived in the area in 1609, and Ft. Orange was established as a fur-trading post. The post, settled by Belgian and French colonists called Walloons, came to be known as Beverwyck. In 1664, the English renamed the comm. Albany—the Scottish title of the Duke of York. (New Amsterdam became NY at this time in honor of the same peer.) Albany was chartered as a city in 1686, when Pieter Schuyler became its first mayor. By 1700, Albany was an established river port and fur-trading center. At the Albany Congress in 1754, Benjamin Franklin, as a representative from PA, submitted his plan of union for the colonies, which although subsequently rejected, was a predecessor of the successful Articles of Confederation and the US Constitution. Albany thus became known as the "Cradle of the Union". In 1797, the city, which had served as a military port, was chosen as the state capital. Following the opening of the Erie Canal in 1825, the city's commercial importance was enhanced since it was located on the distribution line between the Hudson River and the Great Lakes. The establishment of the state's first RR, the Mohawk & Hudson, in 1831 between Schenectady and Albany further contributed to the development of the city. Throughout the 19th and 20th centuries, the city continued to grow steadily as a center of commerce, govt. and finance.

GOVERNMENT. Albany has a mayor-council form of govt., and is the second oldest city in the US still operating under its original (1686) charter. The mayor and the pres. of the council are elected at large, while each of the 16 councillors is elected by residential ward. All members serve four-year terms.

ECONOMY AND INDUSTRY. Albany, the center of govt. of the state of NY, is also a financial and commercial center. Fed., state and local govt. provide jobs for approx. 30% of the city's workers. Approx. 200 manufacturing firms in the city employ about 20% of the total labor force. Major industrial products are electrical equipment, dental products, aspirin, cement, softballs, brake linings, dyes, broad woven fabrics, structural and specialty steel and organic and inorganic drugs. The port of Albany handles approx. 9.1 million metric tons annually. There are several large banking and insurance companies in the city. The total labor force of the greater met. area, was 376,500 in June, 1979, while the rate of unemployment was 4.6%.

Downtown Albany, New York

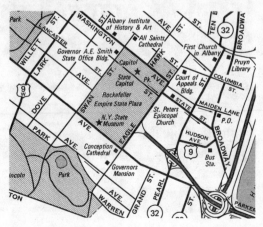

BANKING. There are 13 commercial banks, five savings banks and two savings and loan assns. in Albany. In 1978, total deposits for the 10 banks headquartered in the city were $3,940,152,000, while total assets were $4,550,669,000. Banks include Albany Savings, State Bank of Albany, Union Natl., Natl. Commercial Bank & Trust, Natl. Savings, Home Savings, City & Co. Savings, Bankers Trust, Manufacturers Hanover Trust and Marine Midland.

HOSPITALS. There are seven hosps. in the city, Albany Medical Center (renowned for kidney and bone marrow transplants), V.A. Medical Center, St. Peter's, Memorial, Child's, St. Margaret's House and Hosp. for Babies and Capital District Psychiatric Center, which opened in 1976.

EDUCATION. There are 10 institutions of higher learning in Albany. State U of NY at Albany (SUNYA), the oldest campus of the state U system, was founded in 1844. Its futuristic campus was completed in 1970. One of only four institutions in the SUNYA system awarding doctorate degrees, SUNYA enrolled more than 15,000 in 1978. It is renowned for solar energy and atmospheric sciences research. Union U contains four professional colleges, Albany Law School, Albany Medical Col., the Albany Col. of Pharmacy (all located in the city) and Union Col., located in nearby Schenectady. Rensselaer Polytechnic Institute (RPI), a private institution located in nearby Troy and famous for its engineering programs, enrolled close to 6,000 students in 1978. Other institutions include Albany Bus. Col., Albany Medical Center School of Nursing, Col. of St. Rose, Jr. Col. of Albany, Maria Col. and Mildred Elley Secretarial School. Russel Sage Col., located in Troy, offers an Evening Division in Albany. There are approx. 30 public schools, enrolling about 10,000, and approx. 35 private schools in the city. Libs. include the Albany Institute of History and Art, Albany Public, NY State (exhibiting the original draft of the Emancipation Proclamation and containing a collection of 50,000 photographs) and NY State Supreme Court Appellate Div.

ENTERTAINMENT. Each May, Albany hosts the Tulip Festival in WA Park, which includes the coronation of a Tulip Queen, a Kinderkermis (children's fair) and Dutch-costumed women scrubbing State St. with long-handled brooms. The Pinksterfest, a festival based on an ancient slave holiday, is also held in May in WA Park. It features displays of crafts as well as entertainment. The annual Winter Carnival, a mid-winter festival held at the Empire State Plaza, features magic, music, puppet shows, snow sculpture and sports and ice skating exhibitions. The Schenectady-Albany Bank-a-thon, held the last Sun. of every Mar., is a 20-mi. foot race. Each summer, usually on Sundays, mini-fests—arts and crafts fairs offering entertainment and ethnic foods—are held in WA Park. Spectator sports activities include autumn semi-pro football and Twilight League softball from May to Sept., both at Bleecker Stadium. Teams of SUNYA, RPI in Troy and Union Col. in Schenectady participate in intercollegiate sports.

ACCOMMODATIONS. There are more than 70 hotels and motels in Albany, including the Sheraton Inn Towne and the Quality, Holiday, Ramada, Northway, Best Western-Turf, Americana and Tom Sawyer Motor inns. Airport accommodations include Sheraton Airport and Holiday inns.

FACILITIES. There are 10 major parks in Albany, containing four outdoor swimming pools, 35 tennis courts, picnic areas and one municipal golf course. Among the largest are WA, Lincoln Academy, Thacher and Swinburne. Ice skating is available at Empire State Plaza, Swinburne Park and numerous ponds throughout the city in winter, while boating and fishing facilities are available at Six Mile Waterworks. Several snow skiing facilities are within a two-hour drive from Albany.

CULTURAL ACTIVITIES. There are numerous symphony orchestras, chamber music groups, jazz ensembles, choruses, ballet companies and modern dance troupes, as well as more than 40 comm. and professional theater groups, in the Albany area. The Albany Symphony Orchestra performs at Albany's Palace Theatre. The Albany City Arts Office provides a variety of performing arts activities for the comm. at large, and children especially. Several of the universities and colleges in the area provide musical and dramatic performances. Cohoes Music Hall, 12 mi. from Albany, hosts professional theater, and is listed on the Natl. Register of Historic Places. Free noontime concerts by the music faculty of SUNYA are presented at Gov. Nelson A. Rockefeller Empire State Plaza, which also hosts a free year-round series of popular music, "Wed. Night at the Plaza". The surface and concourse levels of Empire State Plaza also exhibit an 80-piece Contemporary Art Collection, as well as sculpture and paintings. The Plaza's Cultural Education Center contains the NY State Museum, the oldest in the state, featuring displays of the Adirondack wilderness and state birds, agriculture and history. The Performing Arts Center at the Plaza, containing a 987-seat theatre and 500-seat recital hall, is the home of the Empire State Youth Theatre Institute and site of opera, chamber music and dance performances. The Albany Institute of History and Art features regional art and history from the Dutch settlement to the present. Cherry Hill, a preserved home occupied by the Van Rensselaer family for 200 years, features collections of paintings, textiles, porcelain and furniture. Quackenbush Sq., site of the oldest house in Albany (1730), contains a museum as well as a park, outdoor cafe and gardens. Ten Broeck Mansion, home of Gen. Abraham Ten Broeck, delegate to the Continental Congress and mayor of Albany, features many Colonial artifacts.

LANDMARKS AND SIGHTSEEING SPOTS. The Gov. Nelson A. Rockefeller Empire State Plaza in downtown Albany, completed in 1976, contains 11 buildings and a .25 mi.-long concourse lined with restaurants, banks, shops and boutiques. Within the complex, the 44-story Tower building, the tallest skyscraper in upstate NY, contains an observation deck on the 42nd floor. The State Capitol, located on the top of State St. Hill, was completed in 1898 after 30 years in construction. First occupied in 1879, it is of French Renaissance style, designed by four architects. It contains the "Million Dollar Staircase", designed by H.H. Richardson and featuring elaborate carvings, as well as beautiful gardens and fountains outside. City Hall, also designed by Richardson and listed on the Natl. Register of Historic Places, features the first municipal carillon in the US, played at noontime concerts. The Court of Appeals, built in 1842, contains interior columns of native Hudson River marble. The courtroom, also designed by Richardson, was originally in the Capitol. The Executive Mansion, built in the mid-1850s as a private residence, was first used as the gov.'s residence after it was bought by the state in 1877. The historic (1762) Schuyler Mansion was the home of Gen. Phillip Schuyler, whose daughter married Alexander Hamilton. The First Church in Albany (Reformed) was founded in 1624, while its present building was completed in 1789. The pulpit, carved in Holland in 1656, is the oldest in the US. St. Peter's Church was founded in 1715, although its Gothic Revival building was completed in 1859. It contains a silver communion service donated by Queen Anne, among other historic artifacts. The Cathedral of All Saints, the first Episcopal

A view of historic Old Town Plaza where Albuquerque was founded, Albuquerque, New Mexico

cathedral in America, contains fine European wood carving, while the Cathedral of the Immaculate Conception, the city's largest church, built in 1852, features beautiful stained glass windows. St. Mary's Church, founded in 1797 and the first Roman Catholic Church in upstate NY, is listed on the Natl. Register of Historic Places. Other attractions include Center Sq., featuring restored 19th-century residences on tree-lined streets, and the Joseph Henry Memorial in Academy Park, the Philip Hooker formal Georgian brownstone (1817), home of the discoverer of electromagnetism. The Arbor Hill School, an open school without walled classrooms, has won architectural awards for innovative design. Robinson Sq., in the Center Sq. district, is a recently-completed complex featuring boutiques, bookstores, antique shops and cafes.

ALBUQUERQUE
NEW MEXICO

CITY LOCATION-SIZE-EXTENT. Albuquerque is located in central NM on the Rio Grande River 62 mi. SW of Santa Fe, at 35°03' N lat. and 106°37' W long. Seat of Bernalillo Co., Albuquerque encompasses 87.7 sq. mi. It is bordered by Sandoval Co. on the N.

TOPOGRAPHY. Albuquerque is situated in the flat, semi-arid valley of the Rio Grande River. Desert grasslands are to the W, where the mesa rises abruptly to the base of a lava escarpment from a row of five small, extinct volcanoes. The rocky 6,300' foothills of the Sandia Mts. are to the E. The mean elev. of the city, one of the highest in the US, is 5,314'.

CLIMATE. The climate of Albuquerque is dry and continental. The sun shines 77% of the time. Monthly mean temps. range from 35.2°F during Jan. to 78.7°F during July, with an annual avg. of 56.8°F. Most of the annual 8.31" of rainfall occurs between June and Sept. in the form of brief, through sometimes heavy, thunderstorms. Most of the 10.5" of annual snowfall occurs from Dec. to Mar. During winter, the Sandia Mts. protect the city from frigid winds sweeping across the plains from the E. The RH ranges from 16% to 69%. Albuquerque is in the MSTZ and observes DST.

FLORA AND FAUNA. Animals native to Albuquerque include mule deer,

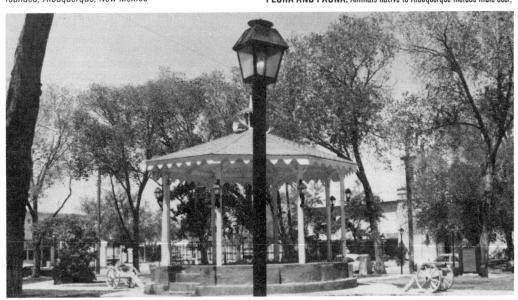

desert cottontail, coyote, bobcat and pronghorn antelope. Common birds include the raven, shrike, W tanager and pinion jay. Coachwhip snakes, skinks, horned lizards and leopard frogs are common, as are several species of venomous rattlesnakes. Typical trees include the pinion pine (state tree), cottonwood, aspen, poplar, willow and juniper. Smaller plants include the yucca (state flower), prickly lettuce, prickly pear cactus and cone flower.

POPULATION. According to the US census, the pop. of Albuquerque (the largest city in the state) in 1970 was 243,751. In 1978 it was estimated that it had increased to approx. 330,000. The median age in the city (1/4 of the pop. of which has resided there five years or less) is 25.

ETHNIC GROUPS. In 1978, the ethnic distribution of Albuquerque was 68.7% Caucasian, 2.6% Black and 28.7% Hispanic.

TRANSPORTATION. Interstate hwys. 25 and 40, US Hwy. 66 and State Hwy. 47 provide major motor access to Albuquerque. AMTRAK and Santa Fe *railroads* serve the city. *Airlines* serving Albuquerque Intl. Airport include CO, FL, TI, TW and AA, as well as several commuter lines. *Bus lines* include Greyhound, Trailways, NM and the local Sun-Tran system. The Sandia Peak aerial Tramway, one of the world's longest at 2.7 mi., operates to the crest of 10,378' Sandia Peak.

COMMUNICATIONS. Communications, broadcasting and print media originating in Albuquerque are: *AM radio stations* KRKE 610 (Indep., Top 40); KDAZ 730 (Indep., Spec. Progsv.); KOB 770 (NBC, MOR, Spec. Progsv.), the first radio station in NM; KQEO 920 (Indep., Btfl. Mus.); KKIM 1000 (UPI, Ed., Christian Mus.-Adult); KUFF 1150 (ABC/E, MOR, Ctry.); KABQ 1350 (Indep., Span.); KRZY 1450 (CBS, Ctry.); KAMX 1520 (Indep., Span.) and KZIA 1580 (ABC/I NBS; Talk, News, Spec. Progsv.); *FM radio stations* KLYT 88.3 (Indep., Ed., Contemp., Christian Mus.); KANW 89.1 (ABC/C, Educ., Top 40); KUNM 90.1 (NPR, Divers., Spec. Progsv.);KIPC 91.5 (NPR, Divers Spec. Progsv.); KRST 92.3 (CBS, AOR); KOB 93.3(NBC, Btfl. Mus.); KRKE 94.1 (Indep., MOR); KHFM 96.3 (Indep., Clas., Jazz); KZZX 99.5 (Indep., MOR, Top 40); KPAR 100.3 (Indep., Btfl. Mus.) and KFMG 107.9 (Indep., Progsv.); *television stations* KOB, Ch. 4 (NBC), the first TV station in NM; KNME, Ch. 5 (PBS); KOAT, Ch. 7 (ABC); KGGM, Ch. 13 (CBS); KMXN, Ch. 23 (Span. TV of NM) and cable; *press*: two major dailies serve the city, the *Journal*, issued mornings, and the *Tribune*, issued evenings. Other publications include the *NM Daily Lobo*, *Health City*, *Sun-News Chieftain*, the *News* and *Albuquerque Consumer Advocate*.

HISTORY. Albuquerque was founded in 1706 by a group of colonists who had been granted permission by King Phillip of Spain to establish a new villa on the banks of the Rio Grande. The settlement was named after the Spaniard Don Francisco Cuervo y Valdez, 13th Duke of Alburquerque (sic) and Viceroy of New Spain (what is now Mexico and NM). Today, it is known as "Duke

City". The first building constructed in 1706 was a church, San Felipe de Neri, around which a plaza developed. The early Spanish settlers established trade with nearby native Americans, as well as farming in the area around the plaza. The settlement developed as a trade and transportation center, since it served as a station on the Chihuahua Trail extension of the Santa Fe Trail between MO and Mexico City. Following the US-Mexican War of 1846 to 1848, Albuquerque became part of the US. Between 1850 and 1880, the settlement was a major supply center for fts. established in the area by the US to protect westward migration. During the Civil War, Albuquerque was occupied for three weeks by Confederate troops who hoped to capture the silver fields of CO. They were shelled by Union forces however, and ended their siege. In 1880, the Santa Fe RR came to the comm., and a "New Town" was established two mi. E of Albuquerque's "Old Town". In 1885, the NM Territorial Legislature chartered Albuquerque as a town. With a pop. of approx. 4,000 in 1891, it was chartered as a city. The city grew steadily throughout the beginning of the 20th century. Between 1950 and 1960, following the city's advent as the atomic energy center of the US (with major R&D facilities located at Sandia Laboratories on Kirtland AFB), the pop. more than doubled. Since then, the city has grown as an R&D, trade, transportation and industrial center of the SW, sharing in the boom of Sunbelt and W cities.

GOVERNMENT. Albuquerque has a mayor-council form of govt. The mayor, elected by the voters at large to a four-year term, is not a member of the council and has no vote. The nine councillors are elected by their respective districts to four-year terms in staggered elections held every two years.

ECONOMY AND INDUSTRY. Albuquerque serves as a major SW center of R&D, finance, insurance, construction, transportation, livestock, medicine and tourism. More than 500 manufacturing firms, primarily of the "clean" type, are located in the city. Products include food processing, electronics, textiles, heavy trailers and industrial heaters. More than 50 firms are directly involved in research, sales and the development and production of space-age and nuclear products. Over six million tourists visit the city each year. In 1979, the labor force for the greater met. area totaled 199,600, while the rate of unemployment was 6.3%. Avg. income per capita in 1977 was $6,820, while the median family income in 1978 was $14,592.

BANKING. There are 12 commercial banks and six savings and loan assns. in Albuquerque. In 1978, total deposits for the 13 banks headquartered in the city were $1,639,144,000, while total assets were $1,936,143,000. Among the banks in the city are Albuquerque Natl., First Natl., Fidelity Natl., Rio Grande Valley, Citizens, Republic, and First N.

HOSPITALS. There are 11 hosps. in Albuquerque including St. Joseph's, Presbyterian and Public Health Service Indian Hosp., The Meson Facility at Los Alamos Scientific Laboratory is involved in cancer treatment. The Bernalillo Co. Medical Center serves as Meson's pre-and post-treatment headquarters. Albuquerque's Lovelace Med. Center, the only major group practice of medicine in the SW, is renowned for having tested the first US astronauts.

EDUCATION. The U of NM, founded in Albuquerque in 1889, is a public coeducational institution enrolling approx. 25,000 students in 1978. It confers bachelor, master and doctorate degrees and contains nine colleges plus schools of law and medicine. The architecture of the U of NM buildings integrates traditional Pueblo with ultra-modern design. The U of NM Medical School operates in conjunction with Bernalillo Co. Medical Center. The U of Albuquerque, a private Catholic col. founded in 1979 and formerly known as "St. Joseph's on the Rio Grande", offers four-year liberal arts

Central Albuquerque, New Mexico

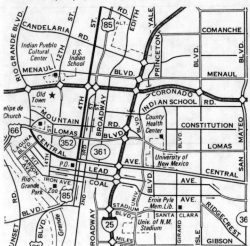

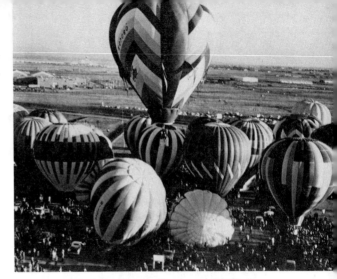

Hot Air Balloon Race in Albuquerque, New Mexico

programs leading to bachelor degrees as well as special two-year courses. Approx. 3,400 enrolled in 1978. Other institutions include the public Albuquerque Technical-Vocational Institute and SW Indian Polytechnic Institute, which offers programs in business, electronics, telecommunications and optical technology to native Americans. The public school system includes 109 schools with approx. 78,000 children enrolled from kindergarten through grade 12. Approx. 6,300 students attend grades one through 12 in 20 private schools. The Albuquerque Public-Lib. system includes a recently completed main lib. and eight branches. Zimmerman Lib. of the U of NM is also available to the public.

ENTERTAINMENT. Dinner theaters in Albuquerque include the Barn and Westgate. The city annually hosts the NM State Fair in Sept., featuring natl. entertainers, rodeos, livestock and horse shows and parimutuel racing. The NM Arts and Crafts Fair is held in the city every year in late June. The SW Arts and Crafts Festival is held one weekend every fall. The Intl. Hot Air Balloon Fiesta is held annually in Oct. The "Hot Air Balloon Capital of the World", as Albuquerque is known, hosts the event featuring the participation of more than 300 balloons. Tingley Coliseum on the NM State Fairgrounds features horse shows, rodeos and circuses year-round. The AAA baseball farm club of the LA Dodgers, the Albuquerque Dukes of the PCL, play at Albuquerque Sports Stadium. The U of NM Lobos participate in collegiate sports in the W Athletic Conf. The city is also the home of the Albuquerque Lasers pro volleyball team. The Natl. Golden Gloves Finals Tournament has also been held in the city in each Mar. Each Christmas, Albuquerque becomes the "City of Little Lights"—the "Luminaria Tour" featuring displays of thousands of candles.

ACCOMMODATIONS. There are 52 motels and hotels in Albuquerque, the Ramada, TraveLodge and Albuquerque inns and the Lorlodge Motels E and W. The Airport Marina and Best Western hotels serve the airport. Howard Johnson's and the Hilton, Holiday, Days, LaQuinta, Royal, Dollar and Rodeway inns are also located in the city.

FACILITIES. Of the 125 municipal parks in Albuqueque, Los Altos is the largest, containing a heated swimming pool, baseball and softball diamonds, tennis courts and a lighted golf course. The 559-acre city park system includes 10 swimming pools, 202 tennis courts, 45 softball fields and numerous bikeways. There are three public golf courses, including Arrova del Oso and Los Altos. "Summer Arts in the Parks" features 75 performances of puppetry, dance, mini theater and music. At the base of 10,378' Sandia Peak in Cibola Natl. Park, which offers skiing, hiking and picnicking facilities, are the public Sandia Stables for horseback riding. The Rio Grande Zoo, is the largest zoological park in NM and features a children's zoo and a breeding program for near-extinct hoofed animals, including a herd of the rare Greater Kudu. The Los Lunas Game Refuge is located nearby, as is Petroglyph Park, nine mi. N of Albuquerque, with 85 acres within city limits. Drawings carved into stone located on a lava flow date from 1100-1600 AD.

CULTURAL ACTIVITIES. The NM Symphony Orchestra of Albuquerque, established in 1932, resides at Lovejoy Hall of the UNM, but also performs throughout the state. Other musical groups based in the city include the Municipal Band, Civic Chorus, Chamber Orchestra of Albuquerque, Albuquerque Lesser Symphony Orchestra and the Youth Symphony. Resident dance companies include the NM Ballet Co., Ballet Folklorico de Albuquerque, Albuquerque Dance Theatre and the NM Dance Works. The Albuquerque Civic Light Opera Assn. presents four performances a year, while the Albuquerque Opera Theatre presents two productions in English. The Albuquerque Little Theatre, a leading comm. theater which performs in the Tiffany Playhouse, presents six shows per season. Other theater groups include the Children's Theatre, Classics Theatre Co., Corrales Adobe Theatre and those of UNM and the U of Albuquerque. The former Kimu Theater houses the Albuquerque Art Center. The new Albuquerque Museum of Art, History and Science, which opened in 1979 in "Old Town", is the first major cultural institution in the US to be solar heated. The Indian Pueblo Cultural Center, operated by the 19 Native American Pueblos of NM, contains an historical museum, arts and crafts market and "Living Arts Program". The Maxwell Museum of Anthropology, Fine Arts Museum and Museum of Geology and Meteoritics are located at the UNM. The Natl. Atomic Museum, the only one of its kind in the US, is located on Kirtland AFB and

features an historical collection of nuclear weapons, including the first two atomic bombs. There are numerous (60 commercial) arts and crafts galleries in the city, many specializing in Native American paintings, pottery, jewelry, rugs and carvings. The Art Gallery at the NM State Fairgrounds is open year-round.

LANDMARKS AND SIGHTSEEING SPOTS. Among Albuquerque's prominent landmarks is San Felipe de Nerl Church, built in the city's historic "Old Town" in 1706. The oldest structure in the city in continuous usage, it has been enlarged and remodeled several times, although the original pueblo walls have been incorporated within the structure. "Old Town" features more than 100 shops on gas lit paths, and includes the city's first (1707) house and first (1881) bank. Rancho de Carnue, an 18th century Spanish rancho in the process of being archaeologically excavated, was the first city land mark placed on the Natl. Register of Historic Sites. The 13' "Hand of Friendship" sculpture, symbolizing the city, is located at the Civic Center.

ALEXANDRIA
VIRGINIA

CITY LOCATION-SIZE-EXTENT. Alexandria, an independent city (with no co. affiliation) in N VA, is situated on the W bank of the Potomac River five mi. S of Washington, DC at 38°48' N lat. and 77°03' W long. The city encompasses 15.75 sq. mi. and is bordered by Fairfax Co. on the W and S and Arlington Co. on the N. The Potomac River separates the city from MD to the E and DC to the NE. Alexandria is part of the Washington, DC greater met. area.

TOPOGRAPHY. Alexandria is situated about 50 mi. E of the Blue Ridge Mts. and 35 mi. W of Chesapeake Bay. In the E part of the city, by the Potomac, the land is flat and close to S L. To the W, the land rises to gently sloping hills and knolls. The mean elev. is 30'.

CLIMATE. The Atlantic Ocean and Chesapeake Bay to the E and the Blue Ridge Mts. to the W influence Alexandria's climate, which is continental and characterized by four well-defined seasons. Monthly mean temps. range from 33°F during Jan. to 76.9°F during July, with an annual avg. of 55.5°F. Most of the avg. annual rainfall of 40.16" occurs during the summer months. Nearly 90% of the annual 19.4" of snowfall occurs from Dec. through Mar. There is occasional flooding in the area, usually caused by the effects of heavy rains in the Potomac basin, hurricanes or a combination of heavy rain and melting snow. The RH ranges from 45% to 91%, and the avg. growing season

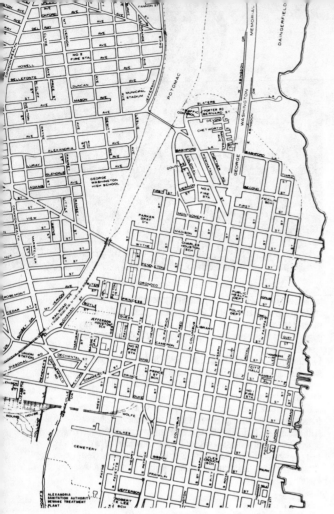

Downtown Alexandria, Virginia

although no *television stations* originate in Alexandria, the city receives broadcasting from nearby Washington, DC; *press:* one daily newspaper is published in the city, the evening *Gazette*, established in 1784, and the oldest daily in the US. Other publications serving the area include the twice-weekly *Alexandria Journal*, the weekly *Alexandria Packet*, the monthly *Alexandrian, Super Stock, Drag Illustrated, Soldiers, Natl. Future Farmer* and *Stock Car Racing.*

HISTORY. In 1669, English colonial Gov. William Berkeley of VA issued a land grant of 6,000 acres, which included the site of present-day Alexandria, along the W bank of the Potomac River for settlement by 120 colonists. The grant was acquired by John Alexander, a pioneer for whom the town was later named. In 1724, John Ramsay, a Scottish merchant considered the founder, settled in the town. A group of Scottish merchants, seeking a port for shipping tobacco, arrived in the area in 1732. The name of the village that developed, Belhaven, was changed to Alexandria in 1748 when the colonial govt. authorized the establishment of a town of 60 acres, which was founded on land owned by the Alexanders. As an apprentice surveyor, George Washington helped lay out the town's streets and lots. Although he lived at Mt. Vernon, S of Alexandria, Washington later frequented the city; he held a pew at Christ Episcopal Church, purchased a fire engine for the town and, in 1754, during the French and Indian War, trained his first troops—about 100 militia men—in Market Sq. During the Revolutionary War, French volunteers for the Continental Army were based near the town, which had become a thriving port, and Hessian prisoners of war were confined there. In 1779, it was incorporated as a town and designated as a Port of Entry to the US, with a Custom House established. The city continued to grow in importance as a seaport and became a center of culture as well as commerce. During the War of 1812, Alexandria, defenseless, surrendered to the British five days after the burning of the White House in Aug., 1814. In 1852, Alexandria was incorporated as a city. From 1861-65, during the Civil War, Alexandria—the transition zone between N and S—was occupied by the Union Army. Although several forts were built in the city as part of the defense of Washington, no fighting occurred. Fed. hospitals were established in the city—the hometown of Confederate Gen. Robert E. Lee—and prison ships anchored in the harbor. The importance of the city as a port diminished in the late 19th century, when sailing ships were replaced by larger steamships, which used the Port of Baltimore. The city continued to grow, however, as a RR center, and the Potomac Yards—one of the largest interchanges on the E Coast—were built by several RR companies. By 1900, the pop. of the city was 15,000. During both WW I and II, a torpedo factory produced munitions. Following WW II, the growth of the fed. govt. attracted thousands of new residents to Alexandria. The city grew through a series of annexations from the adjoining counties of Arlington and Fairfax. Today, Alexandria is a commercial and residential city.

GOVERNMENT. Alexandria has a council-mgr. form of govt. Seven council members, including the mayor as a voting member, are elected at large to three-year terms. The mayor presides over meetings and is the ceremonial head of govt. A city mgr., who is responsible for the city's administration, is appointed by the council, which also selects one of its members to serve as vice-mayor.

ECONOMY AND INDUSTRY. Fed. govt., trade and service are the major employers in Alexandria. Electronics is

is 180 days. Alexandria lies in the ESTZ and observes DST.

FLORA AND FAUNA. Animals native to Alexandria include the raccoon, muskrat and opossum. Common birds include the catbird, mockingbird, brown thrasher, robin and cardinal (the state bird). Cricket frogs, American toads, salamanders, kingsnakes, fence lizards and mud turtles, as well as the venomous copperhead, cottonmouth and rattlesnake, are found in the area. Typical trees include the oak, maple, elm, cherry, sassafras and ash. Smaller plants include the VA pepperweed and flowering dogwood (the state flower).

POPULATION. According to the US census, the pop. of Alexandria in 1970 was 110,938. In 1978, it was estimated that it had increased to approx. 116,900.

ETHNIC GROUPS. In 1978, the ethnic distribution of Alexandria was approx. 74.1 Caucasian, 22% Black and 3.9% other.

TRANSPORTATION. Interstate hwys. 95, 395 and 495, US Hwy. 1 and state hwys. 7, 27, 120, 236 and the George Washington Memorial Pkwy. provide major motor access to Alexandria. *Railroads* serving the city are the Baltimore & OH, Chesapeake & OH, Southern, Delaware & Hudson, ConRail and Richmond, Fredericksburg & Potomac. Nearby Washington Natl. (adjacent to NE Alexandria), Dulles Intl. and Baltimore-Washington Intl. airports are served by all major *airlines*. *Bus lines* serving the city include Greyhound, Trailways and the local Met. Area Rapid Transit (METRO) system, which also provides rail transit. The city, a seaport, is linked to Chesapeake Bay by the 24' deep Potomac River channel. Three riverfront piers handle ocean cargo.

COMMUNICATIONS. Communications, broadcasting and print media originating from Alexandria are: *AM radio station* WPIK 730 (ABC/E, Mod. Ctry.) and *FM radio station* WXRA 105.9 (ABC/E, Mod. Ctry.);

the major industry, followed by research. The largest property owner in the city, Richmond, Fredericksburg & Potomac RR Co., employs approx. 500 people. The 1978 labor force totaled 58,290, while the unemployment rate was 3.8%. In 1976, the avg. per capita income was $9,929, while the median family income was approx. $15,500.

BANKING. There are nine commercial banks and four savings and loan assns. in Alexandria. In 1978, deposits at the one bank headquartered in the city were $60,045,000, while total assets were $65,720,000. Banks include United VA, VA Natl., Burke & Herbert and Dominion Natl.

HOSPITALS. There are three hosps. in the city. Alexandria Hosp., a comm. acute-care facility, was established in 1871. Jefferson Memorial, a private gen. hosp., was established in 1965. Circle Terrace, established in 1970, is a medical-surgical personal care hosp.

EDUCATION. The Alexandria campus of N VA Comm. Col., founded in 1973, is a two-year institution offering associate degrees. In 1978, more than 10,000 students enrolled. The N VA Center—School of Continuing Education of the U of VA is also located in the city. The VA Theological Seminary (Episcopal), founded by Francis Scott Key among others, enrolled more than 300 in 1978. Luther Rice Col., a two-year coeducational Baptist institution established in 1967, offers associate degrees. Alexandria Hosp. maintains a School of Nursing. The public school system consists of 11 elementary (K-6), two jr. high schools (7-9), one high school (10-12), one secondary occupation center and one trainable children's center. The enrollment in 1978 was close to 12,000. There are also 10 private and parochial schools in the city. Lib. facilities include the Alexandria Public (from the 18th century until 1937 a subscription lib.), its two branches and Rare Book, Manuscript and Archives divisions housed in the restored Lloyd House. Other libs. include the Atlantic Research Corp. Defense Documentation Center, the US Army Technical Lib., the Human Resources Research Organization and several that are church-affiliated.

ENTERTAINMENT. The 200-year-old Old Town section of Alexandria, located downtown, features restaurants, historical ambience and musical entertainment. The cruise ship *Dandy* features lunch, and dinner with a live orchestra and dancing, while sailing on the Potomac. Alexandria Days, held annually in July to celebrate the city's birthday, features special sales, concerts, games and other activities in Market Sq. The George Washington Birthday Celebration, the largest annual parade in the US honoring the first pres., is held in Feb. A parade through Old Town features fife and drum corps, floats and bagpipe bands. Robert E. Lee's birthday is commemorated each Jan. with Candlelight Tours of the Lee Boyhood Home and of the Lee-Fendall House. Among annual historic reenactments are those of the 1755 meeting of Gen. Edward Braddock with five of the colonies' Royal Governors, presented in Apr.; the July, 1864 Civil War Battle of Ft. Stevens; a day in the life of a Revolutionary War Encampment, held at Ft. Ward Park each Feb., and Washington's 1798 Review of the Troops each Nov. outside of historic Gadsby's Tavern. The VA Scottish Games, held in July, feature Scottish bagpipes, highland dances, fiddling and Scottish athletic games. The Scottish Christmas Walk, with a parade of bagpipe bands and Scottish Clan Chieftains, is held each Dec. The Gunston Hall Car Show in Sept. features antique, classic and sports cars in competition. The Azalea Festival of Arts and Crafts, with German food and music, is held each year in Apr. at Ft. Ward Park. A Memorial Day Jazz Festival is held annually in Market Sq., while a tour of 18th, 19th and 20th century homes is conducted each Sept. The Annual Juried Art Show is held at the Athenaeum Museum every spring. The Spring Volkslauf, held in May, is a 6.2-mi. people's run. The Autumn Volkslauf and Oktoberfest is held in Oct. The five-mi. Turkey Trot road race is held in Nov. The Alexandria Independents, a professional minor league baseball team of the CRL, play in the city.

ACCOMMODATIONS. Among the 11 hotels and motels in Alexandria are the Guest Quarters, Towers Hotel, Towne Motel, Charter House Motor Hotel, Olde Colony and Howard Johnson's motor lodges and Ramada and Holiday Inns.

FACILITIES. There are 469 acres of public recreational land in Alexandria and four principal park areas, Ft. Ward, the Potomac waterfront, Four-Mi.

Run and Cameron Run. Ft. Ward is both a picnic park and a war memorial, with a Civil War Museum and a fortress, as well as an amphitheater. Three mi. of the Potomac River waterfront on the E edge of the city include the federally-owned Jones Point peninsula, which provides facilities for fishing, hiking and soccer, and Daingerfield Island, with a marina, picnic area and other facilities. Four-Mi. Run and Cameron Run parks are not yet complete. Four-Mi. Run will be a combined swimming, concert and ice-skating facility, while Cameron Run will be the largest park complex in the city, offering tennis, playing fields, a nursery, golf course and archery ranges. The system includes six swimming pools, 50 tennis courts, 26 playing fields and 19 mi. of bike/jogging trails, with 57 mi. planned. The city is also a member of the N VA Regional Park Authority, which includes Bull Run Park and Marina and Pohick Bay Regional Park. Facilities include two public golf courses, swimming pools, nature trails and accommodations for canoeing and sailing.

CULTURAL ACTIVITIES. Members of the Alexandria Performing Arts Council, an assn. of all local non-profit cultural groups formed in 1976, include the Alexandria Symphony (founded in 1944), Little Theatre of Alexandria (established in 1934), Royal Scottish Country Dance Society (established in 1923), Performing Arts Assn. of Alexandria, Port City Playhouse, Seaport Players, Quiet Fire Repertory Co., Alexandria Citizens Band (founded in 1913), Alexandria Harmonizers (organized in 1948), City of Alexandria Pipes and Drums (the city's official band), Alexandria Choral Society (established in 1970), Alexandria Comm. Singers, Alexandria Sweet Adelines, American Puppetry Assn. and the Hauoli Hula Dancers. The Torpedo Factory Art Center, a former munitions plant purchased by the city in 1970, contains studios, galleries and art and drama schools. The Athenaeum, an historic Greek Revival building, is an art museum and headquarters for the N VA Fine Arts Assn. Other museums include the City Ft. Hotel (1792), Ft. Ward Museum (and a partial restoration of a Civil War ft.), the Stabler-Leadbeater Apothecary Shop (a museum and antique shop, built in 1790) and the George Washington N VA Information Center and Museum (which depicts early Alexandria and VA). There are more than 20 art galleries in the city.

LANDMARKS AND SIGHTSEEING SPOTS. There are more than 1,000 restored and preserved 18th and 19th century buildings, including 13 in-city historical landmarks, in Alexandria. The 18-block Old Town Walking

Boyhood Home of Robert E. Lee, Alexandria, Virginia

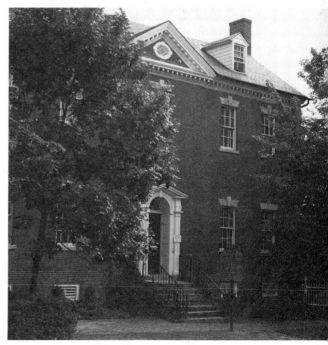

Tour includes stops at the Ramsay House (1724, the oldest in the city), Carlyle House (1752, where Gen. Braddock met five British governors, who proposed the 1755 Stamp Act), Tavern Sq. and Gadsby's Tavern (which Martha and George Washington frequented), the home of Gen. "Light Horse Harry" Henry Lee and the boyhood home of his son, Robert E. Lee, Christ Church Episcopal (1773, where Washington and Lee worshipped), Confederate Monument and Old Presbyterian Meetinghouse (1774, containing the Tomb of the Unknown Soldier of the Revolutionary War). Other attractions include Captain's Row, where sea captains lived during the city's prosperous port days, the Friendship Fire Co. (1774), of which Washington was an early member, the 333' George Washington Masonic Natl. Memorial and, eight mi. S, Mt. Vernon, the home of Washington from 1754 until his death in 1799.

ALLENTOWN
PENNSYLVANIA

CITY LOCATION-SIZE-EXTENT. Allentown is located in E central PA in the Lehigh River Valley at 40°39' N lat. and 75°26' W long. The seat of Lehigh Co., the city encompasses 17.8 sq. mi., 53 mi. NW of Philadelphia. The Allentown-Bethlehem-Easton met. area extends into parts of Carbon and Northampton counties to the NE and N and, in the S, overlaps the greater Philadelphia met. area.

TOPOGRAPHY. Situated on gently rolling terrain which contains many small streams, Allentown is bounded on the N by Blue Mt. and on the S by South Mt. The mean elev. is 364'.

CLIMATE. The climate of Allentown is characterized by moderate temps., averaging 51°F annually, and ample precip. Monthly mean temps. range from 27.5°F in Jan. to 74°F in July. Rainfall is fairly evenly distributed throughout the year and avgs. 44.14" annually. Most of the 32.2" avg. annual snowfall occurs from Dec. through Mar. The RH ranges from 50% to 89%. The growing season avgs. 177 days. Allentown is in the ESTZ and observes DST.

FLORA AND FAUNA. Animals native to Allentown include the raccoon, whitetail deer, groundhog and muskrat. Common birds include the warbler, woodpecker, cardinal, mockingbird and wren. During migration, other birds

Downtown Allentown, Pennsylvania

move through the area as they travel along the Appalachian Mts. or to the Atlantic Coast. Some salamanders, frogs and turtles are found in the area as well as the venomous N copperhead and timber rattlesnake. Typical trees include the Norway maple, red oak, horse chestnut, little leaf linden, white ash walnut, hickory and birch. Smaller plants include the mt. laurel (the state flower of PA), meadowrue, chickweed and partridgeberry.

POPULATION. According to the US census, the pop. of Allentown in 1970 was 109,527. In 1978, it was estimated that it had decreased to 105,069.

ETHNIC GROUPS. In 1978, the ethnic distribution of Allentown was approx. 97.2% Caucasian, 1.8% Black, .7% Hispanic, .2% Asian and .1% other.

TRANSPORTATION. US hwys. 22 and 222, State Hwy. 309 and the NE Extension of the PA Tnpk. provide major motor access to Allentown. Four *Railroads* serving the city are the Reading, DL & Hudson, Lehigh Valley and ConRail. *Airlines* serving Queen City and Allentown-Bethlehem-Easton airports include EA, UA, US Air, Altair and Suburban. *Bus lines* include Trailways, Tri-City, Trans Bridge and Greyhound.

COMMUNICATIONS. Communications, broadcasting and print media originating from Allentown are: *AM radio stations* WAEB 790 (Indep., Contemp.); WKAP 1320 (ABC/I, Adult Contemp.); WSAN 1470 (NBC, Progsv.) and WHOL 1600 (Indep., C&W); *FM radio stations* WMUH 89.7 (Indep., Var.); WZZD 95.1 (Indep., Progsv., Top 40); WFMZ 100.7 (Indep., Btfl. Mus.) and WXKW 104.1 (Indep., Ctry.); *television stations* WLVT Ch. 39 (PBS) and WFMZ Ch. 69 (Indep.); *press*: three major dailies serve the city, the *Evening Chronicle* and the *Morning Call*, which combine in the Sun. *Call-Chronicle* and the *Globe-Times*. Other publications include the *Today Magazine* and *Lehigh Valley Motor Club News.*

HISTORY. Originally called Northampton Towne, Allentown was founded in 1762 by William Allen, who served as a member of the Continental Congress, mayor of Philadelphia and Chief Justice of the provincial Supreme Court from 1730 to 1774. Many of the early settlers were of German descent. During the Revolutionary War, Allentown became known as "The Armory of the Revolution" for the munitions that were produced in the city, and "The Hospital to the Continental Army", since the sick and wounded were treated in many of its public buildings in the winter of 1776. After the battle of Brandywine in 1777, as the British prepared to seize Philadelphia, Gen. Washington sent the Liberty Bell to Allentown. It was concealed beneath the floorboards of the Zion Reformed Church for safekeeping. In 1811, the town was incorporated as the Borough of Northampton.

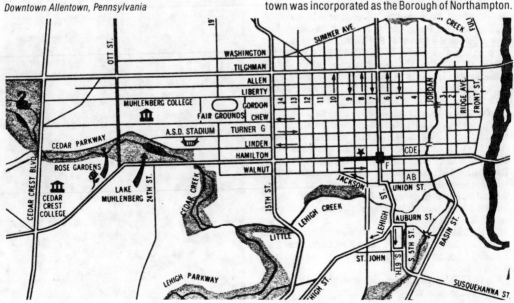

Later, the name "Allentown" came into popular usage, and was officially adopted in 1838. A series of catastrophes from 1839 to 1849, the "Disastrous Decade" which saw major floods, fires and business failures, detracted from the city's growth. The Industrial Revolution resulted in a rapid increase in the city's pop.— from less than 4,000 in 1850 to nearly 14,000 in 1870—to more than 35,000 at the turn of the century. A series of annexations between 1901 and 1911 more than doubled the city's land area and pushed the pop. over 50,000. Growth slowed during the Depression, but following economic recovery, the pop. rose quickly. The city became a major manufacturing center with more than 300 industries contributing to its prominence in the economy of PA.

GOVERNMENT. Allentown has a mayor-council form of govt. consisting of a mayor and seven council members who are elected at large to four-year terms. The mayor, not considered a member of the council, votes only to break a tie. In 1975, Allentown received the All-America City Award for accomplishing three major projects: a new form of city govt., a regional hosp. and a city-center shopping mall.

ECONOMY AND INDUSTRY. Allentown ranks third behind Philadelphia and Pittsburgh in PA manufacturing regions. Of the 300 manufacturing industries operating in the city, electronics is the largest, followed by textiles and steel. Research, meat packing, cement and metal products are also significant. The headquarters of Mack Truck and PA Power and Light are located in the city, which is known as "The Trucking Capital of the World". In June, 1979, the total labor force of the Allentown-Bethlehem-Easton met. area was 299,900, while the rate of unemployment was 6.5%.

BANKING. In 1978, total deposits of the two banks headquartered in Allentown were $1,148,224,000, while assets totaled $1,296,510,000. Banks include First Natl., Merchants, Industrial Valley, First Valley, Bank of PA and American.

HOSPITALS. There are six hosps. in the city, Allentown Gen., Allentown-Sacred Heart, Hosp. Center, Good Shepherd, Osteopathic, Allentown State and a V.A. Clinic.

EDUCATION. Two liberal arts colleges established over a century ago are located in Allentown. Muhlenburg Col., founded in 1848, affiliated since 1867 with the E PA Synod of the Lutheran Church in America and exclusively a men's col. until 1957, enrolled more than 1,800 in 1978. Cedar Crest Col., a private liberal arts col. for women founded in 1867 and affiliated with the United Church of Christ, enrolled more than 650 in 1978. The Allentown Campus of the PA State U System is a two-year pre-baccalaureate institution offering technical courses. Other institutions in the area include Allentown Col. of St. Francis de Sales and United Wesleyan Col., a col. of the Christian ministry. Libs. include the Allentown Public Lib. and the E side and S side branches, the Lehigh Co. Law Lib. and the Scott Trexler Memorial Lib. of the Lehigh Co. Historical Society.

ENTERTAINMENT. The Applause Dinner Theatre is located in Allentown. The Allentown Fair, featuring top entertainers, is celebrated annually in late summer. The Allentown Jets, a semi-professional E Basketball Assn. team, the Wings, a baseball team, and the PA Stoners, an NASL soccer team, are based in the city. The Muhlenburg Col. Mules participate in intercollegiate sports. Bicentennial Park hosts both local and natl. fast-pitch softball competitions.

ACCOMMODATIONS. The hotels and motels in Allentown include the Sheraton Inn and the Traylor, Americus and Walp's hotels.

FACILITIES. More than 1,600 acres of parkland, consisting of 18 parks, four parkways and 35 playgrounds, are available to the residents of Allentown. Within the city are Trexler, Union Terrace, South Mt. Reservoir, Keck, Hamilton and West parks, as well as the Lehigh, Cedar Creek and Trout Creek pkwys. They feature 21 tennis courts, six swimming pools, an 18-hole municipal golf course, bridle paths, nature trails, a rose garden and a year-round "fish-for-fun" area near Lil-Le-Hi Trout Nursery. Eight

single handball courts, 13 school gyms and 12 sledding hills are also located in the city. Boating, fishing, hiking and picnicking areas are available outside the city at Leaser Lake. Just NW of Allentown is the Hawk Mt. Sanctuary, where hawks ride the currents along the mt. ridges. Dorney Park, rated as one of the nation's top 20 amusement parks, is located in the city.

CULTURAL ACTIVITIES. The Allentown Art Museum, ranked as one of the most outstanding small art museums in the US, the Municipal Opera Co. and the Allentown Symphony Orchestra contribute to the city's cultural life. The Allentown Band, organized in 1829, and four other professional bands are responsible for Allentown's title of "Band City USA". The Lehigh Valley Youth Symphony also provides musical entertainment. Museums in the city include Trout, Liberty Bell Shrine and the Lehigh Co. Historical Museum. Art exhibits are shown at the Alma Perlis, Continental, Sam Toff, Hess's and Chmielewski galleries. The Civic Little Theatre, J.I. Rodale Theatre and the summer Guthsville Playhouse present dramatic performances.

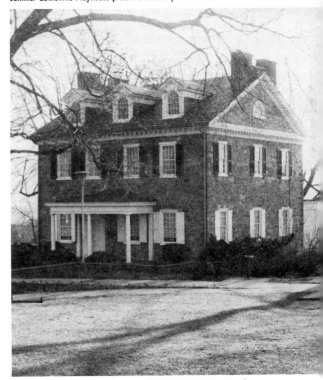

Trout Hall is home of Lehigh County Historical Society, Allentown, Pennsylvania

LANDMARKS AND SIGHTSEEING SPOTS. Many landmarks in Allentown, home of the PA Dutch, reflect the role the city played in American Colonial and Revolutionary War history. The Liberty Bell Shrine features a full-size replica of the bell as well as a mural depicting its journey. Trout Hall was the home of James Allen, son of the city's founder. Just outside the city are the Troxell-Steckel House (in Egypt) and the George Taylor Mansion (in Catasauqua), a Natl. Historic Landmark. Homes of early area settlers, they are both administered by the Lehigh Co. Historical Society. King George Inn, a pre-Revolutionary building .25 mi. outside of the city, is listed on the Natl. Register of Historic sites. Other historic landmarks include the Haines Mill Museum (a restored grist mill), the Old Allentown Cemetery (the town's first burial ground) and several covered bridges in the area, which is known as the "Covered Bridge Capital of the World". The Lil-Le-Hi Trout Nursery, containing 30,000 brook, rainbow and brown trout, is open daily. Hamilton Mall, a shopping-theater-business district located on four blocks in downtown Allentown, features canopied sidewalks, trees, planters, benches and a park-like atmosphere.

AMARILLO
TEXAS

CITY LOCATION-SIZE-EXTENT. Amarillo, located in the heart of the nation's largest cattle-feeding region, is in the center of the panhandle area of N TX at 35°14' N lat. and 101°42' W long. The seat of Potter Co., it occupies 80.06 sq. mi. of land 65 mi. E of NM and 85 mi. S of the OK panhandle region. The greater met. area extends throughout both Potter and Randall counties. There are several lakes in the area, including Meredith, Greenbelt, McKenzie and Rita Blanca.

TOPOGRAPHY. Amarillo is situated in the High Plains of the Llano Estacado region. The "Llano", which signifies "prairie"in Spanish, is an area characterized by extremely flat, nearly treeless grasslands. The landscape is dissected by gaping canyons and carved by numerous creeks, rivers and shallow lakes, which are often dry. The terrain, sloping gradually downward to the E, gradually rises to the W and NW of the city. The mean elev. is 3,657'.

CLIMATE. The climate of Amarillo is typically arid and continental, with wide variations in the weather occurring seasonally. During the winter, cold fronts sweeping across the plains at 40 m.p.h. may cause temps. to drop 50°F to 60°F within a 12-hour period. High winds, low humidity and abundant sunshine are also characteristic of the city's climate. Monthly mean temps. range from 36°F in Jan. to 78°F in July, with an annual avg. of 57°F. Temps. of 100° or higher occur an avg. of three days per year, while temps. of 0°F or lower occur on an avg. of two days per year. The annual rainfall of 20.44" occurs mainly during summer thunderstorms. The annual snowfall of 14.6" usually melts within a few days after falling. Although severe storms are rare, thunderstorms with damaging hail, lightning and wind, as well as tornadoes, occur. The RH ranges from 31% to 80% and occasionally drops below 20% in spring. The growing season avgs. 202 days. Amarillo is in the CSTZ and observes DST.

FLORA AND FAUNA. Animals native to Amarillo include the prairie dog, cottontail, jackrabbit, skunk, mule deer, ground squirrel, porcupine, raccoon, fox, opossum, bobcat, aoudad sheep and coyote. Common birds include the dove, duck, goose, pheasant, quail, turkey, scissortailed flycatcher, meadowlark and mockingbird (the state bird). Lizards, frogs and snakes, including the venomous rattlesnake, are found in the area. Typical plants are mesquite, cottonwood, prickly pear cactus, sagebrush, prairie flower and yucca.

POPULATION. According to the US census, the pop. of Amarillo in 1970 was 127,010. In 1979, it was estimated to have increased to 156,308.

ETHNIC GROUPS. In 1978, Amarillo's ethnic distribution was approx. 89.6% Caucasian, 4.7% Black and 5.7% Hispanic.

TRANSPORTATION. Interstate hwys. 27 and 40 and US hwys. 60, 66, 87 and 287 pass through Amarillo. The city is served by three *railroads*, Burlington Northern, Rock Island and Santa Fe. *Airlines* serving Tradewind and Amarillo Intl. airports are NB, CO, SW, TI, FL and TW. The *bus lines* providing service are Greyhound, Trailways, T.N.M.&O., NM Transportation and the local Amarillo Transit System.

COMMUNICATIONS. Communications, broadcasting and print media serving Amarillo are: *AM radio stations* KGNC 710 (CBS, MOR, Farm); KIXZ 940 (Indep., Contemp.); KDJW 1010 (CBS); KZIP 1310 (ABC/E, C&W); KQIZ 1360 (MBS, MOR) and KPUR 1440 (Indep., Contemp. rock); *FM radio stations* KAVC 89.9 (Indep., Divers.); KQIZ 93.1 (Indep., Top 40); KBUY 94.1 (Indep., Contemp.); KGNC 97.9 (Indep., Btfl. Mus.); KFRN 98.7 (Indep., Gospel)

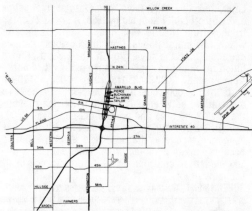

Amarillo, Texas

and KWAS 101.9 (Indep., MOR, Gospel); *television stations* KAMR, Ch. 4 (NBC); KVII, Ch. 7 (ABC); KFDA, Ch. 10 (CBS) and cable; *press*: two major dailies serve the area, the *Amarillo Globe- Times*, issued evenings, and *Amarillo Daily-News*, issued mornings. Other publications include the *Ranger, Accent* and *Quarter Horse Journal.*

HISTORY. Amarillo was settled in 1887 by members of the J. C. Berry Co. of Abilene at the site of an intersection of two RRs that were expected to be built across the Panhandle plains. Sixty residents of Potter Co., many of whom lived on the LX Ranch, became the first lot-owners of the Amarillo townsite. With only 56 legal voters, the comm. was incorporated in 1899. Its RRs, cattle and merchandising formed the basis of Amarillo's industrial growth. By the early 1900s, the city had become the world's greatest cattle shipping market. In the beginning of the 20th century, the first wheat was planted in what was to become one of America's major wheat belts. In 1918, the discovery of oil and natural gas led to the development of a number of industries producing carbon black, petrochemicals and helium.

GOVERNMENT. In 1913, Amarillo became the first city in the SW to adopt a council-manager form of govt. Five commission members, including the mayor—who is the presiding officer and official head of the city—are elected at large by the voters to two-year terms. The commission appoints a city mgr., who, as administrative head of the municipal govt., supervises all city depts. and offices and directs the enforcement of laws and ordinances. The city mgr. advises the commission on urgent policy matters.

ECONOMY AND INDUSTRY. Amarillo is the commercial center of the TX Panhandle. The area's most important industry is petrochemicals. The world's largest helium processing plant is also located here, the "Helium Capital of the World". A RR shipping center for cattle, wheat and other goods, Amarillo's other industries include meat packing, textiles, helicopter parts, farm machinery, chemical refining and food processing. The 1978 labor force totaled 86,130, while the unemployment rate was 4.1%. The median income for 1978 was $6,753.

BANKING. There are 10 commercial banks and five savings and loan assns. located in Amarillo. In 1978, total deposits for the eight banks headquartered in the city were $1,011,804,000 while total assets were $1,223,687,000. Banks serving the city include the Bank of the SW, First Natl., Amarillo Natl., American Natl., Tascosa Natl., Western Natl. and N State banks.

HOSPITALS. There are more than 30 gen. and special care hospitals and clinics in Amarillo. Twelve facilities are located in the 417-acre Amarillo

Area Foundation Medical Center, including High Plains Baptist and V.A. hosps., Psychiatric Pavilion, Children's Rehabilitation Center, Killgore Children's Psychiatric Center and Hosp., Amarillo State Center for Human Development, TX A&M Veterinary Medicine Diagnostic Laboratory, TX Tech U Regional Academic Health Center (operated by the TX Tech School of Medicine), Bivins Memorial Nursing Home, the Amarillo Col. Bio-Medical School and TX A&M Research and Extension Center. Other major hosps. within met. Amarillo include St. Anthony's, Northwest TX General, SW Osteopathic and Palo Duro.

EDUCATION. Among the universities and colleges in the Amarillo area is the three-campus Amarillo Col., a public two-year institution offering academic and vocational comm. programs. Founded in 1929, Amarillo Col. confers AA and AS degrees and has an enrollment of over 21,000. West TX State U (WTSU), located on a 120-acre campus in Canyon, 20 min. SW of Amarillo, has an enrollment of approx. 7,000 and offers 16 degrees at the bachelor and master levels. The U also provides research facilities for students and faculty at the Killgore Research Center, Computer Center, Panhandle-Plains Historical Museum and the WTSU Ranch. Other institutions in Amarillo include the TX State Technical Institute, which has an enrollment of approx. 1,000, and Northwest TX Hosp. School of Nursing. The Amarillo Independent School District consists of 32 elementary schools—including one for special education—one regional school for the deaf, eight jr. high schools, four high schools and an alternative high school, with a total enrollment of over 26,000 in 1978. Fourteen private schools, including three high schools, enroll an additional 2,000 students. Lib. facilities include the Amarillo Public Lib., with the N, SW and SE branches and more than 240,000 vols., and the Cornett Lib. of WTSU.

ENTERTAINMENT. There are two dinner theaters in Amarillo, the Country Squire and Frenchy McCormick's. In Jan., the city hosts The Amarillo Stock Show. "The World's Largest Cattle Auction", at which cattle are auctioned in the local arena, is held several times a year. The Tri-State Fair, held in Sept., features nationally known performers, exhibits, livestock competitions and a giant midway. Amarillo is also the site of the Will Rogers Range Riders' Rodeo and the Greater SW Music Festival held in Apr. The Amarillo Gold Sox, a farm club of the San Diego Padres baseball team, competes in the AA TX League. The city hosts Golden Gloves pro boxing, and the Intl. Hot Rod Assn. World Natl. Finals. At the collegiate level, the Buffaloes of WTSU compete in football, basketball, golf, and track in the MO Valley Conf., while the Amarillo Col. Badgers compete in the Western Jr. Col. Conf. in basketball.

ACCOMMODATIONS. There are more than 70 hotels and motels in Amarillo, including the Best Western-Sands and Villa, Trade Winds, Royal, TraveLodge and Howard Johnson's, as well as the American, Hilton, Holiday, Lexington, Quality, Ramada and Rodeway inns.

FACILITIES. There are 54 public parks in Amarillo, encompassing over 2,240 acres of land. Memorial, Martin Road, Ellwood, Southeast and Southwest parks and the largest, Thompson, contain four swimming pools, 145 tennis courts, one amusement park, one zoo, one 36-hole golf course, 130 softball and baseball fields and three small stocked lakes. Picnic grounds, jogging trails and horseback riding are available S of Amarillo at Palo Duro Canyon State Park, the largest in the TX state park system with over 16,000 acres. The canyon itself stretches for 125 mi. across the High Plains and offers hiking, camping and a scenic miniature RR, the Sad Monkey. Big and little game and varmint hunting is available in the area, although aoudad sheep and antelope can be hunted by permit only. There are a number of ski clubs in the city, and ski instruction is available at Amarillo Col. Swimming, fishing, boating and water skiing are available at nearby lakes Meredith, Greenbelt, Conchas and McClellan. The Amarillo Garden Center provides horticultural instruction.

CULTURAL ACTIVITIES. The 90-member Amarillo Symphony Orchestra,

The musical drama "Texas" performed on the open air stage at the Palo Duro Canyon, Amarillo, Texas

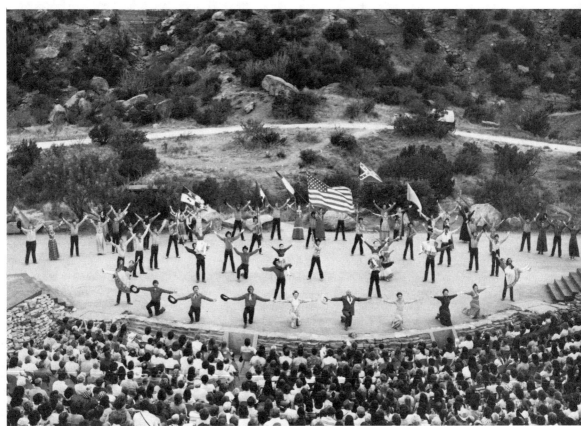

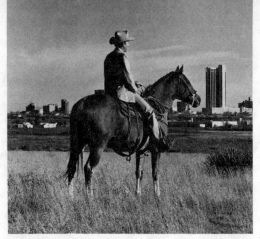

THE ENCYCLOPEDIA OF AMERICAN CITIES

Amarillo's skyline as seen from the western countryside of the Texas panhandle, Amarillo, Texas

established in 1922, the Civic Ballet and the Amarillo Jr. League, which presents a season of dramatic productions, perform at the Amarillo Civic Center. The Amarillo Little Theatre, founded in 1927, presents at least five major productions each season and four children's plays, while sponsoring a Theatre Academy and Peter Piper Players youth performing company. A presentation of the musical "Texas", a history of the struggle to settle the Panhandle Plains in the 1880s, is offered every summer at the Pioneer Amphitheatre in Palo Duro State Park. There are three dance companies in the city, as well as several museums in the Amarillo area. These include the Nielsen Memorial Museum, the Panhandle-Plains Historical Museum on the WTSU campus—selected by the UN as one of America's outstanding museums for its collection of Western art and artifacts—the Amarillo Art Center Museum on the campus of Amarillo Col. and the Intl. Helium Monument and Museum. The Don Harrington Discovery Center contains an ecosphere, similar to a planetarium, a Discovery Hall of Health and a Discovery Hall of Science and Technology. The Sq. House Museum features artifacts and displays from prehistoric Indian culture to the time of the "oil boom".

LANDMARKS AND SIGHTSEEING SPOTS. The six-story high, stainless steel Intl. Helium Monument, dedicated in 1968 to commemorate the centennial anniversary of the discovery of helium, symbolizes the need for conservation of all energy resources. The monument consists of four columns designed to hold artifacts selected by the Smithsonian Institute, which will be opened in 25, 50, 100 and 1,000 years. The only natl. monument in TX, the Alibates Flint Quarries Natl. Monument, is located 30 mi. NE of Amarillo near Lake Meredith. Some 15,000 years ago, Paleo-Indians gathered flint from the quarry, which, to date, has yielded 16,000 artifacts from a 66-room pueblo. A 100-room pueblo has yet to be excavated. Six Gun City, a site for the filming of Hollywood westerns, is open to the public as an amusement center. Wonderland Amusement Park, Storyland Zoo and the American Quarter Horse Assn. headquarters, soon opening a museum, are all popular sightseeing spots in the area.

ANAHEIM
CALIFORNIA

CITY LOCATION-SIZE-EXTENT. Anaheim, located in SW CA at 33°5' N lat. and 117°56' W long., is the largest city in Orange Co. It encompasses approx. 40 sq. mi. on the banks of the Santa Ana River, just W of the Santa Ana Mts. It is located 27 mi. SE of LA and 20 mi. E of the Pacific Ocean. The greater met. area consists of Anaheim and Santa Ana to the S and Garden Grove to the SE and borders LA Co. on the N.

TOPOGRAPHY. Anaheim is located in the flat S CA coastal plain area bordered by the Pacific Ocean on the W and the Santa Ana Mts. on the E. Its terrain is characterized by flat land along the Santa Ana River

which rises to hills in the N, E and S. The mean elev. is 160'.

CLIMATE. The Pacific Ocean and the S Coastal Mt. Range influence the climate of Anaheim, which is characterized by mild year-round temps. Monthly mean temps. range from 52°F in Jan to 72°F in July, with an avg. annual temp. of 64°F. Daily temps. may vary as much as 30°F, resulting in warm to hot days during the summer and cool to cold nights during the winter. Some 85% of the avg. annual rainfall of 15" occurs during the months of Jan. through Apr., while summer rainfall is rare. Snowfall is also rare. The RH ranges from 45% to 52%. The growing season is year-round. Anaheim lies in the PSTZ and observes DST.

FLORA AND FAUNA. Animals native to Anaheim include the coyote, mule deer and bat. Common birds include the hummingbird, scrub jay, house finch, swallow, goldfinch and W kingbird. Several species of reptiles, as well as the venomous S rattlesnake, are present. Typical trees are the pine, willow and CA white oak. Smaller plants include the chaparral shrubs and prickly pear cactus.

POPULATION. According to the US census, the pop. of Anaheim in 1970 was 166,701. In 1978, it was estimated that it had increased to 204,800. Anaheim is the eighth most populous city in CA.

ETHNIC GROUPS. In 1978, the ethnic distribution of Anaheim was approx. 98.3% Caucasian, .1% Black, 10.5% Hispanic, 1.3% Asian and 1.2% other races (a percentage of the Hispanic total is also included in the Caucasian total).

TRANSPORTATION. Interstate hwys. 5 (Santa Ana Frwy.) and 91 (Anaheim/Riverside Frwy.) and state hwys. 22 (Garden Grove Frwy.) 55 (Newport Frwy.) and 57 (Orange Frwy.) provide major motor access to Anaheim. *Railroads* serving the area include the S Pacific, Santa Fe and Union Pacific. All major *airlines* serve nearby Fullerton (6 mi. N), John Wayne/Orange Co. (15 mi. S), Long Beach Municipal (15 mi. W), Ontario Intl. (33 mi. N) and LA Intl. Airport. *Bus lines* include Greyhound, Trailways and the local Orange Co. Transit District and S CA Rapid Transit District.

COMMUNICATIONS. Communications, broadcasting and print media originating from Anaheim are: *AM radio station* KEZY 1190 (Indep., Top 40) and *FM radio station* KEZY 95.9 (Indep., Progsv.); no *television stations* originate from Anaheim, which receives broadcasting from 10 stations including LA, Glendale, Santa Ana and Huntington Beach; *press:* the major daily newspaper published in the city, is the *Anaheim Bulletin,* issued evenings; two daily newspapers serve the city, the *Santa Ana Register* and the *LA Times* (Orange Co.

Anaheim, California

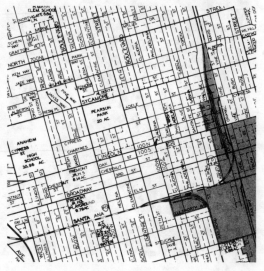

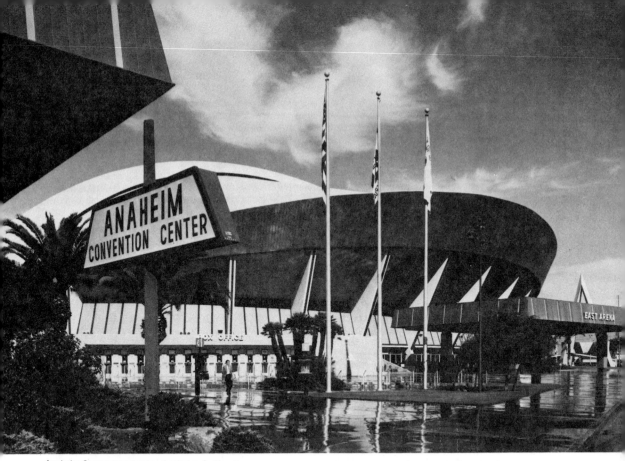

Anaheim Convention Center, Anaheim, California

Edition); other publications include the *Business Digest, Hills News-Times, Anaheim Independent, Trucking Magazine* and *Street Rodder.*

HISTORY. The site of present-day Anaheim was part of a large land grant from Spain to the San Gabriel Mission of the Roman Catholic Church in the late 17th Century. In 1834, after Mexico had gained its independence from Spain and secularized Church holdings in CA, Juan Pacifico Ontiveras acquired 35,970 acres, which included the present sites of Anaheim, Brea, Fullerton and Placentia, and created Rancho San Juan Cajon de Santa Ana. In Sept., 1857, nine years after CA had become a US territory and seven years after it had achieved statehood, John Frohing and George Hansen, two German immigrants, purchased 1,165 acres from Ontiveras. Members of the LA Vineyard Society, a group of about 50 German immigrants who lived in San Francisco and sought to establish a wine-producing comm. in S CA, Hansen and Frohling also acquired a strip of land which included water rights to the Santa Ana River and which could support a canal with the capacity to irrigate 1,200 acres. A colony was established, and Hansen, elected superintendent surveyed 50 20-acre lots. Native Americans constructed the main irrigation canal and ditches to each lot, planted 400,000 vines and built 50 houses on 40 central acres. In 1858, the Society named the comm. "Annaheim" (later changed to Anaheim), for the Santa Ana River and the German word for home, "heim". In Sept., 1858, most of the first colonists arrived by boat from San Francisco. In 1860, the first schoolteacher, Fred Kuelp, began teaching a class of nine children. Although the first school building was destroyed by a flood in 1862, J. M. Guinn, who had begun teaching 20 students in 1869, drafted a bill in 1877, which set a precedent in the US. In

1878, the CA Legislature approved authorization for the school district to issue bonds for the construction of Central School. Anaheim was incorporated as a city in 1870, when its pop. was 8,881 and the first paper in Orange Co., the *Anaheim Gazette,* was published. Unable to afford maintaining the streets, the citizens requested revocation of the incorporation in 1872. In 1875, the S Pacific RR arrived in the city, and, in 1876, following the arrival of a group of Polish settlers, including actress Madame Helen Modjeska and writer Henry Steinklewicz, the city was incorporated again. Soon after, the first oranges were planted, and by 1884, 50 wineries—the grapes harvested by native Americans, Mexicans and Chinese from San Francisco—produced 1,250,000 gallons of wine. In 1887, the Santa Fe RR came to the city. By 1888, a virus with no known cause which had infected the vineyards in 1881 (called Pieroe's or Anaheim disease) had killed most of the vines. Valencia oranges, however, became the most successful commercial crop, from which most of Anaheim's income derived. As late as 1938, massive flooding from the Santa Ana River caused much damage, and, as a result, the Prado Dam was built on the stream. Although the comm. was primarily agricultural until 1950, manufacturing and tourism, especially since the opening of Disneyland in 1955, have become the major industries. The pop. of the city, only 1,456 in 1900, has increased from annexations and immigration. Between the US census of 1950 and 1960, the area grew in sq. mi. from 4.4 to 27.34, while the pop. boomed from 14,556 to 104,184.

GOVERNMENT. Anaheim has a council-manager form of govt., consisting of five council members, the city mgr., the mayor and the mayor pro tempore. The council members are elected at large to four-year terms in staggered-year elections. The council members are the legislative and policy-making members of govt. The city mgr. is a full-time executive, appointed by the Council to an indefinite term, who heads the administrative functions. By a charter amendment of April 9, 1974, the mayor is now elected by direct vote for a two-year term. The mayor, who presides at all meetings, is the official, ceremonial head of the city and may make motions and vote, but has no veto power. The mayor pro tempore is elected annually by the council members.

ECONOMY AND INDUSTRY. Disneyland (which, since 1970, has been visited by more than 10 million people per year), Anaheim Stadium and the convention center are the major tourist attractions. There are more than 600 manufacturing plants in the area, employing about 25% of the total work force. Major products include electronic data processing equipment, automobile batteries, locks, sound equipment and medical instruments. In June, 1979, the total labor force for the greater met. area was estimated to be 1,069,700, while the rate of unemployment was 4.4%.

BANKING. There are 15 commerical banks and 11 savings and loan assns. in Anaheim. In 1978, total deposits for the three banks headquartered in the city were approx. $79,990,000, while total assets were approx. $88,315,000. Banks include Heritage, El Camino, Pacific Natl. and United CA.

HOSPITALS. There are eight gen. hosps. in Anaheim including Anaheim Memorial, W Anaheim Comm., Anaheim Gen. and Martin Luther.

EDUCATION. Anaheim is part of the N Orange Co. Comm., or Fullerton Jr., Col. District founded in 1913. It is the oldest col. in continual operation in CA, comprised of the Fullerton and Cypress campuses. In 1979, approx. 13,000 enrolled at the Fullerton campus, while approx. 7,800 enrolled at the Cypress campus, which was established in 1966. Pepperdine U School of Law, American Col. of Law, S CA Col. of Medicine and Dental Assts., Bryman School, Sawyer Col. of Business and Melodylana School of Theology (Disciples of Christ) are also located in Anaheim. The Anaheim Union (public) School District, consisting of three special, 16 jr. and 8 sr. high schools, enrolled approx. 36,000 in 1978. There are also 24 private and parochial schools in the city. Libs. include Anaheim Public, with three branches and bookmobiles and Rockwell Intl., the US Borax and Northrop Corp. libs.

ENTERTAINMENT. There is one dinner theater, Sebastian's, located in Anaheim. Among the annual events are the Halloween Festival (begun in 1920s), which features a costume parade every Oct., the Carrousel of Anaheim, highlighting cultural activities; the Jack Cope Memorial baseball tournament and the Penny Carnival both held in Aug., and the Anaheim Holiday Fair, featuring arts and crafts, held each year in Nov. at La Palma Park. Anaheim Stadium, which became the home of the CA Angels pro baseball team of the AL in 1966, also hosts the CA Surf pro soccer team of the NASL and, beginning with the 1980 season, the Rams pro football team of the NFL-NFC.

ACCOMMODATIONS. There are about 60 hotels and motels in Anaheim, a major tourist and convention center. Among these are the Anaheim Motor Lodge, Disneyland Hotel, Inn at the Park, Grand Hotel, Howard Johnson's, Hyatt House and Quality, Sheraton and Holiday inns.

FACILITIES. In 1978, Anaheim's Parks, Recreation and Comm. Services Dept. won the Natl. Recreation and Parks Assn. Natl. Gold Medal award for excellence in park and recreation management. There are 10 comm. and 34 neighborhood parks in the city. Among the largest are Charles A. Pearson and La Palma, which contain public area, herb gardens, lily ponds, baseball fields, tennis courts and swimming pools. There are two public golf courses in the city, the H. G. "Dad" Miller and the Anaheim Hills. Anaheim's Action Trail, or parcourse, the first public facility of its kind in the US, combines a jogging trail and exercise stations along a 1.1 mi. course at Peralta Canyon Park.

CULTURAL ACTIVITES. The Anaheim Cultural Arts Center, operated by the Anaheim Foundation for Culture and the Arts, contains an art gallery, performing arts room and auditorium for various exhibits and performances. Among the city's musical groups are the Anaheim Comm. Band, which is Music Under the Stars concerts in Pearson Park in the summer, Sweet Adelines, Ana-belle Singers, Syncopaters and Memory Melodears, a sr. citizens chorus. E/E Showcase Productions is a summer series of music,

dance, variety showcase and comm. performances held in Edison and Reid parks. Theatrical groups include the Ana-Modjeska Players, who perform at the Anaheim Cultural Arts Center, and Little People's Productions, which presents storybook theatre.

LANDMARKS AND SIGHTSEEING SPOTS. The 180-acre Disneyland, Walt Disney's "Magic Kingdom", features six theme-related areas: Tomorrowland, Frontierland, Fantasyland, Adventureland, Bear Country and New Orleans Sq. Charles A. Pearson Park features the Madame Modjeska Statue, commemorating the internationally-acclaimed Polish actress who settled in the city in 1876. Several other landmarks and attractions are located in nearby Orange Co. cities, as well as LA.

ANCHORAGE
ALASKA

CITY LOCATION-SIZE-EXTENT. Anchorage, the largest comm. in AK, is located in the S central part of the state on a peninsula of the Cook Inlet. It is bordered on the NW by the Knik Arm of the inlet and on the SW by the Turnagain Arm, and is N of the Kenai Peninsula. Situated at 61°10' N lat. and 150°01' W long., it is located as far W as the Hawaiian Islands and further N than Helsinki, Finland. The Municipality of Anchorage encompasses approx. 1,900 sq. mi.

TOPOGRAPHY. Anchorage, surrounded on three sides by arms of the Cook Inlet, is situated on a high bluff containing several lakes and creeks. Among the largest lakes are Hood, Otis, Goose, Sand, Jewel and Spenard. Some 85% of the E part of the municipality is uninhabited, consisting largely of mts., glaciers and lakes. The Chugach Mts., with elevs. reaching 10,000', border the city on the S and E, and approx. 35 mi. N is the Matanuska Valley. The Talkeetna Mts. of the AK Mt. Range are approx. 100 mi. to the N, while the Kenai Mts. are to the W across the Turnagain Arm. The mean elev. of Anchorage, which is located on a seismically active zone extending along the entire N American Pacific coast, is 118'.

CLIMATE. The climate of Anchorage is maritime, continental/moderate coastal and semi-arid. It is influenced by the Chugach Mt. Range, which prevents warm, moist air and thus rain from the Gulf of AK to the SE from reaching the city, as well as the AK Mt. Range, which serves as a barrier to very cold air from the N and therefore maintains warmer temps. Monthly mean temps. range from 12°F in Jan. to 58°F in July, with an avg. annual temp. of 35°F. Although there are four definite seasons, winters last from mid-Oct. to mid-Apr., with the sun shining five hours and 28 min. on the shortest day of the year. The weather alternates between cold, clear days and cloudy, often foggy, mild days. Spring, following the "break-up" of ice, lasts from mid-Apr. to June, while summer consists of a dry season (June to mid-July and a wet season (mid-July to early Sept.), with the sun shining 19 hours and 23 min. on the longest day of the year. Fall is the remaining period from early Sept. to mid-Oct. Most of the 14.74" avg. annual rainfall occurs during late summer and early fall, while most of the 70.4" avg. annual snowfall occurs during late fall and winter. Occasionally, damaging SE "Chugach" winds funnel down the creek canyons of the Chugach Mts. reaching speeds of 80-100 m.p.h. The RH ranges between 50% and 83% and the avg. growing

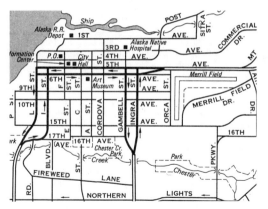

Anchorage, Alaska

season is 124 days. Anchorage is located in the AK-HITZ and observes DST.

FLORA AND FAUNA. Animals native to Anchorage include the moose, dall sheep, black and grizzly bear, snowshoe hare, wolf, wolverine, lynx, fox, coyote, beaver and muskrat. Common birds are the raven, gull, bald eagle, snowy owl, eider duck, magpie and chickadee. Many migratory birds pass through the area and the breeding grounds of numerous waterfowl are located nearby. The cold climate supports very few reptiles and amphibians, although wood frogs are found here. Typical trees include the white birch, larch, aspen, cottonwood, alder, sitka spruce, mt. ash and black spruce. Smaller plants include the greenalder bush, sedge, crowberry, blueberry, raspberry and lingonberries.

POPULATION. According to the US census, the pop. of Anchorage in 1970 was 126,385. In 1979, it was estimated that it had increased to 204,809. Approx. 45% of the state's pop. lives in the city.

ETHNIC GROUPS. In 1978, the ethnic distribution of Anchorage was approx. 89.5% Caucasian, 3% Black, 4.2% Alaskan and Native American, and 3.4% other.

TRANSPORTATION. State hwys. 1 and 3 provide major motor access to Anchorage. The 1,422 mi. long AK Hwy. passes through Anchorage, entering the city from the N as Glenn Hwy. and exiting on the S as Seward Hwy. The AK *Railroad* serves the area. Anchorage Intl. Airport is served by major domestic and foreign *airlines*, including AS, PA, CO, NW, BN, WA and WE. Known as "The Crossroads of the Air World", the city is a major fueling stop for intl. flights between Europe and the Orient, as well as the US and the Orient. The largest float plane base in the world is located on Hood and Spenard lakes, which are joined by a canal. Merrill Field is used for private and charter flights. *Bus lines* include Yukon Motor Coaches, Grayline, AK Sightseeing, Kenai Adventures and the local People Mover System. The Port of Anchorage, the deepwater port farthest N in the US, received cargoes of 441 ships in 1978. The AK Marine Hwy. System, which provides ferry transportation, is served by several cruiseship lines.

COMMUNICATIONS. Communications, broadcasting and print media serving Anchorage are: *AM radio stations* KENI 550 (ABC/C, Top 40); KHAR 590 (APR, Btfl. Mus.); KYAK 650 (MBS, Mod. Ctry.); KBYR 700 (ABC, CBS, AK Broadcasting System, MOR); KFQD 750 (APR, Contemp., Golden) and KANC 1080 (NBC/Mutual Blk., Jazz, Progsv., Top 40); *FM radio stations* KHVN 100.5 (APR, Relig.); KGOT 101.3 (Indep., Contemp., Rock); KJZZ 102.1 (APR, Stereo); KSKA 103.1 (NPR, AK Pub. Radio, Divers.); KKLV 103.9 (Indep., Soft Rock) and KNIK 105.5 (Indep., Btfl. Mus.); *television stations* KENI Ch. 2 (NBC); KAKM Ch. 7 (PBS); KTVA Ch. 11 (CBS) and KIMO Ch. 13 (ABC); *press*: two major dailies serve the area, the *News*, published mornings and the *Times* printed evenings; other area publications include the weekly *AK Journal of Commerce*, *Chugiak-Eagle River Star* and *Greatlander*; the monthly *AK Industry* and the quarterly *AK Geographic*.

HISTORY. Native Americans of the Tanaina tribe of the Athapaskan tribal nation of interior Alaska inhabited the area of present-day Anchorage long before the first white men. Russian explorers and fur traders (the first of whom was Vitus Bering), arriving in the 18th century became the only governing power in AK. By the 1850s, however, fur-trading had declined, and in 1867, US Secy. of State William H. Seward negotiated the purchase of AK from Russia. Although it was known as "Seward's Folly,"and "Seward's Icebox", the area saw development of the fishing industry in the 1870s, and, from 1880, a gold rush. In 1912, the territory of AK was created. The comm. of Anchorage originated in 1914 when several men, sent there to survey land for the federally-owned AK RR (the construction of which was to begin the next year to handle the gold discovered) arrived. Selected as headquarters for the new RR, Anchorage, previously called the "outlet on the inlet", "Ship Creek", around which the first arrivals settled, and "Tent City", since its first residents did not construct homes until July, 1915, received its name in Aug., 1915. The name "Anchorage" was chosen since ships bringing supplies had to anchor offshore near the mouth of Ship Creek before a dock was built in 1917. For years, the AK RR was the principal employer in Anchorage, which was incorporated as a city on Nov. 23, 1920. Anchorage remained a small town until the 1940s, when, after the territory's strategic significance was recognized, Ft. Richardson AFB was established. The pop. of the town, 3,495 in 1940, grew to 30,060 by 1950, as Anchorage became a N US defense center. In 1964, five years after AK achieved statehood, one of the worst earthquakes on record in N America, measuring 8.5 on the Richter scale, caused extensive damage in the city. In 1964, the greater Anchorage Area Borough was created to provide govt. and services to areas beyond the city limits. However, because duplication of efforts resulted, the two govts. were unified in the Muncipality of Anchorage on Sept. 16, 1975. The 798-mi. trans-AK pipeline, built by the Alyeska Pipeline Service Co., a consortium of eight oil companies headquartered in Anchorage, was completed in 1977. Today, the city is the center of the state's commerce, education, culture, govt. and transportation.

GOVERNMENT. The municipality of Anchorage has a mayor-assembly form of govt. consisting of a mayor, who is not a voting member of the assembly, and 11 assembly members. The mayor is elected at large and the assembly members by district, all to three-year terms.

ECONOMY AND INDUSTRY. Govt., including fed., state and municipal, employs approx. 50% of the total Anchorage labor force, which in June, 1979, was approx. 80,430. Although the city is the center of the state's commerce and transportation as well, manufacturing forms only a small part of its economic base. Major industries include oil and gas production, transportation, mining, logging, fishing and tourism. The rate of unemployment in June, 1979, was 8.6%.

BANKING. There are 11 commercial banks and four savings and loans assns. in Anchorage. Total deposits for the nine banks headquartered in the city, including the state's largest (Natl. Bank of AK) and smallest (Security Natl.), were $1,385,846,000 in 1978, while assets totaled $1,684,693,000. Other banks headquartered in the city are First Natl. Bank, AK Mutual Savings, AK State, AK Bank of Commerce, AK Pacific, United Bank AK and Peoples Bank and Trust.

HOSPITALS. There are four hosps. in Anchorage, Providence (administered by the Sisters of Providence), AK Hosp. and Medical Center (supported by the health and welfare trust fund of the AK Teamsters Union), the AK Psychiatric Institute and the AK Native Hosp.

EDUCATION. The state-supported U of AK at Anchorage offers associate,

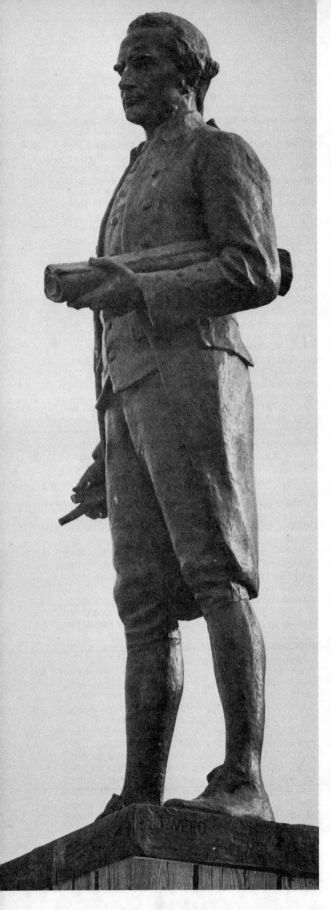

bachelor and master degrees and enrolled more than 4,300 in 1978. Anchorage Comm. Col., a public two-year institution offering associate degrees, enrolled approx. 7,500 in 1978. AK Methodist U, a private liberal arts col. affiliated with the United Methodist Church and founded in 1959, enrolled 160 in 1978. The public school system, consisting of several elementary and 10 jr. high schools, enrolled approx. 38,000 in 1979. Libs. include the AK Municipal (Z. J. Loussac), AK Higher Education Consortium and Heritage Lib. operated by the Natl. Bank of AK.

ENTERTAINMENT. The "Alaska Story" is presented nightly in Anchorage at the Capt. Cook Hotel's dinner show. The Renaissance Open Aire Pleasure Faire at Campbell Creek Park is a two-day annual festival featuring medieval dress, crafts and entertainment. The annual Mayor's Marathon is a 26-mi. run through the Anchorage area. The AK Festival of Music, held annually during two weeks in June, features concerts, recitals, theater, jazz, dance, opera, film and visual arts presentations. The annual Anchorage Fur Rendezvous and World Championship Sled Dog Race, held annually in Feb., commemorates the time when trappers sold their winter caches of fur. Eighty events, including three consecutive days of sled-dog races with 25 mi. heats, music, art, sports, a carnival and the Miners and Trappers Ball, are featured. During June, July, Aug. and Sept., the Indian House on Turnagain Arm hosts the Salmon Bake nightly. The Campbell Creek Classic, or Whacky Regatta, is also an annual summer event in which girls compete in a canoe race. The Anchorage Glacier Pilots, a baseball team, plays in a summer league at Mulcahy Baseball Park. The U of AK-Anchorage Sea Wolves participate in sports at the collegiate level. Concerts-in-the Park is a summer series of band presentations held every Thurs. evening.

ACCOMMODATIONS. There are approx. 15 hotels and motels in Anchorage, including the Anchorage Intl., the Best Western-Barratt, the Holiday, Inlet, Ramada, Sheraton, Travelers and Rodeway inns, Anchorage TraveLodge, Anchorage-Westward Hilton, the Capt. Cook, Voyager and Palace Hotels, Red Ram Motor Lodge, Sheffield House and the Alaska, Arctic Inn, Merrill, Mush Inn and Thunderbird motels.

FACILITIES. There are more than 20 parks encompassing 8,000 acres in Anchorage providing tennis courts, playing fields, nine-hole golf courses and hiking trails, as well as facilities for picnicking and overnight camping. A 70-mi. system of trails is used for jogging, cross-country skiing and bicycle riding. Among the parks are Russian Jack Springs, Goose Lake, Jewel Lake, Resolution, Chester Creek, Centennial, Lynnary and Earthquake. The 495,000-acre Chugach State Park, the largest in the US, is situated on the E and S sides of Anchorage. Swimming is available at Goose, Jewel and Spenard lakes. Fresh- and salt-water boating and sailing are available at several lakes and creeks, including Jewel and Sand lakes and Westchester Lagoon. The AK Zoo contains 35 species of primarily native animals. Seventeen local lakes are annually stocked with rainbow trout, landlocked coho (silver salmon) and grayling. Big game hunting is also available nearby.

CULTURAL ACTIVITIES. The AK Repertory Theatre, the main threatrical group in Anchorage, performs at Sydney Laurence Auditorium. The city has a symphony orchestra and a natl. award-winning comm. chorus. There are several museums in the city, including Anchorage Intl. Art Institute, Anchorage Historical and Fine Arts Museum and AK Arctic Indian and Eskimo Museum, which feature native arts, crafts and history. The Ft. Richardson Wildlife Center and Elmendorf AFB Wildlife Museum display native AK species of birds and animals. The Visual Arts Center of AK, containing studios, is one of the 20 galleries in the city that features native arts and crafts, including ivory, wood and bone carving and sculpture. Art is also displayed at City Hall, the AK RR Station, Boney Memorial Courthouse and several banks.

LANDMARKS AND SIGHTSEEING SPOTS. The City of Anchorage Greenhouse features displays of tropical plants, birds and fish. The Centennial Rose Garden, open in summer, is the northernmost garden of its kind on the N American continent. A 139' AK-grown Sitka spruce flagpole is located on the grounds of City Hall, while inside is the William H. Seward Memorial, with carvings on AK marble, commemorating the centennial of the AK Purchase. The old Fed. Building, built in the

Capt. James Cook Statue, Resolution Park, Anchorage, Alaska

1930s, is listed on the Natl. Register of Historic Places. The Pioneer Schoolhouse, the first school in the city, has been preserved, while two period log cabins are located at Ben Crawford Memorial Park. A 23' statue of a blue whale stands in front of the Carr-Gottstein Building, while a 7.5' statue of Capt. James Cook, who explored Cook Inlet in 1778 in his ship *Resolution*, stands in Resolution Park. A monument inscribed with the legend of Mt. Susitna (sleeping lady), which can be seen across the Knik Arm, is located on the park's wooden deck and walkway. Fourth Ave. is an interesting landmark—during the 1964 earthquake, its N site fell an avg. of 20'. The 15,000-acre Potter Tidal Marsh on the Turn Again Arm, created as a result of the 1964 earthquake when the area dropped and flooded, is a state refuge for birds and waterfowl and a popular site for bird-watching.

ANN ARBOR
MICHIGAN

CITY LOCATION-SIZE-EXTENT. Ann Arbor is located on the Huron River in the lower peninsula of SE MI, 35 mi. W of Detroit, at 42°17' N lat. and 83°54'6" W long. It is the seat and largest city of Washtenaw Co. The city encompasses 24 sq. mi. and is bordered by Wayne and Jackson counties. Its met. area includes Ypsilanti, and is within Detroit's greater met. area.

TOPOGRAPHY. Most of Ann Arbor is situated on descending slopes that were once the banks of a large glacial river. The terrain consists of gently sloping hills, with a broad plateau high above the river bed. The city is surrounded by farmland and contains many streams and ponds. The Huron River flows through the N part of the city. The mean elev. is 850'.

CLIMATE. Although Ann Arbor is situated in the path of major summer and winter storm tracks which create diverse climatic conditions, the Great Lakes exert a moderating influence on the weather. Summers are warm and sunny, with temps. exceeding 90°F an avg. of eight days per year, while winters are relatively cold and cloudy, with temps. reaching 0°F or below an avg. of four days per year. The avg. annual temp. of 50°F ranges from a Jan. mean of 27°F to a July mean of 74°F. Most of the 30" avg. annual rainfall occurs during Apr. and May. The 35" avg. annual snowfall occurs mainly from Nov. to Mar. The RH ranges from 50% to 90% and the length of the growing season is 163 days. Ann Arbor lies in the ESTZ and observes DST.

FLORA AND FAUNA. Animals native to Ann Arbor include the whitetail deer, chipmunk, fox squirrel, raccoon and opossum. Common birds include the robin, warbler, wren, hawk and owl. Salamanders and frogs, as well as the venomous massasauga (a pygmy rattler) and timber rattlesnake, are found in the area. Typical trees include the apple, green ash, burraud white oak, basswood and sugar maple. Smaller plants include the blackberry, sunflower, prickly lettuce and pepperweed.

POPULATION. According to the US census, the pop. of Ann Arbor in 1970 was 100,036. In 1978, it was estimated to have increased to approx. 107,000.

ETHNIC GROUPS. In 1978, the ethnic distribution of Ann Arbor was approx. 89% Caucasian, 9% Black, .5% Hispanic, 1% Asian and .5% Native American.

TRANSPORTATION. Interstate Hwy. 94 and US Hwy. 23 provide major motor access to Ann Arbor. *Railroads* serving the city include AMTRAK and ConRail. Commuter *airlines* serve Willow Run and Ann Arbor Municipal airports, while 13 major airlines serve Detroit Metro Airport. The local Ann Arbor Transportation Authority and Brooks, Greyhound and N Star *bus lines* provide service to the city.

COMMUNICATIONS. Communications, broadcasting and print media

originating from Ann Arbor are: *AM radio stations* WPAG 1050 (ABC/I, MOR) and WAAM 1600 (ABC/E, MOR); *FM radio stations* WCBN 88.3 (Indep., Divers.); WUOM 91.7 (NPR, Fine Arts); WIQB 102.9 (ABC/FM, AOR); and WPAG 107.1 (Indep., MOR, C&W); no *television stations* operate from Ann Arbor, which receives broadcasting from Detroit stations; *press*: two dailies serve the area, the *Ann Arbor News*, issued evenings, and the *MI Daily*, published weekday mornings; other publications include the monthly *Ann Arbor Observer*, the quarterly *Ann Arbor Scene*, UM student publications, issued five days per week, the *Chronicle* and the *Education Digest*.

HISTORY. Native Americans of the Huron, Chippewa and Potawatomi tribes inhabited the area of present-day Ann Arbor before the first white settlers arrived. In 1821, John Allen of VA and Elisha Walker Rumsey of NY left the fur-trading outpost of Detroit and founded the settlement they called "Annarbor" in honor of their wives, Ann Allen and Mary Ann Rumsey. More settlers arrived following the completion of the Erie Canal in 1825, and Ann Arbor was incorporated as a village in 1833. The pop. continued to grow with the beginning of stagecoach runs, the opening of a RR line in 1839 and the establishment of the U of MI in the village to which it had moved from Detroit, in 1837. Many of the early settlers were from Germany and Ireland. The U influenced the growth of Ann Arbor, as well as the development of its economy, in the years which followed. Ann Arbor was incorporated as a city in 1851, and, in 1861, annexed "Lower Town", the comm. N of the Huron River. The city became known not only as a center of education, but also one of research, light industry, medicine and science.

GOVERNMENT. Ann Arbor has a mayor-mgr.-council form of govt. The council consists of the mayor, elected at large, a voting member with veto power, as well as 10 councillors, two elected from each of the city's five wards. All serve two-year terms and appoint a city administrator.

Built in the 1800's, this building now houses the Women's Equal Rights Movement, Ann Arbor, Michigan

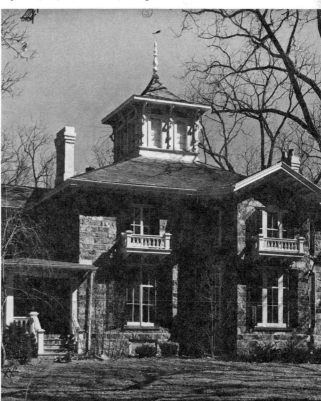

ECONOMY AND INDUSTRY. Among the most important industries in Ann Arbor are research, electronics and scientific instruments. More than 50 manufacturing firms are located in the city. In 1978, the avg. per capita income was $5,690. In June, 1979, the labor force totaled 58,050, while the unemployment rate was 3.6%.

BANKING. There are eight major banking institutions in Ann Arbor, as well as 39 branches. In 1978, total deposits for the four banks headquartered in the city were $622,522,000, while total assets were $686,170,000. Banks Include Ann Arbor Bank & Trust, Natl. Bank & Trust, Huron Valley Natl., and Ann Arbor Trust.

HOSPITALS. There are four hosps. in Ann Arbor, St. Joseph Mercy, U Medical Center (associated with the U of MI Medical School), Mercywood Neuropsychiatric and V.A. Medical Center.

EDUCATION. The U of MI at Ann Arbor is consistently ranked among the top 10 research universities in the US. Established in 1817 and moved from Detroit to Ann Arbor in 1837, it enrolled 36,740 in 1978 at the bachelor, master and doctorate degree levels. Other institutions of higher education in the city are Concordia Lutheran Jr., established in 1962 and enrolling more than 600; Washtenaw Comm. Col., established in 1965 and enrolling more than 7,000, and MI Technical Institute. Research institutions include the Mid-American Research Institute, Kelsey Hayes R&D Center, MI Research Group, Ann Arbor Biological Center, Highway Safety, Research Institute and Space Research Center. Phoenix Memorial Laboratory of the U of MI is devoted to research for peaceful uses of atomic energy. There are 31 public schools in the city including 25 elementary and four jr. and two sr. high schools, as well as six private schools, including two Catholic, two Lutheran and one Seventh Day Adventist. Total public school enrollment is approx. 18,500. Libs. include the Ann Arbor Public, the Huron Valley Lib. for the Blind and the Rudolf Steiner House, as well as the Hatcher Grad. Lib. and William L. Clements Lib. of the U of MI, which houses noted collections of Americana, original manuscripts, maps and rare books.

ENTERTAINMENT. Ann Arbor hosts the Music Festival, Art Fair, Winter

Ann Arbor, Michigan

Art Fair, Ethnic Festival and Greek Festival each year. The U of MI Wolverines participate in intercollegiate sports in the Big Ten Conf., while the Warriors of Washtenaw Comm. Col. and the Falcons of Concordia Col. also play at the collegiate level. The U of MI stadium, with a seating capacity of 101,000, is the largest col. stadium in the US. The professional teams of nearby Detroit also provide spectator sports entertainment.

ACCOMMODATIONS. There are 12 hotels and motels in Ann Arbor, including Ann Arbor Campus, the Wolverine, Weber's, Howard Johnson, and the Holiday, Marriott, Ramada and Hilton inns.

FACILITIES. There are several public parks in Ann Arbor, including Buhr, Veterans' Memorial, West, Leslie and Galup, as well as several public golf courses including Huron, Washtenaw Co. and Ann Arbor. A jogging track is available at Park Washtenaw. Matthaei Botanical Gardens, seven mi. NE of the center of town, features plants from throughout the world in indoor gardens with changing seasonal displays along outdoor nature trails.

CULTURAL ACTIVITIES. Among the performing groups in Ann Arbor are the Ann Arbor Federation of Music, A & A Production and Ann Arbor Symphony. Musical and dramatic performances are presented at the U of MI Power Center for the Performing Arts. The U of MI School of Music presents weekly recitals and concerts. Museums include the U of MI Museum of Art, featuring W Art from the 6th century to the present, near and far E and African art and 20th century prints and drawings; the U of MI Exhibit Museum, containing displays of fossils, minerals, astronomy, MI wildlife, biology and anthropology, as well as a planetarium; and the Kemp House Historical Home. Theaters include the Mendelssohn and Michigan, while the U of MI presents a Professional Theater Program. There are several galleries in the city including Dreyfuss, Valentine, Gallery One and Union Gallery. Concerts and operas are held at Hill Auditorium.

LANDMARKS AND SIGHTSEEING SPOTS. Among the landmarks in Ann Arbor is the Burton Memorial Tower of the U of MI, housing the Baird Carillon of 55 bells, ranging in weight from 12 pounds to 12 tons. Weekly concerts are presented in Spring and Summer. A radio telescope, located 16 mi. NW of the city at Peach Mt., holds three open houses during the summer. Another historic landmark is the Cobblestone Historical Building.

ARLINGTON
TEXAS

CITY LOCATION-SIZE-EXTENT. Arlington lies between Dallas to the E and Ft. Worth to the W in N central TX at 32°44'2" N lat. and 97°6'8" W long. The city occupies 99 sq. mi. in Tarrant Co. and is bordered by Dallas Co. on the E and Ellis and Johnson counties on the S. The W fork of the Trinity River flows through the N part of the city. Arlington is located in the greater Dallas-Ft. Worth met. area, known as the Metroplex.

TOPOGRAPHY. Arlington's topography is characterized by low, rolling hills. The city lies in the transition area between the N central plains region to the W and the gulf coastal plain region to the E. Lake Arlington lies on the W side of the city. The mean elev. is 616'.

CLIMATE. The climate of Arlington is humid and continental, with wide ranges in temp. extremes. The 66°F avg. annual temp. ranges from a mean of 45°F during Jan. to 85°F during July. The 32" avg. annual rainfall occurs mainly in May and Oct. Yearly variations in rainfall range from less than 20" to more than 50". Snowfall avgs. 3.5" annually. The RH ranges from 45% to 88%. The growing season avgs. 250 days. Arlington lies in the CSTZ and observes DST.

FLORA AND FAUNA. Animals native to Arlington include the beaver, nutria, skunk, raccoon, opossum, gray fox and coyote. Common birds are the mockingbird (the state bird), cardinal, crow, vulture, meadowlark and

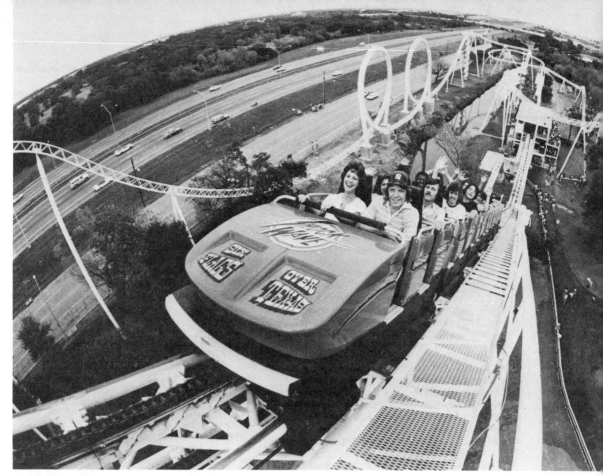

Six Flags Over Texas, Arlington, Texas

grackle. Frogs, lizards, turtles and snakes, including the venomous cottonmouth, copperhead, coral snake and rattlesnake, inhabit the area. The oak, pine and pecan (the state tree) are common trees. Wildflowers include the bluebonnet (the state flower), Indian paintbrush and evening primrose.

POPULATION. According to the US census, the pop. of Arlington in 1970 was 90,643. In 1978, it was estimated to have increased to 168,000.

ETHNIC GROUPS. In 1978, the ethnic distribution of Arlington was approx. 93.5% Caucasian, 2.6% Black, 2.5% Hispanic and 1.4% other.

TRANSPORTATION. Interstate hwys. 20 and 30, US hwys. 157, 303 and 360 provide major motor access to Arlington. *Railroads* serving the city include Great SW, MO Pacific and TX Pacific. Arlington Municipal and nearby Dallas-Fort Worth Regional airports are served by all major *airlines*. The city is served by Suntran, Trailways and TX Motor Coach *bus lines*.

COMMUNICATIONS. Communications, broadcasting and print media originating in Arlington are: *FM radio stations* KWJS 94.9 (Indep., Progsv.) and KPLX 99.5 (ABC/Indep., MOR); there are no *AM radio stations* or *television stations* in the city, which receives broadcasting from nearby Dallas-Ft. Worth; *press*: one major daily serves the city, the *Daily News*, published evenings; other area publications include the *Shorthorn*, the *Citizen-Journal*, the *Urbanite*, *Dairy Men's Digest*, *Arlington Woman* and the quarterly *Arlington Magazine*.

HISTORY. Native Americans of the Caddo tribe inhabited the Arlington area, situated in the natural N-S trailway called the E Cross Timbers belt, before the arrival of white settlers. By the 1830s, the area was considered one of the last strongholds of the native Americans in the new republic of TX. Their hunting grounds jeopardized, the Native Americans continued to confront the TX Rangers and settlers before Pres. Sam Houston arranged the Grand Council of Indians in the hope of negotiating a peace treaty. Several native Americans, as well as TX Rangers, were killed in the battle of Village Creek in May, 1841. Held at Marrow Bone Spring, an ancient Indian campsite in present-day Arlington, the Grand Council resulted in the signing of a treaty on Sept. 29, 1843, by Gen. Edward H. Tarrant, namesake of the co., and subsequently, Marrow Bone Spring became the location of Trading Post #1 of the Republic of TX in 1845 and, in 1846, the outpost of the TX Rangers under the command of Col. Middleton Tate Johnson, considered the "Father of Arlington", as well as the site of his home. The white settlement of the 1840s grew into a stage stop known as Johnson's Station. In 1872, the comm. was relocated NE on the TX & Pacific RR line. Named Johnson by RR surveyors, the community's name was changed to Arlington, in honor of Robert E. Lee's VA. home. Since it conflicted with Johnson's Station three mi. S, Arlington was incorporated as a city on Mar. 18, 1884. It experienced steady growth as a family town, the economy of which was based on agriculture, trade and later, education (Arlington Col. was established in 1895). In the 20th century, the automotive industry contributed to the growth of the city, which was also enhanced by the development of Six Flags Over TX, a major entertainment complex, and Arlington Stadium, home of the TX Rangers professional baseball team.

GOVERNMENT. Arlington has a mayor-mgr.-council form of govt. The seven council members, including the mayor, are elected at large to two-year terms.

ECONOMY AND INDUSTRY. The largest planned industrial development in the US, the Great SW Industrial District, is located in Arlington on the site of the former

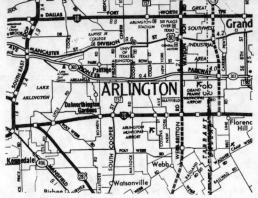

Central Arlington, Texas

Arlington Downs Race Track, which operated in the 1930s until parimutuel betting was made illegal in TX. The city's economy is largely based on industry, distribution, education and entertainment. Major industrial products include cans and containers, oil field equipment, food products, farm equipment, plastics, tool parts, steel, insecticides, trailers, campers, rubber products, printing products, aircraft, electronic components, road equipment and photographic products. The unemployment rate in 1978 was 3.2%. In 1977, avg. household income was $22,520, and the total labor force was 26,229.

BANKING. In 1978, total deposits for the seven banks headquartered in Arlington were $389,724,000, while total assets were $436,095,000. Banks in the city include Arlington Bank and Trust, First City Natl., Arlington Bank of Commerce, Arlington Natl., First City Central and Metroplex Natl.

HOSPITALS. Hosps. in Arlington include Sunrise, Arlington Memorial and Arlington Comm.

EDUCATION. The U of TX at Arlington, which offers associate, bachelor, master and doctorate degrees, enrolled more than 17,000 in 1978. Established as the two-year Arlington Col. in 1895, it became four-year Arlington State Col. in 1959, and part of the UT System in 1967. Arlington Baptist Jr. Col. is also located in the city as is a "fashion" col. More than 32,000 are enrolled in the city's public school system. There are an additional 29 private schools in the city. Lib. facilities are available at the Arlington Public and UT-Arlington libs.

ENTERTAINMENT. The Arlington 200 Art Sale is an annual city event, as is the Arts and Crafts Fair. The Cow Bell Indoor Rodeo, in which the audience participates, is held every Sat. night. The TX Rangers, an AL baseball team, is based in the city. Arlington participates in sports at the col. level. The professional and collegiate sports organizations of the Dallas-Fort Worth area, as well as dinner theaters, festivals and annual events, are easily accessible to residents of Arlington.

ACCOMMODATIONS. Hotels and motels in Arlington include the Inn of the Six Flags, Caravan Hotel, and Rodeway, Quality, King's, Holiday, Day's, Ramada, Metro Park and Great SW inns.

FACILITIES. The 1,345-acre Arlington park system consists of 33 parks, some of which are not yet completely developed. Among the larger parks are Randol Mill, Veterans' Lake Arlington Spillway, Vandergriff and Meadowbrook. The parks contain seven swimming pools, four recreation centers, one comm. center, one 18-hole golf course (Lake Arlington), one nine-hole golf course, 61 ball fields and 26 lighted tennis courts, as well as natural woodlands with hiking trails and camping facilities. Also included in the park system are 22 playgrounds, a 55-acre motorcycle riding area, two paved model airplane fields and 112 acres of picnic area. Dalworthington Gardens is also located in the city, as is the Arlington Entertainment Complex, containing Arlington Stadium, Seven Seas and Six Flags Over TX.

CULTURAL ACTIVITIES. Six Flags Over TX, although an amusement park, features the history of TX under the flags of Spain, France, Mexico, the Republic of TX, the US and the Confederate States of America. The Watson Cabin, built about 1854, was restored in 1976 as the Bicentennial-Centennial project of the Arlington Historical Society. It is located in the Middleton Tate Johnson Cemetery, which also contains the restored 1854 Melear Cabin. Cultural activities of the Dallas-Ft. Worth Metroplex are available to residents of Arlington.

LANDMARKS AND SIGHTSEEING SPOTS. A tour of historical sites

of Arlington includes a stop at Bird's Ft., the first in the area, established in the winter of 1840-41 by Jonathan Bird and volunteer soldiers. Marrow Bone Springs, the site of the Grand Council of Indians and the site of the Battle of Village Creek, where members of the TX militia attacked an Indian village in 1841, are also included on the tour. The homes of early settlers, including the 1878 Cooper home now occupied by the Arlington Woman's Club, have been maintained, as have the Watson and Middleton Tate Johnson Family cemeteries. The site of M. T. Johnson's plantation home, which later became a Stagecoach Inn of the settlement of Johnson's Station, is also on the tour. The Arlington Mineral Water Well was dug in 1891 to serve as the town well. It was initially considered unfit for human consumption, but later sought-after for its "curative" powers. It may now be tasted from a fountain.

ATLANTA
GEORGIA

CITY LOCATION-SIZE-EXTENT. Atlanta, the capital and largest city of the state and seat of Fulton Co., is located in N central GA at 33°39' N lat. and 84°25' W long. The city encompasses 131.5 sq. mi., 250 mi. N of the Gulf of Mexico and 250 mi. W of the Atlantic Ocean. The greater met. area includes all of Fulton and DeKalb counties to the E and extends throughout 15 counties including bordering Cobb and Douglas to the W, Cherokee to the N and Gwinnet to the NE.

TOPOGRAPHY. The terrain of Atlanta, which is situated on the Piedmont plateau in the foothills of the S Appalachian Mts., ranges from gently rolling to hilly, sloping downward toward the E, W and S. The city lies S of the Blue Ridge Mts. and E of the Chattahooche River, while Lake Lanier is to the NE and Allatoona Lake to the NW. The mean elev. is 1,000'.

CLIMATE. The climate of Atlanta, influenced by the Atlantic Ocean, Bermuda high pressure area, the Gulf of Mexico and the Appalachian Mts., is characterized by warm, humid summers and mild winters. The annual avg. temp of 61.4°F ranges from a Jan. mean of 43.2°F

Central Atlanta, Georgia

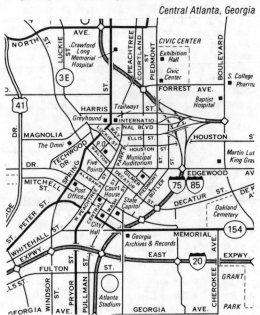

to a July mean of 78.4°F. The 48.5" avg. annual rainfall ranges from an Oct. mean of 2.5" to a Mar. mean of nearly 6". The avg. annual snowfall is 1.5". Tornadoes occasionally result from severe local thunderstorms, which occur frequently from Mar. through May. The RH ranges from 50% to 91%. The avg. growing season is 230 days. Atlanta lies in the ESTZ and observes DST.

FLORA AND FAUNA. Animals native to Atlanta include the fox, raccoon, opossum and whitetail deer. Common birds are the cardinal, wren, chimney swift, chuck-will's-widow and red-eyed vireo. Bullfrogs, tree frogs, mud turtles, green anole lizards and water snakes, as well as the venomous rattlesnake and coral snake, are found in the area. Typical trees include the magnolia, redbud, red and white oak, pine, hickory and sweetgum. Smaller plants include the chicory, lobelia, mayweed and honeysuckle.

POPULATION. According to the US census, the pop. of Atlanta in 1970 was 495,039. In 1978, it was estimated that it had decreased to 456,200.

ETHNIC GROUPS. In 1978, the ethnic distribution of Atlanta was approx. 38.7% Caucasian, 60.3% Black and 1.0% Hispanic (a percentage of the Hispanic total is also included in the Caucasian total).

TRANSPORTATION. Interstate hwys. 20, 75, 85 and 285 provide major motor access to the city. *Railroads* serving the city include AMTRAK, Burlington N, ConRail, FL E Coast, Central Gulf, Santa Fe, S Pacific and Union Pacific. *Airlines* serving Hartsfield Intl. Airport include BN, DL, EA, FL, NA, GW, PI, OZ, PA, Sabena, Airlift Intl., SO, TW, NW Orient and UA. Other airports serving the city are Charlie Brown and DeKalb Peachtree. *Bus lines* serving the city include Greyhound, Trailways, N GA and the local Met. Atlanta Rapid Transit Authority (MARTA). A 53-mi. rapid rail and bus transit system is under construction.

COMMUNICATIONS. Communications, broadcasting and print media serving Atlanta are: *AM radio stations* WPLO 590 (ABC/I, C&W); WRNG 680 (UPI, CBS, News); WBS 750 (NBC, Var.); WQXI 790 (APR, Contemp., Top 40); WXAP 860 (GA News, C&W); WGST 920 (ABC/I, GA APR, News); WKLS 970 (Indep., MOR); WGUN 1010 (Indep., Relig., C&W); WGKA 1199 (GA, Clas.); WIGO 1340 (ABC/C, Mut. Blk.); WAOK 1380 (Natl. Blk., R&B) and WYZE 1400 (GA, Blk.); *FM radio stations* WRAS 88.5 (GA, Progsv.); WRFG 89.3 (Indep., Var., Spec., Progsv.); WABE 90.1 (WETV-TV, Jazz); WREK 91.1 (UPI, Progsv.); WCLK 91.9 (Indep., Progsv.); WZGC 92.9 (Indep., Contemp.); WPCH 94.9 (Indep., Btfl. Mus.); WKLS 96.1 (CBS/FM, Progsv.); WSB 98.5 (WSB-TV, Btlf. Mus); WLTA 99.7 (Indep., MOR) and WVEE 103.3 (ABC/FM, Disco); *television stations* WSB Ch. 2 (NBC); WAGA Ch. 5 (CBS); WXIA Ch. 11 (ABC); WTCG Ch. 17 (Indep.); WETV Ch. 30 (PBS); WATL Ch. 36 (ABC, CBS, NBC) and WANX Ch. 46 (Indep.); *press:* two major dailies serve the city, the morning *Constitution* and the evening *Journal;* other publications include the morning *World*, the weekly *Inquirer, Business Chronicle* and *Emory Wheel*, the monthly *Atlanta Magazine* and *Business Atlanta*, the bi-monthly *Economic Review* and the quarterly *Emory Magazine*.

HISTORY. Native Americans of the Creek tribe, living in a village called Standing Peachtree, inhabited the area of present-day Atlanta before the first white settlers arrived. During the War of 1812, Ft. Peachtree was established near the original Creek Village, connected to another ft. 30 mi. distant by Peachtree Rd (from which Main St. and 23 others in present-day Atlanta take their names). In 1821, the Creeks ceded the site of the city to GA, and in 1837, the comm. of Terminus was established at the terminal point of the W and Atlantic RR. The settlement was incorporated as a town in 1843, at which time its pop. was 200, and was renamed Marthasville in honor of the daughter of Gov. Lumpkin, whose efforts had led to the establishment of a RR. By 1845, three RR ran through the center of town and, upon the suggestion of Edgar Thompson, a RR engineer, its name was changed to Atlanta, in honor of W and Atlantic RR. Chartered as a city on 1847, it became a transportation center and the seat of Fulton Co. in 1853. By 1854, its pop. reached 6,000, and, by the 1860s, 10,000. In 1864, during the Civil War, Union Gen. William Sherman reduced the Confederate supply center to a smoking ruin, with only 400 of the original 4,500 houses and buildings still standing. Rapidly rebuilt, Atlanta was designated the state capital in 1868, and the pop. of the city doubled between 1865 and 1870. Several fairs held during the 1880s attracted famous industries to the city, including Coca-Cola in 1886, which influenced the subsequent growth of the pop. By 1900, it reached nearly 90,000. A fire in 1917 destroyed 2,000 buildings

The Stone Mountain Memorial carving some 300 feet up on the sheer north face of Stone Mt., honors confederate heroes, Atlanta, Georgia

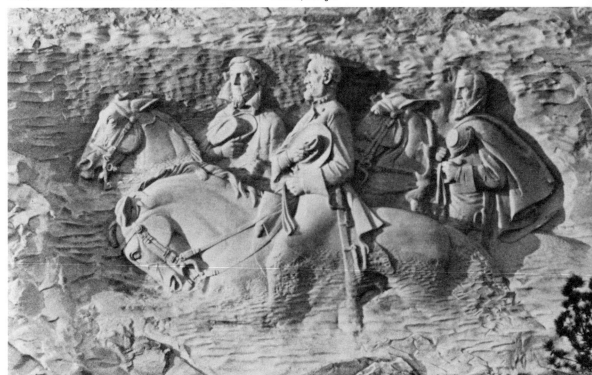

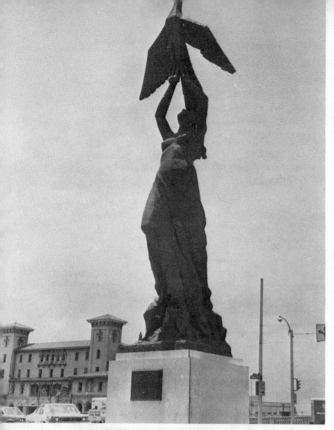

"Atlanta from the Ashes" depicts Atlanta's rise from the ashes
of the Civil War, Atlanta, Georgia

temporarily inhibiting the development of the city,
which grew substantially during WW I with the influx of
farm workers arriving to work in newly established,
defense-related industries. By 1950, the city's pop.
reached 330,000 and territory annexed in 1952 contributed to the growth of pop. to 487,000 by 1960. During the
1960s, the city's public schools were peacefully integrated. An active campaign begun in 1961 to attract
more new industries resulted, by 1970, in a boom in
construction. By 1970, the pop. exceeded 495,000.

GOVERNMENT. Atlanta has a mayor-council form of govt., consisting of
18 council members and the mayor, who may only serve two consecutive,
four-year terms. The mayor and six council members are elected at large
while the remaining 12 are elected by district to staggered four-year terms.

ECONOMY AND INDUSTRY. Atlanta is the distribution,
manufacturing and transportation center of the SE.
Textiles is the oldest and most important industry,
followed by the production of aircraft, automobiles,
furniture, chemicals, communications equipment, food,
paper products, fertilizer, iron and steel products and
soft drinks. Coca-Cola is headquartered in the city.
Office, manufacturing or warehouse facilities of the 500
largest industrial firms in the US are located in the city.
More than 25% of the total work force is employed in
wholesale and retail trade. In June, 1979, the total labor
force of the greater met. area was approx. 919,900,
while the rate of unemployment was 5.3%. In 1977, the
median per capita income was $6,121.

BANKING. There are 16 commercial banks and two savings and loan
assns. in Atlanta. In 1978, total deposits for the six banks headquartered in
the city were $4,322,870,000, while assets were $6,022,287,000. Banks
include First Natl., Fulton Natl., Natl. of GA, Trust Co. Bank, First GA and
Citizens First.

HOSPITALS. There are approx. 50 hosps. in Atlanta, including Grady
Memorial, GA Baptist, Piedmont, Emory U, Crawford W. Long and Doctors
Memorial. The US Center for Disease Control is also located in the city.

EDUCATION. Among the institutions of higher learning in the city are
Atlanta U, which enrolled more than 1,700 in 1978; Emory U, which enrolled
nearly 7,600 in 1978; Morehouse Col., which enrolled more than 1,500;
Morris Brown Col., which enrolled more than 1,600; Oglethorpe Col., which
enrolled nearly 900; and Spelman Col., which enrolled 1,300 in 1978. Atlanta
U Center, an affiliation of six colleges, forms the largest predominantly
black educational complex in the US. Other institutions include the state
controlled GA State U, the largest in the area, established in 1913 and
enrolling nearly 21,000 in 1978; GA Institute of Technology, established in
1885 and enrolling more than 10,100; Atlanta Col. of Art; Atlanta Jr. Col.;
Clark Col.; Mercer U in Atlanta and its School of Pharmacy; the
Interdenominational Theological Center and the S Center for Intl. Studies.
There are more than 150 public elementary and high schools in the city, with
a 1978 enrollment exceeding 100,000. Lib. facilities include the Atlanta
Public Lib., and the US Center for Disease Control Lib.

ENTERTAINMENT. Atlanta hosts a number of annual festivals,
including the Mayor's Week of the Arts, the Piedmont Arts Festival, the
Greek Festival and the Dogwood Festival, held each Apr. The annual Peach
Bowl takes place in the city in Dec. Among the dinner theaters in the city are
the Barn Dinner Theatre, the Midnight Sun, the Harlequin and the Manhattan
Yellow Pages. Professional sports entertainment is provided by the Atlanta
Braves, an NL baseball team and the Atlanta Falcons, an NFL-NFC football
team who play at the Atlanta-Fulton Co. Stadium. The Atlanta Flames, an
NHL hockey team and the Atlanta Hawks, an NBA basketball team,
play in the Omni Coliseum. The Emory U Eagles, the GA Tech. Yellowjackets
of the Atlanta Coast Conf. and the Atlanta Christian Col. Chargers
participate in collegiate sports.

ACCOMMODATIONS. There are several hotels and motels in Atlanta,
including the Hyatt Regency, Colony Sq., Omni, Peachtree Center
Plaza, the tallest hotel in the world, Stadium, Dunfey and Biltmore hotels,
as well as the Marriott, Sheraton, Hilton, Red Carpet, Best Western, Master
Host, Howard Johnson's, TraveLodge and Ramada, Holiday, Rodeway and Day's
inns.

FACILITIES. There are 5,000 areas of municipal and co. parks in
Atlanta providing playgrounds, athletic fields, recreation centers, golf
courses and more than 200 tennis courts. Major parks include Chastain,
Adams, Piedmont, Southside and Grant, which contains the Atlanta Zoo.
Fishing, hunting and boating are available throughout the parks—the city
is considered to be one of the largest inland boating centers in the US.

CULTURAL ACTIVITIES. There are more than 45 performing arts
organizations and several museums in Atlanta. The Atlanta Symphony
Orchestra, the Alliance Theatre, Children's Theatre, Atlanta Opera, Atlanta
Ballet and Atlanta Theatre Co. perform in the Atlanta Memorial Arts Center,
dedicated to the 122 Atlanta Arts Assn. members killed in a Paris airplane
crash in 1962. Other dramatic groups are Academy Theatre, Theatre Under
the Stars, which presents summer musicals, while the S Ballet of Atlanta
and the Ruth Mitchell Dance Co. are other dance organizations. Concert and
other cultural events are held at the Fox Theatre, which is listed on the Natl.
Register of Historic Places. The High Museum of Art, located on the main
floor at the Memorial Arts Center, features French Impressionist paintings
and prints from the Kress Collection. Archives and a museum featuring
displays of the history, architecture, art and music of the city are housed in
the Atlanta Historical Society Headquarters. The GA Archives and Records
Building contains Civil War and state documents, as well as historical
exhibits. The GA State Museum of Science and Industry, located at the GA
State Capitol, displays rocks, minerals, fossils and native American
artifacts. The Fern Bank Science Center contains the third largest
planetarium in the world. The Toy Museum contains 100,000 antique toys.

LANDMARKS AND SIGHTSEEING SPOTS. Historical landmarks in
Atlanta include the Kennesaw Mt. Battlefield Park located at the site of the
Civil War Battle of Atlanta, the Zero Mile Post, scarred "Flame of the
Confederacy Lamppost" which survived the Civil War. The Atlanta
Historical Society maintains the Tullie Smith House, built in 1840, as well as
the Swan House, which typifies a wealthy 20th century lifestyle. Wren's
Nest was the home of Joel Chandler Harris, author of the Uncle Remus
stories, while the Henry W. Grady Monument is a bronze statue of the GA
Civil Orator. Located in Grant Park are Old Ft. Walker and Civil War

breastworks. The tombstone of Martin Luther King, located in the Ebenezer Baptist Churchyard, bears the inscription "free at last, free at last, thank God Almighty, I'm free at last". The Gov.'s Mansion, Peachtree Center, Peachtree Plaza and Peachtree St. are popular attractions, as is Omni Intl., a shopping, food and entertainment complex.

AURORA
COLORADO

CITY LOCATION-SIZE-EXTENT. Aurora, situated 7 mi. E of Denver, is located at 39°44'4" N lat. and 104°52'1" W long. The third largest city in CO, it encompasses 60 sq. mi. in Arapahoe and Adams counties in the N central

FLORA AND FAUNA. Animals native to Aurora include the mule deer, prairie dog, jack rabbit, seven-stripe ground squirrel, chipmunk and coyote. Common birds include the crow, jay, eagle, chickadee, mt. bluebird, woodpecker, magpie and redwing blackbird. Garter snakes, horned and fence lizards and the venomous prairie rattlesnake are found in the area. Typical trees are the cottonwood, willow, box elder and Dutch elm. Smaller plants include the tumbleweed, buffalo grass, grama grass, prickly pear cactus, rose thistle and yucca.

POPULATION. According to the US census, the pop. of Aurora in 1970 was 75,000. In 1978, it was estimated to have increased to 146,000. Aurora is the fastest-growing city of all those in the US with pops. of 100,000 or more.

ETHNIC GROUPS. In 1978, the ethnic distribution of Aurora was approx. 94% Caucasian, 2% Black, 2% Hispanic, 1% Asian and 1% other.

TRANSPORTATION. Interstate hwys. 25, 70 and 225 and US hwys. 36, 40 and 287 provide major motor access to Aurora. *Railroads* serving the

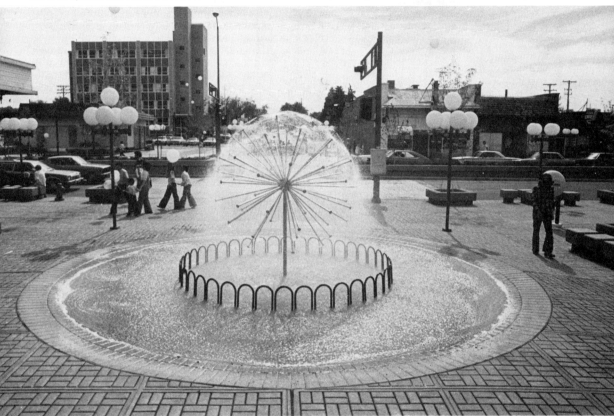

part of the state, 20 mi. E of the Rocky Mts. The city of Aurora, part of the Denver greater met. area, is bordered by Denver.

TOPOGRAPHY. Aurora lies in the high plains region of CO on the E slope of the Rocky Mts. Quincy Reservoir is located in the city. The mean elev. is 5,375'

CLIMATE. Aurora's climate is sunny and semi-arid. The Rocky Mts. modify the effects of prevailing W winds. Monthly mean temps. range from 30°F during Jan. to 73°F during July, with an avg. annual temp. of 50°F. Most of the 14.5" avg. annual rainfall occurs during the months of Mar. through Oct., when there is an avg. of 1.5" per month. Some 37% of the 50" avg. annual snowfall occurs in Mar. and Apr. The RH ranges from 35% to 70%. The growing season avgs. 166 days. Aurora lies in the MSTZ and observes DST.

A redeveloped area of the old business district, Colfax Concourse, Aurora, Colorado

area include Burlington N, CO S, Denver & Rio Grande, Rock Island, Sante Fe, Union Pacific and AMTRAK. *Airlines* serving Stapleton Intl. Airport include ZV, PX, BN, CO, DL, FL, NC, OZ, SO, TI, TW, RW, UA, WA, TransAmerica, Mexicana and Rocky Mt. Arapahoe Co. and Buckley Air Natl. Guard airports also serve the city. *Bus lines* include Trailways, Greyhound, Denver-Boulder and the Regional Transportation District (RTD).

COMMUNICATIONS. Communications, broadcasting and print media located in Aurora are: *AM radio station* KOSI 1430 (Indep., Btfl. Mus.) and *FM radio station* KOSI 101.1 (Indep., Btfl. Mus.); no *television stations* broadcast from Aurora, which is served by five Denver met. area TV stations; *press*: the *Sun* is published each Thurs. in Aurora, which is served by the daily *Denver Post* and *Rocky Mt. News* and the weekly *Village Squire* and the bi-weekly *Sentinel*.

HISTORY. The Aurora area was first settled by white

men in the latter part of the 19th century. The largest of the early landowners was the Union Pacific RR, which eventually sold parcels of its holdings to settlers attracted by precious metal mining in moutains. The town of Aurora, originally called Fletcher, was established between 1885 and 1891. It was named in 1890 after Donald Fletcher, a real estate developer from Denver who reinvested some of his profits in a comm. to the E. In 1889, William Smith, a farmer, donated an acre of land for the area's first school (which burned in 1892). Aurora's first high school was named after Smith, who served as secretary of the school district for 50 years. The Aurora subdivision, located on the E edge of the early comm. of Fletcher, was the largest in the town when Fletcher was incorporated in Apr., 1891. In 1897, the citizens of Fletcher voted to annex to Denver, but no action was taken. In 1902, Arapahoe Co. was divided into five parts and the town of Fletcher was split down the middle, with half in new Adams Co. and half in new S Arapahoe Co. The first Town Hall, completed in 1906, was built on land donated by Myron Van Buren. The town's first newspaper, also established in 1906, was the *Democrat-News*. In Feb., 1907, when the pop. of Fletcher was less than 300, the name of the town was changed by citizen petition to "Aurora". In 1908, electricity came to Aurora. By 1920, its pop. was still less than 1,000. Since then, however, the city has steadily grown. Between 1970 and 1978, its pop. experienced a boom and more than doubled.

GOVERNMENT. Aurora has a council-mgr. form of govt. Nine councillors, including the mayor as a voting member, are elected to four-year overlapping terms in elections held every two years. Four are elected at large, four by district, while the city mgr. is appointed.

ECONOMY AND INDUSTRY. Aurora is experiencing a period of rapid growth in industry as well as pop. In 1979, 21 firms located or expanded within the city. Major industries in the city are brewing and ceramics; electronics; rock drills and air tools; rubber belts and hoses; magnetic tape and sub systems; mining and milling equipment; luggage, furniture and toys; aircraft accessories; contracting; telephone equipment and fishing accessories and equipment. The avg. income per family in the city in 1978 was $20,500, while the

Central Aurora, Colorado

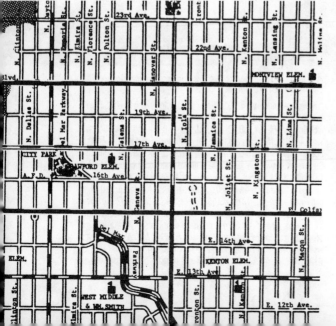

median family income was $17,500. The total labor force was 49,641, while the unemployment rate was 3.4%

BANKING. There are seven commercial banks and 16 savings and loans assns. in Aurora. In 1978, total deposits for the 12 banks headquartered in the city were $188,870,000, while total assets were $212,527,000. Banks include United Bank of Aurora, Peoples Bank and Trust, Aurora Natl., Citizens Natl., Aurora Mt. and Buckingham Natl.

HOSPITALS. Two hosps. are located in Aurora, Presbyterian Medical Center and Aurora Comm.

EDUCATION. The U of CO, CO State U, N CO and Met. State Col. offer extension courses in Aurora. The public Arapahoe Jr. Col. located in the city opened in 1966 and enrolled more than 4,000 in 1978. The Comm. Col. of Denver at Aurora is also located in the city, while the CO School of Mines, Loretto Heights Col., CO Women's Col., Regis Col. and the U of Denver are located nearby. The public school system, consisting of 23 elementary (K-5), six middle (6-8), one alternative high and four high (9-12) schools, enrolled more than 21,000 in 1978. Lib. facilities are available at Aurora Public Lib.'s Main Lib., S Branch and bookmobile.

ENTERTAINMENT. Aurora hosts the annual Gateway to the Rockies Parade. An annual summer concert series is also presented in the city. The Denver Broncos of the NFL and the CO Rockies of the NHL are regionally-oriented sports teams. There are a variety of professional sports organizations, dinner theaters and annual events accessible in nearby Denver.

ACCOMMODATIONS. There are 48 hotels and motels in Aurora, the Hilton, Best Western, Aurora Hotel and the Holiday, Wolf's and La Quinta inns.

FACILITIES. There are close to 4,000 acres of park and recreational facilities in Aurora, as well as 70 mi. of trails for jogging, hiking and horseback and bicycle riding. UT Park, the largest, contains an outdoor swimming pool, four baseball fields, four lighted handball courts and football, soccer and lacrosse fields. Three golf courses, 57 tennis courts, 42 playing fields and eight swimming pools are located throughout the city at several other parks, including Seven Hills, Springhill, Meadow Hills and Aurora Hills. Numerous ski areas are located nearby.

CULTURAL ACTIVITIES. Among the cultural organizations in Aurora are the Civic Ballet Co., Civic Chorus and Aurora Borealis Jazz Band. The Bicentennial Recreation Center, under the auspices of the city and the Arts and Humanities Council, is devoted to arts-related activities. There are several art galleries in the city, including the Columbine. An historical museum is scheduled to be completed at the beginning of 1980.

LANDMARKS AND SIGHTSEEING SPOTS. The William Smith Home, one of the oldest in Aurora, was built in the 1880s. The old Town Hall, completed in 1906, was the first public building in the comm. besides a school which burned in 1892. Aurora's oldest church, the First Presbyterian, was built in 1907.

AUSTIN
TEXAS

CITY LOCATION-SIZE-EXTENT. Austin, capital of the state and seat of Travis Co., is located in S central TX on both sides of a great bend in the CO River where it crosses the Balcones Escarpment separating the TX Hill Country of the Edwards Plateau to the W from the Black Prairie region to the E at 30°17' N lat. and 97°44' W long. The city encompasses 106 sq. mi. Its greater met. area consists of the counties of Travis and Hays to the SW and Williamson to the N and includes the cities of Round Rock, Taylor, Granger, Florence and Georgetown (in Williamson Co.) as well as San Marcos (in Hays Co.) and Pflugerville and Manor in Travis Co.

TOPOGRAPHY. The terrain of Austin ranges from grass

covered plains in the S and E to hills in the NW part of the city and contains numerous creeks and lakes, including Lake Austin and Town Lake. The Highland Lakes chain of seven lakes, which stretches 150 mi. to the NW, begins within the city limits. The city is the gateway to the TX Hill Country. The elev. ranges from 425' at lakeside to 1,000' in the hills. The mean elev. is 632'.

CLIMATE. The climate of Austin is humid, subtropical, characterized by hot summers and avgs. 300 days of sunshine annually. The 68.1°F avg. annual temp. ranges from a Jan. mean of 50.1°F to a July and Aug. mean of 82.40°F. The 32.49" avg. annual rainfall is fairly evenly distributed throughout the year. The avg. annual snowfall is 1". The RH ranges from 53% to 84%. The avg. growing season is 270 days. Austin lies in the CSTZ and observes DST.

FLORA AND FAUNA. Animals native to Austin include the whitetail deer, armadillo, raccoon and opossum. Common birds include the dove, quail, cardinal, mockingbird (the state bird) and scissortailed flycatcher. Salamanders, alligator lizards, tortoises and snakes, including the venomous copperhead, rattlesnake, water moccassin and coral snake are found here. Typical trees are the oak, cedar, madrone, walnut, mesquite, juniper and elm. Smaller plants include the Indian paintbrush, hackberry, crocus and bluebonnet (the state flower).

POPULATION. According to the US census, the pop. of Austin in 1970 was 25,808. In Apr., 1978, it was estimated that it had increased to 331,577. Austin, the fastest-growing city in TX, ranks as one of the 25 fastest-growing in the US.

ETHNIC GROUPS. In 1978, the ethnic distribution of Austin was approx. 78.7% Caucasian, 9.2% Black and 12.1% Hispanic.

TRANSPORTATION. Interstate Hwy. 35, US hwys. 183 and 290 and State Hwy. 71 provide major motor access to Austin. *Airlines* serving the Mueller Municipal Airport are BN, TI, EA, DL, CO, Tejas, SW, Eagle and Chaparral. There are also two private airports in the city. *Railroads* serving the city are MO Pacific, Pacific and AMTRAK. *Bus Lines* include Trailways, Greyhound, Kerrville, Arrow and the local Austin Transit System.

COMMUNICATIONS. Communications, broadcasting and print media

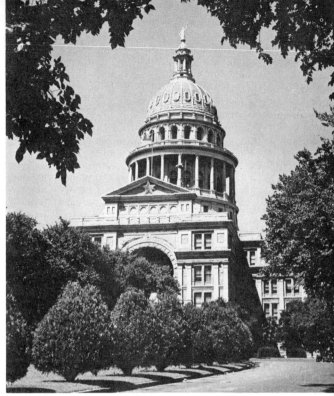

State Capitol, Austin, Texas

serving Austin are *AM radio stations* KLBJ 590 (CBS, C&W, News); KIXL 970 (ABC/E, Relig.); KVET 1300 (Indep., C&W); KOKE 1370 (TX State, C&W) and KNOW 1490 (Indep., Top 40); FM radio stations KMFA 89.5 (Indep., Clas.); KUT 90.7 (ABC/E, MBS, Mtl. Blk., NPR, TX State, Divers.); KLBJ (Indep., Progsv.); KOKE 95.5 (TX State, C&W); KHFI 98.3 (ABC/C, Top 40, Disco); KASE 100.7 (Indep., Btfl. Mus.); KMXX 102.3 (Indep., Span.) and KSCW 103.7 (ABC/FM, Contemp.); *television stations* KLR Ch. 18 (Indep.); KVUE Ch. 24 (Indep.,); KTVV Ch. 36 (NBC); KTCB Ch. 70 (CBS) and cable; *press:* two major dailies serve the city, the morning and

The LBJ Library on Campus of U of Tx., Austin, Texas

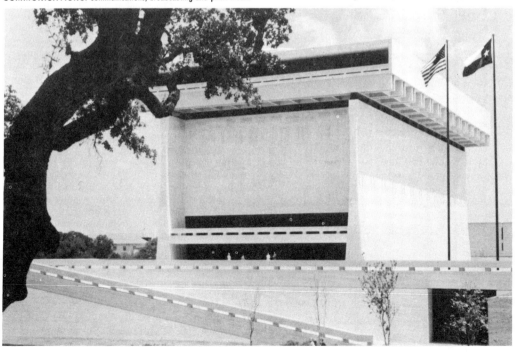

evening *American Statesman*, and the *Citizen*, issued Mon. through Fri.; other publications include the *Business Review, Sun, Capital City Argus, Country Gazette, Austin TX Monthly, Home/Garden, Hill Country News, Libertarian, Round Rock Leader, The Williamson County Sun, Westlake Picayune* and *Villager Newspaper.*

HISTORY. The area of present-day Austin was first inhabited by native Americans of the Tonkawa, Comanche and Lipan Apache tribes. The first white settler of the area, Jacob Harrell, pitched a tent in 1835 on the S bank of the CO River at the present site of downtown Austin. He was joined, in 1838, by three families, and the comm. was named Waterloo. In 1839, the settlement was selected to be the site of the state capital, was renamed in honor of Stephen F. Austin, the "Father of Texas", and surveyed by Edwin Waller, who became the first mayor. In Dec., 1839, the city was incorporated in the Republic of TX. When Mexican troops marched into TX in Mar., 1842, the capital was moved to

Downtown Austin, Texas

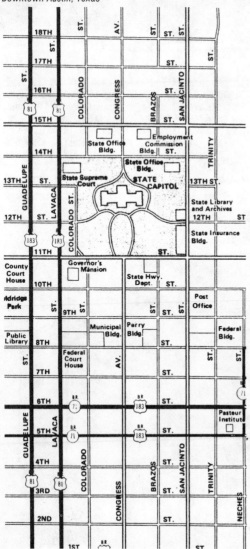

Houston and, shortly thereafter, to Washington-on-the-Brazos. Following waves of protest, however, the location of the capital was permanently returned to Austin in 1846, after TX entered the Union. By that time, the pop. of the city had reached 629. The growth of the city, slow at first, accelerated after the Civil War. Between 1871 and 1910, the city grew as industry and transportation developed and became a distribution center. In 1881, the U of TX was established in the city, which became a center for education as well as govt. After fire razed the capitol building, which had been built in 1855, a new capitol, constructed of pink granite obtained from Granite Mt. in Marble Falls, TX, was completed in 1888. Floods in 1900 and 1935 resulted in the construction of a series of dams, which created the Highland Lakes. Scientific and research industries which had begun to develop in the 1950s, boomed in the 1960s. Between 1960 and 1970, the pop. of the city grew approx. 35%, from 186,545 to 251,808.

GOVERNMENT. Austin has a council-mgr. form of govt. consisting of seven council members, including the mayor as a voting member. The council members, elected at large to two-year terms, appoint a city mgr.

ECONOMY AND INDUSTRY. Austin is a center of state and local govt., education, state and natl. assns. and R&D. There are 120 state and 62 fed. agencies, the headquarters of about 30 state and natl. assns. and organizations and home offices of 33 insurance companies in the city, as well as approx. 450 manufacturing establishments, for the most part of the "clean" type (e.g., scientific, electronics and other high technology). The city is also the shopping and distribution center for a 20-co. trade area, as well as the home of Bergstrom AFB, headquarters of the 12th AF. Poultry, dairy, cotton and grain are major agricultural products. Tourism is another major industry. In 1978, close to 1,100 conventions were held in the city. In 1978, avg. household income for the met. area was estimated to be $18,685, while the avg. per capita income, in 1976, was approx. $5,234. In June, 1979, the labor force of the greater met. area totaled approx. 245,300, while the rate of unemployment was 3.5%.

BANKING. There are 20 commercial banks and eight savings and loan assns. in Austin. In 1978, total deposits for the 18 banks headquartered in the city were $2,056,252,000, while assets were $2,471,386,000. Banks include Austin Natl., Capital Natl., City Natl., American Natl., TX State, N Austin State, Bank of Austin, Citizens Natl. and U State.

HOSPITALS. There are nine hosps., in Austin, including St. David's, Shoalcreek, Westminister, Holy Cross, Brackenridge, Seton and Bailey Surgical Center.

EDUCATION. The U of TX at Austin, which opened in 1883, a state supported institution, is the leading U in the S and ranked eighth nationally. A significant research institution, UT contains the LBJ School of Public Affairs, founded by the late Pres., and has recently installed the largest computer system in the US, a particle accelerator laboratory and a plasma physics and thermonuclear research center. In 1978, approx. 43,100 enrolled. Huston-Tillotson Col., the oldest institution in the city (Tillotson Col. was founded in Austin in 1875, while Samuel Huston Col. was founded in 1876 in Dallas), enrolled approx. 650 in 1978. Other institutions in the city include St. Edward's U, a coeducational institution founded in 1885 and enrolling approx. 1,200, Concordia Lutheran Col., St. Stephen's School, Austin Presbyterian Theological Seminary, American Col. of Musicians, the Episcopal Theological Seminary of the SW and the Institute for Organizational Behavior and Human Resource Development. Austin Comm. Col., a public two-year institution which opened in 1973, enrolled nearly 7,800 in 1978. There are 70 elementary, 18 jr. and 10 sr. high schools, enrolling more than 58,000, in the public school system. There are about 25 private schools as well. Lib. facilities include the State Archives and Lib.,

Austin Public Lib., U of TX Lib. (a major natl. research center) and Lyndon Baines Johnson Lib.

ENTERTAINMENT. Austin annually hosts the 10-day Aqua Festival, which begins the first Fri. of each Aug. Begun in 1962, the Aqua Festival has developed into one of the 10 largest festivals in the US. It includes nine fest nights featuring ethnic foods. Aerofest is an aerial display of the Bergstroms AFB Thunderbirds that features canoe, sailboat and drag boat races achieving speeds in excess of 200 m.p.h., a lighted night water parade and fireworks, motorcycle and auto races, the Twilight Land Parade, a beauty pageant featuring lands and floats, a "day at the races", musical entertainment and a W dance. Other annual events are the Highland Lake Arts and Crafts Fiesta, held each fall, the Highland Lakes Bluebonnet Trail, held each spring, the Sheriff's Posse Rodeo, an annual Jazz Festival, the two-day Laguna Gloria Arts and Crafts Fiesta, held each May and the Austin Livestock Show. The U of T Longhorns participate in intercollegiate sports in the SW Conf.

ACCOMMODATIONS. There are about 40 hotels and motels in Austin including the Alamo, Driskill, Marriott, Stephen F. Austin and Chariot Inn Motor, and the Sheraton Crest, Lakeway, Hilton, World of Resorts, La Quinta, Ramada and Holiday inns.

FACILITIES. The Highlands Lakes, a chain of seven lakes (two within the Austin city limits) formed by the damming of the once turbulent CO River, offers more than 700 mi. of shoreline for hunting, fishing, hiking, swimming, boating, camping and water skiing. Recreational areas within the city include 12 major parks and 100 playgrounds, encompassing nearly 7,700 acres and containing 205 swimming pools (including Barton Springs, which maintains a temp. of 68°F), 47 tennis courts, 17 playing fields and four public golf courses. Among the larger parks are the 39.4-acre Zilker, containing Barton Springs, Zilker Garden and the Austin Area Garden Center, Lake Austin City, Pease, Lake Walter F. Long and Eilers, which contains a Natural Science Center. The city has set aside 1,102 acres along the hills of Lake Austin for future park development. The Hike and Bike Trail at Town Lake is part of the Natl. Recreational Trail System and provides 12.5 mi. along the lake for jogging, bicycling and horseback riding.

CULTURAL ACTIVITIES. There are several museums and more than 50 art galleries in Austin. The Elisabeth Ney Museum exhibits 19th century sculpture and architecture, conducts formal tours and offers a variety of art classes, including sculpture. The O. Henry Museums, a Victorian cottage, once the home of the writer, has been preserved along with some of his possessions and 19th century memorabilia. Creative writing classes and special events are offered throughout the year. The TX Memorial Museum features dioramas of oil field developments, displays of prehistorical fossils, native American relics, gun collections and TX historical, geological and wildlife items. The Daughters of the Confederacy and Daughters of the Republic museums, located on the grounds of the Capitol, exhibit historical relics, including items and guns used by early settlers and flags of the Confederacy and of the Republic. The Laguna Gloria Art Museum, an old estate built in the style of a Mediterranean villa, features changing art exhibitions, art classes, films, lectures, tours and concerts. The LBJ Lib. contains the papers of the 36th Pres., as well as exhibits of gifts from heads of state, life in the White House and a replica of the Oval Room. Among the comm. theaters in Austin is the Zachary Scott Theatre Center, formed in 1921 as the Austin Civic Theatre, which sponsors a "Fun Theatre" for children, as well as acting and theater classes. The B. Iden Payne Theatre, named in honor of a leading authority on Shakespeare, hosts a Shakespearian classic production every spring. The Paramount Theatre for the Performing Arts, built in the early 1900s and recently restored, hosts varied productions at the Mary Moody Theatre, while the U of TX presents dramatic, musical and dance performances and features museums and galleries. The Austin Symphony Orchestra, conducted by Akira Endo, hosts great artists each season, while an opera is performed each spring. The Austin Civic Ballet Theatre, as well as several other dance companies, including Spectrum Deaf Dance Theatre, frequently perform. The Civic Chorus also presents musical performances.

LANDMARKS AND SIGHTSEEING SPOTS. The TX State Capitol Building is one of Austin's major attractions. Built from red TX granite, the cross-shaped Capitol was begun in 1882, and completed in 1888. Its 309'8" dome is seven feet higher than the US Capitol and its terrazzo floor depicts the history of TX under the flags of six nations, Spain, France, Mexico, The Republic of TX, The Confederacy and the USA. The Gov.'s Mansion, built in 1856, contains a gallery running the entire length of the front of the white brick mansion and six massive Ionic columns, made of cedar logs hauled from Bastrop, TX. In it are the Sam Houston Room, containing the bed of the former Pres. of the Republic of TX and Gov. of the State of TX and the mahogany desk of Stephen F. Austin. The French Legation, built of handsawn lumber from Bastrop, TX, in 1841, for Alphonse de Saligny, Ambassador to the Republic of TX, is located on a hill in E Austin. The restored Neill Cochran House, built by Abner in 1853, exemplifies the TX version of the Greek Revival style of architecture which became popular in the S. It has been used as an Institute for the Blind, a hosp. for fed. prisoners and a social center. Other points of interest include the Santa Rita No. 1, the first rig to drill oil on land owned by the U of TX in the W part of the State; the State Cemetery, which contains the graves of Stephen F. Austin, seven govs. and more than 2,000 Confederate veterans and their wives; St. David's Episcopal Church, built in 1854, and the Bremond Block, featuring restored homes of early Austin. The restored Sixth St. now features unique shops, restaurants, theaters and a comedy workshop. Moonlight Towers, a series of several mercury vapor lamps on 165' high iron frames dating from 1895, form the Lone Star of TX and cast a blue moon-fire glow over the city.

BALTIMORE
MARYLAND

CITY LOCATION-SIZE-EXTENT. Baltimore, the largest city in the state and eighth largest in the US, is an independent city (with no co. affiliation) in N MD W of Chesapeake Bay at the mouth of the Patapsco River at 39°11' N lat. and 74°40' W long. The city encompasses 18.3 sq. mi. about 40 mi NE of Washington, DC. The greater met. area extends throughout Baltimore Co. to the N and E and parts of Anne Arundel Co. to the S and Howard and Carroll counties to the E.

TOPOGRAPHY. The terrain of Baltimore, which lies on the Atlantic plain, is characterized by flat land and gently rolling hills. Major inlets of Baltimore Harbor, formed where the Patapsco River empties into Chesapeake Bay, are Curtis and NW bays and Middle Branch. The mouth of the Black River, which flows through the N part of the greater met. area, is NE of the city. There are several lakes in the area. The mean elev. is 32'.

CLIMATE. The climate of Baltimore is continental,

Inner Harbor, Baltimore, Maryland

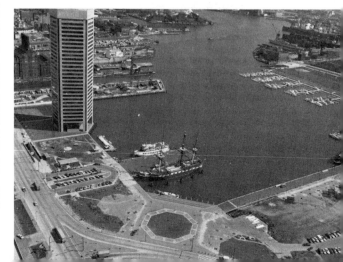

influenced by its position midway between the more rigorous climate of the N and the milder climate of the S, and moderated by Chesapeake Bay and the Atlantic Ocean to the E and ranges of the Appalachian Mts. to the W. Frequent shifts in wind direction contribute to the changeable character of the weather. Summer weather is influenced by the Bermuda High, a high pressure system in the Atlantic Ocean which brings warm humid air from the S. Monthly mean temps. range from 32.6°F during Jan. to 76.8°F during July, with an avg. annual temp. of 55°F. The avg. annual rainfall of 41.49" is fairly evenly distributed throughout the year. Some 94% of the avg. annual 22" of snowfall occurs from Dec. through Mar. The RH ranges from 51% to 85%. The avg. growing season is 194 days. Baltimore lies in the ESTZ and observes DST.

FLORA AND FAUNA. Animals native to Baltimore include the raccoon, opossum, muskrat, mink and whitetail deer. Common birds include the osprey, gull, tern, marsh hawk, heron and bald eagle. Snapping turtles, tree frogs, salamanders, Fowler's toads, skinks and brown snakes, as well as the venomous copperhead and cottonmouth, are found here. Typical trees are the oak, maple, elm, cherry and ash. Smaller plants include marsh grass, sedge, cattails, and blue phlox.

POPULATION. According to the US census, the pop. of Baltimore in 1970 was 905,787. In 1979, it was estimated that it had decreased to approx. 830,000.

ETHNIC GROUPS. In 1978, the ethnic distribution of Baltimore was approx. 53% Caucasian, 46.4% Black and 0.9% Hispanic (a percentage of the Hispanic total is also included in the Caucasian total).

Washington Monument, Baltimore, Maryland

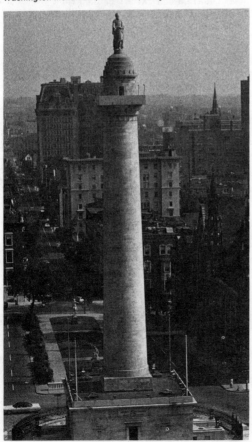

TRANSPORTATION. Interstate hwys. 46, 70, 83, 95, 495 and 695, US hwys. 40, 50 and 302 and state hwys. 3, 24, 25, and 100 provide major motor access to Baltimore. *Railroads* serving the city include AMTRAK and Chessie System. *Airlines* serving the Baltimore-Washington Intl. Airport, 10 mi. S of the city, are AA, US Air, DL, EA, NA, PI, TI, TW and UA. *Bus lines* include Greyhound, Trailways and a local met. system. A major US port, the city is located on one of the largest natural harbors in the world, consisting of 45 mi. of waterfront. The Chesapeake Capes and the Chesapeake-Delaware Canal to the N provide shipping access to Baltimore Harbor from the Atlantic Ocean.

COMMUNICATIONS. Communications, broadcasting and print media serving Baltimore are: *AM radio stations* WCAO 600 (ABC/C, Top 40); WCBM 680 (ABC/E, MOR); WBMD 750 (Indep., C&W); WAYE 860 (Indep., Rock); WSID 1010 (Indep., Blk.); WBAL 1090 (NBC, MOR); WITH 1230 (Indep., Btfl. Mus.); WFBR 1300 (ABC/I, Adult Contemp.); WEBB 1360 (MBS, Blk) and WWIN 1400 (Indep., AOR); *FM radio station* WSPH 88.1 (Indep., Var.); WBIC 91.5 (ABC/FM, Var.); WLPL 92.3 (Indep., Contemp. Rock/Top 40); WPOC 93.1 (Indep., Hit Ctry.); WRBS 95.1 (Indep., Relig.); WBAL 97.9 (NBC, All News); WLIF 101.9 (Indep., Btfl. Mus.); WXVY 102.7 (Indep., Disco) and WMAR 106.5 (Indep. MOR); *television stations* (WMAR Ch. 2); WBAL Ch. 11 (NBC); WJZ Ch. 13 (ABC); WBFF Ch. 22 (Indep.) and WMPB Ch. 67 (PBS); *press:* two major dailies serve the area, the *News American*, printed evenings and the *Sun*, printed mornings and evenings; other publications include *Daily Records*, issued daily, the weekly *Guide*, *Enterprises Labor Herald* and *Jewish Times* and the monthly *Baltimore Magazine, Baltimore Purchaser* and *Baltimore Engineers.*

HISTORY. Native Americans of the Susquehanna tribe inhabited the area before white settlers arrived in the area of present-day Baltimore in 1661. In 1729, Baltimore Town was founded by an act of the MD Gen. Assembly, the colonial govt., and named in honor of the Lords Baltimore, the family which founded and managed the MD colony. Established as a trading center for tobacco farmers in S MD, Baltimore Town grew as a shipping center for other agricultural products. In 1790, it became the seat of the first Roman Catholic diocese in the US. During the Revolutionary War, it served for two months as a natl. capital (after Washington D.C. was burned). In 1797, with a pop. of 20,000, it was incorporated as a city. By 1800, its pop. was 35,000. During the War of 1812, a British attack on the city in 1814, although resisted, inspired Francis Scott Key to write "The Star-Spangled Banner" while he was on a ship in the harbor within site of the bombarded Ft. McHenry. The first RR passenger and freight station in the US was built in Baltimore in 1830, and the first RR, the Baltimore & OH, began operating from the city the same year. In 1844, the first telegraph communication ("What Hath God Wrought") was received there. In the 1840s and 1850s, many European immigrants arrived in the city, and by 1860, it was the third largest in the US with a pop. of more than 212,000. Though MD remained in the Union during the Civil War, many of the city's citizens were Confederate sympathizers. After Union troops passing through the city were attacked in Apr., 1861, the mayor and other city officials were imprisoned as S supporters from May, 1861, until May, 1865, during the Union occupation of the city. Johns Hopkins U, established in the city in 1876, and Johns Hopkins Hosp., founded in 1889, were named in honor of the merchant who, in 1873, left millions to build them. The city grew steadily as a commercial center in the 1800s, and, by 1900, the pop. approached 509,000, swollen by a second wave of European immigrants. The Great Baltimore Fire occurred in Feb., 1904, and raged for two days, destroying every major downtown building. Damage was repaired by 1914, and by WW II, the economy of the city, benefiting from the expansion of industry, was prosperous once again. During the 1940s, many S blacks and Appalachian whites immigrated to the city to work and settled around the central business district. Since 1950, when the pop. of the city reached nearly 950,000, the inner city experienced a decline in both pop. and services as the suburbs have grown. During the 1960s and 1970s, the city instituted urban renewal and inner-city revitalization programs, including the Charles Center Project and the redevelopment of the Inner Harbor.

GOVERNMENT. Baltimore has a mayor-council form of govt. consisting of 19 council members and the mayor, who are elected to four-year terms. Three council members are elected from each of the city's six districts, while the council pres. and mayor are elected at large. An independent city with the same powers as a co., Baltimore sends representatives to the state legislature.

ECONOMY AND INDUSTRY. Baltimore, the educational, industrial and commercial center of MD is a major world port, ranking sixth in the US in tonnage of cargo handled annually. It is the fourth largest industrial

City Hall, Baltimore, Maryland

employer on the E Coast. There are more than 2,000 manufacturing plants in the greater met. area. Major industrial products include steel, electrical machinery, transportation equipment, food products and apparel. In June, 1979, the labor force for the greater met. area totaled 1,080,100, while the rate of unemployment was 6.3%.

BANKING. There are nine commercial banks and eight savings and loan assns. in Baltimore. In 1978, total deposits for the nine banks headquartered in the city were $7,789,307,000, while assets were $9,798,627,000. Banks include MD Natl., First Natl. of MD, Equitable Trust, Union Trust of MD and Savings of Baltimore.

HOSPITALS. There are more than 25 hosps. in Baltimore including the internationally-renowned Johns Hopkins Hosp. and Natl. Institute of Health. The U of MD Hosp., Psychiatric Institute and schools of Dentistry, Medicine, Nursing, Pharmacy and Social Work are located in the city. In 1979, the first implantation of an artificial metal spine in a human occurred at the U of MD Hosp. Other hosps. include Sinai, Baltimore City, Bon Secours, Franklin Sq., Children's Lutheran, V.A. and John F. Kennedy Institute.

EDUCATION. Johns Hopkins U, a private institution founded in Baltimore in 1876, and known for outstanding programs in intl. studies and medicine, enrolled nearly 10,000 in 1978. The U of Baltimore, a private institution founded in 1925, enrolled nearly 5,500 in 1978, while the U of MD at

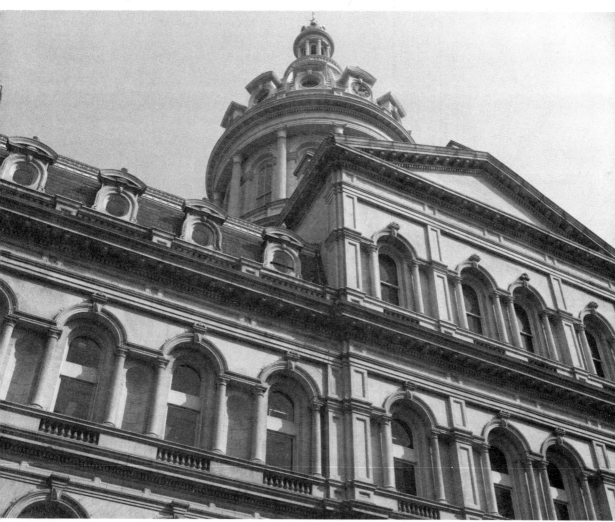

Baltimore, established in 1966, enrolled more than 5,300 in 1978. Other institutions include Morgan State U, one of the nation's oldest black institutions, which enrolled more than 6,000 in 1978, Baltimore Hebrew Col., Baltimore Comm. Col., the MD Institute of Art and the Peabody Conservatory of Music. 200 public elementary and high schools enrolled approx. 200,000. There are approx. 60 private and parochial schools enrolling another 28,000. Lib. facilities include the Enoch Pratt Free Lib., founded in 1882, and its 28 branches as well as the Walters Art Gallery, MD Historical Society and Baltimore Bar Assn. libs.

ENTERTAINMENT. There are several dinner theaters in the city, including Minnick's Perucci's Main Street and New Bolton. Preakness Festival Week, held in Baltimore each spring, features a variety of events preceding the running of the Preakness Stakes, one of the Triple Crown events in horse racing. The Futurity, Pimlico Cup and other races also take place each spring at Pimlico Racetrack, the oldest in MD. Each June, the city hosts Flag Day ceremonies at the Star-Spangled Banner Flag House, while in Sept. it holds the Baltimore City Fair. The Baltimore Colts NFL-AFC football team and the Baltimore Orioles AL baseball team plays at Memorial Stadium. The Clippers EHL hockey team plays at the Civic Center. The Johns Hopkins U Blue Jays and the U of MD Retrievers participate in collegiate sports.

ACCOMMODATIONS. There are several hotels and motels in Baltimore

Central Baltimore, Maryland

including the Baltimore and Intl. hotels, and the Sheraton, Hilton, Ramada, Holiday and Quality inns.

FACILITIES. There are approx. 70 parks, encompassing nearly 6,000 acres in Baltimore. The largest, the 686-acre Gwynns Falls and Leakin Parks System (one of the largest natural parks within the limits of a US city, contains several historical mansions. The 140-acre Druid Hill Park contains the Baltimore Zoo, which includes a Children's Zoo, a Conservatory housing rare plants, zoological Gardens, playing fields, tennis courts and picnic areas. Golf courses and jogging and bicyling paths are available in Carroll, Clifton, Herring Run and Forrest parks. Other parks include Cylburn, a 176-acre wild flower preserve and garden center; Fed. Hill, site of a Civil War ft. and offering views of the Inner Harbor; Freedom, containing a memorial to ethnic groups who have suffered oppression; Patterson, a city park; the seven-acre Sherwood Gardens, containing displays of tulips, azaleas and flowering shrubs; Mt. Pleasant and Harlon. Fishing and boating are available in Chesapeake Bay and the Atlantic Ocean, through the Chesapeake-DL Canal.

CULTURAL ACTIVITIES. The Baltimore Museum of Art features 19th and 20th century French, contemporary, decorative and American fine art. Of particular interest is the Cone Collection of French Impressionist paintings. Sculpture, paintings, illuminated manuscripts and decorative art spanning 6,000 years are on display at the Walters Art Gallery. The Peale (Municipal) Museum, built in 1814 by the portrait painter and scientist Rembrandt Peale—the first building in the US designed as a museum— contains prints and historical portraits. The Lovely Lane Methodist Church and Museum, the "Mother Church of American Methodists" exhibits historical religious materials. Cylburn Mansion houses a nature museum and horticultural lib. The Original manuscript of "The Star-Spangled Banner" is displayed at the MD Historical Society, and a collection of early RR cars and engines is housed in the Baltimore & OH Transportation Museum. Other museums include the Babe Ruth birthplace and Museum, Baltimore Maritime Museum, Baltimore Streetcar Museum and MD Science Center and Planetarium. The Baltimore Symphony Orchestra and the Baltimore Opera Co. perform in the Lyric Theatre, which is also the home of the MD Ballet. The Morris A. Mechanic Theatre presents Broadway plays and the Center Stage Repertory Co. performs a series of plays each year. The Arena Players is an outstanding theater co. The city's center for avant-garde theater, the Theater Project, features musicians, acting companies, poets and mimes.

LANDMARKS AND SIGHTSEEING SPOTS. The Ft. McHenry Natl. Monument and Historical Shrine, constructed in 1790, commemorates Francis Scott Key's penning of "The Star-Spangled Banner" and is listed on the Natl. Register of Historical Places. The first US Navy ship, the US frigate *Constellation*, completed in 1797, is docked at Pier 1 in Baltimore Harbor. It also is a Natl. Historical Landmark. Battle Monument, the first war monument erected in the US, is a tribute to lives lost in the 1814 Battle of Baltimore against the British. The 178' high Washington Monument, the first major monument in the US dedicated to George Washington (1830), stands near the central business district. The Star-Spangled Banner Flag House was the home of Mary Pickersgill, who sewed the flag which inspired the writing of our natl. anthem. The Basilica of the Assumption, the first major Roman Catholic Cathedral in the US, was dedicated in 1821. Oherbein Methodist (1785) is the oldest church in Baltimore. City Hall features French Revival architecture and a cast iron dome. The Edgar Allen Poe House offers visitors a glimpse into the life of the famed writer, who lived there from 1832 to 1835. The Edgar Allen Poe Monument stands in the Westminister Presbyterian Church Cemetery (W Burying Grounds), where Poe's grave was relocated through penny donations made by Baltimore schoolchildren. Mount Clare (1754), the oldest house within city limits, was the home of Charles Carroll (1815) while the Carroll Mansion was the last home of Carroll, a signer of the Declaration of Independence. Old Shot Tower, built in 1828 for the production of shot, is the only one of its kind remaining in the US. At Lexington Market, established in 1803, many of the food, meat and produce stalls are run by members of the original families. Dickeyville, a preserved comm. originally built in 1772 as residences for employees of nearby flour and cotton mills, is maintained as an historical and architectural district. Tyson St. is a quaint block of preserved 19th century homes. Fells Point, one of Baltimore's oldest port-side neighborhoods dating to 1730, is an historical district with 350 original homes currently being restored. In the areas of Otterbein and Stirling St., homesteaders are restoring houses they have bought for one dollar. Notables such as Johns Hopkins, Enoch Pratt, Betsy Patterson and John Wilkes Booth are buried in Greenmount Cemetery (1838).

BATON ROUGE
LOUISIANA

CITY LOCATION-SIZE-EXTENT. Baton Rouge, the state capital, is located on the E bank of the MS River in S central LA at 30°32' N lat. and 91°08' W long. The seat of E Baton Rouge Parish, the city encompasses 48.7 sq. mi. 80 mi. NW of New Orleans and 60 mi. inland from the Gulf of Mexico. Bordered by W Baton Rouge Parish across the MS River to the W, the city's greater met. area extends into that parish, as well as into neighboring Ascension, Iberville and Livingston parishes to the E and S.

TOPOGRAPHY. Baton Rouge lies on the first series of bluffs N of the coastal plain of the MS River delta. The land is characterized by low, rolling hills with intermittent creeks, rivers, lakes and bayous. Lake Pontchartrain lies approx. 33 mi. SE of the city. The elev. ranges from 25' to more than 100', with a mean of 57'.

CLIMATE. Although the climate of Baton Rouge is humid subtropical, it is influenced by polar air masses during the winter. The prevailing winds from the Gulf of Mexico moderate extremes of summer heat, shorten winter cold spells and provide abundant moisture and substantial rainfall. The avg. annual temp. of 67.6°F ranges from a Jan. mean of 52.5°F to a July mean of 81.9°F. The 56.73" avg. annual rainfall is fairly evenly distributed throughout the year. Although snowfall is negligible, hurricanes, hailstorms, tornadoes and wind storms occasionally occur. The RH ranges from 52% to 92%. The avg. growing season is 273 days. The city lies in the CSTZ and observes DST.

FLORA AND FAUNA. Animals native to Baton Rouge include the muskrat, S, bayou/gray and fox squirrels, swamp rabbit, otter, raccoon, opossum and whitetail deer. Common birds include the mockingbird, heron, quail, woodcock, dove, egret, bluejay, cardinal, and grackle. Sirens; bull frogs, Gulf Coast toads and water snakes, as well as the venomous rattlesnake, coral snake, copperhead, and cottonmouth, are found here. Typical trees are the oak, cypress and pine. Smaller plants include the water hyacinth, honeysuckle, blue-eyed grass, morning glory, iris and magnolia (the state flower).

POPULATION. According to the U.S. census, the pop. of Baton Rouge in 1970 was 165,963. In 1978, it was estimated that it had increased to 219,754.

ETHNIC GROUPS. In 1978, the ethnic distribution of Baton Rouge was approx. 72.9% Caucasian, 28.7% Black, and 1.7% Hispanic. (A percentage of the Hispanic total is also included in the Caucasian total.)

TRANSPORTATION. Interstate hwys. 10 and 12 and US hwys. 61 and 190 provide major motor access to Baton Rouge. *Railroads* serving the city include IL Central Gulf, MO Pacific, Santa Fe and TX & Pacific. The Port of Baton Rouge, ranked seventh among US ports and second in LA, is the farthest inland deepwater port on the Gulf of Mexico, lying some 230 water mi. from the mouth of the MS River. Approx. 70 million tons were handled at the port facilities in 1977. The Baton Rouge Barge Canal and Terminal, on the 1,400 mile Gulf Intracoastal Waterway, provided barge connections to points N, S, E, and W of the city. *Airlines* serving Ryan Airport include DL,

SO, and TI. *Bus lines* serving the city include Greyhound and Trailways.

COMMUNICATIONS. Communications, broadcasting and print media serving Baton Rouge include: *AM radio stations* WLCS 910 (UPI, Top 40); WJBO 1150 (NBC, MBS, APR, MOR); WLBI 1220 (MBS, Ctry.); WAIL 1260 (Indep., MOR); WIBR 1300 (APR, Top 40); WYNK 1380 (ABC/E, C&W); WXOK 1460 (Mut., Blk.) and WLUX 1550 (ABC/E, UPI, Relig.); *FM radio stations* WAFB 98.1 (ABC/C, MOR); WQXY 100.7 (Indep., Btfl. Mus.); WYNK 101.5 (ABC/E, APR, C&W) and WFMF 102.5 (ABC/FM, Progsv.); *television stations* WBRZ Ch. 2 (ABC); WAFB Ch. 9 (CBS); WLPB Ch. 27 (PBS); and WRBT Ch. 33 (NBC); *press:* two major dailies serve the area, *The Advocate*, issued mornings, and *State Times*, issued evenings; other publications include the weekly *Catholic Commentator* and *Digest* and the quarterly *S Review*.

HISTORY. Native Americans of the Bayou Goula and Houma tribes lived in the area of present-day Baton Rouge when French explorers arrived in 1699. D'Iberville called the area "Istrouma" or "Red Stick"—in French, "Baton Rouge"—in reference to large red poles, probably cypress trees, which separated the hunting grounds of the two tribes. In 1719, the comm. was founded by French soldiers as a military post. Nine flags have flown over Baton Rouge: the *fleur-de-lis* of France and those of England, Spain, the W FL Republic, the tricolor of France, the Sovereign State of LA, the Confederate States of America and the Stars and Stripes. In 1763, the area was transferred to England in the treaty of Paris and LA became part of W FL. During this period, the settlement was known as New Richmond. In 1779, the Spanish captured the area from the English, and by 1781, all of W FL was under Spanish rule. Spain controlled the W FL parishes until 1810, when Spanish rule was overthrown. The 1,000 people who lived in the Baton Rouge area declared themselves independent and renamed the territory the W FL Republic. Soon, however, the area was annexed by LA and became E Baton Rouge Parish. The town of Baton Rouge was incorporated in 1817, five years after LA achieved statehood, and, in 1849, replaced New Orleans as the

Old State Capitol Building, Baton Rouge, Louisiana

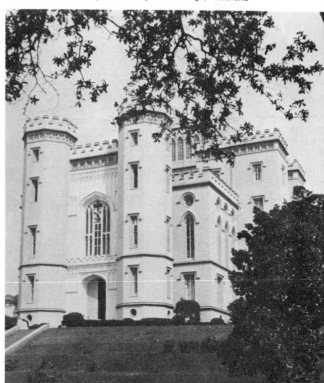

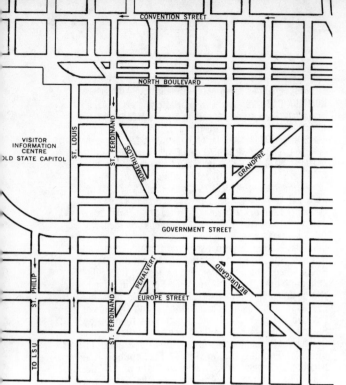

Downtown Baton Rouge, Louisiana

capital of the State. During the Civil War (1861-65), Baton Rouge was occupied by Union forces, except for a brief time in 1862 when the LA capital was moved from Opelousas to Shreveport. Baton Rouge remained under fed. control until 1877, and became the capital again in 1882, at which time the pop. was approx. 7,200. The original Capitol building, built in 1849 and then destroyed, was rebuilt the same year. Commerce and trade gradually resumed during the late 1800's and the city began a period of new growth as a port. By 1900, its pop. reached about 11,300. During the early 1900's, the discovery of oil and gas nearby attracted chemical companies to the area. Rubber first began to be produced from petroleum in the city in the 1930's. In 1932, a new Capitol building—the tallest in the US—was completed during the governorship of Huey Long, one of the most influential politicians in the history of the State. Long was assassinated in the Capitol in 1935. During WW II, the city became a center of the petro-chemical industry. During the 1940's, and as a result of industrial expansion, the pop. of Baton Rouge more than tripled, from 34,719 in 1940 to 125,629 in 1950. Throughout the 1950's and 1960's, the city continued to grow as a center of industry, govt. and education.

GOVERNMENT. Baton Rouge and E Baton Rouge Parish have a mayor-council form of govt. The Mayor-Pres. and 12 council members are elected at large to four year terms.

ECONOMY AND INDUSTRY. Baton Rouge is located at the N end of the "Chemical Strip", an enormous chemical and petroleum complex extending along the MS River. Exxon, the second largest refinery in the US (located in Baton Rouge since 1909) produces more than 700 petroleum products. Other industries include food and kindred products, printing and publishing, lumber and wood products, stone, clay and glass products and fabricated metal products. Major non-industrial employers include govt. (employing approx. 28% of the labor force), wholesale and retail trade (approx. 21%), services (approx. 14.1%) and contract construction (approx. 13%). In June, 1979, the labor force of the greater met. area totaled approx. 202,500, while the rate of unemployment was approx. 7.2%. In 1978, the median household income was $12,192.

BANKING. There are six commercial banks and two savings and loan assns. in Baton Rouge. In 1978, total bank deposits for the six banks headquartered in the city were $1,870,597,000 and assets were $2,284,858,000. Banks serving the city include City Natl., Fidelity Natl., LA Natl. and Capital, Baton Rouge, and American Bank and Trust companies.

HOSPITALS. There are four gen. hosps. in Baton Rouge, Baton Rouge Gen., Doctors Memorial, Our Lady of the Lake Medical Center and Rhodes J. Spedale Gen. The LA State Hosp. is also located in the city. The US Public Health Service facility located in nearby Carville, is the only facility for the treatment of leprosy in the US.

EDUCATION. The Baton Rouge Campus of LA State U and Agricultural and Mechanical Col. is the headquarters of the LSU System. Founded in Pineville in 1855 as the LA State Seminary of Learning and Military Academy, it moved to Baton Rouge in 1869, and later merged with the Agricultural and Mechanical Col. The U offers grad. and professional, as well as undergrad. degrees, and enrolled more than 25,000 in 1978. Other institutions of higher learning include Southern U Agricultural and Mechanical Col., main campus of one of the largest predominantly black U systems in the US. Established in 1880, the public U offers associate, bachelor and master degrees, and enrolled close to 8,300 in 1978. There are 77 elementary, 16 jr. and 15 sr. high schools in E Baton Rouge Parish, with a total enrollment of approx. 75,000. Approx. 12,000 attend private and parochial schools in the city. Area libs. include the LA State Lib. and the E Baton Rouge Parish Lib.

ENTERTAINMENT. The Aubin Lane Dinner Theater is located in Baton Rouge. Among the annual events is Tourism Appreciation Day, sponsored by the Baton Rouge Convention and Visitors Bureau. The LSU Fighting Tigers participate in SE Conf. sports while the Southern U Jaguars participate in collegiate sports in the SWAC.

ACCOMMODATIONS. There are approx. 25 hotels and motels in Baton Rouge, including the Admiral Benbow, Bellemont Oak Manor and Capitol House hotels, and the Holiday, Hilton, Prince Mucat, Sheraton, Day's, Rodeway, and Ramada Inns.

FACILITIES. There are six city parks, including four with public golf courses in Baton Rouge. The 16-acre Cohn Memorial Arboretum contains more than 200 varieties of trees and shrubs, each labeled for indentification, and a greenhouse for the growth exhibition of rare and exotic plants. The 140-acre Greater Baton Rouge Zoo houses more than 500 animals from four continents. A zoo train and sidewalk tram are available for tours. Fishing and hunting are available in bayous in and around Baton Rouge.

CULTURAL ACTIVITIES. The Baton Rouge Symphony Orchestra, Baton Rouge Little Theatre, numerous art galleries and several museums are located in Baton Rouge. Museums located on the campus of LSU are the Anglo-American Art Museum, Museum of Natural Science, featuring an exhibit of more than 350 native birds, and the Museum of Geoscience which displays archological finds from the state's pre-historic Bayou Jasmin site, as well as items of local folklore and Indian culture. The LSU Rural Life Museum, located on the Burden Research Plantation, is an outdoor complex of 19th century buildings of the rural S. The LSU Art Gallery, S Art Gallery and Baton Rouge Gallery feature permanent and changing exhibits. The LA Arts and Science Center, located in the Old Gov.'s Mansion, features a planetarium. The Arts and Science Center Museum features an Acadian house, restored train and MS River exhibits. The LA Art Commission maintains a small gallery on the second floor of the Old State Capitol.

LANDMARKS AND SIGHTSEEING SPOTS. The Old State Capitol, built in 1849, is one of Baton Rouge's landmarks that is listed on the Natl. Register of Historic Places. A Gothic Revival Workman-type castle, it stands on a bluff overlooking the MS River and houses the Baton Rouge Area Convention and Visitors Bureau. Close to the Old Gov.'s Mansion, which has been restored to the period of the 1930's, when it was built, is the MS River Observation Deck an elevated platform providing a clear view of the river and its traffic. The LA Gov.'s Mansion is a modified Greek Revival Structure that was completed in 1963. The LA State Capitol, completed in 1932, features steps commemorating the 50 states leading to its entrance, an observation deck on the 27th floor and 2 acres of formal gardens. A statue marks the grave of Gov. Huey D. Long, in whose administration the Capitol was built. St. Joseph's Cathedral, built in 1853, is the oldest church in the city. Although burned and rebuilt several times, the original structure still stands. Magnolia Mound Plantation House, built in the late 1700's, is also listed on the Natl. Register of Historic Places. The "Red Stick" monument at Southern U was designed by Sculptor Frank Hayden while the Battle Monument marks the site of the two-hour conflict of Aug. 5, 1862. Among the restored homes in the city are the Pino-charlet House (a classical-mode cottage built in Spanish Town in 1823), the Stewart-Dougherty House (an urban mansion built in 1848), the Potts House (built between 1846 and 1850) and the Warden's House (a classical revival structure built between 1837 and 1840).

BEAUMONT
TEXAS

CITY LOCATION-SIZE-EXTENT. Beaumont, seat of Jefferson Co., is located in the Sabine-Neches Piney Woods area of E TX, along the S border of the Big Thicket at 30°4' N lat. and 94°5' W long. It lies on the W bank of the Neches River 25 mi. NW of the Gulf of Mexico and approx. 85 mi. NE of Houston. The city encompasses 71.7 sq. mi. in the "Golden Triangle" area—its greater met. area includes the cities of Orange and Port Arthur to the E and SE as well as the smaller cities of Vidor, Orangefield, Bridge City, Port Neches, Nederland, Groves and Port Acres. Beaumont is bordered by Hardin and Orange counties to the N and E.

TOPOGRAPHY. The terrain of Beaumont, which lies on the flat coastal plain, includes marshes, predominantly pine forest and bayous. Pine Island Bayou flows through the city, while Sabine Lake lies approx. 20 mi. to the SE. The mean elev. is 23'.

CLIMATE. The climate of Beaumont is moderate marine, characterized by long, hot summers and short, mild winters. The avg. annual temp. of 68.8°F ranges from a Jan. mean of 25°F to a July and Aug. mean of 82.7°F. Its location close to the Gulf of Mexico results in an avg. annual rainfall of 53", which is fairly evenly distributed throughout the year. The RH ranges from 64% to 91%. The snowfall avgs. 5" per year. The avg. growing season is 300 days. Beaumont lies in the CSTZ and observes DST.

FLORA AND FAUNA. Animals native to Beaumont include the fox, opossum, muskrat and nutria. Salamanders, frogs, lizards, alligators, and snakes, including the venomous copperhead, cottonmouth, water moccasin and rattlesnake, are found here. Typical trees include the pine, cypress and oak. Smaller plants include the bluebonnet (the state flower) and azalea.

POPULATION. According to the US census, the pop. of Beaumont in 1970 was approx. 126,000. In 1978, it was estimated that it had increased to 129,990.

ETHNIC GROUPS. In 1978, the ethnic distribution of Beaumont was approx. 63.4% Caucasian, 30.7% Black, 5.5% Hispanic and 0.4% other.

TRANSPORTATION. Interstate Hwy. 10, US hwys. 69, 90, 96 and 287 and state hwys. 105, 124 and 347 provide major motor access to Beaumont. *Railroads* serving the city are Kansas City S, MO Pacific, Gulf, CO & Santa Fe and S Pacific. *Airlines* serving Jefferson Co. Airport are DL, TI, SW and Metro, while private and charter plane facilities are available at Beaumont Municipal Airport. *Bus Lines* serving the city are Trailways, Greyhound and the intracity Beaumont Municipal Transit. The 400' wide, 40' deep Neches River Ship Channel connects the city to the Gulf of Mexico and the Intracoastal Waterway. The city's port, the eighth largest in the US, includes 12 public wharves and the 3.5 million bushel grain elevator handles approx. 49 million tons annually.

COMMUNICATIONS. Communications, broadcasting and print media serving Beaumont are: *AM radio stations* KLVI 560 (UPI, Mod.); KTRM 990 (ABC/I, C&W); KJET 1380 (Mutual Blk.) and KAYC 1450 (Indep., Top 40);

Port of Beaumont, Texas

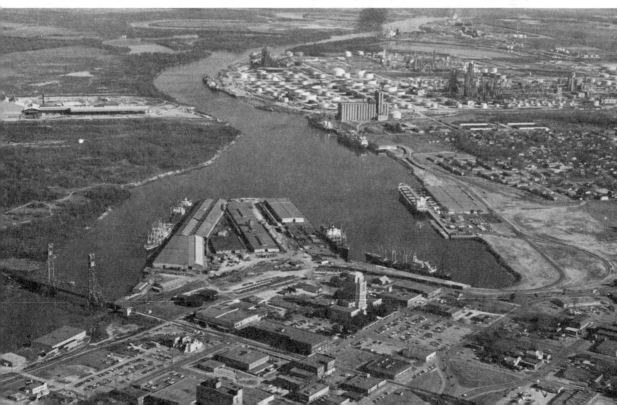

FM radio stations KVLU 91.3 (Lamar U); KOXY 94.1 (NBC, Btfl. Mus.); KALO 95.1 (Natl. Blk.); KAYD 97.5 (Indep., Top 40) and KWIC 107.7 (ABC/FM, Top 40); *television stations* KJAC Ch. 4 (NBC); KFDM Ch. 6 (CBS); KBMT Ch. 12 (ABC) and cable; *press:* the *Enterprise and Journal* is issued mornings and Sun. *(Enterprise)* and evening *(Journal)*; other publications include *Consumer's Beacon, Hardin Co. News, Jefferson Co. Court News, Midcountry Chronicle Review and Shoppers Guide, Orange Leader, Port Arthur News* and the *Victorian.*

HISTORY. One of the first white families to arrive in the area of present day Beaumont was that of Noah Tevis from TN, who settled part of a Mexican land grant on the W bank of the Neches River. Beaumont's permanent settlers included French and Spanish fur-trappers and explorers. In 1835, Tevis sold part of his 2,214-acre grant to Samuel Rogers, Henry Millard and others. This land became the original townsite of Beaumont, which

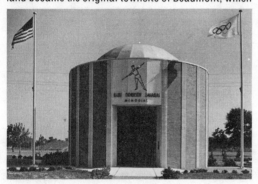

Babe Didrikson Zaharias Memorial, Beaumont, Texas

was organized later that year from Tevis Bluff, or the Neches River Settlement, as the settlement was known. The derivation of the name Beaumont has been variously attributed to Millard's brother-in-law, Jefferson Beaumont; a slight elev. SE of the city called "beau mont"—French for "beautiful hill"—and to a local pioneer family of Beaumont. The town of Beaumont was officially organized in the summer of 1837. By Jan, 1838, it became the seat of Jefferson Co., which had been organized the month before. The town was incorporated in the Republic of TX in Dec., 1838. During the 1840s, the lumber and rice industries became established and began to develop. At the same time, many settlers began to arrive in the town, attracted by offers of free land by the Republic. With the arrival of RR's in the 1850s, the comm. developed as a shipping center for cattle, cotton and sugar cane, among other commodities. In 1881, it was chartered as a city and was a sawmill town. World-wide attention was directed toward Beaumont as the birthplace of the modern oil industry, and, within 30 days of the historic oil strike, the pop. had soared to 30,000. The subsequent construction of refineries included those of the largest oil companies in the world.

GOVERNMENT. Beaumont has a council-mgr. form of govt. Five council members, including the mayor, are elected at large to two-year terms, and a city mgr. is appointed.

ECONOMY AND INDUSTRY. An enormous refining and petrochemical complex is located in Beaumont. Other industries include the production of medical instruments, offshore drilling rigs, precision industrial equipment, valves, heat exchangers, navigation equipment, optical lenses, farm implements, industrial electronics,

machine tools, refrigeration equipment, concrete pipe, steel pipe, wire rod and fabricated steel products. About 25% of the labor force is employed in manufacturing. Other major industries are iron and brass foundries; lumber; pulp and paper mills, rice mills and food processing plants. Raw materials include hydrocarbons, petrochemical feedstock, brine, salt, sulfur, timber, clay, limestone and natural gas. Port-related activity is also important—the city ranks second among TX ports in total ship tonnage handled. Among significant agricultural products are rice, soybeans and cattle. In June, 1979, the labor force totaled approx. 164,700, while the rate of unemployment was 6.9%.

BANKING. There are 18 banks and 10 savings and loan assns. in Beaumont. In 1978, total deposits for the 10 banks headquartered in the city were $657,688,000, while assets were $761,606,000. Banks include First Security Natl., American Natl., Beaumont State and Gateway Natl.

HOSPITALS. There are three gen. and four specialized hosps. in Beaumont, Baptist Hosp. of SE TX, Beaumont Medical Surgical Hosp., St. Elizabeth Hosp., Douglas Hosp. Clinic, Angie Nall Children's Hosp., Beaumont Remedial Clinic and Beaumont Neurological Center. Specialized clinics include the Beaumont State Center for Human Development, the Cerebral Palsy Center and a V.A. clinic.

EDUCATION. Lamar U, a state-supported institution enrolling approx. 12,800 in 1978, offers associate, bachelor, master and doctorate degrees. It also includes a Col. of Technical Arts and an Oil and Gas Drilling Institute. The Beaumont public school system includes 25 elementary, nine jr. and six sr. high schools, as well as a school for the deaf enrolling approx. 29,000 in 1978. There are five Catholic schools including one high and four elementary schools, as well as one Episcopal (K-7) school. Libs. include the Beaumont Public Lib. and two branches, Tyrrell Historical Lib., and Mary and John Gray Lib. of Lamar U.

ENTERTAINMENT. The Beaumont Art Museum sponsors Kaleidoscope, a nationally-renowned, arts and crafts festival, each May. The Neches River Festival, a five-day celebration in Apr., features a beauty pageant, parade, dancing, carnival, boat racing and water skiing. Every Oct., the S TX State Fair is held at Fair Park. The Beaumont Charity Horse Show is a three-day event held in early May. The Young Men's Business League Rodeo takes place in early June. Because so many men from the area have participated in professional football, the US Senate has proclaimed the city the "Pro Football Capital of the World". The Lamar U Cardinals participate in collegiate sports in the Southland Conf.

ACCOMMODATIONS. There are approx. 20 hotels and motels in Beaumont, including the Best Western-Americana Motor Inn, Castle Motel, Lark Hotel, Crown Motel, Rivera Hotel, Ridgewood Motor Hotel and the Ramada, LaQuinta and Red Carpet inns.

FACILITIES. There are 36 parks in Beaumont, encompassing approx. 1,000 acres and containing tennis courts (at 13 parks), swimming pools (at 3 parks), wading pools (at 16 parks), picnic areas, playing fields and golf courses. The 500-acre Tyrrell Park includes an 18-hole golf course, several mi. of jogging and bridle trails, an archery range, picnic and camping facilities, a garden center, a botanical garden and a special garden for the blind. Fresh and salt-water fishing and water fowl and small game hunting are available nearby.

CULTURAL ACTIVITIES. The Beaumont Art Museum, located in the S Regency Mansion of the V. Cooke Wilson Family, features a permanent collection of paintings, sculpture and mixed media. The Spindletop Museum on the campus of Lamar U houses documents and artifacts from the early days of the oil industry and commemorates the Lucas gusher and the Spindletop Field. The Brown and Scurlock galleries offer changing exhibits and art classes. The Beaumont Comm. Players and Beaumont Civic Ballet perform frequently, while musical events are presented by the Beaumont Symphony Orchestra and Beaumont Civic Opera. A Distinguished Artist Series is sponsored by the Beaumont Music Commission.

LANDMARKS AND SIGHTSEEING SPOTS. The French Trading Post, built in 1845 by John J. French of CT, who used it as a tannery, is the oldest historical landmark in Beaumont. Restored in 1969, it is a museum which commemorates the earliest times of Beaumont. Gladys City, a replica of the Spindletop Boomtown which resulted when oil was discovered at the Lucas Well, four mi. S of Beaumont, in 1901, is a complex of 15 buildings constructed for the US Bicentennial. It includes typical clapboard buildings of the early 1900s, oil derricks, wooden storage tanks and displays of early oilfield equipment. The Lucas Gusher Monument, a Natl. Historic Landmark, is a 58' granite shaft commemorating the discovery of oil at Spindletop. The 1863 Civil War Battle of Sabine Pass is marked by the Clifton Walking Beam Monument, while the Temple to the Brave, a small Gothic chapel-like shrine, is a memorial to soldiers of all wars. The (Mildred) Babe Didrikson Zaharias Memorial houses the many trophies and memorabilia of the Olympic Champion and women's professional golfer. St. Anthony's Cathedral, built in 1909 and completely restored in 1972, is a church of Romanesque-style architecture noted for its stained glass windows. The O'Brien Oak, a natural landmark, was the first Jefferson Co. court and site of early day meting out of justice.

BERKELEY
CALIFORNIA

CITY LOCATION-SIZE-EXTENT. Berkeley is located along the E shore of San Francisco Bay, about 12 mi. E of San Francisco, at 37°54'4" N lat. and 122°16' W long. The city encompasses 10.6 sq. mi. in Alameda Co. It is bordered by Emeryville on the SW, Albany on the NW, Piedmont and Oakland on the S and El Cerrito in Contra Costa Co. on the N and is part of the E Bay Greater Met. Area.

TOPOGRAPHY. Berkeley, situated on a peninsula of the San Francisco Bay, is W of the Great or Central Valley Region of CA. It contains low, often steep hills of the CA Coastal Mt. Range, which extends across the Bay to the W, as well as to the E of the city. The terrain consists of flat coastal shoreline and in the E, hills. The city lies 10 mi. E of the San Andreas Fault, a region of active earthquakes. The elev. ranges from SL to 1,300', with a mean of 152'.

CLIMATE. Berkeley's climate is characterized by year-round mild temps., fog (often heavy), overcast mornings and winter rains. Monthly mean temps. range from 48°F during Jan. to 64°F during Sept., with an avg. annual temp. of 57°F. Some 90% of the 23" avg. annual rainfall occurs from Oct. through Apr. Snowfall is rare. The RH ranges from 64% to 85%. The avg. growing season is 307 days. Berkeley is in the PSTZ and observes DST.

FLORA AND FAUNA. Animals native to Berkeley include the opossum, fox squirrel, deer and bat. Common birds include the house finch, scrub jay, acorn woodpecker, W kingbird and W bluebird. Among the water fowl are the seagull, Pacific pelican, coot, great blue heron and duck. Garter snakes, alligator and fence lizards, Pacific treefrogs, CA toads and newts and the venomous N Pacific rattlesnake are also found in the area. Typical trees include the redwood, pine, spruce, eucalyptus and camphor. Wild flowers include the blue lupine, CA golden poppy (the state flower), shooting star, wild iris, Johnny-jump-up, wild sweetpea and scotchbroom.

POPULATION. According to the US census, the pop. of Berkeley in 1970 was 114,091. In 1978, it was estimated that it had decreased to 112,000.

ETHNIC GROUPS. In 1978, the ethnic distribution of Berkeley was approx. 60.5% Caucasian, 25.5% Black, 5.5% Hispanic, 8.7% Asian and .5% other races (a percentage of the Hispanic total is also included in the Caucasian total).

TRANSPORTATION. Interstate hwys. 80 and 580 and state hwys. 13, 17, 24 and 123 provide major motor access to Berkeley. *Railroads* serving the area include AMTRAK, ConRail, Santa Fe, S Pacific and Union Pacific. Nearby Oakland and San Francisco intl. airports are served by all major *airlines*. *Bus lines* include Trailways, Greyhound, Peerless Stages, Bonanza, Trans Cal, AC Transit and the regional San Francisco Bay Area Rapid Transit (BART).

COMMUNICATIONS. Communications, broadcasting and print media originating from Berkeley are: *AM radio stations* KRE 1400 (ABC/E, Contemp. Jazz, Blk., R&B); *FM radio stations* KPFB 89.3 (Indep.); KALX 90.7 (Indep., Progsv., Educ.); KPFA 94.1 (Indep., Var.) and KRE-FM 102.9 (Indep., Contemp. Jazz, R&B); although no *television stations* are located in Berkeley, the city receives broadcasting from nearby San Francisco and Oakland; *press:* two major dailies serve the area, the evening *Daily Californian* and the *Independent and Gazette;* other publications include the *Barb, Berkeley Monthly, Press, Post, Express, Spectator, E Bay Review of the Performing Arts, Grassroots* and *Plexus Bay Area Women's Newspaper.*

HISTORY. Berkeley developed around the new campus of the U of CA, which opened in 1873 N of Oakland. Chartered as a city in 1878, it was named for George Berkeley, an early 19th century Anglican bishop, philosopher, idealist and educator. The city became a major center of education, and industries soon developed. In 1964, the first major col. protest demonstration in the US, organized by the Free Speech Movement, occurred at UC-Berkeley.

GOVERNMENT. Berkeley has a council-mgr. form of govt. consisting of nine council members, including the mayor, elected at large to four-year terms. The city mgr. is appointed by the council and administers city affairs.

ECONOMY AND INDUSTRY. The U of CA at Berkeley is one of the major employers in the city. The headquarters of the state U system is also located in the city. Industries

The Mathewson House, Berkeley, California

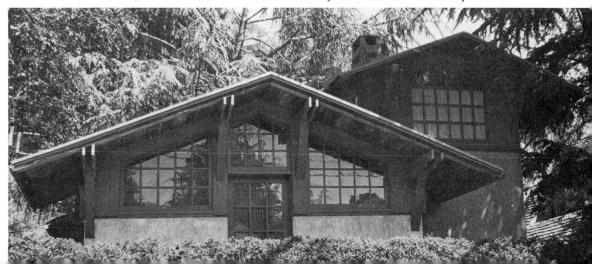

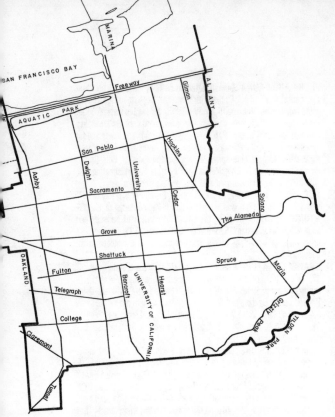

Berkeley, California

manufacture a variety of products, including chemicals, fluorocarbons, plastics, books, steel products, valves and instruments. The total labor force in Aug., 1979, was 61,585, while the unemployment rate was 8.6%. The median household income in 1978 was approx. $13,593.

BANKING. There are nine commercial banks and nine savings and loan assns. in Berkeley including the Bank of CA, United CA, Security Pacific Natl., Crocker Natl., Bank of America, First Enterprise, Security Natl., Wells Fargo and Central.

HOSPITALS. There are three gen. hosps. in Berkeley, Alta Bates, Ashby Geriatric and Herrick Memorial. There are also three convalescent hosps. in the city, Elmwood, Claremont and Berkeley Hills.

EDUCATION. The U of CA at Berkeley (UC-Berkeley), established by the State Legislature in 1866 as a state agricultural, mining and mechanical col., was founded in 1853 as the Contra Costa Academy, in Oakland by the Rev. Henry Durant. In 1855, its name became the Col. of CA. Instruction at the U, chartered in 1868, began on the new campus in 1873. The main campus of the U of CA system, it enrolled approx. 30,000 undergrad. and 10,000 at the grad. level in 1978. The Graduate Theological Union (GTU) was founded in the city in 1962 and includes nine participating institutions, as well as an affiliated center. These are the Dominican School of Theology; the Jesuit School of Theology (founded in 1934) and the Franciscan School of Theology, all of which are Catholic; the American Baptist Seminary of the West, the Starr King School for the Ministry (Unitarian), the Church Divinity School of the Pacific (Episcopal), the San Francisco Theological Seminary (Presbyterian), the Pacific Lutheran Theological Seminary (founded in 1948) and the Pacific School of Religion (founded in 1866 and comprised of Methodist, United Church of Christ-Congregational, and Christian Church-Disciples of Christ denominations); and the affiliate is the Center for Judaic Studies. Grad. students of the GTU, which enrolled approx. 1,400 in 1979, may cross-register at UC-Berkeley. Other institutions include Armstrong Col. (founded in 1918), CA School of Professional Psychology, Nyingma Institute, Vista Col., CA School for the Deaf and CA School for the Blind. There are 20 elementary and five secondary public schools with an enrollment of more than 13,000 in 1978. Libs. include the Berkeley Public, the UC-Berkeley (the largest U lib. in CA), the Bancroft Lib. at UC (containing collections of rare American W materials) and two libs. at the Judah L. Magnes Memorial Museum.

ENTERTAINMENT. Dinner theaters, festivals and annual events are also accessible throughout the San Francisco Bay area. The Golden Bears of UC-Berkeley participate in collegiate sports in the Pac Ten Conf. The professional sports teams of San Francisco and Oakland play nearby.

ACCOMMODATIONS. There are 15 hotels and motels in Berkeley, including the Best Western-Berkeley House Motor and Durant hotels, TraveLodge and the Berkeley Campus, Capri, Plaza, Flamingo and Golden Bear.

FACILITIES. Charles Lee Tilden Regional Park, in the NE part of Berkeley, is a 2,065-acre comm. playground. It contains a nature area, botanical garden, public golf course, picnic area, hiking and bridle trails and tennis courts, and features swimming in Anza Lake, pony rides and a miniature RR which is a replica of a coal-burning engine. Aquatic Park, a mi.-long salt water lake, provides facilities for water sports and model yacht racing. A public fishing pier is available at the Berkeley Marina, which maintains a large private charter boat fleet. The Berkeley Municipal Rose Garden features numerous varieties of roses.

CULTURAL ACTIVITIES. UC-Berkeley presents a performing arts series; its Music School also presents public performances. There are several theatrical groups in the city, including the Berkeley Theatre, Berkeley Stage Co., Black Repertory Group, American Fantasy Theatre, Poetry Playhouse, Berkeley Shakespeare Festival and UC Theater. Museums in the city include the Judah L. Magnes Memorial Museum (the Jewish Museum of the W), which features ceremonial art; the Bade Institute of Bible Archaeology, located at the Pacific School of Religion, which houses exhibits of the Holy Land from 3,500 B.C. to the Christian era; the Pacific Film Archive, which houses a large collection of films; the UC-Berkeley Art Museum and Lawrence Hall of Science, which both feature exhibits, and the Robert H. Lowie Museum of Anthropology in Kroeber Hall at UC.

LANDMARKS AND SIGHTSEEING SPOTS. A large stained-glass window occupies an entire wall of the chapel at the Pacific School of Religion, which also features the Howell Bible collection. The 30-acre UC Botanical Garden, located in Strawberry Canyon, features labeled plants that bloom throughout most of the year. Tours are conducted at the Lawrence-Berkeley Laboratory on the campus of the U of CA.

BIRMINGHAM
ALABAMA

CITY LOCATION-SIZE-EXTENT. Birmingham, the seat of Jefferson Co. and largest city in the state is located 300 mi. N of the Gulf of Mexico in N central AL at 33°34' N lat. and 86°45' W long. The city encompasses 89.76 sq. mi. in Jones Valley. The greater met. area includes all of Jefferson Co., Walker Co. on the N, Shelby Co. on the S and St. Clair Co. on the E.

TOPOGRAPHY. Birmingham, located in Jones Valley between a ridge of hills extending from the NE to the W and the Red Mt. range, which extends from the E to the SW, is situated in the Appalachian Ridge and valley region of AL. The city stretches for 15 mi. along the valley, which is two to four mi. wide. The Red Mt. Range reaches a height of 600' above the valley, where the elev. is as low as 585'. Rolling terrain extends SW and W of the city. The hills which extend to the NE and N are the foothills of the Appalachian Mts. and the Cumberland Plateau. The mean elev. is 620'.

CLIMATE. The hilly terrain of Birmingham causes low winter temps. and prevents the growth of vegetation that would otherwise occur in a subtropical location. Monthly temps. range from a Jan. mean of 45.6°F to a July mean of 80°F, with an avg. annual temp. of 63°F.

Most of the avg. annual rainfall of 53" occurs during the winter months and July (when it falls during thunderstorms). Snowfall, although negligible, occasionally exceeds 2". The RH ranges between 50% and 85%. The avg. growing season is 228 days. Birmingham lies in the CSTZ and observes DST.

FLORA AND FAUNA. Animals native to Birmingham include the opossum, raccoon and whitetail deer. Common birds are the red-eyed vireo, catbird, Carolina wren and cardinal. Bullfrogs, cricket frogs, snapping turtles, skinks, narrow-mouthed toads, water snakes and king snakes, as well as the venomous coral snake, copperhead, rattlesnake and cottonmouth, are found in the area. Typical trees include the oak, pine, dogwood, magnolia, willow and mulberry. Smaller plants are the pokeweed, sunflower and honeysuckle.

POPULATION. According to the US census, the pop. of Birmingham in 1970 was 310,530. In 1978, it was estimated that it had decreased to 278,000.

ETHNIC GROUPS. In 1978, the ethnic distribution of Birmingham was approx. 57.8% Caucasian, 41.3% Black, 0.4% Hispanic and 0.5% other.

TRANSPORTATION. Interstate hwys. 20, 59 and 65 and US hwys. 31, 78 and 280 provide major motor access to Birmingham. *Railroads* serving the city include AMTRAK, Southern Railway, Louisville, Nashville, Seaboard Coast, IL Central Gulf and St. Louis-San Francisco. *Airlines* serving Birmingham Municipal Airport include DL, US Air, EA, Republic and UA. *Bus lines* include Birmingham-Jefferson Co. Transit Authority, Greyhound, Trailways and Vestavia.

COMMUNICATIONS. Communications, broadcasting and print media serving Birmingham are: *AM radio stations* WSGN 610 (Indep., Contemp.); WVOK 690 (ABC/E, Mod. Ctry.); WYDE 850 (ABC/I, C&W); WATV 900 (Indep., Blk.); WERC 960 (APR, MOR); WAPI 1080 (NBC, MOR, Btfl. Mus.); WCRT 1260 (MBS, MOR, Btlf. Mus.); WENN 1320 (Indep., Blk.) and WJLD 1400 (Indep., Blk.); *FM radio stations* WBHM 90.3 (NPR, Clas.); WVSU 91.1 (Indep., Divers.); WDJC 93.7 (Indep., Relig.); WAPI 94.5 (Indep., Btfl. Mus.); WQEZ 96.5 (Indep., Btfl. Mus.); WRKK 99.5 (Indep., Progsv.); WZZK 105 (ABC/FM, C&W); WKXX 106.9 (Indep., Top 40) and WENN 107.7 (Indep., Blk.); *television stations* WBRC Ch. 6 (ABC); WBIQ Ch. 10 (PBS); WAPI Ch. 13 (NBC) and WBMG Ch. 43 (CBS); *press:* two major

dailies are published in the city, the *News*, issued evenings, and the *Post Herald*, issued mornings; other publications include the bi-weekly *Crimson*, the monthly *Progressive Farmer, Birmingham, Southern Living,* and *Southern Medicine.*

HISTORY. Native Americans of the Cherokee, Choctaw and Chickasaw tribes hunted in Jones Valley before the first white settlement was established in 1813. During the Civil War, small furnaces and ironworks, all of which were destroyed by the Union Army before the war's end, were built in iron ore-rich Jones Valley by Confederate forces to produce cannonballs and rifles. The city was founded and incorporated in 1871, at the junction of two RR's by the Elyton Land Co., a group of bankers and investors who hoped to produce steel from the area's rich deposits of coal, iron ore and limestone, and named for the large steel-producing city in England. In 1873, a depression and a cholera epidemic detracted from industrial and city growth, but rapid expansion followed implementation of blast furnaces in 1880. Between 1900 and 1920, the pop. increased tremendously—from 38,415 to 132,685—and Birmingham became known as "Magic City". From 1920 to 1930, the pop. grew from 178,806 to 259,678. The city was particularly affected by the Depression, but an increased demand for steel during WW II contributed to Birmingham's emergence as a leading industrial center of the S by the 1950s. In the 1960s, violent confrontations between whites and blacks, relating to the issue of integration, resulted in intervention by Pres. John F. Kennedy in 1963. Later that year, four black girls were killed by a bomb explosion in a church, but integration of public places and many schools resulted. In response to the pop. of the inner city, new construction and development programs were initiated in the 1970s. In 1971, more than 20 plants were closed by the fed. govt and more effective pollution control requirements were instituted. In 1979, Richard Arrington was elected the first black mayor of Birmingham.

GOVERNMENT. Birmingham has a mayor-council form of govt.,

Aerial view of central Birmingham, Alabama

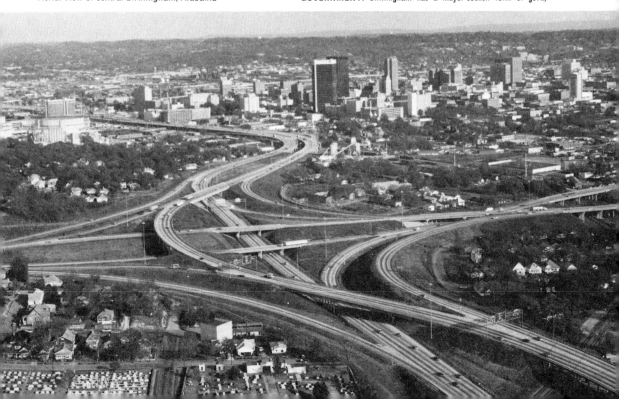

consisting of a mayor, who has no council vote, and nine council members. Every two years, five council members are elected at large—four to four-year terms, and the one receiving the fifth highest number of votes to a two-year term. The mayor is elected at large to a four-year term.

ECONOMY AND INDUSTRY. There are approx. 900 manufacturing firms in the Birmingham area. Major products include iron, steel, or primary metals and fabricated metals. Other industries include textiles, lumber and paper and food processing. Major areas of employment are steel, education, utilities, local govt. and health. Major agricultural products include dairy, livestock and poultry. Of the 1978 total met. area labor force of approx. 372,400, 83,800 were employed in retail and wholesale trade, 68,600 in manufacturing, 62,300 in services and 52,900 in govt. (44,400 state and local). In 1979, the rate of unemployment was 5.8%.

BANKING. There are 14 commercial banks and one savings and loan assn. in Birmingham. In 1978, total deposits for the banks headquartered in the city were approx. $3,311,369,000, and the total assets $4,105,604,000. Among the banks serving the city are Birmingham Trust Natl., First Natl., City Natl., First AL and Central.

HOSPITALS. There are 15 gen. and one children's hosp. in Birmingham, including the U of AL in Birmingham (UAB) Medical Center complex with various research and treatment facilities. Other hosps. are Baptist Medical Center, Carraway Methodist Hosp. and Norwood Clinic, V.A., Cooper Green, S Highland, St. Vincent's E End Memorial and Brookwood Medical Center. The S Research Institute (SRI) is engaged in experimentation with drugs used in the treatment of cancer and other diseases.

EDUCATION. THE U of AL in Birmingham (UAB), a state-supported coeducational institution established in 1964 as a branch campus of the U of AL, includes schools of medicine, dentistry, nursing, as well as hosps. and clinics, and offers bachelor, master and doctorate degrees. In 1978, more than 12,500 enrolled. Other institutions are Birmingham S Col., Miles Col., Samford U, Theodore A. Lawson State Comm. Col., a two-year institution with close to 1,800 enrolled in 1978, Jefferson State Jr. Col. (a state institution enrolling nearly 6,900 in 1978), Birmingham School of Law, Alverson-Draughon Col., Booker T. Washington Bus. Col. and SE Bible Col. The S Research Institute (SRI) conducts research projects relating to

Central Birmingham, Alabama

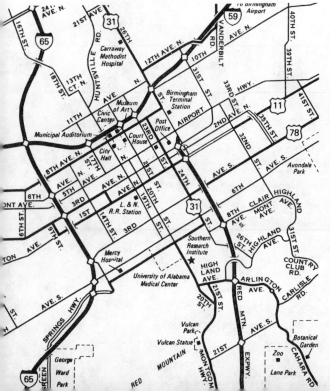

drug therapy, air pollution control equipment and high temp. materials. The public school system, consisting of approx. 80 elementary and 15 high schools, enrolled approx. 49,000 in 1978. There are about 30 private and parochial schools as well. Libs. include the Birmingham and Jefferson Co. Free Lib. and 16 branches.

ENTERTAINMENT. The Celebrity Dinner Theatre is located in Birmingham. The city hosts the AL State Fair every Oct., as well as an annual Arts and Crafts Fair, which features art, crafts, music and dancing, every summer. In late Apr. or early May, a marked route highlights the roses and dogwood trees for which the city is noted. The Birmingham Bulls are a pro WHA hockey team, while the UAB Blazers and the Birmingham S Col. Panthers (NJTL) participate in intercollegiate sports. The Natl. Jr. Tennis League Tournament is held every Aug. in the city.

ACCOMMODATIONS. There are about 50 hotels and motels in Birmingham. Among these are the Best Western-Kahler Plaza, Birmingham Motel, Hyatt House, Holiday Inn-Civic Center, TraveLodge, and the Hilton, Sheraton, Ramada and Rodeway inns.

FACILITIES. There are about 65 public parks, encompassing close to 1,600 acres, in Birmingham. Among them are Fountain Heights, N Birmingham, Central, Willow Wood, Woodrow Wilson, Harrison, Ensley, King, Hawkins and Memorial parks. Public golf courses, tennis courts at 30 of the parks and 14 swimming pools, offering lessons and team competition, are featured. The 67-acre Botanical Garden features a Japanese garden with a teahouse, as well as a conservatory containing more than 500 varieties of rare plants. Jimmy Morgan Zoo, the city's zoological park and one of the largest in the S, displays birds, reptiles and mammals in their natural setting.

CULTURAL ACTIVITIES. Among the cultural organizations in Birmingham are a symphony orchestra, ballet companies and theater groups. The Greater Birmingham Arts Alliance sponsors summer programs featuring music, dance, art, crafts and drama. The Birmingham Museum of Art features a permanent exhibit of a portion of the renowned Kress collection of Italian paintings, as well as native American art and artifacts and art of the old W.

LANDMARKS AND SIGHTSEEING SPOTS. The Arlington Antebellum Home and Gardens, built in 1822, is an old AL mansion furnished with antiques and featuring 19th century gardens. The 55' "Vulcan", one of the largest cast-iron statues in the world, sculpted by Giuseppe Moretti from area pig iron, is a re-creation of the Roman god of fire, symbolizing the city's heritage of iron- and steel-making, stands atop Red Mt. in Vulcan Park. The flame of Vulcan's torch, usually green, burns red for 24 hours in the event of a traffic fatality. An elevator runs to the top of the statue and affords a view of the entire city.

BOISE
IDAHO

CITY LOCATION-SIZE-EXTENT. Boise, the capital of ID and seat of Ada Co., is situated on the Boise River in the SW part of the state at 43°34' N lat. and 116°13' W long. The city encompasses 39 sq. mi. in the Treasure Valley region, 50 mi. E of OR.

TOPOGRAPHY. Boise lies in the Columbia plateau region of ID. The city's topog. is characterized by the gently sloping, heavily wooded land of the Boise River Valley and Snake River plain. The terrain rises to the foothills of the Salmon River and Sawtooth Mt. ranges (of the Rocky Mts.) to the N and E. Within eight mi. of the city, mts. rise to heights of 5,000' to 6,000'. To the S of the "City of Trees" is a sagebrush desert area. Numerous rivers and lakes are in the area, as are Arrowrock, Lucky Peak and Anderson Ranch reservoirs. The mean elev. is 2,838'.

CLIMATE. The climate of Boise is temperate and dry;

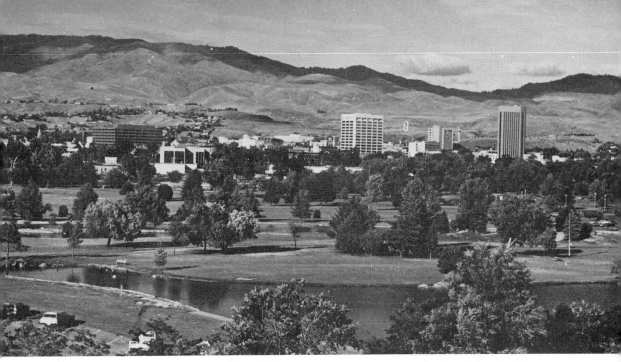

Aerial view of Boise City, Idaho

irrigation from reservoirs upstream has moistened the basically semi-arid area somewhat. Weather variations occur when modified air masses from the Pacific Ocean alternate with atmospheric developments from other directions. The 51.3°F avg. annual temp. ranges from a Jan. mean of 29.9°F to a July mean of 74.5°F. Temps. higher than 100°F occur an avg. of three days per year, although longer periods of extremely cold temps. occur during winter. Most of the avg. annual rainfall of 11.96" occurs during Feb. and Mar., while most of the avg. annual 21.3" of snowfall occurs during the months of Dec. through Feb. An avg. of four hailstorms per year causes occasional damage over small areas. The RH ranges from 22% to 81%. The avg. growing season is 160 days. Boise lies in the MSTZ and observes DST.

FLORA AND FAUNA. Animals native to Boise include the mule deer, bighorn sheep, antelope, Rocky Mt. goat, cottontail rabbit, black bear, porcupine and elk. Common birds are the jay, crow, golden eagle, mt. bluebird and chickadee. Lizards, frogs and snakes, including the venomous Great Basin rattlesnake, are found here. Typical trees include the pine, Norway maple and juniper. Smaller plants include the burning brush and rose.

POPULATION. According to the US census, the pop. of Boise in 1970 was 74,990. In 1978, it was estimated that it had increased to 110,000. Boise is the largest city in ID.

ETHNIC GROUPS. In 1978, the ethnic distribution of Boise was approx. 97.1% Caucasian, 1.1% Black, 1.5% Hispanic and .3% Asian.

TRANSPORTATION. Interstate hwys. 80, US hwy. 30 and state rtes. 20, 21 and 44 provide major motor access to Boise. The city is served by AMTRAK and Union Pacific *railroads. Airlines* providing service to the municipal Boise Air Terminal/Gowen Field are RW, UA, FL, Big Sky, Air OR, Cascade and Mt. W. Another airport serving Boise is Strawberry Glenn. *Bus lines* providing service are Greyhound, Trailways, NW Stage, Boise-Winnemucca Stage and the intracity Boise Urban Transportation System.

COMMUNICATIONS. Communications, broadcasting and print media originating in Boise are: *AM radio stations* KFXD 580 (Indep., UPI Audio, Top 40); KIDO 630 (MBS, Western); KBOI 670 (NBC, MOR/Upbeat); KYME 740 (Indep., Jazz); KSPD 790 (MBS, UPI Audio-All News); KBRJ 950 (Indep., C&W), KGEM 1140 (ABC/I, C&W) and KAIN 1340 (MBS); *FM radio stations* KBSU 90.1 (Indep., Progsv., AOR, Spec.); KBBK 92.3 (Indep., C&W); KBXL 94 (Indep., Good Mus.); KFXD 94.9 (Indep., Top 40); KBOI 97.9 (NBC, Btfl. Mus.) and KNFR 104.3; *television stations* KBCI Ch. 2

(CBS); KAID Ch. 4 (PBS); KIVI Ch. 6 (ABC) and KTVB Ch. 7 (NBC); *press:* the daily *Idaho Statesman*, issued mornings, and the weekly *Journal of Commerce, Advertiser* and *Meridian Times News* serve the Boise area; other publications include the quarterly *Boise Magazine*, the *ID Register, ID Wood Growers' Bulletin* and *ID Farmer-Stockman*.

HISTORY. The settling of Boise occurred in 1862, at the time of the gold rush in ID, which resulted in the discovery of one of the NW's richest mining districts—the Boise Basin, 40 mi. NE of present-day Boise. French trappers were among the first white settlers of the area in the early part of the 19th century. Ft. Boise was established as a British trading post in 1834. The town, whose name is derived from the French "les bois", meaning "the woods", was founded in July, 1863, by Tom and Frank Davis and H.C. Riggs as a townsite adjacent to a planned US military outpost. It served as both a distribution center for the mines in the area and an irrigation center for farms nearby. Boise was incorporated as a city on Dec. 12, 1864, by the ID Territorial Legislature, which also selected the city as the territory's capital and the permanent seat of govt. (which it remained following ID's achievement of statehood in 1890). Ada Co. was also established at this time with Boise as the county seat. Because the surrounding mts. and deserts reinforced Boise's isolation, the city experienced slow growth throughout the remainder of the 19th century, especially after the gold rush ended. With the recent boom in the pops. of W states, however, Boise—as the commercial and distribution center of SW ID—has also grown. Since 1960, and following annexations of neighboring areas, its pop. has more than tripled.

GOVERNMENT. Boise has a mayor-council form of govt. consisting of a mayor and six council members, elected at large to four-year terms. Three council members are elected every two years to overlapping terms. The mayor votes only in the event of a tie.

ECONOMY AND INDUSTRY. Boise is the commercial center of SW ID, E OR and N NV. Wholesale and retail trade, manufacturing, service and govt. are the major employment areas. The manufacturing industries are

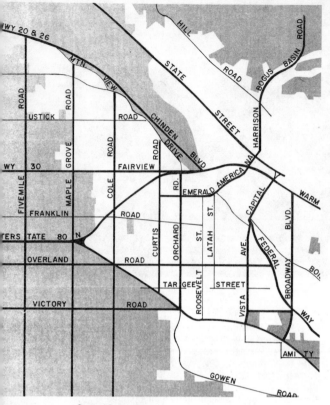

Central Boise, Idaho

largely dependent on the forest and agricultural resources of the area, with lumber, food processing, electronics and meat packing the major industries. The labor force totaled approx. 90,500 in June, 1979, with approx. 3,600, or 4%, unemployed. In 1977, the avg. income per capita was $5,760, while the household avg. was $14,890.

BANKING. There are six commercial banks and five savings and loan assns. in Boise. In 1978, total deposits for the five banks headquartered in the city were $2,717,132,000, while total assets were $3,304,634,000. Banks serving the city are First Security Bank of ID, ID First Natl., Bank of ID, ID Bank and Trust, Citizens Natl. and American Bank of Commerce.

HOSPITALS. There are five hosps. in Boise, St. Alphonsus, established in 1894 and operated by the Sisters of the Holy Cross, serves as the emergency hosp. for the entire comm.; St. Luke's is a gen. hosp., established in 1902 and affiliated with the Episcopal Church; Mt. States Tumor Institute, established in May, 1971, specializes in the field of cancer; V.A. Hosp. and Elks Rehabilitation Center.

EDUCATION. Boise State U (BSU), established in 1932 as Boise Jr. Col., became Boise Col. in 1965 and Boise State Col. in 1969, before achieving its present status in 1974. Offering undergrad. and grad. (in education, business and public administration) degrees, it enrolled more than 10,000 in 1978. Boise Bible Col. is another institution of higher learning located in the city, as are two business, one barber, three beauty and two nursing schools. Boise Center for Urban Research, a joint venture of BSU and the City of Boise, has provided research and data services since 1975. There are 19 kindergartens and 27 elementary, six jr. and three sr. high schools in the Boise public school system, enrolling close to 23,000. Approx. 2,000 additional students are enrolled in the city's seven parochial schools, which include one high and four elementary Roman Catholic schools, one Seventh-Day Adventist elementary school and one Christian school for grades one through 12. Lib. facilities are available at

Boise Public and Information Center, ID State, ID State Historical Society and Archives, ID Genealogical and ID State Law libs.

ENTERTAINMENT. There are two dinner theaters in Boise, the Dinner Theatre and Country Playhouse. Each year in early May, Boise Music Week is held in the city. The first city in the US to present a free, all-comm. Music Week, Boise began hosting the annual event in 1918. Parades, comm. sings, operas, musical comedies, folk festivals and variety programs are featured. The W ID Fair is held each year in late Aug. and early Sept. Horse racing and parimutuel betting are featured annually each summer at Les Boise Park at the W ID Fairgrounds. Yearly raft races down the Boise River are held by various groups while the Kiwanis Jr. High Rodeo and the Christmas Concert in the Capitol Rotunda in mid-Dec. are other annual events. The BSU Broncos participate in sports at the collegiate level in the Big Sky Conf., while the Boise Blades participate in hockey.

ACCOMMODATIONS. There are 48 hotels and motels in Boise including the Rodeway, Holiday, Sheraton Downtowner, Best Western-Vista, Red Lion, Intl. Dunes, Statehouse, Ramada, Quality, Safari, Owyhee Plaza, TraveLodge and Boisean.

FACILITIES. There are 53 public park areas in Boise, encompassing approx. 1,700 acres and containing 12 playgrounds, softball fields, tennis courts, picnic areas, equestrian areas, pools and the Boise City Zoo—the largest in ID—located in Julia Davis Park. The zoo, established in 1916, contains animals of the NW, Bengal tigers, the only two Steppe cats in captivity in the US, a S American rhea and various monkeys, apes and birds. The 86-acre Julia Davis Park, the oldest in Boise and located on the river, contains a boating lagoon, bandshell, historical museum, art gallery, amusement center, tennis courts, rose garden, pioneer village, "Big Mike" (a steam locomotive) and picnic areas. The 153-acre Ann Morrison Park, the largest in the city and dedicated in 1959, features picnic areas, ballfields, tennis courts, "Candy Cane City" playground and a bridle path. The five-acre Shoshone Park contains two tennis courts and a jogging path, while numerous other parks, including Municipal, Camel Back, Cassia, Hillside and Winstead, offer arts and crafts, swimming, archery, tennis and horseback and bicycle riding facilities, among others. There are two public golf courses in the city, including the 18-hole Municipal Golf Course completed in 1972, which offer golfing 300 days of the year. The Boise River Greenbelt, Lake Lowell and Lucky Peak and Arrowrock reservoirs offer canoeing, tubing, rafting, water skiing, swimming, boating and other recreational facilities. Bogus Basin, located 16 mi. from downtown Boise, offers the longest illuminated ski run in the US.

CULTURAL ACTIVITIES. The 60-member Boise Philharmonic Orchestra, established in 1948, presents six major performances as well as Youth Concerts. The Kings of Swing are another musical group. Theatre in a Trunk, a comm. theater established in 1972, presents various dramatic performances, as do Boise Little Theater, ID Public Theatre and BSU theatrical groups. The Oinkari Basque Dancers is a group of American-born Basques which performs locally. The Boise Gallery of Art, located at Julia Davis Park, sponsors lectures and special events such as the annual two-day outdoor Art Fair in early Sept. and the Artist of ID Annual, a juried exhibition of works of ID artists which is one of the major visual arts events in the state. The ID State Historical Museum, also located in Julia Davis Park, features displays of ID and NW history. Galleries in the city include the Boise, Ochi, Fritchman's and Tuesday's Child.

LANDMARKS AND SIGHTSEEING SPOTS. O'Farrell Cabin, the oldest pioneer building in Boise, First United Methodist Church or the "Cathedral of the Rockies", a huge Gothic structure with beautiful stained glass windows, and Ft. Boise, established in 1834, are among the city's historic landmarks. The State Capitol is the most impressive of Boise's landmarks. Built in 1905, but first used in 1912, it was constructed of native sandstone as well as marble from AK, GA and VT and features exhibits of agricultural, mineral and timber products. Many of the trees on the grounds were planted by US presidents. Julia Davis Park, with an amusement park, zoo, art gallery, Platt Gardens, Pioneer Village and historical museum, is a popular attraction. There are numerous natural scenic wonders in the area as well. The old penitentiary, built in 1870, is located five mi. E of Boise and features a museum. Walking tours of the former state prison and grounds are conducted daily.

BOSTON
MASSACHUSETTS

CITY LOCATION-SIZE-EXTENT. Boston, the state capital, seat of Suffolk Co. and the largest city in the NE, is situated in E MA on the S bank of the Charles River, and W of Boston Harbor on MA Bay. The city encompasses 49.4 sq. mi. at 42°22' N lat. and 71°02' W long. and includes the Harbor Islands, a group of more than 30, including Spectacle, Moon, Long, Georges, Lovell, Gallups, Rainsford, Casier, the Brewsters and the Graves. The greater met. area includes 92 cities and towns and extends into bordering Middlesex and Norfolk counties to the NE and SW, as well as Essex Co. to the NE and Plymouth Co. to the SW.

TOPOGRAPHY. Boston lies on hilly terrain on the Atlantic coastal plain between the Atlantic Ocean to the E and the Berkshire Hills 100 mi. to the W. The Blue Hills rise to an elev. of 635' 8 mi. S of the city. Rivers in the area include the Chelsea, Mystic and Charles to the NE, N and NW and the Neponset River to the SE, which all empty into Boston Harbor. Dorchester Bay is a large inlet of Boston Harbor at the mouth of the Neponset River. Ponds in the area include Jamaica, Turtle and Back Bay Fens. The mean elev. is 15'.

CLIMATE. The variable climate of Boston is influenced by its lat. The low pressure systems and the Atlantic Ocean moderate temp. extremes during the summer and winter. The avg. annual temp. of 50.4°F varies from a Jan mean of 28.8°F to a July mean of 72.6°F. Most of the avg. annual rainfall of 41.50" occurs from May through Aug., while most of the annual 43.1" of snowfall occurs from Dec. through Mar. The RH ranges from 52% to 80%. Heavy fog occurs on an avg. of two days per month. The avg. growing season is 165 days. Boston lies in the ESTZ and observes DST.

FLORA AND FAUNA. Animals native to Boston include the deer and racoon. Common birds include the thrush, warbler, robin, blue jay, tanager, sparrow and gull. Salamanders, frogs, turtles and snakes, including the venomous timber rattlesnake and copperhead, are found here. Typical trees are the red oak, maple, beech and elm. Smaller plants include the viburnum, mt. laurel, chicory, daisy, holly and Queen Anne's lace.

POPULATION. According to the US census, the pop. of Boston in 1970 was 641,071. In 1978, it was estimated that it had decreased to 638,000. The city ranks 23rd in the US.

ETHNIC GROUPS. In 1978, the ethnic distribution of Boston was approx. 72% Caucasian, 21% Black, 6% Hispanic, .5% Asian and .5% other.

TRANSPORTATION. Interstate hwys. 90 (the MA Turnpike), 93 and 95 (the Central Artery, or Fitzgerald Expressway), US hwys. 1 and 20 and state rtes. 2, 3 (the SE Expressway), 9, 28 and 138 provide major motor access to Boston. *Railroads* serving the city are AMTRAK, Boston & ME and NY,

Paul Revere House, the oldest home in Boston, Massachusetts

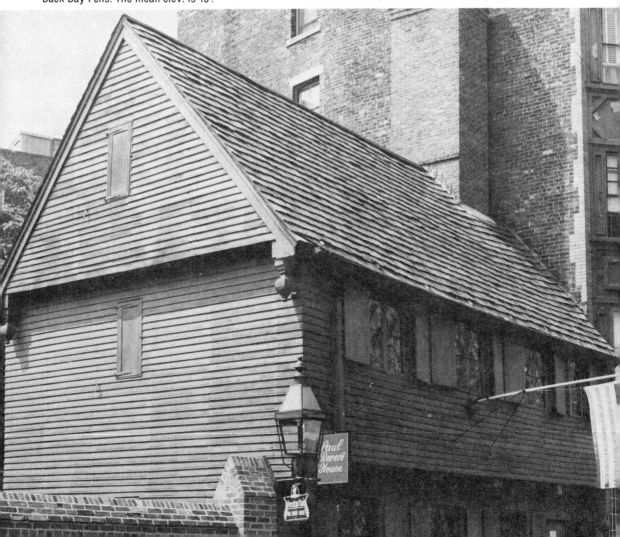

New Haven & Hartford. *Airlines* serving Logan Intl. Airport, the eighth busiest in the world, include the domestic AA, US Air, DL, EA, FL, NA, NC, CO, BN, NW Orient, PI, PA, NE, TW, NW and UA, and the intl. Air Canada, Aer Lingus, Alitalia, British Airways, Lufthansa, Swissair, Aeromexico and Caribbean. *Bus lines* serving the city include Almeida, Peter Pan, Michaud, Greyhound and Trailways. The MA Bay Transportation Authority (MBTA) provides bus, streetcar, subway, train and trolleycar service with 80 mi. of rapid transit streetcar lines, 291 mi. of commuter rail and 3,500 mi. of bus rtes. There are three privately-owned commuter boat lines, and the MA Port Authority oversees harbor operations.

COMMUNICATIONS. Communications, broadcasting and print media originating from Boston are: *AM radio stations* WBZ 103 (Indep.); WEEI 590 (CBS, APR, News); WRKO 680 (APR, Top 40); WHDH 850 (ABC/E, UPI, Contemp., MOR); WROL 950 (Indep., Talk, Relig.); WILD 1090 (MBS, Blk.); WACQ 1150 (ABC/C, UPI, Adult Contemp.); WEZE 1260 (ABC/I, Relig.) and WITS 1510 (NBC, MOR); *FM radio stations* WERS 88.9 (Indep., Var., Spec., Progsv.); WGBH 89.7 (NPR, EPRN, Clas., Educ., Jazz); WBUR 90.9 (NPR, Concert, Jazz, Pub. Affairs); WRBB 91.7 (ABC/I, Divers.); WHRB 95.3 (Indep., Var.); WCOZ 94.5 (Indep., Progsv.); WJIB 96.9 (Indep., Btfl. Mus.); WOR 98.5 (ABC/FM, MOR); WHUE 100.7 (ABC/C, UPI, Progsv.); WEEI 103.3 (Indep., Adult Contemp., MOR); WBCN 104.1 (Indep., Progsv.); WVBF 105.7 (APR, Top 40) and WBZ 106.7 (Indep., Rock, Spec., Progsv.); *television stations* WGBH Ch. 2 (PBS); WBZ Ch. 4 (NBC); WCVB Ch. 5 (ABC); WNAC Ch. 7 (CBS); WSBK Ch. 38 (Indep., Secondary Affil. ABC, CBS, NBC); WGBX Ch. 44 (PBS) and WLVI Ch. 56 (Indep.); *press:* three major dailies serve the city, the *Globe*, issued daily mornings and evenings and weekend mornings, the *Herald-American*, issued daily and weekend mornings, and the natl. *Christian Science Monitor*, issued daily mornings; other publications include the weekly *Boston Phoenix, NE Journal of Medicine, Away* and *Family;* and the bi-monthly *Bankers and Tradesman, MA CPZ Review, Apothecary* and *Harvard Business Review.*

HISTORY. The peninsula between the Charles River and Boston Harbor, on which Boston was founded, was called "Shawmett" by the native Americans of the MA tribe who were inhabiting the area when the first white settlers arrived in the early 1600s. In 1630, John Winthrop and a group of 800 Puritan colonists, who had first settled in Charlestown across the Charles River, accepted an offer of land from the Rev. William Blackstone who lived on what is now Beacon Hill. On Sept. 7, 1630, the name of the settlement was changed to Boston, in honor of the town in England from which many of the colonists had come. In 1634, Blackstone sold back to the Puritans the 50 acres of land they had allotted him. The parcel, which is known as the "Common", was reserved for public use. In 1632, Boston became the capital of the MA Bay Colony. It was a closely-knit village of farmers, craftsmen and ministers who drove out those of differing beliefs and permitted only Puritans to vote and hold office. One of the city's nicknames, "Beantown", originated at this time. Since cooking on Sun. was prohibited by the Puritans, women prepared pots of baked beans on Sat. evenings for Sun. dinner. The early growth of the town derived from its position as a seaport—it became the principal port for the colonies. In 1720, its pop. had reached 12,000, and, by the mid-18th century, it had become a

Downtown Boston, Massachusetts

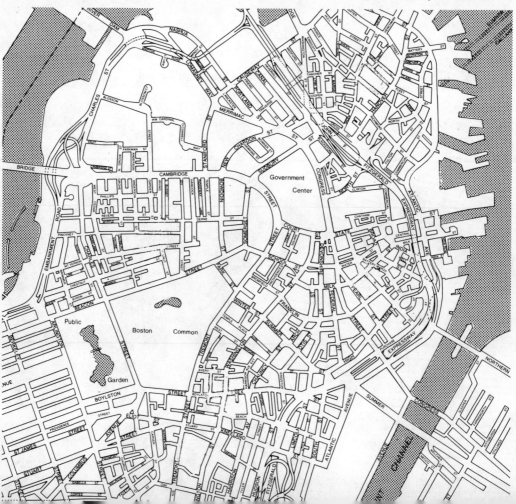

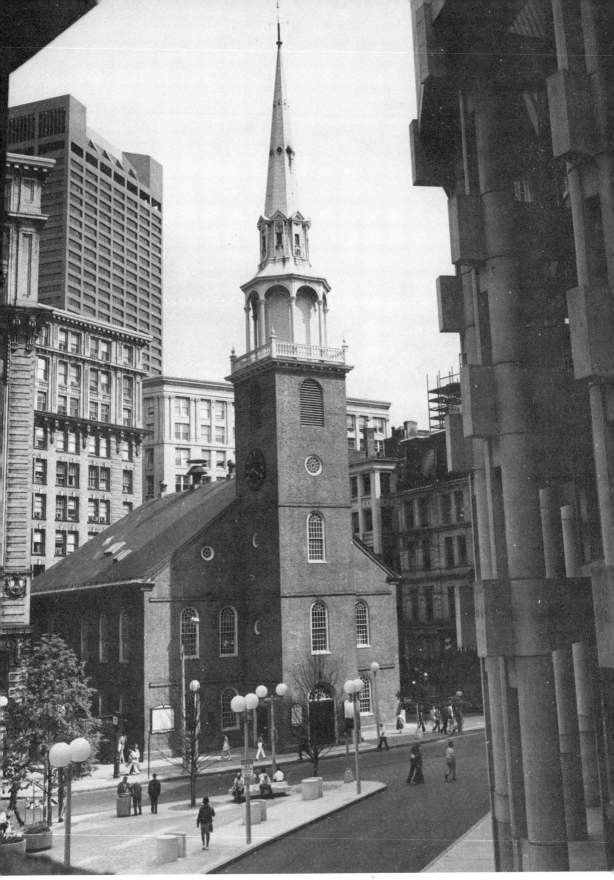

Old South Meeting Hall (Built 1729), Boston, Massachusetts

leading commercial, fishing and shipbuilding center. Boston, the "cradle of Liberty" and "Birthplace of the Revolutionary War", played a significant role in the Revolution against British rule. In 1770, the "Boston Massacre" occurred when six citizens were killed by British troops. In 1773, the "Boston Tea Party" and the subsequent British closure of the port took place. On Apr. 19, 1775, when the British attempted to seize the colonial military stores at Concord, Paul Revere made his now famous ride, calling the Minutemen to arms. The first major battles of the Revolutionary War occurred at Lexington and Concord. American efforts to fortify Charlestown led to the Battle of Bunker Hill. On Mar. 17, 1776, Gen. George Washington mounted cannons on Dorchester Heights and drove out the British, winning the first major colonial victory of the Revolution. After the war, Boston continued to grow as a cultural and commercial—especially whaling and shipping—city. The first town in MA to become a city, Boston was chartered on Mar. 4, 1822. In 1831, the city became the center of the abolitionist movement begun by William Lloyd Garrison and his *Liberator*, and strong anti-secession feelings encouraged some 160,000 MA men to join the Union Army during the Civil War. Following the War, industry and trade expanded, and, between 1880 and 1914, a large influx of immigrants from Italy, Canada, Lithuania and Poland arrived in the city. Many more immigrants, particularly from Ireland, arrived between 1845 and 1847. In 1897, the first subway in the US began operating in the city. By 1900, the pop. had reached 560,000. The city continued to grow as the center of business, finance, govt. and transportation, as well as culture (it became known as the "Hub of the Universe" and "Athens of America") in N.E. during the 20th century. During the 1950s, the inner city experienced deterioration and a decline in pop., but large-scale urban development programs were begun in the 1960s. Since 1970, the city (especially downtown) has experienced revitalization and a pop. increase. In 1974, racial tension erupted in violence after a fed. court ordered the desegregation of public schools and busing of students.

GOVERNMENT. Boston has a mayor-council form of govt. consisting of the mayor, elected at large to a four-year term, and nine council members, elected at large to two-year terms. Five school committee members are also elected at large to two-year terms.

ECONOMY AND INDUSTRY. Boston is the largest industrial, retail and wholesale trade center in the N.E., the ninth largest industrial center in the US, as well as the regional center for govt., finance and transportation. There are more than 5,000 manufacturing plants in the greater met. area. Major products include machinery, medical instruments, fabricated metal products, processed foods, seafood, printing and publishing, apparel and production of mini-computers. Other major employers include services, communications, higher education, science, R&D, port-related activities, tourism and entertainment. Health, business, insurance (the headquarters of 20 companies are located in the city), banking and education (the col. student pop. exceeds 100,000) are the major service-related industries. The city is the largest market of the wool, shoe and leather industries in the US. In June, 1979, the labor force for the greater met. area totaled approx. 1,413,800, while the rate of unemployment was 5%. In 1978, the median income was $7,227.

BANKING. There are 44 banks and savings and loan assns. in Boston,

which ranks second to NYC as a financial center. In 1978, bank deposits for the 35 banks headquartered in the city totaled $17,637,320,000, while total assets were $22,814,622,000. Banks in the city include First Natl., Shawmut, N.E. Merchants Natl., State St. Bank and Trust, Provident Institution for Savings and Boston Five Cents Savings. The First Fed. Reserve District Bank is also located in the city.

HOSPITALS. There are 32 hosps. in Boston, which is renowed as a medical research center, including Boston U Medical Center, Tufts N.E. Medical Center and Harvard U-affiliated hosps. Other hosps. include Peter Bent Brigham, Robert E. Brigham and Boston Hosp. for Women (divisions of Affiliated Hosps. Center) MA Gen., Boston City, Beth Israel, Bournewood, Carney, Children's Medical Center, Charles River, St. Margaret's for Women, St. John of God, St. Elizabeth's, N.E. Deaconess, N.E. Baptist, Faulkner, Glenside, Kennedy Memorial for Children, Huntington Gen., Shriner/Burns, Joslin Clinic, Sidney Farber Cancer Institute, Lakey Clinic, MA Eye and Ear Infimary and MA Mental Health Center. There are also 10 neighborhood health centers in the city.

EDUCATION. There are approx. 30 colleges and universities in Boston. Boston U (BU), the oldest institution of higher education in the city, was founded in 1839 as a theological seminary, moved to Boston in 1867 and was established as a U in 1869. A private nonsectarian institution, BU enrolled more than 24,400 in 1978. Boston State Col., founded in 1852 as Boston Normal School and renamed in 1960, is a public institution enrolling approx. 11,400 in 1978. Northeastern U (NU), established in 1898 as a privately-endowed nonsectarian institution, offers a cooperative education program enabling students to integrate practical experience with studies. In 1978, it enrolled more than 34,000. Other institutions in the city include the U of MA Boston Campus, which was established in 1965 and enrolled nearly 8,400 in 1978; Wentworth Institute, established in 1904 and enrolled approx. 2,200 in 1978; MA Col. of Pharmacy (MCP), a five-year private col. established in 1936 and offering undergrad. and grad. courses enrolled approx. 1,600 in 1978; Suffolk U established in 1906, with a 1978 enrollment of approx. 6,001 and Emerson Col., a private institution enrolling approx. 1,000. Other institutions located in the city are the N.E. Conservatory of Music, the oldest in the US, established in 1867, with a 1978 enrollment of 445; Berklee Col. of Music, established in 1962 and enrolling approx. 2,500 in 1978; Emmanuel Col., enrolling approx. 1,500 in 1978; Harvard U Schools of Medicine and Business; Tufts Medical and Dental Schools; School of the Museum of Fine Arts, with a 1978 enrollment of approx. 900; MA Col. of Art, established in 1873 enrolling approx. 1,700 in 1978; Simmons Col., established in 1899 enrolling approx. 950 in 1978; N.E. Col. of Optometry, with a 1978 enrollment of 350 and N.E. School of Law, which enrolled approx. 900 in 1978. Boston Col., the third largest Catholic Jesuit institution and the largest Catholic U in the US, is located on the SW edge of the city in Newton. Established in 1863, it enrolled approx. 14,000 in 1978. Jr. cols. include Newbury, enrolling approx. 2,300 in 1978; Fisher, with an enrollment of nearly 2,100 in 1978; Laboure, enrolling approx. 400; Bay State Col. of Business and Chamberlayne, both with 1978 enrollments of more than 700; Charleston Comm. Col. and Bunker Hill Comm. Col. The N.E. Institute of Applied Arts and Sciences and the Franklin Institute are also located in the city. The first public secondary school in America, Boston Latin School, was opened in 1635. The public school system consists of approx. 250 public schools with a total enrollment of approx. 85,000 in 1978. There are 75 Catholic and several private schools in the city. Lib. facilities include the Boston Public Lib., founded in 1854 as the first major free lib. in the US, with 26 branches, including a business branch, the Kirstein Public Lib. The Boston Athenaeum, a privately-supported lib., contains books once owned by George Washington. Other libs. include those of the MA State House Archives, the MA Historical Lib., JFK Lib. at U MA-Boston, the MA Horticultural Society Lib. and those at universities, colleges and museums throughout the city.

ENTERTAINMENT. The Boston Marathon, instituted in 1897 is a 26-mi. (42-km.) run from the suburb of Hopkinton to Back Bay held annually on Apr. 19 (Patriots Day). Other annual events celebrated in the city are the Chinese Festival of the Aug. Moon, the religious feast day of Saints Rocco and Joseph (July), as well as Anthony (Aug.), held in the N End featuring processions and festivals, and the annual Fourth of July celebration featuring fireworks displays in the Inner Harbor. First Night, celebrating the New Year, annually takes place at Boston Common and in the Back Bay. Summerthing, a city-sponsored summertime program founded in 1968, features eight weeks of concerts, plays and events for children. The St. Botolph Street Festival, a celebration featuring culture of the W Indies, is held each summer, as is the Charles Street Fair. The annual mid-summer Harbor Islands Week features seven days of historical, educational and recreational activities, while Bunker Hill Day is celebrated in Charlestown on June 17. Professional sports teams include the Boston Tea Men, an NASL soccer team, the N.E. Patriots, an NFL-AFC football team which plays in suburban Foxboro; the Boston Red Sox, an AL baseball team which plays in Fenway Park; the Boston Bruins, an NHL hockey team—both of whom play at Boston Garden. Col. teams include the Boston State Col. Warriors, the Boston U Terriers, the N.E. Huskies and the BC Eagles. Suffolk Downs Racetrack in E Boston features horse racing, while the Wonderland Dog Track in Revere features greyhound racing. St. Patrick's Day-Evacuation Day Parades are held on Mar. 17 in S Boston.

ACCOMMODATIONS. There are approx. 20 hotels in Boston, more luxury-class hotels than any other large city. Hotels include the Sheraton, Boston Park Plaza, Copley Plaza, Colonnade, Bradford, Parker House, Logan Airport Hilton, Copely Square, Ritz-Carlton, Eliot, Fenway Motor, Howard Johnson and the Holiday and Ramada inns.

FACILITIES. The Boston Met. Park System was created in the 1890s by Charles Eliot, who promoted the concept of preserving natural areas in "reservations". There are more than 30 parks in the city encompassing more than 4,500 acres, as well as nine public beaches with 17 mi. of shoreline. The largest park, Franklin, contains a zoo, a children's zoo and a rose garden. Other parks are the 265-acre Arnold Arboretum in Jamaica Plain, containing 6,000 labeled trees and shrubs; the 48-acre Boston Common (the oldest park in the US, dating from 1634); the Public Garden, featuring swan boat rides; the Back Bay Fens; the Charles Bank Park-Esplanade on the Charles River Basin, with a lagoon, boat haven and Hatch Memorial Shell, used for performing arts; Stony Brook Reservation; Neponset Reservation and Columbus, Savin Hill, Ronan and Dorchester parks. Swimming at seven pools, tennis at 15 courts, golf at two courses, skating at 14 rinks, jogging and bicycling trails, fresh and salt water springs and sailing and boating are also available to the public. Boston Harbor Island State Park provides picnic areas, nature trails, beaches, docks and camping facilities. The 25-mi. Charles River bicycling, jogging path, named in honor of the later Dr. Paul Dudley White, flanks both sides of the Charles River from Watertown Sq. to the Charles River Dam.

CULTURAL ACTIVITIES. The Boston Symphony Orchestra, directed by Seiji Ozawa, and the Boston Pops Orchestra, performing popular and classical music, founded in 1885 and directed by the late Arthur Fiedler from 1930 until his death in 1979, play at Symphony Hall in Boston. Other musical groups are the Handel and Haydn Society (the oldest choral group in the US, founded in 1815), Boston Philharmonic Orchestra, the Boston Opera Co., the N.E. Regional Opera, the Civic Symphony of Boston, Associated Artist Opera, Chorus Pro Musica, the Camerata Players, who perform Renaissance and Baroque music with instruments from the Museum of Fine Arts collection, the Natl. Center of Afro-American Artists (NCAAA) Music Program and the N.E. Conservatory of Music. Free chamber music concerts and recitals are performed at the Isabella Stewart Gardner Museum. Dance groups include the Boston Ballet Co. which performs chiefly at the Music Hall and the NCAAA Dance Program consisting of three performing companies—the Dance, Children's Dance and Primitive Dance companies. The NCAAA Drama Program consists of the Natl. Center and the Elma Lewis Children's Theater companies. The NCAAA, under the direction of Elma Lewis, was named the "National Symbol of the Arts Made Meaningful in Current History" by the American Revolutionary Bicentennial Administration in Washington, DC. Other theatrical groups are the Boston Repertory Theater, Charles Playhouse and Cabaret, Pocket Mime Theatre, Stage 1-Next Move Theatre and Theatre Co. of Boston, specializing in abstract and theater of the absurd. The Boston Center for the Arts, consisting of five theaters, three restaurants and an art gallery, provides facilities for a number of cultural organizations, including the Theatre Workshop Boston-OM Theatre, an experimental group. The Colonial, Wilbur and Shubert theaters feature

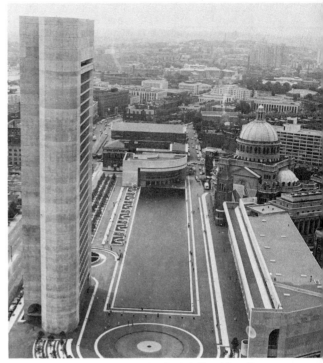

Christian Science Center Complex, Boston, Massachusetts

Broadway and pre-Broadway performances. There are 100 public and private art galleries in Boston, including the Museum of Fine Arts, the largest in Boston, exhibiting Asian, Egyptian, Classical, European and American painting and sculpture. The Isabella Stewart Gardner Museum features Renaissance paintings and sculpture displayed in a mansion, including Titian's "The Rape of Europa", one of the 36 surviving Vermeers in the world. Other museums and galleries include the Institute of Contemporary Art, the Museum of Afro-American History, the Museum of Science and Charles Hayden Planetarium, the Children's Museum, the Boston Tea Party Ship and Museum and the USS *Constitution* Museum.

LANDMARKS AND SIGHTSEEING SPOTS. The 1.5-mi. "Freedom Trail" walking tour of Boston from downtown to the N End, part of the Boston Natl. Historic Park, includes 16 historic sites. The Central Burying Ground on the NW side of Boston Common contains the graves of composer William Billings and artist Gilbert Stuart, among others. The gold-domed State House designed by Charles Bulch in 1798, houses historic colonial documents in its Archives. Declaration of Independence signers Samuel Adams, Robert Treat Paine and John Hancock are buried in the Granary Burying Ground, as are Paul Revere, the parents of Benjamin Franklin, victims of the Boston Massacre and Peter Faneuil. Park Street Church (1809) was the site of William Lloyd Garrison's first anti-slavery speech in 1829, while King's Chapel (1754) contains gifts of silver and vestments from the British rule of Queen Anne and George III. After the Revolution, the chapel became the first Unitarian church in the US. America's first public school, the Boston Latin School, was built in 1635. The Old Corner Bookstore (1712) was a meeting place for Hawthorne, Holmes, Emerson and other literary greats. Colonists discussed the tea tax and initiated the Boston Tea Party at the Old S Meeting House (1729). Called the "Cradle of Liberty" by John Adams, Faneuil Hall, built by Peter Faneuil in 1742, served as a meeting and market place. Now restored, the 19th century Faneuil Hall Marketplace, a shopping, eating and entertainment complex, is a major attraction. The oldest standing structure in downtown Boston is Paul Revere's House, built in 1670 and bought by Revere in 1775. The Old N Church (1723), from which Revere flashed his "one if by land, two if by sea" signal of British invasion, is the oldest standing church in the city. The 221' high Bunker Hill

Monument marks the site of the famous 1775 battle of the Revolutionary War. The USS *Constitution* ("Old Ironsides") is the oldest commissioned warship in the US, berthed at the Charlestown Navy Yard in the Inner Harbor. The ship, which never lost a battle, was launched in Boston in 1797 and restored in the 1970s. Dating from the 18th century, Long Wharf, next to Waterfront Park, is adjacent to the N.E. Aquarium, which contains 450 species of fish. The Boston Harbor Island Park includes Ft. Warren on George's Island, which was used as a prison during the Civil War, and Ft. Independence on Castle Island. Other attractions include the Dorchester Heights Natl. Historic Monument, the Skywalk at the 52-story Prudential Tower and the Observation Deck at the 60-story John Hancock Tower.

BRIDGEPORT
CONNECTICUT

CITY LOCATION-SIZE-EXTENT. Bridgeport, seat of Fairfield Co., is located in SW CT at the mouth of the Pequonnock River on LI Sound. It encompasses 17.5 sq. mi. 60 mi. SW of Hartford, the capital of CT, and 60 mi. NE of NYC at 41°10' N lat. and 73°08' W long. The greater Bridgeport met. area, situated between New Haven to the NE and Stamford to the SW, consists of the towns of Stratford, Trumbull, Fairfield, Monroe, Easton, Shelton and Milford.

TOPOGRAPHY. The terrain of Bridgeport, flat along LI Sound, and in the SE section, marshy, rises in gently rolling hills to the N and NW as it approaches the foothills of the Berkshire Hills, 30 mi. N, and the Catskill Mts., 70 mi. NW, of the city. The mean elev. is 20'.

CLIMATE. The continental climate of Bridgeport, modified by sea breezes from LI Sound, is characterized by warm to moderately hot summers and cool, snowy winters. Temps. range from a Jan. mean of 28.4°F to a July mean of 73.3°F, while the mean annual temp. is 51.1°F. The avg. annual rainfall of 43.94" is evenly distributed throughout the year, while most of the avg. annual snowfall of 27.7" accumulates during Dec. and Jan. The RH ranges from 52% to 84%. Bridgeport is in the ESTZ and observes DST.

FLORA AND FAUNA. Animals native to Bridgeport include the raccoon and opossum, while common birds are the gull, tern, flycatcher, cardinal and willet. Several types of salamanders, turtles, frogs and snakes, as well as the venomous copperhead and timber rattlesnake, are found in the area. Common trees are the birch, hemlock, white ash and tupelo. Smaller plants include the rhododendron, goldenrod, aster and Queen Anne's lace.

POPULATION. According to the US census, the pop. of Bridgeport in 1970 was 154,547. Although it was estimated in 1978 that it had decreased to 148,000, the city is still the most populous in the state.

ETHNIC GROUPS. In 1979, the ethnic distribution of Bridgeport was approx. 67% Caucasian, 20% Black and 13% Hispanic. According to the US Census Bureau, the pop. of Bridgeport is more highly diversified in terms of ethnic derivation than any other city in N.E.

TRANSPORTATION. Interstate Hwy. 90 (the CT Tnpk.) and state rtes. 8, 15 (the Merritt Pkwy.) and 25 provide major motor access to Bridgeport. *Railroads* serving the city include ConRail and AMTRAK. The municipal airport, I.A. Sikorsky Memorial, located 5 mi. NE in Stratford, is served by two commuter *airlines*, Pilgrim and Altair. Ferry service is provided by Port Jefferson Steamboat Co., while hovercraft commuter service is available between Bridgeport and LI. A 36' channel enables the city's main harbor, a deepwater port with 35 wharves and piers, to handle 20% of CT's seaborne shipping. *Bus lines* serving the city include Greyhound, Trailways and the local Bridgeport Auto Transit, Park City, Cross Country, Valley, Chestnut Hill and Stratford.

COMMUNICATIONS. Communications, broadcasting and print media serving Bridgeport are: *AM radio stations* WICC 600 (Indep., MOR); WNAB 1450 (ABC/I, MBS, APR, MOR, Talk) and WDJZ 1530 (ABC/E, Clas.); *FM radio stations* WPKN 89.9 (ABC/E, Var.) and WEZN 99.9 (Indep., Btfl. Mus.); *television station* WEDW Ch. 49 (PBS); the city also receives broadcasting from TV stations in NYC, New Haven and Hartford; *press*: two major dailies are published in the city, the *Post*, issued evenings, and the *Telegram*, issued mornings; other publications include the *Scribe*, a weekly col. newspaper, the monthly *Jewish Digest* and the *Fairfield Co. News*.

HISTORY. Native Americans of the Pequonnock tribe inhabited the site of present-day Bridgeport, the area at the mouth of the Pequonnock River. In 1639, English colonists from the older settlements of Fairfield and Stratford purchased the bulk of the land comprising the present city from the Pequonnocks. Originally called Newfield, it was later, until 1800, called Stratfield, when the borough of Bridgeport was incorporated and named for the first drawbridge erected over the Pequonnock River. In 1821, it was incorporated as a town and in 1836, as a city. During the first 200 years of Bridgeport's existence, it had grown from a small village into a thriving seaport, with whaling the major industry. The RR came to the city in 1840, and, later, electric trolleys. In the mid-1800s, the pop. of the city was about 3,000. After the Civil War, commercial activity shifted from the wharves to water-powered mills, which produced textiles, guns, tools, machinery and metals, as well as the first gramophones and sewing machines produced in the US. The city flourished as an industrial center, since it was close to foreign

Downtown Bridgeport, Connecticut

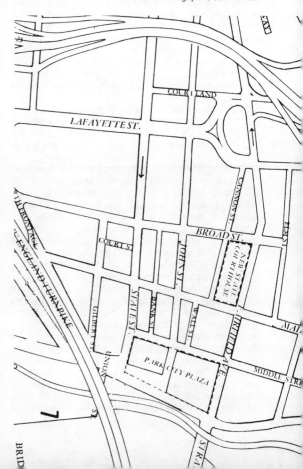

shipping routes, inland waterways and RRs. By 1920, Bridgeport had grown so large that suburbs developed around it, resulting in the met. region known as the "Greater Bridgeport Area". From the mid-19th century, with the first wave of Irish immigrants that arrived in 1845, until 1960, with the recent arrivals of Spanish-speaking Americans, the growth of Bridgeport has been largely attributable to immigration and industry.

GOVERNMENT. Bridgeport has a mayor-council form of govt. The council, called the Board of Aldermen, consists of 20 members. Two are elected from each of the city's 10 districts, while the mayor is elected at large, and votes only to break a tie. All serve two-year terms.

ECONOMY AND INDUSTRY. Bridgeport, the "Industrial Capital of CT" has the highest concentration of industrial employment in the state, which has in gen. experienced a long-term decline. Some 500 industrial firms located in the city produce electrical products, metal products, steel, firearms and ammunition, machine tools, helicopters, tank engines, valves, petroleum products, business machines and clothing. Since 1977, 63 manufacturing firms have begun operating in the city. Retail and wholesale trade rank second to manufacturing. In June, 1979, the labor force totaled approx. 188,900, while the rate of unemployment was 6.0%. Fairfield Co. is the highest per capita income area in the US.

BANKING. There are nine commercial banks and four savings and loan assns., as well as several other financial institutions, located in Bridgeport, the banking center of S CT. In 1978, the seven banks headquartered in the city (including three of the six largest in the state) had total deposits of $4,122,231,000 and resources of $4,671,297,000. Banks serving the city include CT Natl., City Savings, State Natl. of CT, Peoples Savings, Mechanics and Farmers Savings, City Trust, Union Trust and Lafayette, Valley and CT Bank & Trust companies.

HOSPITALS. There are four major hosps. in Bridgeport, Bridgeport, Milford, Park City and St. Vincent's. Dinan Memorial Center is a special chronic disease and convalescent hosp.

EDUCATION. The privately-supported, coeducational U of Bridgeport, founded as a jr. col. in 1927, enrolled approx. 7,300 at the associate, bachelor and master degree levels in 1978. Sacred Heart U, an independent, non-sectarian institution established in 1963, enrolled close to 2,900 in associate, bachelor and master degree programs in 1978. The Bridgeport Engineering Institute, located on the campus of Sacred Heart U, enrolled more than 400 in 1978, while Housatonic Comm. Col., a public, coeducational institution founded in 1967, enrolled approx. 2,600 the same year. Fairfield U, a Jesuit institution founded in 1945, enrolled close to 3,000 in 1978. These five institutions are members of the Higher Education Center for Urban Studies, a consortium which formulates plans for the comm. The public school system consists of 34 elementary, four middle and three high schools, in which close to 25,000 are enrolled. The Bridgeport Public Lib., considered to be one of the best public libs. in the state, maintains four branches. Fairfield Co. Law Lib. is also available, as are those at the local colleges and universities.

ENTERTAINMENT. The Scenario presents dinner theater in Bridgeport, while the Barnum Tent Theatre, the largest round theater in CT, is the site of the week-long P.T. Barnum Festival held each year in July, the second largest parade-float festival in the US. Concerts in the Park is a summer series of musical presentations. The U of Bridgeport Purple Kings and the Housatonic Comm. Col. Hawks participate in sports at the collegiate level.

ACCOMMODATIONS. Hotels and motels in Bridgeport include the Bridgeport Motor and Holiday inns, as well as the Arcade Hotel.

FACILITIES. There are 1,400 acres of recreational land in Bridgeport, known as "Park City", including 25 parks, 37 playgrounds and a marina. The 225-acre Beardsley Park, the largest in the city, is located along the Pequonnock River. Among its facilities are tennis courts, ballfields and a zoo, the largest in CT. Swimming and fishing are also available. Two 18-hole golf courses are located at the public Fairchild-Wheeler Golf Course, while swimming, boating, fishing and waterskiing are available in LI Sound. Two-mi. long Seaside Park is the most extensive salt water beach in the state. The newest city park is Waterfront, located downtown.

CULTURAL ACTIVITIES. The Greater Bridgeport Symphony, Greater Bridgeport Ballet Co., Downtown Cabaret Theater, Polka Dot Players and Youth Bridge, a dance troupe, are among the performing arts organizations in Bridgeport. The P.T. Barnum Museum of Science and History, given by Barnum to the Historical and Scientific societies of Bridgeport in 1893, features circus props., a model circus of 50,000 hand-carved pieces, a 100-year-old miniature Swiss village with 20,000 moving parts and the clothes of the 28" Tom Thumb, who was born in the city. The Museum of Art, Science and Industry (containing a planetarium) and Wheeler Mansion Museum are also located in the city. The renowned American Shakespeare Festival Theatre is located in nearby Stratford.

LANDMARKS AND SIGHTSEEING SPOTS. Bridgeport's Seaside Park contains three monuments: a soldiers and sailors monument, a statue of Elias Howe, the inventor of the sewing machine which the city began to produce, and one of showman P.T. Barnum, who lived in the city. McLevy Hall is another city landmark. University Sq., a shopping, entertainment and dining complex in the S end of the city that has been restored in 19th-century style, contains the largest factory outlet in the world.

Aerial view of central Bridgeport, Connecticut

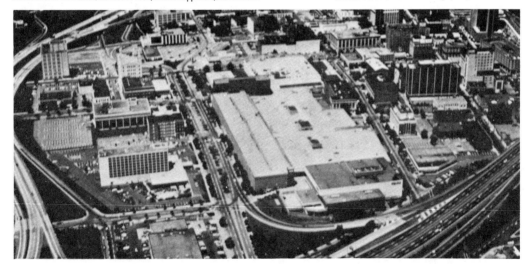

BUFFALO
NEW YORK

CITY LOCATION-SIZE-EXTENT. Buffalo, the seat of Erie Co., is located in NW NY on the shores of Lake Erie at the mouth of the Niagara River. The city encompasses 41.3 sq. mi. at 42°56' N lat. and 78°44' W long. Its greater met. area consisting of all of Erie Co.and most of Niagara Co., is bordered on the S by Cattaraugus Co. and on the E by WY and Genesee counties. Buffalo, located across the Niagara River from Ontario, Canada, is SE of Niagara Falls.

TOPOGRAPHY. The terrain of Buffalo, low and level in the W part of the city by Lake Erie and the Niagara River, consists of gently rolling hills in the S and E sections of the city. Within 15 mi. of the city to the S and E are much higher hills. The mean elev. is 600'.

CLIMATE. The climate of Buffalo is continental. The weather is changeable, influenced by Lake Erie and the interplay of warm and cold air masses. The 47.3°F avg. annual temp. ranges from monthly means of 24.9°F during January to 70.3°F during July. The 90'' avg. annual snowfall occurs from Nov. to Mar. and the avg. annual rainfall is 35.5''. The RH ranges 55% to 83%. Buffalo is located in the ESTZ and observes DST.

FLORA AND FAUNA. Animals native to Buffalo include the muskrat, opossum and raccon. Common birds include the gull, warbler, thrush, heron, cormorant and bittern. Frogs, salamanders, turtles and snakes, as well as the venomous timber rattlesnake and massasauga (a pygmy rattler), are found here. Typical trees include the red oak, maple, birch, hemlock and spruce. Smaller plants include the dogwood, elder, violet and bunchberry.

POPULATION. According to the US census, the pop. of Buffalo in 1970 was 462,768. In 1978, it was estimated that it had decreased to 368,000.

ETHNIC GROUPS. In 1978, the ethnic distribution of Buffalo was approx. 78.8% Caucasian, 20.4% Black and 0.8% Hispanic.

Buffalo, New York

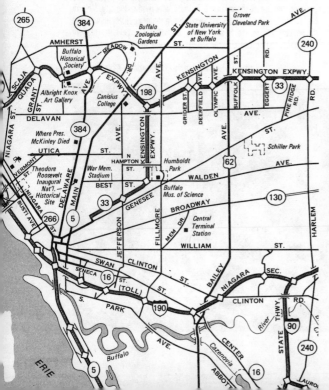

TRANSPORTATION. Interstate hwys. 90 and 190, US hwys. 62 and state hwys 5, 33, 130, 198, 240, 264, 265 and 384 provide major access to Buffalo. The 559-mi. Gov. Thomas Dewey Thruway, the longest toll superhighway in the world, also serves the city. The 4,400'-long Peace Bridge spanning the Niagara River, links the city with Ontario, Canada. The Port of Buffalo, the largest inland port in NY, handles about 15 million short tons (13.6 million metric tons) of cargo annually. *Railroads* serving the city include the Chessie System, ConRail, Erie Lackawanna, Southern and MO Pacific. *Airlines* serving Buffalo Intl. Airport include AA, US Air, EA and UA. *Bus lines* include Greyhound, Trailways and the local (NFT) Niagara Frontier Transit.

COMMUNICATIONS. Communications, broadcasting and print media serving Buffalo are: *AM radio stations* WGR 550 (ABC/E, MOR); WBEN 930 (CBS, MOR); WEBR 970 (NPR, All News); WWOL 1120 (NBC, C&W); WYSL 1400 (ABC/C, Contemp.) and WKBW 1520 (Indep., Top 40); *FM radio stations* WBFO 88.7 (NPR, Var.); WBUF 92.9 (ABC/FM, AOR); WNED 94.5 (NPR, Clas.); WBNY 96.1 (Indep., Btfl., Mus.); WGRQ 96.9 (ABC/E, Progsv.); WDCX 99.5 (Indep., Relig.); WBEN 102.5 (Indep., Rock); WPHD 103.3 (Indep., Contemp.); WWOL 104.1 (ABC/I, C&W) and WADV 106.5 (MOR, Personality); *television stations* WGR Ch. 2 (NBC); WIVB Ch. 4 (CBS); WKBW Ch. 7 (ABC) and WNED Ch. 17 (PBS); *press:* two major dailies serve the city, the *Courier-Express*, issued mornings, and the *Evening News*, printed weekday evenings and weekend mornings; other publications include the *Volksfreund, Record, S Buffalo Review, Law Journal, Christian Inquirer Criterion, The Griffin, Jewish Review, W NY Magazine* and *W NY Motorist*.

HISTORY. The area of present-day Buffalo was the site of a thriving Indian culture over 4,000 years ago, and, more recently, was inhabited by Iroquois Indians before the arrival of white men. The first white settlers were French fur trappers, who established prosperous fur trading posts, following the path chartered by the French explorer, LaSalle, in 1628. Dutch businessmen comprised the next influx of settlers; under the auspices of the Holland Land Co., they established a settlement at the site of present-day Buffalo in 1803, at the bend of an important Indian trail. By 1810, about 1,500 people lived there. Although called New Amsterdam, the community's official name became Buffalo in 1816, and was possibly derived from the Indian mispronunciation of the French Father Hennepin's reaction of "Beau Fleuve" (beautiful river) upon first sight of the Niagara River. During the War of 1812, Buffalo was seized and burned by the British and Indians, but was rebuilt within two years. It was incorporated as a village in 1816 and became the seat of Erie Co. in 1821. Buffalo grew rapidly after the opening of the Erie Canal in 1825, which provided an important link in an all-water route between NYC and the Great Lakes, thus lowering the cost of transporting goods. Buffalo's success as a transportation center was also due to the establishment of an express service to and from the W, Wells Fargo & Co. (later American Express). The city became a major transfer point for people moving from the E to the W, as well as the final stop for slaves fleeing N toward freedom on the "underground RR". In 1832, when it was incorporated as a city, the pop. of Buffalo was 10,000. In 1840, the world's first grain elevator was built in Buffalo, and the first steam-operated grain elevator, built in Buffalo in 1843, made the city the leading grain-handling port of the U.S. By 1850, it ranked as the nation's number-one milling hub. During this time, thousands of European immigrants settled in the city and, by 1860, the pop. had reached more than 81,100. After large-scale production of electric power began at Niagara Falls in 1896, industry grew rapidly, attracting steel plants and other industries that used large amounts of electricity. By 1900, the pop. had reached approx. 352,400. The 1901 Pan American Exposition held in Buffalo brought intl. recognition as well as natl. tragedy to the city. In Sept., Pres. William McKinley was shot there and died in the city eight days later. Theodore Roosevelt was then sworn into office in Buffalo. Two other presidents lived and held office in Buffalo, Millard Fillmore, who died there in 1874, and Grover Cleveland, who served as mayor of the city in 1881. During WW I and II, Buffalo's industries contributed great amounts of food, weapons, and supplies to the Allies. The opening of the St. Lawrence Seaway, in 1959, enabled ocean-going ships to reach Buffalo and made the city a world port. Today, the city is a mix of light and heavy industry. At present, Buffalo is engaged in extensive urban-renewal programs to reverse its pop. decline—from a record high of more than 580,100 at the 1950 census it decreased to approx. 532,800 in 1960 and to approx. 462,800 in 1970—chiefly because of a trend toward suburban living.

GOVERNMENT. Buffalo has a mayor-council form of govt. consisting of 15 council members and a mayor. Six council members are elected at large to four-year terms, while nine are elected by district to two-year terms. The mayor, who is not a member of the council and has no vote, is elected at large to a four-year term.

ECONOMY AND INDUSTRY. There are close to 2,000 manufacturing plants employing approx. 200,000 in Buffalo. Major manufacturers include iron and steel products and transportation equipment. Other important industries include chemicals, fabricated metal products, paper products, food and kindred products, and electronics. Approx. three billion pounds of flour are produced annually. In June, 1979, the greater met. area labor force totaled 586,500, while the rate of unemployment was 5.7%.

BANKING. There are seven commercial banks and eight savings and loan assns. in Buffalo. In 1978, total deposits for the seven banks headquartered in the city were $19,805,601,000, while total assets were $24,101,744,000. Banks serving the city include Bank of NY, Buffalo Savings, Liberty Natl., Erie Co. Savings, Manufacturers and Traders Trust, Marine Midland, W NY Savings and Chase Manhattan.

HOSPITALS. There are 16 gen., acute-care and specialized hosps. in Buffalo, including Mercy, Buffalo Gen., Lafayette Gen., Millard Fillmore, Sheehan Memorial, St Francis, Sisters of Charity, Deaconess, Edward J. McGee Memorial, Buffalo Psychiatric Center, Roswell Park Memorial Institute, an internationally-known cancer research and treatment center, Children's Hosp., which has the largest Pediatric Dental center in the US, and one V.A. hosp., where the pacemaker was invented.

City Hall, Buffalo, New York

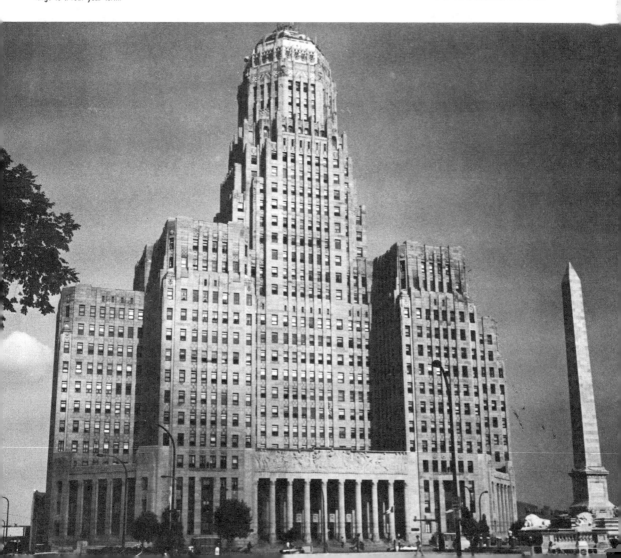

EDUCATION. The State U of NY at Buffalo (SUNYB), originally founded in 1846 as the private U of Buffalo by Millard Fillmore, became part of SUNY in 1960. It is the largest single unit and most comprehensive grad. center in the SUNY system, and includes schools of medicine, dentistry, law and architecture. In 1978, approx. 11,260 enrolled. Other institutions include Medaille, D'Youville, Canisius, Villa Marie, Daemen and Trocaire colleges. There are approx. 85 elementary and 15 high schools in the city, enrolling approx. 15,000. There are about 70 private and parochial schools as well. There are 43 libs. in the city, including the Buffalo and Erie Co. Public Lib., with several branches, and Acres American Engineering Lib.

ENTERTAINMENT. Events include the Easter flower display and autumn mum show held at the Buffalo Botanical Gardens, Edwardian greenhouses featuring exotic plants and fruits. The Canisius Col. Golden Griffins participate in sports at the collegiate level, while four pro sports teams provide spectator entertainment. The Buffalo Bills of the NFL-AFC play football at Rich Stadium. The Buffalo Sabres of the NHL and the Jr. Sabres of the NYPMHL play hockey, and the Buffalo Stallions of the NASL play soccer at the War Memorial Auditorium. The Buffalo Bisons, an AA pro baseball team in the EL, play at Memorial Stadium.

ACCOMMODATIONS. There are many hotels and motels in met. Buffalo, including the Statler and Airways hotels, Howard Johnson's, TraveLodge, Park Plaza, Best Western and Executive Motor inns.

Buffalo Psychiatric Center, Buffalo, New York

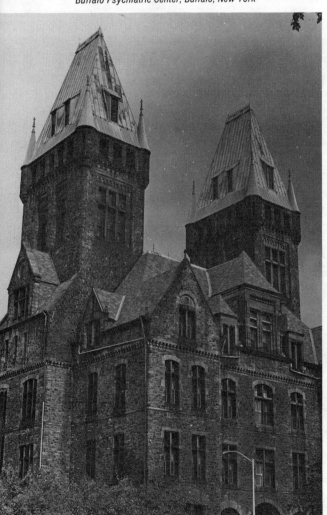

FACILITIES. The Buffalo Park System, designed by Frederick Law Olmsted, encompasses 1,500 acres and includes 75 parks and playgrounds. The 365-acre Delaware Park, the largest, contains the Buffalo Zoological Gardens, a lake accommodating ice skating, boating and facilities for tennis, golf and bicycling. The Buffalo Zoo, the second largest zoo in the US, contains about 850 animals of 350 species and features a children's zoo. A conservatory at South Park features exhibits of rare species of plants, while the 264-acre Tifft Farm Nature Preserve features plants, animals and nature trails.

CULTURAL ACTIVITIES. Kleinhans Music Hall, the home of the Buffalo Philharmonic Orchestra, is the site of concerts, dance and music recitals. The refurbished Sheas Buffalo Theatre, built in 1926, presents a wide variety of entertainment, while the Studio Arena (the foremost legitimate theater in NY outside Manhattan) presents several plays and musicals from Oct. through May. The Albright-Knox Gallery contains works of art completed nearly 5,000 years ago, and a large collection of modern art, including the works of such modernists as Picasso, Mondrian and Rothko. The Buffalo and Erie Co. Historical Museum, which is the only surviving structure of the 1901 Pan American Exposition, is a columned Greek-revival building which features details of the Indian way of life in the region, as well as a replica of an old waterfront street. One of the first Pierce-Arrow automobiles manufactured is enshrined here—Pierce was a Buffalo resident. The Historical Society of the Tonawandas, originally a brick RR station built in 1870, is now a museum and research center. The Louis Siller Museum is in the Prudential Building (one of the first skyscrapers in the US), built in 1896, and designed by Sullivan. The Charles Burchfield Art Center, named after Buffalo's most famous artist, is located on the campus of Buffalo State Col. Buffalo's Museum of Science, established in 1861, contains a dinosaur reconstructed from ancient bones, as well as exhibits of recent advances relating to outer space.

LANDMARKS AND SIGHTSEEING SPOTS. The Forest Lawn Cematary in Buffalo, established about 1850, contains tombs and monuments of such people as Millard Fillmore and Red Jacket, chief of the Seneca native American tribe. Buildings of interest include the Old Post Office, a massive French-Gothic building dedicated in 1901; City Hall/ Observation Tower; the Martin and Boston House (listed on the Natl. Register of Historic Places), which are examples of Frank Lloyd Wright's "prairie architecture"; the Old Co. Hall, built in 1872, and recently restored with 100-year-old clock-works in the clock tower; the St. Louis Church, built in 1876, with a congregation dating to 1829; Butler Hall, an historic mansion designed and built shortly before the turn of the century by Stanford White; the Colt House, the oldest building in Buffalo (1815); the Roosevelt Inaugural Natl. Historic Site, located in the Ansley Wilcox Mansion, which is restored with period furniture in some rooms, including the library where Roosevelt was inaugruated upon McKinley's death and the Buffalo Psychiatric Center, designed by H. H. Richardson and listed in the Natl. Register of Historic Places. Along DL Avenue, where many of the city's most prominent citizens made their homes during the 19th century, many of the houses are still standing, among them the Pratt House, Butler Hall, the Katherine Pratt Horton House and the Dorsheimer House. The Trinity Episcopal Church, built in 1886, and noted for its stained glass windows designed by Tiffany and LaFarge, is also located on DL Avenue. The Peace Bridge, gateway to Canada, commemorates 100 yrs. of peace between the US and Canada. Monuments of interest include the Soldiers and Sailors Monument (a Civil War Memorial located on Lafayette Sq.) and in Niagara Sq., an obelisk erected in memory of Pres. McKinley. At another site, a bronze tablet set in a rock marks the spot where McKinley was shot. Red Jacket monument honors the famous Seneca Indian Chief who lived in the Buffalo area.

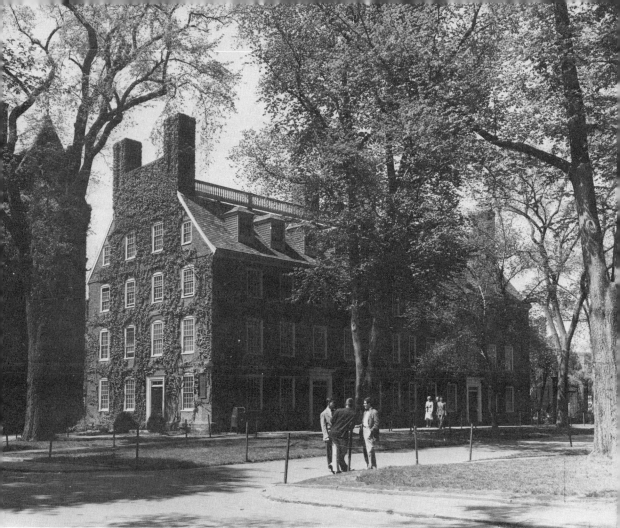

Harvard University in Cambridge, Massachusetts

CAMBRIDGE
MASSACHUSETTS

CITY LOCATION-SIZE-EXTENT. Cambridge, the seat of Middlesex Co., lies on the NW bank of the Charles River in E MA at 42°21'9" N lat. and 21°06'3" W long. The city encompasses 6.25 sq. mi. It is bordered by Somerville and Arlington on the N and Watertown and Belmont on the SW, while the Charles River is a natural four-mi. long boundary between Cambridge and Boston to the E. The city is in the greater Boston met. area.

TOPOGRAPHY. Cambridge is situated on low, hilly terrain in the Atlantic Coastal Plain region. There are numerous brooks and ponds in the area, including Fresh Pond. The mean elev. is 20'.

CLIMATE. The Atlantic Ocean moderates Cambridge's continental, variable climate. Monthly mean temps. range from 29°F in Jan. to 73°F in July, with an annual avg. of 50.4°F. The avg. annual rainfall of 41.5" is well distributed throughout the year, while more than 50% of the annual 43" of snowfall occurs in Jan. and Feb. The RH ranges from 53% to 82% and heavy fog occurs on an avg. of 25 days per year. The avg. growing season is 165 days. Cambridge is located in the ESTZ and observes DST.

FLORA AND FAUNA. Animals native to Cambridge include the opossum and raccoon. Common birds include the blue jay, cardinal, robin, sparrow and starling. Bullfrogs, leopard frogs, spring peepers, dusky salamanders, turtles, red-spotted newts and snakes, including the venomous timber rattlesnake and copperhead, are also found here. Common trees include the red oak, sycamore and American elm. Smaller plants include chicory, pondweed, daisy, lily of the valley and wood sorrel.

POPULATION. According to the US census, the pop. of Cambridge in 1970 was 100,361. In 1978, it was estimated that it had increased to 101,300.

ETHNIC GROUPS. In 1978, the ethnic distribution of Cambridge was approx. 91.4% Caucasian, 6.8% Black and 1.9% Hispanic (a percentage of the Hispanic total is also included in the Caucasian total).

TRANSPORTATION. Interstate hwys. 93 and 95 and state hwys. 2 and 16 provide major motor access to Cambridge. *Railroads* include the Boston & Maine and Fitchburg. All major natl. and intl. *airlines* serve nearby Logan Intl. Airport in E Boston. The MA Bay Transportation Authority (MBTA) provides local commuter rail and bus service, while Greyhound and Trailways *bus lines* also serve the area.

COMMUNICATIONS. Communications, broadcasting and print media originating from Cambridge are: *AM radio station* WCAS 740 (Indep., Progsv., Folk/Rock); *FM radio stations* WTBS 88.1 (Indep., Var.); WHRB 95.3 (Indep., Var.) and WJIB 96.9 (Indep., Btfl. Mus.); no *television stations* broadcast from Cambridge, which is served by the media of neighboring Boston; *press:* two weekly newspapers are published in the city, the *Chronicle-Sun*, issued Thurs., and the *Real Paper*, issued Sun. Other publications published in the city include the daily *Harvard Crimson*, *Radcliffe Quarterly*, *Harvard Educational Review*, *Harvard Independent*, *Harvard Magazine*, *Technology Review* and *Sky and Telescope*.

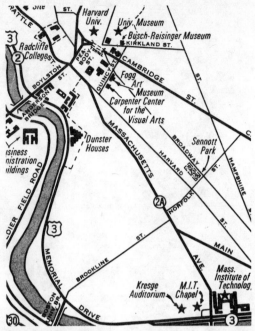

Cambridge, Massachusetts

HISTORY. Cambridge was established as a fortified town in 1630 by the founders of the MA Bay Colony, a group of Puritans who settled further W along the Charles River from Boston. Originally called "Newtowne", the village was located on a small defensible hill between the river and the path from Charlestown and Watertown. The first col. in the US, Harvard, was established in the comm. in 1636. The city's present name was adopted in 1638 in honor of Cambridge U in England. A meetinghouse and marketplace were established in the center of the comm., surrounded by houses and common land for grazing animals, and, further out, farms and pastures. The first book printed in the colonies, *The Bay Psalm Book*, was published in Cambridge in 1640. In July, 1795, following the outbreak of the Revolutionary War, Gen. George Washington took command of the Continental Army, which had gathered on the Cambridge Common, and headquartered in the town through the siege of Boston, until Mar., 1776. A convention was held in the city in 1779 to draft the MA constitution. For more than 150 years, from its founding until the opening of the W Boston (now Longfellow) Bridge in 1793, Cambridge remained a quiet Harvard-oriented semi-rural settlement. The new bridge, however, created a major transportation link between Boston and Cambridge as well as all the settlements to the W, and contributed to the development of the city as a commercial center. Cambridge was incorporated as a city in 1846. During the mid-1800s, several famous writers, including Oliver Wendell Holmes and Henry Wadsworth Longfellow, lived in the city. Much of the city's area was created by land-fill operations of the Charles River tidal marshes. The city grew steadily throughout the mid-19th and 20th centuries as an industrial, residential and academic center, and became known as "University City".

GOVERNMENT. Cambridge has a council-mgr. form of govt. consisting of nine council members including the mayor as a voting member. The councillors, elected every two years, select one of the council members to serve a two-year term as mayor.

ECONOMY AND INDUSTRY. The major industries in Cambridge include the production of electronic equipment, rubber products, technical products and services, electrical hardware, scientific instruments and food products. The economy of Cambridge, part of the greater Boston met. area, is reflected in the economic data of that city.

BANKING. There are nine savings and loan assns. and one commercial bank in Cambridge. In 1978, total deposits for the seven banks headquartered in the city were $1,247,851,000, while assets totaled $1,449,420,000. Banks include Cambridge Savings, Baybank Harvard Trust, Cambridgeport Savings, Shawmut, E Cambridge Savings, Cambridge Trust and Charles Bank Trust.

HOSPITALS. There are five gen. hosps. in Cambridge, Cambridge, Otis, Mt. Auburn, Sancta Maria and Youville Rehabilitation and Chronic Disease. The renowned medical facilities of nearby Boston are accessible to residents of Cambridge.

EDUCATION. Harvard U, established as Harvard Col. in 1636, is a private, nonsectarian coed institution, consisting of the undergrad. Harvard (men's) and Radcliffe (women's, founded in 1878) colleges. In 1978, Harvard U enrolled more than 22,000 at the bachelor, master and doctorate degree levels. MA Institute of Technology (MIT), chartered in 1861 and established in Cambridge in 1916, is a private, highly ranked institution which enrolled more than 8,700 in 1978. Other institutions include Lesley Col., the Episcopal Divinity School, Arthur D. Little Management Education Institute, Goddard-Cambridge Grad. Program, Antioch Grad. Center/Institute of Open Education and Weston Col. of Theology. Tufts U, founded in 1852, is located NW of the city in nearby Medford. It enrolled nearly 7,000 in 1978. There are more than 20 public and private schools in the city, enrolling more than 10,000 in 1978. Lib. facilities include the Cambridge Public Lib. System, including five branches, and the Middlesex Co. Law Lib. of Cambridge. Col. and university libs. available for research include Harvard's Harry Elkins Widener Memorial Lib., one of the largest in the world, containing a Gutenberg Bible, Shakespeare Folios and important historical and literary collections. Houghton Lib. houses a collection of rare preserved books. The Schlesinger Lib., housed in the Radcliffe Institute, contains major collections of the works of Harriet Beecher Stowe, Susan B. Anthony and Julia Ward Howe. MIT's Charles Hayden Memorial Lib. is also available to the public.

ENTERTAINMENT. The Harvard Crimson of the Ivy League, the MIT Beavers and the Tufts' Jumbos participate in sports at the collegiate level. Dinner theaters, professional sports, annual festivals and events are accessible to Cantabrigians in nearby Boston.

ACCOMMODATIONS. The eight hotels and motels in Cambridge include the Fenway Howard Johnson's, Harvard Motor House, Hotel Sonesta, Hyatt Regency, Sheraton Commander and the Holiday, Chalet Suisse and Homestead Motor inns.

FACILITIES. There are 45 public playgrounds in Cambridge offering handicrafts, band concerts, story telling and folk dancing programs, as well as tennis tournaments and track meets. Indoor swimming pools and a public beach as well as 10 (six lighted) flooded areas for ice skating are also available. The bank of the Charles River provides facilities for picnics and sunbathing, as well as boating and sailing. The 315-acre Fresh Pond Reservation contains a nine-hole municipal golf course and a 166-acre lake, while the Alewife Brook Reservation contains 115 acres of open space maintained as a natural area.

CULTURAL ACTIVITIES. There are several museums located on the campuses of Harvard U and MIT in Cambridge. Harvard's Busch-Reisinger Museum displays Germanic sculpture, paintings and decorative arts; the Carpenter Center for the Visual Arts (the only building in the US designed by Swiss architect Le Corbusier) houses studios and exhibits of visual communications and design; the Fogg Art Museum contains ancient and oriental art, as well as Romanesque, Italian and French sculpture, paintings, drawings and prints; the Peabody Anthropological Museum features one of the finest collections of Mayan artifacts in the US, as well as Iron Age exhibits from central Europe, and the U Museum houses the Geological and Mineralogical Museum, Ware Collection of Glass Flowers and Museum of Comparative Zoology. MIT's Hayden Gallery features exhibits of contemporary art, while the Frances Russell Hart Nautical Museum traces the development of marine engineering through engine and ship models. The Museum of Science is partially located in E Cambridge. There are several art galleries in the city. Performing arts groups include the Cambridge Ensemble, Caravan Theater, People's Theater, the Proposition and the Harvard-affiliated Hasty Pudding Theatricals. Harvard U and Brandeis U (located in Waltham, a suburb of Boston) sponsor the Loeb Drama Festival each year, as well as the Springold Theater series.

LANDMARKS AND SIGHTSEEING SPOTS. On the S side of historic Cambridge Common, first reserved for public use in 1631, is a bronze tablet and scion of the "Washington Elm" commemorating the site where Gen. George Washington took command of the Continental Army. The Longfellow House, a Natl. Historic Site on Brattle St. and part of the Longfellow Historic District, is a 1759 Georgian Colonial mansion which served as the headquarters for Washington, and from 1837 until his death in 1882, served as the home of Henry Wadsworth Longfellow while he was a professor at Harvard. His books, manuscripts, furniture and pictures are on display. Mt. Auburn Cemetery, established in 1831, contains the graves of Longfellow, James Russell Lowell, Oliver Wendell Holmes, Mary Baker Eddy and Edwin Booth. The 1811 "Village Smithy", about which Longfellow wrote, is now a restaurant. Other prominent landmarks include the Wadsworth House, Stoughton House and the 1761 Christ Church (located next to the Burying Ground), the oldest church building in Cambridge. Harvard Yard contains the 1815 U Hall, designed by Charles Bulfinch (architect of the Boston and US Capitol buildings) and Austin and Sever halls. The 1814 Old Superior Courthouse of Middlesex Co. is another of Bulfinch's works. The Putnam School, built in 1877, stands on the site of old Ft. Putnam.

CANTON
OHIO

CITY LOCATION-SIZE-EXTENT. Canton, the seat of Stark Co., encompasses 18.99 sq. mi. in E central OH, 24 mi. S of Akron, at 40°48' N lat. and 81°23' W long. Its greater met. area, which overlaps that of Akron, extends into portions of Wayne and Columbiana Counties.

TOPOGRAPHY. The terrain of Canton consists of deep valleys and high hills, between which the land is flat to rolling. There are several small lakes in the area. The highest points reach nearly 1,300', while the mean elev. is 1,065'.

CLIMATE. The climate of Canton is continental. It is influenced by Lake Erie, which modifies cold air masses from the N, delays the arrival of spring, effects humid, moderately warm summers and causes considerable morning fog during the fall. Monthly mean temps. range from 27°F during Jan, to 72°F during July, with an annual avg. of 50°F. The avg. annual rainfall of 36" is well-distributed throughout the year. Nearly 45% of the annual 48" of snowfall occurs during Dec. and Jan. The RH ranges from 50% to 85%. The avg. growing season is 170 days. Canton lies in the ESTZ and observes DST.

FLORA AND FAUNA. Animals native to Canton include the woodchuck, striped skunk, grey and E red fox squirrel, opossum, raccoon, E chipmunk and whitetail deer. Common birds are the ruffed grouse, mourning dove, cardinal, blue jay and crow. Frogs, salamanders, turtles, toads, lizards and snakes, including the venomous copperhead, E massasauga (a small rattlesnake) and timber rattlesnake, are found in the area. Common trees include the red oak, white pine, silver maple, elm, black cherry, American beech, dogwood and birch. Smaller plants include the pepperweed, honeysuckle and meadow rue.

POPULATION. According to the US census, the pop. of Canton in 1970 was 110,053. In 1978, it was estimated that it had decreased to 101,852.

ETHNIC GROUPS. In 1978, the ethnic distribution of Canton was approx. 87.1% Caucasian, 12.5% Black and 1.3% Hispanic (a percentage of the Hispanic total is also included in the Caucasian total).

TRANSPORTATION. Interstate Hwy. 77, US hwys. 30 and 62 and state hwys. 800, 43, 153 and 687 provide major motor access to Canton. *Railroads* serving the city are AMTRAK, Baltimore and OH, ConRail and Norfolk and W. *Airlines* serving Akron-Canton Airport are US Air, UA and Conair. *Bus lines* include Greyhound, Trailways and the local Canton Regional Transit Authority.

COMMUNICATIONS. Communications, broadcasting and print media originating from Canton are: *AM radio stations* WNYN 900 (Indep., C&W); WQIO 1060 (Indep., Blk., Top 40); WHBC 1480 (ABC/C, MOR) and WNIW 1520 (ABC/C, Contemp., Rock); *FM radio stations* WHBC 94.1 (ABC/E, Btfl. Mus.); WTOF 98.1 (UPI, Relig.) and WOOS 106.9 (Indep.); *television station* WJAN Ch. 17 (Indep.); *press:* one major newspaper is published in the city, the *Repository*, issued evenings and Sun. morning; other publications include *Stark Jewish News*, *Jackson Journal*, *Perry Post* and *Plain Tribune*.

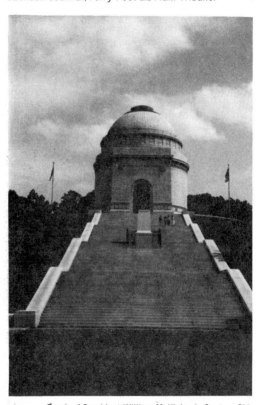

Tomb of President William McKinley in Canton, Ohio

HISTORY. In 1769, the site of present-day Canton was bequeathed by a native American of the DL tribe to a white man, who in turn sold it to Bezaleal Wells, a surveyor from Steubenville. In 1806, Wells surveyed the first plot in the comm. and later sold lots. The first store was established in 1807, the Post Office in 1809, the first schoolhouse in 1811 and the first newspaper in 1815. Wells named the settlement for trader John O'Donnell's Baltimore estate, which was called Canton after the Chinese city. Canton was incorporated as a village in 1828 and as a town in 1834, and in 1854 was chartered as a city. Former US Pres.

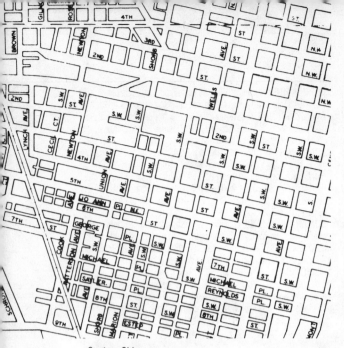

Canton, Ohio

William McKinley lived in the city, and is buried there. In 1920, the American Professional Football Assn. was established in the city, with Jim Thorpe of the Canton Bulldogs as pres. The growth of the city, located in an important agricultural and steel producing area, was and is based on industry.

GOVERNMENT. Canton has a mayor-council form of govt. consisting of 14 council members, elected to two-year terms, and the mayor, elected at large to a four-year term.

ECONOMY AND INDUSTRY. There are nearly 300 manufacturing plants in Canton, producing alloy steel, tapered roller bearings, household appliances, safes and bank vaults, streetlight standards, water softeners, meat products, rubber products, bakery products, internal combustion engines and paper products. In June, 1979, the labor force of the greater met. area totaled approx. 183,200, while the rate of unemployment was 5.5%.

BANKING. There are four commercial banks and four savings and loan assns. in Canton. In 1978, total deposits for the four banks headquartered in the city were $958,897,000, while assets totaled $1,136,320,000. Banks

Stark County Historical Center houses the McKinley Museum, Canton, Ohio

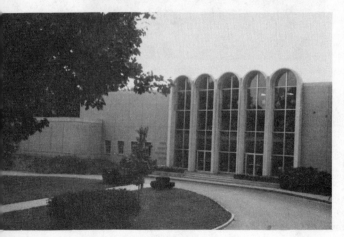

include Harter Bank and Trust, Central Trust of NE OH Natl., AmeriTrust and United Natl. Bank and Trust.

HOSPITALS. There are two hosps. in Canton, Aultman and Timken Mercy.

EDUCATION. Kent State U-Stark Co. Regional Campus established in Canton in 1946, a state-supported institution offering associate degrees, enrolled approx. 2,200 in 1978. Malone Col., a four-year liberal arts col. established in 1892 and affiliated with the Religious Society of Friends, enrolled approx. 800 in 1978. Walsh Col., established in ME in 1958 as La Mernais, a men's col., before moving to Canton in 1968, is a private coeducational liberal arts institution affiliated with the Roman Catholic Church. In 1978, more than 600 enrolled. State-controlled Stark Technical Col, which offers associate degrees, enrolled more than 1,900 in 1978. The public school system consists of 20 elementary, four jr. high and two sr. high schools in the city. Lib. facilities include the Canton Public Lib., Stark Co. district Lib. and Stark Co. Law Assn. Lib.

ENTERTAINMENT. Canton annually hosts induction ceremonies of the Professional Football Hall of Fame, as well as exhibition football games. Dinner theater, festivals and other annual events are accessible in nearby Akron.

ACCOMMODATIONS. There are several hotels and motels in Canton, the Imperial House Motel, TraveLodge and the Sheraton, Red Roof and Holiday Inns.

FACILITIES. There are 42 municipal parks encompassing 860 acres in Canton, including about 31 playgrounds and recreational areas, public golf courses, public tennis courts, playing fields and jogging, bicycling and bridle trails. Mother Gooseland, Clearwater, Lake O'Springs and Sandy Valley comm. are among area parks.

CULTURAL ACTIVITIES. The Culture Center for the Arts in Canton features the Players Guild, Art Institute, Symphony Orchestra, Ballet and Civic Opera. The Stark Co. Historical Center contains the McKinley Museum, Historical Museum, Hall of Science and Industry, and the Hoover-Price Planetarium. The Canton Jewish Center hosts plays of the Urban Arts Program. The Canton Playhouse Performers provide theatrical entertainment. The Classic Car Museum displays about 30 automobiles.

LANDMARKS AND SIGHTSEEING SPOTS. The Professional Football Hall of Fame, a complex established in Canton in 1963, features a statue of football great Jim Thorpe at its entrance, three exhibition areas, a football action movie theater, a research lib. and enshrinement halls, which display mementos of great football players. The McKinley Monument contains the graves of the former US Pres., his wife and two children, while the Church of the Savior United Methodist features four memorial windows presented by Mrs. McKinley. The Garden Center and the John F. Kennedy Memorial Fountain, with an eternal flame, are other attractions. The Hoover Historical Center, featuring preserved 19th century buildings, was the home of Daniel Hoover and his family. William H., one of his sons, founded the vacuum cleaner co. Models of early and recent vacuum cleaners and cleaning devices are on display.

CEDAR RAPIDS
IOWA

CITY LOCATION-SIZE-EXTENT. Cedar Rapids, the seat of Linn Co., is located in E central IA on the E and W banks of the Cedar River, 75 mi. W of IL and 106 mi. S of MN at 91°40' W lat. and 41°59' N long. The city encompasses 53.61 sq. and its greater met. area extends throughout Linn Co. and into Johnson Co. on the S, and includes its sister city of Marion to the N.

TOPOGRAPHY. The terrain of Cedar Rapids which is situated in a transition area between the Young Drift region to the N and the Dissected Till Plains Region to the S, is characterized by flat terrain with rich top soil, as well as low rolling hills and ridges. The Cedar River, flowing through the middle of the city, divides it into the E and W sections. The mean elev. is 730'.

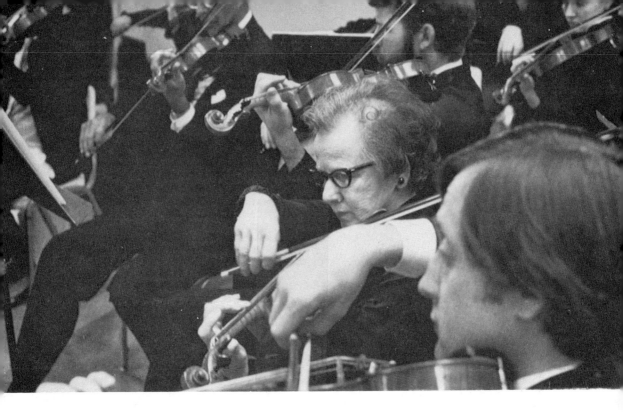

CLIMATE. The climate of Cedar Rapids is continental, with wide seasonal variations in both temp. and precip. The avg. annual temp. of about 50°F ranges from a Jan. mean of 20°F to a July mean of 75°F. Most of the avg. annual rainfall of 31" occurs from Apr. through Sept., While 70% of the avg. annual snowfall of 29" occurs from Dec. through Feb. The RH ranges from 53% to 60%. The avg. growing season is 185 days. Cedar Rapids lies in the CSTZ and observes DST.

FLORA AND FAUNA. Animals native to Cedar Rapids include the whitetail deer, grey squirrel, raccoon, opossum and muskrat. Common birds are the red-tailed hawk, yellow-billed cuckoo, yellow-headed blackbird and meadowlark. Tiger salamanders, bullfrogs, American toads, mud turtles, skinks and milk snakes, as well as the venomous timber rattlesnake and E massasauga (a pygmy rattler), are found in the area. Typical trees include the maple, basswood, ash and elm. Smaller plants are the Canada mayflower, field daisy, butter-and-egg and green foxtail.

POPULATION. According to the US census, the pop. of Cedar Rapids in 1970 was 110,682. In 1978, it was estimated that it had decreased to 110,400.

ETHNIC GROUPS. In 1978, the ethnic distribution of Cedar Rapids was approx. 98.3% Caucasian, 1.6% Black and .8% Hispanic (a percentage of the Hispanic total is also included in the Caucasian total).

TRANSPORTATION. Interstate Hwy. 380, US hwy. 30, 218, and 151 and state hwys. 84, 94, 13, 149, 150 and 382 provide major motor access to Cedar Rapids. *Railroads* serving the city include the Chessie system, ConRail, Burlington N, Rock Island and Santa Fe. *Airlines* serving Cedar Rapids Municipal Airport are UA, OZ and MVA. *Bus lines* include Greyhound, Trailways, MO transit, IA Coaches, Jefferson Lines and Linn Transit System.

COMMUNICATIONS. Broadcasting, communications and print media serving Cedar Rapids are: *AM radio stations* WMT 600 (CBS, Var.); KHAK 1360 (MBS, Mod. Ctry.); KLWW 1450 (APR, Top 40, Contemp.) and KCRG 1600 (ABC/C, Top 40); *FM radio stations* KCCK 88.3 (NPR, Clas., Jazz, Educ.); KWMR 88.9 (Indep., Var.); KOJC 89.7 (SBN, Var.); KCOE 90.3 (MBS, UC, Educ. Progsv., Jazz); WMT 96.5 (CBS, Var.); KHAK 98.1 (MBS, Mod. Ctry.); KQCR 102.9 (Indep. Top 40) and KTOF 104.5 (MBS, Relig.); *television stations* WMT Ch. 2 (CBS); KWWL Ch. 7 (NBC); KCRG Ch. 9 (ABC) and KIIN Ch. 12 (Educ.); *press:* the city's daily newspaper, the *Gazette,* is published evenings weekdays and mornings weekends; other

Cedar Rapid's Symphony Orchestra, the oldest symphony west of the Mississippi River, Cedar Rapids, Iowa

publications include *Construction Equipment Operation and Maintenance, Westside Penny Saver, Cosmos Coa* and *Buildings.*

HISTORY. Roving bands of the Sac, Fox, Mesquakie and Winnebago native American tribes inhabited the area of present day Cedar Rapids before the first white settlers arrived. In 1838, Osgood Shepard built a log cabin on the bank of the Cedar River. Other settlers arrived the following year, and in 1841 a brush dam was built across the river to harness power. Gristmills and sawmills were soon in operation, and the settlement developed in 1844 as a trade center after the first steam boat arrived. Originally called "Rapids City", since it was established at the swift surging rapids of the river, the comm. was later resurveyed and, in 1849, incorporated as a town under its present name. In 1856, it was incorporated as city, and, in 1859, the first RR arrived. Following the Civil War, people and industry were attracted to the city. In 1871, a packing plant (now Wilson Foods Corp.) was established, and, the next year, N Star Oatmeal Mill (now the Quaker Oats Co.) began operating. Later in the 1800s and early 1900s, other industries settled in the area. In 1905, the worst fire in the history of the city occurred but, populated by hard-working Scottish, English, Irish, German and Czechoslovakian people, it continued to develop. In 1959, an urban renewal program was begun. Today Cedar Rapids is the principal industrial city of E Central Iowa as well as the heart of a rich agricultural area.

GOVERNMENT. Cedar Rapids has a commission form of govt., consisting of five commission members, including the mayor as a voting member. All members are elected at large to two-year terms.

ECONOMY AND INDUSTRY. Approx. 200 industries are located in Cedar Rapids, including Quaker Oats, the largest cereal plant in the world. Other major industries besides food processing are telecommunications and electronic equipment, gymnastic equipment, road building and mining machinery, truck parts, steel fabricating, casting of ferrous and non-ferrous metals and pharmaceuticals. Insurance and utilities are other major employers, and the city is also a convention and meeting center. In 1979, the labor force totaled 87,300, while the rate of unemployment was 2.9%. The per capita income was $9,215.

BANKING. There are two natl. and six state banks in Cedar Rapids. In 1978, total deposits for the eight banks headquartered in the city were $543,545,000, while total assets were $648,810,000. Among the banks serving the city are Merchants Natl., First Trust and Savings and Peoples Bank and Trust.

HOSPITALS. There are two hosps. in Cedar Rapids, St. Luke's, the largest acute care facility in the state, maintains a cooperative blood bank program with Mercy Hosp.

EDUCATION. Among the universities and colleges in the Cedar Rapids area are Coe Col., an independent coeducational liberal arts institution founded in 1851 as the Cedar Rapids Collegiate Institution, with approx. 1,200 enrolled in 1978. Mercy Col., a four-year institution enrolling more than 1,000 and Kirkwood Comm. Col. established in 1966 and enrolling more than 4,000 are also located in the city. The public school system consisting of 28 elementary, 26 jr. high and three sr. high schools, enrolled approx. 21,900 in 1978. In addition, 13 parochial schools at the elementary and high school levels serve the city. Lib. facilities include the Cedar Rapids Public Lib., with branches in the SE and NW, and the Iowa Masonic Lib. and Museum with 100,000 volumes.

ENTERTAINMENT. The 125 acre Hawkeye Downs hosts horse shows, guns and antique shows, farm shows, natl., regional, state and district cattle and swine shows, sq. dancing and a variety of trade shows throughout the year, as well as the Hawkeye Downs Speedway which features weekly NASCAR stock car races from May through Sept. The All IA Fair promotes the state livestock and farm industry and serves as a showcase for various creative projects during the week of July Fourth. The Giants, a MWL minor league (A) baseball team of the Reds, and teams of Coe Col. provide sports entertainment in the city.

ACCOMMODATIONS. There are approx. 20 hotels and motels in Cedar Rapids, including Stouffer's Five Seasons Hotel, Roosevelt Royale, Western-Town House and Holiday Inn.

FACILITIES. There are 62 parks encompassing more than 3,600 acres in

Central Cedar Rapids, Iowa

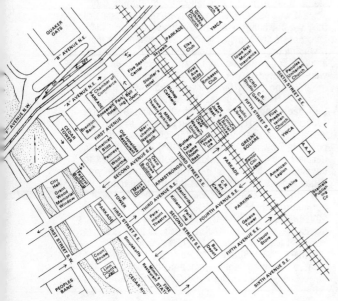

Cedar Rapids. Facilities include five outdoor swimming pools, seven public golf courses, four ice skating rinks, one toboggan run, tennis courts, playing and archery fields, public areas and boating facilities. Bever Park and Zoo, containing Old MacDonald's Farm, operates from May to Oct.

CULTURAL ACTIVITIES. The Cedar Rapids Symphony Orchestra performs at the Paramount Theater for the Performing Arts, while the 60-piece Cedar Rapids Municipal Band performs in city parks during the summer. The Comm. Concert Assn. sponsors four guest artist concerts per year. The Coe Col. Chamber Music Jazz Band and Chorus and the music depts. at Mt. Mercy and Kirkwood Comm. Colleges also perform on a regular basis. Cedar Rapids Comm. Theatre and Studio presents at least five major stage productions each year, while four children's plays are produced each season by the Childrens Theatre of Cedar Rapids. The drama depts. of Coe, Kirkwood Comm. and Mt. Mercy colleges also perform during each academic year. Both ethnic dance and classical ballet are performed by the Dieman-Bennett Dance Theatre at the Hemisphere. In addition to colonial, foreign and native American exhibits in its gen. museum, the IA Masonic Lib. and Museum houses the most complete Masonic collection in the US. A permanent Grant Wood exhibit and other displays are featured at the Cedar Rapids Art Center.

LANDMARKS AND SIGHTSEEING SPOTS. The Cedar Rapids govt. center located on Mays Island on the main channel of the Cedar River, includes the Linn Co. Court house, City Hall and Veterans Memorial Coliseum. Five Seasons Center, completed in 1979, is an entertainment complex featuring various events. Czeck Village is an historical section which preserves the area's ethnic history.

CHARLOTTE
NORTH CAROLINA

CITY LOCATION-SIZE-EXTENT. Charlotte, the seat of Mecklenburg Co., and largest city in the Carolinas encompasses 29.3 sq. mi. in S NC 10 mi. NE of the SC border, at 35°13' N lat. and 80°56' W long. Its greater met. area extends into the bordering counties of Union to the SE, Cabarrus to the NE and Gaston to the NW.

TOPOGRAPHY. The terrain of Charlotte, which is situated in the S Piedmont region—an area of transition between the Atlantic Coastal Plain to the SE and the Blue Ridge Mts. of the Appalachian range to the W—is rolling, rising toward the mts. to the W, N and SW, and descending toward the coastal plain to the E and SE. Several lakes and creeks are located in the area including Stewart, Irwin and Sugar Creek, while the Catawba River forms the city's W border. The mean elev. is 700'.

CLIMATE. The climate of Charlotte is moderate, characterized by cool winters (influenced by the mts. to the W which buffer cold winds from the NW, and occasional seabreezes from the Atlantic Ocean) and warm summers. The avg. annual temp. of 60.5°F ranges from a Jan. avg. of 41.8°F to a July avg. of 78.7°F. The annual avg. 75" of rainfall is fairly evenly distributed throughout the year. The avg. annual snowfall is 5.4". The RH ranges from 47% to 90%. The avg. growing season is 216 days. Charlotte is located in the ESTZ and observes DST.

FLORA AND FAUNA. Animals native to Charlotte include the deer, weasel, muskrat and S flying squirrel. Common birds are the bluebird, red-eyed vireo, robin, brown thrasher, catbird and cardinal. Green anoles, box turtles, bullfrogs, American toads and ribbon snakes, as well as the venomous coral snake, copperhead, rattlesnake and cottonmouth, are found in the area. Common trees include the oak, pine and elm. Smaller plants include the sumac, holly, wild buckwheat and pickerelweed.

POPULATION. According to the US census, the pop. of Charlotte in 1970

was 274,640. In 1978, it was estimated that it had increased to 325,000.

ETHNIC GROUPS. In 1978, the ethnic distribution of Charlotte was approx. 69.5% Caucasian, 26.6% Black, 0.6% Hispanic and 3.3% other.

TRANSPORTATION. Interstate hwys. 77 and 85, US hwys. 29, 21 and 521 and state hwys. 24, 27, 16, 49 and 160 provide major motor access to Charlotte. *Railroads* serving the city include Central Gulf, Rock Island, Seaboard Coast, Southern, ConRail, AMTRAK and Frisco. *Airlines* serving Douglas Municipal Airport are DL, EA, FL, PI, SO and UA. *Bus lines* providing service include Greyhound, Trailways, Piedmont and the local Charlotte Transit System.

COMMUNICATIONS. Communications, broadcasting and print media originating from Charlotte are: *AM radio stations* WAYS 610 (Indep., Contemp.); WSOC 930 (NBC, MBS, All News); WBT 1110 (MOR, Contemp.); WIST 1240 (CBS, Top 40); WHYN 1310 (MBS, Christian); WAME 1480 (MBS, Mod. Ctry.); WRPL 1540 (ABC/C, Progsv.) and WGIV 1600 (Natl. Blk., APR); *FM radio stations* WFAE 90.9 (Univ., Clas., Educ., Jazz); WROQ 95.1 (Indep., Adult Rock); WSOC 103.7 (ABC/I, Mod. Ctry); WEZC 104.7 (APR, EZ List., Btfl. Mus.) and WBSY 107.9 (Btfl. Mus.); *television stations* WBTV Ch. 3 (CBS); WSOC Ch. 9 (NBC); WCCB Ch. 18 (ABC); WRET Ch. 36 (Indep.) and WTVI Ch. 42 (PBS); *press:* the major dailies serving the city are the *News*, issued evenings and Sun. morning, and the *Observer* issued mornings; other publications include *Charlotte Magazine*, *Weekly-East, Mecklenburg Times, Carolina Woman, Go, Post, American Jewish Times, Southern Textile News, Star of Zion, Textile Equipment* and *This Week In Charlotte*.

HISTORY. Native Americans of the Catawba tribe inhabited the area of present day Charlotte when the first settlers arrived in the 1740s. In 1748, the first permanent settlement was established by Scotch and Irish farmers from PA, who named the comm. in honor of Queen Charlotte of Mecklenburg-Stelitz, wife of King George III of England. Charlotte was incorporated as a city in 1768. The Mecklenburg Declaration of Independence, declaring the area free of British rule and considered to be the forerunner of the later version of Thomas Jefferson's, was signed in Mecklenburg Co. in May, 1775. During the Revolutionary War the city was occupied by British forces under Gen. Cornwallis. who called it a "hornet's nest" because of annoying patriotic activities. The mining of gold became an important area industry when it was discovered nearby in 1799. Until the 1849 CA gold rush, the more than 50 Piedmont region mines produced a majority of the nation's gold. In 1865, Confederate Pres. Jefferson Davis convened his full cabinet for the last time in the city, which served as a Confederate military post during the Civil War. Industrial growth in the 1900s and after WW II contributed to an increase in the pop. of the city from slightly more than 18,000 in 1900 to nearly 83,000 in 1930, and about 201,500 in 1960. In 1970, the Charlotte-Mecklenburg Co. school system initiated a major busing program.

GOVERNMENT. Charlotte has a council-mgr. form of govt. consisting of 11 council members and a mayor. The mayor and four council members are elected at large, while seven council members are elected by district. All serve two-year terms.

ECONOMY AND INDUSTRY. The Piedmont region in which Charlotte is located leads the US in textile production. Other industrial products include machinery and food products, while printing and publishing are also important. The city is also the area center of banking, insurance, retail and wholesale trade and distribution. In June, 1979, the labor force of the greater met. area totaled approx. 337,500, while the rate of unemployment was 3.2%.

BANKING. There are seven commercial banks and seven savings and loan assns. in Charlotte. In 1978, total deposits for the five banks headquartered in the city were $5,646,630,000, while assets were $7,261,832,000. Banks include NC Nat'l., First Union Natl., Wachovia Bank and Trust, City Natl., Republic Bank and Trust, Metrolina Natl. and NW First Citizens Bank and Trust.

The Hezekiah Alexander Home built in 1774, is the oldest dwelling in Charlotte, North Carolina.

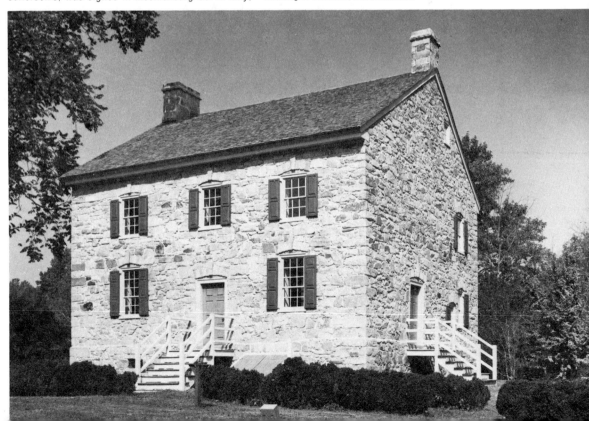

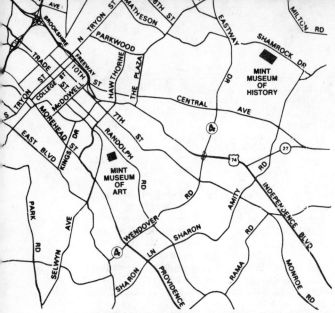

Charlotte, North Carolina

HOSPITALS. There are four gen. and several specialized hosps. in Charlotte including Charlotte Comm., Charlotte Memorial, Mercy, Presbyterian, Charlotte Eye, Ear and Throat, Charlotte Rehabilitation and Orthopedic. Charlotte Treatment Center and Wilmith Hosp. specialize in the treatment of alcoholism.

EDUCATION. Johnson C. Smith U, a private liberal arts col. and theological seminary in Charlotte enrolling more than 1,500 in 1978, was established in 1867. It is affiliated with the United Presbyterian Church. Queens Col., a private women's liberal arts institution also affiliated with the Presbyterian Church and established in 1851, enrolled approx. 750 in 1979. Central Piedmont Comm. Col., a state controlled institution established in 1963, enrolled 15,000 in 1978 in programs leading to associate degrees. King's Col.-Charlotte, a private col. established in 1901 and offering associate degrees, enrolled more than 400 in 1978. The U of NC at Charlotte, established in 1965, enrolled approx. 8,500 in 1978 in programs leading to associate, bachelor and master degrees. The Charlotte Mecklenburg Co. public school system enrolled more than 82,000 in 1978. Lib. facilities include the Public Lib. of Charlotte and Mecklenburg Co., the Metrolina Lib. for the Blind and Physically Handicapped and the Mint Museum of History Lassiter Lib.

ENTERTAINMENT. Annual events in Charlotte include the Carolina Carousel in Nov., Festival in the Park in Sept., the Natl. 500 Auto Race in Oct. and the World 600 Auto Race in May. The Charlotte Orioles, a professional minor SL baseball team and teams of the U of NC at Charlotte 49'ers provide sports entertainment.

ACCOMMODATIONS. There are several hotels and motels in Charlotte including the Radisson Plaza Hotel, Best Western-Coliseum, Howard Johnson's, Golden Eagle, Holiday, Quality and Sheraton inns.

FACILITIES. There are 100 public parks in Charlotte, as well as 17 comm. centers, including 12 public golf courses, tennis courts, playing fields, swimming pools, picnic areas, jogging and bicycle trails.

CULTURAL ACTIVITIES. Among the performing arts groups in Charlotte are the Charlotte Symphony, a 75-member regional orchestra, the Charlotte Opera and the Charlotte Regional Ballet which performs at Spirit Sq. Discovery Place, scheduled to be completed in the early 1980s, will be a science center. The Charlotte Nature Museum and Planetarium feature exhibits which visitors are invited to touch and handle. The Mint Museum of Art, operated as a Branch of the US Mint from 1837 to 1861 and from 1867 to 1913, was remodeled in 1933 to serve as an art and history museum. The Mint Museum of History, established in 1976 as the first historical museum in the city, features displays of American history, costume and ceramic collections.

LANDMARKS AND SIGHTSEEING SPOTS. The ultramodern Charlotte Coliseum features one of the largest steel, aluminum and precast concrete domes in the world. At the entrance of the Co. Courthouse, which is of Greek architectural design, stands a monument to the 1775 signers of the

Mecklenburg Declaration of Independence. The location of the original courthouse, built about 1765, is marked by a tablet in Independence Sq. It contains the "Rockhouse" built in 1774 from stone of nearby quarries. The oldest dwelling still standing in Charlotte's Mecklenburg Co., the Hezekiah Alexander Homesite, is listed on the Natl. Register of Historic Places. Alexander was a comm. leader and one of the signers of the Mecklenburg Declaration of Independence. The Capt. James Jack Monument honors "the Paul Revere of the South" who carried the Mecklenburg Declaration on horseback to the Continental Congress in Philadelphia. The 78-acre Fourth Ward Historic District, the first in the city, is a re-creation of an 18th century Charlotte neighborhood. The birthplace of Billy Graham is another popular attraction.

CHATTANOOGA
TENNESSEE

CITY LOCATION-SIZE-EXTENT. Chattanooga, the seat of Hamilton Co., lies in the Great Valley region of SE TN on the Moccasin Bend of the TN River. It is situated between the Cumberland and Appalachian mts. at 35°02' N lat. and 85°12' W long. The city encompasses 126.9 sq. mi. Its greater met. area extends throughout Hamilton Co. and into Marion Co. on the E, Bradley Co. on the W and the GA border on the S.

TOPOGRAPHY. Chattanooga is located in the S portion of the Great Valley of TN, an area of the TN River between the Cumberland Mts. to the W and the Appalachian Mts. to the E. Most of the city lies S of the TN River, where the terrain is hilly, with a number of small valleys and ridges. In the N and SW sections of the city, the terrain rises abruptly to elevs. of approx. 1,200'. Man-made Lake Chickamauga is six mi. from downtown Chattanooga, whose mean elev. is 685'.

CLIMATE. The climate of Chattanooga is moderate, characterized by cool winters and warm summers. The city's weather is influenced by the Cumberland Mts. to the W and the Appalachian Mts. to the E. The avg. annual temp. of 60.3°F ranges from a Jan. mean of 41°F to a July mean of 79°F. Approx. 40% of the annual rainfall of 52" occurs from Dec. through Mar. The annual avg. snowfall is 4" and the RH ranges from 49% to 91%. The avg. growing season is 228 days. Chattanooga is located in the ESTZ and observes DST.

FLORA AND FAUNA. Animals native to Chattanooga include the black bear, fox, whitetail deer and opossum. Common birds are the robin, cardinal, blue jay, thrasher and vireo. Turtles, frogs, lizards and snakes, as well as the venomous timber rattlesnake and N copperhead, are found here. Typical trees are the magnolia, redbud, tulip poplar, red and white oak, pine, dogwood, hickory and sweetgum.

POPULATION. According to the US census, the pop. of Chattanooga in 1970 was 119,923. In 1978, it was estimated that it had increased to 170,046.

ETHNIC GROUPS. In 1978, the ethnic distribution of Chattanooga was approx. 64.4% Caucasian, 25.5% Black, 0.4% Hispanic and 9.7% other.

TRANSPORTATION. Interstate hwys. 24, 59, 75 and 124, US hwys. 11, 27, 41, 64, 72, 76 and 127 and state hwys. 17, 27, 58, 148 and 153 provide major motor access to Chattanooga. *Railroads* serving the city are S Railway System, Family Lines System, Central of GA, and TN, AL & GA. *Airlines* serving Lovell Field include DL and SO. Collegedale Park and Dallas Bay Skypark airports also serve the city. *Bus lines* include Trailways, Greyhound and the intra-city Chattanooga Area Regional Transportation Authority (CARTA). Chattanooga is a port on the inland waterway system. TVA locks and dams create a navigable nine-ft. channel on the TN River. The TN-Tombigbee Waterway is scheduled to be opened in 1985.

COMMUNICATIONS. Communications, broadcasting and print media serving Chattanooga are: *AM radio stations* WGOW 1150 (Indep., Top 40); WNOO 1260 (Mut. Blk., APR, Blk.); WDEF 1370 (CBS, MOR); WMDC 1450 (APR, MOR, Relig.) and WDXB 1490 (NBC, MOR); *FM radio stations* (ABC, Easy List.) WOWE 105.5 (MBS, Divers.) and WSKZ 106.5 (Indep., Top 40) (ABC, Easy Lis.) WOWE 105.5 (MBS, Divers.) and WSKZ 106.5 (Indep., Top 40) *television stations* WRCB Ch. 3 (NBC); WTVC Ch. 9 (ABC); WDEF Ch. 12 (CBS); WTCI Ch. 45 (PBS) and WRIP Ch. 61 (Indep.); *press:* two major dailies serve the city, the *News-Free Press*, issued evenings, and the *Times*, issued mornings; other publications include the *Hamilton Co. Herald*, *University Echo*, *Labor World* and *Pulpit Helps*.

HISTORY. Native Americans of the Cherokee nation inhabited the area of present-day Chattanooga when Spanish explorer Hernando de Soto arrived in 1540. In 1761, the first white settlers, French fur-traders, established a store at the base of Signal Mt. About 1770, Scotsman John McDonald established a trading post on S Chickamauga Creek. On Sept. 20, 1782, John Sevier and his frontier militia won what has become known as "the last battle of the American Revolution" against native Americans of the Chickamauga tribe on the slopes of Lookout Mt. TN became the 16th state of the Union on June 1, 1796. A couple of years later, Daniel Ross built a home on Chattanooga Creek. About 1815, his son, John Ross—a trader—built a log warehouse on the TN River at the present site of Chattanooga and established a ferry service. The name of the settlement, known as Ross' Landing, was changed in 1838 to Chattanooga, a word believed to be Cherokee for "rock rising to a point", describing Lookout Mt. In 1836, 13,149 Cherokees were expelled from their land and forced on a long march that became known as the "Trail of Tears" to resettle in OK in accordance with terms of a treaty generally considered fraudulent. In Dec., 1939, the town of Chattanooga was incorporated. It became a center for trading, farming and river and railway transportation and was chartered as a city in 1851. By the time of the Civil War, the pop. of the city was 2,500. The citizens of the city, although divided in their sympathies, voted to secede in 1861. In Sept., 1863, Union troops led by Gen. William Rosecrans entered Chattanooga but were defeated by Confederate Gen. James Longstreet in a bloody battle at Chickamauga Creek that preceded the famous Battle of Chattanooga. Union Gen. George Thomas—the "Rock of Chickamauga"—prevented the Union defeat from becoming a rout. Confederate Gen. Braxton Bragg failed to take advantage of the situation, and the Union forces reassembled in Chattanooga under Gen. U.S. Grant and later Gen. William Tecumseh Sherman. The Confed. siege broken, the Union supplies and reinforcements arrived before the three-day battle of Chattanooga, which "sealed the fate of the Confederacy", was won in Nov. After the Civil War, the city grew as former Union soldiers settled there, contributing to the growth of new industry. Although an epidemic of yellow fever struck in 1878, business and industry continued to thrive and the city became known as the "Dynamo of Dixie". The U of Chattanooga opened in 1886, and industry, including the first Coca-Cola bottling operation in the US, steel and textiles, diversified. In the 1930s, the harnessing of the TN River by the TVA for electrical power gave Chattanooga the name "Electric Center of the Nation" and resulted in more rapid industrial expansion.

GOVERNMENT. Chattanooga has a commission form of govt. consisting of four commission members and the mayor, who is a voting member. The mayor and commission members are elected at large to four-year terms.

ECONOMY AND INDUSTRY. More than 600 manufacturers employing approx. one-third of the area's work force, are located in the Chattanooga met. area, which is a major industrial center. Products include primary metals, chemicals, textiles, food products, apparel, fabricated metals and paper products. The headquarters of the TVA Power System—the largest in the US—are located in the city, which is the geographic center of the TVA area. The city receives benefits of flood control, navigation and power production, as well as development of land resources, from the TVA. Tourism is also a major industry with over 12 million people visiting the "Scenic Center of the South." The city also ranks second in TN in terms of foreign trade exports. In June, 1979, the labor force totaled approx. 190,700, while the rate of unemployment was about 6%.

BANKING. There are 18 commercial banks and five savings and loan assns. in the Chattanooga met. area. In 1978, total deposits for the five banks headquartered in Chattanooga were $1,064,166,000, while total assets were $1,869,725,000. Among the banks serving the city are First Fed.,

Ruby Falls, Chattanooga, Tennessee

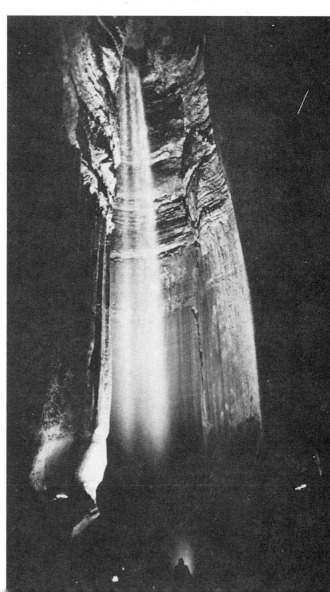

Cherokee Valley Fed., American Natl. Bank and Trust, First TN Natl., Pioneer, United and Commerce United of Chattanooga.

HOSPITALS. There are 13 hosps. in Chattanooga including Baroness, Erlanger, E Ridge Comm., John L. Hutcheson Memorial, Tri-County, Medical Park, Memorial, Downtown Gen., Tepper Pediatric, T.C. Thompson Children's, Wildwood Sanitarium, Orange Grove and Siskin Memorial Foundation.

EDUCATION. The U of TN at Chattanooga, a state-supported institution, awards bachelor and master degrees and enrolled more than 7,100 in 1978. Other institutions include Chattanooga State Technical Comm. Col., Covenant Col., S Missionary Col., Temple Baptist Theological Seminary, TN Temple Bible School and TN Temple Col. The U of TN Clinical Education Center provides training for interns and residents at affiliated Erlanger and T.C. Thompson Children's hosps., as well as continuing education for physicians, pharmacists and other health-field professionals. The public school system includes 38 elementary, 13 jr. and nine sr. high schools, as well as a technical high school and a high school for adults, enrolled more than 49,300 in 1978. There are also 22 parochial schools which enrolled approx. 6,400 in 1978, and five private schools, with a 1978 enrollment of about 2,400, in the city. Libs. include the Chattanooga-Hamilton Co. Bicentennial Lib., with three branches and two bookmobiles, and the E Ridge City Library at City Hall.

ENTERTAINMENT. The Back Stage Playhouse offers dinner theater entertainment in Chattanooga. Among the festive and annual events in the city are art festivals, sq. dancing events, rock, country or bluegrass concerts held downtown and boat cruises through the Cumberland Mts. to view autumn foliage, which culminate in a three-day mt. festival of music, art autumn foliage, which culminate in a three-day mt. festival of music, arts Engel Stadium, while the U of TN at Chattanooga Moccasins participate in collegiate sports. The Indians are a minor SL baseball team.

ACCOMMODATIONS. There are approx. 25 hotels and motels in Chattanooga including the Admiral Benbow, Days, Choo-Choo Hilton, Sheraton, Holiday, Quality, Ramada and Rodeway inns.

FACILITIES. The 34,500-acre Chickamauga Lake, with 810 mi. of shoreline, provides Chattanooga residents with facilities for boating, fishing, camping, picnicking, swimming and waterskiing. Two state, two co. and four municipal parks are located on the lake. Nearby 10,730-acre Nickajack Lake, with 192 mi. of shoreline, offers water sports facilities at Nickajack Dam Reservation. There are 10 city parks and playgrounds in the city, including Orchard Knob and Warner, containing playing fields, bicycle trails, 90 tennis courts and seven public golf courses, including Brainerd, Brown Acres, Concord, Eastgate, Hickory Valley and Moccasin Bend. Zooville and a Rose Garden are located at Warner Park.

CULTURAL ACTIVITIES. Among the cultural organizations in Chattanooga are the Symphony Orchestra, Opera Assn., Civic Chorus, Opera Workshop and Boy's Choir. The U of TN at Chattanooga Drama Dept. and the

Chattanooga, Tennessee

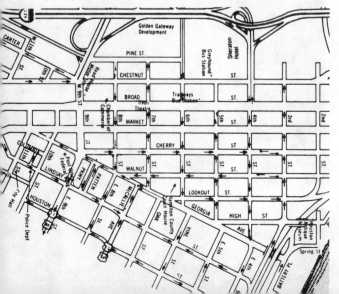

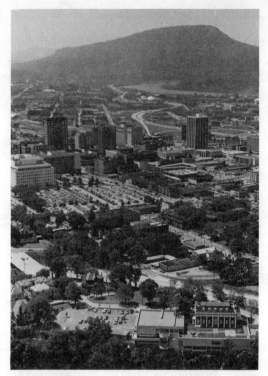

A view of Chatttanooga with the Civil War battlefield in the background. Chattanooga, Tennessee

Little Theatre present theatrical performances, while Miller Park is the site of weekly musical and dramatic presentations during the spring, summer and fall. The Hunter Museum of Art, TN Valley RR Museum, Fuller Gun Museum, Houston Antique Museum and Hall of Presidents Wax Museum are located in the city. The Harris Swift Museum of Religious Art contains artifacts representative of several religions. Galleries include Galbraith and Notchwood.

LANDMARKS AND SIGHTSEEING SPOTS. The 8,092-acre Chickamauga and Chattanooga Natl. Military Park is located in GA and TN and is the oldest and largest of the natl. military parks administered by the US Park Service. The Natl. Cemetary in Chattanooga contains the graves of 25,000 veterans of US wars, including those of men who fought in the battles on Chickamauga Creek, Missionary Ridge, Brainerd Ridge, Lookout Mt. and Chattanooga. Craven House, built by Robert Cravens in 1856, was used as a Confederate field hosp. during the Civil War and occupied by both Confederate and Union troops. It is located in the 2,126'-high Lookout Mt. in the SW section of the city. Ruby Falls and Lookout Mt. Caves, 45' falls located 1,120' underground, are located at Lookout Mt. The Clarence C. Jones Observatory is also a popular attraction. The original Chattanooga Choo Choo Train, which, when it made its first run on Mar. 5, 1880, was the first major link in public transportation between the N and S, is on display at the Chattanooga Choo Choo and Terminal Station in the city. It is the center of a complex of Victorian-era shops and restaurants.

CHESAPEAKE
VIRGINIA

CITY LOCATION-SIZE-EXTENT. Chesapeake, an independent city in the Tidewater Region of SW VA, encompasses 353 sq. mi. at 36°49' N lat. and 76°17' W long. It is bordered on the N by Norfolk and Portsmouth, on the E

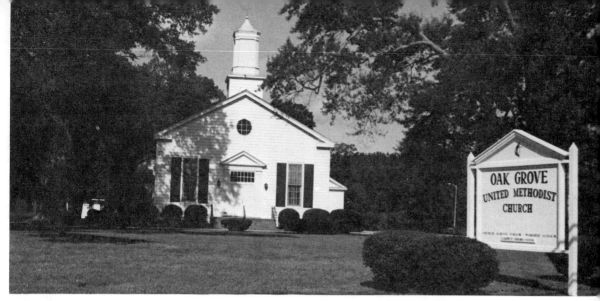

Chesapeake's historic Old Grove Methodist Church built in 1852, Chesapeake, Virginia

by VA Beach, on the W by Suffolk and on the S by the state of NC. It is part of the Norfolk-Chesapeake-Portsmouth greater met. area.

TOPOGRAPHY. The terrain in Chesapeake, situated on the coastal plain of the Tidewater Region of VA, is flat in shoreline areas and marshy in the S and W. There are nine mi. of shoreline on Hampton Roads, a natural harbor N of the city, while Dismal Swamp and Lake Drummond are in the W part of the city. The Dismal Swamp Canal links the Chesapeake Bay with Albemarle Sound via Deep Creek. Chesapeake & Albemarle Canal and Locks link the N Landing River with Deep Creek and Elizabeth River. The NW River flows through the SW part of the city. The mean elev. is 12'.

CLIMATE. The climate of Chesapeake is modified marine, characterized by warm summers and pleasant weather during spring and fall. Monthly mean temps. range from 41°F during Jan to 77°F during July with an avg. annual temp. of 60°F. Most of the 45" avg. annual rainfall occurs during the summer months, while most of the 7.2" avg. annual snowfall occurs in Jan. and Feb. The RH ranges from 50% to 87% and the avg. growing season is 244 days. Chesapeake lies in the ESTZ and observes DST.

FLORA AND FAUNA. Animals native to Chesapeake include the raccoon, mink, otter, opossum, muskrat, whitetail deer and harvest mouse. Common birds are the gull, tern, mockingbird, cormorant and grebes. Salamanders, gray treefrogs, spring peepers, narrow-mouthed toads, cricket frogs, skinks and green snakes, as well as the venomous rattlesnake and coral snake, are found in the area. Typical trees include the maple, Atlantic white cedar, redbud, oak, pine, dogwood and cypress. Smaller plants are the holly, crepe myrtle, hawthorn, sow thistle, foxglove, wild rose, begonia and honeysuckle.

POPULATION. According to the US census, the pop. of Chesapeake in 1970 was 89,580. In 1978, it was estimated that it had increased to 111,896.

ETHNIC GROUPS. In 1978, the ethnic distribution of Chesapeake was approx. 76.7% Caucasian, 23.1% Black and 0.5% Hispanic. (A percentage of the Hispanic total is also included in the Caucasian total.)

TRANSPORTATION. Interstate hwys. 64, 264 and 464, US hwys. 17, 58, 460 and 13 (connecting to the E shore of VA via the Chesapeake Bay Bridge-Tunnel) and state rtes. 165, 168, 190 and 191 provide major motor access to Chesapeake. *Railroads* serving the area are the Norfolk & Western, Southern the Seaboard Coast Line, AMTRAK and ConRail. Commuter *airlines* serve Chesapeake and Chesapeake-Portsmouth Airports, while other airlines serve nearby Norfolk Intl. and S Norfolk airports. *Bus lines* include Trailways and the local Tidewater Regional Transit System. Chesapeake is a port city with a 35'-40' channel.

COMMUNICATIONS. Communications, broadcasting and print media originating from Chesapeake are: *AM radio station* WCPK 1600

(NBC/VA, Btfl. Mus.) and *FM radio stations* WFOS 90.5 (Indep., Var., Educ.) and WJLY 92.1 (Indep., Top 40, Oldies); although no *television stations* originate from the city, Chesapeake receives TV broadcasting from nearby Tidewater cities; *press:* two major daily newspapers are published in the city, *The Ledger Star,* issued evenings and Sun. mornings, and the morning *Virginian-Pilot;* other publications include the *Tidewater Virginian, Metro Magazine, The VA Observer* and the weekly *Chesapeake Post.*

HISTORY. Native Americans lived in the area of present-day Chesapeake when English explorers Capt. John Smith and Capt. Ralph Lane sailed up the Elizabeth River in 1585. The first English settlements, in what is now Chesapeake, were established in 1620, along the banks of the Elizabeth River near the site of the native American village called Ski-coak. In 1643, when the colony of VA was divided into shires, Norfolk Co. (which comprised much of contemporary Chesapeake) was formed. The area thrived due to the cultivation of tobacco, cotton and corn and lucrative trade with the W Indies. On Dec. 9, 1775, during the Revolutionary War, American troops defeated British forces, led by Royal Gov. Lord Dunmore in the historic Battle of Great Bridge. This confrontation resulted in the subsequent bombardment and destruction of Norfolk by Dunmore. However, by 1800, the area was once again prosperous and, in 1801, work began on Dismal Swamp Canal. In 1828, the inland waterway opened to traffic and attracted even more revenue to the area. Although progress was disrupted by the Civil War, the development of industry, especially lumber milling, continued in the latter part of the 19th century and into the 20th century. The area is the largest producer of fertilizer in the world. In 1963, the city of Chesapeake was created when Norfolk Co. merged with the city of S Norfolk (which had incorporated in 1921). Today, it is known as "VA's Finest City".

GOVERNMENT. Chesapeake has a council-mgr. form of govt., consisting of nine council members elected at large for four-year terms. The mayor is selected by and from the council.

ECONOMY AND INDUSTRY. There are 50 manufacturing plants in Chesapeake employing about 15% of the total work force. Major construction industries include automotive assembly, steel fabrication, fertilizer, construction materials, chemicals and manufactured sailboats. The city's nine-mi. waterfront supports nine oil terminals, six chemical plants, two cement plants and two grain elevators. Transportation, the fed. govt. (military) and agriculture are other major employers. Chesapeake is the state's leading producer of nursery and greenhouse products and is an important area for the production of corn, soybeans and wheat. In June, 1979, the labor force totaled 46,086 while the unemployment rate was 5.5%. In 1977, the avg. per capita income was $9,644, while the median family income in 1978 was approx $13,750.

BANKING. There are nine commercial banks and savings and loan assns. in Chesapeake. In 1978, total deposits for the two banks headquartered in the city were $33,367,000, while assets were $37,225,000. Banks include People's of Chesapeake, Chesapeake Bank and Trust, VA Natl., First Merchants Natl. of Tidewater, Dominion Natl. of Tidewater, Fidelity American and UVB/Seaboard Natl.

HOSPITALS. There is one hosp., Chesapeake Gen. (which opened in 1976), in the city, as well as a public health center facility. Nine hosps. in the surrounding met. area also serve the city.

EDUCATION. The Chesapeake campus of The Tidewater Comm. Col, a two-year public institution awarding associate degrees, enrolled more than 1,000 students in 1978. The public school system consists of 35 elementary, jr. and sr. high schools with an enrollment of approx. 28,000, as well as four special schools. The Chesapeake Public Lib. System consists of the Civic Center Lib. and four branches.

ENTERTAINMENT. Dinner theaters, festivals, annual events and spectator sports are available in nearby Tidewater cities.

ACCOMMODATIONS. Hotels and motels in Chesapeake include the Sunset Manor Motel and the Virginia Reel Motor Lodge.

FACILITIES. More than 20,000 acres of the 50,000-acre Dismal Swamp Natl. Wildlife Refuge, the largest natural open space in the Tidewater Region, are located in Chesapeake. The city maintains Great Dismal Swamp Park and Campgrounds. The city, which leases the Great Bridge Locks and Deep Creek parks from the US Army Corps of Engineers, has also developed six picnic areas and one boat-launching site on the Dismal Swamp Canal. The 763-acre NW River Park features picnicking, canoeing, fishing, boating, hiking, camping and bicycling and bridle trails. There are 30 mi. of canoe trails on the Intracoastal Waterway, which runs through the center of the

city. Norfolk owns the 100-acre Indian River Park on which Chesapeake has developed some facilities. The public park system includes 21 playgrounds, five day camps, one nature camp and three multipurpose comm. centers.

CULTURAL ACTIVITIES. The Chrysler Museum in Chesapeake exhibits art and provides facilities for various cultural activities coordinated by the Tidewater Arts Council, including performances by the Chrysler Chamber Ballet and Broadway productions. The Chesapeake Little Theater presents dramatic performances. A Planetarium is located in the Civic Center.

LANDMARKS AND SIGHTSEEING SPOTS. The Dismal Swamp Canal in Chesapeake, an important link in the Intracoastal Waterway which skirts the Atlantic Seaboard and permits boat trips as far S as FL, is the oldest artificial waterway in the US

CHICAGO
ILLINOIS

CITY LOCATION-SIZE-EXTENT. Chicago, the largest city in IL, the second largest city in the US and the seat of Cook Co., is located in NW IL on two branches of the Chicago River along the W shore of Lake MI at 41°50' N lat. and 87°37' W long. The city occupies all of Cook Co. (222.8 sq. mi.)—the second largest co. in the US. The greater met. area extends into N and E IL and into IN on the S and includes the counties of Lake to the N, McHenry to the NW, DuPage and Kane to the W and Will to the SW.

TOPOGRAPHY. The terrain of Chicago, which is situated in the Great Lakes Plains region of the Central Plains, is characterized by predominantly flat land interspersed with small hills, lakes and marshes in the N and W parts of the city. Lake MI once covered the entire area, and the flow of the Chicago River, which originally emptied into Lake MI, was reversed in 1900 to prevent pollution of the lake. The Chicago Sanitary & Ship and the IL & MI canals are major shipping canals, while

Chesapeake Bay Area, Virginia

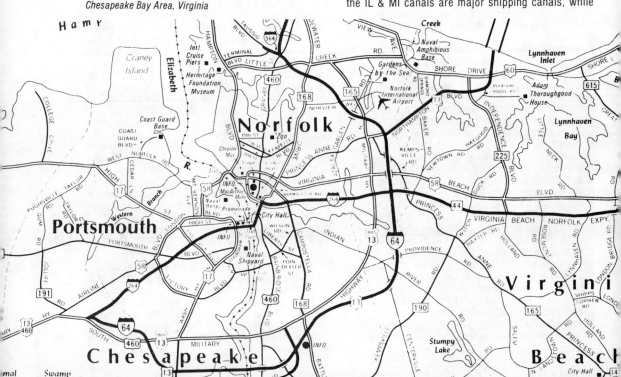

lakes in the city include Calumet and Wolf. The mean elev. is 578'.

CLIMATE. The continental climate of Chicago, characterized by hot summers and cold winters, is influenced by the Great Lakes, especially Lake MI, which modifies air masses that approach the city from the NW and NE. Although the channeling of winds between the tall buildings of the Central Business District contributes to Chicago's nickname, "Windy City", the avg. wind speed in most parts of the city is much lower. The annual avg. temp. of 49.5°F ranges from a Jan. mean of 22.5°F to a July mean of 73.3°F. Most of the annual 33.5" of rainfall results from air masses originating in the Gulf of Mexico. More than 50% of the 40.95" of snowfall occurs during Dec. and Jan. The RH ranges from 53% to 85%. Air pollution restricts visibility more during the winter than during the summer. The avg. growing season is 135 days. Chicago lies in the CSTZ and observes DST.

FLORA AND FAUNA. Animals native to Chicago include the muskrat, opossum, raccoon and whitetail deer. Common birds include the purple martin, blue jay, black tern, spotted sandpiper and killdeer. Spiny softshell turtles, tiger salamanders, Fowler's toads, chorus frogs and milk snakes, as well as the venomous E massasauga (a pygmy rattler) and timber rattlesnake, are found in the area. Common trees include the cherry, red bud, elm, white oak and beech. Smaller plants are the sumac, geranium, buttercup and nutsedge.

POPULATION. According to the US census, the pop. of Chicago in 1970 was 3,369,357. In 1978, it was estimated that it had decreased to approx. 2,940,000. About 60% of the pop. of IL resides in or around the city.

ETHNIC GROUPS. In 1978, the ethnic distribution of Chicago was approx. 66% Caucasian, 32.7% Black and 7.4% Hispanic (a percentage of the Hispanic total is also included in the Caucasian total).

TRANSPORTATION. Interstate hwys. 55 (the Adlai Stevenson Expressway), 57, 80, 90 (the Dwight D. Eisenhower Expressway), 94 (the John F. Kennedy Expressway on the N and the Dan Ryan Expressway on the S) and 294, US hwy. 41 (the Edens Expressway) and the E-W and N IN toll roads provide major motor access to Chicago. The 18 major *railroads* serving the city, which is a major US shipping center, utilize approx. 50% of the US railway system. Among these are AMTRAK, Union Pacific, Southern, ConRail and MO Pacific. RR cars and trucks transport more goods to and from Chicago than any other city in the US. St. Lawrence Seaway, opened in 1959, links the Great Lakes to the Atlantic Ocean and handles approx. 46 million short tons of cargo annually. Navy Pier, located downtown in Chicago Harbor, includes two of the 18 terminals in the city handling cargo ships and barges. River barges use the Chicago Sanitary & Ship Canal, which links Chicago with the MS River, giving the city access to the Gulf of Mexico and points E and W. Chicago-O'Hare Intl. Airport, the busiest in the world, is served by major domestic and intl. *airlines*, including AA, US Air, BN, CO, DL, EA, FT, FL, NC, NW, OZ, PA, PI, RD, SO, TW and US. Private and commuter lines serve Chicago Midway Airport and Meigs Field. *Bus lines* serving the city include Greyhound, Trailways and the local Chicago Transit Authority (CTA), a system of elevated and subway trains and buses as well as six commuter rail lines, which became part of the Regional Transit Authority (RTA) in 1974.

COMMUNICATIONS. Communications, broadcasting and print media originating from Chicago are *AM radio stations* WIND 560 (ABC/E, Talk. News); WMAQ 670 (NBC, C&W); WGN 720 (Indep., MOR, Talk, Sports, Farm); WBBM 780 (CBS, APR, UPI, News); WAIT 820 (Indep., Btfl. Mus.); WLS 890 (ABC/I, Contemp.); WJPC 950 (Natl. Blk., Contemp.); WCFL 1000 (Indep., Adult Contemp.); WMBI 1110 (Indep., Relig., Educ.); WJJD 1160 (ABC/I, C&W); WSBC (Indep., Ethnic), WCRW (Indep., Span., Greek, MOR) and WEDC (Indep., Span.) 1240 (they share time) and WVON 1390 (ABC/E, Blk.); *FM radio stations* WUIC 88.1 (Univ., Divers.); WZRD (Univ., Var.) and WHPK (Indep., Divers.) 88.3 (they share time); WBHI 88.5 (Indep., MOR, Btfl. Mus.); WCYC 88.7 (NPR, Divers.); WOUI 88.9 (Indep., Jazz); WKKC 89.3 (Univ., Divers.); WMBI 90.1 (Indep., Relig., Educ.); WBEZ 91.5 (UPI, NPR, Jazz, Divers.); WXRT 93.1 (Indep., Progsv.); WLAK 93.9 (Indep., Btfl. Mus.); WDAI 94.7 (ABC/FM, AOR); WMET 95.5 (APR, Top 40); WBBM 96.3 (CBS/FM, Mellow Contemp.); WNIB (Indep., Clas.); WEFM 99.5 (Indep., Top 40); WLOO 100.3 (Indep., APR, Adult Contemp.); WJEZ 104.3 (ABC/I, Contemp., Ctry.); and WGCI 107.5 (Indep., MOR) ; *television stations* WBBM Ch. 2 (CBS); WMAQ Ch. 5 (NBC); WLS Ch. 7 (ABC); WGN Ch. 9 (Indep.); WFLD Ch. 38 (Indep.) and WSNS Ch. 44 (Indep.); *press*: three major newspapers are published in the city, the *Tribune*, published mornings and evenings, the morning *Sun-Times*, and the evening *News*; other publications serving the area include the *Daily Defender, Beverly Review, Bilingual News, Blue Island-Calumet Park Index, Daily Law Bulletin, Bridgeport News, Community Reporter, El Manana, Independent Bulletin, El Informador, New*

The Art Institute of Chicago, Illinois

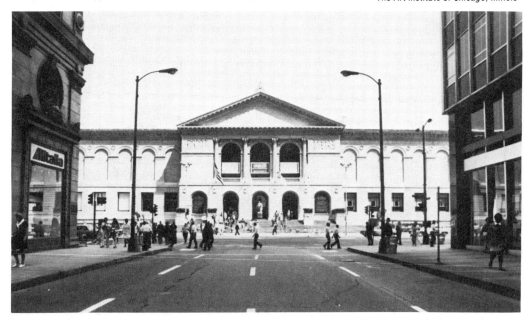

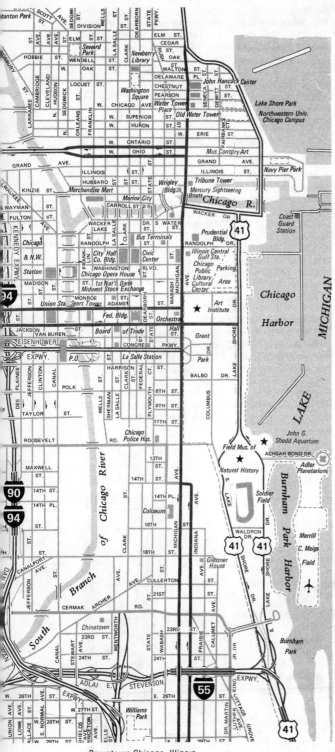

Downtown Chicago, Illinois

Crusader, *N Loop News, N Town News, NW Herald, NW Passage, NW Side Press, Observer, Portage Park Passage, Reporter, Skyline, S Suburban Opinion, South-* town *Economist Chicago Edition, SW News Herald, Star, Sun. Boaster, Suburbanite, Economist, W Side Times, Draugas, Dziennik Zwiazkowy, Hlastal Herald* and *Naujienos News.*

HISTORY. The area of present-day Chicago was first settled by native Americans around 3000 BC. The name of the city is derived from the "Chicagou" River, around which the peaceful Potawatomi tribe lived in the 1600s. The first white men to arrive in the area were French explorer Louis Joliet and Jesuit priest Jacques Marquette, who stopped in 1673 en route to Canada. French fur traders and missionaries followed until the Native Americans of the Fox tribe, located S of the area, closed the passage at the end of the century. About 1770, a black New Orleans fur trader, Jean Baptiste Point du Sable, established a prosperous business on the N bank of the mouth of the Chicago River. The trading post was the basis of one of the first permanent settlements in the area. Conflict between Native Americans and whites in the late 1700s led to the establishment of a blockhouse, Ft. Dearborn, on the river in 1803. Burned when the War of 1812 began, it was rebuilt again in 1816. The pop. of the settlement was 150 in 1833 when it was incorporated as a village, but reached 4,000 after local tribes were forced to leave the region for reservations in KS. In 1837, Chicago was incorporated as a city. Between 1848 and 1856, the city's RR system grew, it became the busiest rail center in the world and its pop. exceeded 100,000. During the Civil War, the economy of the city benefited from the development of the livestock, grain and manufacturing industries. By 1870, the pop. of the city had reached 300,000, aided by an influx of Polish, German and other European immigrants after the war. Chicago also became the lumber capital of the world—and most of its buildings were constructed of wood. The Great Fire of 1871, occurring after an unusually dry summer, burned for 24 hours. Supposedly set when Mrs. Patrick O'Leary's cow kicked over a lighted lantern in a barn, the fire destroyed the downtown section, took the lives of more than 300 people and left 90,000 homeless. In the aftermath, much of the city was redesigned by some of the most talented architects in the US. In 1884, William Le Baron Jenney built the first skyscraper in the world in the city. In 1886, the Haymarket Riot resulted from immigrant workers protesting their squalid living conditions. In 1889, Jane Adams and Ellen Starr founded the Hull House to help them adjust to city living. By 1890, 80% of the one million inhabitants were immigrants, or descended from immigrants, and the city was second only to NY in pop. The city hosted the 1893 World's Columbian Exposition, which drew attention to its enterprise and attracted 27 million visitors—nearly 50% of the US pop. During WW I, industry expanded to meet wartime needs, and many blacks moved to the city from the S. The largest race riot in the history of the city occurred in 1919. During the Roaring Twenties the city prospered, and was the home of many US artists, including writers Carl Sandburg and Upton Sinclair and jazz musicians Louis Armstrong and Benny Goodman. Prohibition contributed to activities such as bootlegging, and violent crime in the city peaked in the 1929 St. Valentines' Day Massacre gangster murders. The 1933 Century of Progress Exposition, celebrating Chicago's 100th anniversary since its incorporation as a village, offset the effects of the Depression. During the 1950s and 1960s, the downtown area experienced a building boom. The economy of the city remained strong, but the poor continued to arrive in increasing numbers as unskilled jobs grew scarce. During the 1960s and 1970s, growing social problems were handled ineffectively—public housing was poorly planned, many of the newcomers required welfare aid, neighborhoods became racially segregated, corrupt ward politics continued and race riots erupted. During the administration of "Boss" Mayor Richard Daley, demonstrating students—supporters of Eugene Mc-Carthy—and members of the media were roughly treated outside the Democratic Natl. Convention by overreacting city policemen. Subsequently, a series of govt. scandals contributed to the splintering of the city's political machine. In 1978, after the sudden death of Mayor Daley, Jane Byrne became the city's first woman mayor.

Exchange, the busiest exchange for future deliveries of agricultural products in the world, are located in the city. Approx. 90% of the nation's grain deliveries are contracted at the Chicago Board of Trade. In June, 1979, the total labor force of the greater met. area was approx. 3,460,100, while the rate of unemployment was 5.7%. In Jan., 1978 the city's labor force totaled 1,250,835, with 121,331 unemployed.

BANKING. There are 81 commercial banks and 23 savings and loan assns. in Chicago. In 1978, total deposits at the 131 banks headquartered in the city were $1,870,597,000, while assets were $2,284,858,000. Banks include Continental IL Natl. Bank and Trust, First Natl., Harris Trust and Savings, Northern Trust, American Natl. Bank and Trust, LaSalle Natl., Central Natl., Chicago Title and Trust and Sears Bank and Trust.

HOSPITALS. There are more than 90 hosps., health care centers and research facilities in Chicago, including Mt. Sinai, Cook Co., St. Luke's, U of

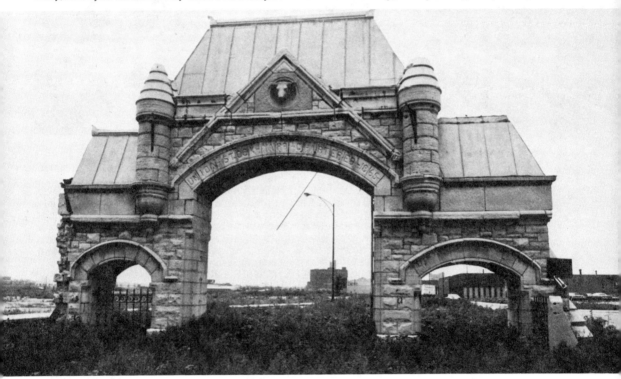

Entrance to Union Stockyards, Chicago, Illinois

GOVERNMENT. Chicago has a mayor-council form of govt. consisting of a 50-member council (the largest in the US) and the mayor, who all serve four-year terms. The councillors are elected by district while the mayor is elected at large. Council or state approval is required for many of the mayor's actions.

ECONOMY AND INDUSTRY. Chicago is the chief industrial, transportation, retail and wholesale trade and financial center of the Midwest. Approx. 14,000 manufacturing plants in the greater met. area employ nearly one million. The area ranks first in the US in the production of iron and steel, electrical equipment and supplies and machinery, as well as in the construction industry. It is also a major center of food production and printing and publishing, as well as a leader in nuclear research, with 1,200 industrial research laboratories located in the area. It is the leading consumer of nuclear power—nuclear power plants produce 30% of the area's electrical power. The Midwest Stock Exchange, the second largest securities market in the US, and the Mercantile

Chicago, NW Memorial, U of IL Medical Center and Rush Presbyterian. The Sonja Shankman Orthogenic School (the site of Bruno Bettelheims' research relating to the treatment of autistic children), La Rabida Institute (a center for research and treatment of childhood diseases) and Children's Memorial (a research and treatment center for children) are located in the city.

EDUCATION. The private U of Chicago, ranked among the top 10 research institutions in the US, was established in 1890 and endowed with $35 million by John D. Rockefeller in the early 1900s. In 1942, research at the U—recognized as the birthplace of nuclear energy—produced the first nuclear chain reaction. Well-known in physics and the biological and social sciences, the U enrolled more than 9,100 in 1978. De Paul U, founded in 1898, is one of the largest Roman Catholic institutions in the US, offering non-traditional programs through the School for New Learning and coopera-tive education in engineering. In 1978, nearly 11,400 enrolled. Chicago State U, established in 1867, offers nontraditional education through its U Without Walls, and enrolled more than 7,000 in 1978. The U of IL-Chicago Circle Campus enrolled close to 21,000 in 1978, and maintains a Medical

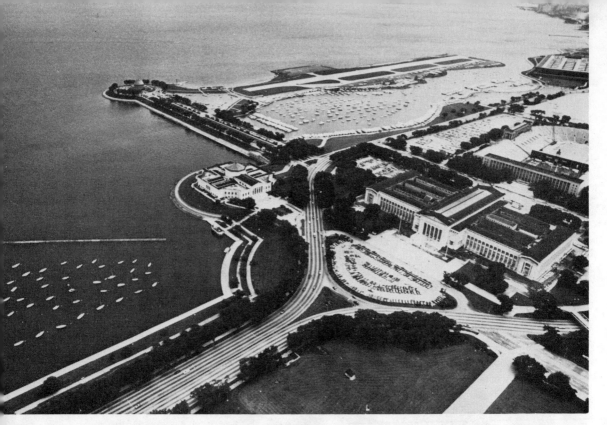

Aerial view of the Chicago waterfront showing Field Museum, Burnham Harbor, Adler Planetarium, Shedd Aquarium and Soldier Field on Lake Michigan, Chicago, Illinois.

Center, which enrolled more than 4,600 in 1978. Loyola U, founded in 1870, consists of six campuses in the Chicago area and one in Rome. More than 13,200 enrolled in 1978. The City Colleges of Chicago, including Chicago City-Wide, Kennedy-King, the Loop, Malcolm X, Olive-Harvey, Richard J. Daley, Truman and Wright colleges offered associate degrees to the nearly 47,800 who enrolled in 1978. Also located in the city are the Art Institute of Chicago, Roosevelt U, the IL Institute of Technology and the Medical, Dental and Law Schools of Northwestern U. The city public school system, third largest in the US, includes 556 elementary and 76 high schools and enrolled nearly 494,900 in 1978. Catholic schools include 238 elementary, enrolling close to 86,200 and 47 high schools, enrolling close to 15,000 in 1978. There are also nine Jewish elementary and two high schools. The Public Lib., the second largest in the US, contains 4,750,000 volumes, two regional and 79 branch libs., the IL Regional Lib. for the Blind and Physically Handicapped, a cultural center and numerous special collections. Other libs. include Newberry, an historical research lib., the Burnham Lib. of Architecture and Ryerson Art Lib. of the Art Institute, the Municipal Reference Lib. in City Hall, the Chicago Academy of Sciences Lib. and the Chicago Historical Society Lib.

ENTERTAINMENT. More than 200 parades are held in Chicago annually, including those on St. Patrick's Day, Memorial Day, Fourth of July, Bud Billiken Day (a variable Sat. in Aug.), Mexican Independence Day (Sept. 15), Chinese Independence Day (Oct. 10), Columbus Day, Veteran's Day and the Sun. after Thanksgiving, heralding the Christmas season. Ethnic celebrations include the Obon Dance Festival, featuring ritual Japanese dances in Old Town in mid-July; the Sicilian feast of St. Joseph, held on a Sun. in mid-Mar. and the German-American Festival for Baron von Steuben in mid-Sept. Other annual events include the Golden Glove Boxing Tournament, the first week in Feb.; World Flower and Garden and Auto shows in Mar.; an all-star football game in early Aug.; the Chrysanthemum Show in Nov. and Easter Sun. Sunrise Service in Soldier Field in Apr. Horse racing takes place in Maywood and Washington parks. The Chicago State U Maroons, U of Chicago Cougars and the U of IL at Chicago Chikas participate in intercollegiate sports. Professional sports teams include the Cubs, an NL

baseball team; the White Sox, an AL baseball team; the Bears, an NFL-NFC football team; the Black Hawks, an NHL hockey team and the Bulls, an NBA basketball team.

ACCOMMODATIONS. There are numerous hotels and motels in Chicago ranging in style from old-world elegance to space-age sophistication to those that are simple and economical. Among them are the Conrad Hilton, Marriott, Drake, Mart Plaza, Hotel Regency, Palmer House, Pick-Congress Hotel, Whitehall, Ritz-Carleton, Howard Johnson's, O'Hare Intl. Hotel, TraveLodge and the O'Hare American, Holiday, McCormick, Hilton, Rodeway, Ramada and Sheraton inns.

FACILITIES. Nearly 20% of the area of Chicago consists of parks and playgrounds—close to 600 parks encompass 6,700 acres. Facilities include 31 beaches on the 250-mi. shore of Lake MI, six golf courses, 669 tennis courts, eight yacht harbors, nearly 4,000 launching ramps, slips and moorings and 72 outdoor and 35 indoor swimming pools. Lincoln Park, the largest in the city, contains a zoo and a children's zoo, conservatory, bird sanctuary, beaches, playgrounds and facilities for golf, tennis, boating and horseback riding. The 200-acre Brookfield Zoo contains the Seven Seas Panorama, with a porpoise show and a children's zoo, featuring baby animals. The Forest Preserve District maintains 60,000 acres of parks along the city waterways and borders. There are approx. 20 mi. of unconnected bicycling and jogging paths along the lakefront. Boating facilities and fishing piers are available on Lake MI.

CULTURAL ACTIVITIES. The Chicago Symphony Orchestra performs at Orchestra Hall, and the Grant Park Symphony presents free concerts each summer. Other musical groups are the Civic Orchestra and the Lyric Opera Co. of Chicago, which performs in the Civic Opera House. The Drama School of the Art Institute presents performances at Goodman Memorial Theater. Second City, a nightclub-theater troupe, presents a syndicated television show. A number of experimental theater groups are based in New Town, on the mid N Side. The Aire Crown Theatre is the site of ballet, concert and theater productions throughout the year. "Theater on the Lake" is a summer series presented by the Park District, while winter theater takes place at Lincoln Park. Natural history exhibits are housed in the Field Museum, while astronomy is covered at nearby Adler Planetarium. The Chicago Academy of Science and the Chicago Historical Society features exhibits of city history. The Museum of Science and Industry includes a display of a working coal mine. The DuSable Museum of African-American History is named in honor of the city's first settler. The Oriental Institute at the U of Chicago contains a museum of ancient Near E civilizations, with exhibits dating from 3000 BC. Polish contributions to the US are chronicled in the Polish Museum of America, while exhibits at the Balzekas Museum of Lithuanian Culture span 800 years of Lithuanian history. The Art Institute of Chicago is noted for its collection of French Impressionist Art and the Jr. Museum, designed exclusively for children. Both the Goodman Children's Theater and the Jack and Jill Theater feature special presentations for children. The Archicenter features architectural exhibits. The Museum of Contemporary Art presents contemporary paintings, sculpture and other visual art forms. Other museums in the city are Ripley's Believe It or Not and the Royal London Wax museums.

LANDMARKS AND SIGHTSEEING SPOTS. The 110-story Sears Tower, the tallest building in the world, has a public observation deck on the 103rd floor. Daley Center Plaza features a five-story sculpture by Pablo Picasso. Other significant art works include an Alexander Calder stabile sculpture in the Fed. Building Plaza and a Marc Chagall ceramic mural, depicting the four seasons on Lake MI, which stands in the First Natl. Bank Plaza. The Board of Trade, one of the oldest and largest commodities exchanges in the world, features a visitor center overlooking the main trading floor. The Elks Natl. Memorial and Headquarters, dedicated to Elks who served in the two world wars, is of classic design, featuring a rotunda and reception rooms adorned with marble, murals, sculpture and wood paneling. Hull House, located on the Chicago Circle Campus of the U of IL, was established by Jane Addams, pioneer social worker and the first American woman to win the Nobel Peace Prize. The John Shedd Aquarium in Grant Park exhibits more than 10,000 fish and sea creatures. The Old Water Tower, completed in 1869, was one of few structures in the city that survived the Great Fire of 1871. The Stephen A. Douglas Historic Site is a 100'-high monument topped by a bronze statue of Douglas, who is buried beneath the memorial. Old Town, a restored German settlement dating from the 1870s, features ethnic architecture and stained glass windows. A 19th century mansion designed by Henry Hobson Richardson, the Glessner House is now headquarters of the Chicago School of Architecture Foundation. Chinatown, with interesting gift shops and restaurants, is another popular attraction.

CINCINNATI
OHIO

CITY-LOCATION-SIZE-EXTENT. Cincinnati, the seat of Hamilton Co., encompasses 78.46 sq. mi. on the N and S banks of the OH River in extreme SW OH, adjacent to KY on the S and IN on the W. at 39°09' N lat. and 84°31' W long. The greater met. area includes Hamilton and Warren counties and part of Clermont Co. to the SE and extends into Kenton, Campbell and Boone counties in KY as well as Dearborn Co. in IN.

TOPOGRAPHY. The terrain of Cincinnati, which is located in the OH River Valley and bisected by Mill Creek is generally hilly N of the OH River and even more rugged to the S. The central part of the city lies in the basin formed by deposits of the Licking River, while the E part of the city lies in the lower part of the Little Miami River Valley. The mean elev. is 550'.

CLIMATE. The climate of Cincinnati is continental, characterized by wide ranges in temp. and frequent weather changes, resulting from cyclonic storms in winter and spring and thunderstorms induced by warm, moist air from the Gulf of Mexico during the summer. The avg. annual temp. of 54°F ranges from a Jan. mean of 30°F to a July mean of 76°F. The avg. annual rainfall of 40" is fairly well distributed throughout the year, while most of the avg. annual 24.6" of snowfall occurs from Nov. through Mar. Major floods

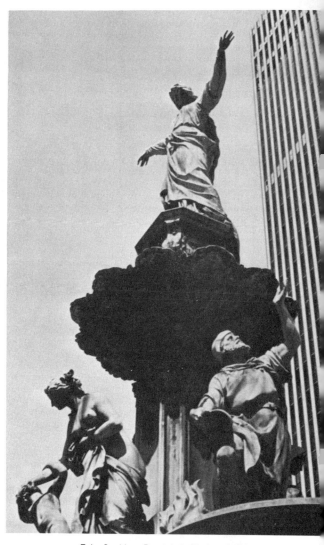

Tyler Davidson Fountain in Cincinnati, Ohio

occur about once in three years. The RH ranges from 53% to 88%. The avg. growing season is 190 days. Cincinnati lies in the ESTZ and observes DST.

FLORA AND FAUNA. Animals native to Cincinnati include the whitetail deer, fox, raccoon and opossum. Common birds are the mockingbird, flycatcher, swallow, bluebird and cardinal. Bullfrogs, pickerel frogs, Fowler's toads, salamanders, skinks, softshell turtles, box turtles and rat snakes, as well as the venomous copperhead, timber rattlesnake and E massasauga (pygmy rattler), are found in the area. Typical trees are the dogwood, sassafras, sycamore, hickory and oak. Smaller plants include buttercup, wood sorrel, elder and blackberry.

POPULATION. According to the US census, the pop. of Cincinnati in 1970 was 453,514. In 1978 it was estimated that it had decreased to approx. 383,000.

ETHNIC GROUPS. In 1978 the ethnic distribution of Cincinnati was approx. 71.8% Caucasian, 27.6% Black and 0.6% Hispanic.

TRANSPORTATION. Interstate hwys. 71, 74 and 75; US hwys. 27, 50, 52 and 127; and state rtes. 4, 16, 17, 19, 28, 125, 177, 264, 561 and 747 provide major motor access to Cincinnati. *Railroads* serving the city include AMTRAK, Chessie System, ConRail, Detroit, Toledo & Ironton, Family Lines, Norfolk and W and Southern. *Airlines* serving Greater Cincinnati Airport

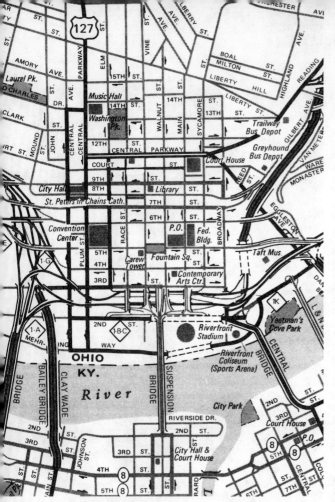

Downtown Cincinnati, Ohio

located S of the city in KY include US Air, AA, PI, DL, NC, EA, TW and Air KY. Lunken Municipal Airport and Blue Ash Field are served by commuter and private aircraft. *Bus lines* serving the city include Greyhound, Trailways and the local Transit Authority of N KY and the Queen City Metro. The port of Cincinnati which contains eight public and 41 private water terminals, handles approx. 10 million tons of cargo annually.

COMMUNICATIONS. Communications, broadcasting and print media serving Cincinnati are: *AM radio stations* WKRC 550 (ABC/E, MOR); WLW 700 (NBC, MOR); WZIP 1050 (UPI, Relig.); WUBE 1230 (Indep., C&W); WCLU 1320 (ABC/E, C&W); WSAI 1360 (ABC/C, Mod. Ctry.); WCIN 1480 (Natl., Blk.) and WCKY 1530 (CBS, ABC/1, Btfl. Mus.); *FM radio stations* WAIF 88.3 (Indep., Divers.); WNSD 90.I (Indep.); WGUC 90.9 (NPR, Clas., Pub. Affairs.); WVXU 91.7 (Indep., Var.); WWEZ 92.5 (Indep., Btfl. Mus.); WAKW 93.3 (UPI, Educ., Relig.); WSAI 94.1 (Indep., Rock); WLVV 94.9 (Indep.); WLWS 96.5 (CBS, Top 40); WLQA 98.5 (MBS, MOR); WHKK 100.9 (Indep., Relig.); WKRQ 101.9 (Indep., Top 40); WEBN 102.7 (Indep., AOR) and WUBE 105.1 (Indep., C&W); *television stations* WLWT Ch. 5.(NBC); WCPO Ch. 9 (CBS); WKRC Ch. 12 (ABC); WXIX Ch. 19 (Indep.) and WCET, Ch. 48 (PBS); *press:* the two major daily newspapers serving the city are the *Enquirer,* mornings, and the *Post,* issued weekday evenings and weekend mornings; other publications include the *Kurier, E Hills Journal, Hilltop News, Cincinnati Magazine, DAV Magazine, W Hills Press, Millcreek Valley News, Clermont Co. Review, Comm. Journal, Forest Hills Journal, Herald, NE Suburban Life, Queen City, Autobody and the Reconditioned Car, Dramatics, Hunting Dog, Modern Machine Shop, Pest Control Technology* and *Signs of the Times.*

HISTORY. Native Americans of the Miami tribe inhabited the area of present day Cincinnati prior to its founding by white settlers who named it Losantiville. Ft. Washington, providing protection for the surrounding

territory, was built in 1789. In 1790, Arthur St. Clair, Gov. of the NW Territory, renamed the settlement in honor of the Society of Cincinnati, an organization of Revolutionary War officers to which he belonged. The area grew rapidly after Gen. Wayne defeated the Miami tribe and the Treaty of Greenville was concluded in 1795. In 1799, the first legislature of the NW Territory met in the village under Gov. St. Clair and elected as its first delegate to Congress, William Henry Harrison, who later became Pres. of the U.S. As traffic on the OH River increased and more settlers arrived to begin farming in the area, the comm. continued to grow and was incorporated as a town in 1801. Steamboat navigation began in 1811, contributing to the town's growth as a trading center, and it was chartered as a city in 1819. The completion of the Miami and Erie Canal, begun in 1825, linked the city with communities in N OH. During the 1840s and 1850s, a large influx of immigrants, especially from Germany and Ireland, resulted in a tripling of the city's pop. when it ranked as the sixth largest in the US. By 1862, it had become the pork-packing center of the US. Such men as William Procter, James Gamble, Nicholas Longworth I, (who founded the local wine industry) and Christian Moerlein (who created the world's first lager beer) contributed to the economic development of the city, while such people as naturalist John James Audubon, painter Frank Duveneck, writers Lafcadio Hearn and Harriet Beecher Stowe and sculptor Clement Barnhorn contributed to its intellectual and cultural life. During the late 1800's, when RRs became the chief form of transportation, much of the city's trade activity was lost to Chicago. In the late 1800's, immigrants contributed to the development of industry in the city, which became the world's leader in machine tool manufacturing. Although the city's economic growth was halted by the Depression of 1929, 100,000 workers were involved in the manufacture of a large variety of products by 1932. During WW II, production of defense-related goods attracted many people from outlying rural areas to the city.

GOVERNMENT. Cincinnati has a council-mgr. form of govt., consisting of nine council members (including the mayor) elected at large to two-year terms. The council appoints a city mgr. and selects a mayor from its members.

ECONOMY AND INDUSTRY. There are about 2,000 manufacturing plants in the greater Cincinnati met. area employing approx. 32% of the total labor force. The world's leading producer of soap and playing cards, the city is also the largest manufacturer of machine tools in the US. Other major industries are automotive assembly and parts, aircraft engines, chemicals, apparel, cosmetics, meat packing and printing and publishing. Since 1967, service industries have grown at the expense of manufacturing. In 1979, the labor force of the greater met. area was 665,900, while the rate of unemployment was 5%.

BANKING. In 1978, total deposits for the six banks headquartered in Cincinnati were $3,244,375,000, while assets totaled $4,311,662,000. Banks include Provident, Central Trust Co. Natl., First Natl., Southern OH, N Side Bank and Trust and Fifth Third.

HOSPITALS. There are 27 hosps. in Cincinnati including Gen. (affiliated with the Medical Center of the U of Cincinnati), Good Samaritan (established in 1852), Jewish (established in 1854), St. Mary's (established in 1858, Bethesda, Christ, Deaconess, Booth Memorial, Christian R. Holmes, Our Lady of Mercy, Providence, St. Francis and V.A. Also located in the city are the Shriner's Burn Institute (one of only three in the US) and Children's Hosp., internationally known for its research center.

EDUCATION. The U of Cincinnati, founded in 1819 as the first municipal U in the US, grants associate, bachelor, master and doctorate degrees and in 1978, enrolled approx. 33,800. Xavier U, founded in 1831, enrolled approx. 6,400 in 1978. St. Gregory's Athenaeum of OH, founded in 1829, is a liberal arts institution for the preparation of candidates for the Roman Catholic priesthood. Other institutions include Edgecliff Col., OH Col., Cincinnati Bible Seminary, Hebrew Union Col. and Jewish Institute of Religion, which offers some programs in conjunction with the U of Cincinnati. The Cincinnati public school system includes about 120 elementary and high schools and enrolled approx. to 50,000 in 1978. Approx. 65 private and parochial schools enrolled an additional 50,000. Lib. facilities include the Public Lib. of Cincinnati and Hamilton Co. with about 40 branches, the Lloyd Lib. and the Cincinnati Historical Lib.

ENTERTAINMENT. Dinner theaters in Cincinnati include La Comedia and Beef 'N Boards. May Music Festival is annually held at the Cincinnati Music Hall. The Summer Fair, another annual event held at Old Coney on the OH River, features exhibits of local artists and craftsmen. The annual OH Valley Kool Jazz Festival is held at Riverfront Stadium which is the home of the Cincinnati Reds, an NL baseball team. The Cincinnati Bengals, an NFL-AFC football team and the Cincinnati Stingers, a CHL hockey team provide pro sports entertainment while the U of Cincinnati's Bearcats and the Xavier U teams participate in intercollegiate sports.

ACCOMMODATIONS. There are several hotels and motels in Cincinnati including the Days, Hilton, Best Western, Sheraton, Kings Island, Kings Point, Marriott, Ramada and Holiday inns and the Imperial House, Howard Johnson's and Stouffer's.

FACILITIES. There are about 100 municipal parks and 10 greenbelt areas, encompassing close to 3,900 acres in Cincinnati, including Mt. Airy, the first municipal forest in the US. The park system features picnic areas, golf courses, swimming pools, tennis courts, hiking and bicycling trails, boating facilities, playing fields and river frontage. The Cincinnati Recreation Commission operates 95 parks and recreation areas covering 2,395 acres, including Mt. Airy Arboretum, Ault Park, Civic Garden Center, Cornelius J. Hauck Botanic Garden, the 164-acre Eden Park, and the Cincinnati Zoo, which specializes in the breeding of endangered species.

CULTURAL ACTIVITIES. The Cincinnati Symphony and the Summer Opera perform at the Music Hall. The Cincinnati Ballet performs under the auspices of the Col. of Conservatory Music of the U of Cincinnati. Dramatic groups include the professional Playhouse in the Park, Edgecliff Col. Theatre, Showboat Majestic (one of the last original floating theaters) and the U of Cincinnati Theatre. The Cincinnati Art Museum features a collection of paintings, sculpture and prints spanning 5,000 years and a Near E collection. Cincinnati Historical Society is also located in the building. Emery Hall at Edgecliff Col. displays the works of student, natl. and intl. artists. The Taft Museum houses an art gallery and hosts concerts and lectures, while the Contemporary Art Center features changing exhibits. Other cultural organizations are the Cincinnati Museum of Natural History, the Cincinnati Nature Center and the Cincinnati Fire Dept. Historical Museum.

LANDMARKS AND SIGHTSEEING SPOTS. The Cincinnati riverfront is the homeport of the *Delta Queen* and *Mississippi Queen* steamboats, the only overnight sternwheelers still operating in the US. The Delta Queen is listed on the Natl. Register of Historic Places. Historic landmarks include the Tyler Davidson Fountain in Fountain Sq., presented to the city in 1871 by Henry Probasco; Elsinore Tower, inspired by a Shakespearean stage set and built in 1883 and originally serving as a valve house for the city waterworks; the Rookwood Pottery Building in which outstanding art pottery was produced from 1892 until the 1940s; Eden Park Water Tower, operated by the waterworks dept. until 1908 and the Melan Arch Bridge, graced by stone eagles and the oldest concrete bridge in the state (built in 1894). The scalloped-arch Springhouse was built in 1905 over a spring reputed to have medicinal values. The largest swinging bell in the world hangs in St. Francis de Sales Church. Historic homes include the Harriet Beecher Stowe House, the home of the author of *Uncle Tom's Cabin* and headquarters of an anti-slavery organization, and the birthplace of Pres. William Howard Taft. Prominent city buildings include City Hall, a Romanesque structure; Carew Tower, a

48-story skyscraper; the Music Hall, more than 100 years old; Union Terminal; St. Peter-in-Chains Cathedral (1841) and the Isaac M. Wise Temple (1865).

CLEVELAND
OHIO

CITY LOCATION-SIZE-EXTENT. Cleveland, the seat of Cuyahoga Co. encompasses 76.5 sq. mi. in NE OH, on the S shore of Lake Erie, at the mouth of the Cuyahoga River, at 42°25' N lat. and 81°52' W long. The lake frontage of the met. area—which extends throughout Cuyahoga Co. and into surrounding Lake, Portage, Geauga, Summit, Medina and Lorain counties—extends for 31 mi.

TOPOGRAPHY. Cleveland is situated on a plateau approx. 100' above lake level, except for an abrupt ridge which rises on the E edge of the city. The Cuyahoga River bisects the city and creates a deep, narrow N-S valley. The mean elev. is 660'.

CLIMATE. Climate in Cleveland is continental, with wide ranging weather conditions. When winds are from the N or W, Lake Erie strongly influences the city's weather. The 50°F avg. annual temp. ranges from a Jan. mean of 27°F to a July mean of 72°F. The 34" avg. annual rainfall is evenly distributed throughout the year. Most of the 50" avg. annual snowfall occurs from Dec. to Mar. Tornadoes occasionally occur in the area. The RH ranges from 57% to 86%. Cleveland lies in the ESTZ and observes DST.

FLORA AND FAUNA. Animals native to Cleveland include the fox squirrel, raccoon, groundhog, whitetail deer, opossum, muskrat and grey squirrel. Common birds are the robin, sparrow, gull, blue jay, swallow and woodpecker. Water birds found on Lake Erie increase in numbers during migration. Bullfrogs, Fowler's toads, tiger salamanders, milk snakes, skinks and soft-shelled turtles and the venomous copperhead, E massasauga (a pygmy rattler), and timber rattlesnake are found here. Typical trees are the maple, oak, juniper, hickory and sycamore. Smaller plants include the viburnum, forsythia, mock orange shrub, dogwood, elder and blackberry bush.

POPULATION. According to the US census, the pop. of Cleveland in 1970

Home of the Cleveland Orchestra, Cleveland, Ohio

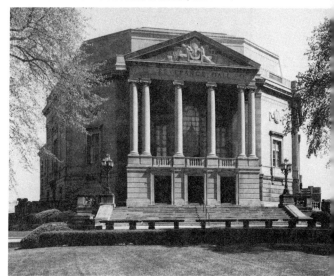

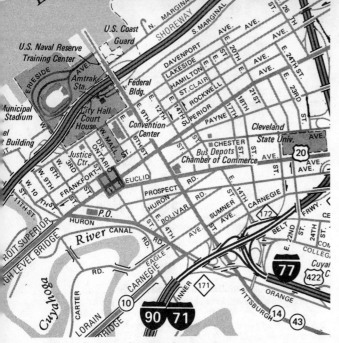

Downtown Cleveland, Ohio

was 750,879. In 1978, it was estimated that it had decreased to 580,000.

ETHNIC GROUPS. In 1978, the ethnic distribution of Cleveland was approx. 61.1% Caucasian, 38.3% Black and 1.9% Hispanic (a percentage of the Hispanic total is also included in the Caucasian total).

TRANSPORTATION. Interstate hwys. 71, 77 and 90, US hwys. 6 and 20 and State Rte. 2 provide major motor access to Cleveland. The city is served by five *railroads*, ConRail, AMTRAK, Chessie System, Norfolk & Western and Newburgh & S Shore. *Airlines* serving Cleveland's Hopkins Intl., Burke Lakefront and Cuyahoga Co. airports include Air Canada, US Air, AA, BN, DL, EA, NC, NW, TW, UA and FW. *Bus lines* providing service include Trailways, Gray Line, Greyhound, Cleveland Transit System (CTS) and the intra-county Regional Transit Authority (RTA), which also provides rail rapid transit. The Cleveland World Port, one of Lake Erie's major ports, serves 40 steamship lines and ships of 150 world ports in 70 countries.

COMMUNICATIONS. Communications, broadcasting and print media serving Cleveland are: *AM radio stations* WJW 850 (CBS, Pers., MOR); WWWE 1100 (NBC, Contemp., Spts.); WGAR 1220 (Natl. Comm., Adult Contemp.); WBBG 1260 (ABC, Talk); WERE 1300 (ABC and Mutual, All News); WHK 1420 (Indep., C&W), the oldest radio station in OH; WJMO 1490 (Natl. Blk., R&B) and WABQ 1540 (Mut. Blk., R&B); *FM radio stations* WCSB 89.3 (Indep., Var.); WBOE 90.3 (Indep.); WRUW 91.1 (Indep., Var.); WZAK 93.1 (Indep., For. Lang.); WCLV 95.5 (Indep., Clas.); WGCL 98.5 (Indep., Top 40); WKSW 99.5 (Indep., Easy List., Inst.); WMMS 100.7 (Indep., Progsv. Rock); WDOK 102.1 (Indep., Easy List.); WQAL 104.1 (Indep., Easy List.); WWWM 105.7 (Indep., Adult Rock) and WZZP 106.5 (Indep., Contemp. Rock, For. Lang.-Sun.); *television stations* WKYC Ch. 3 (NBC); WEWS Ch. 5 (ABC); WJKW Ch. 8 (CBS); WVIZ Ch. 25 (PBS) and WUAB Ch. 43 (Indep.); *press:* the major daily newspapers are the *Press*, published evenings and Sun., *Plain Dealer*, issued mornings and Sun., and *Daily Legal News;* other publications include *Call and Post* (a Blk. weekly), *Industry Week, S End News, Journal* (weekly), *Sun* (weekly), *Foundry Management* and *Technology, Govt. Product News, Hydraulics* and *Pneumatics, Machine Design, Materials Engineering, Midwest Purchasing, New Equipment Digest, OH Farmer, OH Motorist, Golf Business* and *Cleveland Magazine.* There are nine nationality papers—six weekly, three semi-monthly.

HISTORY. Cleveland was established July 22, 1796, at the mouth of the Cuyahoga River by Gen. Moses Cleaveland, head surveyor of the CT Land Co., a private firm which undertook the settlement of the town. Incorporated as a village in 1814, Cleveland remained a frontier village for some 30 years. By 1832, however,

with the opening of the Erie Canal, it emerged as a manufacturing and business center for N OH. In 1836, it was granted a city charter. Its mills and factories, which served the Midwest's new settlers, continued to expand. During the Civil War, machinery and equipment were in increased demand, and the accessibility of iron ore from the Lake Superior region and coal from OH and PA resulted in the city's emergence as an important iron and steel producing center. In 1870, John D. Rockefeller established Standard Oil Co. in Cleveland and the city became the chief refining center for much of PA's oil. Between 1850 and 1870, its pop. increased from approx. 17,000 to more than 145,000. During the latter part of the 1800s, the city's rapid industrial growth attracted many immigrants, chiefly from E Europe and Russia. The city's steel manufacturing industry benefited from the development of the automobile industry in the early 1900s. In both WW I and II, large quantities of armaments were produced in Cleveland. Because of the availablility of work, many people—especially blacks—immigrated to the city from throughout the US. In the 1950s, the trend to suburban living resulted in a decrease in the city's pop. A series of racial problems during the 1960s was moderated by the election of Carl B. Stokes, the first black mayor of a major US city, in 1967.

GOVERNMENT. Cleveland has a mayor-council form of govt. The mayor, elected at large to a two-year term, neither votes nor is a member of the council. The 33 council members, elected by each of the city's 33 wards to two-year terms, select one member to act as council pres.

ECONOMY AND INDUSTRY. The headquarters of 28 of the 1,000 largest industrial corporations in the US (based on sales) are located in Cleveland. Because the economy is based strongly on industry, the city is vulnerable to economic slumps. Cleveland is a major intl. center for diversified manufacturing, including steel, non-electrical machinery, fabricated metal products and primary metals, transportation equipment, electric and electronic equipment, chemicals and allied products and printing and publishing. In 1977, nearly 130,000 people were employed in the manufacturing sector. The same year, the total labor force was 256,000, with 21,000 unemployed. The shipping port has a tremendous impact on the economy of the area, handling 800,000 tons of cargo annually. It provides more than 500 jobs on the waterfront and another 10,000 jobs in the transportation and distribution of the cargoes. Port-related industries account for another 89,000 jobs. Greater Cleveland is also a center for foreign investment, with 80 foreign-owned or joint-venture operations located in the area. Recently, there has been an increase in the construction of residential apartments and office buildings in the downtown area. By the end of 1978, more than five million sq. ft. of space had been added.

BANKING. There are 11 commercial banks and 22 savings and loan assns. in Cleveland. In 1978, total deposits for the eight banks headquartered in the city were $13,390,218, while assets totaled $10,030,458. Banks include Cleveland Trust, Natl. City, Euclid Natl., Central Natl., Society Natl., Midwest Bank and Trust, First Natl. Bank, Union Commerce and Fed. Reserve Bank.

HOSPITALS. Hospitals serving Cleveland include St. Vincent Charity (noted for one of the first aortic heart valve transplants and refinements in the heart-lung machine), St. John's, Fairview Gen., V.A., Cleveland Met. Gen., St. Luke's, St. Alexis, Mt. Sinai Hosp. of Cleveland and Lutheran Medical Center. World-renowned health science institutions such as the U Hosps. (a complex of seven hosps. and one of only three Cystic Fibrosis Institutes in the US), Case W Reserve U Schools of Medicine, Dentistry and Nursing and

Cleveland Clinic (one of the largest group-practice medical complexes in the world and a pioneer in diagnostic and surgical techniques for coronary artery disease) are located in the U Circle area.

EDUCATION. Case W Reserve U (CWRU), a private indep. school formed in 1967 by the federation of W Reserve U (established in 1826) and Case Institute of Technology (founded in 1880) offer bachelor, master and doctorate degree programs and enrolled approx. 8,500 in 1978. Cleveland State U (CSU), established in 1965, enrolled more than 18,000 students at the bachelor, master and doctorate degree levels in 1978. Other institutions in the city include OH Col. of Podiatric Medicine, which enrolled more than 500 in 1978; Cleveland Institute of Art, enrolling over 500 in 1978 and granting the BFA degree; Cleveland Institute of Music, enrolling 350 and granting the bachelor degree; Dyke Col., enrolling 1,700 and granting the AS and BS degrees; and Cuyahoga Comm. Col., a two-year institution, enrolling a total of approx. 27,000 at all three campuses. The public school system includes approx. 180 schools, with a total enrollment of almost 150,000. Another 150,000 attend more than 250 parochial and private schools in the city. The Cleveland Public Lib., which operates over 35 branches, was one of the first in the nation to adopt the open-stacks plan, allowing the public to select books directly from shelves. The Freiberger Lib. at CWRU and the gen. and law libs. at CSU are also available to the public.

ENTERTAINMENT. Dinner theaters in Cleveland include the Playhouse Sq. Palace and You Are Cabaret. The city hosts the annual Home and Flower Show, art shows, All Nations Festival held downtown in the spring and the Natl. Air Show in the summer. The Cleveland Browns, one of the NFL's oldest football teams, competes in the AFC. The Cleveland Indians baseball team plays in the AL, while the Cleveland Cavaliers compete in the NBA. The Cleveland Cobras is a professional soccer team which plays summer, while the Force plays winter professional soccer. The Competitors is a professional softball team. The Cuyahoga Comm. Col. Cougars, the CSU Vikings and the CWRU Spartans participate in intercollegiate sports.

ACCOMODATIONS. Among the hotels and motels in downtown Cleveland are the Cleveland Plaza and Bond Court hotels, the Hollenden House, Stouffer's Inn on the Sq., Park Plaza, Sheraton Hopkins, Swingo's Keg and Quarter, Howard Johnson's and Holiday, Charter House, Marriott, TraveLodge and Ramada inns.

FACILITIES. There are several parks in downtown Cleveland, including Chester Commons, Willard Park, Donald Grey Gardens, Huron Road Mall and Hanna Fountain Mall. Other city parks are Lakefront, Brookside and Rockefeller. Heritage Park, a one-acre parcel of land on the Cuyahoga River, about 400' from the site where Moses Cleaveland landed in the city on July 22, 1796, commemorates the origins of Cleveland. It was a comm. contribution to the US bicentennial celebration. A unique aspect of the Cleveland area is its 17,000-acre Metroparks system, often referred to as "The Emerald Necklace", which offers such recreational facilities as a zoo, tennis courts, horseback riding, golf courses, bike paths, playgrounds, picnic areas and wildlife sanctuaries. The Cuyahoga Valley Natl. Recreation Area, located between Cleveland and Akron, contains the Boston Mills ski area. Public golf courses include Highland Park, Shawnee Hills, Sleepy Hollow, Seneca, Mastic Woods and the Rocky River courses. The city maintains numerous swimming pools, both indoor and outdoor. Both swimming and boating facilities are provided on the shores of Lake Erie, where there are 1600 boat slips at public and private marinas. There are several jogging tracks located in the area, at Tremont Valley, Woodland Hills and the 13th St. Racquet Club.

CULTURAL ACTIVITIES. The internationally-acclaimed Cleveland Symphony Orchestra, which performs in Severance Hall, the Cleveland Ballet Co., which performs in Hanna Theatre, and the Opera Theatre contribute to Cleveland's cultural life. Playhouse Sq. contains several theaters, Hanna, Allen, Ohio, Front Row, State and Palace, in which dramatic and musical performances are presented. Professional repertory theater is performed at the Cleveland Playhouse and Centerep Theatre. The Shakespeare Festival Theatre is also located in the city. Karamu House, an experimental theater with integrated casts, opened in 1915 as a means of promoting racial understanding. Other performances are held at the

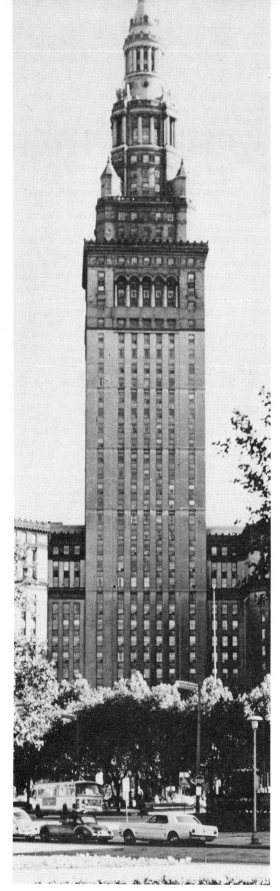

Terminal Tower, Cleveland, Ohio

Cleveland Public Auditorium and Kulas Hall at the Cleveland Institute of Music. "Peoples and Cultures", an organization which promotes folk art and life, was formed in Cleveland, in 1971, to enhance ethnic and racial harmony. The Cleveland Museum of Art features one of the world's finest collections of oriental art. Other museums include the Dali Museum, presenting several of Salvadore Dali's works, the Cleveland Museum of Natural History, Howard Dittrick Museum of Historical Medicine, Cleveland Health Museum, Dunham Tavern Museum (built in 1824 as a stopping place on an old stage road), W Reserve Historical Society (containing historical and auto-aviation museums) and the Garden Center of Greater Cleveland. There are approx. 30 art galleries, including Nova, New, Mayer, Bonfoey and Vixseboxe, in the city.

LANDMARKS AND SIGHTSEEING SPOTS. The Cleveland Arcade, built in 1890, is an historic landmark which features a five-story, glass-roofed gallery of more than 100 shops. The 40-plus story Terminal Tower located downtown was the tallest building outside of New York City when built in 1928. The 125' high Soldiers-Sailors Monument, built of black granite, stone and bronze, stands in Public Sq. as a symbol of the Civil War. The Old Stone Church, first erected in 1834 and later destroyed by fire in 1853, is a Presbyterian church reconstructed in 1855, with stained glass windows designed by Louis Tiffany. Union Commerce Bank has the largest bank lobby in the US, and the Cleveland Trust Co. features a 61'-in-diameter Tiffany glass dome in its rotunda. The masterpiece version of the famous painting "Spirit of '76" (the first version of which was executed in the city in 1876) is displayed in the rotunda of Cleveland City Hall. The Moses Cleaveland Landing and the Moses Cleaveland Statue are two landmarks commemorating the city's founding. Other landmarks are the Erie Street Cemetery, a mass grave of the city's first residents, and the Garfield Monument in Lakeview Cemetery, containing the tomb of Pres. James A. Garfield. The Lorenzo Carter Cabin Site, which served as an early trading post and meeting house, was rebuilt at Heritage Park under the High Level Bridge in 1976. Mall Plaza, adjacent to the Convention Center, contains the beautiful Hanna and War Memorial fountains. The NASA Lewis Research Center and the Cleveland Aquarium are two popular sightseeing spots. Settler's Landing in "The Flats" on the E and "Ohio City" on the W sides of the Cuyahoga River contain restored and original homes and buildings. Cruises on the river and around the harbor are conducted on the 500-passenger *Goodtime II*.

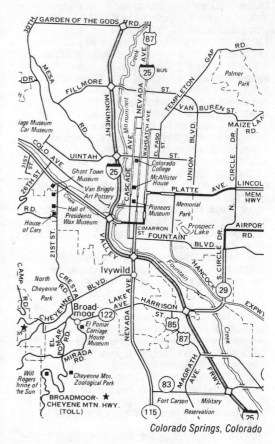

Colorado Springs, Colorado

COLORADO SPRINGS
COLORADO

CITY LOCATION-SIZE-EXTENT. CO Springs, the seat of El Paso Co. and second largest city in the state, encompasses 85.3 sq. mi. in central CO at 38°49' N lat. and 104°50' W long. Located 70 mi. S of Denver, the city is located in the AR River drainage basin. The 14,100' Pikes Peak of the Rocky Mt. Range is located about 10 mi. W of the city on US 24 through Ute Pass. The greater met. area extends N into Douglas Co. and W into Teller Co.

TOPOGRAPHY. The terrain of CO Springs, which is situated on a semi-arid plateau on the E slope of the Rocky Mts., is relatively flat. The mts. to the W rise abruptly above the plateau to avg. heights of 11,000'. Gently rolling prairie lies to the E of the city, while to the N the land slopes upward towards the Palmer Lake Divide. The mean elev. is 6,145'.

CLIMATE. The climate of CO Springs is continental, influenced by the Rocky Mts. to the W which protect the area from temp. extremes and the high elev. which ensures cool, although sunny summers. The sun shines an avg. of 310 days per year. The avg. annual temp. of 48.3°F ranges from a Jan. mean of 29°F to a July mean of 70.8°F. Some 80% of the avg. annual 15" of rainfall occurs from Apr. to Sept., primarily during thunder-

storms. The avg. annual snowfall is 40", while the RH ranges from 34% to 70%. The avg. growing season is 149 days. CO Springs lies in the MSTZ and observes DST.

FLORA AND FAUNA. Animals native to CO Springs include the mule deer, porcupine, otter, black bear and coyote. Common birds are the golden eagle, snipe, scrub jay, phoebe and mt. bluebird. Leopard frogs, box turtles and bull snakes, as well as the venomous rattlesnake, are found in the area. Typical trees are the white fir, ponderosa pine and willow. Smaller plants include the penstemon, lupine, gilia and wild thistle.

POPULATION. According to the US census, the pop. of CO Springs in 1970 was 135,060. In 1978, it was estimated that it had increased to 200,000.

ETHNIC GROUPS. In 1978, the ethnic distribution of CO Springs was approx. 85% Caucasian, 5.2% Black, 8.5% Hispanic and 1.3% other.

TRANSPORTATION. Interstate hwy. 25, US hwys. 24, 85 and 87 and state hwys. 1, 2, 4, 27, 83, 94, 115 and 122 provide major motor access to CO Springs. *Railroads* serving the city include the Denver & Rio Grande, Rock Island, Santa Fe and Burlington. *Airlines* serving CO Springs Municipal Airport include BN, CO, TW, FL and Rocky Mt. *Bus lines* include Greyhound, Trailways and CO Springs Coach.

COMMUNICATIONS. Communications, broadcasting and print media originating from CO Springs are: *AM radio stations* KSSS 740 (NBC, Mod. Ctry.); KRDO 1240 (MBS, MOR); KVOR 1300 (ABC/E, MOR); KYSN 1460 (UPI, Top 40); KXXV 1530 (ABC/E, Progsv., Top 40) and KPIK 1580 (ABC/C, Intermt., C&W); *FM radio stations* KRCC 91.5 (NPR, Clas., Jazz, Var.); KVOR 92.9 (ABC/E, MOR); KILO 93.9 (Indep.); KRDO 95.1 (MBS, Btfl. Mus.); KKFM 96.5 (Indep., AOR); KINX 101.9 (Indep., Contemp.) and KEPC 90.5 (ABC/FM, Educ., Var.); *television stations* KOAA Ch. 5 (NBC); KTSC Ch. 8 (PBS); WKTV Ch. 11 (CBS) and KRDO Ch. 13 (ABC); *press*: two major dailies serve the city, the *Sun* issued mornings, and the *Gazette*

Telegraph, issued mornings and evenings; other publications include the *Falcon News, Mountaineer, Aerospace Observer, Rampart Review, Sparkles, Numismatist, Western Horseman* and *Bookstore Journal.*

HISTORY. The site of present-day CO Springs lies along a trail used by native Americans of the Arapahoe tribe before the first white settlers arrived in the area. In 1858, gold seekers from KS laid out the town of El Paso, meaning "the pass", in a narrow two-mi.-long strip of land along the trail at Ute Pass by Fountain Creek. Named El Dorado (meaning "the gold") City in 1859, it was renamed CO City in 1866, and has, since 1917, been known as "Old Town", or W CO Springs. The town of Fountain Colony was planned to the E of CO City by Civil War hero Gen. Willam J. Palmer, who came from Philadelphia, PA, and a promoter of the Denver and Rio Grande W RR. Incorporated in 1871 as a health resort for wealthy Easterners, Fountain Colony was later renamed CO Springs for the mineral springs located six mi. away at Manitou. The planning of broad avenues, expansive parks and lots for schools and churches, as well as the promotion of the area by the RR as a scenic wonderland and health resort and the establishment of tubercular sanitariums by physicians, attracted many wealthy immigrants to the city. Among them were numerous Englishmen, for whom the city received its nickname of "Little London". In 1873, the city became the co. seat and, in 1874, CO Col. was established. Productive gold mines at nearby Pikes Peak contributed to the stability of the economy. Between 1900 and 1910, it was claimed that the city was the wealthiest per capita in the US and its pop., including wealthy artists and writers who contributed to the high standard of living, increased from 11,000 to nearly 20,000. The mt. parks system, created in 1907, received the famous Garden of the Gods two years later when it was bequeathed to the city. During the Depression, increasingly high gold prices enabled the city to maintain a strong economic base. The establishment of Camp Carson in 1941, Peterson Field in 1948, NORAD in 1957, the USAF Academy nearby in 1958, continual annexations, and the city's dry mt. air constantly attracted tourists and clean industry contributed to the growth of its pop. from nearly 45,500 in 1950 to approx. 70,200 in 1960. Since 1960, its pop., which continues to boom, has more than doubled.

GOVERNMENT. CO Springs has a council-mqr. form of govt. Five of the nine council members, including the mayor, are elected at large, while the remaining four are elected by district. All serve four-year terms and appoint a city mqr.

ECONOMY AND INDUSTRY. Trade, govt., services and manufacturing are the major employers in CO Springs.

Colorado Springs with Buena Vista and The Pikes Peak in the background, Colorado Springs, Colorado

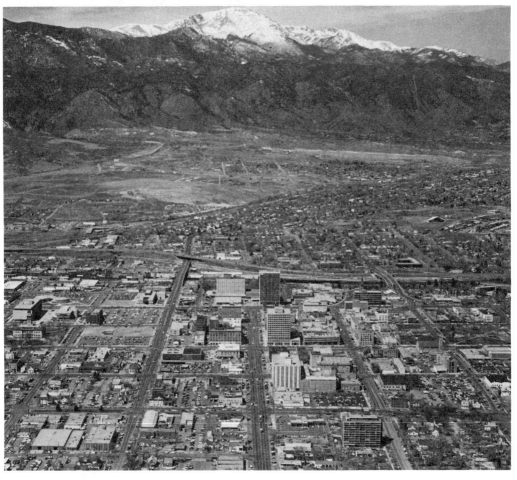

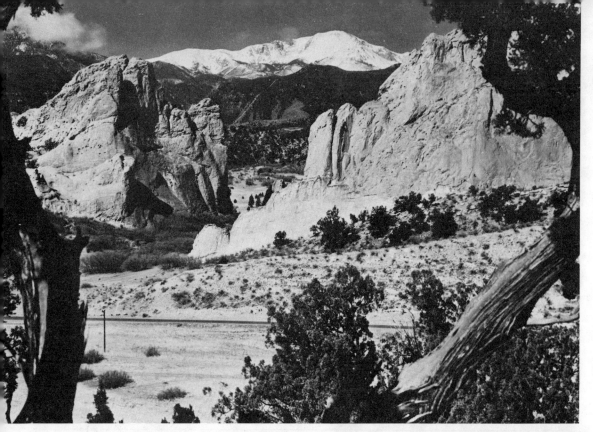

Natural rock formation in Colorado Springs, Colorado

Beet sugar products, mining equipment, mini computers, electronic equipment, construction material, agricultural irrigation, greeting cards and stationery, medical products, hand tools, locks, security equipment and automobile accessories are among the major manufacturers. In 1978, the labor force totalled 114,230, while the rate of unemployment was 4.5%. In 1977, the median household income was $12,697.

BANKING. In 1978, total deposits for the 21 banks headquartered in CO Springs were $716,164,000, while assets totaled $815,361,000. Among the banks serving the city are First Natl., Exchange Natl., CO Springs Natl., United, Central, American Heritage, W Natl. and Pikes Peak Natl.

HOSPITALS. There are nine hosps. in CO Springs including CO Springs Comm., St. Francis, Memorial, Penrose, Eisenhower Osteopathic and Emory John Brady.

EDUCATION. The U of CO at CO Springs, established in 1965, enrolled approx. 3,100 undergrad. and 1,300 grad. students in 1978. The USAF Academy, established in 1958, enrolled approx. 4,150 in 1978, while Pikes Peak Comm. Col., a two-year institution established in 1967, enrolled approx. 4,950 in 1978. CO Col., established in 1874, enrolled approx. 1,900 in 1978. Other institutions in the city are Nazarene Bible Col., Blair Business Col., CO Springs Col. of Business, CO Technical Col., Natl. Col. of Business and Technical Trades Institute. The public school system, consisting of 83 elementary and jr. and 10 high schools, enrolled approx. 43,650 in 1978. In addition, four private high schools, including one parochial school and the Springs School for the Deaf and Blind, are located in the city. Lib. facilities include the CO Springs Penrose Lib. which maintains bookmobile service to outlying areas.

ENTERTAINMENT. Among the dinner theaters in CO Springs include the Iron Springs Chateau and Playhouse and the Flying W Chuckwagon Suppers and Western Show. The headquarters of the Professional Rodeo Cowboys Assn.(PRCA) which sanctions 600 rodeos per year, as well as that of the US Olympic Commitee and Training Center, are located in the city. Annual events held in the city include the Natl. Sports Festival, featuring approx. 30 different sports events and 3,000 participants; the Fine Arts Festival,

held at Miramont Castle every Memorial Day; Graduation Week at the USAF Academy; and Little Britches Rodeo in June and on July 4. Pikes Peak Auto Climb and the Range Riders Street Breakfast are held downtown. The Pikes Peak or Bust Rodeo, featuring top stock and nationally ranked cowboys, is held in Aug., while a display of fireworks on the top of Pikes Peak is featured for New Years Eve. The Broadmoor ice review features natl. and intl. figure skating champions in performance at the World Arena. Teams of the U of CO, CO Col. and the USAF Academy participate in intercollegiate sports.

ACCOMMODATIONS. There are several hotels and motels in CO Springs, including the Antlers Plaza and Broadmoor hotels, the Garden Valley, Four Seasons and Embers motels, Palmer House, Sheraton, Hilton, Holiday and Ramada inns

FACILITIES. There are 76 public parks and playground areas emcompassing more than 4,000 acres in CO Springs. The Garden of the Gods, located NW of the city and part of the mt. parks system, features the Cathedral Spires and other rock formations of red sandstone inside the massive Gateway Rocks. High Drive, also part of the city's mt. park system, leads up the mts. via N Cheyenne Canyon and down through Bear Creek canyon. Other parks include Straton Park, Pikes Peak Natl. Park and the 700-acre Palmer Park on Austin Bluffs. Facilities include two public golf courses, tennis courts, picnic areas and hiking, bicycling and jogging trails. Swimming, fishing and skiing facilities are also located nearby.

CULTURAL ACTIVITIES. There are 13 major museums and galleries in CO Springs as well as several cultural organizations, including the Broadmoor Intl. Center, CO Springs Symphony, CO Springs Civic Theatre, CO Springs Fine Arts Center and the CO Col. Theatre. Among the museums are the Manitou Cliff Dwellings Museum and outdoor museum which depicts the lives and architectural achievements of Native Americans of the SW during the Great Pueblo Period (1,100-1,300 A.D.). The May Natural History Museum which exhibits invertebrates from remote jungles of the world and contains the Golden Eagle Safari Campgrounds and resort; the Buffalo Bill Wax Museum, which features wax figures of W pioneers; the Hall of Presidents Wax Museum, which contains displays of all the US presidents and some first ladies; the Pioneers' Museum which features historical and archeological collections; the Natl. Carvers Museum, which features woodcarvings; the Doll and Carriage Museum, at the entrance to the Garden of the Gods, which features a collection of 1,300 dolls and carriages dating from 1858; the El Pomar Carriage House Museum, which displays old vehicles, saddles and other riding accessories and the House of Cars Museum, which features restored antique and classic automobiles. The Fine Arts Center houses an art gallery, museum, theater, studios and art school. The Ghost Town Museum features buildings of the past while the W Museum of Mining and Industry displays machinery used in hardrock mining for gold and silver.

LANDMARKS AND SIGHTSEEING SPOTS. There are several natural and man-made landmarks in CO Springs. Miramont Castle features nine different types of architecture, including Gothic, Romanesque and Tudor. The 1.25-mi.-long Mt. Manitou Scenic Incline Railway, the longest in the US, leads to the top of Mt. Manitou, while the Pikes Peak Cog Railway, the highest in the US, travels to the top of Pikes Peak. The USAF Academy, which contains a planetarium, features a visitors center, and tours are conducted daily. Seven Falls, which can be seen from Eagle's Nest, is illuminated in summer. Tours 2.5 hours in duration are also conducted daily through the N American Air Defense Command (NORAD), which maintains a 24-hour alert to warn against air attack. Cave of the Winds, noted for its high alt. (7,000') and colorful rock formations, may be reached via Serpentine Drive through Williams Canyon, a spectacular scenic drive, as are the 36-mi.-long Gold Camp Road over the roadbed of the old Cripple Creek Short Line RR and the Broadmoor-Cheyenne Mt. Highway. At the top of this hwy., which winds up the E face of Cheyenne Mt., are the Cheyenne Mt. Zoological Park and, at an elev. of 8,000', the Shrine of the Sun, a granite tower memorial to Will Rogers. Santa's Workshop on Pikes Peak Hwy. in N Pole, CO, features Santa, his reindeer, toymakers, glassblowers, potters and candlemakers at work. Other landmarks include the McAllister House, built in 1873 of bricks from Philadelphia, PA, and containing period furnishings; a bronze statue of Gen. Palmer, the city's founder, sitting on a horse and gazing W toward Pikes Peak, and the Professional Rodeo Hall of Champions, featuring a display of 50 years of world champions which opened in 1979.

COLUMBIA
SOUTH CAROLINA

CITY LOCATION-SIZE-EXTENT. Columbia, the state capital and seat of Richland Co. and largest city in the state, encompasses 108.6 sq. mi. in central SC on the E bank of the Congaree River, S of the junction of the Broad and Saluda rivers, at 33°57' N lat. and 81°7' W long. The greater met. area includes the cities of W Columbia, Cayce and Forest Acres and extends throughout Richland Co. and into Lexington Co. to the SW.

TOPOGRAPHY. The terrain of Columbia, which is situated near the division between the Piedmont region and the Atlantic coastal plain, is characterized by rolling sandy hills sloping from an elev. of 250' in the N part of the city to 200' in the SE part. The Saluda and Broad rivers join in the NW part of the city to form the Congaree River, which constitutes the W border of the city. It is also part of the Santee River System, which provides access to the Atlantic Ocean. Gills Creek runs through the E portion of the city. The mean elev. is 259'.

CLIMATE. The climate of Columbia is relatively temperate, characterized by long, warm summers and short, mild winters. The avg. annual temp. of 64°F ranges from a Jan. mean of 46°F to a July mean of 81°F. The temp. exceeds 100°F an avg. of six days per year, the temp. reaches 20°F or less an avg. of five days per year. About 33% of the avg. annual rainfall of 45.26" occurs during the summer. Snowfall is negligible—the avg. annual amount is 1.7". The RH ranges from 43% to 94%. The avg. growing season is 217 days. Columbia lies in the ESTZ and observes DST.

FLORA AND FAUNA. Animals native to Columbia include the opossum, raccon, whitetail deer and fox squirrel. Common birds include the robin, bluebird, catbird, red-eyed vireo and cardinal. Spring peepers, bullfrogs, chorus frogs, cricket frogs, treefrogs, narrow-mouthed toads, salamanders, lizards, turtles and snakes, including the venomous coral snake, rattlesnake, copperhead and cottonmouth, are found in the area. Common trees include the ash, Carolina buckthorn, magnolia, oak and hickory. Smaller plants include the yarrow and bluet.

POPULATION. According to the US census, the pop. of Columbia in 1970 was 113,542. In 1978, it was estimated that it had decreased to 109,600. The greater met. area is, however, one of the fastest growing in the S.

ETHNIC GROUPS. In 1978 the ethnic distribution of Columbia was approx. 69.4% Caucasian, 29.9% Black and 1.8% Hispanic (a percentage of the Hispanic total is also included in the Caucasian total).

TRANSPORTATION. Interstate hwys. 20, 26, 77 and 126 and US hwys. 1, 21, 76, 176 and 378 provide major motor access to Columbia. *Railroads* serving the city are Columbia, Newberry and Laurens, Seaboard Coast Line, Southern and AMTRAK. *Airlines* serving Columbia Met. Airport are DL, EA, PI and SO. Owens Field Airport provides private aircraft facilities. *Bus lines* serving the city include Greyhound, Trailways and the local SC Electric and Gas Co. System.

COMMUNICATIONS. Communications, broadcasting and print media originating from Columbia are: *AM radio stations* WIS 560 (NBC, MOR); WNOK 1230 (CBS, MOR); WOIC 1320 (Natl. Blk., Contemp.); WCOS 1400 (Indep., Contemp.) and WQXL 1470 (ABC/E, Blk.); *FM radio stations* WMHK 89.7 (Indep., Educ., Relig.); WLTR 91.3 (NPR, SC Educ. Radio Network, Clas., Educ., Oldies); WUSC 91.9 (Indep., Progsv., Educ.); WXRY 93.5 (Indep.,

Town Theater, Columbia, South Carolina, one of the oldest little theaters in the US, operating continuously since 1919

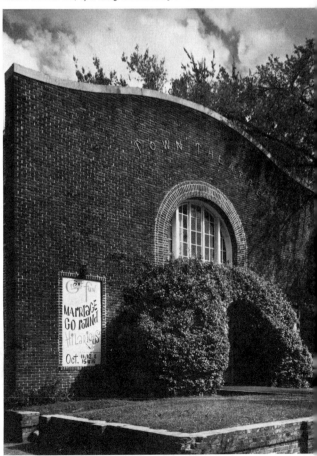

Btfl. Mus.); WCOS 97.9 (Indep., C&W); WSCQ 100.I (APR, Personality) and WNOK I04.7 (ABC/C, MOR); *television stations* WIS Ch. 10 (NBC); WLTX Ch. 19 (CBS); WOLO Ch. 25 (ABC); WRLK Ch. 35 (ETV) and cable; *press:* two daily newspapers serve the city, the *State* and the *Record*. Other publications include the *Journal*, published twice weekly, and the *Star Reporter*, *St. Andrews News*, *Richland NE*, *Black on News*, *Richland Chronicle*, *Ft. Jackson Leader*, *Twin City News* and *Dispatch News*, all published weekly.

HISTORY. In the mid-18th century, a frontier ft. called the Congarees was established in the area of present day Columbia, on the W bank of the Congaree River at the head of navigation on the Santee River System. In 1754 a ferry was established by the SC colonial govt. to connect the ft. with growing settlements on the higher ground of the E bank. One of the earliest planned towns in the US, Columbia was carefully constructed and surveyed after the SC legislature selected it as the site of the state capital in 1786. The legislature governed Columbia until 1805. SC Col. (now the U of SC) was established in 1801. By 1816, the pop. of the capital had reached 1,000. As it gained access to the RRs, the town grew larger. In 1842, it was linked to Charleston, SC and, by 1850, it had become an important RR center of the SE. The city was incorporated in 1854. Its growth was halted by the Civil War, however, and the city was crowded with war refugees fleeing other parts of the state. Gen. William T. Sherman and his Union troops, continuing their march through the S, reached Columbia on Feb. 17, 1865, and destroyed 84 of the 124 city blocks by fire. Within a few years, though, the city was rebuilt, and suburban areas began to be annexed in the 1870s. Although there were "street crossings" to prevent pedestrians from having to wade through seas of mud between wooded sidewalks, there were no paved streets in the city until 1908. Ft. Jackson, established

Childhood home of Woodrow Wilson, built about 1870, maintained as the Woodrow Wilson Memorial Museum since 1930, Columbia, South Carolina

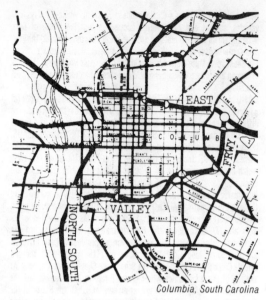

Columbia, South Carolina

nearby during WW I, became one of the largest military bases in the US. Businesses and industrial plants continued to locate in the city, which proceeded to grow steadily in both area and pop. The city is now the center of a large met. area of 373,000 people.

GOVERNMENT. Columbia has a council-mgr. form of govt. The five council members, including the mayor as a voting member, are elected at large to four-year staggered terms. The city mgr. is appointed by the council.

ECONOMY AND INDUSTRY. Columbia is the business, financial, education and transportation center of SC. A service center for growing industry throughout the state, 70% of the labor force is employed in services and 18% employed in manufacturing. Fed., state and

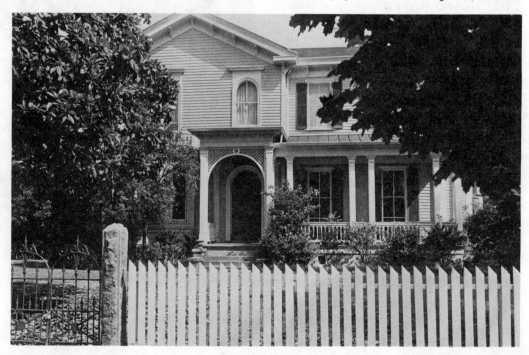

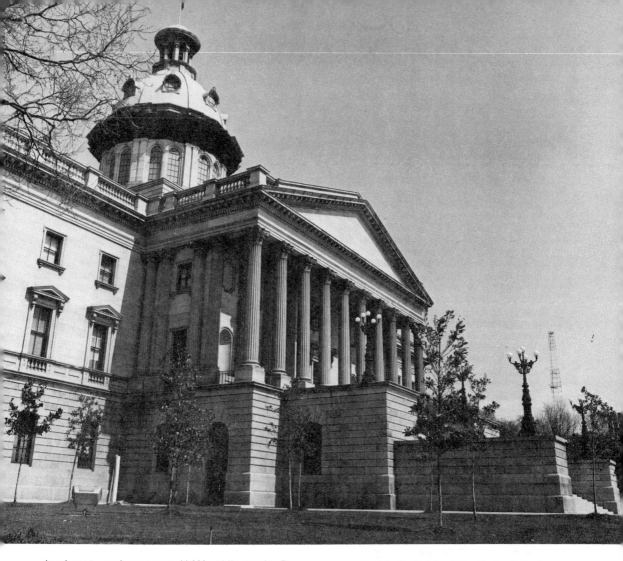

State Capitol Building, Columbia, South Carolina

local govt. employ approx. 44,000, while nearby Ft. Jackson, one of the largest training centers of the Army, trained approx. 60,000 soldiers in 1978. There are more than 250 industrial plants in the city, producing fertilizer, concrete, electronic components, lumber, metal products, food products and textiles. Printing and publishing are also major industries. The city is a principal farm market for the SE—the State Farmer's Market is also located in the city. Major agricultural products include livestock and poultry, which are increasing at the expense of such traditional products as peaches and cotton. In June, 1979, the total labor force for the greater met. area was approx. 174,900, while the rate of unemployment was 4.4%. In 1977, the median household income was $18,282, while the per capita income was $5,437.

BANKING. In 1978, total deposits for the six banks headquartered in Columbia were $1,498,836,000, while assets were $1,803,877,000. Banks include First Natl., Bankers Trust, First Citizens Bank and Trust, First Palmetto State Bank and Trust, Republic Natl. and Victory Savings.

HOSPITALS. There are nine hosps. in Columbia, including Richland Memorial, a gen. hosp. established in the early 1900s, Providence, SC State, William S. Hall Psychiatric Institute, James F. Byrnes Clinic Centers, V.A., Health center, Craft-Farrow State and Midland Center.

EDUCATION. The coed U of SC at Columbia, established in 1801, is one of the oldest state-supported institutions in the US. Offering bachelor, master and doctorate degrees, it enrolled nearly 23,600 in 1978. Benedict Col., a private institution offering bachelor degrees, was established in 1870. In 1978, more than 2,000 enrolled. Midlands Technical Col., established in 1974, is a two-year institution under state/local control offering associate degrees. In 1978 nearly 5,600 enrolled. Columbia Commercial Col., a private institution established in 1935, offers associate degrees. In 1978, approx. 1,400 enrolled. Other institutions in the city include Allen U (affiliated with the African Methodist Episcopal Church), Columbia Bible Col., Columbia Col. (affiliated with the United Methodist Church) and Lutheran Theological Seminary (affiliated with the Lutheran Church in America). In 1977, approx. 72,000 students enrolled in the greater met. area public school system. An additional 5,200 students were enrolled in private and parochial schools. Lib. facilities include Richland Co. Public Lib., with six branch libs. and the U of SC McKissick Memorial Lib., which houses a large collection of SC historical material.

ENTERTAINMENT. The SC State Fair is annually held in Columbia during the third week of Oct. The U of SC Fighting Gamecocks and the teams of Benedict and Columbia colleges participate in intercollegiate sports.

ACCOMMODATIONS. There are several hotels and motels in Columbia including the Carolina Townhouse, Howard Johnson's and the Quality, Holiday, Days, Downtowner Motor, Golden Eagle Motor, Tremont Motor and Vagabond inns.

FACILITIES. There are 25 city parks in Columbia which include swimming pools, tennis courts, playing fields, a nine-hole and an 18-hole golf course and playgrounds. The 150-acre Riverbanks Zoological Park, opened in 1974, contains 185 animals, including the only three Amur leopards in captivity in the US and 600 birds in a natural habitat. It specializes in the breeding of endangered species. The Birdhouse, the only rain forest exhibit in the SE, presents simulated rainstorms complete with thunder and lightning. The park also contains nature trails, botanical gardens and the ruins of SC's first textile mill. Facilities for camping, hunting, fishing and water sports are available at nearby Lake Murray to the W.

CULTURAL ACTIVITIES. The Columbia Music Festival Assn., composed of six branch organizations—the Columbia City Ballet, the Columbia Philharmonic Orchestra, the Columbia Youth Orchestra, the Columbia Lyric Theatre (which presents six operas a year), the Columbia Choral Society and the Women's Symphony Assn.—promotes performing arts in the city. The U of SC and Columbia Col. drama depts. present annual productions of musicals, plays and ballets. There are two comm. theaters in the city, the Town Theater, established in 1919 and the oldest comm. theater in continuous existence in the US and the Workshop Theater, which annually performs eight plays. The Township and Carolina Coliseum are performing arts facilities presenting Broadway plays and concerts. The Columbia Museum of Art features the Kress Collection of Italian Renaissance paintings. The Science Museum, which also contains Gibbes Planetarium features natural history dramas and physical science and aquatic displays. The Confederate Museum is located in the State Archives Building, which also houses state records spanning three centuries. The Jackson Museum features exhibits of more than 200 years of American history. Other cultural organizations are the Columbia Art Assn., the Guild of SC Artists and the SC Arts Commission. McKissick Museums at the U of SC is a center containing museums, an art gallery and archives.

LANDMARKS AND SIGHTSEEING SPOTS. The Historic Columbia Foundation maintains three historic homes, open to the public for tours: the restored Hampton Preston House (1820), which is the former home of Wade Hampton; the Mann Simmons Cottage, which was built in 1850 by a black woman who had bought her freedom and walked to Columbia; the Robert Mills House, which was designed by that native of SC, who was also the architect of the Washington Monument; the boyhood home of Woodrow Wilson, which was built in 1872; and the Governor's Mansion, containing many antiques. Modeled after the US capitol, the SC State House survived Sherman's march through Columbia, as did the Trinity Episcopal Cathedral, built in 1846. Its churchyard contains the graves of six SC governors, while the parents of Woodrow Wilson are buried in the graveyard of the First Presbyterian Church. The First Baptist Church, constructed in 1859, served as the meeting place of the 1860 Secession Convention. Most of the structures on the campus of the U of SC were built prior to 1850.

COLUMBUS
GEORGIA

CITY LOCATION-SIZE-EXTENT. Columbus, the seat of Muscogee Co., is situated on the E bank of the Chattahoochee River across from Phenix City, AL in extreme W GA. Located approx. 225 mi. W of the Atlantic Ocean and 170 mi. N of the Gulf of Mexico at 32°31' N lat. and 84°57' W long., the city encompasses 220 sq. mi. The greater met. area extends into Harris and Talbot counties on the N, Marion Co. on the E and Chattahoochee Co. on the E and S.

TOPOGRAPHY. The terrain of Columbus, which is located in the Chattahoochee River valley on the fault line between the Piedmont region and the Atlantic coastal plain, is characterized by rolling hills. Two lakes, Oliver and Walter F. George, are located in the city. The mean elev. is 445'.

CLIMATE. The humid SE climate of Columbus is influenced by both continental and maritime effects. The avg. annual temp. of 64.8°F ranges from a Jan. mean of

47.3°F to a July mean of 81°F. The 51.48'' avg. annual rainfall is fairly evenly distributed throughout the year, with greater amounts falling in Mar. and July. Snowfall is rare. The RH ranges from 48% to 91%. The avg. growing season is 221 days. Columbus lies in the ESTZ and observes DST.

FLORA AND FAUNA. Animals native to Columbus include the raccoon, opossum, whitetail deer and fox. Common birds are the red-eyed vireo, warbler, shrike, orchard oriole and summer tanager. Snapping turtles, frogs, salamanders, king and water snakes, as well as the venomous coral snake, rattlesnake, copperhead and cottonmouth, are found in the area. Typical trees are the honey locust, dogwood, sycamore, sweet gum, witch hazel, magnolia, willow, oak and pine. Smaller plants include the hawthorn, sumac, aster, azalea and yellow jasmine.

POPULATION. According to the US census, the pop. of Columbus in 1970 was 167,377. In 1978, it was estimated that it had increased to approx. 170,000.

ETHNIC GROUPS. In 1978, the ethnic distribution of Columbus was approx. 73.9% Caucasian, 24.2% Black, 1.7% Hispanic and 0.2% other.

TRANSPORTATION. Interstate Hwy. 185, US hwys. 27, 80, 280, 431 and state rtes. 22, 85, 103 and 357 provide major motor access to Columbus. *Railroads* serving the city are Southern, L & N, Seaboard Coast and Central of GA. *Airlines* serving Columbus Met. Airport are DL and Atlanta-Southeastern. *Bus lines* providing service are Greyhound, Trailways and the local city-operated METRA. The GA Port Authority maintains an inland terminus in the city to accommodate barges navigating the Chattahoochee River from the Gulf IntraCoastal Waterway to Columbus.

COMMUNICATIONS. Communications, broadcasting and print media serving the Columbus area are: *AM radio stations* WDAK 540 (ABC/I, Top 40); WHYD 1270 (APR, Relig.); WOKS 1340 (Mut. Blk., Natl.); *FM radio stations* WEIZ 100.1 (Indep., Btfl. Mus.); WVOC 102.9 (Indep., Blue Grass); WFXE 104.9 (ABC, Soul/Disco) and WCGQ 107.3 (Indep., Top 40); *television stations* WRBL Ch. 3 (CBS); WTVM Ch. 9 (ABC); WJSP Ch. 28

Columbus, Georgia

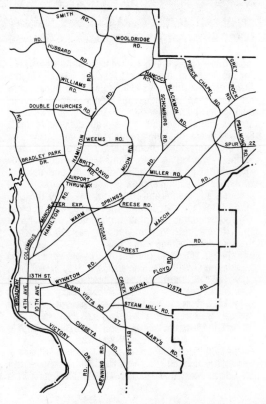

(PBS); WYEA Ch. 38 (NBC) and cable; *press*: two daily newspapers serve the city, the morning *Enquirer*, and the *Ledger*, issued weekday evenings and weekend mornings; other publications include the weekly *Bayonet* and *Times*.

HISTORY. Native Americans of several "Lower Creek" tribes inhabited the area of present-day Columbus before the first Spanish and English settlers arrived in the area in the 17th century. Although trade agreements were established with the tribes, some conflict between native Americans and Anglo newcomers resulted from westward migration after the Revolutionary War. After the War of 1812, most of the Creek lands were either ceded or sold. Muscogee Co. was created by the GA legislature on Dec. 11, 1826, and, in 1828, Edward Lloyd Thomas was appointed to survey and plan a city in extreme W GA. Established as a trading center, Columbus was incorporated as a town in Dec., 1828. Its strategic riverside location contributed to the development and prosperity of the town. Aided by power from the river, many textile and related industries began to develop by the 1840s and, by the time of the Civil War, Columbus was a shipping, commercial and manufacturing center. In the mid-19th century the RRs replaced steamboats and signaled the end of river transport. The city became one of the leading suppliers of war materials to the Confederacy, ranking second only to Richmond in armament production. It was seized by Fed. troops on Apr. 16, 1865, in one of the final battles of the war. The establishment of Ft. Benning, an Army base, in 1919, and diversification of industry throughout the century, contributed to the economy and development of the city. It is now the second-largest textile producing center in the country.

GOVERNMENT. In 1971, the govts. of Columbus and Muscogee Co. merged (the first in GA to do so) into a mayor-mgr.-council form of govt. consisting of 10 council members and a mayor. The mayor and six council members are elected at large, while four are elected by district. All serve four-year terms.

ECONOMY AND INDUSTRY. Ranging from towels to denim, cotton textile manufacturing is the most important industry in Columbus, followed by food products (including soft drinks, candy and peanut products), metals and machinery (including farm implements). Stone, clay and glass products, lumber and wood products and chemicals are also produced. Fort Benning, the largest infantry training center in the US, employs more than 500 civilians and 20,000 military personnel. The city is also the retail trade center for 26 surrounding counties. In 1979, the labor force for the greater met. area totaled approx. 88,200, while the rate of unemployment was 7.4%. In 1978, per capita income was approx. $12,460.

BANKING. In 1978, total deposits for the four banks headquartered in Columbus were $478,743,000, while assets were $547,823,000. Banks serving the city include Columbus Bank and Trust, First Natl., Natl. Bank and Trust, and Trust Co. of Columbus.

HOSPITALS. There are three gen. hosps. in Columbus, St. Francis, Doctors' and Columbus Medical Center. Ft. Benning Army Hosp. is also located nearby.

EDUCATION. Columbus Col., established in 1958 and elevated to sr. col.

Fort Benning Infantry School in Columbus, Georgia

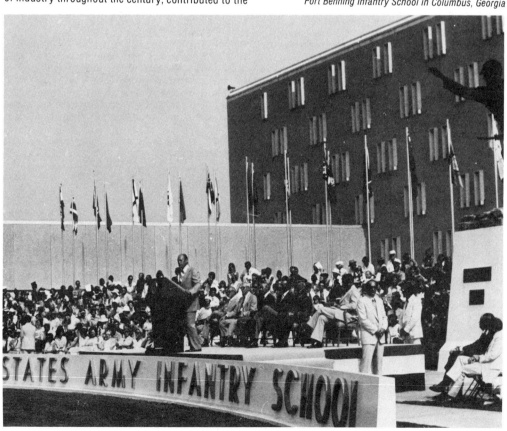

status in 1970, is the fastest-growing unit of the U of GA system. Offering associate, bachelor and master degrees, it enrolled more than 5,100 in 1978. Auburn U, one of the largest institutions in the S, is located nearby. In 1978, nearly 18,000 enrolled. The Muscogee Co. School District, consisting of 40 elementary, nine jr. and eight sr. high schools, enrolled approx. 32,700 in 1978. Seven private schools enrolled approx. 1,800 in 1978. A wide range of special education programs are available. The Bradley Lib. serves the Chattahoochee Valley region.

ENTERTAINMENT. Columbus annually hosts the PGA Southern Open Tournament, held at the Green Island Country Club, in Sept. In Feb., the Columbus Exchange Pancake Club sponsors a Jamboree, held at the Municipal Auditorium, and Columbus Col. sponsors a student art exhibition. The Salisbury Fair, held annually in late Apr. and early May at Salisbury Park in the Historic District, features arts, crafts, musical performances, food and children's games. Ft. Benning annually celebrates the birthday of the Army on June 14 with various activities. Other annual events include the Miss GA Pageant and Heritage Ball in June, the Chattahoochee Valley Exposition (a fair held in Oct.) and a Christmas Parade. The Columbus Astros, a SL baseball team, is based in the city. The Columbus Col. Cougars and the SE Conf. teams of Auburn U participate in intercollegiate sports.

ACCOMMODATIONS. Hotels and motels in Columbus include the Quality and Holiday inns, Heart of Columbus and Sheraton. A Columbus Hilton is scheduled to be opened in 1982.

FACILITIES. There are 20 public parks in Columbus, encompassing more than 2,000 acres and containing 18 swimming pools, 27 tennis courts, three golf courses, jogging tracks, numerous playgrounds, one marina, several fishing ponds and other recreational facilities. Parks include Flat Rock, Cooper Creek and Chattahoochee Promenade, Bull Creek and Cooper Creek. Fishing and other water sports are available at Lake Oliver.

CULTURAL ACTIVITIES. The Springer Opera House in Columbus, an example of 19th century theater architecture and a Natl. Historic Landmark, is the home of the GA State Theatre. The Springer Theatre Co. presents five productions each year. A special children's theater and ballet guild are also active in the city. The Columbus Symphony often performs at the Fine Arts Building of Columbus Col., while the Three Arts League sponsors dance, musical and dramatic performances at the Three Arts Theatre. There are several museums in Columbus. The Confederate Naval Museum houses the salvaged gunboats, *Chattahoochee* and *Muscogee*. Ft. Benning's Infantry Museum, depicting the evolution of the infantry from the French and Indian War to the present, displays artifacts, weapons, uniforms, flags and medals. The Columbus Museum of Arts and Sciences exhibits jewelry, prehistoric native American artifacts and Yuchi materials.

LANDMARKS AND SIGHTSEEING SPOTS. The Historic District of the city, an area encompassing 26 blocks and a variety of architectural styles, is a 19th century Victorian residential area. Included in this area are the Pemberton House and Apothecary Shop, the home of the originator of Coca-Cola, and the Walker-Peters-Langdon House, the oldest in the city. A distinctive feature of the District is the former site of the Columbus Iron Works, an 1840 structure now housing the Convention and Trade Center. Other points of interest include the Folly, the only house in the US shaped like a double octagon, the Rankin House, an historic home (and museum) of the 1850 to 1870 period, and Rankin Sq., a city block of restored old brick commercial buildings.

COLUMBUS
OHIO

CITY LOCATION-SIZE-EXTENT. Columbus, the state capital and seat of Franklin Co., is located on both sides of the Scioto River in central OH at 40° N lat. and 82°53' W long. Encompassing 173.2 sq. mi., 125 mi. SW of Cleveland, it is the largest city (in area) in OH. The greater met. area extends throughout Franklin Co. and into Pickaway Co. on the S, Fairfield Co. on the SE,

Delaware Co. on the N, Licking Co. on the E and Madison Co. on the W and includes the cities of Whitehall to the E, Gahanna to the NW and Upper Arlington to the W.

TOPOGRAPHY. The terrain of Columbus is characterized by gently rolling hills typical of the OH River drainage area. Four nearly parallel streams, the Scioto and Olentongy rivers and the Alum and Big Walnut Creeks create gorgelike areas throughout the city. Hoover Reservoir is approx. 10 mi. N of the city. The mean elev. is 780'.

CLIMATE. The continental climate of Columbus is influenced by cool air masses from central and NW Canada during autumn and winter and by tropical air masses from the Gulf of Mexico during spring and summer. The avg. annual temp. of 52°F ranges from a Jan. mean of 29.1°F to a July mean of 74.8°F. The avg. annual rainfall of 36.94" is evenly distributed throughout the year. Most of the 28.4" avg. annual snowfall occurs during the months of Dec. through Mar. The RH ranges from 52% to 87%. The avg. growing season is 190 days. Columbus lies in the ESTZ and observes DST.

FLORA AND FAUNA. Animals native to Columbus includes the fox, whitetail deer and raccoon. Common birds include the bobwhite, mourning dove, robin, blue jay and crow. Frogs, salamanders, turtles, lizards, toads and snakes, including the venomous copperhead, timber rattlesnake and E massasauga (a pygmy rattler), are also found here. Typical trees include the red oak, maple, birch, hickory and elm. Smaller plants include the blackberry, honeysuckle and dogwood.

POPULATION. According to the US census, the pop. of Columbus in 1970 was 540,025. In 1978, it was estimated that it had decreased to 529,000. The city ranks second largest in the state in pop.

ETHNIC GROUPS. In 1978, the ethnic distribution of Columbus was approx. 81% Caucasian, 18.4% Black and 0.6% Hispanic.

TRANSPORTATION. Interstate hwys. 70, 71 and 270 and US hwys. 23, 33, 40 and 62 provide major motor access to Columbus. *Railroads* serving the city include ConRail, Norfolk & Western, Chessie System and AMTRAK. *Airlines* serving Port Columbus Intl. Airport are AA, US Air, DL, EA, FW, NC, PI, TW and VA. Private and commuter airlines serve Don Scott Field at OH State U, the municipally-operated Bolton Field and Columbus SW Airport. *Bus lines* serving the city include the local Central OH Transit Authority (COTA), Greyhound and Trailways.

COMMUNICATIONS. Communications, broadcasting and print media serving Columbus are: *AM radio stations* WTVN 610 (ABC/E, MOR); WOSU 820 (NPR, Educ., News); WRFD 880 (APR, UPI, Personality, MOR); WMNI 920 (MBS, C&W); WCOL 1230 (UPI, MOR); WBNS 1460 (APR, ABC/I, MOR) and WVKO 1580 (Mut., Blk.); *FM radio stations* WOSV 89.7 (Indep., Btfl. Mus.); WCBE 90.5 (NPR, News, MOR); WXGT 92.3 (Indep., Top 40); WVKO 94.7 (Indep., Jazz); WLVQ 96.3 (Indep., Top 40); WBNS 97.1 (Indep., Btfl. Mus.); WRMZ 97.9 (MBS, Adult Contemp.); WNCL 97.9 (ABC/C, Top 40) and WMNI 99.7 (Indep., MOR); *television stations* WCMH Ch. 4 (NBC);

Downtown Columbus, Ohio

WTVN Ch. 6 (ABC); WEBNS Ch. 10 (CBS) and WOSO Ch. 34 (PBS, CEN); *press*: two major dailies serve the city, the *Citizen-Journal*, published mornings, and the *Dispatch*, issued evenings and weekend mornings; other publications include the *Reporter, Booster, Lower NE News, Upper Arlington News, Buckeye Farm News* and *Jersey Journal*.

HISTORY. Native Americans of the DL and Wyandot tribes inhabited the area of present-day Columbus before the first white settlers established the village of Franklinton at the confluence of the Scioto and Olentongy rivers in 1797. Columbus, named for explorer Christopher Columbus, was founded across the Scioto River from Franklinton in 1812 by German settlers, when it was proposed by the state legislature as the site of the capital. The pop. of the town reached 700 by 1816, when the state capital was moved from its temporary site in Chillocothe to its permanent location in Columbus. In 1824, it became the co. seat. The town became a center of transportation and commerce following the 1831 opening of the OH and Erie Canal and the 1833 arrival of the Natl. Hwy. By the time of its incorporation as a city in 1834, its pop. had reached 3,500. The first RR arrived in 1850 and, within 20 years, five RRs were serving the city. During the Civil War, the city served as a major military center—an arsenal and the largest Confederate prisoner-of-war camp in the N (Camp Chase) were established in the city. By 1900, Columbus had become the manufacturing center of central OH, with buggy manufacturing a major industry. In 1913, nearly 100 people died when the Scioto River flooded; a waterfront reconstruction program followed. During the 1940s, the city began to attract many industries. The consequent expansion was reflected in a pop. growth from 290,500 in 1930 to more than 471,000 in 1960. In addition, the city began to pursue an active policy of annexation and urban renewal during the 1950s. By the 1970s, it had become the largest city in area in the state, as well as the second most populous.

GOVERNMENT. Columbus has a mayor-council form of govt. consisting of seven council members and the mayor, all of whom are elected at large to four-year terms.

ECONOMY AND INDUSTRY. There are approx. 1,000 manufacturing firms in the greater Columbus area employing about 25% of the total work force. Major products include electronics, aircraft, household appliances, automotive hardware, roller bearings, steel castings, glassware and coated fabrics. Printing and publishing is also a major industry. Fed., state and local govts. employ about 20% of the total work force, as do wholesale and retail trade. The headquarters of more than 40 insurance companies and the largest non-profit research laboratory in the world, Battelle Memorial Institute, are also located in the city. In June, 1979, the total labor force for the greater met. area was 544,700, while the rate of unemployment was 5.1%.

BANKING. There are eight commercial banks and five savings and loan assns. in Columbus. In 1978, total deposits for the eight banks headquartered in the city were $3,480,049,000, while assets were $4,360,692,000. Banks include OH Natl., Huntington Natl., City Natl. Bank and Trust, OH State, Society, Franklin, Columbus Trust and First Trust.

HOSPITALS. Some of the 15 hosps. in Columbus include Grant, Mt. Carmel, Mercy, Children's, Riverside Methodist, St. Ann's, St. Anthony's and OH State U. Research at Children's Hosp. has produced significant

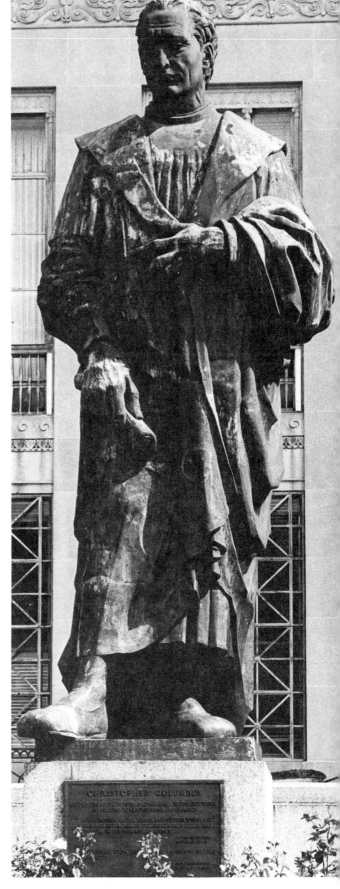

Statue of Christopher Columbus stands outside City Hall in Columbus, Ohio

contributions in such areas as cancer, cystic fibrosis and epilepsy in children, as well as birth defects.

EDUCATION. OH State U (OSU) in Columbus, established in 1890 as the OH Agricultural and Mechanical Col., enrolled more than 51,000 in 1978. In 1922, OSU founded WOSU, the first educational radio station in the US. Pontifical Col. Josephinum, the only seminary in the W hemisphere admininstered directly by the Holy See, enrolled approx. 960 in 1978. Capital U, established as the Evangelical Lutheran Theological Seminary in Canton, moved to Columbus in 1950 and became a U. Supported by the American Lutheran Church, it offers "The U Without Walls" (courses on a self-directed basis), as well as programs leading to bachelor's and master's degrees. Other institutions include OH Dominican Col., Franklin U, OH Institute of Technology, Columbus Col. of Arts and Design and Columbus Technical Institute. The first state school for the blind in the US opened in the city in 1837, while the first jr. high school in the US opened here in 1904. The public school system consists of 118 elementary, 29 jr. high and 17 sr. high schools with a 1978 enrollment of approx. 180,000. In addition, there are 66 private schools in the co. with an enrollment of approx. 16,500. Lib. facilities include the Columbus Public Lib. with 21 branches, the OH Historical Society Lib. and the various U libs.

ENTERTAINMENT. The Country Dinner Playhouse in Columbus offers dinner theater entertainment. The OH State Fair, held annually in late Aug. or early Sept., is one of the largest in the US. The Festival of Arts, featuring displays of arts and architecture as well as dance and dramatic performances, is held each June in Capitol Sq. The OH State U Buckeyes, consistently top-ranked in the Big Ten Conf., and the Capital U Crusaders participate in intercollegiate sports. The Columbus Clippers, a minor league (AAA) baseball team of the NY Yankees organization, play at Franklin Co. Stadium. Horse racing takes place at Scioto Downs and Beulah Park. The Pacesetters, a women's pro football team, and the Stringers, a men's minor league pro football team are based in the city, which is also the site of the annual Memorial Golf Tournament, hosted by Jack Nicklaus, Borden's LPGA Tournament, Wendy's Intl. Tennis Classic and the Buckeye Cup Speedboat Regatta.

ACCOMMODATIONS. There are numerous hotels and motels in Columbus including the Christopher, Sheraton and Holiday inns, Neil House and the Southern Hotel.

FACILITIES. There are 100 parks and playgrounds in Columbus, encompassing nearly 5,500 acres, offering facilities for swimming, water sports, golfing (five public courses), tennis, ball playing, bicycling, jogging and horseback riding. The Columbus Zoo features a children's zoo. Parks include Alum Creek, Big Run, Big Walnut, Blacklick Woods Met., Fairwood, Goodale, Jonson, Lincoln, Lower Scioto, Nelson, Schiller, Westgate, Wolfe and Whetstone. Franklin Park Conservatory, featuring displays of tropical flowers, is situated in one of the oldest city parks. Bicentennial Riverfront Park, part of the redevelopment of the city's riverfront, features fountains and flags of the 50 states, while the Park of Roses exhibits approx. 36,000 rose plants.

CULTURAL ACTIVITIES. The Columbus Symphony Orchestra and the Kenley Players perform in the Veterans' Memorial Auditorium, located downtown. Concerts and plays are presented at the OH Theatre, a restored 1928 structure, and on the State House lawn in summer, while OH State U and Capital U present experimental theater. (The largest theater lib. in the US is located at OH State U.) Capital U and Ballet Met., a professional ballet co. performing in the city, plans to become a touring co. The works of George Bellows, a native of Columbus known for his oil paintings of boxing matches and of his family, are exhibited in the Columbus Gallery of Fine Arts. A city arts and craft center, the Cultural Arts Center, is located in the renovated Natl. Guard Armory, constructed in 1868. The Center of Science and Industry features the Battelle Planetarium, Hall of History, a Foucault Pendulum, a simulated coal mine and Durell Street of Yesteryear, a replica of a 19th century street. Orton Museum, on the campus of OH State U, features geological displays, while the US Fine Arts Building contains galleries and a sculpture court. Archaeological and natural history displays are featured at the museum of the OH Historical Center.

LANDMARKS AND SIGHTSEEING SPOTS. The 551' Leveque-Lincoln State Tower, the tallest building in Columbus, stands on the E shore

of the Scioto River. A 20' high bronze statue of Christopher Columbus, donated to the city by Genoa, Italy, in 1955, stands in City Hall Plaza, which is also located on the riverfront. The State Capitol, a limestone, Grecian Revival structure completed in 1861, is situated in the 10-acre Capitol Park in downtown Columbus, and features portraits of the govs. of OH. The 233-acre German Village, a restored German settlement of 500 homes dating from 1840 to 1860, features a Haus and Garten Tour held annually on the last Sun. in June. OH Village, a reconstruction of a 19th-century OH co. seat, is a complex of period buildings featuring similarly costumed inhabitants. The Olentangy River Caverns, limestone caves 55' to 105' underground, were used by Wyandot Native Americans as shelters, while OH Frontier Land, a replica of an old frontier town containing a ft., features simulated gunfights. Camp Chase Confed. Cemetery contains the graves of 2,260 Confederate soldiers.

CORPUS CHRISTI
TEXAS

CITY LOCATION-SIZE-EXTENT. Corpus Christi is located on Corpus Christi Bay, an inlet of the Gulf of Mexico, in SE TX at 27°46' N lat. and 97°30' W long. The seat of Nueces Co., it encompasses 105 sq. mi. of land and 221 sq. mi. of water. The city lies 145 mi. SE of San Antonio and 160 mi. N of the Mexico border. The greater met. area extends throughout Nueces Co. and into neighboring San Patricio Co.

TOPOGRAPHY. Corpus Christi is situated on flat to gently rolling terrain of the Black Prairie region and the low flat Gulf Coastal Plain. The Nueces River, Lake Corpus Christi and numerous bays are located in the area. The mean elev. is 35'.

Beach in Corpus Christi, Texas

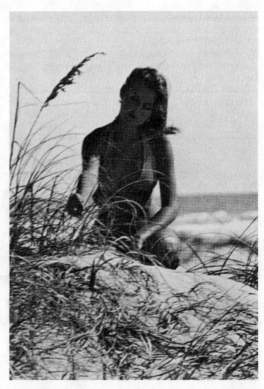

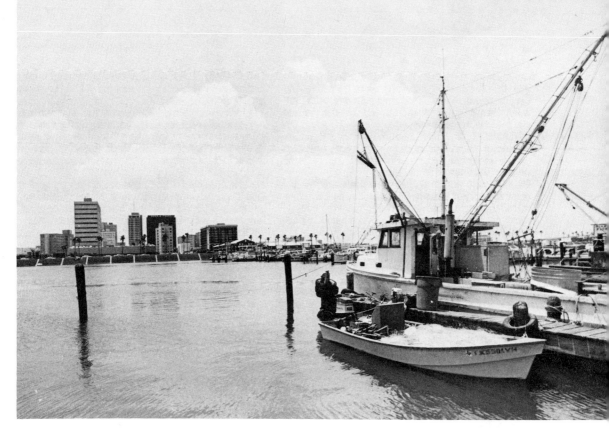

The Port of Corpus Christi

CLIMATE. The climate of Corpus Christi is humid subtropical. The avg. annual temp. of 71°F ranges from a Jan. mean of 56°F to a mean during July and Aug. of 83°F. Summers are typically long and warm, while winters are short and mild. Most of the avg. annual rainfall of 27" occurs in May and Sept. Snowfall is negligible. Hurricanes and tornados occur infrequently. The RH ranges from 58% to 93%. Corpus Christi lies in the CSTZ and observes DST.

FLORA AND FAUNA. Animals native to Corpus Christi include the armadillo, cottontail and jack rabbit, peccary, raccoon, opossum and whitetail deer. Common birds are the laughing gull, mockingbird, cardinal, grackle, blue jay, heron, tern, ibis, pelican, wild turkey and quail. Several species of reptiles, as well as the venomous cottonmouth, copperhead, rattlesnake and coral snake, are found in the area. Common trees include the palm oak, ash, goldenrod, magnolia and mimosa. Smaller plants include the yucca, bluebonnet, orchid, cactus, mesquite, buttercup, phlox and Confederate jasmine.

POPULATION. According to the US census, the pop. of Corpus Christi in 1970 was 204,525. In 1978, it was estimated that it had increased to approx. 225,000.

ETHNIC GROUPS. In 1978, the ethnic distribution of Corpus Christi was approx. 40.18% Caucasian, 5.65% Black, 54.02% Hispanic, .07% Asian and .08% Native American.

TRANSPORTATION. Interstate Hwy. 37, US hwys 77 and 181 and state hwys. 9, 43, 44, 286, 357, 358 and 685 provide major motor access to Corpus Christi. *Railroads* serving the city are MO Pacific, Southern Pacific and TX-Mexican. The Port of Corpus Christi, at 45' the deepest on the Gulf of Mexico and the ninth largest in the US in terms of tonnage handled, served 43 steamship agencies representing 320 cargo carriers and 43 barges on the Intracoastal Canal. *Airlines* serving the Corpus Christi Intl. Airport are BN, EA, SW, TI and Tejas. *Bus lines* providing service are Trailways, Greyhound and intra-city service.

COMMUNICATIONS. Communications, broadcasting and print media serving Corpus Christi are: *AM radio station* KCTA 1030 (NPR, Relig. Span.); KCCT 1150 (Indep., Span.); KSIX 1230 (CBS, Btfl. Mus.); KRYS 1360 (ABC/I, MOR); KUNO 1400 (Indep., Span.); KEYS 1440 (TX Rep., Contemp.); KROB 1510 (MBS, C&W); KIKN 1590 (Indep., C&W); *FM radio station* KQIV 91.9, KEXX 93 (NBC, Contemp.); KSIX 93.9 (Indep., Btfl. Mus.); KZFM 95.5 (ABC/C, MOR); KIOU 96.5 (Indep., Btfl. Mus.); KROB 99.9 (MBS, C&W); KNCN 101 (AOR) and KOUL 103 (NPR, C&W); *television station* KIII Ch. 3 (ABC); KRIS Ch. 6 (NBC); KZTV Ch. 10 (CBS); KEDT Ch. 16 (PBS) and KORO Ch. 28 (Intl. Network-Span.); *press:* one major newspaper serves the area, the *Caller-Times* issued mornings and evenings on weekdays and mornings on weekends.

HISTORY. The Karankawa Indians inhabited the area of present day Corpus Christi when Spanish explorer Alvarez Alonzo de Pineda arrived in Corpus Christi Bay in 1519 and named it on the Festival Day of Corpus Christi. Later, Spanish, Portuguese, English and French ships anchored in the bay and, and it was said, pirates took haven there. In the winter of 1838-39, adventurer Col. Henry Lawrence Kinney established a trading post on the bay called Kinney's Trading Post or Kinney's Ranch, to serve area ranchers. The small settlement remained obscure until 1845, when US troops commanded by Gen. Zachary Taylor arrived, remaining until the following year before the outbreak of the Mexican War. In 1847, Nueces Co. was formed, named for the Nueces ("nuts" in Spanish) River, which was lined with pecan trees. In 1848, the community was named Corpus Christi and, in 1852, it was incorporated as a city. During the Civil War, the city was blockaded by Union gunboats and captured in 1864. By 1900, the pop. of the city was approx. 4,700. The area's first natural gas well, which was uncontrollable, was discovered in 1913. The 1923 development of a well and the 1926 opening of the port contributed to a growth in pop. from 10,522 in 1920 to 27,741 in 1930. Oil deposits discovered nearby in 1930 formed the basis of the area's oil industry and resulted in an increase of the city's pop. to more than 57,300 by 1940. During World War II, more than 40,000 fliers were trained at the Corpus Christi Naval Air Training Station. After the war, increased gas production attracted new industries and a tourist trade developed.

GOVERNMENT. Corpus Christi has a council-mgr. form of govt. The seven council members, including the mayor as a voting member, are elected to two-year terms. Four councillors are elected by district, while two councillors and the mayor are elected at large.

ECONOMY AND INDUSTRY. Petrochemicals are the primary industry in Corpus Christi, followed by manufacturing, port-related activity, agriculture, fishing, ranching, tourism and the fed. govt. Other manufactures include primary metals, stone, clay and glass products, fabricated metals, apparel and electronic components. In June, 1979, the labor force. of the greater met. area totaled approx. 135,100, while the rate of unemployment was approx. 5.9%.

BANKING. There are 13 commercial banks and eight savings and loan assns. in Corpus Christi. In 1978, total deposits for the 13 banks headquartered in the city were $962,797,000, while assets were $1,164,051,000. Banks include Corpus Christi Natl., Corpus Christi Bank and Trust, Citizens State Bank of Corpus Christi, Guaranty Natl. Bank and Trust, Parkdale State, First State of Corpus Christi, Mercantile Natl. and American Natl.

HOSPITALS. There are 10 hosps. in Corpus Christi. The largest, Memorial Medical Center, is supported by Nueces Co. and handles both private and indigent care needs. Other hosps. are Spohn, Doctors Central, Doctors N, Physicians and Surgeons Gen., Corpus Christi Osteopathic, Ada Wilson Crippled Children's, Driscoll Foundation Children's and Robstown Riverside Hosp. and Clinic.

EDUCATION. Del Mar Jr. Col. in Corpus Christi is a public comm. col. offering associate degrees in liberal arts and technical fields at the E campus and in vocational and adult education at the W campus. Founded in 1935, the institution enrolled more than 1,000 students in 1978. Corpus Christi State U awards bachelor and master degrees. Established in 1971, it enrolled close to 2,500 students. In 1978, the U of TX Institute of Marine Science, Engineering and Resources offers graduate courses at nearby Port Aransas. The TX A&M U Research and Extension Center is located between Corpus Christi and Robstown. The Corpus Christi Minor Seminary is also located in the city. The public school enrollment is 49,607. The city has five districts, the largest of which is the Corpus Christi Independent School District, with 38 elementary, 11 jr. high and five sr. high schools. Several private and parochial schools also serve the city. Lib. facilities include La Retama Lib., and three branch libs., Parkdale, Greenwood and Parker Memorial Park.

ENTERTAINMENT. Since 1935, Corpus Christi has celebrated the annual Buccaneer days during late Apr. and early May. A music festival, art jamboree, carnival and parade are featured. Other annual events include the S TX Traditional Art, China and Antique show in Feb., and yacht races in June. The annual TX Jazz Festival, the Port Aransas Bill Fish Tournament and the Deep Sea Roundup are held in July. Area tennis tournaments include the Corpus Christi Collegiate Team Tournament, the SW Conf. championships, the USTA 21 and under Natl. Hardcourt tennis championships and the TX Sectionals.

ACCOMMODATIONS. There are more than 70 hotels and motels in Corpus Christi. These include the Airport Hilton, Best Western-Master Host, Holiday-Emerald Beach, La Quinta Royale Motor, Sheraton Marina, Quality-Bayfront and Ramada inns and the Padre Island Beach Hotel.

FACILITIES. There are 160 parks in Corpus Christi, ranging in size from one to 80 acres and featuring picnic areas, basketball facilities, playing fields, fishing piers, swimming pools, bicycle trails and playground facilities. Among the largest are the 28-acre Cole Park, the 42-acre Greenwood Park, the 18-acre Cullen Park and the 80-acre W Guth Park. A municipally-operated marina in the central bayfront area provides slips for some 420 boats. There are two public golf courses in the city, as well as three tennis centers, including 16 lighted courts at the H.E. Butt Municipal Tennis Center. Fishing is available along the bays and shore waters of the city. Beach areas, including Nueces Co. Park and Padre Island. Natl. Seashore, offer skin diving, water skiing, boating, sailing, surfing, swimming, fishing and shell hunting.

CULTURAL ACTIVITIES. The Japanese Art Museum, which houses art, artifacts, dolls and masks depicting Japanese culture, is located in Corpus Christi. The Corpus Christi Museum contains wildlife, historic and educational exhibits, while the Art Museum of S TX exhibits contemporary art. The Art Comm. Center contains studies and galleries for local artists. The Little Theatre of Corpus Christi is a comm. theater which performs at the Harbor Playhouse and Bayfront Plaza Auditorium. The Corpus Christi Symphony Orchestra occasionally performs in the Cole Park Amphitheater during the summer, overlooking Corpus Christi Bay and sponsors a Young People's Concert Series, opera and ballet.

LANDMARKS AND SIGHTSEEING SPOTS. Among the attractions of Corpus Christi is Padre Island Natl. seashore, part of a 131-mi. long stretch of beach formed by Padre and Mustang islands. The port channel is spanned by the 640'-long Corpus Christi Harbor Bridge, at 235' the highest in TX. Ocean Drive Scenic Route and Circle Drive around Corpus Christi Bay offer magnificent views of the bay area. Several historic homes are located in the city. The 19th-century Sidbury and Lichtenstein homes are currently being restored by the Jr. League. The restored Centennial House, built around 1850, is the oldest existing structure in the city. Mercado Del Mar is an old town entertainment complex consisting of shops, galleries and restaurants. The 850,000-acre King Ranch, 40 mi. SW of the city, is the largest in the US. Established in 1845, the ranch developed the first breed of cattle originating in the nation, the Santa Gertrudis.

Corpus Christi, Texas

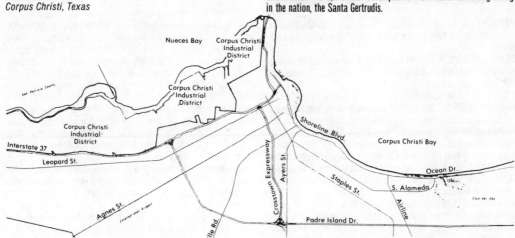

DALLAS
TEXAS

CITY LOCATION-SIZE-EXTENT. Dallas, the second largest city in the state, seventh largest in the US and seat of Dallas Co., encompasses 378 sq. mi., including 45 sq. mi. of lakes, in N central TX at 32°54' N lat. and 97°02' W long. Its greater met. area extends into the counties of Collin to the NE, Denton to the NW, Ellis to the S and Rockwall and Kaufman to the E. With the greater met. area of Ft. Worth, which lies 20 mi. W, it is part of the SW Metroplex, which also includes the cities of Arlington and Irving to the W and Richardson and Garland to the N.

TOPOGRAPHY. The terrain of Dallas, which is situated on the rolling land of the great plains region of TX, consists primarily of prairie. The headwaters of the Trinity River, including Elmfork and the White Rock, Prairie and Five Mile rivers, as well as several lakes, including Dallas, Mt. Creek, White Rock, Ray Hubbard, and Bachman, are located in the area. The mean elev. is 468'.

CLIMATE. The climate of Dallas is continental, characterized by wide variations in weather conditions. Monthly mean temps. range from 45°F during Jan. to 84°F during July and Aug., the avg. annual temp. is 65.7°F. The avg. annual rainfall is 32" and the avg. annual snowfall is 3.5". The RH ranges from 45% to 88% and the avg. growing season lasts 250 days. Dallas lies in the CSTZ and observes DST.

FLORA AND FAUNA. Animals native to Dallas include the whitetail deer, opossum, armadillo and raccoon. Common birds include the cardinal, blue jay, grackle, mockingbird, scissor-tailed flycatcher and ruby-throated hummingbird. The red-eared turtle, bullfrog, green anole lizard, garter snake and the venomous cottonmouth, coral snake, rattlesnake and copperhead are also found in the area. Common trees include the oak, pine, pecan, elm, mesquite, mimosa and red bud. Smaller plants include the bluebonnet (the state flower), Indian paintbrush and fleabane.

POPULATION. According to the US census, the pop. of Dallas in 1970 was 844,400. In 1979, it was estimated that it had increased to approx. 898,000.

ETHNIC GROUPS. In 1978, the ethnic distribution of Dallas was approx. 74.3% Caucasian, 24.9% Black and 8.0% Hispanic. (A percentage of the Hispanic total is also included in the Caucasian total.)

TRANSPORTATION. Interstate hwys. 20, 30, 35, 45 and 635, US hwys. 67, 75 (the Central Expressway), 77, 80 (the Ft. Worth Pike) and 175 and state hwys. 12 (encircling the city), 78, 114, 183, 244, 289, 352 and 408 provide major motor access to Dallas. *Railroads* serving the city are MO-Pacific, MO-KS-TX, S Pacific, St. Louis-San Francisco and the Atchison, Topeka & Santa Fe. *Airlines* serving Dallas/Ft. Worth Regional Airport include AA and BN, the world headquarters of which are currently under construction, as well as CO, DL, EA, FT, FL, OZ, PA, RD and TI. Love Field and

"Old Ned" Country Courthouse in Dallas, Texas

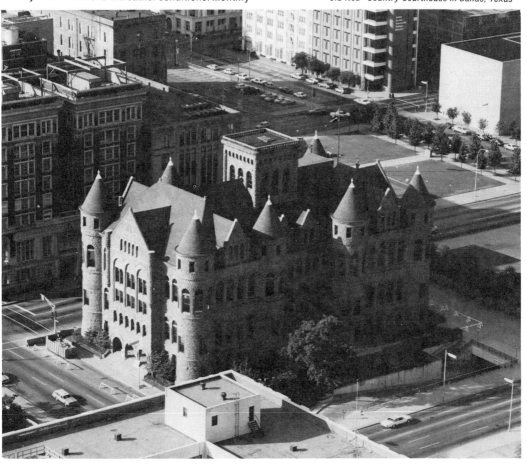

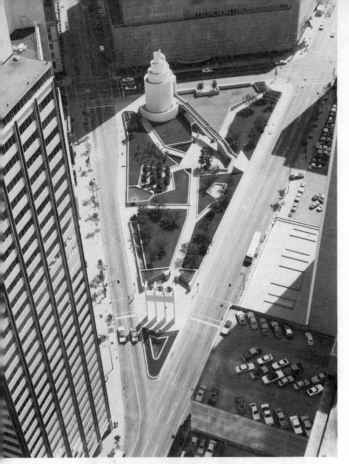

Thanksgiving Square, Dallas, Texas

Redbird airport are also located in the city. *Bus lines* include Trailways, Greyhound and the local Dallas Transit System.

COMMUNICATIONS. Communications, broadcasting and print media originating from Dallas are: *AM radio stations* WFAA 570 (CBS. MOR); KSKY 660 (Indep., Blk., Relig.); KPBC 1040 (Indep., Relig.); KRLD 1080 (ABC/C, All News); KVIL 1150 (ABC/C, MOR); KLIF 1190 (UPI, Top 40) and KBOX 1480 (UPI, C&W); *FM radio stations* KCBI 89.3 (Indep., Var., Educ.,); KERA 90.1 (NPR, Var.); KCHU 90.9 (Indep., Var.); KVTT 91.7 (Indep., Educ.); KAFM 92.5 (CBS/FM, Progsv., C&W); KZEW 97.9 (Indep., Rock); KNUS 98.7 (ABC/FM, Rock); KMEZ 100.3 (Indep., Btfl. Mus.); WRR 101.1 (Indep., Clas.); KMGC 102.9 (UPI, Relig.); KKDA 104.5 (Indep., Easy List.) and KOAX 105.3 (Indep., Btfl. Mus.); *television stations* KDFW Ch. 4 (CBS); KXAS Ch. 5 (NBC); WFAA Ch. 8 (ABC); KTVT Ch. 11 (Indep.); *press:* two major dailies serve the city, the morning *News* and the *Times-Herald*, issued weekday evenings and weekend mornings; other print media include the *Journal of Air Law and Commerce, Journal of Petroleum Technology, Oak Cliff Tribune, Ocean Resources Engineering, Petroleum Engineer, Intl. Pipeline & Gas Journal, TX Business, TX Contractor, TX Homes Magazine, TX Methodist/United Methodist Reporter, D Magazine* and *Dallas.*

HISTORY. In 1841, John Neeley Bryan settled on the banks of the upper Trinity River, site of present-day Dallas, and established a trading post. When Dallas Co. was organized in 1846, the settlement became the co. seat. It is believed to have been named for George Dallas, who served as VP under Pres. James Polk from 1845 to 1849. In 1855, a cooperative community was established near the town by a group of French intellectuals, many of whom moved to Dallas when their venture failed. Dallas was incorporated as a town in 1856. It served as a stage stop and later as a crossroad for cattle drives. In the early 1870s, when two RRs arrived, Dallas began to grow as a commercial

center and it was incorporated as a city in 1871. By 1886, six RRs and a thriving trade in cotton, wheat, wool, sheep and cattle existed, and, by 1890, the pop. of the city exceeded 38,000. That year, Dallas replaced Galveston as the largest city in TX, but in turn was replaced by Houston in 1930. The 1930 development of the E TX oilfield near Dallas boosted its economy and resulted in an influx of new industries. During WW II, the city's manufacturing plants produced military equipment. Later, the manufacture of aircraft, electrical and electronic equipment gained importance. Between 1940 and 1970, when industry expanded tremendously, the pop. of the city grew by 500,000. The city of Dallas responded to the decline of its urban pop. and its downtown businesses during the 1960s with civic improvements. On Nov. 22, 1963, Pres. John F. Kennedy was assassinated in the city and Lyndon B. Johnson took the presidential oath of office there aboard AF 1, the presidential airplane. The city, the transportation center of the SW, is a major US retail, manufacturing and financial center as well.

GOVERNMENT. Dallas has a council-mgr. form of govt. The 11 council members, including the mayor as a voting member of the council, serve two-year terms. Eight are elected by district and three, including the mayor, are elected at large. The council appoints a city mgr., who carries out council policies, prepares the budget and appoints dept. heads.

ECONOMY AND INDUSTRY. Dallas is a major natl. center of banking, fashion, manufacturing, trade and transportation. Principal manufactures are electronic and electrical equipment, aircraft, missile parts, and apparel. There are more than 2,500 factories in the city, employing approx. 20% of the work force. Other important industries include the production of nonelectrical machinery, food and food products and printing and publishing. The city is one of the world's leading cotton markets. Some 75% of the known oil reserves in the US are within 500 mi. of the city, in which more oil firm headquarters are located than any other US city. In addition, there are more insurance company headquarters in the city than in any other. Tourism is a significant factor in the economy. In June, 1979, the labor force of the Dallas-Ft. Worth Metroplex was approx. 479,000, while the rate of unemployment

Dallas, Texas

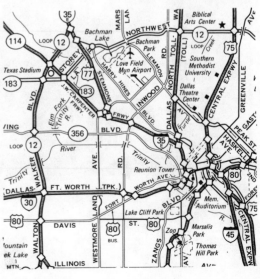

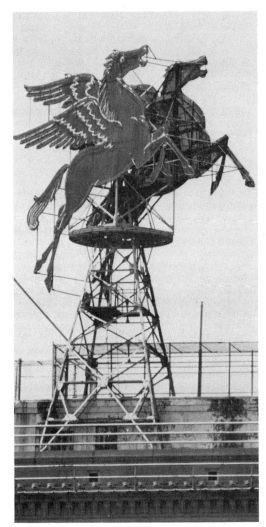

Mobile Building with Pegasus Flying Horse, Dallas, Texas

was 4.0%. The avg. per capita income in 1978 was $7,277.

BANKING. There are 55 commercial banks and five savings and loan assns. in Dallas. In 1978, total deposits for the 56 banks headquartered in the city were approx. $15,123,424,000, while assets were $19,792,948,000. Banks include Republic Natl., First Natl., Mercantile Natl., First City, Natl. Bank of Commerce, Preston State, Lakewood Bank and Trust, TX AM Bank of Dallas N, Oak Cliff Bank and Trust and Citizens' Natl.

HOSPITALS. There are more than 30 hosps. in Dallas, including Baylor U Medical Center, U of TX Health Services Center, Brookhaven Medical Center, Dallas Court District-Parkland Memorial, Methodist, Presbyterian, St. Paul, TX Scottish Rite Hosp. for Crippled Children, Timberlawn Psychiatric and V.A.

EDUCATION. S Methodist U in University Park, a privately supported, coeducational U founded in 1911, is the largest and oldest institution in the Dallas area. Affiliated with the United Methodist Church, the U grants bachelor, master and doctoral degrees and enrolled nearly 8,700 in 1978. The U of Dallas, founded in 1956, is a privately supported, coeducational, Roman Catholic U which awards bachelor, master and doctoral degrees. Located in Irving, a Dallas suburb, it enrolled more than 1,900 in 1978. Bishop, Dallas Baptist, Centro, Richland and Mountainview cols., the Col. of Professional Assistants, TX Institute, and Dallas Theological Seminary are

also in the city. There are 182 elementary and secondary schools in the Dallas public school system, which enrolled approx. 170,000 in 1978, while 38 church-supported schools enrolled more than 12,000. Lib. facilities include Dallas Public Lib., which maintains 17 branches, and Dallas Co. Lib., as well as the libs. of the various cols. and universities.

ENTERTAINMENT. Dinner theaters in Dallas include the Windmill, Country and Granny's. Annual events in the city include the TX State Fair, held two weeks in Oct., and Cotton Bowl Week, which runs from Dec. 26 to Jan. 1 and which highlights the Cotton Bowl on New Year's Day. Professional sports entertainment is provided by the Dallas Cowboys, an NFL-NFC football team which plays in neighboring Irving, the Tornadoes, an NASL soccer team, and the Blackhawks, a CH hockey team. The S Methodist U Mustangs of the SWC compete in intercollegiate sports.

ACCOMMODATIONS. There are numerous hotels and motels in Dallas, including the Fairmont, Hyatt Regency, Adolphus, Marina, Howard Johnson's, Le Baron, Travelodge and the Holiday, Sheraton, LaQuinta, Rodeway, Ramada, Day's and Best Western inns.

FACILITIES. There are many parks in Dallas, encompassing 14,000 acres, with numerous public golf courses, tennis courts and swimming pools. The two major parks are Old City and State Fair Park, which features 10 permanent exposition buildings and an amusement park. The Marsalis Zoo is also located in the city.

CULTURAL ACTIVITIES. There are many performing arts organizations in Dallas, which is known as the "Cultural Center of the SW." The Dallas Civic Opera and the Dallas Symphony perform at Fair Park Music Hall. The Chamber Music Society, Civic Chorus, Civic Ballet Society and Met. Ballet also present regular performances. Dramatic groups include the Dallas Repertory Theater, Theater Onstage and Theater Three. Several companies are also housed in the Theater Center, the only theater designed by American architect Frank Lloyd Wright. American and European paintings and sculpture are displayed at the Dallas Museum of Fine Arts. Other museums include the Dallas Health and Science Museum; the Dallas Museum of Natural History; the TX Historical Museum; and the John F. Kennedy Museum.

LANDMARKS AND SIGHTSEEING SPOTS. The John Fitzgerald Kennedy Memorial is a white, concrete monument near Dealey Plaza, designed as a place of meditation which commemorates the Pres., who was assassinated in Dallas in 1963. There is also a memorial plaque in Dealey Plaza, near the site of the assassination. Old City Park downtown contains several original and reconstructed buildings depicting 19th century pioneer life in N TX, including a train depot, doctor's office, log cabin, gen. store and the Millermore Mansion. The 50-story Reunion Tower of Dallas is topped by a three-level geodesic dome and features an observation deck. Wax World, a wax museum, features scenes from the administration of each Pres. The Hall of State, built in 1936 for the TX Centennial Exhibition, features a huge, gold medallion in its Hall of Six Flags.

DAVENPORT
IOWA

CITY LOCATION-SIZE-EXTENT. Davenport, the seat of Scott Co. and third largest city in the state, is located in extreme E IA at the junction of the Rock and MS rivers at 41°32' N lat. and 90°36 W long. Davenport is the principal city of the greater metropolitan area known as "Quint Cities"—which includes Bettendorf, IA and Rock Island, Moline and E Moline as well. Encompassing 63 sq. mi., Davenport is 60 mi. SE of Cedar Rapids and 160 mi. W of Chicago on the IL state line.

TOPOGRAPHY. The terrain of Davenport, which is situated in the dissected till plain region of IA, is characterized by low, rolling hills and rocky ridges containing many streams. The mean elev. is 700'.

CLIMATE. The continental climate of Davenport is marked by wide variations in seasonal weather conditions. Monthly mean temps. range from 22°F in Jan. to 75°F in July, with an annual avg. of about 50°F. The avg. annual rainfall is 33". Most of the avg. annual snowfall of approx. 30" occurs in Dec., Jan. and Feb. The RH ranges from 55% to 85%. The avg. growing season is 185 days. Davenport is located in the CSTZ and observes DST.

FLORA AND FAUNA. Animals native to Davenport include the whitetail deer, opossum, and raccoon. Common birds are the meadowlark, house wren, barn swallow, red-tailed hawk, great horned owl, E phoebe and

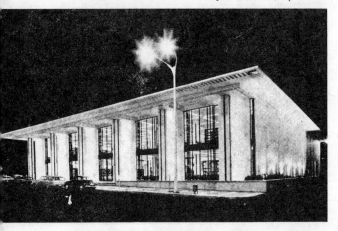

Davenport Public Library, Davenport, Iowa

mourning dove. Bullfrogs, mud turtles, box turtles, American toads, tiger salamanders, skinks and milk snakes, as well as the venomous timber rattlesnake and E massasauga (a pygmy rattler), are found in the area. Ccmmon trees are the maple, elm, ash, sycamore and oak. Smaller plants include the green foxtail, field daisy, violet, yellow orchid and chicory.

POPULATION. According to the US census, the pop. of Davenport in 1970 was 98,469. In 1978, it was estimated that it had increased to 101,800.

ETHNIC GROUPS. In 1978, the ethnic distribution of Davenport was approx. 95.5% Caucasian, 4.2% Black and 2.0% Hispanic. (A percentage of the Hispanic total is included in the Caucasian total.)

TRANSPORTATION. Interstate hwys. 74, 80 and 280 and US hwys. 61, 67 and 150, and state hwys. 22 and 130 provide major motor access to Davenport. The city is served by three *railroads*, the Burlington Northern; the Chicago, Milwaukee, St. Paul and Pacific, and the Chicago, Rock Island and Pacific. OZ, UA, Britt and MVA *airlines* serve Quad City Airport.

COMMUNICATIONS. Communications, broadcasting and print media serving Davenport are: *AM radio stations* KSTT 1170 (ABC/C, Contemp.); WOC 1420 (NBC, MOR) and KWNT 1580 (ABC/E, C&W); *FM radio stations* KALA 90.1 (NPR, Educ.); KIIK 103.7 (Indep., Rock, Contemp.) and KRVR 106.5 (Indep., Btfl. Mus.); *television stations* WHBF Ch. 4 (CBS); WOC Ch. 6 (NBC) and WQAD Ch. 8 (ABC); *press*: the Quad *City Times*, a daily published in morning and evening editions, is the area's major newspaper. Other publications include the *Catholic Messenger, International Review of Chiropractic* and *IA Bird Life.*

HISTORY. Native Americans of the Sac tribe inhabited the area of present day Davenport prior to settlement by white men in 1808. White encroachment on Sac lands caused bitter conflicts, and, in 1823 the Sacs were directed to move westward. When Chief Blackhawk and some of his people refused, the resulting tensions, aggravated by cruel white aggression, led to bloodshed and war. His followers killed, wounded or scattered. Blackhawk was captured in the fall of 1832. On Sept. 30, 1832, a treaty was concluded with Blackhawk, resulting in the acquisition by the US of six million acres of land

W of the MS River known in history as the Blackhawk Purchase. In 1833, land in what is now the S part of Davenport was claimed by interpreter Antoine LeClaire, who also bought parcels of other claimants. In the fall of 1835, a group of men met at the home of fur trader George Davenport on Rock or Arsenal Island and agreed to form a company to survey a town. The area previously purchased by LeClaire was sold to the company and surveyed into lots for the new town of Davenport in the spring of 1836. The city was incorporated in 1839. In 1854, the first RR from the E reached the MS River S of the city and the first bridge over the river was constructed in 1856. City growth through the late 1800s and into the 1900s was based on shipping and light and heavy manufacturing industries.

GOVERNMENT. Davenport has a mayor-council-mgr. form of govt. It consists of a mayor and ten council members, called aldermen, who appoint a city administrator. The mayor and two of the aldermen are elected at large, while eight are elected by ward. All members serve two-year terms.

ECONOMY AND INDUSTRY. The principal manufactures of Davenport include aluminum, cement, flour, locomotives, electronic equipment, men's clothing and iron and steel products. In 1979, a huge roller gate dam, largest of its type in the US, regulates the waters of the MS River at Davenport as part of the US govt.'s canalization project of the upper MS. In 1979, the labor force of the greater met. area totaled about 69,900, while the unemployment rate was 3.6%. Avg. household income was $17,308.

BANKING. There are four commercial banks and three savings and loan assns. in Davenport. In 1978, deposits at the four banks headquartered in the city totaled $561,044,000, while assets totaled $680,527,000. Among the banks are Davenport Bank and Trust, First Natl. Bank of Davenport, First Trust and Savings and Northwest Bank and Trust.

HOSPITALS. There are three hosps. in Davenport, Davenport Osteopathic, Mercy and St. Lukes.

EDUCATION. Ten institutions in IA and IL including Marycrest Col., located in Davenport are affiliated with the Quad-Cities Grad. Study Center. Organized in 1969, the Center coordinates programs and awards master degrees. In 1978, approx. 5,000 enrolled. Marycrest Col., a liberal arts institution, enrolled approx. 1,200 in 1978. Palmer Jr. Col., a two-year institution offering associate degrees, enrolled approx. 600 in 1978. St. Ambrose Col., a four-year liberal arts institution, enrolled approx. 1,700 in 1978. Other colleges in the city include E IA Comm. and Palmer Col. of Chiropractic. The public school system consists of 27 elementary, five jr. and two sr. high schools and had an enrollment of

Davenport, Iowa

23,000 students in 1978. There are seven parochial elementary schools and one private high school in the city as well. Davenport Public Lib. maintains one branch.

ENTERTAINMENT. The Bix Beiderbecke Memorial Jazz Festival is held in LeClaire Park in Davenport each summer. Day and night concerts feature traditional jazz bands. The Bettendorf Intl. Folk Fetival, another annual summer event, features customs, handicrafts and foods of more than 25 nations. The Handel Oratorio Society performs "The Messiah" at Christmas. The city supports the Quad City Cubs baseball team of the MWL.

ACCOMMODATIONS. Among the hotels and motels in Davenport are the Clayton House, Crest, Bronze Lantern, Blackhawk Hotel and the MS, Town House, Tallcorn, Quality, Holiday and Ramada inns.

FACILITIES. There are 23 parks and playgrounds in Davenport containing a children's zoo, picnic areas, golf courses, tennis courts, playing fields, swimming pools and bridle paths. Rose Park Gardens in Vander Veer Park contains approx. 2,500 species of roses. Fishing and boating facilities are available on the MS and Rock rivers.

CULTURAL ACTIVITIES. The Davenport Municipal Art Gallery contains American, Mexican and European art, as well as the permanent Grant Wood exhibit of the works of one of the foremost artists of IA. The art gallery is adjacent to the Putnam Museum, which houses natural science and historical exhibits as well as relics of native American mound-builders, and the original Blackhawk Treaty. The John M. Browning Memorial Museum, located on Arsenal Island, contains one of the most complete weaponry displays in the US. A museum featuring agricultural machinery is located in the John Pure Administration Center. The Tri-City Symphony Orchestra, founded in 1914, presents six concerts each year, while the Youth Symphony performs under its auspices. The Friends of Chamber Music presents a season of five programs and concerts and workshops are conducted by the American Guild Organists. The Playcrafters, the Bettendorf Community Theater, the Quad-City Music Guild and the Davenport Theater present a variety of stage productions, while the Genesis Guild performs Greek and Shakespearean plays. The Broadway Theater League sponsors Broadway road shows for the Quad-City area.

LANDMARKS AND SIGHTSEEING SPOTS. Interesting buildings in the city include the Davenport City Hall, the original structure of which was built in 1895; a restoration of the central portion of the home of Col. George Davenport, on Arsenal Island, where he is also buried; a replica blockhouse of Ft. Armstrong, built on the original (1816) Rock Island site of the outpost and the Judge James Grant Lib. in the Scott Co. Courthouse, which preserves the lib. of the highest paid lawyer in the US during his era. The John F. Dillon City Foundation was dedicated in 1914 in memory of Judge Dillon, an early Davenport jurist. Little Bit O'Heaven, the collection of world traveler Dr. B. J. Palmer, is displayed in a conservatory at the Palmer Col. of Chiropractic. Soldiers Monument was erected in 1850 in memory of Scott Co. men who died in the Civil War. Confederate soldiers who died while imprisoned at Rock Island Arsenal during the Civil War, as well as Union soldiers, are buried at the Arsenal Cemetery on Arsenal Island.

DAYTON
OHIO

CITY LOCATION-SIZE-EXTENT. Dayton, seat of Montgomery Co., encompasses 49.30 sq. mi. in W OH in the Miami River Valley, 45 mi. SW of Cincinnati, at 39°54' N lat. and 84°12' W long. The greater met. area extends W into Preble Co., N and W into Montgomery Co., N into Miami Co. and E into Greene Co.

TOPOGRAPHY. The terrain of Dayton, which is situated on a plain of the Miami River Valley, 50' to 200' below the gen. elev. of the adjacent rolling areas, is nearly flat. Three Miami River tributaries, the Mad and Stillwater rivers and Wolf Creek, enter the city from the N and join the Miami River within the city limits. Terrain N

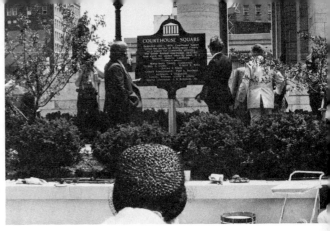

Courthouse Plaza in downtown Dayton, Ohio

of the city rises gradually towards the highest point in OH, while S of the city, the terrain slopes downward to the point where the Miami meets the OH River. The elev. ranges from 715' to 965', with a mean elev. of 757'.

CLIMATE. The climate of Dayton is continental, influenced by the Great Lakes to the N as well as by its position in the Miami River Valley, and characterized by moderate temps. Monthly mean temps. range from 28.6°F in Jan to 75°F in July, with an annual avg. of 52.4°F. The annual avg. rainfall of 36" is fairly evenly distributed throughout the year, while most of the annual avg. snowfall of 28.6" occurs from Dec. to Mar. The RH ranges from 54% to 86%. The avg. growing season is 185 days. Dayton lies in the ESTZ and observes DST.

FLORA AND FAUNA. Animals native to Dayton include the opossum, weasel and chipmunk. Common birds include the mourning dove, swallow, blue jay and cardinal. Frogs, salamanders, toads, lizards, turtles and snakes, including the venomous timber rattlesnake, E massasauga (a pygmy rattler) and copperhead, are found in the area. Common trees are the hickory, elm, oak, birch, maple, buckeye and redbud. Smaller plants include the honeysuckle, wood sorrel, blackberry and hepatica.

POPULATION. According to the US census, the pop. of Dayton in 1970 was 244,560. In 1978, it was estimated that it had decreased to 197,000.

ETHNIC GROUPS. In 1978, the ethnic distribution of Dayton was approx. 69% Caucasian, 30.4% Black and 0.6% Hispanic.

TRANSPORTATION. Interstate hwys. 70, 75 and 675, US hwys. 25,35 and 40 and state hwys. 4, 48 and 49 provide major motor access to Dayton. *Railroads* serving the city include the Chessie System and ConRail. *Airlines* serving James M. Cox Dayton Intl. Airport are US Air, AA, DL, NC, TW and UA. *Bus lines* serving the city include Greyhound, Trailways, Dayton & SE, Dayton Valley, Dayton-Xenia, Miami Valley Regional Transit Authority (RTA), Day-Brook and W Milton-Dayton.

COMMUNICATIONS. Communications, broadcasting and print media originating from Dayton are: *AM radio stations* WONE 980 (Indep., C&W); WAVI 1210 (ABC/E, Talk, News); WHIO 1290 (CBS, MOR) and WING 1410 (UPI, Contemp.); *FM radio stations* WGKM 88.1 (Indep., Divers.); WWSU 88.5 (Indep., Divers.); WCXL 88.7 (Indep., Divers.); WHIO 99.1 (Indep., Btfl. Mus.); WTUE 104.7 (Indep., AOR) and WDAO 107.7 (ABC/C, Mut. Blk., Soul); *television stations* WDTN Ch. 2 (NBC); WHIO Ch. 7 (CBS); WPTD Ch. 16 (PBS, CEN, OEB) and WKEF Ch. 22 (ABC); *press*: two major dailies serve the city, the *Journal Herald*, published mornings, and the *Daily News*, issued evenings and Sun. mornings; other publications include the weekly *Black Press* and *Sky Writer*, the bi-monthly *Educational Dealer* and *Manager*, the monthly *Today's Catholic Teacher* and *Jet Stone News*.

HISTORY. Native Americans of the Miami and Shawnee tribes inhabited the area of present-day Dayton before the first white settlers arrived. In 1795, the site of the settlement was purchased by four men, including Gen. Jonathan Dayton, who served under Revolutionary War hero Gen. Lafayette. The following year, settlers from Cincinnati arrived, attracted by the convergence of three major rivers—the Mad, the Miami and the Stillwater—and named the comm. in honor of land-owner Dayton. In 1805, two years after OH achieved statehood, Dayton was incorporated as a village. The construction of the Miami-Erie Canal contributed to the importance of the town as a transportation and trade center, and, from 1810 to 1840, its pop. grew from nearly 400 to more than 6,000. In 1841, Dayton was incorporated as a city. During the latter part of the 19th century, various industries were established in the city, and its pop. reached 30,000 by 1870. Orville and Wilbur Wright first experimented with airplanes in their bicycle shop in the city, known as the "Birthplace of Aviation", at the end of the 1800s. By 1910, its pop. exceeded 116,500. In 1913, the city was devastated and more than 300 people killed in the flooding of the Mad, Miami and Stillwater rivers. To prevent future flooding, the Miami Conservancy District was established in 1915. One of the most effective flood control systems in the world, it consists of five dams built between 1918 and 1922, funded exclusively by local monies. Through-out the 1900s, the city continued to grow as a manu-facturing center, largely based on the development of the airplane industry. Later, the Wright-Patterson AFB was established in the city.

GOVERNMENT. After the great 1913 flood, Dayton became the first US city with a pop. exceeding 100,000, to adopt the commission-mgr. form of govt. Five council members, including the mayor, are elected at large to four-year terms.

ECONOMY AND INDUSTRY. There are 800 manufacturing plants in Dayton, employing nearly 30% of the total work force. Products include aircraft equipment, scien-tific instruments, rubber, chemical and plastic goods, carbon steel products, automotive parts and motors, electrical equipment, computer systems and printed materials. The headquarters of NCR Corp., the world's chief producer of cash registers, is located in the city. Wright-Patterson AFB is the largest single employer. In 1979, the total labor force for the met. area was approx. 392,400, while the rate of unemployment was 6.8%

BANKING. There are 10 commercial banks and nine savings and loan assns. in Dayton. In 1978, deposits at the six banks headquartered in the city totaled approx. $1,517,452,000, while assets totaled approx. $1,827,305,000. Among the banks serving the city are Central Trust Co. of Montgomery Co., Farmers & Merchants, First Natl., First OH State, Trotwood and Unity State.

HOSPITALS. There are several hosps. in Dayton, including Miami Valley, St. Elizabeth, Good Samaritan, Charles F. Kettering Memorial, Grandview Osteopathic, Wright-Patterson AFB, Dayton State, V.A., Dayton Children's Psychiatric and Children's Medical Center.

EDUCATION. The U of Dayton, a private Roman Catholic institution founded more than 100 years ago, offers associate, bachelor and master degrees. In 1978, full-time enrollment exceeded 9,600 and included nearly 2,700 grad. students. Wright State U, a state-supported institution established in 1964, awards associate degrees, bachelor and master degrees and includes a medical school. In 1978, approx. 13,750 enrolled. Other institutions include Miami-Jacobs Col. of Business, AF Institute of Tech., Sinclair Comm. Col. (which enrolled nearly 13,800 in 1978), Intl. Broadcasting School, OH Institute of Photography and United Theological Seminary. There are 28 elementary and secondary schools, as well as two vocational schools, enrolling more than 38,100 in the public school system. In addition, there are 37 private elementary and secondary schools. Lib. facilities include the Dayton-Montgomery Co. Public Lib.

ENTERTAINMENT. Local sports entertainment in Dayton is provided by the Wright State U Raiders, the U of Dayton Flyers and the Sinclair Comm. Col. Tartans, who participate in intercollegiate sports.

ACCOMMODATIONS. There are several hotels and motels in Dayton, including the Daytonian, Stouffer's Hotel, Imperial House, Howard Johnson's and the Sheraton, Holiday, Ramada, Quality and Days inns.

FACILITIES. There are several public parks in Dayton, including Deeds, Madden, Five Oaks, Belmont, Eastwood, Triangle, De Weese and Princeton. Facilities include public golf courses, tennis courts, picnic areas, swimming pools and bicycling, horseback riding and jogging trails.

CULTURAL ACTIVITIES. The Dayton Civic Ballet, which is nationally-recognized, and the Dayton Philharmonic Orchestra are among the performing arts organizations in the city. The Kenley Players, OH Ballet and other visiting groups also perform in the city at the Victory Theatre, Memorial Hall, Dayton Convention and Exhibition Center, Hara Arena and the U of Dayton Field House. The Dayton Art Institute houses Oriental and European art, a pre-Columbian collection and two medieval cloisters. The Dayton Museum of Natural History features small animal and reptile exhibits, as well as native American relics and a planetarium. The Montgomery Co. Historical Society Old Courthouse Museum houses historical and cultural exhibits and devotes a section to the Wright Brothers. Aviation exhibits are located at the USAF Museum. It features displays on space travel, the atomic bomb and the history of aviation.

LANDMARKS AND SIGHTSEEING SPOTS. Carillon Park in Dayton features the 40-bell Deeds Carillon, a transportation exhibit and the Newcom Tavern, the oldest structure in the city. The Wright Brothers Memorial, located N of Wright Field, commemorates the early aviators. Historic homes in the city include the Dunbar House, home of poet Paul Lawrence Dunbar and a state historic site, and the Patterson Homestead, built in 1816 by Revolutionary War hero and Lexington, KY founder Col. Robert Patterson. It is furnished with 18th-century items, portraits and family memorabilia. The OR District, one of Dayton's earliest communities, features renovated homes, shops and restaurants.

Dayton, Ohio

DENVER
COLORADO

CITY LOCATION-SIZE-EXTENT. Denver, the seat of Denver Co. and capital of the state, is located in N central CO, approx. 50 mi. E of the Continental Divide and about 10 mi. E of the Rocky Mts., at 39°43' N lat. and 104°58' W long. The city encompasses 115.08 sq. mi. Its greater

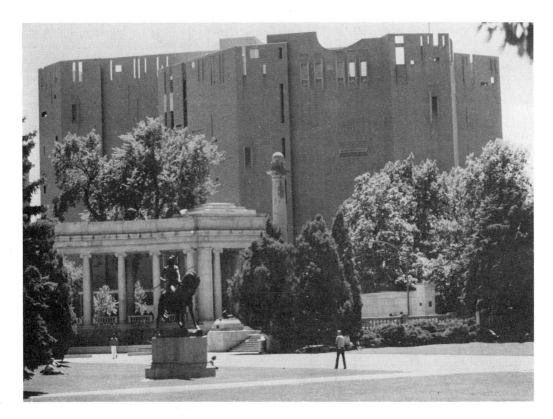

Denver Art Museum, Denver, Colorado

met. area extends into Adams Co. on the N and E, Arapahoe Co. on the S and E and Jefferson Co. on the W and includes the cities of Aurora to the E, Englewood and Lihrton to the S, Lakewood and Golden to the W and Arvada and Commerce City to the N.

TOPOGRAPHY. Denver, bordered on the E by the Great Plains, is located in the foothills of the Rocky Mts. The terrain is characterized by rolling high plains broken by drainage ditches, many of which carry water only during times of heavy run-off from melting snow. The S Platte River divides the W third of Denver from the E two-thirds of the city. Other bodies of water in the city are Cherry Creek, Bear Creek, Marston Lake, Sloan Lake and Johnson Reservoir. The mean elev. of the "Mile High City" is 5,283'.

CLIMATE. The mild, sunny, semi-arid climate of Denver is due largely to its location at the foot of the E slope of the Rocky Mts. in the path of prevailing westerlies. The weather is also influenced by air masses from Canada and AK, warm, moist air from the Gulf of Mexico and warm, dry air from Mexico and the SW. The avg. annual temp. of 50.2°F ranges from a Jan. mean of 30.1°F to a July mean of 72.7°F. The avg. annual rainfall is 14.5", while the avg. annual snowfall is 59". The RH ranges from 35% to 71%. Denver lies in the MSTZ and observes DST.

FLORA AND FAUNA. Animals native to Denver include the mule deer, bighorn sheep, elk, antelope, jackrabbit and seven-striped ground squirrel. Common birds are the mt. bluebird, crow, magpie, scrub jay, redwinged blackbird and golden and bald eagles. Lizards, frogs and snakes, including the venomous prairie rattlesnake, are found here. Typical trees include the Dutch elm, spruce, pine, willow, box elder and cottonwood. Smaller plants include the yucca and ivy.

POPULATION. According to the US census, the pop. of Denver in 1970 was 514,678. In 1978, it was estimated that it had increased to 516,000.

ETHNIC GROUPS. In 1978, the ethnic distribution of Denver was approx. 60% Caucasian, 14.2% Black, 23.3% Hispanic, .6% Asian and 1.9% other.

TRANSPORTATION. Interstate hwys. 25, 70, 76 and 225, US hwys. 6, 40, 87, 285 and 287 and State Hwy. 95 provide major motor access to Denver. *Railroads* serving the city are the Rio Grande, Union Pacific, CO & S, Burlington N and AMTRAK. *Airlines* serving Stapleton Intl. Airport are UA, CO, TW, WA, FL, BN, TI, OZ, PX and Mexicana. *Bus lines* serving the city are Trailways, Greyhound and the Regional Transportation District.

COMMUNICATIONS. Communications, broadcasting and print media serving Denver are: *AM radio stations* KLZ 560 (ABC/E, MOR); KHOW 630 (ABC/E, MOR); KERE 710 (Indep., C&W); KOA 850 (CBS, Gen.); KPOF 910 (Indep., Spec. Progsv.); KIMN 950 (Indep., Top 40); KRKS 990 (Keystone Rep., MOR); KAAT 1090 (MBS, Relig.); KWBZ 1150 (Indep., talk); KBNO 1220 (MBS, Span.); KTLK 1280 (ABC, Contemp.); KDEN 1340 (ABC/I, News); KFML 1390 (Indep., Free) and KLAK 1600 (Indep., CUW); *FM radio stations* KCFR 90.1 (NPR, Gen.); KXKX 95.7 (Indep., Top 40); KXMN 98.5 (Indep., top 40); KVOD 99.5 (Indep., Clas.); KLIR 100.3 (Indep., Clas.); KOSI 101.1 (Indep., Btlf. Mus.); KOZQ 103.5 (Indep., Adult Rock); KADX 105.1 (ABC, Jazz); KBPI 105.9 (Indep., Progsv.) and KAZY 106.7 (Indep., AOR); *television stations* KWG Ch. 2 (WGN); KOA Ch. 4 (NBC); KRMA Ch. 6 (PBS); KGMH Ch. 7 (CBS) and KBTV Ch. 9 (ABC); *press:* two major dailies serve the area, *the Post*, published weekday evenings and weekend mornings, and *Rocky Mt. News*, issued mornings; other publications in the area include the *Denver Weekly*, *Daily Journal*, *Industry and Commerce*, *Denver Magazine* and *Rocky Mt. Journal*.

HISTORY. Denver was founded in the gold rush that followed the discovery of gold first by native Americans of the Cherokee nation and then by a group of GA miners, led by W. Green Russell, in Dry Creek, in 1858.

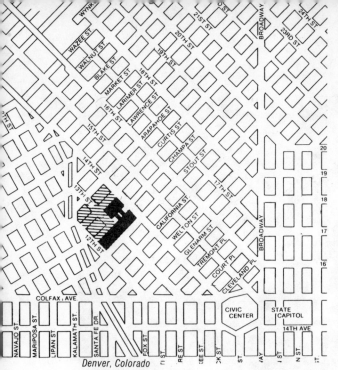

Denver, Colorado

ECONOMY AND INDUSTRY. Major industries in Denver include energy development, research, electronics, food processing, petrochemicals and exports. The fed. govt., aerospace, military installations and tourism are also important to the city's economy. The US Mint in Denver, which has been operating since 1906, produces four billion coins annually and is one of the only two remaining mints in the US. In 1978, the median family income in Denver was estimated at $14,400, while the total labor force was estimated to be 326,000. In Apr., 1978, the rate of unemployment was approx. 5.2%.

BANKING. There are 56 banks headquartered in Denver. In 1978,total deposits for the banks headquartered in the city were approx. $4,918,308,000, while total assets were $6,116,847,000. Among the banks are American Natl., Central, CO Natl., First Natl., and United.

HOSPITALS. The Natl. Asthma Center, CARISH, is located in Denver. There are approx. 20 hosps. in the city, among them Beth Israel, Children's, U of CO

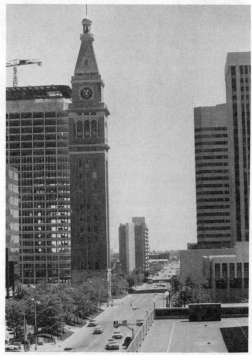

The D and F "Tilting" Tower of Denver, built in 1910, seems to be tilting but does not. Denver, Colorado.

Medical Center, Porter Memorial, Rocky Mt. Osteopathic, St. Anthony, St. Joseph, St. Luke's, Spears Chiropractic, Denver Gen., Ft. Logan Mental Health Center, Mercy Medical Center, Mt. Airy Psychiatric Center, Natl. Jewish Hosp. and Research Center, Rose Med. Center and Spalding Rehabilitation Center.

EDUCATION. The U of Denver, a private institution established in 1864 offers undergrad. and grad. courses. In 1978, it enrolled close to 7,800. The publicly supported U of CO at Denver, established in 1956, enrolled more than 8,800 in 1978. Also located in the area are Loretto Heights Col., established in 1918, Regis Col. (established in 1877), CO Women's Col. (established in 1888), Col. of Denver, CO School of Mines, CO Institute of Art, Barnes Business Col., Denver Inst. of Technology and Parks School of Business. The public school system consists of 93 elementary schools, 18 jr. high and nine sr. high schools and several special facilities. There are also more than 690 private schools in the city. The Denver Public Lib., founded in 1889, was the first in the US to initiate a children's lib. and is noted for its

The first settlement, known as MT City, was moved to the junction of the S Platte River and Cherry Creek, when it became known as Auraria Town Co. In Nov., 1858, a group of prospectors from KS organized a co. town on the E bank of Cherry Creek opposite Auraria, and named it in honor of James W. Denver, then Gov. of KS Territory, in which the area was located. Denver became a supply and service center for the gold fields. Incorporated as a CO territorial city in 1861, Denver became, in 1877, the capital of CO, after it had achieved statehood. The arrival of the RR in 1870 at which time the pop. was less than 4,800, increased the city's importance as a distribution point. Irrigation contributed to the development of the city as a successful ranching and farming community, and a silver boom in the 1880s and 1890s benefited the city's economy as well. By 1890, its pop. had reached 106,713. With the adoption of the gold standard in 1893, the silver market collapsed and the city experienced a depression. It recovered however, when gold was again discovered at Cripple Creek, 100 mi. S, at the end of the century. A new charter in 1902 created a combined city-county form of govt. for Denver and six adjoining towns. The city pursued a development and beautification program, and emerged from a prairie town. Although the city's progress slowed during the Depression, the pop. soared during WW II as the rate of fed. employment increased. The post-war years saw the migration of former military personnel stationed there. Under the auspices of the fed. govt., a major expansion of technological activities, including the aerospace industry, occurred in the greater met. area. At the same time, the discovery of oil in the Dakotas and S Canada attracted petroleum management, research and exploration companies to Denver from OK and TX. Most recently, local, state and fed. agencies have been involved in conservation of the environment while industries have expanded and major anti-pollution and urban renewal projects have been initiated.

GOVERNMENT. Denver has a strong mayor-council form of govt. consisting of 13 council members and a mayor with complete appointive and budgetary powers. The mayor and two council members are elected at large, while 11 councillors are elected by district. All serve four-year terms.

W history dept. and conservation lib. It maintains 14 branch libs., seven store-front libs. and two bookmobiles. Other libs. are available at area colleges and universities and the State Heritage Center.

ENTERTAINMENT. There are several dinner theaters in Denver, including the County Dinner Playhouse and Eugene's Dinner Theatre. The oldest continuous summer stock theater in the US, founded in 1891, performs at Elitch Gardens. The Denver Opera Foundation annually presents the "Post Opera" in a free public performance. Auto racing events include the Continental Wheelstander Championships, the Annual Rocky Mt. Funny Car Championship, the annual Indy Rocky Mt. 150 Road Race, the High Alt. Natls. and the Fuel Dragster and Pro Stock Review. The Natl. W Livestock Show and Rodeo is held in the city every Jan. The Denver Bears, an AA League baseball team, and the Denver Broncos, an NFL-AFC football team, play at the Mile-High Stadium. The Denver Nuggets, an NBA basketball

CULTURAL ACTIVITIES. Among the museums and art galleries in Denver are the Denver Art Museum, which features permanent and loan collections of ancient Mediterranean, Gothic, Renaissance, Impressionistic, American and Oriental art; the galleries of CO Women's Col., the Denver Artists Guild and the Denver Public Lib; the Museum of Natural History; the CO State Historical Museum, featuring exhibits of the early W and models of native American life; and the CO School of Mines Geology Museum. Specialized museums include the Buffalo Bill Cody Memorial, CO RR, Forney Transportation and CO Transportation Museums, as well as the House of Carvings, displaying the work of the late Dr. Niblack. The Denver Symphony Orchestra, conducted by Gaetano Delogu, performs at the Boettcher Concert Hall, part of the Denver Center (a performing arts complex) and also presents outdoor concerts. Other musical organizations are the Brico Symphony conducted by Dr. Antonia Brico, the Denver Concert Band, the

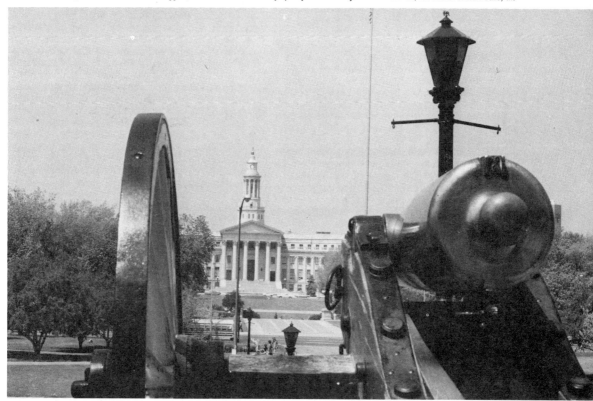

City and County Building, Denver, Colorado

team, and the CO Rockies, an NHL-Campbell Conf. hockey team, play at McNichols Sports Arena. The Caribous, an NASL soccer team, the Comets, an Intl. Volleyball Assn. team, and the Racquets, a WTT tennis team, also play in the city, while teams of the U of CO participate in intercollegiate sports in the Big Eight Conf.

ACCOMMODATIONS. Among the hotels and motels in Denver are the Brown Palace Hotel, Hilton, Marina, Executive Tower, Radisson Denver, Denver Plaza, Stapleton Plaza, Fairmont, Stouffer's, Writer's Manor Hotel, Country Village, TraveLodge, and the Kipling, Regency, Sheraton, Holiday, Ramada, Rodeway, LaQuinta and Quality inns.

FACILITIES. There are 180 city parks in Denver encompassing close to 4,200 acres, 46 parkways totaling 77.7 mi. in length and 27 mt. parks in neighboring counties encompassing 13,500 acres. Major parks include City, Berkeley, Chessman and Washington. The park system contains seven public golf courses, playing fields, tennis courts, ice skating rinks, swimming facilities and more than 100 mi. of hiking-bicycling and jogging trails (including a 12-mi. trail along the Platte River Greenway). The Denver Zoo in City Park includes a children's zoo. The Botanical Gardens house a conservatory and horticultural hall.

Friends of Chamber Music and the Central City Opera House Assn. and Classic Chorale, which also perform at the Denver Center. Recitals are given by the Met. State Col. and U of Denver Lamont School of Music. The Munt-Brooks Dancers, the CO Concert Ballet and the Denver Civic Ballet are also based in the city as are approx. 20 theater groups, including the Denver Center Theatre Co. (a regional professional repertory group), the Bonfils Theatre (a comm. arts theater), the Co. of Players Children's Theatre and the Theatre Under Glass Children's Theatre.

LANDMARKS AND SIGHTSEEING SPOTS. The Denver State Capitol Complex houses the State Capitol, State Services and State Office buildings, State Capitol Annex and State Historical Museum. The Capitol is a Corinthian style structure of CO granite. The 13th step on the W side is exactly one mi. above SL. Nearby is the Civic Center and outdoor Greek Theatre. Larimer Sq., a 19th-century restored historic and commercial area, contains shops, restaurants, nightspots and galleries in a mid-Victorian setting. In this block was the site of the first drugstore, the first US Post Office and the first book store in Denver. The D&F tower, focal point of the city's skyline, is fashioned after the bell tower of St. Mark's Cathedral in Venice. Built in 1910, it is listed on the Natl. Register of Historic Places. The "Molly Brown House" has been preserved in tribute to the memory of the legendary heiress, Molly Brown, who survived the sinking of the Titanic. Sakura Sq., a Japanese Cultural Center, is a block of oriental restaurants, shops and businesses surrounded by Japanese gardens.

DES MOINES
IOWA

CITY LOCATION-SIZE-EXTENT. Des Moines, the capital and largest city of the state and seat of Polk Co., encompasses 64.3 sq. mi. in central IA on the Des Moines River at 41°32' N lat. and 93°39' W long. The greater met. area extends throughout Polk Co. and into Dallas Co. to the W and Warren Co. to the S.

TOPOGRAPHY. The terrain of Des Moines, which is situated in the interior lowland region of N America, is gently rolling and contains numerous rivers and lakes, including Gray's. Case's, Dean and Lake Easter. The Raccoon River enters the city from the W and joins with the Des Moines River (in the central part of the city), which flows through the E part of the city. The mean elev. is 815'.

CLIMATE. The climate of Des Moines is continental, characterized by cold winters and warm summers. The avg. annual temp. of 50°F ranges from a Jan. mean of 20.5°F to a July mean of 76.1°F. Most of the 31.5" avg. annual rainfall occurs during spring and summer, while nearly 70% of the 33.4" avg. annual snowfall occurs from Dec. through Feb. The RH ranges from 53% to 84%. The avg. growing season is 190 days. Des Moines lies in the CSTZ and observes DST.

FLORA AND FAUNA. Animals native to Des Moines include the fox, opossum, shrew and raccoon. Common birds are the barn swallow, starling,

Downtown Des Moines, Iowa

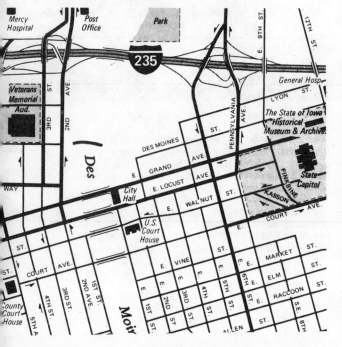

yellow-billed cuckoo, E gold finch (the state bird), mourning dove and cardinal. Bullfrogs, skinks, tree frogs, painted turtles and hognose snakes, as the well as the venomous E massasauga (a pygmy rattler) and timber rattlesnake, are found in the area. Common trees include the maple, elm, ash, oak (the state tree) and sycamore. Smaller plants include the wild rose (the state flower), violet, yellow orchid, chicory, mulberry, crab apple and pepperweed.

POPULATION. According to the US census, the pop. of Des Moines in 1970 was 201,104. In 1978, it was estimated that it had decreased to approx. 189,200.

ETHNIC GROUPS. In 1978, the ethnic distribution of Des Moines was approx. 93.8% Caucasian, 5.7% Black, 1.3% Hispanic, .1% Asian and .3% other (a percentage of the Hispanic total is also included in the Caucasian total).

TRANSPORTATION. Interstate hwys. 35, 80, and 235, US hwys. 6, 65, 69 and 163 and state hwys. 5, 28, 46, 90, 401 and 415 provide major motor access to Des Moines. *Railroads* serving the city include AMTRAK, Burlington Northern, Des Moines Union, Santa Fe and Union Pacific. *Airlines* serving Des Moines Municipal Airport include AA, BN, OZ and UA. *Bus lines* include Jefferson, Greyhound and Trailways, as well as the local Airport Transit Authority and Des Moines Met. Transit Authority.

COMMUNICATIONS. Communications, broadcasting and print media serving Des Moines are: *AM radio stations* KIOA 940 (Indep., Rock); WHO 1040 (NBC, Var.); KRNT 1350 (CBS, Contemp.); KCVC 1390 (ABC/C, All Music) and KSO 1460 (ABC/E, C&W); *FM radio stations* KMGK 93.3 (Indep., Rock); KGGO 94.9 (Indep., Top 40); KDMI 97.3 (NBC, Relig., News); KLYF 100.3 (Indep., Btfl. Mus.) and KRNQ 102.5 (Indep., Rock); *television stations* WOI Ch. 5 (ABC); KCCI Ch. 8 (CBS); KDIN Ch. 11 (PBS) and WHO Ch. 13 (NBC); *press:* two major dailies serve the city, the *Register*, issued mornings, and the *Tribune*, issued evenings; other publications include the *Lee Town News*, *Highland Park News* and *Better Homes and Gardens*.

HISTORY. Native Americans of the Sac and Fox tribes inhabited the area of present-day Des Moines before the first white settlers arrived. In 1842, a treaty was signed in which the Sacs and Foxes relinquished their rights to the area. The following year, Des Moines was established as a US military garrison at the junction of the Des Moines and Raccoon rivers, with the purpose of preserving peace and protecting the Sac and Fox from the hostile Sioux, as well as from unscrupulous whites. The name is derived from the French corruption of the native American word "moingona", meaning "river of the mounds". In 1845, the region was opened to white settlers, and, although the ft. was abandoned by the military the following year, the 127 area settlers remained. Later that year, Ft. Des Moines became the seat of Polk Co. By 1853, when Ft. Des Moines was incorporated as a town, its pop. had reached approx. 500, and, by 1857, when it was designated the state capital and renamed the city of Des Moines, the pop. had grown to 3,500. Its economy benefited from its establishment as the capital, and, by 1890, the pop. had reached 50,000 and the municipal boundaries were extended. The city became a military training center and was the site of a Natl. Guard Camp in 1898, during the Spanish American War. In 1902, a cavalry post was established, and, during both WWs I and II, the city was the site of a major troop training facility. By 1950, the pop. of the city, which became the chief manufacturing center of the state, had grown to nearly 178,000.

GOVERNMENT. Des Moines has a council-mgr.-ward form of govt. consisting of seven council members, including the mayor as a voting member. The mayor and two council members are elected at large, while four members are elected by ward, to four-year terms. The council hires a city mgr., who is responsible for the administration of the govt.

ECONOMY AND INDUSTRY. The manufacturing plants in the Des Moines area, which is the chief manufacturing and commercial center of IA, annually produce more than 500 different products, including chemicals, pharmaceuticals, apparel, tools, machinery, automotive accessories, rubber products and agricultural equipment. Printing and publishing is also a major industry. More than 700 wholesale and 20,000 retail firms as well as the headquarters of over 60 insurance companies, are located in the area. In June, 1979, the total labor force for the greater met. area was approx. 183,300, while the rate of unemployment was 3.2%.

BANKING. There are 25 commercial banks, with 32 associate offices, and 10 savings and loan assns., with 16 branch offices, in Des Moines. In 1978, total deposits for the 12 banks headquartered in the city were $1,607,604,000, while total assets were $2,133,527,000. Banks serving the city include Bankers Trust, Central Natl., IA Des Moines Natl. and Valley Natl.

HOSPITALS. There are seven hosps. in Des Moines, including Des Moines Gen., Broadlawns, IA Lutheran, IA Methodist, Mercy, NW Comm. and V.A.

EDUCATION. Drake U, a private institution located in Des Moines, enrolled nearly 6,600 in 1978. Other institutions include the Col. of Osteopathic Medicine and Surgery, Grand View Col., Des Moines Area Comm Col., American Institute of Business and Open Bible Col. The Des Moines public school system, consisting of six sr. high, 13 jr. high, 49 elementary and four special schools, enrolled approx. 35,500 in 1978. Lib. facilities include the Des Moines Public Lib. which maintains 18 branches.

ENTERTAINMENT. There are two dinner theaters in Des Moines, the Purple Cow and Charlie's Showplace. The IA State Fair, held each Aug. at the State Fairgrounds, features agricultural and industrial exhibits. The Drake Relays, held each Apr., is a major track and field event. Other festivals and annual events are Horse and Buggy Days, Art in the Park, Victorian Weekend, Future Farming Days, Old Fashioned Fourth, Two Rivers Festival, Homemade Pie Festival, State Plowing Matches, IA Corn Days, Old Wheels Day and the Home and Flower Show.

ACCOMMODATIONS. There are many hotels and motels in Des Moines, including the Hotel Fort Des Moines, the Savery, Howard Johnson's and the Hilton, Ramada and Holiday inns.

FACILITIES. There are several public parks in Des Moines, featuring three golf courses, tennis courts, swimming pools, playing fields and the Des Moines Children's Zoo, which houses 150 varieties of animals and a reptile exhibit and offers elephant and burro rides. An amusement park and Botanical Center are also located in the city.

CULTURAL ACTIVITIES. The Des Moines Symphony Orchestra, Des Moines Civic Ballet, Des Moines Comm. Playhouse, Des Moines Civic Music Association, the Drama Workshop, Drake U Theater and the Theater for Young People are among the performing arts organizations located in the city. Works by Rodin, Goya and contemporary artists are displayed in the Des Moines Art Center, which was designed by architects Eliel Saarinen and J.M. Pei. The Des Moines Center of Science and Industry features a Foucault Pendulum and a display of computer technology, among other exhibits. Native American artifacts, minerals and fossils are included in the extensive collection of the Historical Building and Museum.

LANDMARKS AND SIGHTSEEING SPOTS. Among the landmarks in

Civic Center, Des Moines, Iowa

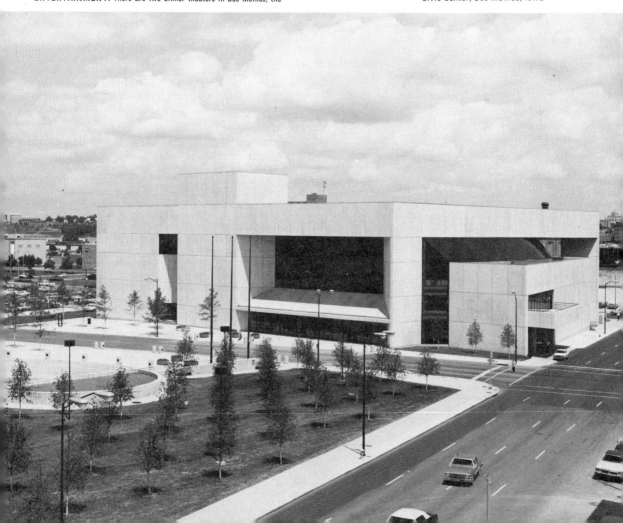

Des Moines is the Salisbury House, a replica of the King's House in Salisbury, England, which houses valuable art objects, a rare book lib. and furnishings of the Tudor Age. Four rooms are open for tours. The State Capitol, featuring a 22-karat gold leaf dome, houses valuable paintings and a collection of war flags. The 80-acre park surrounding the hill-top Capitol contains several memorial monuments. Terrace Hill, the Victorian "Prairie Palace of the West", donated to the state of IA by the Hubbell family estate, is now the residence of the Gov. A new Botanical Garden on the river bank opened in Dec., 1979

DETROIT
MICHIGAN

CITY LOCATION-SIZE-EXTENT. Detroit, the seat of Wayne Co., sixth largest city in the US and largest border city in the world, encompasses 139.6 sq. mi. in SE MI on the Detroit River and St. Lawrence Seaway at 42°25' N lat. and 83°01' W long. The only major city in the US from which one looks into neighboring Canada, Detroit is located across the Detroit River from Windsor, Ontario. Its greater met. area, the fifth largest in the US, includes the cities of Dearborn to the SE, Livonia to the W and Warren and Pontiac to the N, and extends into the counties of Livingston to the NW, and Oakland, Washtenaw to the SW, Macomb to the NE and Monroe to the S.

TOPOGRAPHY. The terrain of Detroit, which is situated in the Great Lakes plain region of the lower peninsula of MI, is nearly flat near the St. Lawrence Seaway, which consists of the Detroit and St. Clair rivers, Lake St. Clair, which borders the city on the E, and the W end of Lake Erie, 20 mi. to the SW. From the Seaway, the land

The Spirit of Detroit Monument, Detroit, Michigan

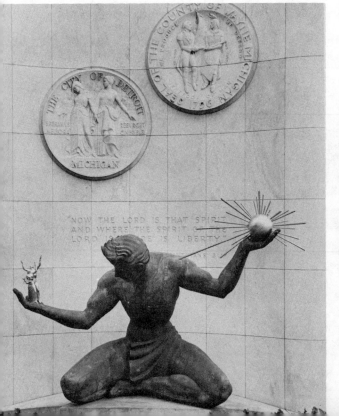

slopes upward to the NW for approx. 10 mi., at which point the terrain becomes increasingly rolling. Numerous small lakes, including Wing, Gilbert, Walnut, Orchard, Cass, Orange, Sylvan and Elizabeth lie approx. 20 mi. NW of the city. The mean elev. is 581'.

CLIMATE. The climate of Detroit is continental, influenced by its location near major storm tracks and the Great Lakes, which warm and moisten arctic air in the winter, while also causing much cloudiness, and moderate weather extremes. The annual mean temp. of 48.9°F ranges from a Jan. mean of 23.8°F to a July mean of 72.4°F. Temps. exceed 90°F an avg. two or three days each summer. The avg. annual precip. of 31.49" falls evenly throughout the year. Approx. 88% of the avg. annual snowfall of 36.1" occurs from Dec. through Mar., while individual snowstorms avg. 3". The RH ranges from 51% to 88%. The avg. growing season is 180 days. Detroit lies in the ESTZ and observes DST.

FLORA AND FAUNA. Animals native to Detroit include the E chipmunk, E cottontail rabbit, red squirrel, muskrat, brown bat and weasel. Common birds are the robin, thrush, brown thrasher, sharp-shinned hawk, herring gull and cuckoo. Salamanders and frogs, as well as the venomous E massasauga (a small rattlesnake) and timber rattlesnake, are found in the area. Typical trees include the oak, pine, maple and elm. Smaller plants are the fern, honeysuckle, rose, blackberry and dogwood.

POPULATION. According to the US census, the pop. of Detroit in 1970 was 1,514,063. In 1978, it was estimated that it had decreased to 1,210,000. More than 50% of the pop. of MI resides in the greater Detroit met. area.

ETHNIC GROUPS. In 1978, the ethnic distribution in Detroit was approx. 55.6% Black, 43.6% Caucasian and 1.8% Hispanic (a percentage of the Hispanic total is also included in the Caucasian total). More than 17,000 Arabic-speaking persons live in the area, the largest such group in the US.

TRANSPORTATION. Interstate hwys. 75, 94, 96 and 696, US hwys. 10 and 12 and state hwys., 1, 3, 5, 53, 85, 97, 102 and 153 provide major motor access to Detroit. *Railroads* serving the city include Burlington Northern, Canadian Natl., Chessie, ConRail, Delray, Detroit Toledo and Ironton, Grand Trunk Western, Milwaukee Road, Norfolk and Western, Santa Fe, and AMTRAK. *Airlines* serving Detroit Met. Airport include AA, US Air, BN, DL, EA, FL, NC, NW, OZ, PA, SO, TW and UA. Detroit City and Willow Run airports also serve the city. *Bus lines* serving the city include Greyhound, Trailways and the local Detroit Dept. of Transportation and SE MI Transportation Authority (SEMTA). The Port of Detroit, one of the busiest waterways in the world provides connections to more than 200 overseas ports and serves approx. 60 shipping lines and nearly 1,000 foreign ships annually. Four shipping terminals handle nearly three million tons of cargo.

COMMUNICATIONS. Communications, broadcasting and print media originating from Detroit are: *AM radio stations* WJR 760 (NBC, APR, Variety); WWJ 950 (CBS, APR, All News); WCX 1130 (ABC/E, MOR); WXYZ 1270 (ABC/C, MOR, Contemp.); WJLB 1400 (Indep., Blk.) and WDEE 1500 (ABC/I, Mod. Ctry.); *FM radio stations* WDTR 90.9 (Indep., Educ.); WTWR 92.3 (Indep., Adult Contemp.); WCRQ 93.1 (Indep., Contemp.); WCZY 95.5 (Indep., Btfl. Mus.); WJR 96.3 (Indep., Btfl. Mus.); WWS 97.1 (Indep., Btfl. Mus.); WMZK 97.9 (Indep., Bi-Lingual); WBFG 98.7 (UPI, Relig.); WABX 99.5 (Indep., Progsv.); WRIF 101.1 (ABC/FM, AOR); WDET 101.9 (NPR, Alter.); WMUZ 103.5 (APR, MOR, Adult Contemp.); WOMC 104.3 (Indep., Contemp.); WQRS 105.1 (Indep., Clas.); WJZZ 105.9 (APR, Jazz); WWW 106.7 (UPI, Progsv.) and WGPR 107.5 (Indep., Blk.); *television stations* WJBK Ch. 2 (CBS); WWJ Ch. 4 (NBC); WXYZ Ch. 7 (ABC); WXON Ch. 10 (Indep.); WTVS Ch. 56 (PBS) and WGPR Ch. 62 (Indep.); *press*: two major newspapers serve the area, the *Free Press*, issued mornings, and the *News*, issued evenings and weekend mornings; other publications include the *MI Chronicle, Building Tradesman, Burroughs Clearing House, Football News, S End, Detroit Business News* and *Hamtramek-N Detroit Citizen*.

HISTORY. The site of present-day Detroit, the oldest city in the Midwest, was originally inhabited by native

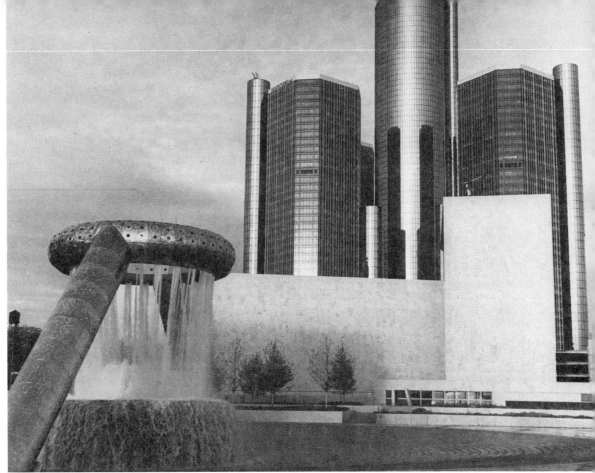

Rennaisance Center (background) and the Horace E. Dodge and Son Memorial Fountain, Detroit, Michigan

Americans of the Wyandot tribe of the Iroquois language group. In 1701, Antoine de la Mothe Cadillac and 100 Frenchmen were sent by King Louis XIV of France to establish a village on the shores of the Detroit River. Since it was surrounded by the river, the village was named Ville d'Etroit or "City of the Strait" by Cadillac. The crude palisade constructed by the men and named Ft. Pontchartrain later became an important fur-trading post. When France and Great Britain struggled for control of N America during the French and Indian Wars, Detroit was the objective of major military campaigns. In 1760, the British captured Ft. Pontchartrain and in 1778, constructed Ft. Lernoult on the site. During the Revolutionary War, British and native American troops attacked nearby American settlements from Detroit. More interested in fur revenues than in colonizing the region, the British retained control of the settlement until 1796, although the Revolutionary War had ended 13 years earlier. In 1802, Detroit was incorporated as a town. Following a fire in 1805, the town was rebuilt and redesigned, modeled after Washington, DC. During the War of 1812, the British regained control of Detroit for a year, but surrendered the city in 1813, after a decisive victory by US Navy Capt. Oliver Perry. Detroit was incorporated as a city in 1815. A flourishing shipping industry was initiated in the city when the first steamship to navigate the Upper Great Lakes, the "Walk-In-The-Water", arrived soon after. The opening of the Erie Canal in 1825 provided a water link with the E US and resulted in an influx of settlers to the area from N.E. and NY. From 1837 to 1847, Detroit served as the capital of MI, and, by 1850, its pop. had reached 21,000. The arrival of the RR two years later further contributed to the development of commerce, while the opening of the Soo Canals in 1855 and the subsequent development of industry resulted in the increase of the pop. of the city to 45,600 by 1860. An important manufacturing center after the Civil War, the city was inhabited by 116,000 by 1880. At the turn of the century, Henry Ford, Ransom E. Olds, Walter Chrysler and John and Horace Dodge were among those who pioneered the automobile industry, which grew rapidly because of the accessibility of raw materials and a large labor pool. Between 1900 and 1910, the pop. of the city increased from more than 285,700 to nearly 465,000. During WW I, defense industries attracted thousands of workers, and, by 1920, the pop. had reached one million. During the 1930s, unemployment was high and, by 1940, the United Automobile Workers Union, created in 1935, was a significant factor in the automotive industry. Blacks and whites from the S US, as well as European immigrants, arrived in the city, which became known as the "Automobile Capital of the World", to work in that industry. During a race riot which paralyzed the city in 1943, 34 persons were killed, while 2,500 fed. troops were called in to restore order. The rapid growth of the city contributed to racial tension, increased crime and overcrowded schools, and during the 1950s and 1960s the city undertook many urban renewal and city programs. By 1960, the pop. declined to approx. 1,670,150, as many of the white middle class moved to suburbs. In July, 1967, the largest civil disturbance in US history occurred in the city. The week of rioting resulted in 43 deaths, millions of dollars in property damage and the ruin of scores of businesses. In 1973, Coleman A. Young was elected the first black mayor of the city, and, in 1977, he was reelected to a second four-year term.

GOVERNMENT. Detroit has a strong mayor-council form of govt.,one of the few full-time city legislative bodies in the US, consisting of nine council members elected to four-year terms and the mayor, elected at large to a four-year term.

ECONOMY AND INDUSTRY. Detroit, the "Industrial Capital of the World", accounts for 2.5% of the US Gross Natl. Product. There are more than 7,000 manufacturing plants in the city employing approx. 33% of the total met. area work force. Nearly 14% of the work force is employed in the Detroit automobile industry which leads the US with 20% of the total annual production of cars and trucks. Other products include business machines, chemicals, hardware, machine tools, pharmaceuticals and paint. The city is also the potato chip manufacturing capital of the world, and the location of the world headquarters of 51 firms (34 of them among the Fortune 500) with annual sales of $100 million or more. Due to the massive retoolment underway for more fuel-efficient vehicles for the 1980s the area is at full employment in the semi-skilled and skilled categories. In 1978, the avg. per capita income in Wayne Co. was $20,731, while Detroit had the highest per capita income in the US. In June, 1979, the total labor force of the greater met. area was approx. 2,085,900, while the rate of unemployment was 7.1%

BANKING. In 1978, total deposits at the eight banks headquartered in Detroit were approx. $16,573,412,000, while assets were $21,092,204,000. Banks include Natl. Bank, Manufacturers Natl., Detroit Bank and Trust, MI Natl., City Natl., Bank of the Commonwealth, First Independence Natl. and Merchants.

HOSPITALS. There are 88 gen. and acute care and 15 osteopathic hosps. in Detroit, including Detroit Gen., Mt. Carmel Mercy, Detroit Receiving, Harper, Grace, Henry Ford, Hutzel, and Children's. The Detroit Medical Center, completed in 1978, consists of several hosps. and clinics as well as the

largest single campus medical school in the US, Wayne State.

EDUCATION. Wayne State U, a state-supported institution offering grad. and undergrad. degree programs in a variety of areas, enrolled nearly 34,400 in 1978. The U of Detroit, founded in 1877 and affiliated with the Society of Jesus, is a coeducational U offering bachelor, master and doctorate degrees. In 1978, approx. 8,350 enrolled. Other teaching and research institutions include Mercy Col., Shaw Col., Merrill-Palmer Institute, Sacred Heart Seminary Col., Detroit Col. of Law, Detroit Institute of Technology, Marygrove Col., Wayne Co. Comm. Col. and Detroit Col. of Business Administration. There are approx. 350 elementary and high schools in the public school system, enrolling 600,000. More than 90,000 students attend more than 150 parochial and private schools. Lib. facilities include Detroit Public Lib., with 30 branches, the Archives of American Art and the Walter P. Reuther Archives, located on the Wayne State U campus and the largest labor lib. in the world.

ENTERTAINMENT. There are several dinner theaters in Detroit, including Somerset Mall and Vittorio's. Some 20 ethnic festivals are held annually each summer. Other annual events include the Automobile Show, held in Jan.; the Boat Show, held in Feb.; the Builders and Flower Show, held in Mar.; the Intl. Freedom Festival, held in July; the State Fair, held in late Aug.; the Meadowbrook Music Festival and the Christmas Carnival, held in Dec. Professional sports entertainment is provided by the Detroit Tigers, an AL baseball team, which plays in Tiger Stadium; the Detroit Lions, an NFL-NFC football team, the Detroit Pistons, an NBA basketball team, and the Detroit Express, an NASL soccer team, all of whom play in the Pontiac Silverdome and the Detroit Redwings, an NHL hockey team, which plays in Joe Louis Arena. The U Detroit Titans and the Wayne State U Tartans participate in intercollegiate sports. Professional wrestling is held at Cobo Arena. Auto racing is offered at MI Intl. Speedway and the Detroit Dragway, while horse racing is available at Northville and Hazel Park among others.

ACCOMMODATIONS. There are 220 hotels and motels in Detroit, including the Hotel Pontchartrain, Radisson Cadillac Hotel, St. Regis, Host Intl., the Holiday, MI, Sheraton and Ramada inns and TraveLodge and Howard Johnson's. The 740' high Detroit Plaza Hotel is the tallest hotel in the world.

FACILITIES. There are several parks in Detroit, including 10 met. parks with facilities for swimming, golfing, boating and ice skating. Major parks are Belle Isle, Palmer, Elisa Howell, Chandler, Rouge and Detroit Zoological. The Detroit Zoo, which contains more than 5,000 animals, an aviary, reptile house, great ape exhibit, tiger den, monkey island and the largest

Detroit, Michigan

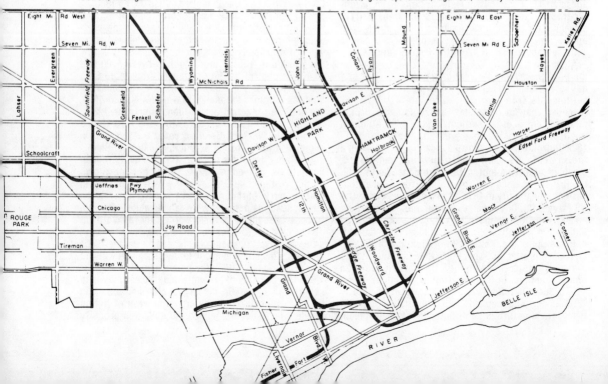

penguinarium in the US, established the first "natural habitat" environment in the US. Belle Isle, the largest island park located within a city in the US, contains a zoo, lagoon, aquarium, nature interpretive center, jogging track, golf course, tennis courts, playing fields, a 1.5 mi. beach, playgrounds, four fishing piers, Scott Fountain, Whitcomb Conservatory, the Peace Tower, Dossin Great Lakes museum and a 30' floral clock. Palmer Park contains the historic Palmer Homestead (a log cabin furnished in pioneer style), golf courses; jogging track and bridle trails and wading pools. The 1,203-acre Rouge Park located along the Rouge River includes a bathhouse, swimming pools, picnic groves, tennis courts, a golf course and facilities for such winter sports as tobogganing, skiing and ice skating.

CULTURAL ACTIVITIES. The Detroit Symphony and Detroit Concert Band, one of the foremost "Sousa" bands in the US, are among the cultural organizations in the city. Popular artists perform at the "Renaissance Live" and "P-Jazz" outdoor concert series. The MI Opera Theatre, as well as intl. touring artists, perform at the Music Hall Center for the Performing Arts, while the Detroit Institute of Arts offers an Early Jazz series and "Brunch with Bach" concerts. Modern ballet performances are offered by the Detroit Dance Co. band. Concerts and performances of the Pine Knob Music Theatre are presented on summer evenings at Belle Isle. Among the theaters in the city are the Fisher Theatre, which presents Broadway hits; the Attic Theater, which stages avant garde productions; the Bonstelle and the Hilberry Classic Theaters at Wayne State U; the Marygrove Theater at Marygrove Col.; the Detroit Repertory Theater and the Detroit Youth Theatre. The Detroit Film Theater presents historical perspectives of famed director works each weekend. The U Cultural Center Assn., affiliated with Wayne State U, consists of the Detroit Insitute of Arts, which houses Diego Rivera murals and an extensive collection of African art; the Intl. Institute, featuring arts and crafts of 43 countries; Your Heritage House, a fine arts museum offering instruction for children; the Children's Museum; the Detroit Historical Museum, featuring displays of the city during the 1800s; and the Scarab Club, an organization of 230 Detroit-area artists who sponsor annual art and photo shows and the Science Center. The Dossin Great Lakes Museum at Belle Isle features displays of the shipping industry. Other museums are the Ft. Wayne Military Museum (a pre-Civil War citadel covering 30 acres, featuring the original stone barracks and powder magazine), the Afro-American Museum and the Wayne State Natural History Museum.

LANDMARKS AND SIGHTSEEING SPOTS. The Detroit Civic Center, encompassing 75 acres along the downtown riverfront, includes Cobo Arena, the City-Co. Building, Vets.' Memorial Building and the Henry and Edsel Ford Auditorium. Trolley car rides are available from Cobo Arena to Grand Circus Park, where a fountain honoring Thomas Edison is illuminated nightly during the summer. A statue of Steven T. Mason, the first gov. of MI, is located in Capitol Park. Old Mariner's Church, originally built in 1849 for seafarers, was moved stone by stone to its present location in 1956. Meadowbrook Hall and Fair Lane, two mansions built from automobile industry fortunes, contain priceless collections of china, furniture and art. The Civil War Soldiers' Monument was erected in 1842. The home of the Model T, the Old Indian Council House, the 1763 Pontiac Uprising, JFK's last appearance in the city and the 1812 Soldiers Burial Ground are indicated by historical markers. The Boston Edison neighborhood is the largest designated historical district in the US. The Pontchartrain Hotel stands on the site of the first permanent settlement established in 1701 by Cadillac and the headquarters of Gen. "Mad Anthony" Wayne, as well as the point from which the city was rebuilt in 1805. The E Market, built in the 1890s on the site of an early hay and wood market, is a colorful patchwork of produce stalls, meat packing houses, fish markets and storefronts. Greektown, one of the oldest neighborhoods in the city, features numerous restaurants and speciality shops. Hart Plaza features a skating rink, amphitheater, covered theater, food booths, gallery and restaurant complex, as well as the Dodge Fountain. The Renaissance Center, part of the city's extensive redevelopment project, is a thriving complex of retail shops, eateries and offices, and the site of the tallest building in MI, the Plaza Hotel. The 440' high Fisher Building, built in 1928 from 40 different types of marble from around the world, encompasses seven acres and elegant shops and galleries and handpainted arcades. The Paul McPharlin Gallery of

Puppets is located at the Detroit Institute of Arts. The Money Museum, located at the Natl. Bank, displays 12,000 coins and primitive money forms such as furs, tobacco and beetle shells. A museum on the first floor of the Fire Dept. Headquarters contains mementos of the early history of the city's volunteer firemen. An antique trolley, still used, features drivers in turn-of-the-century uniforms.

DURHAM
NORTH CAROLINA

CITY LOCATION-SIZE-EXTENT. Durham, the seat of Durham Co. and fifth largest city in the state, encompasses 40.57 sq. mi. in N central NC 20 mi. NW of Raleigh at 35°60' N lat. and 78°54' W long. It also extends W into Orange Co., and with Raleigh and Wake Co. to the SW, forms the met. area.

TOPOGRAPHY. The terrain of Durham, which is situated in the transitional zone between the Atlantic coastal plain and the Piedmont plateau regions of NC, is rolling to hilly, rising gradually to the W. The Eno River flows through the city. The mean elev. is 399'.

CLIMATE. The climate of Durham is moderate continental, due to its central location between the Blue Ridge Mts. to the W (which inhibit the movement of cold air masses from the continent) and the Atlantic Ocean to the SE. Monthly mean temps. range from 41°F in Jan. to 78°F in July, with an avg. annual temp. of 60°F. The 45" avg. annual rainfall is fairly evenly distributed throughout the year. Snowfall avgs. 7" per year. The RH ranges from 47% to 93%. The growing season avgs. 205 days. Durham lies in the ESTZ and observes DST.

FLORA AND FAUNA. Animals native to Durham include the opossum, whitetail deer and raccoon. Common birds include the thrasher, cardinal, catbird, red-eyed vireo, warbler and blue jay. Frogs, salamanders, turtles and snakes, including the venomous cottonmouth, copperhead, rattlesnake and coral snake, are found in the area. Typical trees include the ash,

Duke University in Greater Durham, North Carolina

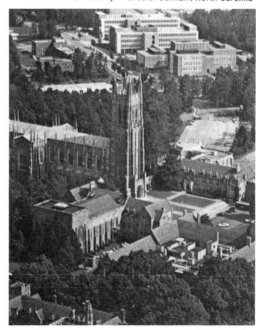

sweetgum, magnolia, elm, oak and pine. Smaller plants include the viburnum, buckthorn, partridge pea, day lily and wood sorrel.

POPULATION. According to the US census, the pop. of Durham in 1970 was 95,438. In 1978, it was estimated that it had increased to 107,000.

ETHNIC GROUPS. In 1978, the ethnic distribution of Durham was approx. 60.9% Caucasian, 38.8% Black and .7% Hispanic (a percentage of the Hispanic total is included in the Caucasian total).

TRANSPORTATION. Interstate hwys. 40 and 85, US hwys. 15, 70 and 501 and state hwys. 54, 55, 98 and 751 provide major motor access to Durham. *Railroads* serving the city are AMTRAK, Durham Southern, Norfolk & Western, Seaboard Coast and Southern. *Airlines* serving Raleigh-Durham Airport include DL, EA, PI and UA. *Bus lines* serving the city are Greyhound, Southern Coach and Trailways.

COMMUNICATIONS. Communications, broadcasting and print media originating from Durham are: *AM radio stations* WDNC 620 (CBS, MOR); WTIK 1310 (MBS, C&W); WSRC 1410 (Natl. Blk.); and WDUR 1490 (ABC/C, Contemp.); *FM radio stations* WAFR 90.3 (NPR, Educ., Blk.); WDCG 105.1 (ABC/E, C&W, Top 40) and WDBS 107.1 (UPI, AOR); *television stations* serving the Raleigh-Durham area are WRAL Ch. 5 (ABC); WTVD Ch. 11 (CBS) and WPTF Ch. 28 (NBC); *press:* two major dailies serve the city, the morning *Herald*, and the *Sun*, issued evenings and Sun. mornings; other publications include *NC Anvil*, *The S Atlantic Quarterly*, *Duke Alumni Register* and *NC Leader*.

HISTORY. Native Americans of the Shocco, Adshysheer and Eno tribes inhabited the area of present-day Durham before the first white settlers arrived. In 1851, a US post office was established in the settlement, which was given the name Durhamville in honor of Dr. Bartlett Snipes Durham, who owned land in the area. In 1854, Dr. Durham offered the NC RR land to be used for a right-of-way. As the Civil War began, the town was an insignificant RR point in which a tobacco factory operated. In 1865, Gen. Joseph Johnston surrendered his Confed. troops to Gen. William Sherman at a farmstead called Bennett Place. Both Union and Confed. soldiers raided the factory and returned home extolling the fine quality of the tobacco. With the manufacture of "Bull Durham", the tobacco industry was established. Durham was incorporated as a city in 1866, and again in 1869, after the US Congress invalidated the statutes of the old Confederacy. By that time, its pop. had reached 258. During the late 1800s, profits from the prosperous tobacco industry were invested in other manufacturing enterprises, including cotton and textile mills. The construction of architecturally significant commercial buildings in the city during the late 1800s and early 1900s resulted in the placement of its business district on the Natl. Register of Historic Places, the first in the

state to be so recognized. Duke U, formerly Trinity Col., was established in 1924, heavily endowed by the tobacco fortunes of the Duke family. Research Triangle Park, the largest research-oriented industrial park in the US, was founded 8 mi. S of Durham, the result of cooperative efforts of state universities and the State of NC.

GOVERNMENT. Durham has a council-mgr. form of govt. consisting of 13 councillors, including the mayor as a voting member. The mayor and six council members are elected at large, while the remaining six are elected by ward in staggered-year elections. The mayor serves a two-year term, while the council members serve four-year terms. The city mgr., the administrative head of govt., is appointed by the council.

ECONOMY AND INDUSTRY. The major industry in Durham is tobacco manufacturing. Other industries produce textiles, machinery, proprietary medicines, furniture, lumber products, building materials, chemicals and food for livestock. Some 85% of the 5,400-acre Research Triangle Park is located in Durham. Nearly 30 research organizations employ approx. 12,000, and their per capita concentration of Ph.D. scientists and engineers is the highest of the 100 largest met. areas in the US. In June, 1979, the labor force of the greater met. area totaled approx. 282,500, while the rate of unemployment was 3.6%.

BANKING. There are nine commercial banks and five savings and loan assns. in Durham. In 1978, total deposits for the four banks headquartered in the city were $464,010,000, while assets totaled $534,005,000. Banks include Central Carolina Bank and Trust, Mechanics' & Farmers', Liberty Bank and Trust and Guaranty State.

HOSPITALS. There are several gen. and special care hosps. in Durham, including Duke Medical Center (ranked among the top five academic health centers in the US), the locally supported Durham Co. Gen. and Watts hosps., Lenox Baker Children's, McPherson and V.A. There are also several clinics in the city in which the ratio of doctors per 1,000 pop. is the highest in the SE US.

EDUCATION. Duke U's Comprehensive Cancer Center, a part of the "Research Triangle of NC" is ranked first among such centers in the US. Founded in 1838 as Trinity Col., Duke U was renamed in 1924 in honor of benefactor James B. Duke. Famed for its Gothic architecture, as well as its professional schools of medicine and law, Duke U enrolled approx. 9,400 in 1978. NC Central U, which was founded in 1910 as a religious training school, later became the first state-supported sr. liberal arts col. for Blacks in the US. Now integrated, its lib. contains many primary materials on Black life and culture. In 1978, the U enrolled approx. 4,800. The Durham Tech. Institute, founded in 1956, is under state/local control. It offers assoc. degrees and, in 1978, enrolled approx. 3,000. Durham Col., a private institution established in 1947, offers assoc. degrees. In 1978, approx. 350 enrolled. The Durham public school system consists of 27 elementary, nine jr. high and five sr. high schools. Six private and parochial schools also serve the city. Libs. include Durham Co. Lib.

ENTERTAINMENT. The Village Dinner Theater provides dining entertainment in Durham. Among the annual events held in the city are the American Dance Festival, a world-renowned summer festival (which takes place at Duke),and the NC Folklife Festival, a three-to-four day celebration of NC culture held in alternate years. The Duke Blue Devils of the Atlantic Coast Conf. and the NC Central U Eagles participate in intercollegiate sports.

ACCOMMODATIONS. There are numerous hotels and motels in Durham, including the Day's, Cricket, Happy, Downtowner Motor, Governor's, Hilton and Ramada Inns, Best Western-Skyland Motel, Washington Duke Motor Inn-Best Western and Howard Johnson's.

FACILITIES. There are several public parks in Durham, including the Eno River City Park, which offers facilities for hiking, rafting, picnicking and canoeing. It also contains an historical recreation of the West Point Mill Comm., featuring a reconstructed working grist mill, which originally operated from 1778 to 1942. The restored McCown Mangum House, also located in the park, features a Visitors' Center and small museum. Five

Downtown Durham, North Carolina

public golf courses and a zoo (at the NC Museum of Life and Science) are also located in the city.

CULTURAL ACTIVITIES. Duke U and NC Central U present musical, dramatic and other performing productions in Durham. The Duke Art Museum features collections of classical, native American, African, medieval and Oriental artifacts. The 78-acre NC Museum of Life and Science features prehistoric relics and aerospace exhibits.

LANDMARKS AND SIGHTSEEING SPOTS. Duke Chapel, located on the U campus in Durham, features 77 stained glass windows, a 210' bell tower with bells weighing from 10 to 11,200 pounds and a $500,000 Flentrop organ. Thousands of irises, daffodils and tulips are featured at the Sarah P. Duke Memorial Gardens on the W campus of Duke. The ornate buildings in the city's commercial district, which is listed on the Natl. Register of Historic Places, feature early 20th-century architecture. Duke Homestead, a state historic site and natl. historic landmark, was the home of one of the early founders of the city's tobacco industry. The site includes the main house, two tobacco factories, a packing house, a curing barn and the Tobacco Museum. Bennett Place, an historic site, commemorates the surrender of Confed. Gen. Joseph E. Johnston to Union Gen. William T. Sherman in 1865. A restored log house is maintained at the location, while picnic areas are located on the grounds. In addition, local tobacco companies offers tours of their plants.

ELIZABETH
NEW JERSEY

CITY LOCATION-SIZE-EXTENT. Elizabeth, the sixth largest city in NJ and seat of Union Co., is located on the Elizabeth River in NE NJ 14 mi. W of NYC at 40°39' N lat. and 74°13' W long. It is bordered on the E by Arthur Kill (a bay inlet separating it from S Staten Island) and Newark Bay. Encompassing 11.7 sq. mi, it is, with the nearby cities of Newark to the N, Jersey City to the NE and Bayonne to the E part of the "inner ring" around Manhattan in the tri-state (NY, NJ and CT) NYC greater met. area.

TOPOGRAPHY. The terrain of Elizabeth, which is situated on the Piedmont Plain of the Atlantic coastal plain region is relatively flat along Arthur Kill and Newark Bay. The terrain slopes upward to the W, rising eventually to the Watchung Mts. Warinanco Lake is located in the city. The mean elev. is 38'.

CLIMATE. The climate of Elizabeth is intermediate continental, influenced by dry winds from the NW and moderating winds from the Atlantic Ocean to the SW. The avg. annual temp. of 54°F ranges from a Jan. mean of 31°F to a July mean of 76°F. The avg. annual rainfall is fairly evenly distributed throughout the year, while most of the avg. annual snowfall of 28" occurs from Dec. through Feb. The RH ranges from 45% to 78%. The avg. growing season is approx. 200 days. Elizabeth lies in the ESTZ and observes DST.

FLORA AND FAUNA. Animals native to Elizabeth include the muskrat, striped skunk, opossum, red and grey fox, raccoon and weasel. Common birds include the starling, sparrow, blue jay and robin. American toads, tree frogs, salamanders, skinks and milk snakes, as well as the venomous copperhead and timber rattlesnake, are found in the area. Typical trees include the Norway maple, pin oak, ailanthus and ash. Smaller plants include the sumac, viburnum, arrowhead, meadowrue and forsythia.

POPULATION. According to the US census, the pop. of Elizabeth in 1970 was 112,654. In 1978, it was estimated that it had decreased to approx. 104,000.

ETHNIC GROUPS. In 1978, the ethnic distribution of Elizabeth was approx. 54% Caucasian, 11% Black, 34% Hispanic and 1% other (a percentage of the Hispanic total is included in the Caucasian total).

TRANSPORTATION. The NJ Tnpk., Garden State Parkway, US hwys. 1 and 9 and State hwys 21, 22 and 27 provide motor access to Elizabeth. *Railroads* serving the city include AMTRAK, ConRail and N Jersey Coast, Jersey Shore. *Airlines* serving Newark Intl. Airport (located partially in the city) include AA, UA, TW, PA, EA, NA, BN, US Air and World Airways. *Bus lines* include Greyhound, Trailways, Transport of NJ and the local Elizabeth Transit. The city, which is a port, is known as the "Container Ship Capital of the World". More than 30% of the containership cargo handled in

Business District, Elizabeth, New Jersey

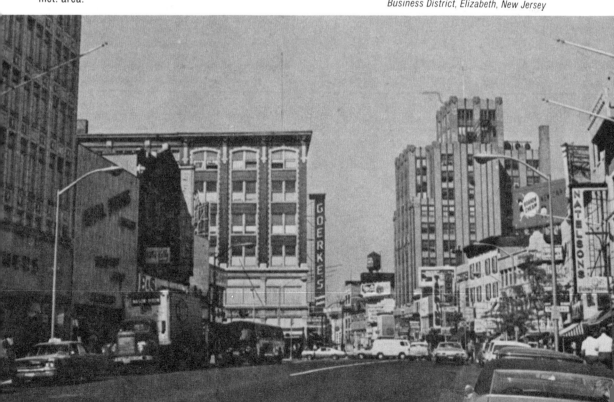

the world is handled by the Elizabeth port facility, which contains a 35' channel.

COMMUNICATIONS. Communications, broadcasting and print media originating from Elizabeth are: *AM radio station* WJDM 1530 (Indep., MOR); although no *FM radio stations* or *television stations* originate from the city, broadcasting is received from nearby Newark and other cities in the NYC met. area; *press*: two daily newspapers serve the city, the *Daily Journal*, and the *Community News*; other publications include the weekly *Citizen Weekly* and *La Voz* and the monthly *Electronic Market/Management*.

HISTORY. The area of present-day Elizabeth was inhabited by native Americans before the first white settlers, John Baker, John Ogden, John Bailey and Luke Watson purchased the land from them on Oct. 8, 1664. The same year, Philip Carteret, the first English gov. of NJ, selected the site, the first English-speaking settlement in NJ, to be the first of the colony. He named it Elizabethtown in honor of Lady Elizabeth, wife of Sir George Carteret, his fourth cousin. From 1668 to 1682, the first Colonial Assembly met in the town, which was incorporated as the Borough of Elizabethtown in 1739. The Col. of NJ, now Princeton U, was established in the borough in 1746 and later relocated to Princeton. On June 7, 1780, during the Revolutionary War, the borough was invaded by the British. Among the early inhabitants of the town were William Livingston, Gov. of NJ from 1776 to 1790; Alexander Hamilton and Aaron Burr, who were educated there; Gen. Winfield Scott, first US officer to receive the Congressional Medal of Honor for meritorious service in the War of 1812; Rev. James Caldwell, the "Fighting Parson", and Elias Boudenot, signer of the Treaty of Peace with Great Britain. By 1835, industrial development began in the town when businessmen from NYC built manufacturing plants on land bordering S Staten Island. Elizabeth was incorporated as a city in 1855, and continued to develop as an important RR center and shipping port. In the latter part of the 1800s, Philip Holland built the first successful

Central Elizabeth, New Jersey

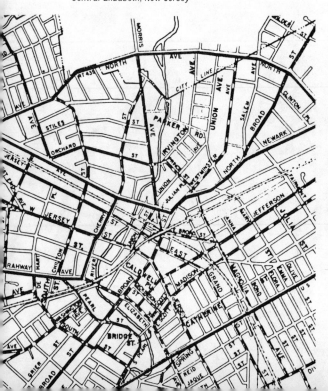

submarine in the city. In 1928, the Goethals Bridge, connecting Elizabeth and S Staten Island, opened, and the city continued to grow as industry diversified. In 1962, a new port facility was completed, contributing to the importance of the city as a shipping center.

GOVERNMENT. Elizabeth has a mayor-council form of govt., consisting of the mayor, who is not a voting member of the council, and nine council members. The mayor and three council members are elected at large, while the remaining six are elected by wards. All serve four-year terms.

ECONOMY AND INDUSTRY. There are more than 600 manufacturing plants in Elizabeth, producing chemicals, steel, petrochemicals, food products, "serving" machines and electronic equipment. Elizabeth is known as the containership capital of the world. The export business is also a major employer. In 1978, the total labor force was approx. 57,200, while the rate of unemployment was 7.4%.

BANKING. There are 19 commercial banks and 24 savings and loans assns. in Union Co., of which Elizabeth is the seat. In 1978, total deposits for the seven banks headquartered in the city were approx. $1,587,502,000, while assets were $1,785,857,000. Banks serving the city include Natl. State, Union Co. Savings, United Counties Trust, City Trust Services Natl., Elizabeth Savings, United Jersey Central and Harmonia Savings.

HOSPITALS. There are three hosps. in Elizabeth, Elizabeth Gen., St. Elizabeth and Alexian Brothers.

EDUCATION. Union Col., located in nearby Cranford, maintains an Urban Campus Concept, by which technical and business courses are offered at two facilities in Elizabeth. There are 27 public schools in the city, enrolling approx. 15,000 in 1978. Lib. facilities include the Elizabeth Free Public Library, which maintains three branches.

ENTERTAINMENT. The Villa Roma offers dinner theater in Elizabeth. Annual events held in the city include the St. Rocco Italian Festival, the Elizabeth Ethnic Festival and the Memorial Day Celebration. The NJ Gems, a women's professional basketball team, plays at the Dunn Sports Center.

ACCOMMODATIONS. There are several hotels and motels in Elizabeth, including the Sheraton and Elizabeth Carteret hotels, the Empress House, the In-Town Motor Lodge and the Polly's Elizabeth and Holiday Inns.

FACILITIES. There are more than 40 public parks in Elizabeth, including Warinanco Lake Park, which contains a jogging track and ice skating rink. Williams Field Track also features a jogging track. Mattano Park, currently being remodeled,will feature recreational sports and other facilities when it is completed in 1981, besides the existing playing fields, tennis courts, pool and picnic areas. Three major recreational facilities, the Arabell Miller, Mickey Walker and Drotar Field Centers, also under construction, will feature gyms, swimming pools, weight training rooms and saunas when completed in 1980.

CULTURAL ACTIVITIES. The Regent Theater in Elizabeth hosts theatrical and operatic performances. The Thomas G. Dunn Convention and Sports Center also contains theater facilities.

LANDMARKS AND SIGHTSEEING SPOTS. There are several historical landmarks in Elizabeth including the First Presbyterian Church, the first church organized in NJ in which services were held in English. Built in 1665, the plain wooden structure was also used for meetings of the Supreme Court, Legislature and First Gen. Assembly of NJ, which convened there in 1668. A new church erected in 1724 was burned by the British in 1780, and the present structure, altered and expanded several times since then, was completed in 1789. The Belcher-Ogden Mansion, built about 1680, was first occupied by an original settler of the city, John Ogden, and later by Jonathan Belcher, Royal Gov. of the Province. George Washington and Gen. Lafayette were both entertained at the house. The Nathaniel Bonnell House, built before 1682, is preserved as a pre-Revolutionary farmhouse. Other historical buildings in the city included the birthplace of Adm. William Halsey and Nicholas Murray Butler, Christ Church, St. Augustine's Church, the Andrew Hampton House, St. John's Episcopal Church, The Elizabeth Carteret Hotel, Hersh Tower and the Boudinot Mansion, or Boxwood Hall, built in the 1760s and now a state-owned historical shrine. Elizabeth Avenue, (formerly Water St.) may be the oldest hwy. in NJ. Later known as the King's Hwy., it became the post and stage route to Philadelphia. The Soldiers' and Sailors' Monument, erected in 1908, commemorates soldiers and sailors who participated in the Civil War. The Union Co. Courthouse, erected in 1903, was built on the site of the former Courthouse and Sherman House. The Boundary Stone on the grounds of the Liberty Square Branch Lib. is another old landmark, containing the chiseled date 1694. It marked the boundary line of the property of Richard Townley and Benjamin Price.

EL PASO
TEXAS

CITY LOCATION-SIZE-EXTENT. El Paso, the seat of El Paso Co., encompasses 239.21 sq. mi. in extreme SW TX on the Rio Grande River at 31°48' N lat. and 106°24' W long. It is bordered by Juarez, Mexico across the Rio Grande to the S, as well as Dona Ana Co., NM, on the N and W.

TOPOGRAPHY. The terrain of El Paso, which is situated in the basin and range, or trans-Pecos, region of TX, consists of a high semi-arid plain. The terrain becomes hilly in the N part of the city in the foothills of the Franklin Mts., a spur of the Rocky Mts., which extends N for about 16 mi. With a mean elev. of 3,762', the city is the lowest all-weather pass through the Rocky Mts.

CLIMATE. The climate of El Paso is arid continental, characterized by an abundance of sunshine throughout the year, high daytime summer temps., low humidity, scant rainfall and a mild winter season. The avg. annual temp. of 64°F ranges from a Jan. mean of 45°F to a July mean of 82°F. Daytime summer temps. frequently rise above 90°F while nighttime temps. fall into the 60°F range. Daytime winter temps. avg. 55°F to 60°F while nighttime temps. drop to near 32°F or below. The avg. annual rainfall is 8.5", with heavier amounts occurring in the month of July and Aug. The avg. annual snowfall is 4.6". Dust and sandstorms are frequent in Mar. and Apr. The RH ranges from 15% to 67%. El Paso lies in the MSTZ and observes DST.

FLORA AND FAUNA. Animals native to El Paso include the shrew, bat, deer, jackrabbit, ground squirrel, kangaroo rat and bobcat. Common birds include the scaled quail, whippoorwill, white-throated swift and brown towhee. There are numerous reptiles and amphibians, including several species of venomous rattlesnakes in the area. Desert plants in the area include ochotilla, mesquite, prickly pear cactus and various other types of cacti.

POPULATION. According to the US census, the pop. of El Paso in 1970 was 322,261. In 1979, it was estimated that it had increased to 395,514.

ETHNIC GROUPS. In 1978, the ethnic distribution of El Paso was approx. 96.6% Caucasian, 2.3% Black, 58.1% Hispanic, .2% Asian, .2% Native American and .5% other (a percentage of the Hispanic total is also included in the Caucasian total).

TRANSPORTATION. Interstate hwys. 10, 25 and 110, US hwys. 80, 180, 62, 54 and 85 and Mexico hwys. 45, the Border Frw. and the N-S Frw. provide major motor access to El Paso. *Railroads* serving the city include Santa Fe, Southern Pacific, Missouri Pacific, Natl. of Mexico, and AMTRAK. *Airlines* serving W TX, El Paso Intl. and Faens airports include Airways of NM, AA, CO, FL, SW and Aeromexico. *Bus lines* serving the city include Greyhound, Trailways, Autobuses Internacionales, NM Transportation, T.N.M.&O. Coaches, Omnibus de Mexico and the local Sun City Area Transit (SCAT).

COMMUNICATIONS. Communications, broadcasting and print media originating from El Paso are: *AM radio stations* KROD 600 (Indep., MOR); KHEY 690 (APR, ABC/I, C&W); KELP 920 (Indep., Top 40); KAMA 1060 (APR, Span.); KISO 1150 (ABC/E, Relig. Spec. Progsv.); KSET 1340 (MBS, MOR); KTSM 1380 (NBC/MBS/APR, News) and KINT 1590 (ABC/C, Top 40); *FM radio stations* KTEP 88.5 (ABC/E, NPR, Pub. Spec. Progsv.);

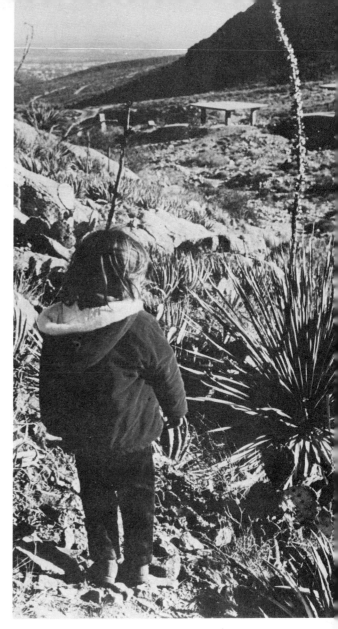

McKelligon Canyon Park, within city limits of El Paso, Texas

KAMA 93.1 (APR, Span.); KPAS 93.9 (MBS, AOR); KSET 94.7 (Indep., C&W); KLAQ 95.5 (Indep., AOR); KEZB 96.3 (Indep., Btfl. Mus.); KINT 97.5 (Indep., Top 40); KTSM 99.9 (Indep., Contemp.) and KLOZ 102.1 (Indep., C&W); *television stations* KDBC Ch. 4 (CBS); KCOS Ch. 7 (PBS); KTSM Ch. 9 (NBC); KVIA Ch. 13 (ABC); KCIK Ch. 14 (CBN, PTL, TBN) and cable; *press:* two major daily newspapers are published in the city, the morning *Times* and the *Herald-Post,* issued evenings and Sun. mornings; other publications include *El Continental,* a Span. publication issued evenings and Sun. mornings, and the monthly *El Paso Today.*

HISTORY. Native Americans of the Manso and Suma tribes inhabited the area of present-day El Paso before the first white settlers arrived. In 1598, an expedition led by Juan de Onate camped on the N and S banks of the Rio Grande and claimed the area for Spain. Onate called the area "El Paso del Rio del Norte", meaning "the crossing of the river of the N", after fording the Rio Grande near what is now the downtown section of the city. In 1680, native Americans of the Giggera tribe, forced out of NM by the Pueblo Revolt, and Spanish

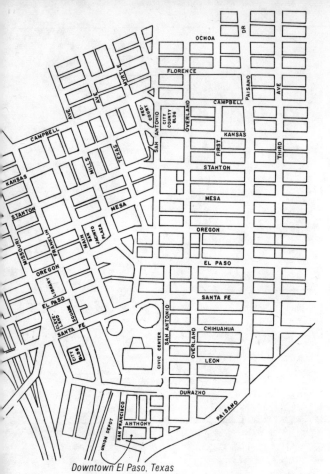

Downtown El Paso, Texas

continued to arrive in the city, its pop. grew from nearly 130,500 in 1960 to almost 276,700 in 1970. During the 1970s, industrial air pollution increased and the city initiated programs to alleviate the problem, as well as to renew the central city.

GOVERNMENT. El Paso has a mayor-council form of govt. Six aldermen, representing aldermanic districts, and the mayor are elected to serve two-year terms. The mayor votes only to break a tie.

ECONOMY AND INDUSTRY. El Paso is the center for a farming and ranching area, the land of which is irrigated by the Rio Grande Project. Major agricultural crops are vegetables, cotton, pecans and grains. The highest producing pecan farm in the US is located in the area. Livestock is also important. In 1979, approx. 20% of the total work force is employed in the 475 manufacturing companies located in the El Paso-Juarez area. The major product is cotton clothing, with 60 plants employing approx. 9% of the work force. Petroleum refining and natural gas distribution, electronics, food processing, smelting and refining of copper and lead, lumber and research are other important industries. Military bases located nearby also employ a large part of the area labor force, which in 1979 totaled 172,600. The rate of unemployment was 9.0%.

BANKING. There are 21 banks in El Paso. In 1978, total deposits for the 19 banks headquartered in the city were approx. $1,405,957,000, while assets totaled $1,620,120,000. Banks include El Paso Natl., State Natl., First City Natl., Bank of El Paso, American Bank of Commerce, First State, Continental Natl., Bassett Natl., First Intl. and Coronado State.

HOSPITALS. There are 15 hosps. in El Paso, including Sun Towers which recently opened a burn care unit, Sierra Medical, Hotel Dieu, Providence and Eastwood. Thomason, a county hosp., is affiliated with TX Tech. School of Medicine. The El Paso Cancer Treatment Center, which opened in 1974 and William Beaumont Army Medical Center, one of the largest in the US Army, are also located in the city.

EDUCATION. The U of TX at El Paso (UTEP), a publicly supported coeducational university with a 1978 enrollment of approx. 15,800, was created by the TX Legislature in 1913 as the TX School of Mines and Metallurgy. In 1919, it became a branch of UT, in 1949, TX W Col. and in 1967, assumed its present name and status. UT offers bachelor and master degrees, in addition to a doctorate in geology. Other teaching and research institutions in the city include El Paso Christian Col., Comm. Col. (enrolling approx. 9,500 in 1978). Durham Business Col., El Paso School of Electronics, Intl. Business Col., TX Tech. U School of Medicine, offering grad. courses and post grad. residency programs, and TX A&M Research Center. The El Paso public school system consists of 95 elementary and 38 secondary schools enrolling more than 110,000 in 1978. Private schools include 16 elementary and seven high schools as well as the Radford School, Lydia Patterson Institute and Loretto Academy. The El Paso Public Lib. and its seven branches are part of the TX Trans Pecos Lib. System.

ENTERTAINMENT. Among the dinner theaters in El Paso is Gillespie's Green Room. Rodeos and rough riding, as well as automobile drag stock car and motorcycle races are seasonal events held each week. Polo matches are held at Armstrong Field of Ft. Bliss on Sun. in autumn, while professional volleyball matches are held at the Civic Center during the summer. Bullfights and horse racing take place throughout the summer in Juarez. Each Feb., the "SW Intl. Livestock Show and Rodeo and Bull and Horse Sales" takes place in the El Paso Coliseum. Other annual events include the Cotton Festival, held in Aug., the Fiesta de Las Flores, held the weekend before Labor Day and Kermezaar Arts and Crafts Show, the County Fair and the SW Sun Carnival all held in the autumn. The Diablos, a farm club of the CA Angels major league team, participate in professional baseball in the TXL, while the UTEP Miners participate in collegiate sports in the WAC. The collegiate Sun Bowl is held each year in the city in Dec.

ACCOMMODATIONS. There are numerous hotels and motels in El Paso, including Plaza, Caballero, TraveLodge and the Holiday, Ramada, Sheraton Rodeway and Hilton inns.

colonists settled within the present city limits. Two years later, Franciscans established what are now the oldest missions in TX in Ysleta (a section of the city). In 1821, settlements in the area were incorporated into the Mexican State of Chihuahua after Mexico gained independence from Spain. By the 1848 Treaty of Guadalupe-Hidalgo, however, the town was divided by the Rio Grande into settlements, one of which became Juarez, Mexico, while the other formed the nucleus of modern El Paso, TX. The same year, a trading post and the US military post that later became Ft. Bliss were established in El Paso. During the Civil War, the town supported the Confederacy, but in 1862, soldiers from CA attacked Ft. Bliss and captured the area for the Union. Later, the town became an important stagecoach station on the Butterfield Overland Mail stage operation. Incorporated as a city in 1873 with a pop. of 173. El Paso experienced a land boom and more rapid development when the RR arrived in 1881. Many workers who came to the city to work on the RR remained and by 1890, the pop. exceeded 10,300. Additional settlers were attracted to the area by the mining and cattle ranching industries. By 1910, nearly 40,000 persons lived in the city, and during the 1920s, the pop. increased with the arrival of many Mexican immigrants. The main gateway for travel between the US and Mexico, the city continued to grow as an increasingly important SW distribution, manufacturing and military center. The long-standing Chamizal boundary dispute, which arose when the course of the Rio Grande changed in 1864, was resolved in 1963, when the US returned 630 acres of land that had originally belonged to Mexico. As industry developed and Mexican immigrants, both documented and undocumented,

FACILITIES. There are 100 parks in El Paso, including Ascarate which has a man-made lake with facilities for boating, fishing and water skiing; McKelligon Canyon, with picnic and barbecue areas and a foot trail to the summit of one of the peaks of the Franklin Mts.; Washington which contains a municipal zoo and gardens; Tom Mays, a picnic area in the Franklin Mts. and Memorial, which contains the Municipal Rose Garden and Garden Center. Three historical parks, City Hall, Cleveland Sq. and Pioneer Plaza, are also located in the city. Other facilities include five public golf courses, 16 tennis courts, 11 swimming pools and an archery range. Hiking, trailriding, camping, fishing, hunting and water and snow skiing are available at nearby lake and mt. areas.

CULTURAL ACTIVITIES. The El Paso Symphony Orchestra, El Paso Pro Musica, Community Concert Assn. and the Music Dept. at UTEP are among the musical organizations located in the city. Local dance companies include Ballet Folklorico and the Civic Ballet. Theatrical groups perform at the El Paso Playhouse, UTEP Fine Arts Playhouse, Civic Center and Amphiteatre. The El Paso Museum of Art features an exhibit from the Kress collection and the Heritage Gallery, while the Ft. Bliss Replica Museum houses historical exhibits spanning 100 years of the old West. Other museums are the Centennial museum at UTEP, the Chamizal Natl. Memorial Museum, the Cavalry Museum and the Bullfight Museum.

LANDMARKS AND SIGHTSEEING SPOTS. Several missions constructed in the 1600s by the Spaniards still stand in El Paso. Among them is the Mission Nuestra Senora del Carmen, established in 1662. The 55-acre Chamizal Natl. Memorial commemorated the peaceful settlement of a century long dispute between Mexico and the US concerning the intl. boundary. The Scenic Drive, a paved road to an overlook on the Franklin Mts., affords a spectular view of El Paso and Juarez, Mexico. Atop Mt. Cristo Rey stands the Sierra de Cristo Rey, a huge statue of Christ overlooking El Paso and neighboring Mexico.

ERIE
PENNSYLVANIA

CITY LOCATION-SIZE-EXTENT. Erie, the third largest city in the state and seat of Erie Co., encompasses 18.9 sq. mi. in NW PA on the SW shore of Lake Erie, 80 mi. SW of Buffalo, NY, at 42°05' N lat. and 80°11' W long. Its met. area extends throughout Erie Co.

TOPOGRAPHY. The terrain of Erie, which is situated in the Erie lowland and Allegheny plateau regions of PA, rises gradually from the W in a series of ridges parallel to the shoreline of Lake Erie. Some 15 mi. inland, the ridges reach a peak of 1,000'. The mean elev. is 731'.

CLIMATE. The climate of Erie is moderate continental. It is influenced by Lake Erie, which moderates cold air masses from the N during the winter, causing excessive cloudiness and frequent snow. The avg. annual temp. of 42°F ranges from a Jan. mean of 27°F to a July mean of 71.3°F. The avg. annual rainfall of 37.5" is well-distributed throughout the year. More than 50% of the 84" avg. annual snowfall occurs in Dec. and Jan. The RH ranges from 61% to 86%. The avg. growing season is 160 days. Erie lies in the ESTZ and observes DST.

The USS Wolverine, America's First Ironhulled Warship, in the Historic District of Erie, Pennsylvania

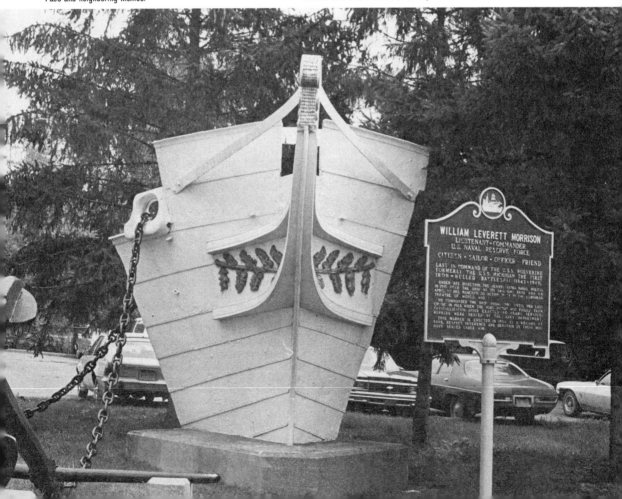

FLORA AND FAUNA. Animals native to Erie include the opossum, raccoon and muskrat. Common birds include the red-winged blackbird, pied-billed grebe, great blue heron, scarlet tanager and woodcock. Salamanders, tree frogs, hognose snakes, snapping turtles, and skinks, as well as the venomous timber rattlesnake, copperhead and massasauga (pygmy rattler), are found in the area. Typical trees include the hemlock (the state tree), maple, elm, hickory, birch, oak, beech, ash, plum and oak. Smaller plants are the pawpaw, witch hazel, aster, spring beauty, chickory and fireweed.

POPULATION. According to the US census, the pop. of Erie in 1970 was 129,265. In 1978, it was estimated that it had decreased to approx. 125,800.

ETHNIC GROUPS. In 1978, the ethnic distribution of Erie was approx. 93.2% Caucasian, 6.6% Black and .2% other.

TRANSPORTATION. Interstate hwys. 79 and 90, US hwys. 19 and 20 and state hwys. 5, 8, 97 and 99 provide major motor access to Erie. *Railroads* serving Erie include AMTRAK, ConRail, E Erie Commercial and Norfolk & Western. *Airlines* serving Erie Intl. Airport include US Air and TW. Nearby Erie Co. Airport provides facilities for private planes. *Bus lines* serving the city include Greyhound and the local Erie Met. Transit Authority (EMTA). The Port of Erie provides access to water transportation via the St. Lawrence Seaway.

COMMUNICATIONS. Communications, broadcasting and print media originating from Erie are: *AM radio stations* WLKK 1260 (CBS, Mod. Ctry); WRIE 1330 (ABC/E, MOR); WJET 1400 (Indep., Contemp.) and WWGO 1450 (ABC/I, MOR); *FM radio stations* WERG 89.1 (ABC/FM, Var.); WQLM 91.3 (NPR, Var.); WLVU 99.9 (Indep., Btfl. Mus.) and WCCK 103.7 (ABC/I, Contemp.); *television stations* WICO Ch. 12 (NBC); WJET Ch. 24 (ABC); WSEE Ch. 35 (CBS) and WQLN Ch. 54 (PBS); *press*: two major dailies serve the city, the morning *News*, and the evening *Times*; other publications include the *Sentinel*, *Lake Shore Visitor*, *Motorist* and *Fraternal Leader*.

HISTORY. A small but fierce nation of native Americans known variously as the Eriez, Eries, Erigas, Eriehonpws, Mas Spirtis and the Cats Nation inhabited the area of Erie long before the first whites arrived. In 1753, the French arrived under the command of Chevalier Pierre Paul Marin, who built Ft. Presque Isle on the site of Erie. Within two years, about 365 families had arrived and established a small village. The fort, which served as a supply base during the French and Indian Wars, was captured by the British in 1759, and in 1763, by native Americans led by Pontiac, who destroyed it. After the Revolutionary War, the state's need for a harbor on Lake Erie led to its purchase, in 1792, of the triangle of land bounded by PA, NY and the lake. Capt. John Grubb was sent to establish an American fort at the site of Presque Isle, and the town was surveyed in 1795. The first American settlers, almost all of them farmers, arrived from E PA, NJ, NY, N.E., Ireland, Scotland and Germany. Early commerce centered on the salt trade, which arrived from NY by boat and was reshipped to Pittsburgh and Louisville. Shipbuilding began in 1798. Erie Co. was established in 1800, and Erie, the co. seat, was incorporated as a borough in

Erie, Pennsylvania

1805. Most of the ships in the fleet of Comm. Oliver Hazard Perry during the War of 1812 were built in Erie. While aboard the *Niagara*, Perry forced the British squadron to surrender. After the War, improved transportation and the advent of the RR led to rapid development of the town. Early mfg. industries were based on agriculture, while heavy industry began in the town with the building of an iron foundry in 1833. In 1844, when the Erie Extension Canal was completed, cheap transportation to the Pittsburgh region was provided. In 1851, Erie was incorporated as a city. Erie entered the 20th century as a mfg. center and major inland port. With the opening of the St. Lawrence Seaway in 1959, the city became a seaport.

GOVERNMENT. Erie has a mayor-council form of govt. consisting of a mayor and seven council members, all of whom are elected at large to four-year terms.

ECONOMY AND INDUSTRY. There are more than 475 industrial plants in Erie Co., employing approx. 35% of the work force. Metal mfg. is the major industry, and includes such products as boilers, engines, power shovels, meters, turbines, castings, forgings, pipe equipment, motors and diesel engines. Plastics and paper are also manufactured. In June, 1979, the labor force of the greater met. area totaled approx. 127,000, while the rate of unemployment was 7.8%.

BANKING. There are four banks and six savings and loan assns. in Erie. In 1978, total deposits for the two banks headquartered in the city were approx. $360,118,000, while assets totaled $457,890,000. Banks include Security People's Trust, Union Bank and Trust, Marine and Security People's Trust and First Natl. of PA.

HOSPITALS. There are eight hosps. in Erie Co., including St. Vincent's, Hamot Medical Center, Erie Osteopathic, Doctor's Osteopathic, V.A. and Shriner's.

EDUCATION. Gannon Col., founded in Erie in 1944, is a private liberal arts institution awarding bachelor and master degrees. Approx. 3,500 enrolled in 1978. PA State U-Behrend Col. offers assoc., bachelor and master degrees and, in 1978, enrolled approx. 1,700. Other teaching and research institutions include Mercyhurst and Villa Maria colleges, Erie Bus. Center and Erie Inst. of Tech. There are 18 elementary, five middle and four high schools in the public school system. Lib. facilities include the Erie City and Co. Lib.

ENTERTAINMENT. The Village Dinner Theatre provides dining entertainment. The Summer Festival of the Arts, a week-long event in June, features exhibits of art, crafts and photographs, as well as musical and dramatic presentations. Sports entertainment in Erie is provided by the Blades, an NEHL hockey team, as well as the Behrend Col. Cubs and collegiate teams from Gannon and Mercyhurst colleges.

ACCOMMODATIONS. There are several hotels and motels in Erie, including the Peninsula, Bel-Aire, Peek & Peak and the Holiday, Hilton and Ramada Inns.

FACILITIES. There are 29 recreational parks, encompassing approx. 500 acres, and a 15-acre zoo in Erie. Facilities include tennis courts, swimming and wading pools, playgrounds and picnic areas. Among the parks are Waldameer and Presque Isle State, which is situated on Presque Isle, a peninsula extending into Lake Erie. It includes lagoons, scenic hiking trails, seven mi. of beach, boat ramps, docking facilities and picnic grounds.

CULTURAL ACTIVITIES. The Erie Arts Council consists of several organizations, including the Erie Philharmonic, Erie Art Center (which presents multi-media exhibits), Erie Civic Ballet, Civic Music, Erie Civic Theatre and the Erie Playhouse, as well as theaters at Gannon, Mercyhurst and Behrend Cols. Lake Shore Railway History Society, a former NY Central passenger depot, displays historical locomotives and RR cars. The Erie Museum and Planetarium features local history and science exhibits and the Firefighters' Historical Museum displays equipment spanning 150 years.

LANDMARKS AND SIGHTSEEING SPOTS. The Perry Memorial House and Dickson Tavern, which was built in 1809, served as a hotel for

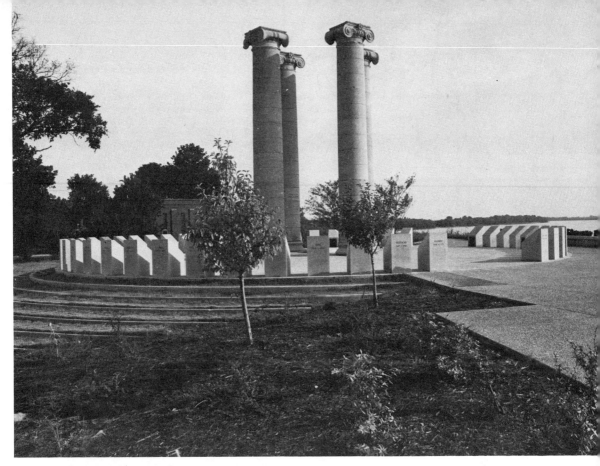

"Four Freedom's Monument" commemorates the Bicentennial, Evansville, Indiana

many notables, including Comm. Perry. The walls contain secret passageways which were used to hide runaway slaves. Other reminders of the Battle of Lake Erie in 1813 are the restored Brig *Niagara*, at the foot of State Street, and the Perry Monument on Presque Isle. The USS *Wolverine*, the Customs House, the Cashier's House and the Wayne Blockhouse, a replica of the house where Revolutionary War "Mad Anthony" Wayne died in 1796, are historical sites in the downtown area. The Sprague Home, built in 1835, was another underground slave station. The Washington Monument at Ft. Le Boeuf is the only known monument of Washington as a young man in a British uniform. The Soldiers' and Sailors' Home, completed in 1886, sits on a bluff overlooking the bay between Lake Erie and the Presque Isle peninsula.

EVANSVILLE
INDIANA

CITY LOCATION-SIZE-EXTENT. Evansville, the seat of Vanderburgh Co., encompasses 37 sq. mi. in extreme SW IN on the N bank of the OH River, just N of KY. The city lies 165 mi. S of Indianapolis, 155 mi. N of Nashville, 125 mi. W of Louisville and 170 mi. E of St. Louis at 28°03' N lat. and 87°32' W long. The greater met. area extends throughout Vanderburgh Co., into Posey Co. to the W, Warrick Co. to the E and across the OH River into Henderson Co., KY on the S.

TOPOGRAPHY. The terrain of Evansville, in the OH River Valley, is characterized by low rolling hills. The OH River forms the S border of the city. The Pigeon River enters the city from the E and joins a great bend of the OH River in the S central portion of the city. The smaller Locust River flows into the Pigeon River from the NW portion of the city. The mean elev. is 385'.

CLIMATE. The climate of Evansville is continental, influenced by prevailing winds from the S, which carry moisture-laden low pressure formations to the area from the W Gulf of Mexico. The avg. annual temp. of 56.7°F ranges from a Jan. mean of 33.4°F to a July mean of 78.8°F. The avg. annual rainfall of 42.27" is fairly evenly distributed throughout the year. Most of the annual 14" of snowfall occurs from Jan. through Mar. The RH ranges from 53% to 88%. The avg. growing season is 199 days. Evansville lies in the CSTZ and observes DST.

FLORA AND FAUNA. Animals native to Evansville include the fox, opossum and deer. Common birds are the blue jay, cardinal, chickadee, tufted titmouse, Carolina wren, woodpecker, brown thrasher, vireo and owl. Broad-headed skinks, five-lined skinks, E box turtles, red-eared slider toads, leopard frogs, hognose snakes, S black racers, gray rat snakes, black and regular king snakes and rough green snakes, as well as the venomous rattlesnake, copperhead and cottonmouth, are found in the area. Typical trees include the elm, maple, pine, sweetgum and sycamore. Smaller plants include the iris, passion flower, spicebush, pawpaw, hazelnut, wildgrape and honeysuckle.

POPULATION. According to the US census, the pop. of Evansville in 1970 was 138,764. In 1978, it was estimated that it had decreased to 130,100.

ETHNIC GROUPS. In 1978, the ethnic distribution of Evansville was approx. 92.7% Caucasian, 7.3% Black and .4% Hispanic (part of the Hispanic total is also included in the Caucasian total).

TRANSPORTATION. Interstate Hwy. 164, US Hwy. 41 and state hwys. 57, 62, 65 and 66 provide major motor access to Evansville. The 12' deep OH River Channel accommodates five barge lines, which move from the seaport of New Orleans, and Mead Johnson terminal handles 700,000 tons of cargo annually. *Railroads* serving the city include ConRail, IL Central Gulf, Louisville & Nashville and S. *Airlines* serving Evansville Dress Regional

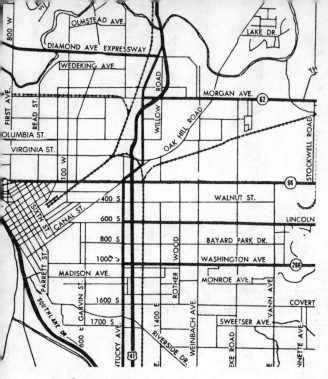

Evansville, Indiana

iron, steel and furniture manufacturers had located in the city, which had also become one of the largest tobacco centers of the US. Nearly 50% of the city's residents were of German descent, and during WW I, when the US declared war on Germany, conflict arose from strong anti-German sentiments. In 1929, oil was discovered in the area, but during the Depression, many manufacturing plants failed. By 1939, however, the city became an important oil producing center, and the idle factories were once again productive. Following WW II, manufacturing expanded considerably, particulary in the automotive, appliance and power generation equipment industries, and, by the 1960s, the pop. of the city approached 140,000.

GOVERNMENT. Evansville has a mayor-council form of govt., consisting of nine council members and the mayor. Six council members are elected by ward, while the remaining three and the mayor are elected at large. All serve four-year terms.

ECONOMY AND INDUSTRY. Some 150 manufacturing firms located in Evansville employ approx. 28% of the total area labor force. Major products include electrical and nonelectrical machinery, household appliances, fabricated metal products, construction material, aluminum, pottery and tile. Wholesale and retail trade, mining and quarrying, contract construction and service are important non-manufacturing industries. The city lies in the heart of a coal producing region which yields 250 million tons annually, as well as in a 36-co. agricultural belt, consisting of more than 31,000 farms totaling approx. 6.25 million acres. In June, 1979, the labor force of the greater met. area totaled 141,900, while the rate of unemployment was 4.7%.

BANKING. There are four commercial banks and six savings and loan assns. in Evansville. In 1978, total deposits for the four banks headquartered in the city were $908,765,000, while assets were $1,070,841,000. Banks serving the city include Old Natl., Citizen's Natl., Natl. City and Peoples Savings.

HOSPITALS. There are three gen. hosps. in Evansville, Deaconess, St. Mary's and Welborn Memorial Baptist, as well as IN State Hosp. and Evansville Psychiatric Children's Center.

EDUCATION. The U of Evansville, a private institution affiliated with the United Methodist Church and established in the city in 1919 (originally 1854), offers associate, bachelor and master degrees as well as a study center in Grantham, England. In 1978, more than 4,900 enrolled. IN State U of Evansville, established in 1965, offers associate and bachelor degrees. In 1978, more than 2,900 enrolled. The IN Vocational Tech. Col. at Evansville, a state supported institution established in 1968, ITT Tech. Institute and Lockyear Col., a two-year business school, offer associate degrees. The public school system consists of 31 elementary schools, which enrolled more than 15,000 in 1978, and five high schools, which enrolled more than 15,000. In addition, Catholic schools, 22 elementary and two high schools enrolled 4,000, two Lutheran high schools enrolled about 350 and the Seventh Day Adventists (one elementary and one high school) enrolled approx. 50 students. Lib. facilities include the Evansville and Vanderburgh Co. Public Lib., Central and Willard Lib., which contains a large collection of out-of-print books as well as a genealogical reference center.

ENTERTAINMENT. Among the annual events held in Evansville are the Mid-States Art Exhibition at which works of regional artists are judged; the OH River Arts Festival, a weekly series of events featuring arts, crafts, music, poetry, drama and film productions; and the Artists Guild Art Fair which features displays and demonstrations of artistic creations. The Freedom Festival, a mid-summer event features a bierstube, sky-diving, hydro-plane racing, a parade and a large fire works display. The Fall Festival, an early autumn week-long event sponsored by the West Side Nut Club, features ethnic food, kiddie rides and street fair activities. The Philharmonic Fair, held each May, includes a tennis tournament, beer can trading, an antique auto show, arts and crafts, exhibits, films and music.

Airport are DL, EA, US Air and Conair. Tri-State Aero and Skyland Airport provide commuter and private aircraft service. *Bus lines* serving the city include Greyhound, Trailways and the local Met. Evansville Transit System.

COMMUNICATIONS. Communications, broadcasting and print media serving Evansville are: *AM radio stations* WIKY 820 (Indep., MOR); WGBF 1280 (APR, Top 40); WJPS 1330 (ABC, Contemp.) and WROZ 1400 (ABC/I, C&W); *FM radio stations* WPSR 90.7 (Indep., Educ.); WUEV 91.5 (Indep., Progsv.); WIKY 104.1 (APR, MOR, Btfl. Mus.) and WVHI 105.3 (MBS, Relig.); *television stations* WTVW Ch. 7 (ABC); WNIN Ch. 9 (PBS); WFIE Ch. 14 (NBC); WEHT Ch. 25 (CBS) and cable; *press*: the two major daily publications serving the city are the *Courier*, issued mornings, and the *Press*, issued evenings, which issue a combined Sun. edition.

HISTORY. Founded in 1812 by Col. Hugh McGary, Evansville was named after Gen. Robert Evans, a territorial legislator who designated the settlement the co. seat of justice in order to ensure its growth. For 20 years, however, no industry developed in the village and founder McGary went bankrupt. Belief that the planned Wabash and Erie Canal would intersect the OH River at Evansville resulted in an increase in the pop. of the town in the 1830s, and a sawmill and cabinet-making shop were established. When the canal finally opened in 1854, only the hasty construction of a RR connecting the town to the canal enabled the merchants to survive. During the 1840s, a large number of Germans seeking work immigrated to the town from NY, and by the time Evansville was chartered as a city in 1847, it ranked as the eighth largest in IN. Agricultural implements, pottery, and iron castings and stoves were being produced in 1856, when the city was designated a river port of entry. Prior to the Civil War, citizens of Evansville secretly aided hundreds of blacks fleeing northward to freedom on the Underground RR. In 1868, coal was discovered near the city, and the establishment of coal mining formed the basis of new economic growth. During the 1870s, the first lumber co. was founded in the town, followed by brick and tile, muslin and cotton yarn factories. Between 1860 and 1890, industrial employment increased from slightly more than 900 to nearly 7,500. By 1900, more than 300

The Goosetown Festival, a block party held in the historic Riverside District features a flea market, auctions, arts and crafts exhibits, games and a tour of the neighborhood. The Vanderburgh Co. 4-H Fair, held in late July and early Aug., features tractor pulls, national performers and horse and livestock shows. The Germania Maennerchor Volkfest, held each Aug., offers German food and entertainment. The Triplets, a professional minor league baseball team and the U of Evansville's Aces, provide spectator sports entertainment.

ACCOMMODATIONS. There are 22 hotels and motels in Evansville including the Jackson House, Arrowhead Lodge, Travelodge, Towne and St. Mary's motels and the Holiday, Executive, Ramada, Williamsburg, Riverboat and Sheraton inns.

FACILITIES. There are 29 parks encompassing 1,700 acres in Evansville, including public golf courses, swimming pools, tennis courts, playing fields, picnic areas, jogging and bicycling trails, boating and fishing facilities and an amusement park. Mesker Park contains a zoo housing hundreds of animals including monkeys which live on a concrete replica of the Santa Maria in the center of a lake. The two hundred-acre Wesselman Park Nature Center features marked trails winding through the virgin forests.

CULTURAL ACTIVITES. The Evansville Philharmonic Orchestra performs in Vanderburgh Auditorium, which also features stage performances by various visiting artists and groups. The Broadway Theater League and Musicians Club of Evansville also sponsor visiting artist performances. The Shanklin Theater of the U of Evansville, award-winner at the American Col. Theater Festival, the Evansville Civic Theatre and six other groups stage dramatic productions in the city. The Evansville Museum of Arts and Science features displays of art as well as historical and scientific exhibits, including Native American rafts and a collection of Civil War weapons. The Koch Planetarium is also located in the building.

LANDMARKS AND SIGHTSEEING SPOTS. The old Vanderburgh Co. Courthouse and Jail (1887), a neo-Baroque structure located in the historic First Street area of Evansville, is listed on the Natl. Register of Historic Places. The Four Freedoms monument, the bicentennial project of the city located on the Bank of the OH River contains columns of native limestone which were originally part of the old Evansville Comm. Center. A RR exhibit featuring a steam locomotive, a 20th-century parlor car and a caboose is located in Sunset Park. On the U of Evansville campus are two reconstructed pioneer lodges and a one-hundred year-old cabin which is currently being restored. The John A. Reitz home (1870), exemplifying a style popular during the Second French Empire is maintained as a house museum. The Downtown Walkway, a reconstruction of the old Main Street shopping district, is open only to pedestrian traffic. Other attractions include Santa Claus Land, the Conrad Baker Center and the Lincoln Heritage Trail and Memorial.

FALL RIVER
MASSACHUSETTS

CITY LOCATION-SIZE-EXTENT. Fall River encompasses 33.0 sq. mi. in SE MA at the mouth of the Fall and Taunton rivers where they empty into Mt. Hope Bay located 20 mi. SE of Providence, RI and 50 mi. S of Boston at 41°42' N lat. and 71°08' W long. It is bordered on the W and S by RI and on the E by Watuppa Pond.

TOPOGRAPHY. The terrain of Fall River, which lies in the Atlantic coastal lowland region, is characterized by rolling hills, small lakes and ponds, including Cook Pond, and short, shallow rivers. The city lies on the W side of a high hill which slopes downward toward Mt. Hope Bay and the Fall River. The mean elev. is 130'.

CLIMATE. The continental climate of Fall River, modified by Narragansett Bay and the Atlantic Ocean to the E, is characterized by mild winters and cool summers. The avg. annual temp. of 50°F ranges from a monthly mean of 30°F in Jan. to 71°F in July. The temp. exceeds 90°F on an avg. of five days per summer. Most of the avg. annual rainfall of 44" occurs from Apr. through Oct., while more than 50% of the avg. annual 33" of snowfall

Battleship Cove is home of a "fleet" of former USN vessels, Fall River, Massachusetts

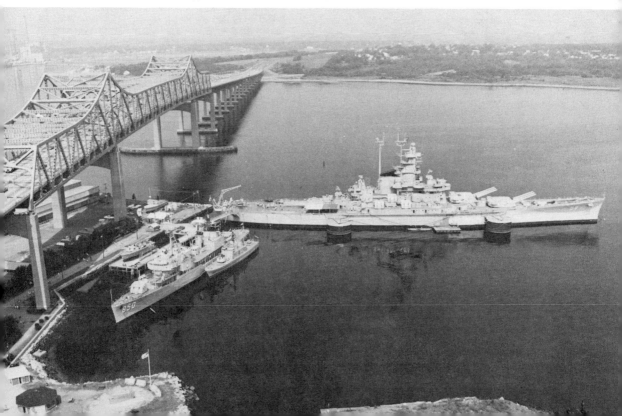

occurs in Jan. and Feb. The avg. growing season is 195 days. The RH ranges from 46% to 84%. Fall River lies in the ESTZ and observes DST.

FLORA AND FAUNA. Animals native to Fall River include the raccoon, weasel, muskrat and fox. Common birds are the gull, barn owl, flycatcher, crow and rail. Tree frogs, leopard frogs, salamanders, toads, box turtles and green snakes, as well as the venomous timber rattlesnake and copperhead, are found in the area. Typical trees include the ash, oak and maple. Smaller plants include the tupelo, rhododendron, holly and bugbane.

POPULATION. According to the US census, the pop. of Fall River in 1970 was 95,898. In 1978, it was estimated that it had increased to 100,430.

ETHNIC GROUPS. In 1978, the ethnic distribution of Fall River was approx. 98% Caucasian, 1% Black and 1% other races.

TRANSPORTATION. Interstate Hwy. 195, US Hwy. 6 and state hwys. 81, 24 and 79 provide major motor access to Fall River. ConRail provides *railroad* service to the city, while Fall River Municipal Airport is served

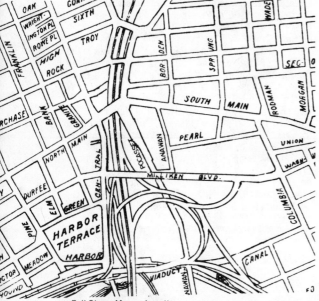

Fall River, Massachusetts

by private aircraft and charter *airlines*. Airports in New Bedford and Providence also provide service. *Bus Lines* include Greyhound, Trailways, Bonanza and the local SE Regional Transit Authority (SRTA). The city's protected inland deep water port is 18 mi. from open sea and has modern facilities.

COMMUNICATIONS. Communications, broadcasting and print media originating from Fall River are: *AM Radio station* WALE 1400 (MBS, Info/Adult Music) and WSAR 1480 (CBS, MOR); no *FM radio station* or *television stations* broadcast from the city, which is served by media from nearby New Bedford Providence and Boston; cable TV, however, is available; *press:* one daily newspaper is published in the city, the *Herald News,* which is issued evenings and Sun. mornings: other publications include the weekly *Anchor,* issued on Thurs.,the *Diocesan Press* and *Jornal De Fall River,* a Portuguese newspaper.

HISTORY. Native Americans of several MA tribes inhabited the area of present-day Fall River when the first white settlers arrived in 1654. The site, known as Freeman's Purchase, was part of a land grant from the Plymouth settlement to the NE. In 1683, it was combined with another tract of land called Pocasset Purchase, and renamed Freetown. In 1778, during the Revolutionary War, local citizens defended the settlement against the British in the Battle of Fall River. In 1803, the village of Freetown was incorporated as the

town of Fall River, after the river on which it was located. The native Americans called the city "Quequechan", translated as "falling water." It was renamed in 1804, and known as Troy for the next 30 years. In 1837, the name of the town was again changed—to Fall River, and it was chartered as a city in 1854. One of the most famous and controversial murder cases in the US was prosecuted in the city in 1892, when Lizzie Borden, a Fall River Woman, accused of killing her parents, was tried and acquitted. An important textile producer during the late 1800s and early 1900s, the city was the major cotton manufacturing center of the US at the turn of the century. The luxurious steamships of the Fall River Line fleet were internationally known. The Credit Union movement started in the city. Although the number of mills decreased after 1929, the economy of the city is still based on textile manufacturing and the garment industry.

GOVERNMENT. Fall River has a mayor-council form of govt. The mayor, who is not a voting member of the council, and the nine council members are elected at large for two-year terms.

ECONOMY AND INDUSTRY. Textile manufacturing employs approx. 75% of the total Fall River labor force. Major products are high-grade cotton, frequently combined with synthetics, and rubber and latex goods. Food and paper products, abrasives and lighting fixtures are among the manufactured products. Other products are boats, chemicals, surgical supplies and electronic equipment. In 1978, the total labor force of Fall River was 50,100, while the rate of unemployment was approx. 7.7%. Avg. income per capita in 1978 was $8,500.

BANKING. There are three commercial banks and six savings and loans assns. in Fall River. In 1978, total deposits for the seven banks headquartered in the city were $589,122,000, while assets were $655,158,000. Banks include Citizens Savings, Fall River Five Cent Savings, Fall River Savings, Fall River Trust, BMC Durfee Trust, Fall River Natl., Union Savings, First Fed. Savings and Fall River Peoples' Cooperative.

HOSPITALS. There are two gen. hosps. in Fall River, St. Anne's and Charlton Memorial, formerly Union-Truesdale. The city is also served by Hanover Clinic, Commonwealth of MA Mental Health Center, ILGWU Health Center and the Dr. John Corrigan Mental Health Center.

EDUCATION. Bristol Comm. Col., a state-supported jr. col. established in 1965, is located in Fall River. In 1978, approx. 5,890 enrolled. The public school system enrolled more than 14,300 in 1978. In addition, 10 Roman Catholic elementary and high schools are located in the city. Lib. facilties include the Fall River Public Lib. and two branches.

ENTERTAINMENT. The Bristol Comm. Col. Knights and the N.E. Patriots, an NFL-AFC professional football team which plays at Schaefer Stadium in Foxboro, 25 mi. N of Fall River, provide spectator sports entertainment. The city sponsors an Ethnic Festival each spring, featuring food, art and entertainment in the tradition of the city's 12 ethnic groups. A Farmer's Market is held twice weekly at Kennedy Park from June to Nov. Additional dinner theaters entertainment are available in nearby Providence and Boston.

ACCOMMODATIONS. Among the hotels and motels in Fall River are the Fall River Inn, Howard Johnson's and Motel Somerset.

FACILITIES. The 22 public parks and recreational areas in Fall River provide tennis courts, two swimming pools, picnic areas, jogging tracks, golf courses, playing fields and ice skating rinks, while fishing and boating facilities are available at Mt. Hope Bay and Watuppa Pond. Camping, picnicking, boating, fishing and swimming facilities are available at 594-acre Horseneck Beach, located 14 mi. S of the city. The Tauton River waterfront includes a Bicentennial Park with a boat launch and fishing pier.

CULTURAL ACTIVITIES. The Fall River Symphony Orchestra, the Little Theater of Fall River and the Summer Street Theater Program are among the performing arts organizations in the city. The history of steamship transportation is depicted through lithographs, paintings, photographs, and model ships at the Marine Museum, while the Fall River Historical Society maintains a collection of historical artifacts.

LANDMARKS AND SIGHTSEEING SPOTS. An historical marker on the Fall River City Hall commemorates the 1778 Battle of Fall River during the Revolutionary War. Battleship Cove harbors US Navy vessels of the 20th century, as well as several which participated in wartime battles in this century. Among these are the *USS Lionfish*, a WW II attack submarine; the *USS Joseph P. Kennedy Jr.*, a destroyer which saw action in Korea, Vietnam and the Cuban missile crisis; the *USS MA (Big Mamie)*, which survived 55 WW II battles and contains a PT boat museum and model aircraft exhibit, and the *PT Boat 796*, one of the remaining operational torpedo boats of WW II. The Lizzie Borden House, the scene of the woman's alleged murder of her parents in 1892, is maintained as a popular attraction. St. Anne's Church and Shrine was constructed in 1906, and is one of 80 churches of architectural interest in Fall River.

FLINT
MICHIGAN

CITY LOCATION-SIZE-EXTENT. Flint, the seat of Genesse Co. and third largest city in the state, encompasses 32.9 sq. mi. in the Flint River Valley in SE central MI 50 mi. NW of Detroit at 42°58' N lat. and 83°44' W long. The greater met. area extends E into Lapeer Co. and W into Shiawassee Co.

TOPOGRAPHY. The terrain of Flint, MI, which lies in the Great Lakes Plain region of the lower peninsula of MI, is generally flat. The land rises in the SE part of the city to a range of hills 15 to 20 mi. away. Lake Huron lies approx. 65 mi. to the E, while Saginaw Bay is approx. 40 mi. to the N. The mean elev. is 750'.

CLIMATE. The climate of Flint is continental, influenced by the Great Lakes, which temper cold waves from the NW, delay spring and prolong warm weather in late autumn. The avg. annual temp. of 47.4°F ranges from a Jan. mean of 22.4°F to a July mean of 70.1°F. Most of the annual 30.51" of rainfall occurs in the spring, summer and fall. Approx. 85% of the annual 45.4" of snowfall occurs from Dec. through Mar. Tornadoes associated with thunderstorms and squall lines occasionally strike the area. The growing season is 180 days. The RH ranges from 55% to 86%. Flint is located in the ESTZ and observes DST.

FLORA AND FAUNA. Animals native to Flint include the fox, squirrel, raccoon and whitetail deer. Common birds are the blue jay, woodcock, robin (the state bird), snipe, bluebird and sapsucker. Wood frogs, salamanders, box turtles, skinks and the venomous E massasauga and timber rattlesnake, are found in the area. Typical trees are the hawthorn, elm, red oak, white pine (the state tree) and cottonwood. Smaller plants include the partridge berry, wintergreen, bluebell and buckwheat.

POPULATION. According to the US census, the pop. of Flint in 1970 was 193,317. In 1977, it was estimated that it had decreased to 163,594.

ETHNIC GROUPS. In 1978, the ethnic distribution of Flint was approx. 60% Caucasian, 38.5% Black and 1.5% Hispanic (a percentage of the Hispanic total is included in the Caucasian total).

TRANSPORTATION. Interstate hwys. 69, 75 and 475, US hwys. 23 and 10 and state hwys. 31, 54 and 56 provide major motor access to Flint. *Railroads* include AMTRAK, Chesapeake & OH and Grand Trunk. Bishop Int. Airport is served by several *airlines* including VA and RP. *Bus lines* include Greyhound, Indian Trails and the Mass Transportation Authority.

COMMUNICATIONS. Communications, broadcasting and print media originating from Flint are: *AM radio stations* WFDF 910 (NBC, MOR); WTAC 600 (ABC/C, Contemp., Top 40); WTRK 1330 (ABC/1, MOR); WKMF 1470 (ABC/E, Ctry.); WAMM 1420 (R&B, Blk.) and WLOB 1570 (MBS, Relig.); *FM radio stations* WFBE 95.1 (NPR, Educ.); WWCK 105.5 (ABC/FM, AOR) and WGMZ 107.9 (Indep., Btfl. Mus.); *television station* WNEM Ch. 5 (NBC); WJRT Ch. 12 (ABC); WEYI Ch. 25 (CBS) and cable; *press:* one major daily serves the city, the *Journal*, issued evenings; other publications are the *Catholic Weekly* and *Flint Spokesman*.

HISTORY. The area of present-day Flint was inhabited by Native Americans, who called the river "the river of flint stones", before the first white settlers arrived. In 1819, Detroit fur trader Jacob Smith established a community on the river which was settled by pioneers from W NY. Originally a farming and lumbering community, Flint was incorporated as a city in 1855. The city became prominent in the carriage-making industry. By 1900, more than 100,000 carriages and wagons were produced in "Vehicle City". In 1902 and 1903, the production of automobiles began in the city, and, in 1904, W.C. Durant, who had been involved in the carriage industry, gained control of the Buick Motor Co. Because of his success, Durant organized Gen. Motors Co. (GM) In 1905. Since that time, the largest concentration of GM employment and production in the world has developed in the city.

GOVERNMENT. Flint has a mayor-council form of govt. The mayor is elected at large to a four-year term, while the nine council members are elected to two-year terms.

ECONOMY AND INDUSTRY. There are approx. 350 manufacturing plants in Flint, employing approx. 35% of the work force. Automobiles and auto parts are the major

Sculpture at Riverbank Park, Flint, Michigan

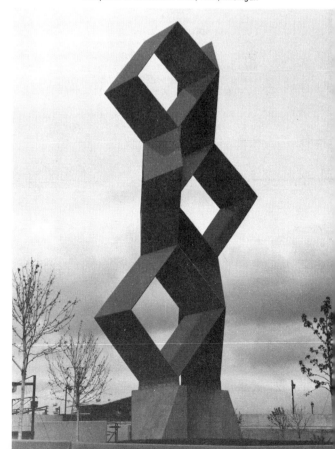

products; the city ranks second to Detroit as the leading automobile manufacturer in the US. Five divisions of GM operate 10 plants in the city. Other products are building materials, chemicals, foundry products, paints and varnishes. In 1979, the labor force for the greater met. area totaled approx. 230,100, while the rate of unemployment was 7.4%.

BANKING. There are 10 banks and five savings and loan assns. in Flint. In 1978, total deposits for the two banks headquartered in the city were approx. $1,545,772,000, while assets totaled $1,763,058,000. Banks include Citizens Commercial & Savings, Genesee Merchant Bank & Trust, MI Natl. and First Fed. and Detroit & N Savings and Loans.

HOSPITALS. There are six hosps. in the city, including Flint Gen., Flint Osteopathic, Genesee Memorial, St. Joseph, McLaren Gen. and Hurley Medical Center.

EDUCATION. The U of MI at Flint, one of three four-year colleges in the U of MI system, awards bachelor and master degrees and enrolled more than 3,900 in 1978. Gen. Motors Institute, a private coeducational engineering and management col. affiliated with GM, enrolled approx. 2,350 in a five-year cooperative program in 1978. Charles S. Mott Comm. Col., established in 1923, enrolled nearly 9,100 in 1978. Other institutions are Baker Jr. Col. of Bus., and Ross Medical Education Center. There are 44 elementary, eight jr. high and four sr. high schools in the public school system, as well as 24 private and parochial schools. There are 23 public libs. in Flint and Genesee Co.

ENTERTAINMENT. Among the annual events held in the city are the Flint Art Fair, which takes place in June, the Olympian Games, held in July, and the CAN USA Games, which take place in Aug. The Flint Generals, an IHL hockey team provide professional sports entertainment.

ACCOMMODATIONS. There are several hotels and motels in Flint, including Howard Johnson's, the Farm, Walli's Motor Lodge, and the Red Roof and Sheraton inns. A Hyatt Regency Hotel will open in 1981.

FACILITIES. There are 26 parks and 27 playgrounds in Flint, encompassing more than 1,500 acres. Facilities include four swimming pools, numerous playing fields, four municipal golf courses, five gymnasiums, 29 tennis courts and 25 ice skating rinks.

CULTURAL ACTIVITIES. The Flint Symphony Orchestra and the Flint Institute of Music present musical performances, while Flint Community Players and the Mott Comm. Col. Players stage dramatic productions in the Bower Theater. The Flint Cultural Center houses the Alfred P. Sloan Jr. Museum, the Flint Institute of Arts and the Robert T. Longway Planetarium. The museum features displays of local history, the automobile industry and

a doll museum, while the Flint Institute of Arts features paintings, sculpture and Renaissance tapestries in the Dewaters Art Center.

LANDMARKS AND SIGHTSEEING SPOTS. Among the attractions in Flint are the Farmers Market and tours of GM, Buick, Chevrolet and Fisher Body manufacturing plants. Crossroads Village, a restored 1860-1880 community, features an operating blacksmith shop, sawmill, leather shop, cider mill, antique-furnished homes, and a gen. store with old-fashioned merchandise. The Huckleberry RR at Crossroads Village features open and closed passenger coaches pulled by a Baldwin locomotive.

FORT LAUDERDALE
FLORIDA

CITY LOCATION-SIZE-EXTENT. Ft. Lauderdale, the seat of Broward Co., encompasses 31 sq. mi. including 165 mi. of inland waterways and beach areas in SE FL on the Atlantic Ocean at 26°07' N lat. and 80°08' W long. Its greater met. area extends throughout Broward Co., S to that of Miami, 25 mi. away, into Palm Beach Co. on the N and includes the city of Hollywood.

TOPOGRAPHY. The terrain of Ft. Lauderdale, situated on the Atlantic coastal plain, is characterized by very flat areas dissected by numerous waterways. The Everglades area lies W of the city while Port Everglades, at the mouth of the Stranahan River, is to the S. The New River flows through the S part of the city and joins the Stranahan River to the SE. The mean elev. is 10'.

CLIMATE. The climate of Ft. Lauderdale is subtropical marine, influenced by the Atlantic Ocean and characterized by long, warm, rainy summers and mild, dry winters. The avg. annual temp. of 75°F includes monthly means of 67°F during Jan. to 83°F during July. Most of the annual rainfall of 59'' occurs during the summer. The RH ranges from 55% to 90%. Ft. Lauderdale lies in the ESTZ and observes DST.

FLORA AND FAUNA. Animals native to Ft. Lauderdale include the fox squirrel, grey fox and whitetail deer. Common birds are the heron, ibis, gull, tern, crow, cardinal, red bellied woodpecker, bluejay, spotted breasted oriole, grackle, screech owl and mockingbird, the state bird. Many species of water fowl winter at the Everglades and Okeechobee Lake. Siren alligators, FL soft-shelled turtles, indigo snakes and swamp snakes as well as the venomous cottonmouth, coral snake and rattlesnake are found in the area. Common trees include the live oak, water locust, mangrove and bald cypress. Smaller plants include the eugenia, paradise tree, seagrape and palmetto.

POPULATION. According to the US census, the pop. of Ft. Lauderdale in 1970 was 139,590. In 1978, it was estimated that it had increased to approx. 156,400.

ETHNIC GROUPS. In 1978, the ethnic distribution of Ft. Lauderdale was approx. 85.2% Caucasian, 14.6% Black and 2.2% Hispanic (a percentage of the Hispanic total is also included in the Caucasian total).

TRANSPORTATION. Interstate Hwy. 95, US hwys. 1, 27 and 441 and state rtes. 84, 91 (the FL tnpk.), 809, 811, 816, 838 and 842 provide major motor access to Ft. Lauderdale. *Railroads* serving the city include FL E Coast, Seaboard Coast and AMTRAK. *Airlines* serving Ft. Lauderdale-Hollywood Intl. Airport include BN, CO, DL, EA, NA, NW, S, TW, UA and WA. In addition, three local airports serve private and commuter aircraft. *Bus Lines* include Greyhound, Trailways and the local Broward Transportation Authority. Port Everglades, the deepest Atlantic seaport S of Norfolk, VA, is the leading intl. cruise ship port in FL, as well as the site of the first foreign trade zone in the state.

COMMUNICATIONS. Communications broadcasting and print media serving Ft. Lauderdale are: *AM radio stations* WAVS 1190 (MBS,

Flint, Michigan

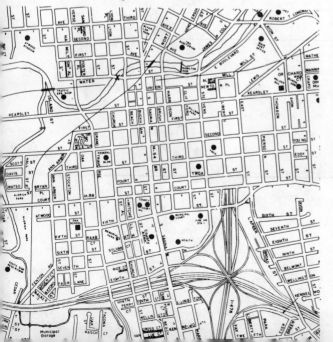

News); WFTL 1400 (ABC/I, MOR); WRBD 1470 (ABC/C, R&B) and WSRF 1580 (Indep., AOR); *FM radio stations* WAFG 90.3 (Indep., Educ.); WHYI 100.7 (Indep., Top 40) and WAXY 105.9 (ABC, Oldies); *television stations* WKID Ch. 51 (Indep.); the city also receives radio and televison broadcasting from nearby Miami; *press:* two major daily newspapers serve the area, the *News,* issued evenings and Sun. morning, and the *Sun-Sentinel* issued mornings Mon. through Sat.; other publications include the *Broward Tribune, High Riser, Side Gazette, Gold Coast of FL, Broward Review and Business Record, Gondolier, Jewish Floridian* and *Intl. Marine Angler.*

HISTORY. Native Americans of the Tequesta tribe inhabited the New River area, site of present-day Ft. Lauderdale, from about 1500 BC to 1763 AD when the first white settlers, the Spanish, arrived. The Treaty of 1763 resulted in the expulsion of the Tequestas by the Spanish to Cuba, and the area subsequently became part of a British settlement. During the Revolutionary War, it was part of a large sanctuary for Loyalists. In the Treaty of 1783, however, Britain relinquished its rights to FL, and the area again was controlled by the Spanish. In the late 18th century, native Americans of the Seminole tribe arrived to live in the area, and, in 1793, the Surla and Frankee Lewis family established a plantation on the New River. By 1835, a settlement of 50 to 60 whites, encouraged to homestead by the Spanish, had been established on the banks of the New River. A successful arrowroot starch-processing plant, founded by William Cooley, was among the first industries of the area, which was evacuated in 1836 following the massacre of the Cooley family and the advent of the second Seminole War. The site, which became the center of hostilities, was to be occupied by US troops on three different occasions in the next 20 years. In 1838, when Maj. William Lauderdale arrived from TN

with 500 volunteers, the first of several forts in the area was constructed and named in his honor. In 1876, the Ft. Lauderdale "House of Refuge", one of a chain maintained at 25 mi. intervals along the E Atlantic coast to shelter shipwrecked sailors and a forerunner of the US Coast Guard, was established. By the time Frank Stranaham, considered the founder of the city of Ft. Lauderdale, arrived in the New River area in 1893, the settlement there was commonly referred to by its present name. In 1896, the first train arrived. After 1900, when its pop. stood at 52, the town grew as a farming community. In 1906, Gov. Napoleon Bonaparte Broward announced a project to reclaim and drain the Everglades, with dredging to begin at the New River. Following initial speculation, the "land boom" which resulted, collapsed and, shortly thereafter, the downtown section was destroyed by fire. By 1911, when Ft. Lauderdale was incorporated as a city, its pop. had reached only 143. A second major land boom collapsed with the Hurricane of 1926, and the city entered into a depression three years earlier than the rest of the nation. The city was a slow-growing retirement and recreation center until WW II began, when it was selected as the site for a Naval Base and military training center. The importance of agriculture to the economy diminished as land development, and subsequently, tourism, became the primary industries. The resultant, rapid growth in pop. contributed to the city's distinction as one of the fastest growing in the US. During the 1960s, col. students began migrating to the area during their spring vacations and natl. attention was drawn to the city. By 1970, its pop. had exceeded 139,000.

GOVERNMENT. Ft. Lauderdale has a commission-mgr. form of govt.,

A view of Bulier Park, Fort Lauderdale, Florida

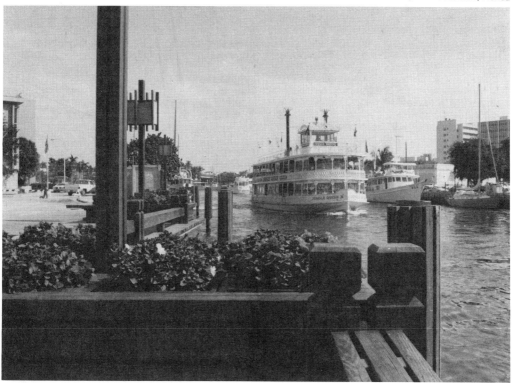

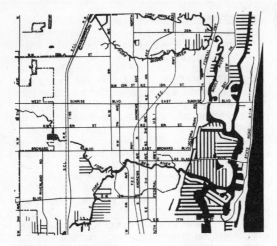

Fort Lauderdale, Florida

consisting of four commission members and a mayor, who are elected at large to three year terms.

ECONOMY AND INDUSTRY. Tourism is the most important industry in Ft. Lauderdale, followed by electronics manufacturing. Other manufactures include surgical instruments, construction materials and yachts. In June 1979, the labor force of the greater met. area totaled approx. 395,000, while the rate of unemployment was 5.3%. In 1978, the median income in Ft. Lauderdale was $12,177.

BANKING. There are 40 commercial banks and 23 savings and loan assns. In Ft. Lauderdale and Broward Co. In 1978, total deposits for the one bank headquartered in the city (SE Bank of Broward) were $325,053, while assets totaled $360,732. Other banks serving the city are American Natl., Century, Landmark First Natl. and Bank of Ft. Lauderdale.

HOSPITALS. There are 25 hosps. in Ft. Lauderdale and Broward Co., including Broward Gen., Ft. Lauderdale, N Ridge Gen., Las Olas, Holy Cross and N Beach.

EDUCATION. Nova U, founded in Ft. Lauderdale in 1967, offers bachelor and master degrees. In 1978, about 8,150 enrolled. Broward Comm. Col., a public two-year col. established in 1959, enrolled nearly 14,400 in 1978. Other institutions in the city are Ft. Lauderdale Col. of Business and Finance and Prospect Hall Col. There are 94 elementary, 27 middle and 20 sr. high schools in Broward Co, enrolling more than 140,000 in 1978, as well as approx. 100 private schools, which enrolled about 25,000 in 1978. Lib. facilities includes Broward Co. Lib., which maintains 11 branches, including one in Ft. Lauderdale.

ENTERTAINMENT. A variety of summertime annual events are held in Ft. Lauderdale, including a pop concert in June, a hot air balloon race and art festivals. Dinner theaters in the city include Showtime and Cypress Creek. The Strikers, an NASL, soccer team, and an FSL minor league baseball team of the NY Yankees provide professional sports entertainment.

ACCOMMODATIONS. There are numerous hotels and motels in Ft. Lauderdale, a major resort, including the Stouffer Hotel and the Bahia Mar. Costa Del Sol, Golden Sands, Pier 66, Marina, Sunrise, Hilton, Holiday, Best Western, Ramada, Howard Johnson's, Sheraton and Quality inns.

FACILITIES. There are several parks in Ft. Lauderdale, including John Lloyd Birch State, Holiday, George English, Stranahan and Snyder. Swimming, boating and fishing facilities are available along the five-mi. of beach, while golf courses, tennis courts, swimming pools, playing fields, scenic areas and jogging and bicycling trails are provided at the city parks.

CULTURAL ACTIVITIES. The Ft. Lauderdale Symphony and the Opera Guild are among the musical organizations which perform in the city. The Encore Theatre and the Parker Playhouse stage dramatic productions, while the Museum of Art maintains both permanent and changing exhibits.

LANDMARKS AND SIGHTSEEING SPOTS. The Intl. Swimming Hall

of Fame in Ft. Lauderdale contains a museum honoring Olympic athletes. Bahia Mar, the site of the House of Refuge built in 1876, is now a recreation-shopping-entertainment complex. Among the historic structures located in the city are the original New River Inn, host to such notables as US Pres. Cleveland, Gov. Broward, Henry Flagler and Henry Ford, which has been restored and operates as a museum; a replica of the 1899 one-room schoolhouse where the first formal class in the community was taught, and the King-Cromartie House, built in 1907, which has been refurnished with period pieces. A sightseeing cruise down New River includes sites of early settlements of the 1800s. Fogg's Memorial is the airfield used in 1926 by Merle Fogg, who aided city residents during the destructive hurricane of that year. Ocean World, another features trained porpoises and sea lions in continuous shows.

FORT WAYNE
INDIANA

CITY LOCATION-SIZE-EXTENT. Ft. Wayne, the seat of Allen Co. and second largest city in the state, encompasses 55.3 sq. mi. at the junction of the St. Mary's, St. Joseph and Maumee rivers in NE IN at 41° N lat. and 85°12' W long. The greater met. area extends into the counties of DeKalb on the N and Wells on the S and approaches the OH border on the E.

TOPOGRAPHY. The terrain of Ft. Wayne, which is situated in the Great Lakes plains region, varies from generally flat in the S and E to rolling in the SW and W and hilly in the N and NW. The St. Mary's and St. Joseph rivers converge within the city, forming the Maumee River. The mean elev. is 791'.

CLIMATE. The climate of Ft. Wayne is continental, influenced by the Great Lakes. Monthly mean temps. range from 25°F in Jan. to 74°F in July, with an avg. annual temp. of 50°F. The avg. annual rainfall is evenly distributed throughout the year. Most of the 31.8" avg. annual snowfall occurs from Dec. through Feb. The RH ranges from 54% to 88%. The growing season avgs. 173 days. Ft. Wayne lies in the ESTZ and does not observe DST.

FLORA AND FAUNA. Animals native to Ft. Wayne include the whitetail deer, fox, weasel, chipmunk and opossum. Common birds include the flycatcher, swallow, blue jay, cardinal and house wren. Frogs, snakes, salamanders, turtles and toads, as well as the venomous E massasauga (pygmy rattler), are found in the area. Typical trees include the elm, oak, maple, walnut and sycamore. Smaller plants include the sumac, wahoo, buckeye, ironweed and chickweed.

POPULATION. According to the US census, the pop. of Ft. Wayne in 1970 was 178,021. In 1979, it was estimated that it had increased to approx. 185,500.

ETHNIC GROUPS. In 1978, the ethnic distribution of Ft. Wayne was

Fort Wayne, Indiana

approx. 89.1% Caucasian, 10.2% Black and 1.6% Hispanic (a percentage of the Hispanic total is also included in the Caucasian total).

TRANSPORTATION. Interstate hwy. 69, US hwys. 24, 27, 30, 33 and 327 and state hwys. 1, 3, 14, 37 and 427 provide major motor access to Ft. Wayne. *Railroads* serving the city include ConRail, Norfolk & Western and AMTRAK. *Airlines* serving Baer Field are DL, UA and Air Wisconsin, a commuter line. *Bus lines* serving the city include IN Motor, Greyhound, Trailways and the local Ft. Wayne Public Transportation Co.

COMMUNICATIONS. Communications, broadcasting and print media originating from Ft. Wayne are: *AM radio stations* WFWR 1090 (ABC/I, Easy List.); WOWO 1190 (APR, Var.); WGL 1250 (CBS, Talk, MOR); WQHK 1380 (APR, Top 40) and WLYV 1450 (ABC/E, C&W); *FM radio stations* WLHT 88.3 (Indep.); WIPU 89.1 (IHETS, Clas., Educ., Jazz); WBCL 93.0 (IHETS, UPI, Clas., Educ., Relig.); WPTH 95.1 (Indep., Top 40); WMEE 97.3 (Indep., Btfl. Mus.); WCMX 101.7 (Indep., AOR) and WXKE 103.9 (NBC, UPI, AOR); *television stations* WANE Ch. 15 (CBS); WPTA Ch. 21 (ABC); WKJG Ch. 33 (NBC); WFFT Ch. 55 (Indep.) and cable; *press*: two major dailies serve the area, the *Journal-Gazette*, issued mornings, and the *News-Sentinel*, distributed evenings and Sun. mornings; other publications include the bi-weekly *Waynedale News* and the semimonthly *Food Executive*.

HISTORY. The site of present-day Ft. Wayne was first settled by native Americans of the Miami tribe when Chief Little Turtle established a village at the strategic junction of the St. Mary's, St. Joseph and Maumee rivers. Later, French fur traders recognized the potential of the site as a trading center. In the mid-18th century, the English established a trading post on the site, calling it Miami Town, but later abandoned it. In 1794, Gen "Mad Anthony" Wayne defeated the Miami and established the first American fort, Ft. Wayne, in the area. After the last Indian War in 1813, the ft. was abandoned and in 1819, Judge Samuel Hanna, called "the Builder of the City", built a log cabin trading post and gristmill there. At a govt. sale of land in 1823, John Barr and John McCorkle purchased the parcel which later became downtown Ft. Wayne. In 1824, the town was designated the seat of newly-organized Allen Co. "Johnny Appleseed" Chapman was buried in the city in the 1830s. The growth of Ft. Wayne, which was incorporated as a city in 1840, was stimulated by the completion of the Wabash-Erie Canal in 1843, and by the arrival of the RR in 1852, which contributed to the city's development as an industrial center. In 1883, the first night baseball game in the US was played in the city under arc-lighting. Throughout the late 19th and 20th centuries, Ft. Wayne continued to grow as an industrial and commercial center.

GOVERNMENT. Ft. Wayne has a mayor-council form of govt. The mayor, who is not a voting member of the council, and three council members are elected at large, while six councillors are elected by district. All serve four-year terms.

ECONOMY AND INDUSTRY. Manufacturing (with approx. 35% of the work force), trade, services and govt. are the major employers in Ft. Wayne. There are more than 150 manufacturing plants in the city. Major manufacturers include electrical, electronic, transportation and mining equipment. The area is the location of a major defense-related industrial complex, containing 42 companies under govt. contract. The city is the distribution center for agricultural products from a large surrounding area. In June, 1979, the labor force of the greater met. area totaled approx. 196,000, while the rate of unemployment was 5.2%.

BANKING. There are five commercial banks and four savings and loan assns. in Ft. Wayne. In 1978, bank deposits at the five banks headquartered in the city totaled approx. $1,647,623,000, while total assets were

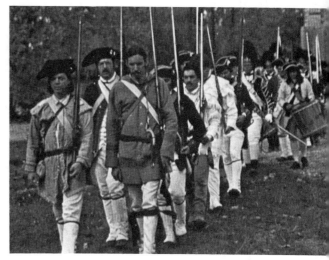

Changing of the Guard at Old Fort, Fort Wayne Indiana

$2,026,975,000. Banks include Ft. Wayne Natl., Lincoln Natl. Bank Trust, IN Bank & Trust, People's Trust and Anthony Wayne.

HOSPITALS. There are several hosps. in Ft. Wayne, including Lutheran, Parkview, St. Joseph's and V.A.

EDUCATION. The publicly-supported IN U-Purdue U at Ft. Wayne, founded as part of IN U in 1917, moved to the campus it currently shares with Purdue in a unique cooperative effort. It enrolled approx. 9,300 in 1978. IN Institute of Technology, a private institution established in 1930, awards bachelor's degrees and offers cooperative (work-study) engineering programs. In 1978, more than 300 enrolled. Other institutions include St. Francis Col., Concordia Theological Seminary, Ft. Wayne Bible Col. and Intl. Jr. Col. of Business. The public school system consists of 66 elementary, 17 jr. high and 13 sr. high schools. There are 17 Catholic and 16 Lutheran schools as well. Lib. facilities include the Ft. Wayne and Allen Co. Public Libs. and the Allen Co. Law Lib.

ENTERTAINMENT. The Arena Dinner Theater offers dining entertainment in Ft. Wayne. Each year, Ft. Wayne hosts the Johnny Appleseed Festival and the Three Rivers Festival, which features more than 100 historical events, displays, parades, the Three Rivers Hot Air Balloon Race and the 26-mi. TV 33/Hooks Marathon. Ft. Wayne is the home of the Komets, an IHL hockey team and of the Ft. Wayne Sports Club, which plays in the IN-OH Soccer League. Collegiate teams include the St. Francis Col. Cougars and the IN U-Purdue U Tuskers.

ACCOMMODATIONS. There are approx. 30 hotels and motels in the Ft. Wayne area, including TraveLodge, Harley, Imperial House, Chalet Suisse Intl. and Hilton, Holiday, Marriott and Ramada inns.

FACILITIES. There are 65 public parks and playgrounds in Ft. Wayne, encompassing 1,800 acres. Among the parks are McMillen, Swinney, Johnny Appleseed, Lawton and Fox Island. Franke Park features a large bird sanctuary, a children's zoo, an outdoor theater and an African veldt zoo. Other city park facilities include eight public golf courses, tennis courts and rose and mum gardens. There are 200 lakes within a 50-mi. radius of the city, offering additional recreational areas.

CULTURAL ACTIVITIES. Performing arts organizations in Ft. Wayne include the Civic Theatre, Philharmonic Orchestra and the Ballet. The Wagon Wheel Playhouse and the Purdue-IN U Theatre present dramatic productions, and various performances are held at the Allen Co. War Memorial Coliseum and the Comm. Center for the Performing Arts. The Ft. Wayne Art School and Museum features a small permanent collection as well as temporary exhibits. Other museums include the Allen Co.-Ft. Wayne Historical Museum, the Abraham Lincoln Lib. and Museum, which contains paintings and photographs of Lincoln, his family and descendants, and the Children's Museum.

LANDMARKS AND SIGHTSEEING SPOTS. The grave of John

"Johnny Appleseed" Chapman, who planted seeds of apple trees across the US, is a popular Ft. Wayne attraction. The Cathedral of the Immaculate Conception features Bavarian stained-glass windows and an intricately-carved wooden altar. The Lincoln Tower Building contains an observation deck on its 22nd floor, and historic river cruises are also offered in the city. Ft. Wayne, a reconstruction of an early 19th-century fort, features artifacts from the original fort, as well as reproductions of soldiers' barracks and officers' quarters.

FORT WORTH
TEXAS

CITY LOCATION-SIZE-EXTENT. Ft. Worth, the seat of Tarrant Co., encompasses 244 sq. mi. in N central Tx on the W fork of the Trinity River at 32°45' N lat. and 97°18' W long. Located 30 mi. W of Dallas, it is part of the Dallas-Ft. Worth Metroplex. Its greater met. area extends into the neighboring counties of Parker to the W, Wise and Denton to the N, Dallas to the E, Johnson to the S and Hood to the SW.

TOPOGRAPHY. The terrain of Ft. Worth, which is situated in the Great Plains region of TX, is characterized by rolling hills ranging in elev. from 500' to 800'. The Clear and W forks of the Trinity River join near the center of the city. There are several lakes in the area, including Lake Worth and Eagle Mt. Lake which form part of the city's NW border, Benbrook Lake, which forms part of the SW border, and Arlington Lake, which forms part of the SE border. The mean elev. is 670'.

CLIMATE. The climate of Ft. Worth is both continental and humid subtropical, due to its N location in the subtropical region. It is characterized by wide variations in annual weather conditions, as well as long, hot summers and short, mild winters. The mean annual temp. of 65.7°F ranges from a mean of 45°F in Jan. to a mean of 85°F in July and Aug. The mean annual precip. is 32", with heavier amounts occurring during Apr. and May. The avg. annual snowfall is 3.5". The RH ranges from 45% to 88%. The growing season avgs. 250 days. Ft. Worth lies in the CSTZ and observes DST.

FLORA AND FAUNA. Animals native to Ft. Worth include the fox, opossum and armadillo. Common birds are the mockingbird (the state bird), cardinal, blue jay, grackle, scissortailed flycatcher and E kingbird. Snapping turtles, red-eared turtles, bullfrogs, toads and green anole lizards, as well as the venomous copperhead, rattlesnake, water moccasin and coral snake, are found in the area. Typical trees are the oak, mimosa, sycamore and mesquite. Smaller plants include the bluebonnet (the state flower), Indian paintbrush and fleabane.

POPULATION. According to the US census, the pop. of Ft. Worth in 1970 was 393,455. In 1979, it was estimated that it had increased to approx. 420,140.

ETHNIC GROUPS. In 1978, the ethnic distribution of Ft. Worth was approx. 82.8% Caucasian, 10.8% Black, 5.8% Hispanic and .6% other.

TRANSPORTATION. Interstate hwys. 820, 20, 30 and 35, US hwys. 81, 80, 18, 377 and 287 and state hwys. 183, 121 and 199 provide major motor access to Ft. Worth. *Railroads* serving the city include AMTRAK, ConRail, Atchison, Topeka & Santa Fe, Chicago, Rock Island & Pacific, Ft. Worth & Denver, TX & Pacific, Burlington N, MO-KN-TX, MO Pacific, St. Louis-San Francisco, St. Louis SW and S Pacific. *Airlines* serving Dallas/Ft. Worth Regional Airport include AA, BN, CO, DL, EA, FL, PA, RD, FT, OZ, TI, Mexicana and Air Canada. Meacham Field, the municipal airport, also serves the city. *Bus lines* include Greyhound, Trailways, TX Motor Coach, Central TX and the local Ft. Worth City Transit Company (CITRAN) and SURTRAN, a joint Ft. Worth-Dallas system. Tandy Center Subway, the only privately-owned subway in the world, operates between a riverfront parking area and a shopping center.

COMMUNICATIONS. Communications, broadcasting and print media originating from Ft. Worth are: *AM radio stations* WBAP 820 (NBC, C&W, MOR); KJIM 870 (SW, C&W); KNOK 970 (Natl. Blk.,) KFJZ 1270 (Indep., MOR, Oldies); KXOL 1360 (UPI, C&W) and KRXV 1540 (MBS, APR, MOR, News); *FM radio stations* KTCU 88.7 (Univ., Relig.); KESS 93.9 (SIS News Net., Span.); KSCS 96.3 (Indep., C&W); KFJZ 97.1 (Indep., Top 40); KPLX 99.5 (Indep., MOR); KTZQ 102.1 (Indep., AOR) and KNOK 107.5 (Indep., Blk.); *television stations* KXAS Ch. 5 (NBC); KTVT Ch. 11 (Indep.) and cable; *press*: one major daily newspaper is published in the city, the *Star Telegram*, issued weekday evenings and weekend mornings; weekly publications include the *Observer*, *Weekly Livestock Reporter*, *Tribune*, *Florist and Nurseryman*, *N Ft. Worth News*, *News Tribune*, *White Settlement Bomber News*, *Church-week*, *Dallas-Ft. Worth TX Jewish Post* and *Metro Cities News*; monthly publications include *TX Metro Magazine*, *SW News*, *Soul Teen*, *Sepia*, *Santa Gertrudis Journal*, *Quarter Racing Record*, *Outdoor Power Equipment*, *Open Road and the Professional Driver*, *Bicycle Journal*, *Bronze Thrills*, *Cattleman* and *Ft. Worth*; other publications include the quarterly *TX Veteran News*, the bi-weekly *Como* and the bi-monthly *Make It With Leather*.

HISTORY. In 1849, TX Ranger Maj. Ripley A. Arnold and his Dragoons from the nearby military post at Arlington founded Ft. Worth to protect white settlers from attacks by Native Americans. Named for Gen. William J. Worth, a Mexican War hero, it was abandoned by the soldiers in 1853, and the settlement became a trading

Kimbell Art Museum in Fort Worth, Texas

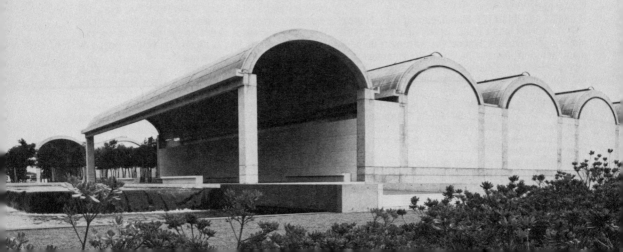

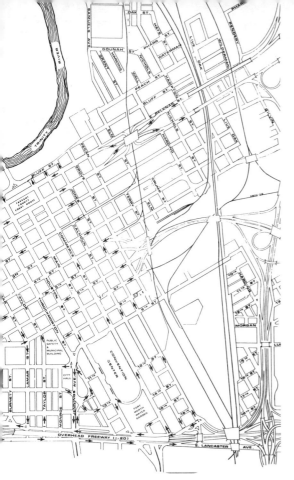

Fort Worth, Texas

post. Located on a primary route of the Chisholm Trail, the village soon became a cattle market known as "Cowtown". In 1860, Ft. Worth became the seat of Tarrant Co., and was incorporated as a city in 1873. In 1876, the TX & Pacific RR arrived in the city, further contributing to the growth of the cattle shipping industry. In 1882, the first flour mill in the city opened, and, as the cattle and grain industries developed, its pop. soared from 500 in 1870, to nearly 26,700 by 1900. Meat packing companies were soon established, and, by 1910, the pop. of the city exceeded 73,300. In 1917, the discovery of oil at Ranger and other oil fields in N and W TX contributed to the diversification of the city's economy and attracted more people to it, so that by 1930, the pop. had reached approx. 163,450. Although immigration to the city slowed considerably during the Depression, the production of military goods and the growth of the defense industry during WW II attracted a large influx of people, a trend which continued after the war ended. By 1960, the pop. of the city approached 356,300. Slowdowns in the defense and oil industries, which had become important elements of the city's economy, affected Ft. Worth's growth during the 1960s and early 1970s, as did the trend toward suburban relocation by residents and businesses. In 1974, the Dallas-Ft. Worth Regional Airport—the result of efforts toward greater cooperation between the traditional rivals—opened. Today, the city is one of the largest livestock centers in the SW.

GOVERNMENT. Ft. Worth has a council-mgr. form of govt. Nine council members, including the mayor as a voting member, serve two-year terms. The mayor is elected at large, while the eight remaining council members are elected by districts. The council appoints the city mgr., who is the chief administrative officer.

ECONOMY AND INDUSTRY. Approx. 50% of the work force of the Ft. Worth area is employed in manufacturing. Major products of the 1,570 industrial plants in the area are food and beverage products, automobile parts, machinery, helicopters, oil field equipment and steel and plastic products. The offices of 35 oil companies, and the headquarters of 40 insurance companies are located in the city, which is also a major SW wholesaling center and leading grain milling and storage center as well. In addition, agriculture-oriented industries, including livestock marketing and agribusiness, are important to the area. In June, 1979, the labor force of the Dallas/Ft. Worth met. area totaled approx. 1,479,000, while the rate of unemployment was 4.0%.

BANKING. In 1970, total deposits for the 24 banks headquartered in Ft. Worth were approx. $3,294,365,000, while assets totaled $4,052,521,000. Banks include Ft. Worth Natl., First Natl., Continental Natl., Ridglea, Bank of Ft. Worth, U Central Bank & Trust, Riverside State and N Ft. Worth.

HOSPITALS. There are 35 hosps. in Ft. Worth, including 18 gen., two children's and four govt. hosps. Among the health facilities are Ft. Worth Public Health Center, Ft. Worth Children's, Duncan Memorial, Tarrant Co., All Saints, St. Joseph's and Harris Hamilton Methodist.

EDUCATION. TX Christian U, affiliated with the Christian Church, is the oldest institution of higher learning in W TX and the largest in Ft. Worth. Founded as the Addran Male and Female Col. at Thorp Springs in 1873, it moved to Ft. Worth in 1911, and now awards bachelor, master and doctorate degrees. In 1978, close to 5,900 enrolled. TX Wesleyan Col., founded in 1891 as Polytechnic Col. and renamed TX Women's Col. in 1914, is affiliated with the Methodist Episcopal Church. It offers bachelor degrees and, in 1978, enrolled approx. 1,500. SW Baptist Theological Seminary, established in 1901, is the largest evangelical seminary in the world and the first seminary of any denomination to be granted membership in the Natl. Assn. of Schools of Music. Its Fleming Lib., with more than 200,000 volumes, is the largest theological lib. in the US. The institution awards bachelor, master and doctorate degrees and, in 1978, enrolled approx. 3,450. Other institutions include Tarrant Co. Jr. Col. and TX Col. of Osteopathic Medicine. The Ft. Worth Independent School District consists of 106 schools enrolling approx. 68,000. There are also five major private and parochial institutions at the primary and secondary levels. The Ft. Worth Public Lib. maintains five bookmobiles and seven branches.

ENTERTAINMENT. Weekly rodeos are held each month except July and Aug. at the Cowtown Coliseum Rodeo in Ft. Worth, which hosted the first indoor rodeo in the US in 1917. The Kow Bell Indoor Rodeo is the only weekly rodeo in the US held year-round. The SW Exposition & Fat Stock Show, which features indoor rodeo, is the oldest (held each Jan. since 1893) and most prestigious of its kind in the US. Other annual events include the SW Farm Show & Tractor Pull and the Natl. Invitational Golf Tournament, one of the most prestigious events on the PGA tour, held at the Colonial Country Club. Circuses, rodeos and horse shows, as well as games of the Ft. Worth Texans, a professional (HL) hockey team, are held at Will Rogers Memorial Center.

ACCOMMODATIONS. There are several hotels and motels in Ft. Worth, including the Caravan Motor Hotel, Howard Johnson's and the Kahler Green Oaks, Hilton, LaQuinta, Ramada, Holiday and Days inns.

FACILITIES. There are several parks in the city, including Ft. Worth Water Garden, Heritage (created as a Bicentennial project), Burnett, Trinity and Forest Parks. Facilities include golf courses, tennis courts and bicycle trails through parks and along the Trinity River and Marine Creek. The 3,400-acre Ft. Worth Greer Island Nature Center and Refuge, a wildlife habitat featuring free-roaming native animals, includes a buffalo and deer enclosure, visitors center with exhibits, marked hiking and horseback riding trails and fishing and picnicking facilities. Ft. Worth Water Garden Park, donated to the city by the Amon G. Carter Foundation in 1974, features three major water displays. Trinity Park houses the 114-acre Botanic Gardens, containing more than 2,150 plants and trees and featuring fragrance and Japanese gardens. The 36-acre Ft. Worth Zoo, with more than 5,000 animals of 900 species, the James R. Record Aquarium, a herpetarium, a children's zoo and a rain forest with rare and exotic birds, is located in Forest Park, which also features amusement rides, one of the longest miniature RRs in the US, two streamlined trains and an old-fashioned steam engine. Six large lakes within 25 mi. of the city provide facilities for water sports and recreation.

CULTURAL ACTIVITIES. The Arts Council of Ft. Worth and Tarrant Co. arranges performance schedules and raises funds to support local cultural groups, including the Ft. Worth Ballet, Ft. Worth Symphony, Ft. Worth Opera Assn., Community Theater, TX Boys' Choir and the Van Cliburn Competition. The William Edrington Scott Theater hosts the Comm. Theatre and special film productions. Casa Manana, the first permanent musical-arena theater in the US, stages Broadway musicals from May to Sept. There are numerous museums in Ft. Worth, including the Kimbell Art Museum, which houses a collection ranging from the prehistoric to Picasso; the Amon Carter Museum of W Art, constructed of TX shell limestone and containing a major portion of the works of two important W artists, Frederick Remington and Charles M. Russell; the Ft. Worth Art Museum, which houses an extensive collection of modern painting and sculptures in addition to old masters, and the Ft. Worth Museum of Science and History, the largest museum for children in the world, which also contains the Noble Planetarium. Lifesized wax figures in authentic settings are featured at the SW Historical Wax Museum, while the Pate Museum of Transportation contains exhibits representing all modes of travel. .

LANDMARKS AND SIGHTSEEING SPOTS. Seven cabins built about 1850, located at Log Cabin Village in Ft. Worth, have been restored and furnished with period antiques. The Ft. Worth Stockyards and Cattlemen's Exchange, where cattle and livestock are auctioned, and special shops offering W apparel and merchandise related to the cattle industry, are located in historic N Ft. Worth. The Tarrant Co. Courthouse, constructed in 1895 as a small-scale replica of the State Capitol, is surrounded by new court buildings. Other buildings of interest include Thistle Hill, the Cattle Baron's Museum, built in 1903 and the last remaining mansion of the city's wealthy cattle barons; the D Van Zandt Cottage, built by Maj. K.M. Van Zandt after the Civil War, which accommodated stagecoach passengers and was frequented by trail bosses; and the Livestock Exchange Building, built in 1902. A bronze statue of Will Rogers, located in front of the Will Rogers Memorial Center, features the late humorist astride his horse "Soap Suds."

FREMONT
CALIFORNIA

CITY LOCATION-SIZE-EXTENT. Fremont, situated on the E side of San Francisco Bay at its S end, is located in central W CA midway between Oakland and San Jose. The largest city in Alameda Co. and fifth largest in CA, in area, Fremont encompasses 96.5 sq. mi. at 37°32'1" N lat. and 121°57'4" W long.

TOPOGRAPHY. The terrain of Fremont varies considerably throughout the city, although much of it is flat and nearly at sea level. San Francisco is 10 mi., and the Pacific Ocean 30 mi., W of the city. Fremont contains the highest mt. peak, 2658', in Alameda Co. and its Bay shoreline is the longest of the cities in the county. The terrain to the E consists of a series of ridges, which rise to heights of 2500' 12 mi. and 3500' 18 mi. E of the city, and within which lie the Livermore Valley. Lake Elizabeth is a man-made lake in Fremont. The mean elev. of the city is 57'.

CLIMATE. Prevailing westerly winds result in mild year-round temps. abundant rainfall during winter and almost no rain during summer in Fremont. The avg.

annual temp. of 57°F ranges from a Jan. mean of 48°F to a Sept. mean of 64°F. Temps. reach above 90°F an avg. of five days per year, while temps. fall lower than 32°F an avg. of 13 days per year. Annual rainfall avgs. approx. 18", while snowfall is rare. The RH ranges between 67% and 85%. Fremont lies in the PSTZ and observes DST.

FLORA AND FAUNA. Animals native to Fremont include the coyote, ground squirrel, badger, pocket gopher and harbor seal. Common birds include the gull, wrentit, Alameda song sparrow, snowy egret, scrub jay, hummingbird and housefinch. Skinks, pond turtles, tree frogs and W toads, as well as the venomous prairie rattlesnake, are also typical. Common trees are the spruce, pine, sycamore and willow. Smaller plants include the blue blossom, yellow clover, toothwort, filaree, CA poppy, CA wild lilac and scotch broom.

POPULATION. According to the US census, the pop. of Fremont in 1970 was 100,869. In 1978, it was estimated that it had increased to 125,345.

ETHNIC GROUPS. In 1978, the ethnic distribution of Fremont was approx. 96.9% Caucasian, .4% Black and 16.4% Hispanic (a percentage of the Hispanic total is also included in the Caucasian total).

TRANSPORTATION. Interstate Hwy. 680 and state hwys. 17, 9, 21, 84 and 238 provide major motor access to Fremont. Southern Pacific and Western Pacific *railroads* serve the city. Fremont and Sky Sailing airports, located in the city, are both private, although Oakland and San Francisco intl. airports (22 and 30 mi. away, respectively) and San Jose Airport (12 mi. away) are served by all major *airlines*. *Bus lines* include the local AC Transit, Greyhound and Peerless. Bay Area Rapid Transit (BART), a monorail system, provides service throughout the San Francisco Bay area.

COMMUNICATIONS. Communications, broadcasting and print media serving Fremont are: *FM radio stations* KOHL 89.3 (Indep., Educ.) and KFMR 104.9 (Indep., Relig., Span.); although no *AM radio stations* or *television stations* operate from the city, it receives broadcasting from nearby Oakland, San Francisco and San Jose; *press*: one daily newspaper is published in the city, the morning *Argus*; *Dollar Saver* is a weekly publication distributed on Wed.

HISTORY. In 1797, Father Fermin Francisco de Lasuen of the Franciscan order established Mission San Jose at the site of present-day Fremont. The mission thrived until 1822, when Mexico obtained its independence from Spain, CA came under Mexican rule and the mission holdings began to deteriorate. Gen. J.C. Fremont, for whom the town was named, was appointed to administer the mission lands, which were granted in part to the Catholic Church. In the mid-19th century, a wave of settlers, including Mormons from NY, immigrants from the Azores and Portugal and Chinese laborers, arrived in the area. They established ranches and built a winery and RR. In the early 1900s, the area became known as the "Northern Hollywood of the Movie Industry"—among others, Charlie Chaplin's "The

Fremont, California

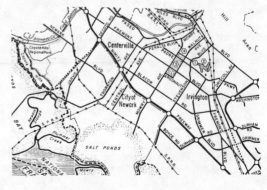

Tramp"was filmed in the Niles district. On Jan., 1956, citizens of five rural unincorporated communities— Centerville, Irvington, Mission San Jose, Niles and Warm Springs—voted to merge in order to avoid annexation by neighboring cities and to maintain control over local affairs, which had been administered from Oakland, the county seat. Fremont, the largest city, at the time, in N CA, and believed to be the only city in the US created from five communities, was thus incorporated. It has since experienced tremendous growth, and a boom in residential development. In 1956, its pop. was approx. 22,000, and, in 1967, 90,000. It is estimated that it will reach 200,000 by 1980.

GOVERNMENT. Fremont has a council-mgr. form of govt. consisting of four council members and a mayor elected by the voters at large to a four-year term and a two year term respectively.

ECONOMY AND INDUSTRY. The largest salt-producing facility and agrl-business industry in Alameda Co. are located in Fremont, which ranks as having the highest per household buying power ($16,489) for cities with populations of 50,000 or more. Major industries include auto assembly, fabricated metal products, electronics and printing. As of Jan., 1979, the total civilian labor force was 44,263, while the unemployment rate was 5.4%.

BANKING. There are 19 commercial banks and 10 savings and loan assns. in Fremont. In 1978, bank deposits for the one bank headquartered in the city were $50,411,000, while total assets were $55,628,000. Banks include Bank of America, CA First, and Crocker Natl.

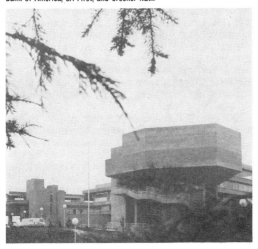

City Government Building, Fremont, California

HOSPITALS. There is one gen. hosp., Washington, in Fremont.
EDUCATION. Ohlone Col., a jr. col. established in 1966, is named for the Native Americans who inhabited the Fremont area before the Spanish arrived. Administered by the Fremont-Newark Comm. Col. District, Ohlone Col. offers programs in occupational and gen. areas and confers associate degrees. Enrollment in 1978 was more than 8,300. There are 33 elementary, six jr. high and seven sr. high schools in the city's public school system. State schools for the Deaf and Blind, serving 500 deaf and 150 blind students, are also located in the city. There are four libs., Fremont Main, with the Irvington, Centerville and Niles branches.
ENTERTAINMENT. Dinner theater, professional sports and annual festivals are accessible to residents of Fremont in nearby San Francisco, Oakland and San Jose.
ACCOMMODATIONS. Among the hotels and motels in Fremont are the Best Western-Thunderbird, TraveLodge, Islander, Mission Peak Lodge, Frontier Hotel and Hotel Irvington.

FACILITIES. Fremont is the only city in Alameda Co. in which a Natl. Wildlife Refuge is located. The 920-acre Central Park, located on Lake Elizabeth, contains a waterfowl refuge, boat house and swim lagoon. There are 25 parks and city playgrounds in Fremont. Warm Springs and Parkway provide public golf courses. A glider port is available at Fremont Airport.
CULTURAL ACTIVITIES. Among the cultural organizations located in Fremont are the Fremont-Newark Philharmonic Orchestra, Fremont Community Theatre, Fremont Ballet Folklorico and the Afro-American Cultural and Historical Society. The Ohlone Col. Drama Dept. performs locally, as does the Sweet Adelines musical group.
LANDMARKS AND SIGHTSEEING SPOTS. The only mission in Alameda Co., Mission San Jose, is located in Fremont. Completed June 11, 1797, the red-roofed adobe building contains a central fountain, workshops, a granary, jail cells and guard quarters. Original statues, documents of the mission's history, prayer books and altar bells are displayed. The Mission San Jose Old Town Complex contains several old buildings; including the 1895 Ehrman Store, the 1895 Solon Building, the 1895 Washington Hotel, the 1900 Steinmetz Harness Shop and the 1895 Sunderer Home. The Niles Town and RR Complex is an historic district which contains a RR depot, commercial buildings, town jail, courthouse and Victorian homes. Shinn Historic Park was the Victorian ranch of James and Lucy Shinn, prominent in the nursery business, who arrived in Niles in 1856. The grounds surrounding the 1850 Sims Cottage and 1876 Shinn Home (constructed during the Gold Rush from portions of derelict ships found in San Francisco Bay) feature formal gardens and orchards. The Park complex was restored by the Mission Peak Heritage Foundation. Coyote Hills Regional Park features ancient Indian shell mounds.

FRESNO
CALIFORNIA

CITY LOCATION-SIZE-EXTENT. Fresno, the seat of Fresno, Co., encompasses 58 sq. mi. on the E central edge of the San Joaquin Valley at 36°46' N lat. and 119°43' W long., 220 mi. NE of LA and 185 mi. SE of San Francisco. The greater met. area extends into the bordering counties of Madera to the N, Kings to the S and Tulare to the SE.
TOPOGRAPHY. The terrain of Fresno, which is located in the E central part of the San Joaquin Valley, is characterized by generally flat land, rising in an abrupt slope 15 mi. E in the foothills of the Sierra Nevada Mt. Range. The San Joaquin River flows N through the city, while the foothills of the Pacific Coastal Range lie about 45 mi. W of the city. There are several lakes in the area including Millerton Lake, located approx. 20 mi. to the SE. The mean elev. is 331'.
CLIMATE. The climate of Fresno is dry continental, characterized by mild winters and warm summers and influenced by winds from the NW. The annual mean temp. of 63°F ranges from a Jan. mean of 45.8°F to a July mean of 81.7°F. During the warmest months, daytime temps. often reach 99°F or warmer, while the more comfortable nighttime temps. may be 35°F lower. Approx. 95% of the avg. annual rainfall of 9.69" falls from Oct. through Apr. with an avg. of approx. 40 days of rain per year. Snowfall is rare. The RH ranges from 23% to 73%. From Nov. through Feb., periods of fog may last two weeks. The avg. growing season is 291 days. Fresno lies in the PSTZ and observes DST.
FLORA AND FAUNA. Animals native to Fresno are the black bear, ground squirrel, coyote, mule deer, porcupine, bobcat and gopher. Common birds include the woodpecker, hummingbird, swallow, Steller's jay and Bewick's wren. Pacific tree frogs, salamanders, fence lizards, garter snakes and the venomous Pacific rattlesnake, are found in the area. Typical trees include the sequoia, spruce, sycamore, white ash, pinion, pine and live oak.

Smaller plants include the yellow clover, evening primrose, yarrow and godetia.

POPULATION. According to the US census, the pop. of Fresno in 1970 was 167,927. In 1978, it was estimated that it had increased to approx. 200,000.

ETHNIC GROUPS. In 1978, the ethnic distribution of Fresno was approx. 70.5% Caucasian, 6.5% Black, 19% Hispanic, 2% Asian and 2% other.

TRANSPORTATION. US Hwy. 99 and State Hwy. 41 provide major motor access to Fresno. *Railroads* serving the city include Santa Fe, Pacific and AMTRAK. *Airlines* serving Fresno Air Terminal include UA, RW, Pacific SW, Air Canada and Swift Aire. Chandler Downtown Airport is served by private and commuter aircraft. *Bus lines* serving the city include Greyhound, Trailways and the local Fresno Transit.

COMMUNICATIONS. Communications, broadcasting and print media serving Fresno are: *AM radio stations* KMJ 580 (NBC, Golden West, MOR); KBIF 900 (Indep., Relig.); KFRE 940 (ABC/I, UPI, MOR); KEAP 980 (MBS, C&W); KYNO 1300 (UPI, Top 40); KMAK 1340 (ABC/E, C&W); KARM 1430 (CBS, News); KIRV 1510 (ABC/I, Btfl. Mus.); KXEX 1550 (Indep., Span.) and KGST 1600 (Indep., Span.); *FM radio stations* KFCF 88.1 (Indep., Univ.); KVPR 89.3 (NPR, Public, Clas., Jazz); KFYE 93.7 (ABC/C, Adult Rock); KYNO 956.5 (Indep., AOR); KMJ 97.9 (Indep., Clas.); KFIG 101.1 (ABC/FM, Btfl. Mus.); KFRY 101.9 (Indep., Btfl. Mus.); KKNU 102.7d (Indep., Btfl. Mus.) and KKDJ 105.9 (Indep., MOR/Adult Pop.); *television stations* KMTF Ch. 18 (PBS); KMJ Ch. 24 (NBC); KMPH Ch. 26 (Indep.); KFSN Ch. 30 (CBS); KJEO Ch. 47 (ABC) and KAIL Ch. 53 (Indep.); *press*: one major newspaper serves the area, the *Bee*, issued mornings; other publications include the *Fresno Guide, CA-AZ Cotton, Hay and Grain Grower*, and *W State Grape Grower, Courier, Central Valley Jewish Heritage, Collegian, Divine Love, Fresno Daily Legal Report, Insight* and *Valley Labor Citizen*.

HISTORY. The area of present-day Fresno, part of a vast desert, was named in the 1830s by Mexican Soldiers in pursuit of a group of bandits, who eluded them by running through groves of white ash trees. During the CA gold rush, several mining towns were established in the area. In 1870, a system of canals was constructed in the area and wheat—the first agricultural crop to be raised—was planted. In 1872, the area attracted the attention of Leland Stanford as a likely site for a station on his Central Pacific RR. Established as a station, the town became the county

Fresno, California

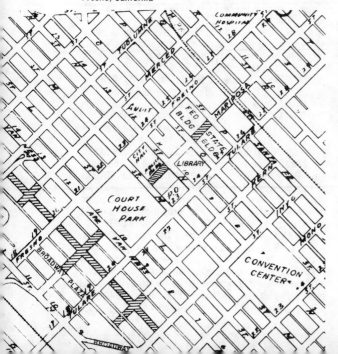

seat in 1874, and in 1885, was incorporated as a city. The next year, experiments with the Smyra fig conducted in the city led to the development of that industry. The great Central Valley Water Project, which dammed the San Joaquin River in the early 20th century, contributed greatly to the growth of Fresno Co. as the most agriculturally productive in the US and to the development of its seat as the marketing and shipping center of the Central Valley. The city has grown at a rapid rate as supporting industries have continued to develop.

GOVERNMENT. Fresno has a council-mgr. form of govt., consisting of seven council members, including the mayor as a voting member elected at large to four-year terms. The council appoints a city mgr.

ECONOMY AND INDUSTRY. Fresno lies in the heart of the agri-business center of the world, which produces more than 200 commercial crops worth more than one billion yearly, led by cotton and grapes ($100 million each). About 385 manufacturing plants in the Fresno area produce food products, farm tools, irrigation products, light machinery, sheet glass, winery equipment, fertilizer and transportation equipment. City industrial facilities include machine shops, iron foundries, nonferrous metal foundries, public warehouses and industrial supply firms. Govt., including regional headquarters of the US Internal Revenue Service, is another major area employer. In June, 1979, the labor force of the greater met. area totaled approx. 267,500 while the rate of unemployment was 6.9%. The avg. income per capita in 1978 was $11,664.

BANKING. There are 50 commercial banks and 33 savings and loan assns. in Fresno. In 1978, total deposits for the three banks headquartered in the city were approx. $100,966,000, while total assets were $112,788,000. Banks serving the city include First Natl., CA Valley, Bank of Fresno, Bank of America, Wells Fargo, Crocker and Security Pacific.

HOSPITALS. There are six hosps. in Fresno, Fresno Community, St. Agnes (operated by the Sisters of the Holy Cross), Sierra, Valley Children's, V. A. and Valley Medical Center.

EDUCATION. CA State U at Fresno, a public liberal arts institution established in 1911, offers bachelor and master degrees. In 1978, nearly 15,500 enrolled. Fresno City Col., a state/locally-controlled institution established in 1910, offers associate degrees. Fresno Pacific Col., a private coeducational institution affiliated with the Mennonite Brethern Church and founded in 1944, offers bachelor and master degrees. In 1978, close to 700 enrolled. Other institutions include the Mennonite Brethern Biblical Seminary, CA Christian Col., W Coast Bible Col. and CA School of Professional Psychology at Fresno. The Fresno Unified School District consisting of 54 elementary, 10 middle, three jr. high and four sr. high public schools, enrolled more than 60,000 in 1978. Catholic schools, including five elementary, enrolling approx. 1,800 and one high school, enrolling approx. 1,700, a Lutheran elementary school, enrolling close to 200 and a Seventh Day Adventist (K-12) school, enrolling approx. 500, are among the private schools in the city. Lib. facilities include the Fresno Co. Lib. which maintains nine branches.

ENTERTAINMENT. There is one dinner theater in Fresno. Roger Rocka's Good Company Music Hall, Eating Establishment & Drinking Emporium. Annual events include the Oban-Odori Festival, featuring Japanese dancing, the Fresno District Fair in Oct., the Camellia Show and the Sun Maid Kennel Club Dog Show in Mar. and the Caballo Club Rodeo. The CA State U at Fresno Bulldogs participate in intercollegiate sports, and the U hosts the W Coast Relays each May. a CA minor league baseball team of the San Franciso Giants provides professional spectator sports entertainment.

ACCOMMODATIONS. There are several hotels and motels in Fresno, including the Hilton, Best Westen, Holiday, Picadilly, Ramada, Smuggler's and Village inns.

FACILITIES. There are several public parks in Fresno. The 160-acre Roeding Park contains the third largest zoo in CA, which features more than

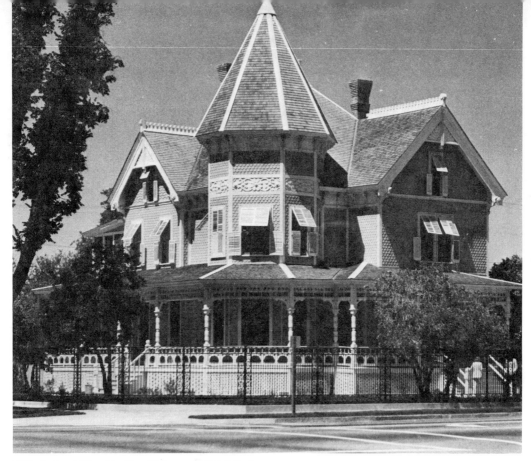

Meux House Museum, Fresno, California

1,000 animals and 250 reptiles. The reptile house, with 35 individually-controlled atmospheres, was the first of its kind in the US. The park also contains eight tennis courts, a square dancing facility, the Homer C. Wilson Camellia Gardens and Storyland, which depicts various well-known children's stories. The 240-acre Woodward Park, located on the S bank of the San Joaquin River, contains a bird sanctuary, picnic area and a five-acre lake. Eighteen playgrounds are jointly operated by the city's park and school system, while there are an additional 11 municipal playgrounds, each occupying 2.5 to 10 acres. The city also operates two 18-hole golf course, three swimming pools and a campground located at Dinkey Creek in the High Sierra Mts.

CULTURAL ACTIVITIES. In addition to a series of regular concerts, the Fresno Philharmonic Orchestra sponsors such musical activities for young people as Youth Concerts, the Jr. Philharmonic, Philharmonic Youth Orchestra, Sierra Music Camp, Young Artist Award and a col. scholarship program. Oldest of the city's cultural organizations, the Fresno Musical Club performs locally and presents a guest artist series of internationally famous performers. The Fresno Community Chorus and Fresno Opera Assn. are volunteer organizations. Under the auspices of the Dance Theatre of Fresno, local jr. and sr. dance companies appear regularly in concerts and in cooperation with other local performing theater groups. The only dance assn. in the US with three distinct categories of dance, the Fresno Dance Repertory Assn. offers programs in classical ballet, contemporary dance and ethnic dance. Students of both Fresno City Col. and CA State U at Fresno present productions and programs in dance, drama and visual arts. The Fresno Arts Center presents a program of creative arts activities and exhibits. Housed in the Discovery Center are natural history, natural science and conservation displays, including Native American relics. The Fresno Downtown Mall features an art collection purchased with funds donated by the business community.

LANDMARKS AND SIGHTSEEING SPOTS. The Kearney Mansion Museum, located in the 250-acre Kearney Park in Fresno, is the restored Edwardian home of a country pioneer in agriculture, housing historical displays and archives containing material of the late 1800s. The Meux House, dating from 1888, has also been restored. It is now a museum and open for tours. The Fort Miller Blockhouse Museum, the oldest structure in the city and built in 1851 contains historical relics of the area. Warehouse Row, an entire downtown block comprised of three major warehouse structures is listed on the Natl. Register of Historic Places. Downtown Fulton Mall is an artistic attraction and one of the highlights of Fresno's extensive urban renewal program.

GARDEN GROVE
CALIFORNIA

CITY LOCATION-SIZE-EXTENT. Garden Grove is located in Orange Co. in SW CA, nine mi. E of the Pacific Ocean. Bordered on the N by LA Co. and on the S by San Diego Co., its met. area includes Anaheim to the NE and Santa Ana to the SE. Encompassing 17.4 sq. mi., Garden Grove is located at 33°46'5" N lat. and 117°54'8" W long.

TOPOGRAPHY. Garden Grove is situated in the Pacific coastal, or LA basin region. San Pedro Bay is to the W and the Santa Ana Mts. to the E. The mean elev. is 85'.

CLIMATE. The weather in Garden Grove is generally pleasant and mild throughout the year. The avg. annual temp. of 64°F ranges from monthly means of 60°F during Jan. to 72°F during Aug. Daily temps. may vary as much as 25°F, resulting in warm days and cold nights in winter, and in summer, hot days and cool nights. Most of the annual rainfall of 12.6" occurs during winter, while summers are practically rain free. Snowfall is rare. The RH ranges from 52% to 85%. Garden Grove lies in the PSTZ and observes DST.

FLORA AND FAUNA. Animals native to Garden Grove include the coyote, pocket gopher, badger and opossum. Common birds include the housefinch, scrub jay, flycatcher, swallow and hummingbird. Bullfrogs, pond turtles,

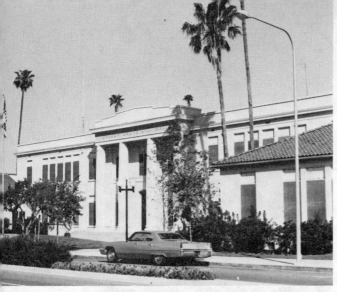

City Hall, Garden Grove, California

spadefoot toads and skinks are also common. Typical trees include the willow and pine. Smaller plants include the chaparral shrub, barnyard grass, sowthistle, laurel, blue blossom and prickly pear cactus.

POPULATION. According to the US census, the pop. of Garden Grove in 1970 was 121,155, when the city was ranked fourth largest in Orange Co. and 17th largest in CA. In 1978, it is estimated to have decreased to 118,454.

ETHNIC GROUPS. In 1978, the ethnic distribution of Garden Grove was approx. 87% Caucasian, .5% Black, 7.5% Hispanic, 2.2% Asian and 2.8% other.

TRANSPORTATION. State hwys. 22 (Garden Grove Frwy.) and 39 (Beach Blvd.), as well as US Hwy. 101 and Interstate Hwy. 5 (Santa Ana Frwy.), provide major motor access to Garden Grove. *Railroads* serving the city include Southern Pacific, Santa Fe and Union Pacific. Nearby Orange Co., Ontario Intl., John Wayne and LA Intl. airports are served by all major *airlines*. *Bus lines* include the local Orange Co. Transit District, S CA Rapid Transit District and Greyhound.

COMMUNICATIONS. Communications, broadcasting and print media serving Garden Grove include: *FM radio station* KORJ 94.3 (Indep., Rock/Jazz, Span., Progsv.); although no *AM radio stations* or *television stations* operate from the city, it receives broadcasting from nearby LA; *press*: major weekly publications serving the city include *Orange Co. News*; other print media in the area are the *Register*, *Anaheim Bulletin*, *Orange Co. Jewish Heritage*, *Anaheim-Fullerton Indep.* and *Huntington Beach Indep.*

HISTORY. The Spanish first occupied the Santa Ana Valley, near the site of present day Garden Grove, in 1769. In 1784, the Garden Grove district, part of a vast land grant to Don Manuel Nieto, became known as Rancho Las Bolsas. Part of Mexico from 1822, when Mexico gained independence from Spain, the Garden Grove district became a territory of the US in 1848 following the war between the US and Mexico. In 1868, rancher and landowner Abel Stearns purchased Rancho Las Bolsas from heirs of Manuel Nieto. In the following years, Stearns' vast holdings were sold in parcels to new settlers, one of whom was Garden Grove's founder, Dr. Alonzo Cook. Having purchased a 160-acre tract in 1875, Dr. Cook donated part of the land for the village's first schoolhouse, which he suggested be called "Garden Grove" along with the village. The growth of the agricultural town, which had a pop. of approx. 200 in 1880, was accelerated by the arrival of the Pacific Electric RR in 1905. Although a flood from heavy rains in 1916 and an earthquake in 1933 detracted from the town's growth, the community continued to develop, especially after WW II, and was incorporated as a city on June 18, 1956. Its pop. boomed from nearly 4,000 in 1950 to more than 120,000 in 1970.

GOVERNMENT. Garden Grove has a council-mgr. form of govt. Five council members, including the mayor as a voting member, are elected at large—the mayor to a two-year term, the four other councillors to four-year terms. The council elects one member to serve as mayor pro tem.

ECONOMY AND INDUSTRY. Prefabricated metals, transportation equipment, electronics, lumber, clothing and chemicals are among Garden Grove's major industries, while strawberries are major agricultural products. The total labor force in 1978 was 49,159, while unemployment was 4.8%. Total wages and salaries in 1978 were $615,863,952, while the avg. per capita income was $5,084.

BANKING. There are nine banking institutions in Garden Grove including the Bank of America, Crocker Natl., Coast, Farmers and Merchants, Mitsubishi Bank of CA, Security Pacific Natl. and United CA.

HOSPITALS. Hospitals serving Garden Grove are Palm Harbor, Kaiser Clinic, Orange Grove Rehabilitation, and Chapman-Harbour Convalescent.

EDUCATION. Among the institutions of higher learning in Garden Grove are the Whitley Col. of Court Reporting and Exacto Tax School. The Garden Grove Unified School District operates 49 elementary and 20 secondary schools. There are five private schools in the city, including St. Paul Lutheran, Bethel Christian and Orangewood Academy. Libs. include Garden Grove Regional Lib., with the Chapman Ave. and W Garden Grove branches, and the Lib. of Vehicles.

ENTERTAINMENT. Garden Grove hosts two annual events: the Garden Grove Strawberry Festival and Garden Grove Gorgeous, an event in which homes are judged. Youth art shows are held every Mar. at the Village Green Cultural Arts Complex. Although no professional sports teams play in the city, the CA Angels (AL baseball) and CA Surf (soccer) play in nearby Anaheim. The many professional and collegiate teams based in LA are accessible to the residents of Garden Grove.

ACCOMMODATIONS. There are several motels located in Garden Grove, including the Tropic, Fiesta, Fire Station, Harbor, Hollandease, Sandman, Pitcairn Motor and Ranch motels, as well as TraveLodge.

FACILITIES. There are several parks in Garden Grove offering recreational and sports facilities. Among them are Eastgate, Faylane, Garden Grove, Gutosky, Magnolia, Morningside, Pioneer, Twin Lakes Freedom, W Grove, W Haven and Woodbury. Village Green Park is a central focal point for the community.

CULTURAL ACTIVITIES. Garden Grove's Village Green Cultural Arts Complex includes the Mills House Visual Arts Complex, which was the former home of Myrtie Fulson and named for her grandfather. The Civic Art Gallery features locally owned collections as well as works of LA artists. Special shows include exhibits of blind artists and works of native Americans. The Gem Theatre, a 200-seat comm. theater featuring the performing arts, was built in the 1920s and recently restored in a 1930s motif. Musicals, plays, informal opera and dance presentations are featured. The annual Aug. Shakespearean Festival is held at the Strawberry Bowl Amphitheatre.

LANDMARKS AND SIGHTSEEING SPOTS. Among the landmarks in the city are the Garden Grove Crystal Cathedral, Bicentennial Monument and Gem Theatre.

Garden Grove, California

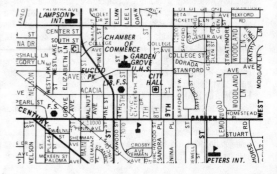

GARLAND
TEXAS

CITY LOCATION-SIZE-EXTENT. Garland is located in N central TX, 12 mi. NE of Dallas at 32°55' N lat. and 96°37' W long. The city encompasses 54.7 sq. mi. in N Dallas Co. It is located in the greater Dallas-Fort Worth met. area, known as the Metroplex.

TOPOGRAPHY. Garland is situated in the Blackland prairie region, which is characterized by flat land and rolling hills that range in elev. from 500' to 800'. The city lies near the headwaters of the Trinity River. White Rock Reservoir is to the SW between Garland and Dallas, while Lake Lavon lies approx. 15 mi. to the NE and Lake Ray Hubbard lies about eight mi. to the SE The mean elev. is 551'.

CLIMATE. The climate of Garland is intermediate between humid subtropical and continental, characterized by hot summers, mild winters and wide seasonal variations in weather conditions. During winters, periods of extreme cold are of short duration, while the highest temps. of summer are accompanied by fair skies, westerly winds and low humidities. The avg. annual temp. of 64°F ranges from monthly means of 45°F during Jan. to 84°F during July. Most of the annual 34" of rainfall occurs during the winter months, while the avg. annual snowfall is 2.1". The RH ranges from 49% to 80%. The avg. growing season is approx. 250 days. Garland lies in the CSTZ and observes DST.

FLORA AND FAUNA. Animals native to Garland include the skunk, raccoon, opossum and fox. Common birds are the chimney swift, bobwhite quail, purple martin, mockingbird (the state bird) and cardinal. Lizards, frogs, turtles, and snakes, including the venomous coral snake, rattlesnake, copperhead and cottonmouth are common. Typical trees include the pine, oak, pecan (the state tree), hackberry, elm, orange, mimosa, and sycamore. Smaller plants include the bluebonnet (the state flower), black-eyed Susan, evening primrose and firewheel.

POPULATION. According to the US census, the pop. of Garland in 1970 was 81,437. In 1978, it was estimated that it had increased to 149,302.

ETHNIC GROUPS. In 1978, the ethnic distribution of Garland was approx. 88.5% Caucasian, 6.1% Black, 4.1% Hispanic and 1.3% other.

TRANSPORTATION. Interstate hwys. 635, 30 and 20, US Hwy. 67 and State Hwy. 78 provide major motor access to Garland. *Railroads* serving the city are AMTRAK, Santa Fe and MO-KS-TX. All major *airlines* serve Dallas-Fort Worth Regional Airport, 34 mi. W of Garland. *Bus lines* serving the city include Greyhound and a Park-and-Ride service operates between Garland and Dallas.

COMMUNICATIONS. Communications, broadcasting and print media serving Garland include *AM radio stations*, *FM radio stations* and *television stations* originating from nearby Dallas and Fort

City Hall , Garland, Texas

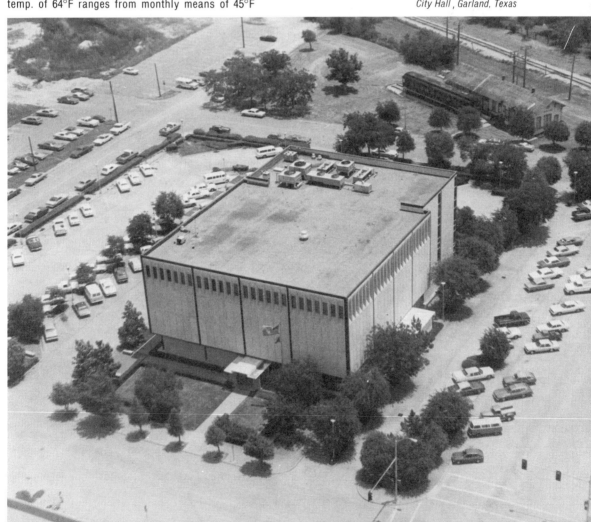

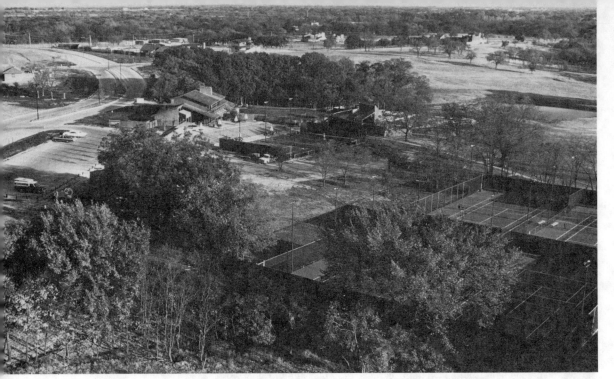

Recreation facilities operated by the city of Garland, Texas

Worth; *press:* one daily newspaper is published in the city, the *News*, which is issued evenings.

HISTORY. Garland evolved from the village of Duck Creek, which had been established in 1874, when a gen. store was built on the W bank of Duck Creek by a merchant named Moles. Additional businesses and homes were built and, in 1878, the village was designated a post office. The extensions of the Santa Fe RR in 1886 and the MO-KS-TX RR somewhat later, passed to the N and E of Duck Creek. Two new settlements developed around the depots of the RRs and, after a fire in Duck Creek, in 1887, a US Congressman decided that the old Duck Creek post office should be moved midway between the two depots, NE of the original site. In 1888, the new town was renamed Garland in honor of A.H. Garland, who was at the time US Atty. Gen. in the administration of Pres. Grover Cleveland. Garland was incorporated as a town in 1891. In 1899, a fire destroyed about 30 businesses, which were, however, rebuilt. The city's growth during the early 1900s was slow—its pop., of 965 in 1910, had increased to 2,200 by 1940. During the 1940s, however, as new industries located in

Downtown Garland, Texas

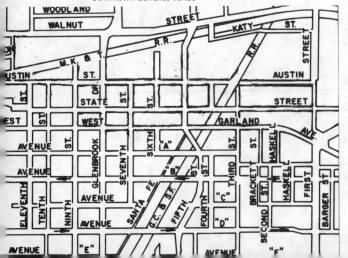

Garland, the city grew, and, by 1950, its pop. reached 10,251. Garland was incorporated as a city in 1951. Since then, the city has attracted a variety of new industries and experienced continuous growth.

GOVERNMENT. Garland has a council-mgr. form of govt. consisting of nine council members and the mayor as a voting member, all of whom are elected at large to two-year terms.

ECONOMY AND INDUSTRY. There are approx. 300 manufacturing plants in Garland. Major industries include electronics, steel, apparel, chemicals, food processing and research. Avg. per capita income in 1977 was $6,558. The total labor force in 1978 was 44,000, while the rate of unemployment was 3.6%.

BANKING. As of Dec. 31, 1978, total deposits for the six banks headquartered in Garland were $229,489,000, while assets were $253,379,000. Banks in the city include First Nat'l., First Security Nat'l., Garland Bank and Trust, TX Bank and Trust and American Nat'l.

HOSPITALS. There are three gen. acute-care hosps. in Garland, Garland Community, Garland Medical Center and Hosp. and Memorial.

EDUCATION. Publicly-supported Eastfield and Richland comm. cols. serve the Garland area. Eastfield Comm. Col., located in nearby Mesquite, grants associate degrees and enrolled approx. 10,000 students in 1978. Richland Comm. Col. also awards associate degrees and, in 1978, enrolled close to 12,000 students. Libs. include the Nicholson Memorial Lib. The Garland Independent School District, consisting of 31 elementary, 10 jr. and four sr. high schools, enrolled close to 31,000 students in 1979.

ENTERTAINMENT. The Garland Art Fair and J.C. Jubilee are among the festivals and annual events occurring in the city. Dinner theaters, other annual events and professional sports entertainment are available in nearby cities of the Dallas-Ft. Worth met. area.

FACILITIES. There are 55 parks in Garland, containing a hot-air balloon port, horseback riding, fishing and boating facilities, nine swimming pools, 43 playing fields, 48 tennis courts, 40 jogging trails and 2,000 acres of landscaped area. Two public boat ramps are located at Lake Ray Hubbard

CULTURAL ACTIVITIES. Among the cultural organizations in the city are the Garland Symphony Orchestra, Garland Civic Theater, Garland Country Music Assn., a ballet-troupe and the Landmark Museum. Garland Community Concerts is a program sponsored by the city.

LANDMARKS AND SIGHTSEEING SPOTS. Several brick stores on the Garland downtown square, which were rebuilt after a fire in 1899, are among the historical landmarks in the city. Historical homes include the Pickett and Sarver houses.

GARY
INDIANA

CITY LOCATION-SIZE-EXTENT. Gary is located in Lake Co. in NW IN at the S tip of Lake MI, 25 mi. SE of Chicago. The city encompasses 42.7 sq. mi. at 41°36' N lat. and 87°20'W long. The greater Gary, Hammond and E Chicago met. area extends throughout Lake Co. into Porter Co. on the E and IL on the W.

TOPOGRAPHY. Gary is situated in the Great Lakes plain region of the central plains. The terrain is flat with low rolling hills. The Calumet River runs through the city. The mean elev. is 599'.

CLIMATE. The climate of Gary is typically continental, although influenced by Lake MI when winds are from the N. Monthly mean temps. range from 23°F during Jan. to 73°F during July, with an annual avg. of 50°F. Most of the annual rainfall of 34" occurs when moisture-laden clouds arrive from the Gulf of Mexico. Almost 50% of the annual 40" of snowfall occurs in Dec. and Jan. The RH ranges from 53% to 85%. Gary is in the CSTZ and observes DST.

FLORA AND FAUNA. Animals native to Gary include the whitetail deer, chipmunk, rabbit, opossum and raccoon. Common birds include the red-shouldered, marsh and sparrow hawk, great blue and green heron, blackbird, mockingbird, swallow, wood thrush, ring-necked pheasant, cardinal and red-headed and downy woodpecker. Bullfrogs, chorus frogs, American toads, mudpuppies, water snakes, skinks and painted turtles, as well as the venomous E massasauga (a pygmy rattler), are also common. Typical trees include the N red oak, tamarac, black oak, sugar maple, American beech, willow and elm. Smaller plants include the sumac, camas, violet, field daisy, orange fringe orchid, cuckoo flower and dune willow.

POPULATION. According to the US census, the pop. of Gary in 1970 was 175,415. In 1978, it was estimated that it had decreased to 171,300.

ETHNIC GROUPS. In 1978, the ethnic distribution of Gary was 46.7% Caucasian, 49.2% Black, and 8.1% Hispanic. (A percentage of the Hispanic total is also included in the Caucasian total.)

TRANSPORTATION. The IN Toll Road, interstate hwys. 65, 80, 90, and 94, US hwys. 12, 20 and 6, and state roads 912, 51, 53 and 55 provide major motor access to Gary. ConRail and S Shore *railroads* provide commuter service. Gary Municipal Airport provides limited service, although all major *airlines* serve Chicago's O'Hare Field. *Bus lines* include the Local Gary Public Transportation, Greyhound and Trailways.

COMMUNICATIONS. Communications, broadcasting and print media originating from Gary are: *AM radio stations* WWCA 1270 (ABC/E, MOR) and WLTH 1370 (MBS, MOR, Talk); *FM radio station* WGVE 88.7 (NPR, Educ.); *television station* Ch. 50 (PBS); *press*: one daily newspaper is published in the city, the *Post-Tribune*, distributed weekday evenings and weekend mornings. Other publications include the *Info, Herald* and *The Gary* and the weekly *Crusader* and the *Review*.

HISTORY. Jesuit priests were the first white settlers in the area of present day Gary. Tradition maintains that Father Marquette camped at the E mouth of the Grand Calumet River, where Gary's Marquette Park is now located. In 1822, fur trader Joseph Bailly settled in the area. Lake Co. was established in 1837 by the IN

Aerial view of Brunswick Village, Gary, Indiana

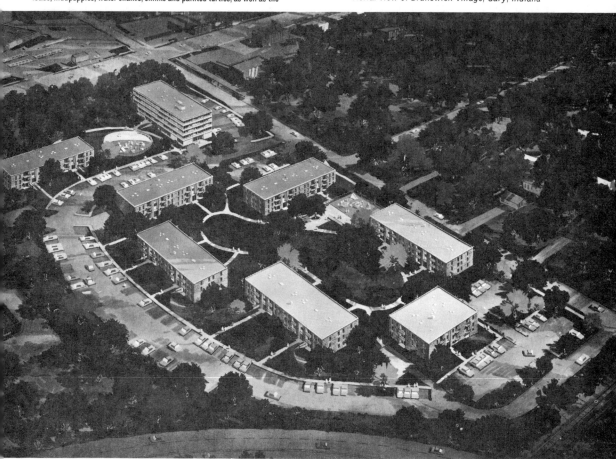

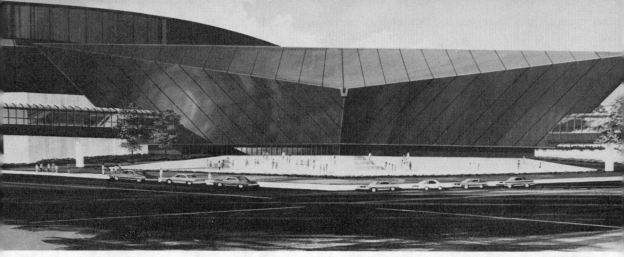

Civil Rights Hall of Fame Building in Gary, Indiana

legislature. In the early 1900s, Judge Elbert H. Gary (for whom the city was named), Chairman of US Steel Corp., dreamed of establishing the world's largest steel mill on the shores of Lake MI. Workmen soon arrived, and Gary, one of the first planned cities in the US, was built on sand dunes and marshes on the S side of the Calumet River. Incorporated on July 17, 1906, the city became known as "Magic City" since it developed quickly to serve as a residential and commercial community for one of the newest industrial centers in the US. The Gary Works of US Steel was completed in 1909, and other companies began to locate in the city in order to use the steel produced there for the manufacture of other products. Gary became an ethnic melting pot, with Slavic, Latin and, especially after WW II, S blacks arriving to work in the city. Between 1910 and 1950, the pop. of the city grew from 16,800 to 133,900, earning Gary the name "City of the Century"—the largest US city of 20th-century origins. In 1967, one of the first black mayors of a large US city, Richard Hatcher, was elected.

GOVERNMENT. Gary has a mayor-council form of govt. The mayor, elected at large for a four-year term, votes only to break a tie. Of the nine council members, who also serve four-year terms, six are elected on a district basis and three are elected at large.

ECONOMY AND INDUSTRY. Gary is part of the industrial area known as the Calumet District, one of the world's greatest steel centers. The US Steel Corp., which employs about 30,000 workers, manufactures a vast

Gary, Indiana

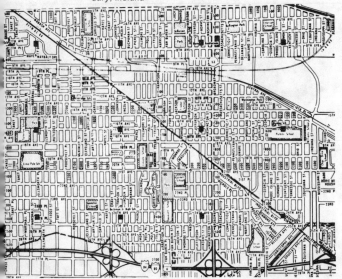

amount of sheet steel, tin plate, coke, gas, cement, steel rails and bridges. There is also a large coke plant in the city. Other manufactured products include clothing, hosiery, bedding, mattresses, refractory brick and lighting fixtures. The city, a large truck freight center, also serves as a shipping center since its harbor lies on Lake MI. The total labor force in Gary in 1979 was 75,000, while the unemployment rate was 6.1%. In 1977, the met. area ranked fifth highest in the US in avg. income per capita. Avg. hourly earnings for production workers in Mar., 1979, was $10.02.

BANKING. In 1978, total deposits for the two banks headquartered in Gary were $683,300,000, while total assets were $814,063,000. Banks include Gary Natl., Bank of IN and First Fed. Savings.

HOSPITALS. There are two hosps. in Gary, Gary Methodist and St. Mary Medical Center.

EDUCATION. IN U-Northwest, established in Lake Co. in 1922, is a public institution located in Gary. Offering undergrad. and grad. degrees, it enrolled approx. 5,000 in 1978. IN Vocational Tech. Col. is also located in the city. There are 30 elementary, six jr. high and eight sr. high schools in the public school system, which has won natl. acclaim for its "Gary School Plan", a work-study-play program developed by William Wirt. He was Gary's first superintendent of schools and a famous work-study educator. There are also one private and 18 parochial schools in the city. The Gary Public Lib. maintains eight branches throughout the city.

ENTERTAINMENT. Dinner theater entertainment and annual festivals are accessible to residents of Gary in nearby Chicago. Professional sports teams of the nearby Chicago area are also available to residents of Gary, who may also follow the IN U-NW Chiefs in intercollegiate sports. Several famous sports-related persons were born in the city. Among them are Oakland A's owner Charles O. Finley, track star Lee Calhoun, football players Alex Karras and Gerald Iron, KC Chiefs coach Hank Stram and middleweight champion Tony Zale. Each year Gary hosts the Sr. Little League World Series which involves teams from four continents.

ACCOMMODATIONS. There are six hotels and motels in Gary, including the Sheraton Suisse Chalet, TraveLodge and La Quinta and Ramada inns.

FACILITIES. There are 28 parks in Gary providing recreational and sports facilities. IN Natl. Lakeshore on Lake MI is one mi. E of the city. There is one 18-hole public golf course in the city, as well as several tennis and swimming centers.

CULTURAL ACTIVITIES. The Greater Gary Arts Council coordinates such performing groups as the Gary Musicians and the NW IN Symphony, while IN U-NW presents dramatic and musical performances. The Artist League sponsors art shows and exhibits. Among the city natives who have excelled in musical or dramatic fields are the Jacksons, opera star James McCracken and actor William Marshall.

LANDMARKS AND SIGHTSEEING SPOTS. The 1822 home of fur trader Joseph Bailly, located eight mi. E of Gary, has been preserved as an historic landmark. Marquette Park commemorates the traditional encampment site of the Jesuit priests. Among the other attractions in the city are the Gary Land Co. Building, the Civil Rights Hall of Fame (scheduled to be completed in 1981) and the Old Miller Town Hall (annexed by Gary in 1918).

GLENDALE
CALIFORNIA

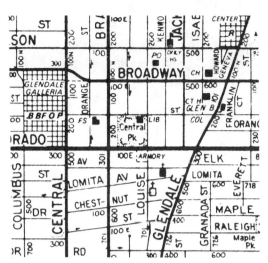

Glendale, California

CITY LOCATION-SIZE-EXTENT. Glendale is located in LA Co. in SW CA, seven mi. NE of LA. Situated in the San Fernando Valley, the city covers 29.2 sq. mi. at 34°9' N lat. and 118°20' W long. It is part of the greater LA met. area.

TOPOGRAPHY. Glendale is nestled in a valley and surrounded on three sides by mts., the San Raphael Hills on the E, the Santa Monica Mts. on the W and, on the N, the Verdugo Mts. The mean elev. is 450'.

CLIMATE. The climate of Glendale is normally mild and pleasant throughout the year. The avg. annual temp. of 64°F ranges from monthly means of 56°F during Jan. to 74°F during Aug. Daily temps. may vary by as much as 30°F, resulting in warm days and cool nights. Nearly 85% of the annual rainfall of 14" occurs during the winter months, while summers are almost rain free. Snowfall rarely occurs. The RH ranges from 40% to 80%. Glendale lies in the PSTZ and observes DST.

FLORA AND FAUNA. Animals native to Glendale include the coyote, mule deer, jackrabbit, pocket gopher and opossum. Common birds include the scrub jay, W kingbird, goldfinch, swallow and hummingbird. Bullfrogs, Pacific treefrogs, fence lizards, pond turtles and skinks occur here, as does the venomous Pacific rattlesnake. Typical trees include the oak, fir, pine and willow. Smaller plants include the CA laurel, blue blossom, CA poppy, vetch and clover.

POPULATION. According to the US census, the pop. of Glendale in 1970 was 132,664. In 1978, it was estimated that it had increased to 134,300, placing the city third largest in pop. of the 78 cities in LA Co.

ETHNIC GROUPS. In 1978, the ethnic distribution of Glendale was approx. 98.4% Caucasian, .1% Black and 10.3% Hispanic. (A percentage of the Hispanic total is also included in the Caucasian total.)

TRANSPORTATION. US hwys. 2, 5, 66 and 118 and the Golden State (5), Ventura (134), Foothill (210) and Glendale (2) frwys. provide major motor access to Glendale. Southern Pacific, Union Pacific and Santa Fe *railroads* serve the city, while AMTRAK offers passenger service. There are no airports in the city. Nearby Hollywood-Burbank (nine mi.) and LA Intl. (24 mi.) airports are served by all major natl. and intl. *airlines*. *Bus lines* include the local S CA Rapid Transit District, Trailways and Greyhound.

COMMUNICATIONS. Communications, broadcasting and print media serving Glendale are: *AM radio station* KIEV 870 (Indep., Talk, Btfl. Mus.) and *FM radio station* KUTE 101.9 (Indep., Progsv.); there are no *television stations* in the city (which receives broadcasting from LA), although cable TV is available; *press:* the *News-Press* is Glendale's only daily newspaper, distributed evenings and Sun. morning. Other publications include the *Star* and *Pacific Union Recorder*, which are weekly newspapers; *Alumni Report* and *Print-Equipment News*, published monthly, and the *Ledger*, published twice each week.

Downtown Glendale with the Verduge Mts. in the background

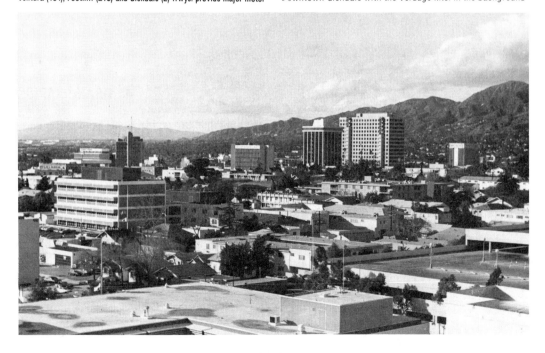

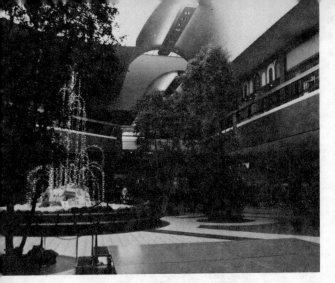

Galleria Shopping Center, Glendale, California

GOVERNMENT. Glendale has a council-mgr. form of govt., consisting of five voting members including the mayor. Council members are elected at large to overlapping four year terms, while the mayor is selected from the council by fellow members for a one-year term. The city mgr. is the chief administrator of the municipal govt.

HISTORY. The area which is now Glendale was originally part of a 36,403-acre parcel of land granted to the Verdugo family by the King of Spain in 1784. The Verdugos, for whom the mt range N of Glendale was named, operated the land as a ranch for many years. In 1847, the Cahuenga Capitulation Treaty, which terminated CA's participation in the Mexican War, was signed on the ranch. In the 1880s, Ranchero de los Verdugos was split into several smaller tracts, which continued to be worked as ranches. The town of Glendale, which emerged to accommodate the ranchers, became known as the "Jewel of the Verdugos". The Southern Pacific RR reached the town in 1883, at which time 13 Anglo families lived there. Glendale was incorporated as a city in 1906. It continued to grow throughout the century as an industrial and residential city, sharing in the tremendous increase in pop. of nearby LA.

ECONOMY AND INDUSTRY. There are approx. 450 industries in Glendale which employ more than 20,000 people. The major manufactured products include electrical/electronic components, medical equipment, ceramics, pharmaceuticals, aircraft and missile parts and commissary products. An approx. equal number of people (more than 20,000) are employed in services and retail trade.

BANKING. There are eight commercial banks and 11 savings and loan assns. in Glendale. In 1978, total deposits for the two banks headquartered in the city were $120,087,000, while total assets were $134,130,000. Among the banks serving the city are Security Pacific, Bank of America, Barclays Bank of CA, and Community Bank.

HOSPITALS. There are six hosps. in Glendale, Glendale Adventist Medical Center, Glendale Community, Memorial Hosp. of Glendale, N Glendale, Pacific Glen Hosp. and Clinic and Verdugo Hills.

EDUCATION. Glendale Comm. Col., a public jr. col. founded in 1927, offers programs leading to associate degrees. In 1978, over 8,000 students enrolled. Other institutions include Glendale Col. of Bus., Glendale U Col. of Law, Kensington U and LA Col. of Chiropractic. There are 27 elementary, five jr. and six sr. high schools in the Glendale Unified School District, enrolling more than 9,000 students. There are seven libs. in the city, including the Main Lib. and the Grandview and Casa Verdugo branches and the Brand Park Lib. and Cultural Center, a former mansion housing a special collection of books and art pieces.

ENTERTAINMENT. The various professional sports teams of nearby LA provide the residents of Glendale with spectator activities. Dodger Stadium is located five mi. from the center of Glendale. The Rose Bowl, also located five mi. from the center of town, is the site of many collegiate sporting events.

ACCOMMODATIONS. There are 10 hotels and 16 motels in Glendale, including the Glendale Town House, the Vagabond, Bell and Golden Key motor hotels and the Astro, Regal Lodge and Sands motels.

FACILITIES. There are 22 parks and 31 playgrounds in Glendale, providing facilities for picnics, hiking, square dancing, games, horseback riding and swimming, as well as instruction in various arts and handcrafts. Among the city's parks are Brand, Carr, E Glenoaks, Casa Adobe, Nibley, Dunsmore, Maple, Emerald Isle, Palmer, Piedmont, Fremont, Verdugo, Scholl Canyon and Pelanconi. Griffith Park contains a public golf course, and there are 45 public tennis courts in the city. Descanso Gardens features camellia, azalea and rose gardens, and is a haven for more than 150 species of birds. The LA Zoo, one of the newest in the US, is located on the SW edge of Glendale. It is arranged in "continental zones" where large animals roam freely in replicas of their natural habitats.

CULTURAL ACTIVITIES. The Glendale Symphony Orchestra, which often performs at the Music Center of LA Co., has, under the direction of Carmen Dragon, received special Emmy awards for musical shows on television. The Glendale Arts Assn. arranges art shows and exhibits. Forest Lawn Memorial Park contains a collection of art and sculpture, including reproductions of all of Michelangelo's greatest works as well as "The Crucifixion", at 195' x 45' the largest religious painting in the world, and "The Last Supper", a stained glass reproduction of Leonardo da Vinci's masterpiece. The Forest Lawn Museum also features a gem collection and the Eaton collection of every coin mentioned in the Bible—originals, not replicas. Brand Park Lib.'s Cultural Center, a 1904 Moorish-style mansion, houses an art collection and contains facilities for art exhibits, studios and dramatic performances. The Theater-in-the-Round also presents musical and dramatic performances.

LANDMARKS AND SIGHTSEEING SPOTS. Griffith Park's Planetarium is a popular sightseeing spot in the Glendale area. The San Fernando and San Gabriel missions, historic old-world churches, are located nearby, while the ancient Casa Adobe San Rafael is a major historic Glendale landmark. Since the city is located close to LA, many of the sightseeing spots in that city are easily accessible to Glendale residents or visitors.

GRAND RAPIDS
MICHIGAN

CITY LOCATION-SIZE-EXTENT. Grand Rapids, the seat of Kent Co., is located in SW MI at the rapids of the Grand River. It is 30 mi. E of Lake Michigan, 147 mi. NW of Detroit and 172 mi. NE of Chicago in the W central portion of MI's lower peninsula. It encompasses 44.9 sq. mi. at 42°53' N lat. and 85°31' W long. Its met. area includes Kent Co. and Ottawa Co. on the W.

TOPOGRAPHY. Grand Rapids is located in the Grand River Valley. It is bisected by the river into E and W sections. The terrain on both sides of the river is flat to gently rolling, while tall bluffs and high hills surround the valley. There are several small lakes in the city, whose mean elev. is 784'.

CLIMATE. The climate of Grand Rapids is influenced by Lake Michigan. In spring, the lake produces a cooling effect which retards the growth of vegetation, while in fall it produces a warming effect which deters frost, allowing crops to mature. During winter, the lake tempers cold air masses from the NW. Monthly mean temps. range from 24.l°F during Jan. to 72.6°F during July, with an annual avg. of 48.4°F. The annual rainfall of 33.23" is fairly evenly distributed throughout the year, while some 85% of the annual snowfall of 77.3" occurs from Dec. through Mar. The RH ranges from 62% to 83%. The avg. growing season is 170 days. Violent storms are infrequent, although gusts have occasionally exceeded 65 m.p.h. during summer thunderstorms. Grand Rapids is in the ESTZ and observes DST.

FLORA AND FAUNA. Animals native to Grand Rapids include the whitetail deer, raccoon, opossum, woodchuck and chipmunk. Common birds are the pheasant, swallow, wood thrush, woodcock, flycatcher and red-tailed hawk. Salamanders, bullfrogs, chorus frogs, milk snakes, painted turtles, box turtles and the venomous E massasauga (a pygmy rattler) are found here. Common trees include the oak, pine, elm, maple, apple, cherry, poplar and beech. Smaller plants include the dogwood, buttonbush, meadowrue, goldenrod and selfheal.

POPULATION. According to the US census, the pop. of Grand Rapids in 1970 was 197,649. In 1978, although the pop. was estimated to have decreased to approx. 190,000, Grand Rapids is the second largest city in MI.

ETHNIC GROUPS. In 1978, the ethnic distribution of Grand Rapids was approx. 87.2% Caucasian, 11.3% Black and 1.5% Hispanic.

TRANSPORTATION. Interstate hwys. 96, 196 and 296, US Hwy. 131 and state hwys. 11, 21, 37, 44, 45 and 50 provide major motor access to Grand Rapids. ConRail, Chessie and Grand Trunk Western *railroads*, as well as AMTRAK, serve the city. Kent Co. Intl. Airport is served by VA, NC and Trans MI *airlines*. There are several private airports in the area, including Lowell, S Kent, Sparta and Wells. *Buslines* serving the city include the local Grand Rapids Transit, Empire, Greyhound and North Star.

COMMUNICATIONS. Communications, broadcasting and print media originating from Grand Rapids are: *Am radio stations* WCUZ 1230 (ABC/I, Ctry.); WOOD 1300 (NBC, MOR); WLAV 1340 (ABC/C, Contemp.); WGRD 1410 (Indep., Contemp.); WMAX 1480 (MBS, News) and WFUR 1570 (Indep.); *FM radio stations* WCSG 91.3 (Indep., Variety); WJFM 93.7 (CBS, Btfl. Mus.); WZZM 95.7 (Indep., Top 40); WLAV 96.9 (ABC/C, AOR); WGRD 97.9 (Indep., Contemp.); WFUR 102.9 (Indep.); WVGR 104.1 (Indep.) and

"La Grande Vitesse" sculpture by Alexander Calder in City-County Plaza, Grand Rapids, Michigan

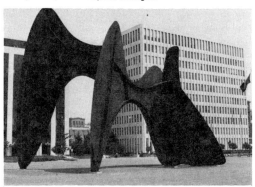

WOOD 105.7 (NBC, Btfl. Mus.); *television stations* WKZO Ch. 3 (CBS); WOTV Ch. 8 (NBC); WZZM Ch. 13 (ABC); WGVC Ch. 35 (PBS); WUHQ Ch. 41 (ABC) and cable, Ch. 10, which broadcasts Chicago and Detroit programming; *press*: the major publication is the daily *Press*, distributed evenings and Sun. morning. Other publications printed in the area include the *Photo Reporter, Wyoming Advocate, Banner, Church Herald, Chimes, Insight, Accent, Grand Rapids* (monthly), the *Collegiate, Sunrise* and *W Michigan Catholic*.

HISTORY. The Hopewell Indians, who inhabited Kent Co. from 300 BC to 300 AD, were replaced by the Ottawa

Indians who, in the late 18th century, established good relations with the early French missionaries and trappers. In Nov., 1826, Louis Campau, a trader, and his family founded Grand Rapids on the banks of the Grand River. Kent Co., named in honor of a NY lawyer, was established in 1831. Grand Rapids was incorporated as a village on Apr. 5, 1838, from that settlement and the neighboring village of Kent, founded in 1831 by Lucius

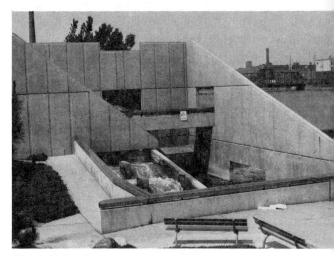

"Fish ladder" sculpture on the Grand River, Grand Rapids, Michigan

Lyon. The furniture industry, for which Grand Rapids later became known as "Furniture City", was established in the village in 1847, since the city was located near MI's great forests. The furniture trade developed rapidly following the Civil War, and an exhibition at the Centennial Exposition in Philadelphia in 1876 established Grand Rapids as world headquarters for fine and artistic furniture. The city was incorporated Apr. 2, 1850. During the late 1800s and early 1900s, Dutch, Polish and Lithuanian people immigrated to the city (35% of the present pop. is now of Dutch descent) to work in the furniture trade. Grand Rapids eventually became the wholesale trade center for W MI. In 1945, it became the first city in the US to add fluoride to its drinking water.

GOVERNMENT. Grand Rapids has operated under a commission-mgr. form of govt. since May 7, 1917. It consists of six commissioners, a mayor and city comptroller. Each of the city's three wards elects two commissioners, while the mayor and city comptroller are elected at large.

ECONOMY AND INDUSTRY. More than 1200 manufacturing firms in the Grand Rapids area produce over 100 products. The region is a major wholesale and distribution center for agricultural and industrial products. The major industries include metal working, electronics, automotive trade and wood working. Of the total work force, 30% is employed in manufacturing. The total labor force in the Grand Rapids area in Apr., 1979 was 295,000, while the unemployment rate was 5.9%. Avg. hourly earnings for industrial workers in Mar., 1979 was $7.29.

BANKING. There are 12 commercial banks and four savings and loan assns. in Grand Rapids. In 1978, total deposits for the four banks headquartered in the city were $1,633,062,000 while total assets were $1,953,811,000. Banks include Union Bank & Trust, Michigan Natl., Old Kent Bank & Trust, First Natl. Bank of Grand Rapids and Grand Valley Natl.

HOSPITALS. There are 12 hosps.—four gen. and eight specialized—in Grand Rapids, which is the major medical center of W MI. Blodgett Memorial, Butterworth, Osteopathic and St. Mary's are gen. hosps., while Booth Memorial, Ferguson-Droste-Ferguson, Forest View Psychiatric, Kent Community, Kent Oaks, Mary Free Bed and Rehabilitation Complex, MI Veteran's Facility and Pine Rest Christian are specialized. The city is known as an important medical service, educational and research center. The city has been in the forefront in plastic surgery, while artificial silicone implants for arthritis victims, as well as a major breakthrough in the diagnosis and treatment of sickle-cell anemia, have been developed by the city's medical community. All of the major hosps. are teaching hosps.

EDUCATION. There are three colleges offering undergraduate and graduate degrees, three two-year cols. and four Bible or religious institutions in Grand Rapids. Aquinas (with an enrollment of 1700), Calvin (4,000) and Grand Valley State (8,000) cols. confer bachelor and master degrees, while Davenport Col. of Bus. (2,000) and Grand Rapids Jr. Col. (7,500), established in 1916 as the first jr. col. in MI, are the two-year institutions. Kendall School of Design enrolls approx. 400 in a three-year program. The cols. that offer Bible or religious training are Grace Bible, Grand Rapids Bible, Grand Rapids School of Bible and Music and Reformed Bible. The U of MI, MI State U and Western MI U offer extension courses leading to bachelor and master degrees in the Grand Rapid City Center. The city is an official campus of MI State U's Col. of Human Medicine, and Grand Rapids Osteopathic Hosp. is associated with MSU's Col. of Osteopathic Medicine. There are also five schools of nursing—Blodgett, Butterworth, St. Mary's, Grand Rapids Jr. Col. and Grand Valley State Cols. There are more than 38,000 students enrolled in the city's public school system, while private schools are operated by Roman Catholic, Lutheran and Seventh Day Adventist denominations. Among the libs. are the Grand Rapids and Kent Co. public. The Grand Rapids Ryerson Lib., containing publications on furniture design and manufacture, as well as a MI room, operates five branches throughout the city.

ENTERTAINMENT. Annual events in the area include the Holland Tulip Festival in May, the Reeds Lake and Vandenburg art festivals in June, the

Grand Rapids, Michigan

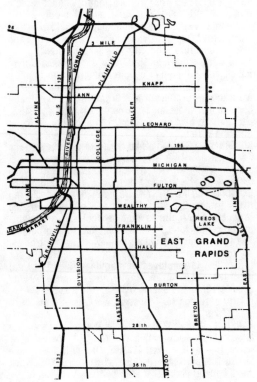

Lowell Showboat and the Ionia Free Fair in July, the Wyoming Rodeo and the raft race on the Grand River in Aug., Greenville Danish Days and the MI Championship Rodeo in Sparta in Sept., Cedar Springs Red Flannel Days in Oct. and the Grand Haven Nativity Scenes in Dec. The 3,000-meter Old Kent River Bank Run is a more recently-established yearly tradition. The colleges of Grand Rapids each participate in intercollegiate sports. Among these teams are the Grand Rapids Jr. Col. Raiders, Aquinas Col. Saints and Calvin Col. Knights. The Grand Rapids Owls is a professional hockey team, and the Wyoming Cobras participate in semi-pro football. Several teams compete in a semi-pro baseball league in the summer.

ACCOMMODATIONS. Among the hotels and motels in Grand Rapids are the Pantlind Hotel, Howard Johnson's, TraveLodge, and the Mr. Pick, Holiday, Ramada, Hospitality, Best Western, Gateway, Beltline, Cascade and Midway motels.

FACILITIES. There are 37 county parks, 86 municipal parks and 35 public or semi-private golf courses in the Grand Rapids area. Eight jogging tracks and several city parks, including Belknap, Highland, Richmond Hills, Garfield and Calder, offer sports and recreational facilities. Sailing, boating, fishing and swimming are available at Reeds Lake, Comstock Riverside Park and Hogdenpyl Park by Fisk Lake. The Blanford Nature Center in the NW part of the city, operated by the Grand Rapids Public Museum, is an outdoor laboratory featuring 105 acres of woods, field and water containing nature trails, live exhibits and a nature museum. The zoo at John Ball Park, which contains picnic and recreation facilities, features 500 mammals as well as reptiles, birds and fish. It is one of the largest in the state.

CULTURAL ACTIVITIES. The 90-member Grand Rapids Symphony Orchestra performs more than 50 concerts annually, including cabaret pop series, young people's and chamber music concerts and the annual spring Mozart festival. Both the Grand Rapids Symphony and Jr. Symphony perform in the city's Civic Auditorium. The Circle-in-the-Park Theater performs during the summer in the pavilion at John Ball Park, while the Grand Rapids Civic Theater performs regular and children's dramatic productions each season. Grand Valley State Cols. also presents dramatic performances during the school year. Opera is performed at St. Cecilia's Hall. There are several museums in the city, including the Grand Rapids Public, one of the first to be accredited by the American Museum Assn. Established in 1854 as the Grand Rapids Lyceum of Natural History, it is now one of the largest and most varied museums in MI, containing displays of the state's animals, plants, native American relics, archaeology and furniture. The adjacent Roger B. Chaffe Planetarium, named for the late astronaut, is a "theater of the sky", simulating space and time travel. The Grand Rapids Art Museum, established in 1844, houses a permanent collection of paintings, sculptures and prints and sponsors lectures, temporary showings and chamber music concerts. The Baker Furniture Co. maintains a private furniture museum which is open to the public. The Gerald R. Ford Presidential Museum is also located in the city. There are several art galleries in Grand Rapids, including Bergsma, Burton Russell, Heffner's and Louis.

LANDMARKS AND SIGHTSEEING SPOTS. "La Grande Vitesse" (the Grand Rapids, or "the great swiftness") is a huge Alexander Calder sculpture located in downtown Grand Rapids. Standing 40' high and weighing 42 tons, it is located on the plaza of Vandenburg Center, the city's redevelopment project. A 127' x 127' painting by the same artist adorns the roof of the nearby county administration building. Another sculpture is the walk-on Kinnebrew fish ladder at the Sixth St. dam, where salmon may be watched leaping the rapids on their annual upstream migration. The "Grand River Queen", an authentic paddlewheel riverboat featuring a Dixieland band, offers 10 mi. excursion trips on the Grand River from June through Oct. "Gaslight Village" near the Public Museum features 1870 to 1900 re-creations of streets paved with cedar blocks, hitching posts and harness-maker, gunsmith and apothecary shops. The Heritage Hill Historic District near downtown Grand Rapids features year-round self-guided walking tours by historic old homes, which are open to the public during MI week in May and on weekends in the fall. A covered bridge built across the Thornapple River in 1867 in Ada, 3 mi. E of the city, is one of only four such bridges remaining in W MI. It is open to pedestrian traffic only.

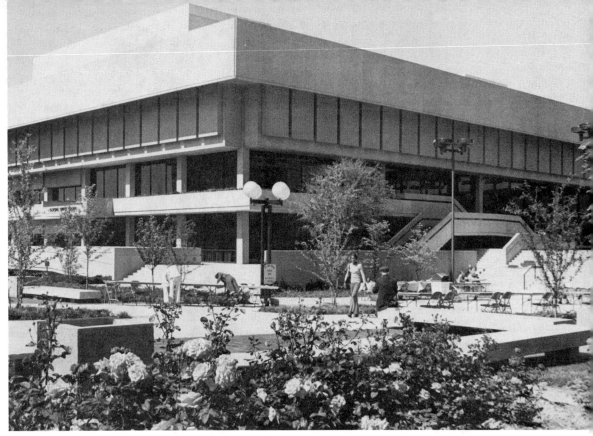

Government Center Complex, Greensboro, North Carolina

GREENSBORO
NORTH CAROLINA

CITY LOCATION-SIZE-EXTENT. Greensboro, the seat of Guilford Co., encompasses 60.6 sq. mi. in N central NC, 25 mi. E of Winston Salem at 36°F 05' N lat. and 79°F 57' W long. Located in the Greensboro-Winston-Salem-High Point met. area, its met. area extends into the counties of Forsyth on the W and Randolph on the S.

TOPOGRAPHY. The terrain of Greensboro, which is located in the N Piedmont region, is characterized by rolling hills. Ridges overlook the Yadkin River to the W and the Dan River to the N, while the Haw River is N and E, and the Deep River, S and W, of the city. Further W, the terrain rises more abruptly toward peaks of the Blue Ridge Mts. The mean elev. is 841'.

CLIMATE. The climate of Greensboro is moderate, influenced by the Blue Ridge Mts. of the Appalachian range, which form a NE-SW barrier to cold air masses from the W. Monthly mean temps. range from 38.7°F during Jan. to 77.2°F during July, with an annual avg. of 58.1°F. The avg. annual rainfall of 42.36" is fairly evenly distributed throughout the year. The avg. annual snowfall of 8.7" occurs during Jan. and Feb. The RH ranges from 48% to 92%. The avg. growing season is approx. 200 days. Greensboro lies in the ESTZ and observes DST.

FLORA AND FAUNA. Animals native to Greensboro are the whitetail deer, opossum, raccoon and fox. Common birds are the cardinal (the state bird) warbler, blue jay, robin, bluebird and thrasher. Box turtles, cricket frogs, narrow-mouthed toads, salamanders, newts and ribbon snakes, as well as the venomous copperhead, cottonmouth, coral snake and rattlesnake, are also found in the area. Typical trees are the pine (the state tree), oak, redbud, mulberry and magnolia. Smaller plants include the holly, crabapple,

purslane herb and milkweed.

POPULATION. According to the US census, the pop. of Greensboro in 1970 was 147,948. In 1979 it was estimated that it had increased to approx. 157,326.

ETHNIC GROUPS. In 1978, the ethnic distribution of Greensboro was approx. 69.0% Caucasian, 30.0% Black, 0.5% Hispanic and 0.5% other.

TRANSPORTATION. Interstate hwys. 85 and 40, US hwys. 29, 220, 421 and 70, and state hwys. 22 and 6 provide major motor access to Greensboro. *Railroads* serving the city include AMTRAK and Southern. *Airlines* serving Greensboro/High Point/Winston-Salem Regional Airport include DL, EA, PL and UA. *Bus lines* serving the city include Greyhound, Carolina Trailways and the local Duke Power Co. and Suburban Systems.

COMMUNICATIONS. Communications, broadcasting and print media originating from Greensboro are: *AM radio stations* WPET 950 (Indep., C&W); WCOG 1320 (ABC/C, Top 40, Contemp.); WGBC 1400 (ABC/I, Contemp.); WGIG 1470 (CBS, Contemp.) and WEAL 1510 (Mut. Blk.); *FM radio stations* WUAG 89.9 (Indep., Educ., Divers); WQDS 90.7 (Col. Var.) WQMG 97.1 (Indep., Blk., MOR, Relig.) and WROK 98.7 (Indep., C&W); *television stations* WFMY Ch. 2 (CBS) and cable; additional broadcasting is received from High Point and Winston-Salem; *press:* two major daily newspapers are published in the city, the *Daily News*, issued mornings and the evening *Record*; other publications include the *Times, Carolina Peacemaker, NC Christian Advocate, Carolina, Democrat, Guilford Gazette, Future Outlook, S Industrial Supplier* and *S Plumbing Heating and Cooling.*

HISTORY. Guilford Co., in which the town of Greensboro was later established, was organized in 1770. The town was named after Revolutionary War Gen. Nathaniel Greene, who successfully commanded the Continental Army against the invading British forces of Lord Cornwallis at the Battle of Guilford Courthouse in 1781. Located six mi. S of the Courthouse, Greensboro was incorporated as a town and designated county seat in 1808. First Lady Dolley Madison and short story writers William Sydney Porter (known as O. Henry) and Wilbur

Daniel Steele were born in Greensboro. In the latter part of the 19th century, the textile industry began to develop in the town which was chartered as a city in 1870 (the centennial of the organization of Guilford Co.). The city continued to grow, and, in the 20th century, became a center of education and insurance as well as manufacturing.

GOVERNMENT. Greensboro has a council-mgr. form of govt. The seven council members, including the mayor as a voting member, are elected at large to two-year terms. The mgr. is appointed as the administrative head of govt.

ECONOMY AND INDUSTRY. Manufacturing, education and insurance are the major employers in Greensboro. Major products are textiles, which include denim, flannel, khaki, rayon and nylon stockings. Other products are metal products, service station equipment, cigarettes, chemicals, pharmaceuticals and electrical and non-electrical machinery. In June, 1979, the labor force of the met. area totaled approx. 426,200, while the rate of unemployment was 4.5%.

BANKING. In 1978, deposits of the three banks headquartered in Greensboro were approx. $61,615,000, while assets totaled $71,356,000. Banks include Gateway, Community of Carolina and Greensboro Natl.

HOSPITALS. There are four hosps. in Greensboro, Moses H. Cone, Wesley Long Community, L. Richardson Memorial and Greensboro.

EDUCATION. The U of NC at Greensboro, established in 1891, awards bachelor, master and doctorate degrees, and in 1978, enrolled approx. 9,900. The NC Agricultural and Technical State U, a publicly-supported institution established in 1891 by the Gen. Assembly of NC, awards associate bachelor and master degrees. In 1978, approx. 5,400 students enrolled. Other institutions in the city include Bennett, Guilford, Jefferson and Greensboro colleges and the Electronic Computer Programming Institute. The public school system consists of 30 elementary, eight jr., four sr. high and six special schools. The State Dept.of Public Institution has approved 11 religious, military and col. preparatory schools in the area. The Greensboro

Central Greensboro, North Carolina

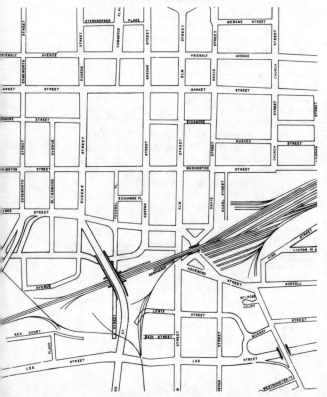

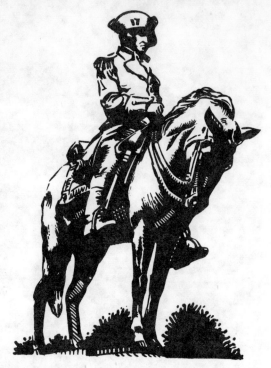

General Nathaniel Greene Monument, Greensboro North Carolina

Public Lib. and its five branches and bookmobiles are among the lib. facilities available.

ENTERTAINMENT. Among the dinner theaters in Greensboro is the Barn. The Greater Greensboro open of the PGA tour, with the third largest purse on the professional circuit, is held every spring in the city. The E Musical Festival is also held annually, as is the four day Festival Arts in spring. The Greensboro Hornets, a professional baseball team, play in Memorial Stadium. The U of NC Spartans participate in collegiate sports in the Atlantic Coast conf.

ACCOMMODATIONS. There are several hotels and motels in Greensboro, including the Albert Pick, Coliseum, Guest Quarters, Howard Johnson's, Cricket, Hilton, Holiday and Ramada inns.

FACILITIES. There are 105 parks and recreational areas in Greensboro encompassing more than 2,600 acres. Facilities include four outdoor and three indoor swimming pools, 13 lighted ballfields, 75 tennis courts, two golf courses and archery range. Greensboro Co., Lanndale Drive, Guilford Courthouse Natl. Military, Old Battleground Road and Hagan-Stone are the largest parks in the area. Nearby Bryan Park Complex, a 600-acre site bordering Lake Townsend, features a wildlife sanctuary, several nature trails, a public golf course and public tennis courts. A zoo is located at Greensboro Co. Park. The three reservoirs of the city's water system provide lakes for sailing, fishing and boating.

CULTURAL ACTIVITIES. Organizations affiliated with the Greensboro Council include the Community Theatre, Greensboro Symphony, Green Hill Art Gallery, the Greensboro Artists' League, Greensboro Arts & Crafts Assn. Greensboro Ballet and the Society for the Preservation of Barbershop Quartet Singing in America. The center for the Performing Arts is housed in the renovated Carolina Theatre. The United Arts Center is the headquarters for the city's art organizations. Among galleries in the city are the U of N Weatherspoon Gallery (known for its contemporary art collection), H.C. Taylor Gallery, and the NC Agricultural and Technical State U Gallery, which features the art of minorities and the third world. On the site of O.Henry's birthplace is the Masonic Temple Museum. Exhibits in the Greensboro Historical Museum trace the development of the Guilford Co. area from prehistoric times to the 20th Century. In addition, the Natural Science Center and Edward R. Zane Planetarium are located in the city.

LANDMARKS AND SIGHTSEEING SPOTS. Guilford Courthouse, six mi. NW of downtown Greensboro, is the site of one of the last battles of the Revolutionary War. The site includes the battlefield, where forces of Gen. Nathaniel Green met British troops of Lord Cornwallis in 1781.

HAMMOND
INDIANA

CITY LOCATION-SIZE-EXTENT. Hammond encompasses 24.1 sq. mi. in Lake Co. in NW IN E of the IL state line at 41°38' N lat. and 87°30' W lat. The city is bordered by Lake MI on the N and the greater met. area, part of the met. areas of Chicago on the W and Gary on the E, extends into Cook Co., IL on the W. Hammond is part of the Calumet District, an industrial center formed by Hammond, E Chicago, Gary and Whiting.

TOPOGRAPHY. The terrain of Hammond, which is situated in the Great Lakes plain region, is characterized by low flat land which rises gently to the E. The mean elev. is 591'.

CLIMATE. The climate of Hammond is continental and influenced by Lake MI which moderates air masses from the N. The mean annual temp. of 50°F ranges from monthly means of 23°F in Jan. to 73°F in July. Most of the avg. annual precip. of 33" occurs during the warmer months. Most of the avg. annual snowfall of 40" occurs during the months of Dec. and Jan. The RH ranges from 53% to 86%. The growing season avgs. 158 days. Hammond lies in the CSTZ and does not observe DST.

FLORA AND FAUNA. Animals native to Hammond include the muskrat, fox, whitetail deer and raccoon. Common birds are the crow, blue jay, flycatcher, swallow and thrasher. Bullfrogs, chorus frogs, salamanders, garter and water snakes, soft-shelled turtles and skinks, as well as the venomous E massasauga (a pygmy rattler), are found in the area. Typical trees are the oak, maple, elm and hickory. Smaller plants include the waterlily, yarrow, thistle, buttercup and spring beauty.

POPULATION. According to the US census, the pop. of Hammond in 1970 was 107,790. In 1978, it was estimated that it had decreased to 102,400.

ETHNIC GROUPS. In 1978, the ethnic distribution of Hammond was approx. 95.4% Caucasian, 4.3% Black and 3.1% Hispanic (a percentage of the Hispanic total is also included in the Caucasian total).

TRANSPORTATION. Interstate hwys. 80, 90, 94 and 294, US hwys. 6, 12, 20 and 41 and state hwy. 141 provide major motor access to Hammond. *Railroads* serving the city include AMTRAK, Baltimore & OH, ConRail, Louisville & Nashville, Norfolk & Western and S Shore. All major *airlines* serve O'Hare Intl. Airport and Midway Airport in Chicago, both within a one-hour drive, while Gary Municipal Airport, also nearby, is served by private and community aircraft. *Bus lines* include Greyhound, Trailways and the local Gary Public Transportation Corp. Nearby port W of IN. Harbor and Lake Calumet Harbor provide water transportation facilities.

Hammond, Indiana and vicinity

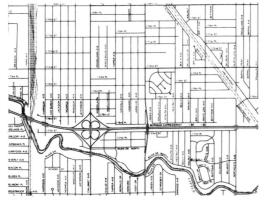

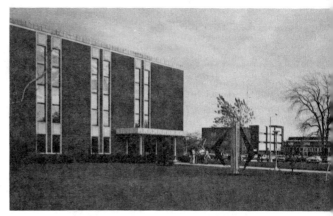

Purdue University, Calumet Campus, Hammond, Indiana

COMMUNICATIONS. Communications, broadcasting and print media originating in Hammond are: *AM radio station* WJOB 1230 (Indep., MOR, Talk) and *FM radio station* WYCA 92.3 (Indep., Gospel); no *television stations* originate in Hammond, which receives broadcasting from the Chicago met. area; *press*: one major daily serves the city, the *Times*, issued weekday evenings and weekend mornings.

HISTORY. Founded in 1868, Hammond was named for entrepeneur G. H. Hammond, who established a meat-packing business in the town in 1869. Incorporated as a town in 1883, Hammond received its city charter the following year. The city's economy, based primarily on meat packing, suffered a major set-back in 1901, when the largest meat-packing plant was consumed in a fire. A major steel company was established in the city in 1912. During the 1950s and 1960s, the trend to suburbanization and the lack of an adequate tax base resulted in a decay of the downtown area. During the 1970s, the "Hammondation" project was instituted to revive the inner city.

GOVERNMENT. Hammond has a mayor-council form of govt. The nine council members and the mayor, who is not a voting member of council, are elected at large to four-year terms.

ECONOMY AND INDUSTRY. Manufacturing is the largest employer in Hammond. Industrial plants make various products, including chemicals, plastics, furniture, cleaning products, food products, transportation equipment, steel, lead, tin and construction equipment. In June, 1979, the labor force for the Hammond-Gary-E Chicago met. area totaled approx. 290,200, while the rate of unemployment was 6.5%.

BANKING. There are three commercial banks and six savings and loan assns. in Hammond. In 1978, total deposits at the three banks headquartered in the city were approx. $481,980,000, while total assets were $561,860,000. Banks include Calumet Natl., Mercantile Natl. and Hoosier State.

HOSPITALS. There is one gen. acute care hosp. in Hammond. St. Margaret's clinic also serves the city.

EDUCATION. The Calumet campus of Purdue U in Hammond offers associate degrees in most areas, and the bachelor degree in its School of Technology. In 1978, approx. 6,900 enrolled. Other institutions include Bishop Noll Institute, IN Col. of Commerce, Sawyer Col. of Business and Calumet Institute of Automation. The public school system consists of 21 elementary, seven middle and five high schools, and offers vocational-technical training. Nine parochial schools, including two high schools, serve the area. Lib. facilities include those at the Hammond Public Lib.

ENTERTAINMENT. The Intl. Culture Festival held annually in Hammond, is a two-day event featuring food, arts, crafts and continuous entertainment by more than 40 ethnic groups. The LaCare Art Fair is another annual event. The Purdue U-Calumet Campus Pipers provide collegiate sports entertainment.

ACCOMMODATIONS. There are several hotels and motels in Hammond, including Holiday Inns and Howard Johnson's Motor Lodges.

FACILITIES. There are 33 municipal parks in Hammond, encompassing 951 acres and including six public swimming pools, numerous baseball and softball diamonds and several tennis courts. In the winter, the city provides 23 ice skating (10 with warming areas) and four hockey rinks. The 400-acre Wolf Lake Park-Beach Complex includes facilities for hiking, boating, fishing and camping. Natural and man-made recreational facilities along the S shoreline of Lake MI are also available.

CULTURAL ACTIVITIES. The Hammond Civic Theatre, Tech Players of Hammond Vocational-Technical High School, IN U Theatre NW and Purdue-Calumet Theatre Co. stage dramatic productions in the city. Hammond Adult Band and the Hammond Young Orchestra, as well as other symphonic and popular groups, also perform in the city. The N IN Assn. schedules cultural events throughout the year.

LANDMARKS AND SIGHTSEEING SPOTS. Many attractions including Chinatown, Morton Arboretum and Adler Planetarium are available to residents of Hammond in nearby Chicago and its met. area.

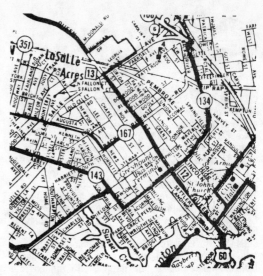

Central Hampton, Virginia

HAMPTON
VIRGINIA

CITY LOCATION-SIZE-EXTENT. Hampton is an independent city located in SE VA in the Tidewater Region at 37°2' N lat. and 76°23'W long. It encompasses 54.7 sq. mi. at the E tip of the VA peninsula between the James and York rivers and Chesapeake Bay. The greater met. area includes Newport News to the W, Poquoson to the N and Williamsburg to the NW, as well as Gloucester, James City and York counties to the NW.

TOPOGRAPHY. The terrain of the Hampton area is characterized by generally low, flat land almost entirely surrounded by water. Chesapeake Bay is N, the Atlantic Ocean is E and Hampton Roads, the largest natural harbor in the world, is SW of the city. The mean elev. is 12'.

CLIMATE. Because Hampton is surrounded by water on three sides, the climate is modified marine, with mild winters and long, warm summers. The avg. annual temp. of 60°F ranges from monthly means of 41°F in Jan. to 79°F in July. Most of the annual 45" of rainfall occurs during the warmer months, while most of the avg. annual 7.2" of snowfall occurs in Jan. and Feb. The RH ranges from 52% to 90% The avg. growing season is 240 days. Hampton lies in the ESTZ and observes DST.

FLORA AND FAUNA. Animals native to Hampton include the muskrat, raccoon, fox, whitetail deer and opossum. Common birds are the osprey, bald eagle, crow, mourning dove, gallinule and tern. Nearby Chesapeake Bay, containing an abundance of blue crabs and oysters, is the wintering ground for numerous waterfowl and shore birds. Water snakes, cricket frogs, bullfrogs, salamanders, newts, yellowbilled turtles and the venomous copperhead, rattlesnake, water moccasin and coral snake, are found here. Common trees include the oak, maple, sweet gum, willow, red bay and ash. Smaller plants include the tupelo and marsh grasses.

POPULATION. According to the US census, the pop. of Hampton in 1970 was 120,779. In 1977, it was estimated that it had increased 8.7% to 131,300. The estimated 1981 pop. is 140,400.

ETHNIC GROUPS. In 1978, the ethnic distribution of Hampton was approx. 74.1% Caucasian, 25.4% Black and 1.3% Hispanic (a percentage of the Hispanic total is also included the Caucasian total).

TRANSPORTATION. Interstate Hwy. 64 and US hwys. 60, 17 and 258 provide major motor access to Hampton. AMTRAK provides passenger *railroad* service to the area. Patrick Henry Airport serves Hampton, Newport News, Williamsburg and York Co., with US Air, NA, PI and UA the *airlines* providing service. *Bus lines* include the local Peninsula Transportation District Commission (PENTRAN) and Greyhound.

COMMUNICATIONS. Communications, broadcasting and print media originating from Hampton are: *AM radio station* WWDE 1490 (Indep., Adult Contemp.): *FM radio stations* WHOV 88.3 (Indep.) and WWDE 101.3 (Indep., Adult Contemp.): no *television stations* are located in Hampton, which receives broadcasting from Norfolk; *press*, the daily *Times-Herald* and *Daily Press* (published in Newport News)serve the area, as do the bi-weekly *Flyer* and the bi-monthly *HamptonScript.*

HISTORY. The friendly Kicotan tribe of native Americans welcomed the first Anglo settlers of the Hampton area. The oldest continuous English-speaking community in the US, Hampton was established in July, 1610 as the Town of Kecoughtan, and was one of the original boroughs. It was later named for the Earl of Southampton, Henry Wriothesley. Although Hampton was settled after Jamestown, it thrived as a trading center when the latter was abandoned. In 1634, the first free school in America was established in the town by Benjamin Syms. In 1775, during the Revolutionary War, the town was pillaged by British forces. Later, during the War of 1812, British forces attacked and burned Hampton. Following the war, the US govt. built Ft. Monroe, known as the "Gibraltar of Chesapeake Bay". Begun in 1819 and completed in 1834, the fort protected Hampton Roads harbor, where the US fleet anchored, and later became the base for the Union army during the Civil War. In Aug., 1861, Hampton was burned again, this time by Confederate soldiers who sought to prevent the town from falling to Union forces. Hampton Roads was the site of the important battle of the ironclads *Monitor* and *Merrimac*, while the first major land battle of the Civil War was fought at Big Bethel, located within the city limits of present-day Hampton. On May 22, 1865, after the war's end, Jefferson Davis (Pres. of the Confederate States of America) was falsely accused of plotting the assassination of Abraham Lincoln and imprisoned by the Union army at Fort Monroe until he was released in 1867. The fishing industry became established, and the city is today a major E coast seafood center. Langley AFB was built in the city during WW I, while NASA's Langley Research Center was established in 1917. Since then, the US govt. has become one of the area's major employers.

GOVERNMENT. Hampton has a council-mgr. form of govt. consisting of seven council members, including the mayor as a voting member. The councillors are elected at large to four-year terms, while the mayor is selected from among the council members to serve a two-year term.

BANKING. There are 10 banking institutions in Hampton. In 1978, total deposits for the two banks headquartered in the city were $62,170,000, while total assets were $67,997,000. Banks serving the city include Dominion Natl., First and Merchants Natl., First VA Bank of Tidewater and United VA.

ECONOMY AND INDUSTRY. The transportation equipment industry employs three of every four persons employed in manufacturing in the greater Hampton-Newport News met. area. The Newport News Shipbuilding and Dry-Dock Co. is VA's largest employer and the world's largest shipyard. Food and kindred products (of which seafood products and beverages are the major categories) rank as the second largest employer in the manufacturing sector of the area. Third and fourth in manufacturing in terms of number employed are chemicals and petroleum, and printing and publishing. Other manufactures include primary and fabricated metals, apparel and textiles, machinery, electrical equipment, lumber and wood products, stone, clay and glass, and instruments. Other leading non-manufacturing industries include the travel trade, medical services, educational services, port related activities, research and development and the state govt. Manufacturing accounts for approx. 40% of the total number of persons employed in the area (about 150,000 in 1979), while the fed. govt. employs approx. 39%. With a total labor force of approx. 158,000 in 1979, the unemployment rate for the Hampton-Newport News area was 5.1%. In 1977, per capita effective buying income was $5,176, while per household median effective buying income was $14,329.

HOSPITALS. Hospitals located in Hampton include Hampton Gen., Bayberry Psychiatric, a USAF hosp. and a V.A. facility.

EDUCATION. Hampton Institute, founded in 1868 primarily for the education of freed slaves (Booker T. Washington was an early alumnus), is a private institution offering programs leading to bachelor and master

Coliseum, Hampton, Virginia

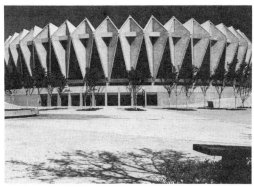

degrees. In 1978, approx. 3,000 enrolled. Thomas Nelson Comm. Col. is also located in the city. Established in 1967, and enrolling more than 4,000 in 1978, the col. offers courses leading to the associate degree. Five other institutions of higher learning are located in the area. The VA School for the Deaf and Blind is a special school in Hampton. The city is served by the Charles Taylor Lib. as well as the lib. facilities of NASA's Langley Research Center.

ENTERTAINMENT. The Coliseum in Hampton is the site of many annual events. including the Coliseum Mall Intl. Tennis Tournament, the Hampton Jazz Festival and the CIAA Basketball Tournament. Hampton Fair Day and

Medley of the Arts are other festivals celebrated in the city. Hampton hosts the Peninsula Phillies, a baseball team in the CRL, while Hampton Institute's Fighting Pirates participate in sports at the collegiate level.

ACCOMMODATIONS. Hotels and motels in Hampton include the Sheraton Inn-Coliseum, Holiday and Strawberry Bank Motor inns.

FACILITIES. There are many areas offering recreational and sports—especially water—facilities in Hampton. Among the parks is Gosnold's Hope Park, containing camping sites, picnic areas, bridle trails and a boat ramp. Buckroe Beach on Chesapeake Bay contains a fishing pier, boating and swimming areas and an amusement park. Grandview Pier offers fishing facilities as well as campgrounds. Bluebird Gap Farm is a zoo featuring domestic animals and 50 types of fowl.

CULTURAL ACTIVITIES. The Hampton Center for the Arts and Humanities, besides featuring an exhibit of artifacts, photos and dioramas of old Hampton, sponsors cultural and artistic events. There are several museums in Hampton, including the Ft. Monroe Casemate Museum, which commemorates the captivity of such famous prisoners as Chief Blackhawk of the Sacs and Foxes and Jefferson Davis of the Confederacy in chambers in the wall of the fort. Converted gun casemates house the US Army Coast Artillery Museum at Ft. Monroe, which is the only active moat-encircled fort in the US, serving as headquarters for the US Army's Training and Doctrine Command. The Syms-Eaton Museum, named for Hampton forefathers Benjamin Syms (who in 1634 established the first free school in America) and Thomas Eaton (who in 1659 willed 500 acres for the same purpose) traces the city's history from its founding to the present. It also features an exhibit of public school education. The Kenneth E. Rice Memorial Museum and Fossil Pit houses the largest collection of fossils in VA. Hampton Institute features an African Museum, containing a display of Congolese artifacts.

LANDMARKS AND SIGHTSEEING SPOTS. The 90-passenger flagship *Kicotan Clipper*, a former oyster boat, conducts tours of the Hampton Roads harbor, sailing by Ft. Monroe and the site of the historic battle of the *Monitor* and the *Merrimac*. Hampton's St. John's Church, established in 1610 and rebuilt for the fourth time in 1728, is the oldest continuous English parish in America. It has survived both British occupation during the War of 1812 and partial burning during the Civil War. Kicotan Indian Village, a reconstructed settlement of the early 1600s, contains replicas of the lodges and huts of the Native Americans who welcomed the first English settlers to the Hampton area. Langley AFB, headquarters for the Tactical Air Command, is the oldest continuously active AFB in the US. Nearby is the NASA Langley Research Center, which served as the training base for the astronauts of Apollo 11. Founded in 1917, it is the oldest continuously active aeronautical research center in the US. Aerospace Park, an "aerospace playground", contains jet aircraft and missile and space vehicle displays.

HARTFORD
CONNECTICUT

CITY LOCATION-SIZE-EXTENT. Hartford, the state capital and seat of Hartford Co., encompasses 16.8 sq. mi. on the W bank of the CT River in central CT., approx. midway between Boston and NYC, at 41°56' N lat. and 72°41' W long. The greater met. area extends E into Tolland Co., W. into Litchfield Co. and S into Middlesex Co. and includes the cities of W Hartford and E Hartford.

TOPOGRAPHY. The terrain of Hartford, which is situated in the CT River Valley, is characterized by gently rolling hills to the W and to the NW, the Berkshire Mts. The mean elev. is 15'.

CLIMATE. The climate of Hartford is moderate continental, characterized by daily weather variations and influenced by continental polar air from the N, which results in cold dry winters; and from the S, maritime air

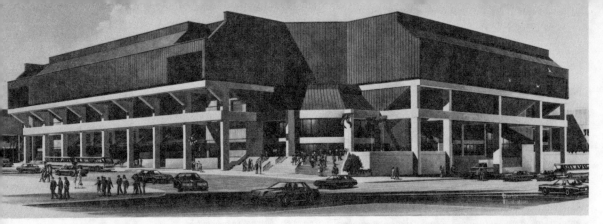

Civic Center Coliseum, Hartford, Connecticut

from the Atlantic Ocean which results in warm summers. The avg. annual temp. of 50°F ranges from monthly means of 26.9°F in Jan. to 73.1°F in July. The avg. annual rainfall of 43.10" is evenly distributed throughout the year. Approx. 94% of the avg. annual snowfall of 54.1" occurs from Dec. through Mar. The RH ranges from 43% to 87%. The growing season avgs. 176 days. Hartford lies in the ESTZ and observes DST.

FLORA AND FAUNA. Animals native to Hartford include the shrew, weasel, mink, vole and fox. Typical birds include the bittern, robin, rail, mourning dove, flycatcher and cardinal. Leopard frogs, bullfrogs, pickerel frogs, salamanders, box turtles and water snakes, as well as the venomous copperhead and timber rattlesnake, are found in the area. Typical trees are the elm, oak, maple and basswood. Smaller plants include the sumac, willow, jewelweed, spring beauty and chickweed.

POPULATION. According to the US census, the pop. of Hartford in 1970 was 158,107. In 1978, it was estimated that it had decreased to approx. 124,000.

Central Hartford, Connecticut

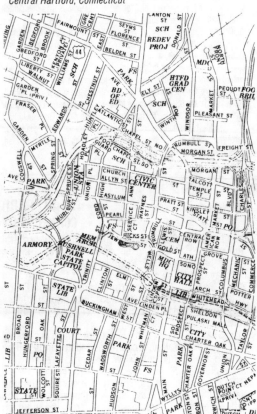

ETHNIC GROUPS. In 1978 the ethnic distribution of Hartford was approx. 71% Caucasian, 27.9% Black, and 7.6% Hispanic, (a percentage of the Hispanic total is also included in the Caucasian total).

TRANSPORTATION. Interstate hwys. 84, 86, 91 and 95 and US Hwy. 44 provide major motor access to Hartford. *Railroads* include AMTRAK and ConRail. *Airlines* serving Bradley Intl. Airport, 14 mi. N of the city, are AA, US Air, DL, EA, TW, UA and commuter lines Altair, Bar Harbor and Pilgrim. Hartford-Brainard Airport is served by private and commuter aircraft. *Bus lines* include the local CT Transit System, Greyhound and Trailways. The city lies at the uppermost navigable point for ocean going vessels on the CT River.

COMMUNICATIONS. Communications, broadcasting and print media serving Hartford are: *AM radio stations* WTIC 1080 (NBC, MOR, Talk); WCCC 1290 (ABC/C, AOR); WDRC 1360 (Indep., Top 40); and WPOP 1410 (CBS, APR, All News); *FM radio stations* WJMJ 88.9 (Indep., Easy List.); WRTC 89.3 (UPI, Divers.); WQTQ 89.9 (UPI); WLVH 93.7 (Indep., Span.); WTIC 96.5 (Indep., Top 40); WDRC 102.9 (Indep., Top 40); WHCN 105.9 (Indep., AOR) and WCCC 106.9 (ABC/C. Progsv.); *television stations* WFSB, Ch. 3 (CBS); WHCT Ch. 18 (Relig.) WEDH, Ch. 24 (PBS); and WVIT Ch. 30 (Indep.); *press*: one major daily serves the area, the *Tribune* issued mornings; weekly publications include the *Advocate Journal Inquirer*, *Trinity Tripod*, *CT Jewish Lodger*, *CT Italian Bulletin* and *Tri-Town Reporter*.

HISTORY. The area of present-day Hartford was inhabited by native Americans of the Suckiag tribe, who called the settlement "Suckiag," meaning "black earth," Before the white settlers, arrived, traders had previously traveled through in 1633. The first settlers established a post called the "House of Hope." In 1636, a Congregationalist minister led a discontented group of English families on foot from the village of Newtowne (now Cambridge), MA and founded the comm., naming it after the English town of Hertford, birthplace of their minister, Samuel Stone. In 1639, the 200 English settlers of the CT Colony met at the Hartford Meeting House and composed the "Fundamental Orders", the first written constitution in history and a forerunner to the later *US Constitution.* One of the oldest newspapers in America, the *Hartford Courant,* was first printed in the town in 1764. In 1784, Hartford was chartered as a city. With New Haven, the city served as the capital of CT from 1701 to 1875, when Hartford became the sole capital. During the late 18th century, the city became a thriving port from which furs, wood and spices departed for Europe and the W Indies, and, in the early 1800s, it was the center of a rum distilling business. During the War of 1812, the British blockaded the city, and following the war, shipping was replaced by insurance as the major industry. In 1835, the Hartford Fire Insurance Co. promptly paid claims for damages resulting from a fire in NYC, and the city gained a reputation for dependable insurance companies. Samuel Colt pioneered experiments in interchangeable firearm parts in Hartford, which led to assembly line production and the area's dominance in precision manufacturing. In 1844, having discovered the anesthetic properties of nitrous oxide, Dr. Horace Wells submitted to its first practical application in dentistry by having one of his teeth pulled while under its influence. In 1877, Col. Albert Pope manufactured the first bicycle in the US in Hartford. Between 1900 and 1920, an influx of European immigrants caused the pop. of the city to nearly double from 79,850 to more than 138,000. By 1950, the pop. had reached nearly 177,400, but during the next decade many residents moved to the suburbs, and an urban renewal program was initiated in the early 1970s. Today, the city is known as both the "Insurance Capital of the US" and a center of manufacturing. It is also the second largest retail center in the N.E. after Boston.

GOVERNMENT. Hartford has a council-mgr. form of govt. The nine city councillors and the mayor are elected on a partisan basis to two-year terms.

ECONOMY AND INDUSTRY. There are approx. 2,200 manufacturing firms in the Hartford area, which is an industrial center. Products include aircraft engines and accessories, helicopters, propellors, fuel control systems, firearms, atomic reactors, electrical supplies, precision machine tools, turbines, recreational products, office equipment, hardware, plastics and food and beverage products. Retailing is the second largest industry in the area, which is also an important wholesale distribution center. Insurance is the third largest employer in the area, engaging approx. 10% of the work force. The greatest concentration of multiple-line insurance underwriting companies in the US are located in Hartford, "The Insurance Capital of the World." Research and agriculture (including tobacco as one of the most important crops) are also important industries. In June, 1979, the total labor force of the greater met. area was approx. 389,000, while the rate of unemployment was 4.9%.

HOSPITALS. There are several hosps. in Hartford, including the Institute of Living, well-known for its mental health care; Hartford Hosp., the seventh largest in the US; Mt. Sinai, St. Francis and V.A. The Burgdorf Health Center combines the ambulatory health services of the city health dept. with the U of CT Health Center outpatient clinics and rehabilitation center.

BANKING. There are eight commercial banks and savings and loan assns. in Hartford. In 1978, total deposits for the eight banks headquartered in the city were $6,480,254,000, while assets were $7,653,817,000. Banks include CT Bank and Trust Co., Hartford Natl. Bank and Trust Co., Mechanics Savings Bank, United Bank and Trust Co., Society For Savings, State Bank for Savings.

EDUCATION. The U of CT Hartford Branch includes Law and Medical-Dental schools., the Col. of Insurance and the School of Social Work. The U of Hartford, a private coed institution, awards bachelor's, master's and doctoral degrees. In 1978, more than 9,400 enrolled. The state-controlled Greater Hartford Comm. Col., which awards associate degrees, enrolled approx. 2,900 in 1978. Other educational institutions include Trinity Col., Hartford Col. for Women, Hartford Grad. Center, St. Joseph Col., Hartford Seminary Foundation and Hartford State Technical Col. The American School for the Deaf, the first school for the handicapped in the W hemisphere, opened in W Hartford in 1817; and in 1893, the CT Institute for the Blind was founded in the city. There are 112 elementary, 34 jr. and 37 sr.

Wadsworth Atheneum in the background of "Stegosauius", a gigantic stabile, Hartford, Connecticut

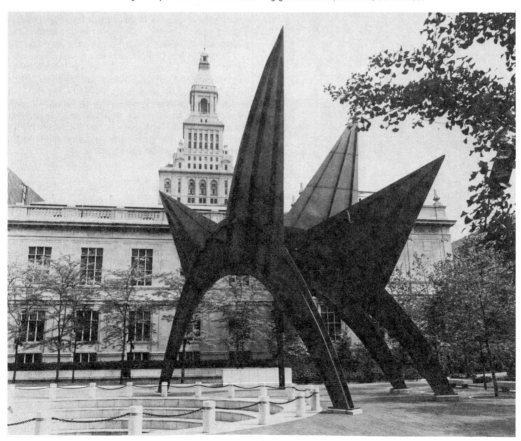

high schools in the greater Hartford area. There are also 10 special education schools for the handicapped and 44 private schools in the area. Lib. facilities include the Hartford Public Lib. and the Ct State Lib., housing state historical documents and a reference collection of Americana.

ENTERTAINMENT. Annual events in Hartford include the nine-day Greater Hartford Civic and Arts Festival held downtown in June; the Festival of Lights, held from late Nov. to early Jan., when 250,000 lights illuminate the Plaza; the House and Garden Tour and the N.E. Fiddle Contest in May; the Jumping Frog Contest in June; the CT Antiques Show in Oct. and the Spring Flower and Garden Show in Mar. Sporting events include the Sammy Davis, Jr. Greater Hartford Open, a golf event; and the Aetna World Cup Pro Tennis Tournament. The N.E. Whalers based in Hartford, play pro hockey in the NHL; and the Boston Celtics, an NBA basketball team, play some of their games at the Hartford Civic Center. Trinity Col.'s Bantams and Hartford Col. for Women's Hawks participate in intercollegiate sports.

ACCOMMODATIONS. Hartford's hotels and motels include the Howard Johnson's Motor Lodges, the Sheraton Hartford Hotel, the Hotel Sonesta, the Summit Motel and the Holiday, Koala, Hilton, Ramada and Suisse Chalet inns.

One of the country's largest elliptical buildings in Hartford, Connecticut

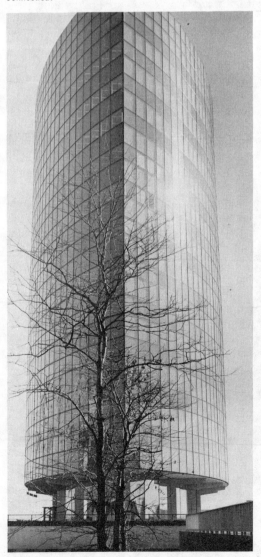

FACILITIES. There are nearly 2,800 acres of public parks and squares in Hartford. In 1853, the 41-acre Bushnell Park became the first public park in the US to be purchased by a city. A registered natl. landmark, it contains some 500 trees of over 150 varieties. Elizabeth Park contains the oldest municipal rose garden in the nation, featuring 1,100 varieties of roses and more than 4,000 rose bushes. A pond located in the park serves as an ice-skating rink during the winter. Keney Park contains Sherwood Forest, a children's zoo. There are two municipal golf courses, while public tennis courts are available at several locations. There are several ski slopes. cross-country skiing and snowmobile trails in the area as well.

CULTURAL ACTIVITIES. The Hartford Symphony Orchestra, CT Opera Assn., Hartford Chamber Orchestra and Artists Collective are among the musical organizations in Hartford. The Hartford Ballet Co. and the Chamber Ballet are also based here. Dramatic productions are staged by the Producing Guild and the Hartford Stage Co. Concerts, operas, ballets, films and theatrical productions are presented at Bushnell Memorial Auditorium. The Wadsworth Atheneum, established in 1842, is the oldest free public art museum in America and includes the Tactile Gallery for the Blind. The CT Historical Society, housed in a mansion on an eight-acre estate, contains a museum as well as displays of 17th and 18th century rooms and an extensive collection of portraits. The Museum of CT History, was constructed in 1910 and contains the original *Royal Charter* and the Colt Collection of Firearms. Fed. architecture, changing exhibits and special displays are featured at the Old State House.

LANDMARKS AND SIGHTSEEING SPOTS. Historic buildings of interest in Hartford include the Butler-McCook Homestead, built in 1782, which contains architecture and furnishings dating from the 18th century to the Victorian period; the Amos Bull House (1788), now the home of the CT Historical Commission; Nook Farms, a 19th century neighborhood, which includes the homes of authors Harriet Beecher Stowe, the author of *Uncle Tom's Cabin*, and Mark Twain; the Day House, housing a collection of memorabilia spanning the years 1840 to 1900; the State Capitol, which became the seat of govt. in 1878 and includes historic displays such as Lafayette's bed and bullet-ridden battle flags; the Old State House, designed by Charles Bullfinch; and Christ Church (1788), the site of the ratification of the *US Constitution* by CT. Thomas Hooker is thought to be buried under the present First Church, which has stood since 1807 and features several windows designed by Louis Tiffany. A brownstone monument, the Civil War Memorial Arch, commemorates the 4,000 Hartford men who served in that war. The Corning Fountain is one of the few memorials in the US commemorating the bravery and heritage of the native Americans. Grave markers in the first public cemetery in the city, the Ancient Burying Ground, date back to 1640. One of the last original merry-go-rounds in existence, the Bushnell Park Carousel was built in 1914.

HIALEAH
FLORIDA

CITY LOCATION-SIZE-EXTENT. Hialeah encompasses 22 sq. mi. in Dade Co. at 29°49' N lat. and 80°17' W long. in S FL adjacent to the NW border of Miami, W of Biscayne Bay on the Atlantic Ocean. It is part of the Miami met. area, which extends N of the city into Broward Co.

TOPOGRAPHY. The terrain of Hialeah, which is located in the Atlantic coastal plain region, is characterized by low, flat land which, although sparsely wooded, contains lush tropical vegetation. The mean elev. is 6'.

CLIMATE. The climate of Hialeah is subtropical, characterized by long, warm, rainy summers followed by short, mild, dry winters. Monthly mean temps. vary little, ranging from 67°F during Jan. to 83°F during Aug., with an annual avg. of 76°F. Most of the avg. annual 59" of rainfall occurs during the warmer months, with heavier amounts occuring in June and Sept. Tropical hurricanes occur most frequently during Sept.

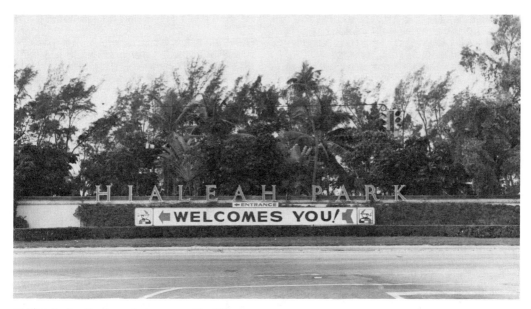

Hialeah Park, Hialeah, Florida

and Oct. Destructive tornadoes are rare. The RH ranges from 53% to 88%. Hialeah is in the ESTZ and observes DST.

FLORA AND FAUNA. Animals native to Hialeah include the fox squirrel, rice rat, gray fox, whitetail deer, raccoon and everglades panther. Common birds are the grackle, egret, heron, ibis, gull, tern, pelican and crow. Coral reefs are abundant in the coastal areas. Alligators, indigo snakes, soft-shelled turtles, pig frogs and the venomous coral snake, rattlesnake and cottonmouth are found in the area. Typical trees are the oak, red mangrove, bald cypress, cabbage palm and Dade pine. Smaller plants include the palmetto, marsh grass, rose gentian and gumbo.

POPULATION. According to the US census, the pop. of Hialeah in 1970 was 102,452. In 1978, it was estimated that it had increased to 138,000.

ETHNIC GROUPS. In 1978, the ethnic distribution of Hialeah was approx. 98.6% Caucasian, 1.1% Black, and 55.0% Hispanic (a percentage of the Hispanic total is also included in the Caucasian total).

TRANSPORTATION. Interstate Hwy. 95, the FL Tnpk. (Homestead Extension), US hwys. 27 and 441 and state hwys. 9 and 826 provide major motor access to Hialeah. *Railroad* service is provided by AMTRAK. All major *airlines* serve nearby Miami Intl. Airport. *Bus lines* serving the city include Greyhound, Trailways and the local Dade Metro Transit Authority.

COMMUNICATIONS. Communications, broadcasting and print media serving Hialeah are: no *AM* or *FM radio* or *television stations* originate from Hialeah, although the city receives broadcasting from neighboring Miami; *press*: two weekly newspapers serve the city, the *Home News* and *Las Noticias de Hialeah*, both issued on Thurs.; *FL Grocer* is a monthly publication; additional print media is published in Miami.

HISTORY. Native Americans of the Tequesta tribe inhabited the area of present-day Hialeah before the first white settlers arrived. Hialeah was settled in 1910 near the still-young Miami, and incorporated as a city in 1925. Original growth was slow and the pop. of the city had not yet reached 20,000 by 1950. Thereafter, however, small industries were established in the city and its pop. expanded to more than 100,000 by 1970. Today, Hialeah is an important Miami suburb, and shares in the growth of that city as a tourist and resort center.

GOVERNMENT. Hialeah has a mayor-council form of govt., consisting of seven council members, elected at large to four-year terms, and the mayor (who is not a member of the council), elected at large to a two-year term.

ECONOMY AND INDUSTRY. Among the products manufactured in Hialeah are coin-operated machines, fiberglass boats, women's sportswear, industrial steel products concrete products and aluminum awnings and sliding doors. The district headquarters of appliance manufacturers, food suppliers and dept. stores are located in the city. Economic data for the city is reflected in greater Miami met. area statistics, for which the June, 1979, labor force totaled 723,100, while the rate of unemployment was 6.0%.

BANKING. There are 11 commercial banks in Hialeah. In 1978, total deposits at the seven banks headquartered in the city totaled $366,639,000, while assets were $423,552,000. Banks include First Natl. Bank of Greater Miami, Hialeah-Miami Springs First State, N Hialeah First State, Popular Bank of Hialeah, SE Bank of Westland, Manufacturers' Natl. and People's Hialeah Natl.

HOSPITALS. The three hosps. in Hialeah include Hialeah, Palmetto Gen. and Palm Springs Gen. The Children's Psychiatric Center is also located in the city.

Central Hialeah, Florida

EDUCATION. The Hialeah School of Health Careers and the Miami Lakes Technical Education Center are both located in Hialeah. The public school system includes four elementary, two jr. high and two sr. high schools. The Hialeah J.F. Kennedy Lib. is among the libs. serving the city.

ENTERTAINMENT. Thoroughbred racing is held from early Jan. to mid-May at the Hialeah Park Race Course. Additional sporting events, festivals and entertainment are available in Miami.

ACCOMMODATIONS. There is a Holiday Inn in Hialeah and other lodging is available in nearby Miami.

FACILITIES. Hialeah Park, the site of the Race Course, features displays of tropical vegetation gardens and scenic drives. In addition, the only flock of pink flamingos ever to propagate in captivity live at the 32-acre Infield Lake. Surfing, skindiving, swimming, waterskiing, boating, fishing and other water sports are available at local beaches, creeks and bays.

CULTURAL ACTIVITIES. Performing arts organizations and museums are available to residents of Hialeah throughout the greater Miami met. area.

LANDMARKS AND SIGHTSEEING SPOTS. Approx. 1.5 million people annually visit Hialeah Race Course in Hialeah Park, located 12 mi. N of downtown Miami.

HOLLYWOOD
FLORIDA

CITY LOCATION-SIZE-EXTENT. Hollywood encompasses 26.9 sq. mi. in Broward County in S FL on the Atlantic coast between Miami and Ft. Lauderdale at 26°00' N lat. and 80°9' W long. It is part of the Ft. Lauderdale-Hollywood met. area, which extends N into Ft. Lauderdale.

TOPOGRAPHY. The terrain of Hollywood, which is located on the Atlantic Coastal Plain region, ranges from very flat near the Atlantic Ocean to gently sloping wooded land further inland in the W part of the city. The mean elev. is 15'.

CLIMATE. The climate of Hollywood is subtropical marine, tempered by winds from the Atlantic Ocean which are active 50% of the time. The avg. annual temp. of 76°F varies little between a Jan. mean of 67°F and an Aug. mean of 83°F. Most of the avg. annual 56" of rainfall occurs during late spring and early fall. The RH ranges from 55% to 90%. Hollywood is located in the ESTZ and observes DST.

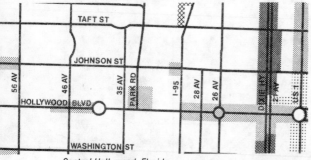

Central Hollywood, Florida

FLORA AND FAUNA. Animals native to Hollywood include the opossum and raccoon. Common birds are the grackle, tern, gull, heron, ibis and blue jay. Softshelled turtles, alligators, tree frogs, leopard frogs, S toads and scarlet and green snakes as well as the venomous cottonmouth, coral snake and rattlesnake are found in the area. Typical trees are the palm, oak and bald cypress. Smaller plants include the palmetto, sawgrass and nutsedge.

POPULATION. According to the US census, the pop. of Hollywood in 1970 was 106,873. In 1978, it was estimated that it had increased to approx. 127,000.

ETHNIC GROUPS. In 1978, the ethnic distribution of Hollywood was approx. 80.2% Caucasian, 3.7% Black, 3.5% Hispanic and 12.6% other.

TRANSPORTATION. Interstate hwy. 95 (the FL Tnpk.), US hwys. 1, 27 and 441 and state hwys. A1A, 820, 822 and 823 provide major motor access to Hollywood. Port Everglades, at the N end of the city, is one of the busiest commercial ports on the Atlantic coast, and a regular port-of-call for several world cruise ships. The first foreign trade zone in FL has been constructed at the port. *Railroads* serving the city include FL E Coast, Seaboard Coast and AMTRAK. *Airlines* serving Ft. Lauderdale/Hollywood Intl. Airport include BN, CO, DL, EA, NA, NW, SO, TW, UA and WA. Miami Intl. Airport, located 18 mi. S, and the smaller N Perry Airport, also provide service. *Bus lines* serving the city include Greyhound, Trailways and the local Broward Co. Transit.

COMMUNICATIONS. Communication, broadcasting and print media originating from Hollywood are: *AM radio station* WGMA 1320 (ABC/E, Mod. Ctry.); no *FM radio* or *television stations* originate from the city, which receives broadcasting from nearby Miami and Ft. Lauderdale; *press:* one major daily serves the city, the evening *Sun-Tattler*; other publications include the *Jewish Floridian & Shofar, Communique, FL Italian Bulletin, Recommend, FL Construction Industry* and *Miami Herald-Broward Edition.*

HISTORY. Native Americans of the Tequesta tribe, and later, Seminoles, inhabited the area of present-day Hollywood before the first white settlers arrived. The town of Hollywood was established in 1921 by Joseph W. Young, a developer who had earlier developed Indianapolis and assisted in the planning of Long Beach and Hollywood, CA. Young built the site from a palmetto jungle and attracted developers and buyers to the area. By 1925, thousands of people had arrived in Hollywood. It was incorporated as a city the same year and Young was elected its first mayor. In Sept., 1926, however, the new city was destroyed by a hurricane. Attempts at rebuilding were hindered by the collapse of the FL land boom and the natl. financial disaster of 1929. Young died in 1936 before seeing his plans for Hollywood realized. The establishment of naval training schools in the city during WW II stimulated its growth, and after the war, many USN personnel returned to the city to settle permanently. Despite the hurricanes of 1947, post-war building took place between the years 1945 and 1950. For the next 20 years, the city continued to be one of the fastest-growing in the US. Today, it is a major tourist center due to its location on the Gold Coast.

GOVERNMENT. Hollywood has a council-mgr. form of govt., consisting of five council members, including the mayor as a voting member, who are elected at large. Councilmen serve four-year terms, while the mayor serves a two-year term.

ECONOMY AND INDUSTRY. Tourism is the major industry in Hollywood. In addition, the city has experienced recent industrial expansion. The 175 manufacturing plants in the city produce aluminum furniture, fishing equipment and electronic components, among others. In June, 1979, the labor force for the Ft. Lauderdale-Hollywood area totaled approx. 395,00, while the rate of unemployment was 5.3%.

BANKING. There are nine commercial banks and two savings and loan assns. in Hollywood. In 1978, total deposits at the six banks headquartered in the city were $326,225,000, while assets totaled $364,831,000. Banks include Atlantic Natl. of Broward, First Natl., Commercial and Hollywood Natl.

HOSPITALS. There are five hosps. in Hollywood. Memorial. Hollywood Medical Center, Doctors, Pembroke Pines Gen. and Comm. of S Broward.

EDUCATION. Heed U in Hollywood offers liberal arts and teaching programs leading to master and doctorate degrees. The 1978 enrollment was approx. 150. The city is also the location of the S campus of Broward Comm. Col., FL Bible Col. and Prospect Hall Col. The public school system consists of 20 schools with a 1978 enrollment of approx. 19,950. The 15 private schools had an enrollment of approx. 3,480. Two branches of the Broward Co. Lib. System are located in the city.

ENTERTAINMENT. Each year, Hollywood hosts the Seven Lively Arts Festival at the Young Circle Bandshell, in Apr., and the Seven Lively Winter Arts Show in Dec. The Hollywood Dog Tracks feature dog racing from mid-May to mid-Apr.

ACCOMMODATIONS. There are numerous hotels and motels in Hollywood, including the Attache Resort, Elms, Mariner, Auberge Sur Le Parc, Colony Club, Riviera, Hollywood Hills, Sunshine, Holiday Inn and Howard Johnson's.

FACILITIES. Among the facilities in Hollywood are charter boats for deep-sea fishing, available at the Municipal Yacht Basin, and small fishing boats which may be rented in the coastal waterways. Fresh-water fishing is available in the streams and canals W of the city. Topeekeegee Yugnee Park features 150 acres for biking and picnicking and a 35-acre lake with boating facilities. The six mi. of public bathing beaches in the city feature the "Boardwalk", a two-mi. long, 24'-wide oceanfront promenade, and picnic area. There are several public golf courses and tennis courts.

CULTURAL ACTIVITIES. The Theatre Under the Stars offers free evening entertainment in Hollywood. The Greater Hollywood Philharmonic Orchestra gives free performances in the Young Circle Bandshell from Jan. through Apr. The city maintains an art museum and gallery, The Art and Culture Center of Hollywood.

LANDMARKS AND SIGHTSEEING SPOTS. The Seminole Okalee Indian Village, near Hollywood, contains thatched-roof huts, arts and crafts exhibits and alligator wrestling. Sightseeing and dinner cruises are available on nearby waters.

HONOLULU
HAWAII

CITY LOCATION-SIZE-EXTENT. Honolulu, the state capital and seat of Honolulu Co., encompasses 83.9 sq. mi. along the beach from Koko Head on the E to Pearl Harbor on the W on the Island of Oahu, one of the Hawaiian Islands in the Pacific Ocean, at 21°20' N lat. and 157°56' W long. It is the largest city and chief port of the islands. Legally, the city and county of Honolulu

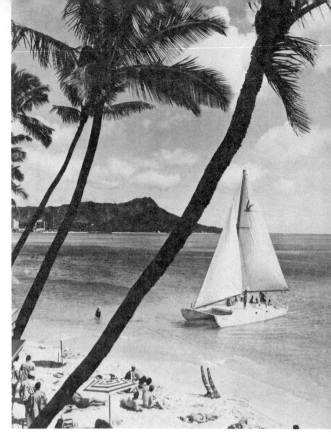

Waikiki Beach, Honolulu, Hawaii

includes most of the NW Hawaiian Islands from Niihau to Kure Atoll, 1,367 mi. from Honolulu, but it is usually defined as the Island of Oahu, a land area of 607 sq. mi. (the other islands and reefs add only three sq. mi. to the total area).

TOPOGRAPHY. The majority of the terrain of Honolulu lies in a coastal plain area, while two mt. ranges parallel the coast, the Koolau on the NE and the Waianae on the W. The mean elev. is 7'.

CLIMATE. The climate of Honolulu is tropical, characterized by prevailing NE trade winds, variability of rainfall over short distances, the suniness of leeward lowland and the infrequency of severe storms. The winds help

The Garden of the Missing at Punchbowl National Memorial Cemetery, Honolulu, Hawaii

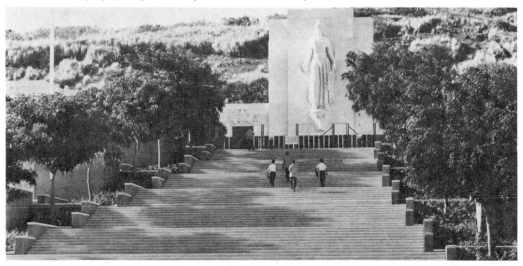

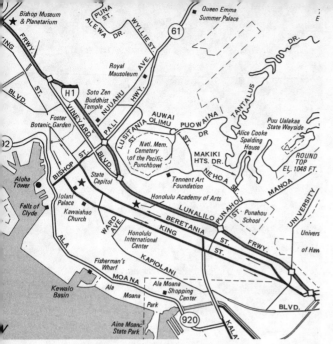

Central Honolulu, Hawaii

maintain a moderate RH, while the consistency of the amount of sun and the tempering effect of the surrounding ocean help to maintain a nearly constant daily and monthly temp. The mean annual temp. of 76.3°F ranges from monthly means of 80°F in July to 72.6°F in Jan. The avg. annual rainfall of 23.38″ occurs almost entirely during the Oct. to Apr. "winter" season. Storms are infrequent. The RH ranges between 51% and 80%. Honolulu lies in the AK-HI time zone and does not observe DST.

FLORA AND FAUNA. Animals native to Honolulu include the HI Monk seal, HI bat and wild boar. Common birds include the apapane, amakihi, elepaio, brown noddy, gray-backed tern, golden plover, short-eared owl, albatross, thrush, honeyeater, hawk and the Nene goose (the state bird). No venomous snakes are found in HI. Common trees include the palm, coconut, koa, ohia, hau and kukui (the state tree). Smaller plants include the hibiscus (the state flower), orchid, ti, plumeria and bird-of-paradise.

POPULATION. According to the US census, the pop. of Honolulu in 1970 was 630,528. In 1978, it was estimated that it had increased to 720,000.

ETHNIC GROUPS. In 1978, the ethnic distribution of Honolulu was approx. 29.1% Caucasian, 26.2% Japanese, 8.9% Filipino, 16.4% Hawaiian and part-Hawaiian, 5.2% Chinese, 9.1% mixed other than part-Hawaiian and 5.1% other (these percentages include 118,000 military personnel and dependents).

TRANSPORTATION. US hwys. 1 and 2 and state hwys. 61, 63, 72, 78, 90 and 92 provide major motor access to Honolulu. Many cargo steamship companies operate through the city. A foreign-trade zone located at the Pt. of Honolulu provides duty-free storage for merchandise. *Airlines* serving Honolulu Intl. Airport are AA, BN, CO, HA, NW, PA, TS, UA and W. Two scheduled airlines, air taxi and charter companies provide inter-Island flights. *Bus lines* include those of the city and co. of Honolulu.

COMMUNICATIONS. Communications, broadcasting and print media originating from Honolulu are: *AM radio stations* KGMB 590 (Indep., MOR, News, Personality); KORL 650 (Indep., Top 40); KKUA 690 (Indep., Variety); KGU 760 (NBC, MOR); KIKI 830 (ABC/C, MOR, Top 40); KAIM 870 (Indep., Relig., Clas.); KHVH 1040 (ABC/E, NBC, CBS, News); KIOE 1080 (Indep., Rock, Contemp.); KOHO 1170 (Indep., Talk, Educ., Relig., Japanese); KZOO 1210 (Indep., Jap.); KNDI 1270 (Indep., Var.); KISA 1540 (Indep., Filipino) and KUMU 1500 (Indep., Btfl. Mus.); *FM radio stations* KTUH 90.3 (NPR., Divers.); KQMQ 93.1 (Indep., MOR); KHUI 93.9 (Indep.); KUMU 94.7 (Indep. Btfl. Mus.); KAIM 95.5 (Indep., Clas., Relig.) and KHSS 97.5 (Indep., Btfl. Mus.); *television stations* KGMB Ch. 9 (CBS); KHET Ch. 11 (PBS); KHON Ch. 2 (NBC); KIKU Ch. 13 (Indep.) and KITV Ch. 4 (ABC); *press*: two major dailies are published in the city, the morning *Advertiser* and the afternoon *Star Bulletin*; other publications include *Snooper, This Week on Oahu, Aloha-The Magazine of HI, HI Business, Waikiki Beach Press, Honolulu Magazine, HI Church Chronicle, HI Hochi, HI Tourist News* and *Sun Press*.

HISTORY. Honolulu was first settled by Polynesians, who arrived in the Hawaiian Islands from Tahiti as early as 1,000 A.D. The Island of Oahu was sighted by the British Captain James Cook in 1778, marking his "discovery" of Hawaii for the world. English Capt. William Brown sailed into Honolulu Harbor in 1794. The following year, King Kamehameha I defeated forces of the Oahu king and added Oahu to his all-island kingdom. Ships began to harbor in Honolulu and, during the 1800s, the comm. became a center for the sandalwood trade. In 1820, missionaries arrived from N.E. In 1845, King Kamehameha III and the Legislature moved to Honolulu from the capital at Lahaina, on Maui, and, on Aug. 31, 1850, the king officially declared Honolulu a city and the capital of the kingdom. In the same year, the first unit of Honolulu's Fire Dept., the Board of Health, and the Chamber of Commerce of Honolulu were established. By the middle of the century, Honolulu had become the main Pacific whaling port. During the late 1800s, the sugar industry was developed,

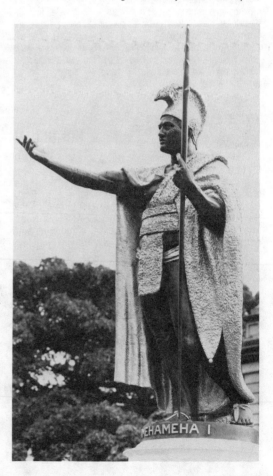

ABOVE—Kamehameha I. Hero of Hawaiians, who united the islands into one kingdom; RIGHT—City of Refuge. a revered site to Hawaiians, once holding the remains of Hawaiian kings

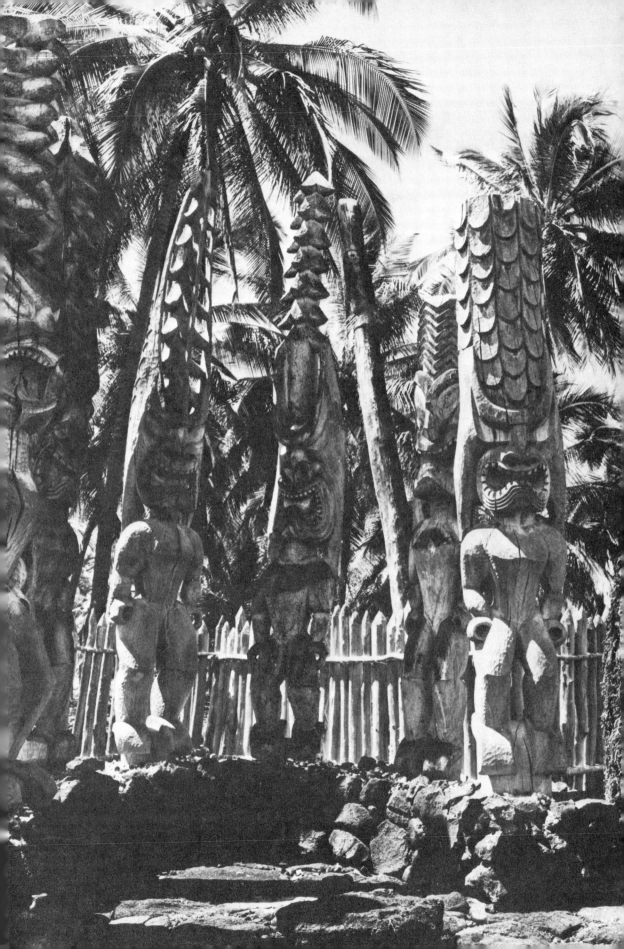

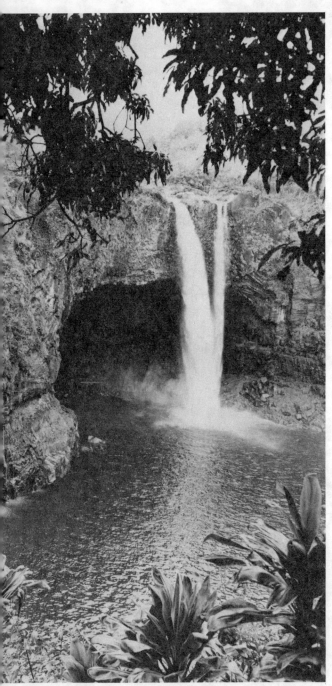

Rainbow Falls near Honolulu, Hawaii

bringing an influx of immigrants, including the Chinese, in 1852, the Japanese in 1868, and later, the Filipinos. The stream of imported labor, lasting until 1946, also brought Koreans, Portuguese and Puerto Ricans. Hawaii became a US territory in 1898, with Honolulu remaining the capital. During the early 1900s, the pop. continued to grow due to expansion in the sugar industry, the development of the pineapple industry and the establishment of military bases in the area. The

first successful non-stop flight from the mainland in 1927 by Army Lt. Lester Maitland and Albert Hegenberger coincided with increased efforts to promote a tourist industry. PA began regular commercial flights to the city in 1936. When the Japanese attacked Pearl Harbor in 1941, Honolulu became a major base for the Allied Pacific war effort. Oahu remained a center of US defense activities. Camp H. M. Smith, near Honolulu, is the headquarters of CINPAC. In 1959, HI became the 50th state of the US with Honolulu as its capital. Tourism flourished during the 1960s and 1970s, while construction boomed as facilities were provided for tourists and for the growing pop. During 1977, more than four million tourists visited Honolulu.

GOVERNMENT. Honolulu city and county are consolidated under a unified mayor-council form of govt., which administers the entire county. Nine members are elected to four-year terms. The mayor has power of veto which may be overridden by a two-thirds majority vote in the council.

ECONOMY AND INDUSTRY. Most of HI's manufacturing is concentrated in Honolulu, with more than 612 companies listed in the city and county. Food processing, including sugar, pineapple and fruit juices, is the largest industry. Heavy manufacturing includes two oil refineries, two cement plants, a steel mill producing reinforcing rods and 19 concrete products plants. Over 20% of the land is agricultural, with pineapple and sugarcane being the major crops. Major employers are the military and tourism. Active R&D fields include oceanography, geophysics and bio-medicine. The June, 1978, Honolulu city and county labor force totaled 315,600, while the rate of unemployment was 7.0%. The per capita income in 1976 was estimated at $7,325.

BANKING. Honolulu is the financial center of HI. Main offices of the state's eight banks, savings and loan assns. and industrial loan companies are located in Honolulu. In 1978, total deposits for the 11 banks headquartered in the city were $3,704,915,000, while assets were $4,211,864,000. Banks include Bank of HI, First Hawaiian, Central Pacific, American Security, Liberty, HI Natl., Bank of Honolulu and City Bank of Honolulu.

HOSPITALS. There are 11 state and private acute-care hosps. in Honolulu, including Kapiolani, Queen's, Kaiser and Leahi. Tripler Army Hosp. provides full care for service personnel and dependents.

EDUCATION. The state-supported U of HI at Monoa, located in Honolulu, was established in 1907 and became the U of HI in 1920. Located on its campus is the EW Center, a natl. institution for technical and cultural interchange with Far East nations. The 1978 enrollment was approx. 20,900. Chaminade U, a private Catholic U, enrolled approx. 2,600 in 1978. Other institutions include HI Pacific Col., HI Loa Col., Brigham Young, U-HI and several comm. cols. The 228 public schools and 128 private schools in the city enrolled approx. 166,250 in 1977-1978. Libs. include the Municipal Reference and the HI State, which is administered by the State Dept. of Education.

ENTERTAINMENT. Annual events in Honolulu include the Hula Bowl in Jan., Cherry Blossom Festival from Feb. through Apr., Kuhio Day, honoring one of the first Hawaiian delegates to Congress, in Mar., Hawaiian Music Festival in May, Hula Festival in Aug., Aloha Week in Sept., the Orchard Show in Oct. and the Intl. Surfing Championships at Makaha Beach in Dec. The Rainbows of the U of HI participate in intercollegiate sports in the WAC. Professional sports entertainment is offered by the HI Islanders AAA baseball team.

ACCOMMODATIONS. There are more than 130 hotels and motels in Honolulu, including Ala Moana Americana, Hawaiian Regent, Hyatt Regency Waikiki, Kahala Hilton, Outrigger, Waikiki-Beachcomber, Gateway, Marina's and several Sheraton hotels and Holiday Inns.

FACILITIES. There are 13 beach parks and one park in a forested mt. area in Honolulu. Major parks include Ala Moana and Kapiolani. Nuuanu Pali

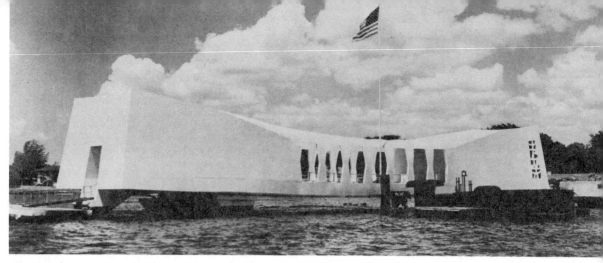

offers the more popular scenic views of Oahu's irregular coastline. The 20-acre Foster Botanic Garden features many botanical displays, including an orchid section. The Waikiki Aquarium contains an extensive collection of colorful tropical fish. Salt water fishing, swimming, surfing, diving and sailing are available at the city's beaches and ocean waters. Several public tennis courts and golf courses are located on the island. A 50,000-seat football-baseball stadium has recently been completed.

CULTURAL ACTIVITIES. The 80-piece Honolulu Symphony Orchestra presents more than 100 concerts and operas annually, including performances for school children. The Royal Hawaiian Band, a city and county group, performs weekly at Iolani Palace, Sky Gate on the Civil Green and Kapiolani Park, except during Aug. Stage productions are presented by the Honolulu Comm. Theatre, the HI Performing Arts Co. and the U of HI Theatre. The Neal S. Blaisdell Center, housing a 2,000-seat Concert Hall, an 8,000-seat Arena and additional display areas, and the John F. Kennedy Theatre at the U of HI provide cultural facilities. Bishop Museum, located in the city, was founded in 1889 and as a center of Pacific-wide ethnological research. It features Pacific art. The Honolulu Academy of Arts is noted for its permanent collection of European, Oriental, and HI art and offers educational programs to foster art appreciation. Mission Houses Museum encompasses such historic buildings as the Chamberlain House, Frame

The memorial to the U.S.S. Arizona in Pearl Harbor, Honolulu, Hawaii

House and Printing House. A replica of the first printing press is located nearby.

LANDMARKS AND SIGHTSEEING SPOTS. Aloha Tower offers a view of the harbor area and downtown Honolulu from its observation balcony on the 10th floor. The Falls of Clyde, docked at pier five, is a four-masted, square-rigged ship constructed in 1878. Fisherman's Wharf harbors the Glass Bottom Boat and other sightseeing boats, which offer tours featuring tropical fish, coral gardens and Polynesian plantlife. Built in 1882, Iolani Palace was the home of HI royalty until Queen Liliuokalani was deposed in 1893. Services are held in both HI and English at Kawaiahao Church, built in 1841. Honolulu's oldest church, it was the royal chapel of HI royalty. HI's greatest ruler is commemorated by the King Kamehameha's Statue, which stands in front of the Judiciary Building. The historic Mission Houses, built by the first missionaries in the area, are located in the civic center. The Natl. Memorial Cemetery of the Pacific contains the graves of more than 14,000 killed in WW II, the Korean and Vietnam conflicts. A

Iolani Palace, where Hawaiian kings lived, houses the only throne room in U.S. territory, Honolulu, Hawaii

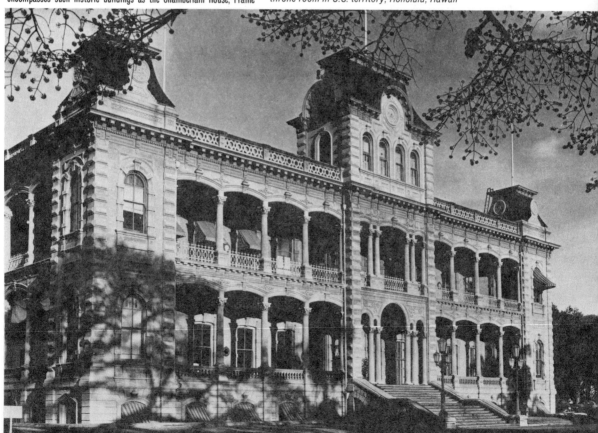

scenic masterpiece is Nuuanu Pali. Seven mi. from Honolulu, this 1,200'-high gap is flanked by cliffs which rise to 3,000' and is the site where Kamehameha defeated the Oahuans in 1795. Our Lady of Peace Cathedral, erected in 1843, was built on the site of HI's first Roman Catholic church. Queen Emma Summer Palace contains memorabilia of the HI monarchy. Royal Mausoleum is the burial ground for the Kamehameha and Kalakaua dynasties. St. Andrew's Cathedral, founded by King Kamehameha IV, was constructed in 1862 of stone brought from England. The Italian-design Soto Zen Buddhist Temple is noted for its ornate altar. Washington Place, a large white colonial house, was formerly the home of Queen Liliuokalani and residence of the gov. Chinatown offers shops, restaurants and markets in downtown Honolulu. The 56-acre Dole's Pineapple Cannery, the world's largest fruit-canning plant, is located in the area. Pearl Harbor, another major attraction, was the site of Japan's surprise air atack on Dec. 7, 1941. Nearby Diamond Head received its name from the volcanic crystals which 19th-century seamen mistook for diamonds.

HOUSTON
TEXAS

CITY LOCATION-SIZE-EXTENT. Houston, the fifth largest city in the US, the seat of Harris Co. and the fastest growing major city in the US, encompasses 556.37 sq. mi. in SE TX, 50 mi. NW of the Gulf of Mexico, at 95°22' W long. and 29°46' N lat. The incorporated area, which includes Lake Houston to the N and the canal linking it to the city, lies in three counties—Harris (549.02 sq. mi.); Ft. Bend (5.15 sq. mi.) and Montgomery (2.2 sq. mi.). The greater met. area includes the cities of Pasadena and Baytown to the E, and extends into the counties of Ft. Bend to the SW, Brazoria to the SE, Liberty to the NE, Montgomery to the N and Waller to the NW.

TOPOGRAPHY. The terrain of Houston, which is situated near the center of the Gulf Coastal Plain, is characterized by flat lands with fertile soil. The mean elev. is 49'.

Downtown Houston, Texas

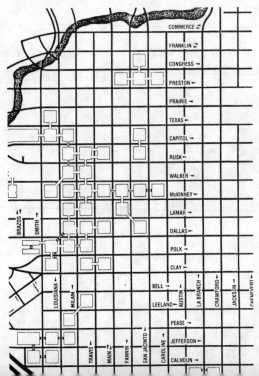

CLIMATE. The climate of Houston is humid-subtropical and marine, influenced by winds from the Gulf of Mexico and characterized by mild winters, hot, humid summers and cool summer nights. Occasional Arctic air fronts produce frost and freezing temps. during winter "blue northers". The avg. rainfall is 46.92", with nearly 50% occurring from May through Sept. The avg. annual snowfall is 0.4". Monthly mean temps. range from 50.4°F in Jan. to 82.4°F in July, with an avg. annual temp. of 67.7°F. The RH ranges from 60% to 91%. The avg. growing season is 305 days. Houston lies in the CSTZ and observes DST.

FLORA AND FAUNA. Animals native to Houston include the opossum, raccoon, deer, armadillo, squirrel and swamp rabbit. Common birds include the mockingbird (the state bird of TX), blue jay, robin, purple martin, cardinal, egret, cedar waxwing, nighthawk, goose and duck. The bullfrog, toad and the venomous coral snake, rattlesnake, copperhead and water moccasin are also found in the area. Common trees include the pecan (the state tree of TX), mulberry, china berry, hickory, pine, magnolia, live oak, palm and elm. Smaller plants are the azalea, black-eyed Susan, dewberry, blackberry, Indian paintbrush, amaryllis and bluebonnet (the state flower of TX).

POPULATION. According to the US census, the pop. of Houston in 1970 was 1,232,802. In 1978, it was estimated that it had increased 31.7% to approx. 1,632,000. The city continues to grow by approx. 70,000 each year.

ETHNIC GROUPS. In 1970, the ethnic distribution in Houston was 60.7% Caucasian, 23.8% Black and 15.5% Hispanic. Since then, many other races have moved into the area.

TRANSPORTATION. Interstate hwys. 10, 45 and 610, US hwys. 59, 75, 90 and 290 and state hwys. 3, 35, 225 and 288 provide major motor access to Houston. *Railroads* serving the city include Burlington N, Katy, MO Pacific, Rock Island, Santa Fe, S Pacific and AMTRAK. *Airlines* serving Houston Intercontinental and Hobby airports include US Air, AA, OZ, RW, TW, RP, BN, PA, TI, CO, DL, EA, NA, SW, Houston Metro, Aeromexico, Air Canada, British Caledonia, KLM, Air France, Cayman, Viasa, Alia, Royale, Rio and Chapparral. *Bus lines* serving the city are Trailways, Greyhound, Kerrville, TX and the local Houtran, part of the Met. Transit Authority (MTA). The port of Houston, the third largest seaport in the US, handled more than 100 million short tons of cargo in 1979. The port ranks second in the US in both volume and value of foreign trade.

COMMUNICATIONS. Communications, broadcasting and print media originating from Houston are: *AM radio stations* KILT 610 (Indep., Top 40); KTRH 740 (CBS, MBS. Talk); KULF 790 (Indep., MOR); KEYH 850 (Indep., Span.); KPRC 950 (NBC, APR, UPI, News, Talk); KLAT 1010 (Indep., Span.); KENR 1070 (APR, Mod. Ctry.); KNUZ 1230 (ABC/I, C&W); KXYZ 1320 (Indep., Relig.); KCOH 1430 (Mut. Blk., R&B, Jazz) and KYOK 1590 (Indep., Blk.); *FM radio stations* KUHF 88.7 (MBS, Var., Spec. Prog.); KPFT 90.1 (NPR, Var., Spec. Prog.); KLEF 94.5 (Indep., Clas.); KIKK 95.7 (Indep., C&W); KAUM 96.5 (ABC/C, Rock); KFMK 97.9 (Indep., Contemp.); KODA 99.1 (Indep., Btfl. Mus.); KILT 100 (Indep., Pop Rock); KLOL 101.1 (CBS, MBS, Progsv.); KQUE 102.9 (ABC/I, MOR); KRBE 104.1 (Indep., Top 40) and KHCB 105.7 (Indep., Relig., Spec. Progsv.); *television stations* KHOU Ch. 11 (CBS); KHTV Ch. 39 (Indep.); KPRC Ch. 2 (NBC); KRIV Ch. 26 (Metromedia); KTRH Ch. 13 (ABC) and KUHT Ch. 8 (PBS); *press:* two major dailies serve the city, the *Chronicle* and the *Post*, issued twice daily and weekends; major weeklies include the *Business Journal*, *Tribune*, *Westside Reporter*, *Jewish Herald-Voice*, *Forward Times* and the *Informer*; monthly publications include *Houston Magazine*, *Houston Home/Garden* and *Houston City Magazine.*

HISTORY. Houston was founded on August 26, 1836, when two brothers, Augustus C. and John K. Allen, paid slightly more than $1.40 per acre for 6,642 acres of land near the headwaters of Buffalo Bayou. The city was named for Gen. Sam Houston first Pres. of the Republic of TX. and commander of TX Army which had gained independence for TX from Mexico at the Battle of San Jacinto fought E of the site of the city on Apr. 21, 1836.

Part of highway system, Houston, Texas

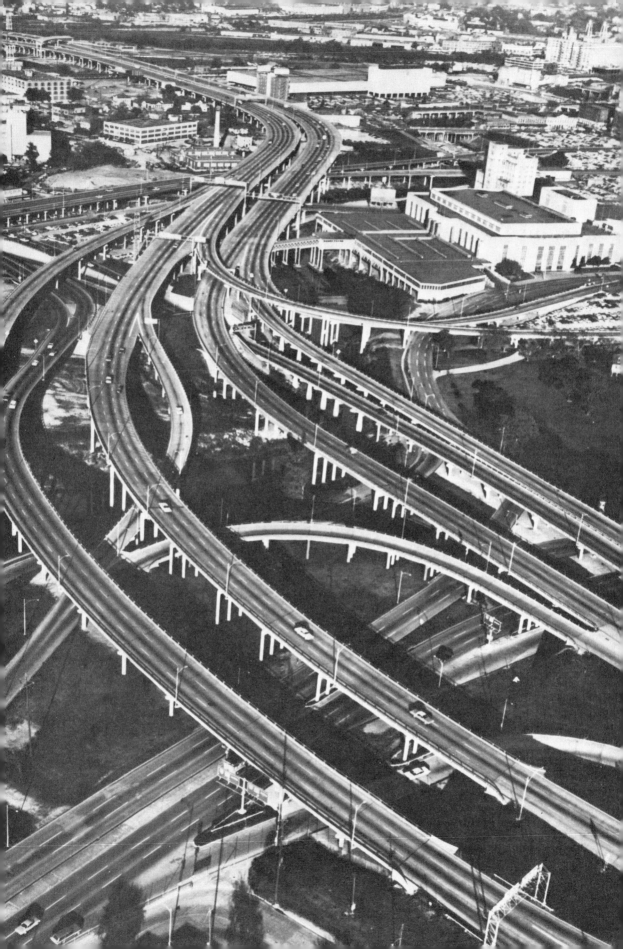

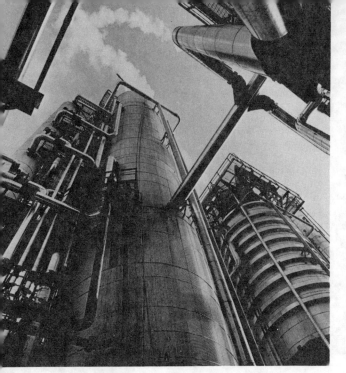

An oil refinery in Houston, Texas

Houston served as the capital of the Republic from 1837 until 1839, and received its city charter in 1839. The first RR in TX began operating in the town in 1853 and one of the first newspapers in the state was published in Harrisburg, now part of Houston. A fire in 1859 destroyed much of the city and, in 1867, a yellow fever epidemic hit the city. Transportation facilities created further growth and, by 1870, the pop. of the city stood at 9,382. The discovery of oil in SE TX at Spindletop in 1901 and the opening of the man-made Houston Ship Channel in 1914 stimulated rapid development of petroleum refining and metal fabricating in the area. In 1930, Houston replaced Dallas as the largest city in TX, with a pop. of 292,352. The manufacture of petro-chemicals on a large scale began during WW II, creating further pop. increases from 384,514 in 1940 to 938,219 in 1960. In the early 1960s, the city became a center of manned spacecraft activities, which earned it the title "Space City". During the 1970s, the city greatly expanded. Numerous major companies were established and the city pursued an active policy of annexation. Recent trends include proliferation of R&D activities and a growing prominence in intl. business.

GOVERNMENT. Houston has a mayor-council form of govt. The 14 council members and the mayor are elected to concurrent two-year terms. Nine members are elected by district, while the remaining five and the mayor, a voting member of the council, are elected at large.

ECONOMY AND INDUSTRY. Major industries in Houston include petrochemicals, chemicals, synthetic rubber, lumber products, salt recovery, metal products, R&D, engineering, space and medical technology, fertilizers, furniture, glass products, electrical machinery and equipment, transportation equipment, technical instruments, apparel and printing and publishing. Important agricultural products, which comprise 50% of the total export tonnage of the Port of Houston, include rice, nursery crops and cattle. In June, 1979, the labor force of the met. area totaled 1,401,500, while the rate of unemployment was 3.9%. In 1977, net per capita income of the met. area was $7,272.

BANKING. There are 199 commercial banks in Houston. In 1978, total deposits for the 111 banks headquartered in the city were approx. $17,171,719,000, while total assets were approx. $21,022,576,000. Banks include Bank of the SW, Houston Natl., First City Natl., Greater S W, TX Bank & Trust and TX Commerce.

HOSPITALS. The medical facilities in Houston are renowned for cancer research and treatment, heart surgery and cardiovascular disease and coronary care. The 230-acre Texas Medical Center, established in 1943, consists of 25 institutions. Major units include Baylor Col. of Medicine, Ben Taub Gen. Hosp., Hermann Hosp., Methodist Hosp., St. Luke's Episcopal Hosp., Shriners Hosp. for Crippled Children, TX Children's Hosp., TX Heart Institute, TX Institute for Rehabilitation and Research, TX Research Institute for Mental Sciences, TX Woman's U School of Nursing, U of TX Health Science Center at Houston, U of TX System Cancer Center at Houston (M. D. Anderson Hosp. and Tumor Institute) and the U of TX System School of Nursing at Houston. The largest hosp. is the V.A. facility.

EDUCATION. There are more than 25 colleges and universities in the Houston area. The publicly-supported U of Houston, the second largest university in TX, includes three major branch campuses. Established in 1927 as a jr. col., it became a four-year institution in 1934 and achieved its present status in 1963. In 1978, approx. 39,000 enrolled. Rice U, a private institution famous for science, engineering and arts programs, was established in 1891 and, in 1978, enrolled more than 3,600. TX Southern U was established in 1947 and, in 1978, enrolled approx. 9,500. Other institutions include Dominican Col., Gulf Coast Bible Col., Houston Baptist U, St. Mary's Seminary, Bates Col. of Law at U of H, S TX Col. of Law, S Bible & Jr. Col., TX Bible Col., U of St. Thomas, Baylor Col. of Medicine and UT Health Science Center. The Houston Independent School District, the seventh largest in the US, consists of 233 schools, including 170 elementary, 31 jr. high, 19 sr. high, five jr.-sr. high and eight alternative, enrolled approx. 107,000 in 1978. Approx. 30,000 are enrolled in numerous private and parochial schools. The Houston Public Lib. System, housing more than 10 million volumes, includes the Clayton Lib. for Genealogical Research, 26 branches, three bookmobiles and the Children's Carousel.

ENTERTAINMENT. There are several dinner theaters in Houston, including Marietta's, Dean Goss' and the Windmill. The Astroworld Amusement Park, located in the Astrodomain, also provides entertainment, as do such annual events as the Houston Livestock Show & Rodeo in Feb., the Westheimer Colony Arts Festival in Apr. and Oct., the Westbury Sq. Arts

The Galleria in Houston, Texas

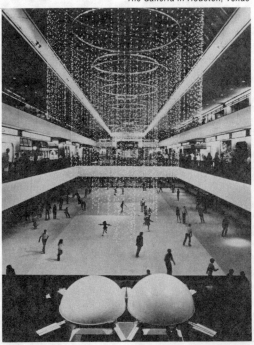

Festival, the Greek Festival and the Italian Festival, both held in Oct. Professional sports entertainment is provided by the Houston Astros, an NL baseball team, the Houston Oilers, an NFL-AFC football team, the Houston Hurricane, an NASL soccer team, the Apollos, a CHL hockey team, the Rockets, an NBA basketball team and the Angels, a WBL basketball team. The Summit Soccer Team competes in MISL soccer. Many local teams compete in intercollegiate sports, including the Rice Owls and the U of Houston Cougars of the SWC and the TSU Tigers of the SWAC.

ACCOMMODATIONS. There are numerous hotels and motels in Houston, including the Warwick, Sheraton, Galleria Plaza, Host Intl., Astro Village, Lamar, Marriott, Stouffer's and Whitehall hotels, Hyatt Regency, Houston Oaks, Shamrock Hilton, Howard Johnson's, TraveLodge and Rodeway, La Quinta, Ramada and Hilton inns.

FACILITIES. There are 271 municipal parks in Houston, encompassing more than 7,600 acres of land and 23,236 acres of water. Facilities include five 18-hole golf courses, 38 swimming pools, three tennis centers with 54 courts, 85 neighborhood tennis courts, 287 playing fields and 52 community recreational centers. Hermann Park contains a children's zoo, Museum of Natural Science, Burke Baker Planetarium, rose garden, golf course, tennis courts, picnic areas and Miller Outdoor Theatre. Golf and picnicking facilities are available at Bear Creek Park, located on land adjacent to the Addicks Reservoir. The 1,052-acre Memorial Park contains a golf course, tennis center, picnic areas, swimming pool, bridle path, playing fields and municipal greenhouse, and the 213-acre Houston Arboretum and Botanical Gardens, which contain nature trails. Eisenhower Park is located on the San Jacinto River below the Lake Houston Dam. Aline McAshan Botanical Hall contains displays of native animals and plants. Three park developments begun as part of the celebration of the US Bicentennial are Tranquillity Park in the Civic Center, the expansion of Allen's Landing Park and the transformation of Buffalo Bayou into a lineal park for outdoor activities.

CULTURAL ACTIVITIES. The Houston Symphony Society, founded in 1913, maintains a 94-member orchestra which presents a full season of concerts in Jones Hall, plus free, open-air, summer concerts at Miller Outdoor Theatre in Hermann Park. Other symphony ensembles are the Houston Civic Symphony, Houston Pops Orchestra, Houston Youth Symphony, Symphony N, Houston All-City (school) Orchestra and the orchestras of Houston Baptist U, TX Southern U and the U of Houston. The Houston Grand Opera, in addition to its regular season, presents an annual free Spring Opera Festival. Theatre Under the Stars presents free summer productions, in addition to its winter indoor season, and operates the Humphreys School of Performing Arts. Other musical groups are the Contemporary Chamber Ensemble, Houston Chamber Orchestra, Lyric Art String Quartet, Shepherd Quartet, Virtuoso Quartet, Woodwinds of Houston, Concert Choral Society of Houston, Houston Symphony Chorale, Tuesday Musical Club, American Guild of Organists—Houston Chapter, Houston Classic Guitar Society, Houston Harpsichord Society and the Music Guild. The Alley Theatre, one of the three oldest resident theaters in the US, stages an extended professional season. Other professional and amateur theatrical organizations include the Equinox Theatre, Channing Players, Hamster Theatre, Houston Shakespeare Society, the Kerygma Players, SW Theatre Guild, TX Comedy Theatre, Theatre Suburbia, Westside Theatre and area university players' groups. The Houston Ballet, founded in 1955, became a professional co. in 1969. Other dance groups are the Houston Jazz Ballet, Houston Contemporary Dance Theatre, Dance Center, Discovery Dance Group, Greater Houston Civic Ballet Co., Houston Allegro Ballet, Met. Concert Ballet Group, Royal Academy Ballet Theatre and the Space Dance Group. The

The Astrodome in Houston, Texas

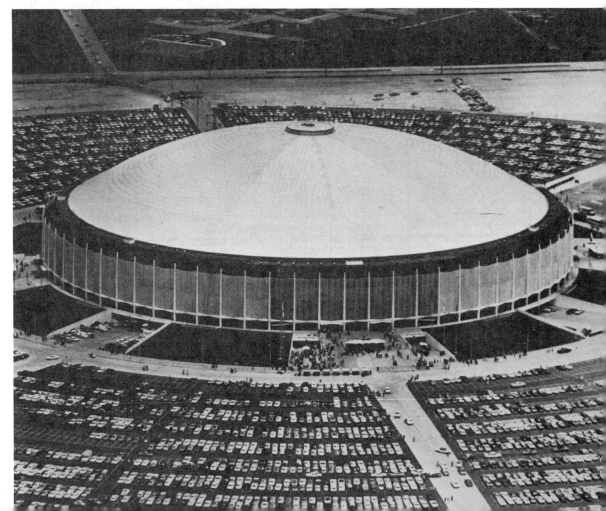

Museum of Fine Arts, including a branch at Bayou Bend, presents a series of major loan exhibitions and conducts a professional art school. Bayou Bend, formerly the Hogg family home and now a museum, features a collection of early American decorative art. The Contemporary Arts Museum exhibits modern works in various media. The Rice Museum, on the Rice U campus, and the Sarah Campbell Blaffer Gallery, at the U of Houston, feature exhibits of major intl. works. Unlike those in most other major US cities, the museums charge no admission. Other museums include the Houston Museum of Natural Science, which contains the Museum of Medical Science, and the Burke Baker Planetarium, all in Hermann Park, and the Johnson Space Center Museum, which features exhibits relating to the Mercury, Gemini and Apollo space flights.

LANDMARKS AND SIGHTSEEING SPOTS. The Astrodomain, consisting of the Astrodome, Astrohall and Astroworld Amusement Park, is a prominent tourist attraction in Houston. Other major attractions include NASA's Lyndon B. Johnson Space Center, the Port of Houston and the Houston Ship Channel, the TX Medical Center and Houston's Civic Center, which includes the Alley Theatre, Jones Hall for the Performing Arts and the Albert Thomas Convention Center, with its Space Hall of Fame. In the 21-acre Sam Houston Historical Park, located downtown, the Harris Co. Heritage and Conservation Society has restored and furnished five early Houston homes and an early church and has reconstructed the historic Long Row Building (the first row of stores in town), including a gen. store, barber shop and the first Houston lending lib.

HUNTINGTON BEACH
CALIFORNIA

CITY LOCATION-SIZE-EXTENT. Huntington Beach encompasses 27.3 sq. mi. in Orange Co. on San Pedro Bay in SW CA, eight mi. SE of Long Beach and 35 mi. SE of L.A., at 33°40' N lat. and 118°05' W long. The greater met. area extends into Seal Beach to the NW, Westminister to the N, Midway City to the NE, Fountain Valley to the E, Costa Mesa to the SE and Newport Beach to the S.
TOPOGRAPHY. The terrain of Huntington Beach, which is situated in the L.A. Basin, is relatively flat. The mts. of

Downtown Huntington Beach, California

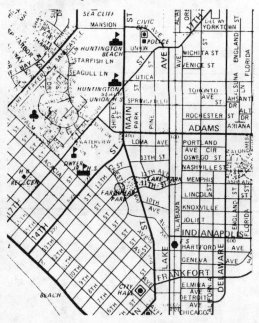

the Los Angeles Ranges lie to the N and E. The mean elev. is 35'.
CLIMATE. The climate of Huntington Beach is normally mild and pleasant throughout the year, characterized by prevailing westerlies from the Pacific Ocean. Monthly mean temps. range from 54°F in Jan. to 69°F in Aug., with an annual mean of 62°F. Most of the avg. annual precip. of 12" occurs during the winter months, with summers virtually free of rainfall. Light fog occurs throughout the year, while heavy fog occurs approx. 25% of winter days and less often during summer. The RH ranges from 55% to 87%. Huntington Beach lies in the PSTZ and observes DST.
FLORA AND FAUNA. Animals native to Huntington Beach include the pocket gopher and opossum. Typical birds are the bull, great blue heron, house finch and scrub jay. Fence lizards, skunks, gopher snakes, and tree frogs, as well as the venomous Pacific rattlesnake, are found in the area. Common trees are the pine and willow. Smaller plants include the blueblossom, CA poppy, mule fat, filaree, bulrush and wild celery.
POPULATION. According to the US census, the pop. of Huntington Beach

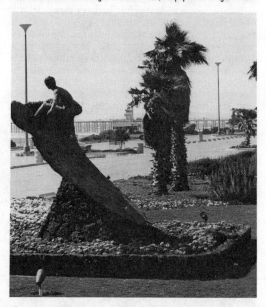

Beach Front, Huntington Beach, California

in 1970 was 115,960. In 1978, it was estimated that it had increased to approx. 164,500.
ETHNIC GROUPS. In 1978, the ethnic distribution of Huntington Beach was approx. 98.1% Caucasian, .1% Black and 8.7% Hispanic (a percentage of the Hispanic total is included in the Caucasian total).
TRANSPORTATION. Interstate hwy. 405 and state hwys. 1 and 39 provide major motor access to Huntington Beach. *Railroads* serving the city include the Santa Fe, S Pacific and Union Pacific. Los Angeles Intl., Long Beach and Orange Co. airports serve the area with flights on all major *airlines. Bus lines* serving the area include Greyhound and Trailways.
COMMUNICATIONS. Communications, broadcasting and print media originating in Huntington Beach are: no *AM* or *FM radio stations* although the city receives broadcasting from nearby L.A.; *television station* KOCE Ch. 50 (PBS); *press:* one major newspaper which serves the area, *News,* issued weekly; other publications include *Pennysaver, Branding Iron* and *New Era Laundry & Cleaning Lines.*
HISTORY. Prior to the Spanish/Mexican Rancho period which spanned from 1784 to 1849, the area of present-day Huntington Beach was inhabited by Indians. The

city is situated on a portion of the Old Los Bolas Rancho, a 3,000-acre Spanish land grant owned by Abel Sterns until the 1880s. In 1889, the town consisted of a small group of settlers. It was known as Shell Beach until 1901, when it became Pacific City. The name was changed again in 1904, to Huntington Beach, in honor of Henry E. Huntington, who sponsored the extension of the Pacific Electric RR to the seaside village. The city became a center for various religious groups, and in 1905, after a large auditorium was constructed for revivals, tents in the surrounding campgrounds led to the nickname "Tent City". Huntington Beach was incorporated in 1909 but remained small until oil was discovered in a rich field nearby in 1920. Nearly every major oil company located in the city during the resulting boom and the pop. grew from 1,500 to 5,000 in less than a month. During the years which followed, Huntington Beach was an oil production center and a truck farming market. Expansion of the city, begun in 1957 with a series of annexations, was followed by industrial expansion in the 1960s with the construction of a generating plant and the opening of a major aerospace facility. Based on commercial and industrial activity, Huntington Beach has grown from a pop. of 11,492 persons in 1960 to over 168,000 today.

GOVERNMENT. Huntington Beach has a council-mgr. form of govt. The mayor is elected by and from the council members to a four-year term, while the remaining seven council members are elected at large to four-year terms. The city administrator, appointed by the council, coordinates city depts. and carries out and recommends council policies.

ECONOMY AND INDUSTRY. Located near one of CA's largest oil fields, Huntington Beach maintains a decreasing, yet still active, oil production. The major industry is aerospace, followed by manufacturing, data and computer research and precision instruments.

BANKING. In 1978, Pacific City Bank and its branches, located in Huntington Beach, had total assets of $44,505,000 and total deposits of $41,544,000. Other banks in the area include Barclay, Crocker and Golden State.

HOSPITALS. The three hosps. located in Huntington Beach are Huntington Inter Comm., Pacific and Co. Gen.

EDUCATION. The two publicly-supported jr. colleges located in Huntington Beach are Golden W Col., which enrolled more than 19,000 in 1978, and Orange Coast Col., enrolling more than 15,000 in 1978. More than 36 elementary and five high schools serve the area. The Huntington Beach Lib. and Cultural Resource Center provides reading centers and bookmobiles.

ENTERTAINMENT. Huntington Beach has hosted a July fourth parade and celebration for approx. 75 years. It also hosts a Spring Festival. The Golden W Rustler provide intercollegiate sports entertainment.

ACCOMMODATIONS. There are several hotels and motels in Huntington Beach, including the Sun 'N Sands and Huntington Shores Motel.

Huntington Beach Pier, Huntington Beach, California.

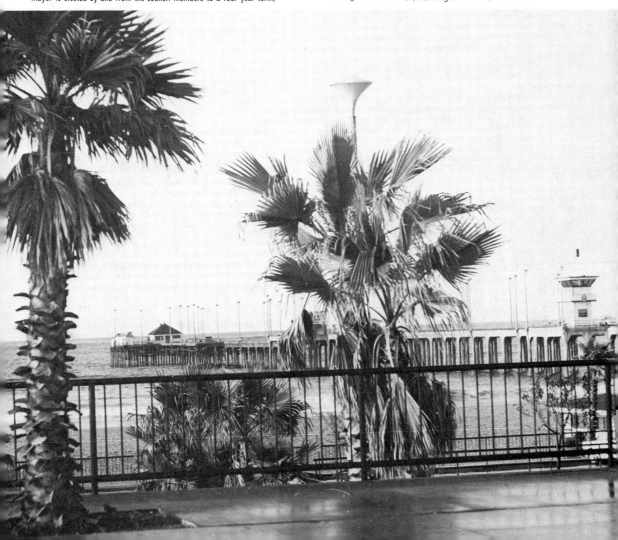

FACILITIES. The 350-acre Huntington Beach park system includes 39 parks. The largest is the 200-acre Central Park, containing Lake Huntington, Lake Talbert, a swamp area and facilities for boating, fishing, picnicking, camping and ball playing. An 18-acre nature center contains nature paths. There are two golf courses and four mi. of beaches providing sunning, surfing, fishing and swimming.

CULTURAL ACTIVITIES. Theatrical and musical performances are presented in Huntington Beach's Memorial Hall, erected in 1923. Many additional cultural events are offered in nearby L.A. and its met. area.

LANDMARKS AND SIGHTSEEING SPOTS. The Newland Historical House is Huntington Beach's most outstanding landmark. The Huntington Beach Pier, the only solid concrete pier in the US, is a focal point of the beaches and home to the US Surfing Championships.

HUNTSVILLE
ALABAMA

CITY LOCATION-SIZE-EXTENT. Huntsville, the seat of Madison Co. and largest city in the state, encompasses 113 sq. mi. at the Big Bend of the TN River in central AL, approx. 85 mi. N of Birmingham, at 34°39' N lat. and 86°46' W long. The greater met. area extends into Limestone Co. to the W, Lincoln Co., TN, to the N, Jackson Co. to the E and Marshall and Morgan counties to the S.

TOPOGRAPHY. The terrain of Huntsville, which is situated in the interior low plateau, varies from the mt. ridges of the Appalachian foothills to flat and gently rolling TN River Valley. The TN River flows seven mi. S of the city, while the Keel, Sharp and Sice mts. lie to the E and Putnam and Hale mts. lie to the NE. The mean elev. is 624'.

CLIMATE. The climate of Huntsville is temperate, characterized by complete seasonal cycles and pleasant spring and fall weather which are caused by tran-

Huntsville Municipal Building, Huntsville, Alabama

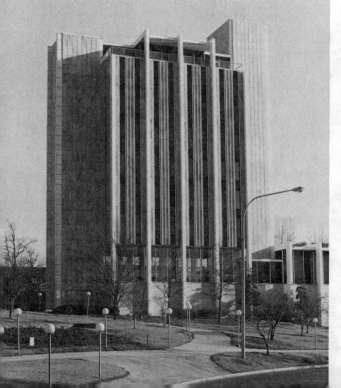

sitions between cool N air masses and more humid air movements from the Gulf of Mexico. The mean annual temp. of 60.7°F varies from a Jan. mean of 40.2°F and a July mean of 79°F. Most of the 55.7" of rainfall occurs from Dec. through March. Snowfall is negligible, though seasonal totals have reached 20". The growing season avgs. 214 days. Huntsville lies in the CSTZ and observes DST.

FLORA AND FAUNA. Animals native to Huntsville include the opossum, fox, squirrel, skunk, muskrat and whitetail deer. Common birds are the purple martin, parala warbler, red-eyed vireo, mockingbird and egret. Bullfrogs, red-ear turtles, water snakes, salamanders and green anole lizards, as well as the venomous copperhead, coral snake, cottonmouth and rattlesnake are found in the area. Common trees include the oak, elm, cedar, pine, hickory and magnolia. Smaller plants include the holly, dogwood, honeysuckle, hawthorn, morning glory and mulberry.

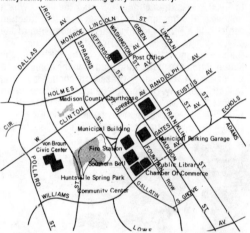

Central Huntsville, Alabama

POPULATION. According to the US census, the pop. of Huntsville in 1970 was 139,282. In 1978, it was estimated that it had increased to 143,500.

ETHNIC GROUPS. In 1978, the ethnic distribution of Huntsville was approx. 87.7% Caucasian, 12% Black and .9% Hispanic (a percentage of the Hispanic total is also included in the Caucasian total).

TRANSPORTATION. Interstate Hwy. 65, US hwys. 72, 231 and 431 and state hwys. 1, 2, 20 and 53 provide major motor access to Huntsville. *Airlines* serving Huntsville-Madison Co. Airport, the "Jetplex", include UA and SO. *Railroads* serving the city include the Louisville & Nashville and the S Railway System. Among the *bus lines* serving the city is Trailways. Water transportation is available on the 30' TN River channel. Access to the pt. of Mobile will be available upon the completion of the TN-Tombigbee Waterway.

COMMUNICATIONS. Communications, broadcasting and print media originating from Huntsville are: *AM radio stations* WVOV 1000 (ABC/C, C&W); WBHP 1230 (ABC/I, C&W); WFIX 1450 (CBS, MOR); WAAY 1550 (Indep., Top 40); WEUP 1600 (Mut. Blk.); *FM radio stations* WLRH 89.3 (NPR, Clas., Jazz, Talk); WNDA 95.1 (MBS, Sacred Mus., Sports, Clas.); WRSA 96.9 (Easy Lis.) and WAHR 99.1 (ABC/FM, Btfl. Mus.); *television stations* WHNT Ch. 19 (CBS); WHIQ Ch. 25 (PBS); WAAY Ch. 31 (NBC) and WYUR Ch. 48 (ABC); *press*: two major dailies serve the area, the evening *Times*, and the morning *News*; other publications include the *Madison Co. Record.*

HISTORY. The "Big Spring" area, now the center of downtown Huntsville, served as the sacred meeting place of native Americans of the Choctaw and Chickasaw nation before the first white settlers arrived. In 1805, John Hunt erected a cabin near the "Big Spring" area, thereby establishing the first English-speaking comm. in what is now the state of AL. It became the co. seat in

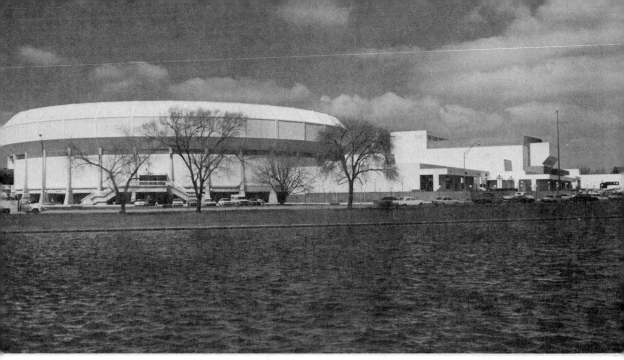

Von Braun Civic Center, Huntsville, Alabama

1810. Originally known as Twickenham, the city was renamed Huntsville after founder Hunt in 1811. The city experienced such a rapid pop. increase that in 1811 the public land office was moved from Nashville to Huntsville and the city became the state's first incorporated town. The following year a newspaper was established and numerous stores were built around the public square. In 1819, the state's first constitutional convention and legislature met in the city. Huntsville was the state's leading cotton market during the early 1800s and the manufacture of flour, shoes, lumber, copper stills and pumps also contributed to its growth. During the Civil War, Huntsville was occupied by Union troops in Apr., 1862, recaptured by Confed. troops in Sept., 1862, and again occupied by Union troops from July, 1863, until the end of the war. Though it sustained considerable damage during the Civil War, Huntsville again prospered as an agricultural center after the war, and was, by 1900, a thriving textile center. Local industry expanded during WW I, but declined during the Great Depression. Before WW II, the federal govt. constructed the Huntsville and Redstone Arsenals for the manufacture of chemical artillery shells. At the peak of WW II production, these arsenals employed approx. 20,000. In 1950, the Army transferred its small group of missile experts, including Dr. Werner von Braun, to Huntsville. After the successful launching of a Jupiter C missile in 1958, the entire US Army Missile Development and Training Program and NASA's Space Vehicle Center were established in the city. The city began annexations of most of the surrounding area and, by 1976, the city limits increased to 112.7 sq. mi. Today, Huntsville is a major commercial center and the state's largest city.

GOVERNMENT. Huntsville has a mayor-council form of govt. The mayor, not a voting council member, and the five council members are elected by the voters at large to four-year terms. The mayor has veto power on ordinances and resolutions passed by the council, although a two-thirds majority of the council can override a veto.

ECONOMY AND INDUSTRY. Major manufactures produced in Huntsville are abrasives, electronic equipment, farm implements, shoes and textiles. The Redstone Arsenal conducts US Army guided missile research and the Natl. Aeronautics and Space Administration operates its Space Flight Center in the area. The median household income of the city was $17,730 in 1978, while the avg. per capita income of $6,295 ranked second in the state. The total labor force for the met. area in June, 1979, was 140,400, while the rate of unemployment was 8.9%.

BANKING. There are six banking institutions in Huntsville. In 1978, total deposits for the five banks headquartered in the city were $386,959,000, while assets were $433,015,000. Banks include First AL, Henderson Natl., Bank of Huntsville, American Natl. and Peoples Natl.

HOSPITALS. There are four hosps. in Huntsville, including Huntsville, Crestwood, Medical Center and the military hosp. at Redstone Arsenal. The U of AL at Huntsville School of Primary Medical Care provides outpatient care.

EDUCATION. AL Agricultural and Mechanical U, located in Normal (which is adjacent to Huntsville), is a coeducational land-grant institution which offers bachelor, master and specialist degrees. A modern Learning Resource Center serves as a lib. and instructional media center for the U and is open to the public. In 1978, the U enrolled more than 4,600. The U of AL in Huntsville, state controlled and established as a branch campus of the U of AL in 1950, awards bachelor, master and doctorate degrees. It is the youngest campus in the U of AL's system. The 1978 enrollment was approx. 4,000. Oakwood Col., a private Seventh-Day Adventist institution established in 1896, awards bachelor degrees. It enrolled more than 1,300 in 1978. Other institutions include Drake State Technical Col. and N AL Col. of Commerce. There are five sr. high, eight middle and 25 elementary school and six special centers in Huntsville, with a total enrollment of approx. 29,500 in 1978. Five private and parochial schools also serve the city. Lib. facilities include the Huntsville-Madison Co. Public Lib., with four branches and two bookmobiles and serving as headquarters for the N AL Cooperative Lib. System; the Huntsville Heritage and Zeitler Rooms, containing materials on genealogy and local S and Civil War history; Redstone Scientific Information Center, administered jointly by the Army and NASA; and the U of AL in Huntsville and Oakwood Col. libs.

ENTERTAINMENT. Annual events in Huntsville include the Spring Arts and Crafts show and the "Pops in the Park" concert in May, the Arts-in-the-Park outdoor festival in June and Fine Arts Week in Apr. The U of AL-Huntsville Chargers and the AL A&M Bulldogs participate in intercollegiate sports.

ACCOMMODATIONS. There are several hotels and motels in Huntsville, including the Sheraton and Best Western Sands hotels and the Hilton, Ramada, Holiday and Century inns.

FACILITIES. There are twelve city parks in Huntsville, including Big Spring Intl., Constitution Hall and Brahan Spring. Brahan Spring Park facilities include tennis courts, two lagoons, several baseball fields, playgrounds and picnic grounds and the Huntsville Natatorium indoor olympic size pool, which is equipped with two three-meter and two one-meter diving boards. The 2,140-acre Monte Sano State Park, most of which lies within city limits, contains picnicking and camping areas and hiking trails. Big Spring Intl. Park features flowers, trees and memorabilia donated to the city by foreign countries. There are two municipal golf courses and 72 municipal tennis courts in the city.

CULTURAL ACTIVITIES. There are approx. 27 performing and participating cultural organizations in Huntsville, including the Youth Orchestra, Comm. Ballet Assn., Fantasy Children's Playhouse, Symphony Orchestra, Comm. Concert Assn., Broadway Theatre League, Assn. of Folk Musicians, Classical Guitar Society, Huntsville Concert Band and Huntsville Little Theatre (one of the nation's oldest Little Theatre groups). In addition, the U of AL in Huntsville, AL A&M U and Oakwood Col. present a variety of cultural presentations. Located in the Von Braun Civic Center, the Huntsville Museum of Art contains exhibition galleries. Atop Monte Sano Mt. is the Burritt Museum, which contains historical items, silver and china, paintings, artifacts and gems. A pioneer homestead has been restored on the grounds. The Depot Museum is planned to contain exhibits related to transportation in Madison Co.

LANDMARKS AND SIGHTSEEING SPOTS. The Twickenberry Historic District, in downtown Huntsville, features antebellum houses, many of which are still occupied by descendants of the original owners. The district is listed on the Natl. Register of Historic Sites. Constitutional Hall Park marks the site where the first state constitutional convention met and where AL was signed into the US in 1819. AL Space and Rocket Center has the world's largest collection of space-related memorabilia. Huntsville's Von Braun Civic Center is a multi-purpose entertainment, convention and sports complex named in honor of Werner von Braun, the "father of modern aeronautics".

INDEPENDENCE
MISSOURI

CITY LOCATION-SIZE-EXTENT. Independence, the seat of Jackson Co., encompasses 67.5 sq. mi. S of the MO River, adjacent to the E border of KC in W central MO, at 39°5.6' N lat. and 94°25' W long. Its met. area is part of the KC greater met. area, and extends E into Lafayette Co.

TOPOGRAPHY. The terrain of Independence, which is situated in the W plains region of MO, varies from flat to gently rolling. The Little Blue River forms part of the city's SE boundary. The elev. is 900'.

CLIMATE. The climate of Independence is continental. The avg. annual temp. of 56°F ranges from monthly means of 29°F during Jan. to 80°F during July. The 37" avg. annual rainfall occurs mainly during the warmer months. The annual avg. snowfall is 20". The RH ranges from 50% to 85%. The avg. growing season is approx. 200 days. Independence lies in the CSTZ and observes DST.

FLORA AND FAUNA. Animals native to Independence include the coyote, fox, opossum, raccoon and whitetail deer. Common birds include the crow, blue jay, catbird, bluebird (the state bird) and cardinal. The bullfrog, snapping turtle, tiger salamander, mudpuppy, red milk snake and the venomous rattlesnake, copperhead and cottonmouth are also found in the area. Typical trees are the oak, dogwood (the state tree), sycamore, elm and E red cedar. Smaller plants include hawthorn (the state flower), foxtail and honeysuckle.

POPULATION. According to the US census, the pop. of Independence in

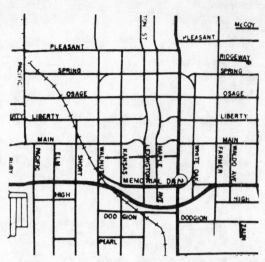

Central Independence, Missouri.

1970 was 111,630. In 1978, it was estimated that it had decreased to approx. 109,700.

ETHNIC GROUPS. In 1978, the ethnic distribution of Independence was approx. 99.1% Caucasian 0.6% Black and 0.9% Hispanic (a percentage of the Hispanic total is also included in the Caucasian total).

TRANSPORTATION. Interstate hwys. 29, 35, 70 and 435, US hwys. 24 and 40 and state hwys 12, 78 and 291 provide major motor access to Independence. *Railroads* serving the city include AMTRAK, IL Central & Gulf, MO Pacific and Santa Fe. All major *airlines* serve nearby KC Intl. Airport. Additional airport facilities are Independence Municipal Airfield and KC Downtown Airport. *Bus lines* serving the city include Greyhound and the local Area Transportation Authority.

COMMUNICATIONS. Communications, broadcasting and print media originating in Independence are: *AM radio station* KCCV 1510 (Indep., Relig.); no *FM radio stations* or *television stations* originate from Independence which receives broadcasting from neighboring KC; *press*: one major daily serves the city, the evening *Examiner*, other publications include the bi-monthly *Doll Talk* and the monthly *Saints' Herald*.

HISTORY. Native Americans of the Osage tribe inhabited the area of present-day Independence when the Lewis and Clark Expedition, sent out by Pres. Jefferson as a frontier defense and trading party, established Ft. Osage approx. 15 mi. E of the present city site. In 1825, the Osage tribe ceded the land by treaty and the ft. was abandoned. Jackson Co. was created in 1826 by the MO Gen. Assembly and 240 acres of high land were chosen as the co. seat and named "Independence", after one of the chief character traits of Gen. Andrew Jackson. The first town lots were sold in 1827. However, for the next 22 years the town had no municipal govt. and was controlled by the co. court. Independence prospered in the early years. Trade increased so that two river ports, the Upper (Wayne City) and lower (Blue Mills) landings were developed. Independence was the take-off point for the Santa Fe Trail and, soon after 1830, the OR and CA Trails. The wealth and the frontier lifestyle of Independence gave it a wild reputation, causing Joseph Smith, Jr., founder and prophet of the Mormon Church, to send three missionaries from Kurtland, OH, in 1831. The "Comm. of Zion" of the Mormons didn't materialize. Instead, in the ensuing "Mormon War", the Mormons were driven out of Independence in 1832. Tales of wealth and excitement continued to attract artists and adventurers from the E and Europe, including such figures as Washington Irving and Count Albert-Alexander de Pourtales, who left Independence for OK in 1832. The city was incorporated in 1849. In the spring of the same year, a cholera epidemic ravaged the city. As more stable families, businesses and churches moved into the city, Independence began to shed its "Wild West" image. The first mayor, William McCoy, was elected in 1849. The first incorporated RR W of the MS linked Independence to its Upper Landing in 1849, signaling the end of the trail business in Independence. The Civil War brought hard times to the area as pro N and pro S sympathizers engaged in guerrilla raids against each other. In order to stop this, Gen. Ewing issued Order Number 11, which involved the jailing of the wives and female relatives of suspected raiders, to pressure the men to give themselves up. Later, after the Civil War, young men like Frank and Jesse James, who had ridden with Quantrill's raiders, roamed through the area robbing trains. Independence contributed two full batteries to the war effort during WW I. Bootlegging flourished in the 1920s, but not at the expense of legitimate business. Harry Truman, "the man from Independence", became the 33rd Pres. of the US In 1945. Independence is the world headquarters of the Reorganized Church of Christ of the Latter-day Saints.

GOVERNMENT. Independence has a council-mgr. form of govt. consisting of six council members and the mayor, a voting member of the council. The mayor and two council members are elected at large, and four are elected by district, all to four-year terms. The council appoints the city mgr.

ECONOMY AND INDUSTRY. Major manufactured products in Independence are small-arms ammunition, harves-ting combines, food products and refined oil. In 1977, the labor force in the city totaled 54,887 and the unemployment rate was 3.9%.

BANKING. There are nine banks and eight savings and loan assns. in Independence. In 1978, total deposits for the seven banks headquartered in the city were $227,835,000, while assets were $273,778,000. Banks include First Natl. of Independence, Noland Road Mercantile, Standard State, Bank of Independence, Chrisman Sawyer, Commerce and Hub State.

HOSPITALS. There are two hosps. in Independence—the Medical Center and the Sanitarium and Hosp.

EDUCATION. Many of the institutions of higher education available to residents of Independence are in neighboring KC. The Truman Campus of the U of MO-KC is located in Independence and offers fully-accredited evening and day classes. The city's public school system consists of 15 elementary, three jr. high and two sr. high schools and enrolled approx. 13,800 students in 1978. Lib. facilities are provided by the Mid-Continent Public and the Harry S. Truman libs.

ENTERTAINMENT. The most important annual event in Independence is the Santa-Cali-Gon Festival, held on Labor Day Weekend, to celebrate the three trails to the W and deriving its name from the trail names Santa Fe, CA and OR. The Festivale Intl., which will begin in May, 1980, in honor of the many nationalities in the area, will feature entertainment, food, crafts and displays. Harry Truman's Birthday, a week-long celebration in May, features the presentation of the Harry S. Truman Public Service Award. A children's Halloween Parade is held each Oct. Collegiate and professional sports are available in neighboring KC.

ACCOMMODATIONS. There are a number of hotels and motels in Independence, including Howard Johnson's and the Ramada and Red Roof inns.

FACILITIES. There are several parks and playgrounds in Independence, including Mill Creek, Charles Richard Long and McCoy parks, featuring facilities for baseball, basketball, football, tennis, golf, swimming and

Truman Library, Independence, Missouri

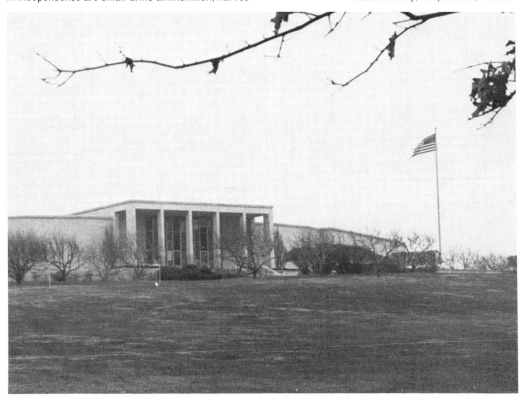

handball. In addition, a public golf course is available at the Chapel Woods Golf Club. The city maintains a Sr. Citizens' Recreation Center.

CULTURAL ACTIVITIES. The Comm. Arts Assn. in Independence formulates artistic events in the city. The museum attached to the Harry S. Truman Lib. houses a replica of Truman's office in the White House and exhibits on the history of the Presidency.

LANDMARKS AND SIGHTSEEING SPOTS. The Truman gravesite is in the courtyard of the Harry S. Truman Lib. and Museum in Independence. There are a number of vintage homes in the city, including the Samuel Woodson House, built in 1866, during the wave of prosperity following the Civil War; the Overfelt-Johnson Home, one of the oldest of the Civil War era where Civil War bullets are still evident in the walls; the Waggoner-Gates estate, once the residence of Caleb Bingham, the painter of "Fur Traders Descending the MO". The Harry S. Truman Historic District reflects different architectural styles in houses in the area where Pres. Truman grew up. The present Jackson Co. Courthouse is a replica of "Independence Hall" in Philadelphia. The restored old Co. Jail House in the late fed. style of architecture, dates back to 1859. Among the more famous inmates of the jail were William Quantrill, Cole Younger and Frank James. The Truman "Summer White House", an 1867 building, served as the Summer WhiteHouse from 1945-1952. Other landmarks include the Church of Christ Temple Lot, dedicated by Joseph Smith, Jr., as site for the temple in the City of Zion, and the Reorganized Church of Jesus Christ of Latter-day Saints Auditorium whose large pipe organ provides daily recitals. Ft. Osage, the first US military outpost in the LA Purchase, is 14 mi. NE, near Old Sibley.

INDIANAPOLIS
INDIANA

CITY LOCATION-SIZE-EXTENT. Indianapolis, the largest city in the state, the largest state capital in the US and the seat of Marion Co., encompasses 379.4 sq. mi. at the NW fork of the White River in central IN at 39°44' N lat. and 86°16' W long. The greater met. area extends into the counties of Boone to the NW, Hamilton to the N, Hancock to the E, Shelby to the SE, Johnson to the S, Morgan to the SW and Hendricks to the W.

TOPOGRAPHY. The terrain of Indianapolis, which is situated in the Till Plain region, slopes gradually toward the White River. The White River runs through the W portion of the city and Little Eagle, Big Eagle and Crooked Creeks join the river from the W. Eagle Creek Reservoir lies in the NW portion of the city. The mean elev. is 792'.

CLIMATE. Indianapolis has a continental climate, characterized by warm summers, moderately cold winters and occasional wide variations in temps., especially during the colder months. The annual avg. temp of 52.6°F ranges from monthly means of 28.2°F in Jan. to 75.7°F in July. The annual avg. rainfall of 39.94" is fairly well distributed throughout the year. Most of the annual 22" of snowfall occurs from Dec. through Mar. The RH ranges from 60% to 91%. The avg. growing season is approx. 183 days. Indianapolis lies in the ESTZ and does not observe DST.

FLORA AND FAUNA. Animals native to Indianapolis include the chipmunk, raccoon and opossum. Common birds include the blue jay, bobwhite, meadowlark, cardinal, mockingbird and house wren. The American toad, gray tree frog, cricket frog, tiger salamander, box turtles, hognose snake and the venomous copperhead, timber rattlesnake and E massasauga (a pygmy rattler) are also found in the area. Typical trees include the poplar, oak, elm and maple. Smaller plants include the honeysuckle, peony, bluots, milkweed and purple coneflower.

POPULATION. According to the US census, the pop. of Indianapolis in 1970 was 742,925. In 1978, it was estimated that it had decreased to approx. 720,000. Indianapolis is the 11th most populous city in the US.

ETHNIC GROUPS. In 1978, the ethnic distribution of Indianapolis was approx. 81.6% Causian, 16.9% Black and .8% Hispanic.

TRANSPORTATION. Interstate hwys. 05, 69, 70, 74 and 465, US hwys. 31, 36, 40, 52 and 136 and state hwys. 37, 67, 135 and 431 provide major motor access to Indianapolis. *Railroads* serving the city incluide Baltimore & OH, Chessie System, Chicago & NW, ConRail, IA Central Gulf, Milwaukee Road, Norfolk & W, Santa Fe, Union Pacific and AMTRAK. *Airlines* include AA, US Air, DL, EA, OZ and TW. Eagle Creek Airpark provides facilities for private aircraft. *Bus lines* serving the city include Greyhound, Trailways and the local Metro Transit.

COMMUNICATIONS. Communications, broadcasting and print media originating from Indianapolis are: *AM radio stations* WATI 810 (Indep., Btfl. Mus.); WXLW 950 (CBS, MOR); WIBC 1070 (APR, MOR); WNDE 1260 (ABC/C, Top 40); WIFE 1310 (Indep., MOR); WIRE 1430 (ABC/E, C&W); WBRI 1500 (UPI, Relig.) and WNTS 1590 (ABC/I, Relig.); *FM radio stations* WICR 88.7 (Indep., Educ., Rock, MOR); WJEL 89.3 (ABC/C, Educ., Top 40) WIAN 90.1 (NPR, Clas., Talk, Educ., Jazz); WEDM 91.1 (UPI, Noncom., Divers.); WRFT 91.5 (Indep., Educ); WBDG 90.9 (NPR, Educ., MOR); WNAP 93.1 (Indep., Top 40); WFBQ 94.7 (ABC/FM, Progsv.); WFMS 95.5 (NBC, Mod. Ctry.); WAJC 104.5 (MBS, Var.); WTLC 105.7 (Indep., Blk.) and WXTZ 103.3 (Indep., Btfl. Mus.); *television stations* WTTV Ch. 4 (Indep.); WRTV Ch. 6 (ABC); WISH Ch. 8 (CBS); WTHR Ch. 13 (NBC); WFYI Ch. 20 (PBS) and WHMB Ch. 40 (Indep.); *press:* three major daily newspapers are published in the city, the morning *Star*, the evening *News* and the *Commercial*, a weekday publication; other publications include the weekly *Topics Newspaper, E Side Herald, N Jewish Post & Opinion, Speedway Edition, Journal, NE Reporter, Westside Enterprise, NW Press, Criterion* and *Spotlight*, and the monthly *IN Rural News, AAU News, Baptist Observer, Buckeye Trucker, Child Life* and *Children's Playmate Magazine.*

HISTORY. Native Americans of the Delaware tribe inhabited the area of present-day Indianapolis when George Pogue and his family, the first white settlers, arrived in the spring of 1820. The Pogues settled at the Fall Creek-White River junction, several mi. S of a trading post

Central Indianapolis, Indiana

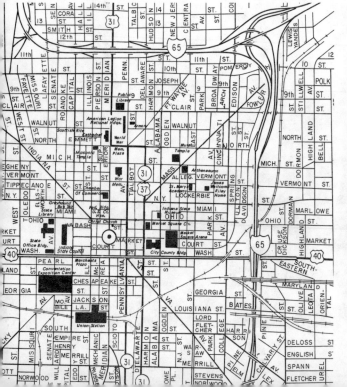

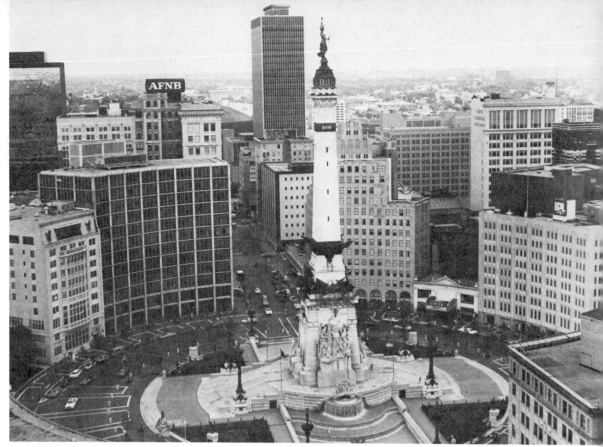

Monument Circle in the center of Indianapolis, Indiana

that had been established by William Conner. More settlers began to arrive from small IN towns such as Andersontown. In the summer of 1820, a state commission selected the settlement as the site of the state capital because of its central location and in the mistaken belief that the White River was navigable. The name Indianapolis was suggested by Supreme Court Judge Jeremiah Sullivan and to Alexander Ralston, one of the assistants of Maj. L'Enfant, who helped plan Washington, DC, and designed the city. The town's first newspaper, the *Gazette*, began publication in 1822. In 1825 the capitol was constructed and the legislature moved to Indianapolis from Corydon, the temporary capital. In 1830, the Natl. Road (now US hwy. 40) reached the town, and its economy and pop. began to grow. By 1830, the pop. approached 1,100. Indianapolis was incorporated as a town in 1836, the same year that German and Irish immigrants began arriving to build the Indianapolis to Broad Ripple Canal which helped encourage industrial growth in the town. Although the canal itself was a failure, growth continued with the arrival of the RR in 1847, and Indianapolis received a city charter the same year. Seven other RRs arrived in the city, and the first Union RR station was opened in 1853. By the time the Civil War began, there were more than 100 manufacturing and industrial companies in the city. Between 1863 and 1873, rapid growth and expansion occurred, due to the installation of the first streetcars. The Indianapolis Stockyards and the Belt RR both were established in 1877, and the discovery nearby of natural gas in the 1880s contributed to further growth. By the early 1900s, the city had become a farm market and the center of the automobile industry. In 1909, the Indianapolis Speedway was built to test-drive automobiles and, in 1911, the first Indy 500 (mi.) race was held. About 1820, Detroit began to replace the city as the leading producer of auto-

mobiles, and by 1937, the manufacture of cars in Indianapolis had ended. The transportation equipment industry, however, expanded before WW II, and, during the war, provided parts for military vehicles. During the same decade, the W Electric Co. built a telephone manufacutring plant in the city, which continued to grow throughout the 1950s and 1960s. The boundaries of the city, which serves as a chief Midwest center of manufacturing, transportation and distribution, now extend throughout much of Marion Co., due to city and co. consolidation effected in 1970.

GOVERNMENT. Indianapolis has a unique, natl. recognized consolidated city and co. met. govt. consisting of a 29-member city-co. council. The mayor, who is not a voting member of council, and four council members are elected at large, while 25 council members are elected by district. All serve four-year terms.

ECONOMY AND INDUSTRY. There are about 1,450 manufacturing firms in the Indianapolis met. area. The manufacture of transportation equipment and automotive parts and bodies is the chief industry, and the city is the world leader in telephone production. Other major products include chemicals, electrical and non-electrical machinery, electronic components, fabricated and primary metals and food products. Printing and publishing and distribution are all major industries. Approx. 15% of the area workforce is employed by govt. agencies. In June, 1979, the total labor force of the met. area was approx. 599,000, and the rate of unemployment was 5.3%. Avg. per capita income in 1977 was $6,404 and median household income was $17,084. Indianapolis consistently ranks among the top five cities in the US in median family income.

BANKING. There are 10 savings and loan assns. in Indianapolis and six banks in Marion Co. In 1978, total deposits at the five banks headquartered in the city were approx. $4,301,157,000, while assets totaled $6,080,556,000.

Banks include American Fletcher Natl. Bank & Trust, First Natl. Bank & Trust, IN Natl., Merchants Natl. Bank & Trust, Midwest Natl. and Peoples Bank & Trust.

HOSPITALS. There are 10 hosps. in Indianapolis including Comm., IN U hosps. (James Whitcomb Riley and R. W. Long), LaRue Carter Memorial, Methodist, St. Vincent's, U Heights, Westview Osteopathic, Wm. W. Wishart Memorial, Winona Memorial, V.A. and Central State.

EDUCATION. IN U-Purdue U Center at Indianapolis, is a publicly supported institution created by their respective boards of trustees awarding degrees ranging from associate to grad./professional, including medical. In 1978, approx. 21,700 enrolled. IN Central U, privately supported and one of three United Methodist Church institutions in the state, offers programs leading to associate, bachelor and master degrees and enrolled approx. 3,350 in 1978. Other institutions in the city include Butler U, Marion, Porter and IN Business cols., Jordan Col. of Art and the Christian Theological Seminary. The public school system, consisting of approx. 175 elementary and 18 high schools, enrolled more than 165,000 in 1978. There are 65 private and parochial schools in Marion Col., enrolling approx. 23,000. The Indianapolis-Marion Col. Public Lib. system consists of a central lib. and approx. 20 branches. The State Lib. and Historical Bldg. in the city specializes in IN history.

ENTERTAINMENT. Among the dinner theaters in Indianapolis are the Beef and Boards and Black Curtain. The most famous annual event held in Indianapolis is the 500 mi. Indy 500 automobile race, held during the Memorial Day weekend at the Motor Speedway and attended by over 300,000 people. The month-long 500 Festival, instituted nearly 30 years ago to celebrate the race, includes many comm.-wide events and is highlighted by the Festival Memorial Parade. Annual events held at the IN State Fairgrounds include the Indianapolis Auto Show in Dec. and Jan., the Indianapolis Home Show and the Custom Auto Show in Feb., the IN Flower and Patio Shows in Mar., the Hoosier Antiques Expositions in Mar., June and Sept., antique shows in Apr. and Oct., the IN State Fair in Aug., the Hoosier "100" Auto Race in Sept., and the Hobby and Gift Show in Nov. Professional sports entertainment is provided by the IN Pacers, an NBA basketball team, an AAA League farm club of the Cincinnati Reds baseball team, and the Checkers, a CHL hockey team. Collegiate sports are provided by the IN U-Purdue U-Indianapolis Metros. Tyndall Armory hosts professional boxing, and harness racing is held at the IN State fairgrounds.

ACCOMMODATIONS. There are numerous hotels and motels in Indianapolis, including the Atkinson, Best Westerns, Marten House, Howard Johnson's, Hyatt Regency and the Marriott, Ramada, Days and Hilton inns.

FACILITIES. There are 187 parks in the Indianapolis park system, encompassing 11,000 acres. The 4,900-acre Eagle Creek Reservoir, the largest municipally-owned lake and park in the US, contains facilities for boating and other water sports, as well as golfcourses and hiking and jogging trails. Other parks are Coffin, Douglas, Pleasant Run, Riverside, S Grover, Broad Ripple and N Eastway. The Indianapolis Zoological Park, located in George Washington Park, includes a children's zoo. The park dept. maintains more than 300 specialized facilities, including more than 100 tennis courts, 155 playing fields, 17 swimming pools and 11 public golf courses. Watersports facilities are also available at Geist Reservoir and Morse Reservoir.

CULTURAL ACTIVITIES. The Showalter Pavilion features the Indianapolis Ballet Theatre, while Broadway shows and touring ballet groups perform at Clowes Memorial Hall. The IN Repertory Theatre presents a season of drama from Oct. to Apr. The Philharmonic Orchestra of IN gives three subscription concerts annually at Marion Col. Other performing arts groups are the Athenaeum Players, Footlight Musicals and the Christian Theological Seminary Repertory Theatre. Art spanning 4,000 years is displayed at the Indianapolis Museum of Art which features Oriental art, 17th century Flemish and Dutch paintings, 18th century French, English and Italian decorative arts and 19th century British and American paintings. The IN State Museum features displays of natural history and paintings by IN artists. The Museum of IN Heritage features exhibits of the cultures of various native American tribes, while the Children's Museum contains displays of natural history, pioneer life, science and transportation.

LANDMARKS AND SIGHTSEEING SPOTS. The Benjamin Harrison

Memorial Home, erected in Indianapolis in 1872, has been restored as a natl. shrine of the 23rd Pres. of the US (1889-93) and features family artifacts and furniture. The Carmelite Monastery, which resembles a medieval castle, and the home of poet James Whitcomb Riley are also located in the city. Other landmarks are the 285 Soldiers and Sailors Monument and the IN World War Memorial. The James Irving Holcomb Observatory and Planetarium on the campus of Butler U houses the largest telescope in the state, while the Scottish Rite Cathedral, a Gothic building, contains a carillon of 54 bells. The IN State Capitol, completed in 1878, is constructed of IN limestone.

IRVING
TEXAS

CITY LOCATION-SIZE-EXTENT. Irving, located in Dallas Co. in N central TX, 8 mi. W of Dallas, is 28 mi. E of Ft. Worth and 250 mi. N of the Gulf of Mexico, and encompasses 63 sq. mi. at 32°48.8' N lat. and 96°56.2' W long.

TOPOGRAPHY. The terrain of Irving, situated on the upper margin of the Gulf Coastal Plains region, near the headwaters of the Trinity River, consists of rolling hills Mountain Lake is S of Irving. The area is rich in petroleum deposits. The elev. ranges from 400' to 800' with a mean elev. of 470'.

CLIMATE. The climate of Irving is humid subtropical and continental, characterized by long, hot summers and relatively short, mild winters, with wide variations in weather conditions from season to season. "Northers" occur about three times each winter month and are often accompanied by sudden drops in temp., but the occasional periods of extreme cold are short-lived. The avg. annual temp. of 66°F ranges from a Jan. mean of 45°F to a July and Aug. mean of 85°F. The avg. annual rainfall of approx. 30" varies seasonally from as low as 20" to as high as 50", and occurs most frequently during the night. Most of the rainfall is from spring thunderstorms. The avg. annual snowfall is a scant 3.5" with an avg. of only one measurable fall occurring annually. The RH ranges from 45% to 88%.

Irving, Texas

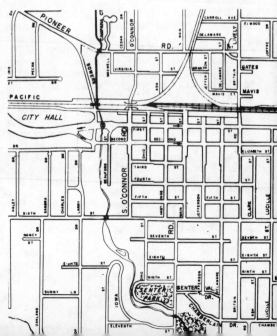

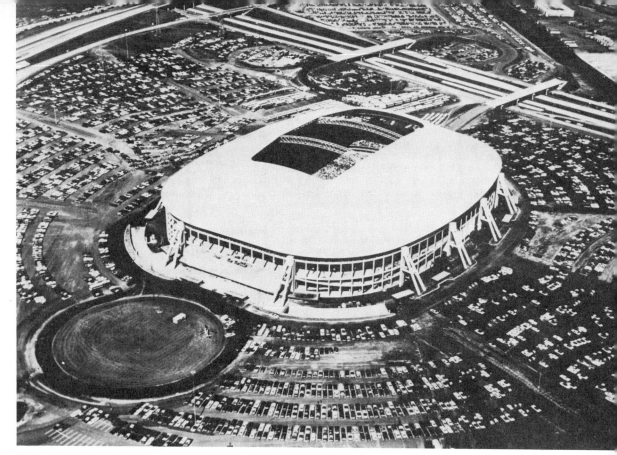

Texas Stadium, home of the Dallas Cowboys, Irving, Texas

The growing season is approx. 250 days. Irving lies in the CSTZ and observes DST.

FLORA AND FAUNA. Animals native to Irving include the opossum, armadillo, whitetail deer and coyote. Common birds are the mockingbird (the state bird), scissortail flycatcher, cardinal, grackle, crow and meadowlark. King snakes, bullsnakes, box turtles and toads, as well as the venomous copperhead, cottonmouth, coral snake and rattlesnake, are found in the area. Typical trees are the oak, cedar and elm. Smaller plants include the bluebonnet (the state flower), paintbrush, aster and primrose.

POPULATION. According to the US census, the pop. of Irving in 1970 was 98,961. In 1978, it was estimated that it had increased to 107,000.

ETHNIC GROUPS. In 1978, the ethnic distribution of Irving was approx. 98.5% Caucasian, 0.9% Black and 4.4% Hispanic (a percentage of the Hispanic total is also included in the total Caucasian total).

TRANSPORTATION. Interstate Hwy. 30 (Dallas-Fort Worth Turnpike), US Hwy. 77 and state hwys. 114, 183 and 356 provide major motor access to Irving. *Railroads* serving the city include the Frisco and Rock Island. All major *airlines* serve the Dallas-Fort Worth Regional Airport in Irving, including TI, PA, OZ, BN, AA, RD and CO, while Love Field in nearby Dallas offers private plane facilities. *Bus lines* serving the city include Trailways and Greyhound.

COMMUNICATIONS. Communications, broadcasting and print media originating from Irving are: no *AM radio stations*, *FM radio stations* or *television stations* originate from Irving, which receives broadcasting from nearby Dallas and Ft. Worth; *press*: one major daily serves the city, the *News*, issued evenings (except Sat.); other publications include the monthly *Mission*, a religious publication.

HISTORY. Irving was founded in 1903 by two RR surveyors, J. O. Schulze and Otis Brown, who were working on a section of a RR extension from Ft. Worth to Dallas and thought a particular parcel of land seemed a likely town site. As partners, they bought 80.2 acres and planned the new town to be called "Irving". In 1903, they held a barbecue and auctioned off 400 lots and in 1914 the city was incorporated. A post office was moved from another town to Irving

and the city thrived in its first year. In 1907, a branch of the Frisco RR N to Carrollton was built and in 1920 a privately-owned telephone system was installed. The city grew slowly and had a pop. of only 2,621 in 1950. Beginning in the mid 1950s, the city experienced phenomenal growth to over 45,000 people in 1960 and 97,260 in 1970. Irving is the new natl. headquarters of the Boy Scouts of America. It is the site of the immense Dallas-Fort Worth Regional Airport, which became operational in 1974.

GOVERNMENT. Irving has a council-mgr. form of govt. consisting of nine council members, including the mayor as a voting member, who are elected to two-year terms.

ECONOMY AND INDUSTRY. There are approx. 150 manufacturing plants in Irving. Major products include electrical equipment, generating systems, heavy equipment, food products, electronic equipment, machine fittings, hydraulic and pneumatic controls and chemicals. The city is a distribution and trucking center due to its accessibility to the Dallas-Ft. Worth area. The avg. disposable household income in 1978 was $23,008. In June, 1979, the total labor force of the Dallas-Ft. Worth met. area, including Irving, was 1,479,000, while the rate of unemployment was 4.0%.

BANKING. There are seven commercial banks and five savings and loan assns. in Irving. In 1978, total deposits for the six banks headquartered in the city were $285,704,000, while assets were $315,337,000. Banks include TX Commerce Irving, SW Bank and Trust Co., American, Citizens', Colinas Natl. of Irving and First Natl.

HOSPITALS. There are four hosps. in Irving, including Comm. Hosp., which participates in LVN, RN and X-ray teaching programs, Physicians' and Surgeons' and Professional Center.

EDUCATION. The U of Dallas, a privately-supported U affiliated with the Roman Catholic Church, was founded in 1956 and offers course work leading from bachelor to doctorate degrees. Enrollment in 1978 was 1,909. N Lake Col., a member of the seven-col. Dallas Co. Comm. Col. District, opened its 276-acre campus in 1977 and offers a full range of two-year degree programs in the liberal arts and sciences, as well as hundreds of Comm. Service Division non-credit courses. Encompassing an area of nearly 50 sq. mi., the Irving Independent School District is comprised of 16 elementary, six middle and three high schools and enrolls 24,253 students. The first pub. school planetarium in N TX provides astronomy instructions, while 18 vocational courses are offered by the Vocational/Technical Education program. The city has five private schools, including four elementary and one jr. high. Libs. include the Irving Pub. Lib. System, with three locations.

ENTERTAINMENT. The Irving Art Assn. presents an annual exhibit and juried show. The 65,000-seat TX Stadium, completed in Irving in 1971 and the home of the Dallas Cowboys, is also used for concerts, rodeos, motorcycle races and other events. Dallas U's Crusaders participate in intercollegiate sports. Additional entertainment is available in the nearby Dallas and Ft. Worth metroplex area.

ACCOMMODATIONS. There are many hotels and motels in Irving, including Day's and LaQuinta, Best Western and Quality, Ramada and Lexington Motor inns.

FACILITIES. The Irving met. park system includes 31 recreational areas encompassing 486.2 acres. These areas include 39 baseball and softball diamonds, 23 soccer and six football fields, 14 supervised playgrounds, 10 tennis courts, and seven recreation centers—three in the city and four used in a joint City-School program. City parks include Cottonwood Creek, Dupree, Hurwitz, Keeler, Lee, MacArthur, Northgate, Senter, Sunrise, Woodhaven and West. Four nearby lakes offer facilities for fishing, swimming and winter sports. Two pub. golf courses, including one at Knollwood Golf Club and one private course, are available. The six municipal pools include locations at Senter, Lee, Lively, NW, and W parks. Fritz Park contains a children's zoo, open during the summer. Lee Park features four handball courts. The Senior Citizens' Center, in E Senter Park, offers recreation to senior citizens and croquet/chuffleboard courts and picnic facilities. Games and crafts for area children are available at the W Irving Improvement Assn. building.

CULTURAL ACTIVITIES. Irving is served musically by a symphony orchestra and community concert assn. During the year the Art Assn. presents an annual exhibit of traveling works. The U of Dallas presents exhibitions, concerts and dramatic events for the community. Irving also has a Garden and Arts Center Assn. for women and a number of garden and book review clubs.

LANDMARKS AND SIGHTSEEING SPOTS. There are several plush dude ranches located in Irving. Historical buildings of interest include the William Smith house, built in 1880 with hand-hewn logs; the Robert H. Power Home, constructed on the original land grant by Sam Houston to Lawrence Hollenbeck in 1857; the Irving Heritage House, the restored 1912 home of C. P. Schultze, Sr., and Hawks Chapel (1906), the first church in the Union Bower Comm. A low, old, ironbridge, the Grawyler Bridge, was built in 1885. The California Crossing is an old water crossing on the Trinity River used during the gold rush, while another old water crossing of the Trinity River, the Record Crossing on the Elm Fork, is now spanned by a bridge.

JACKSON
MISSISSIPPI

CITY LOCATION-SIZE-EXTENT. Jackson, the state capital, largest city in the state and one of two seats of Hinds Co., encompasses 105.38 sq. mi. in central MS on the W bank of the Pearl River, 195 mi. S of Memphis, TN at 32°19' N lat. and 90°05' W long. The greater met. area extends into Rankin Co. to the SE and Madison Co. to the NE.

TOPOGRAPHY. The terrain of Jackson, which is located in the E Gulf coastal plain region of MS, is character-

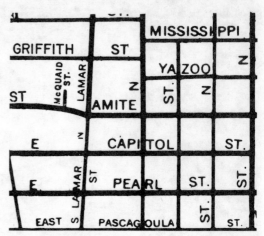

Central Jackson, Mississippi

ized by rolling hills, prairie and lowland areas near the Pearl River. The mean elev. is 294'.

CLIMATE Jackson's climate is humid during most of the year, with S winds from the nearby Gulf of Mexico prevalent during the long warm season, and polar and arctic air masses common in the short cold season. The avg. annual temp. of 65.4°F ranges from a Jan. mean of 48°F to a July and Aug. mean exceeding 81°F. Most of the annual precip. of 51" occurs during the winter, spring and summer, while the relatively dry autumn receives 2" to 3" monthly. The avg. annual snowfall is 1.2". The RH ranges from 54% to 94%. The growing season avgs. 235 days. Jackson lies in the CST7 and observes DST. **FLORA AND FAUNA.** Animals native to Jackson include the opossum, raccoon, whitetail deer, fox, muskrat and armadillo. Common birds are the cardinal, blue grosbeak, summer tanager, mockingbird (the state bird) and warbler. Snapping turtles, red ear turtles, bullfrogs, leopard frogs, Fowler's toad, green anole lizards, garter snakes and salamanders, as well as the venomous coral snake, rattlesnake, cottonmouth and copperhead, are found in the area. Typical trees are the magnolia (the state tree), oak, elm and sweetgum. Smaller plants include the iris, waterlily, pokeberry, honeysuckle and holly.

POPULATION. According to the US census, the pop. of Jackson in 1970 was 162,380. In 1978, it was estimated that it had increased to more than 210,000.

ETHNIC GROUPS. In 1978, the ethnic distribution of Jackson was approx. 60.3% Caucasian, 37.6% Black, 0.3% Hispanic and 1.8% other.

TRANSPORTATION. Interstate hwys. 55, 20 and 220, US hwys. 49, 51, 80 and state hwys. 18 and 25 provide major motor access to Jackson. *Railroads* serving the city include AMTRAK and IL Central Gulf. *Airlines* serving Jackson Municipal Airport are DL, SO, TI and US Air. *Buslines* serving the city include Trailways and Greyhound.

COMMUNICATIONS. Communications, broadcasting and print media originating in Jackson are: *AM radio stations* WSNY 600 (ABC/I, MOR); WJDX 620 (NBC, Adult Contemp.); WSLI 930 (Indep., MOR); WOZN 970 (Indep., Gospel); WRBC 1300 (ABC/I, MBS, MOR); WVOJ 1320 (NBC, Mod. Ctry.); WERD 1400 (MBS/Blk., R&B); WPDQ 1460 (ABC/I, MOR) and WWUN 1590 (Indep., C&W); *FM radio stations* WJSU 90.7 (Univ., Educ.); WFAM 91.1 (Indep., Divers.); WVLS 91.5 (Indep., Divers.); WKWI 94.7 (Natl. Blk.); WLIN 95.5 (Indep., Btfl. Mus.); WJFR 96.3 (Indep.); WJMI 99.7 (Indep., Btfl. Mus.) and WZZQ 102.9 (Indep., Rock); *television stations* WAPT Ch. 16 (ABC); WTTV Ch. 12 (CBS); WLBT Ch. 3 (NBC) and WMAA Ch. 29 (PBS); *press*: two major dailies serve the city, the *Clarion-Ledger*, issued mornings, and the *News*, issued evenings; other publications include *Baptist Record*, *MS Today*, *MS United Methodist Advocate*, *Jackson Magazine*, *Cattle Business*, *Northside*

Sun, MS Educator, MS Legionnaire, Pulpit Digest and *MS Farm Bureau News.*

HISTORY. The first inhabitants of the present-day Jackson area were Native Americans of the Choctaw and Chickasaw tribes. In 1792, French-Canadian trader Louis LeFleur established a trading post, known as LeFleur's Bluff in the area. Because of its central location the settlement was chosen as the site for the state capital in 1821, and named in honor of Andrew Jackson. In 1822, the state legislature moved to its new location and Jackson was incorporated as a city in 1833. During the Civil War, Gen. William T. Sherman's armies destroyed most of the city, and what remained was called "Chimneyville". Before the Battle of Vicksburg, Gen. Ulysses S. Grant occupied the city. Rebuilding after the war was slow, although during the late 1800s the growth of transportation and trade resulting from the arrival of RRs contributed to the city's nickname "Crossroads of the S". In the 1930s, Industrial development was stimulated by the discovery of a natural gas field near the city. In the 1960s and 1970s, a program for economic development was instituted by the city and numerous new factories located there. This program, as well as a policy of annexation begun in 1971, increased the area of the city from 64 sq. mi. to 105 sq. mi. and resulted in a significant increase in the pop. during the 1970s.

GOVERNMENT. Jackson has a commission form of govt. The three commission members, including the mayor as a voting member, are elected at large to four-year terms.

ECONOMY AND INDUSTRY. The 357 manufacturing plants in Jackson produce electrical machinery, food products, furniture and fixtures, primary metals, fabricated metal products, apparel and stone, clay and glass products. A number of oil and gas companies are also headquartered in the city. In June, 1979, the total labor force of the greater met. area was approx. 149,300, while the rate of unemployment was 3.8%.

BANKING. There are seven banking institutions in Jackson. In 1978, total deposits for the six banks headquartered in the city were $2,238,434,000, while total assets were $2,696,164,000. Banks include Deposit Guaranty Natl., First Natl., MS, Consumer Natl. and Guardian Trust.

HOSPITALS. There are 10 hosps. in Jackson, including Doctors, Hinds Gen., MS Baptist Medical Center, MS Methodist Rehabilitation Center, Rankin Gen., Riverside, St. Dominic-Jackson Memorial, U Medical Center, V.A. and Women's. The Jackson Mental Health Center also serves the city.

EDUCATION. Jackson State U, a state institution formerly operated by the American Baptist Home Mission Society, was founded at Natchez in 1877. In 1882, the col. moved to its present site and, in 1940, became a state teachers' col. It awards bachelor and master degrees, with an approx. enrollment (1978) of 7,800. Hinds Jr. Col., a public two-year institution awarding vocational/technical and academic programs, enrolled more than 5,700 in 1978. Other institutions include Belhaven Col., the U of MS Medical School, Millsaps Col., Phillips Col., Reformed Theological Seminary and Draughon Business Col. There are more than 55 public and 30 private elementary and secondary schools. Lib. facilities include the Jackson Lib. with several branches, and the MS State Lib.

ENTERTAINMENT. Annual events in Jackson include the MS State Fair in Oct., the Jr. League Carnival Ball and the Dixie Natl. Livestock Show and Rodeo in Feb. and the MS Arts Festival in Apr. MS State U and the U of MS, both of the SE Conf., and the Jackson State Col. Tigers of the SWAC participate in intercollegiate sports.

ACCOMMODATIONS. There are several hotels and motels in Jackson, including the Hilton, Coachlight, Howard Johnson's and the Passport, Sheraton, Ramada, Downtowner and Holiday inns.

FACILITIES. The 3,000-acre Jackson park system includes 45 parks. The Jackson Zoological Park houses birds, mammals and reptiles in natural surroundings. Mynelle Gardens features azaleas, camellias, magnolias and water plants. The city operates three public golf courses and 43 public tennis courts. The nearby Barnett Reservoir provides facilities for water sports.

CULTURAL ACTIVITIES. The Jackson Symphony Orchestra, MS Opera Assn., Jackson Ballet Co., Opera S, New Stage, MS Art Assn., Little Theater, Jackson Music Assn., Children's Comm. Theater and local colleges present performing arts productions throughout the year. The MS Arts Center-Russell C. Davis Planetarium opened in 1978. MS's Old Capitol Museum, containing state historical displays, the Museum of Natural Science, containing live and still exhibits of native wildlife and the city-maintained

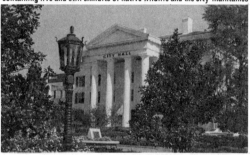

City Hall, Jackson, Mississippi

Municipal Art Gallery are among the city's museums. Others are the MS Museum of Art, MS Military Museum and Dizzy Dean Baseball Museum. The Museum of Agriculture and Forestry was established by the State Legislature in 1978.

LANDMARKS AND SIGHTSEEING SPOTS. The Oaks, an antebellum cottage erected in 1846 and occupied by Gen. Sherman during his siege of Jackson during the Civil War, is the oldest house in the city. City Hall was built in 1854 by slave labor. The Governor's Mansion, Civil War headquarters for Generals Grant and Sherman, was completed in 1842. The Old Capitol, built in 1833, served as the seat of MS govt. until 1903, when the New Capitol was constructed.

JACKSONVILLE
FLORIDA

CITY LOCATION-SIZE-EXTENT. Jacksonville, located in NE FL on the St. Johns River 30 mi. from the GA border, encompasses 840 sq. mi. at 30°30' N lat. and 81°42' N long. The largest city in area in the 48 contiguous states, Jacksonville extends from the Atlantic Ocean to 40 mi. inland. Its greater met. area covers all of Duval Co. and extends into the cos. of Clay and Johns to the S, Baker to the W and Nassau to the N.

TOPOGRAPHY. The terrain of Jacksonville, situated on the Atlantic Coastal Plain region, is flat. Within the city, the Arlington and Trout rivers meet the St. Johns River, which flows into the Atlantic Ocean. The mean elev. is 19'.

CLIMATE. The climate of Jacksonville is humid subtropical, influenced 40% of the time by E winds from the Atlantic Ocean which modify the summer heat and winter cold. The avg. annual temp. of 67.9°F ranges from monthly means of 54.7°F in Jan. to 80.4°F in July. Approx. 60% of the avg. annual rainfall of 51.54" occurs from July to Sept. The RH ranges from 47% to 90%. Jacksonville lies in the ESTZ and observes DST.

FLORA AND FAUNA. Animals native to Jacksonville include the opossum, armadillo, raccoon, mink and whitetail deer. Common birds are the heron, egret, gull, grackle, crow, chuck-will's-widow and mockingbird (the state bird). Narrow-mouthed toads, tree frogs, dwarf salamanders, newts, turtles and alligators and green and garter snakes as well as the venomous cottonmouth, rattlesnake, coral and copperhead are also found here. Typical trees are the basswood, cypress, oak, elm, magnolia and redbud. Smaller plants include the palmetto, holly, pyracantha, yaupon, bumelia, azalea and meadow beauty.

POPULATION. According to the US census, the pop. of Jacksonville in 1970 was 528,865. In 1978, it was estimated that it had increased to 539,000.

ETHNIC GROUPS. In 1978, the ethnic distribution of Jacksonville was approx. 77% Caucasian, 22.3% Black and 6.3% Hispanic (a percentage of the Hispanic total is also included in the Caucasian total).

TRANSPORTATION. Interstate hwys. 10, 75, 95 and 295, US hwys. 1, 17, 90 and 301 and state rtes. 10, 13, 105, 111 and 115 provide major motor access to Jacksonville. *Railroads* serving the city include FL E Coast Railway, Seaboard Coast Line RR-Louisville & Nashville RR, S Railway and AMTRAK. *Airlines* serving Jacksonville Intl. Airport include Air FL, DL, EA, NA and SO. *Bus lines* serving the city include Greyhound, Trailways and the local Jacksonville Transportation Authority. Navigable waterways are the St. Johns River, with a channel depth of 38', and the Inland Waterway, with a 12' deep channel. There are 20 public and private pt. terminals and 26 steamship agents.

COMMUNICATIONS. Communications, broadcasting and print media originating from Jacksonville are: *AM radio stations* WAPE 690 (Indep., Top 40); WCMG 1090 (MBS, C&W); WEXI 1280 (Indep., Contemp.); WCGL 1360 (Indep., Btfl. Mus.); WJQS 1400 (CBS, C&W); WJXN 1450 (MBS, Relig.) and WCRJ 1530 (Indep., Relig.); *FM radio stations* WJCT 89.9 (NPR, Clas.); WJAX 95.1 (Indep., Contemp.); WKTZ 96.1 (Indep., Btfl. Mus.); WAIV 96.9 (Indep., AOR); WQIK 99.1 (ABC/E, C&W); WIVY 102.9 (Indep., Top 40) and WJEE 107.3 (Indep., Btfl. Mus.); *television stations* WJXT Ch. 4 (CBS); WJCT Ch. 7 (PBS); WTLV Ch. 12 (NBC) and WJKS Ch. 17 (ABC); *press:* two major dailies serve the city, the *FL Times-Union* and the *Journal*, both issued mornings; other publications in the area include the weekly *Herald* and *FL Baptist Witness*, the monthly *Both Sides Now*, *FL Grower and Rancher*, *FL Truck News*, *Journal of the FL Medical Assn.* and *Seafarer* and the bi-monthly *Jacksonville Magazine* and *Metropolitan*.

HISTORY. The site of present-day Jacksonville was first inhabited by native Americans of the Timuqua tribe. In

Central Jacksonville, Florida

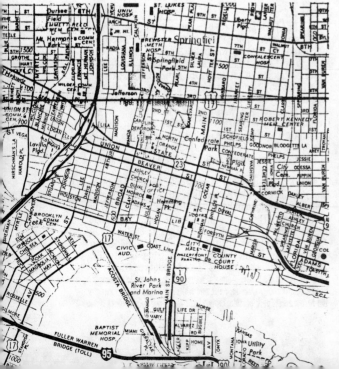

1565 a band of French Hugenot protestants led by Jean Ribault arrived at the mouth of the St. John River, claimed the area for France and built Ft. Caroline, the first European settlement in the US. In this ft. the first white child in the US was born. However, the settlement posed a threat to Spanish power and was destroyed by a Spanish expedition from Ft. St. Augustine. In 1816, Zacharia Hogans became the area's first American settler. In 1822, Isaiah D. Hart, a GA plantation owner, bought 18 acres in the area and led a movement to build a settlement there. The town of 15 was known as Cowford, a translation of "Wacca Pilatka", the Indian name for the area. In 1832, the town was renamed Jacksonville in honor of Andrew Jackson, then the state territorial gov. Jacksonville developed rapidly, but had numerous problems to contend with during its first 40 years. The seven-year war with Native Americans of the Seminole tribe ended in 1850, the same year the city received a steamship and a RR line. In 1854, fire almost leveled the village. During the Civil War, Union troops occupied the city four times, burning it twice. Still, by 1888, Jacksonville was the nation's leading winter resort. Disaster struck again when a yellow fever epidemic caused a mass exodus from the city and some 427 deaths. Another fire destroyed more than half of the city in 1901, but a massive reconstruction job was initiated at once and the city developed into a met. area. Jacksonville became the leading commercial center of FL as many banks, industries, insurance and transportation firms moved in. In 1968, Jacksonville citizens adopted a new consolidated govt. with home-rule authority to tackle problems in the entire co. area.

GOVERNMENT. Jacksonville and Duval Co. govts. combined to form a unified city-co. govt. in 1968. The mayor, who is not a member of the council, is elected at large to a four-year term, as are the 19 council members, five of whom are elected at large and 14 by district. The council is the chief legislative body and must approve many of the mayor's actions, including appointments.

ECONOMY AND INDUSTRY. Jacksonville is the financial, industrial, transportation and commercial center of FL. The largest naval storage yard and wholesale lumber market as well as the second largest coffee importation port on the S Atlantic coast are located in the city. A regional distribution center, Jacksonville is FL's second busiest port, handling 15,108,032 tons of cargo in 1977. Industries include insurance, banking, food processing, the production of lumber, paper products, chemicals and fertilizers, cigar manufacturing, petroleum refining, glass manufacturing, port operations and construction. The USN is a major employer in the area. Per capita income in the Jacksonville met. area in 1976 was below the natl. avg. of $5,890. Retail sales for that year were $2 billion and effective buying income was $2,694,086,000. In June, 1978, the labor force for the greater met. area was 317,700, while the rate of unemployment was 6.1%.

BANKING. In 1978, total deposits for the 25 banks headquartered in Jacksonville were $1,835,601,000, while assets were $2,264,588,000. Banks include Atlantic Natl., FL First Natl., Jacksonville Natl., American Natl., Flagship, Barnett of Murray Hill and SE First.

HOSPITALS. There are numerous hosps. in Jacksonville, including Baptist Medical Center, Memorial, Riverside Gen., St. Lukes, St. Vincents, Jacksonville Gen., and Hope Hanen Childrens. The Jacksonville City Health Center offers services in all branches of public health, such as the T.B. Regional Control Center, the V.D. Control Clinic, Dental Clinic, Environmental Health Services, Public Health Nursing and Nutrition and Mental Health.

EDUCATION. The U of N FL, a publicly-supported coeducational, upper level U created in 1965 by the FL Legislature, opened in 1972 and enrolled 24,269 in 1978. Jacksonville U is privately supported and offers coursework leading to bachelor and master degrees. Enrollment was 2,163 in 1978. Other teaching and research institutions include Edward Waters Col., Jones Col., FL Jr. Col., FL Col. of Med. and Dental Assistants, Jacksonville Business Col., U Hosp. of Jacksonville and Baptist Memorial Hosp. There are approx. 135 public elementary and high schools in Jacksonville enrolling some 126,000. Appox. 15,000 students attend the city's 55 private and parochial schools. Jacksonville's public lib., the Haydon Burns Lib., consists of a main branch located in the city and eight branches. A bookmobile service is also available.

ENTERTAINMENT. Each Dec., Jacksonville hosts the Gator Bowl football match and Festival. The Gator Bowl is also the scene of the traditional FL-GA gridiron clash in early Nov. The city also hosts the Jacksonville Intl. Invitational Tennis Tournament. Sports entertainment is offered by the professional Firebirds and Suns and the amateur Jacksonville Rugby Club, the Royals of the SL play baseball, while Jacksonville U's Dolphins and the Waters Col. Tigers participate in intercollegiate sports. Dining entertainment is available at the Alhambra Dinner Theater.

ACCOMMODATIONS. Jacksonville hotels and motels include the Jacksonville Hilton, Jacksonville TraveLodge and Rodeway, Gator Bowl, Skycenter, Holiday and Ramada inns.

FACILITIES. The Jacksonville met. park system includes more than 200 parks and approx. 102 playgrounds and play areas. Main parks include Hanna, Memorial and Treaty Oak. St. Johns Park and Marina, located downtown, provides docking and service facilities for 20 boats up to 108' in length. Hanna Park features one and one-half mi. of sandy beach, 60 acres of fresh-water lakes, nature trails, 300 campsites with water and power, 50 acres of primitive campsites, picnic areas and hot showers. Several mi. of clean beaches are available for surfing, swimming, fishing and shelling. Jacksonville Beach provides a 1,200-foot fishing pier and a municipal golf course. There are also several other public golf courses and tennis courts available for use in the city. An amusement park operates in season and lifeguards are on duty during summer months. The zoo is a home for 225 species of animal life and a collection of rare water fowl. The park system also provides 96 softball and baseball diamonds, 13 basketball playing sites, nine swimming pools and 76 sq. mi. of water available for water skiing.

CULTURAL ACTIVITIES. Jacksonville is served musically by a symphony orchestra, an opera group and the Civic Music Assn. Concerts and other musical programs are presented in the Gator Bowl and the Coliseum. Dramatic productions are staged by four local comm. theater groups, and the city also is home of a ballet company. Museums include the Cummer Gallery of Art, featuring works dating from the 5th century, B.C. to the present in addition to a collection of European and American paintings, tapestries, furniture and sculpture and the Jacksonville Museum of Arts and Sciences, which houses a planetarium as well as African, Oriental, pre-Columbian and modern art exhibits.

LANDMARKS AND SIGHTSEEING SPOTS. Treaty Oak, the oldest tree on the E coast of the US, was so named because under this tree local Indians concluded a peace treaty with early white settlers. A replica of Ft. Caroline and a museum stand at the original site of the Hugenot settlement as a national memorial to the earliest white settlers in the US. Another memorial to the Hugenot venture is the Jean Ribault Overlook, located on a bluff that affords a view of the St. Johns River, named for the Hugenot leader. The Kingsely Plantation on Ft. George Island has survived from the late 1700s, when it was the center of a large slave trading network. The plantation house and slave quarters stand intact. Friendship Fountain in downtown Jacksonville sends 17,000 gals. of water to a height of 120' each minute. Towering 37 stories above the waterfront is Independent Square, the home of Independent Life Insurance and the tallest structure in FL.

Aerial view of downtown Jacksonville, Florida

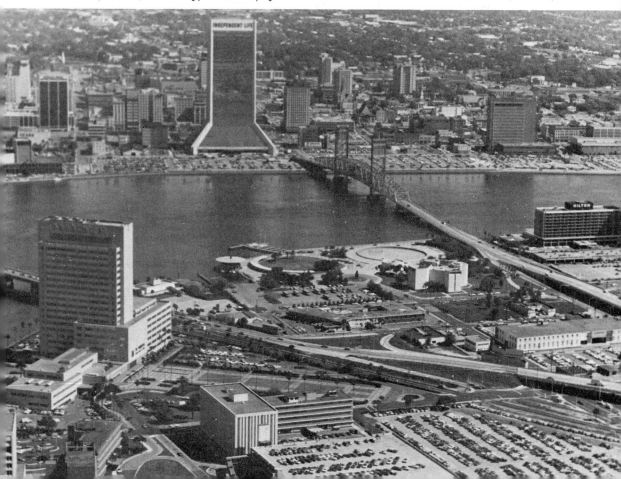

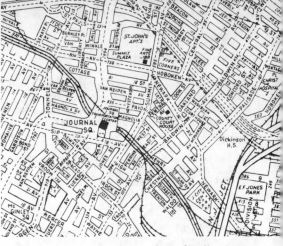

Jersey City, New Jersey

JERSEY CITY
NEW JERSEY

CITY LOCATION-SIZE-EXTENT. Jersey City, the seat of Hudson Co. and second largest city in the state, is located in NE NJ across the Hudson River from lower Manhattan to the E, to which it is linked by the Holland Tunnel. The city encompasses 16.6 sq. mi. between the Hudson and Hackensack rivers at 40°44' N lat. at 74°4' W long. Its met. area consists of Hoboken, Weehawken and Union City to the N, and is part of the greater NYC met. area. Newark is to the W and Paterson is to the NW, while Essex and Harrison counties are to the W and Bergen Co. is to the N.

TOPOGRAPHY. Parts of Jersey City are located in the flood plain and Palisades Hill regions of NJ. The terrain ranges from flat, low land to gently rolling hills. The Hackensack River flows into Newark Bay W of the city while the Hudson River empties into upper NY Bay on the E. Staten Island lies to the S of the city, where NY Bay joins the Atlantic Ocean. The mean elev. is 11'.

CLIMATE. The climate of Jersey City is continental, influenced by prevailing winds from the W and characterized by extremes in temp. during the summer and winter. Monthly mean temps. range from 32°F during Jan. to 76°F during July, with an annual avg. of 54°F. The avg. annual rainfall is 43". More than 50% of the annual snowfall of 29" occurs during Jan. and Feb. The RH ranges from 51% to 79% and the avg. growing season is 200 days. Jersey City lies in the ESTZ and observes DST.

FLORA AND FAUNA. Animals native to Jersey City include the opossum, cottontail rabbit and raccoon. Common birds are the cardinal, thrush, sparrow, pigeon and jay. Salamanders, frogs, turtles and snakes, including the venomous timber rattlesnakes and N copperheads, are found in the city. Common trees include the maple, cottonwood, elm and red cedar. Smaller plants include the bayberry, pickerel weed, selfheal, violet and aster.

POPULATION. According to the US census, the pop. of Jersey City in 1970 was 260,350. In 1978, it was estimated that it had decreased by 6.2% to 244,200.

ETHNIC GROUPS. In 1978, the ethnic distribution of Jersey City was approx. 56% Caucasian, 27% Black, 12% Hispanic, 4% Asian and 1% other.

TRANSPORTATION. Interstate hwys. 95, 78 and 495 (also the Lincoln Tunnel), US hwys. 1 and 9 and State Rte. 440 provide major motor access to Jersey City. *Railroads* serving the city include PATH and ConRail. All major *airlines* serve nearby Newark, LaGuardia and John F. Kennedy Intl. airports. The city is served by 20 independent *bus lines*, including Hudson, Transport of NJ (TNJ), as well as Greyhound and Trailways.

COMMUNICATIONS. Although no *AM radio*, *FM radio* or

The Old Berger Church Jersey City, New Jersey

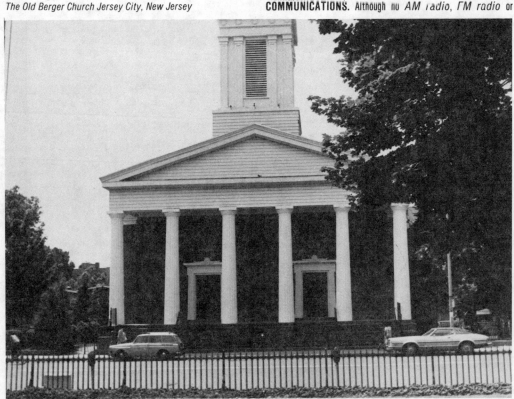

television stations originate from Jersey City, the city receives broadcasting from nearby NY and Newark; *press*: two daily newspapers are published in the city, the evening *Jersey Journal* and the *Hudson Dispatch*. Publications include the weekly *Jersey City*, the bi-monthly *Hudson*, the *Jewish Standard*, the *Journal of Critical Analysis, Pauw Wow* and *Svoboda*.

HISTORY. Prior to the 1620s, when a trading post was established by the Dutch, the site of Jersey City was inhabited by Native Americans of the Delaware tribe. In 1630, Michael Pawles, considered the founder, established a trading post in the area, and the settlement which developed became known as Pawles Hook. In 1664, the English gained control of the community and named it in honor of Jersey, the largest island in the English Channel. The community was incorporated as the town of Jersey City in 1804, and as a city in 1820. Two RRs arrived in the city in 1834, and, the same year, a treaty established the middle of the Hudson River as the boundary between NJ and NY. Thus, Jersey City was able to develop its waterfront and industry began to thrive. Between 1850 and 1860, the pop. of the city increased fourfold, from about 6,900 to 29,200. Jersey City and NYC were linked by the Hudson Tubes, the first RR tunnel between the cities; in 1909, and the Holland Tunnel opened in 1927. By 1950, the pop. of the city had reached 299,000, but thereafter experienced a steady decline as businesses and people moved to the suburbs. Urban renewal projects have since been initiated.

GOVERNMENT. Jersey City has a mayor-council form of govt. consisting of nine council members and a mayor, who votes only in the event of a tie. All are elected to four-year terms.

ECONOMY AND INDUSTRY. Jersey City is a major port and industrial and transportation center. Approx. 600 manufacturing plants produce electronic equipment, steel, food products, petrochemicals, lumber products and textiles. Govt. is a major employer. In 1978, the labor force was approx. 106,000, while the rate of unemployment was approx. 8%.

BANKING. In 1978, total deposits for the five banks headquartered in Jersey City were $3,042,187,000, while assets totaled $3,566,101,000. Banks serving the city include Hudson City Savings, First Jersey Natl., Provident Savings and Commercial Trust Co. of NJ.

HOSPITALS. There are five major hosps. in Jersey City, Medical Center, Christ, St. Francis, Greenville and Jewish.

EDUCATION. Jersey City State Col., a public institution established in 1927, offers bachelor and master degrees and enrolled more than 9,700 in 1978. Hudson Co. Comm. Col., a public two-year institution awarding associate degrees, enrolled more than 900 in 1978. St. Peter's Col., a four-year liberal arts institution affiliated with the Roman Catholic Church, was chartered in 1872 and became coeducational in 1966. Enrollment in 1978 was 4,430. Other institutions include Jersey City Technical Institute and Rutgers U Extension. Libs. include the Jersey City Public Lib. and the Hudson Co. Bar Assn. Lib.

ENTERTAINMENT. The city annually hosts the Jersey City Cultural Arts Festival, a July 4th celebration held at Liberty Park, and Sun. concerts. The Gothics of Jersey City State Col. and teams of St. Peter's Col. participate in intercollegiate sports.

ACCOMMODATIONS. Hotels and motels in Jersey City include the Starlite, Skyway, Hudson Motor Lodge, Holiday Inn and Hotel on the Square.

FACILITIES. Among the parks in Jersey City are Liberty State, Lincoln, Washington, Bayside and Pershing Field. Jogging tracks, a public golf course and ice skating facilities are available at Pershing Field and Lincoln Park, while playing fields, tennis courts and swimming pools are also provided in the city.

CULTURAL ACTIVITIES. The Jersey City Museum and Jersey City State Col. Symphony Band are among the cultural organizations located in the city. There are several art galleries, including the Upstairs Gallery and Studio 81.

LANDMARKS AND SIGHTSEEING SPORTS. Three historic districts, Pawles Hook, Van Vorst and Hamilton Park, containing 20 Natl. Historic Landmarks, are located in Jersey City. A tour of the Van Vorst brownstone house is annually conducted. Liberty State Park, which includes the Statue of Liberty and Ellis islands, is a popular attraction. Other landmarks within the city are the Old Firehouse, Ionic House, St. Paul's Church, Grace Van Vorst Church, Old Bergen Church (completed in 1660), the Old Hudson Co. Courthouse and Speer Cemetery. The Colgate Clock, with a dial 50' in diameter and a 2,200-lb. minute hand that moves 23" every minute, is one of the largest clocks in the world.

City Hall in Jersey City, New Jersey

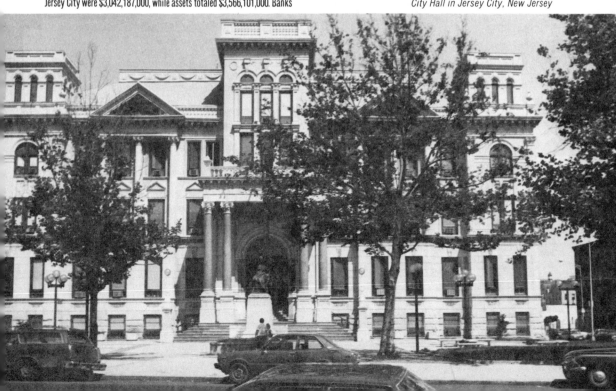

KANSAS CITY
KANSAS

CITY LOCATION-SIZE-EXTENT. KC, the seat of Wyandotte Co., encompasses 111 sq. mi. in NE KS at the junction of the KS and MO rivers at 39° 7' N lat. and 94° 37.5'N long. The greater met. area is shared with KC, MO, which borders the city to the E, and extends into the MO counties of Platte to the W, Clay to the NE and Jackson to the E and the KS counties of Leavenworth to the W and Johnson to the S.

TOPOGRAPHY. The terrain of KC, which is situated in an area of transition between the dissected Till plains and the SE Plain regions of KS, is gently rolling, with a few low hills. The mean elev. is 744'.

CLIMATE. The climate of KC is continental, characterized by rapid weather changes and excessive winds which sweep from all directions. The avg. annual temp. of 56°F ranges from monthly means of 29°F in Jan. to 80°F in July. Nearly 70% of the 37" avg. annual rainfall occurs during Apr. through Sept. Snowfall avgs. 20" annually. The RH ranges from 50% to 86%. The growing season avgs. approx. 200 days. KC lies in the CSTZ and observes DST.

FLORA AND FAUNA. Animals native to KC include the raccoon, coyote, opossum and fox. Common birds are the blue jay, meadowlark, mockingbird, vulture, cardinal and indigo bunting. Toads, salamanders, and snakes, including the venomous copperhead, rattlesnake and water moccasin, inhabit the area. Typical trees are the oak, cottonwood, elm,

Kansas City, Kansas

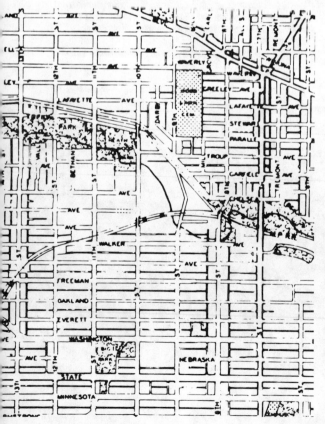

sycamore and willow. Smaller plants include the native sunflower, evening primrose, clover and broomsedge.

POPULATION. According to the US census, the pop. of KC in 1970 was 178,889. In 1978, it was estimated that it had decreased to 170,708.

ETHNIC GROUPS. In 1978, the ethnic distribution of KC was approx. 79.3% Caucasian, 19.2% Black and 3.2% Hispanic (a percentage of the Hispanic total is also included in the Caucasian total).

TRANSPORTATION. Interstate hwys. 35 and 70, US hwys. 69 and 73 and state hwys. 5, 10, 32 and 132 provide major motor access to KC. *Railroads* serving the city include AMTRAK, Burlington N, Chessie, Chicago & N Western, ConRail, Frisco, IL Central Gulf, KC Southern, MO-KS-TX, Rock Island, Santa Fe and Union Pacific. All major *airlines* serve KC Intl. Airport, N of the city. Fairfax Municipal and KC Downtown airports, both NE of the city, offer private and charter plane facilities. *Bus lines* serving the city include Greyhound, Trailways and the local Met. Transit Authority.

COMMUNICATIONS. Communications, broadcasting and print media originating from KC are: *AM radio stations* KCKN 1340 (Indep., C&W); *FM radio stations* KCKN 94.1 (Indep., 25% AM Simulcast) and KUDI 98.1 (ABC/I Mellow Rock); no *television stations* originate from KC, which receives broadcasting from neighboring KC, MO; *press:* one major daily serves KC, *The Kansan*, issued evenings; other publications include the *E KS Register, Wyandotte Echo, Wyandotte W, KC Globe, Call Newspaper* and *KC Voice.*

HISTORY. The KC area was first inhabited by native Americans of the KS tribe, who departed by the 1820s as the result of a govt. treaty. In 1818 the area was made a Delaware Indian Reservation, and settled in 1843 by the Wyandot Indians from OH, who bought the land from the Delaware Indians and established a comm. called Wyandot City. The Wyandots built the first free school in KS, a council house and opened a comm. school. Whites, who outnumbered the native Americans by the 1850s, renamed the settlement Wyandotte. In 1859, a convention met in Wyandotte to write the constitution of KS. Wyandotte opposed slavery during the Civil War and after it ended some blacks settled there. An influx of European immigrants in the area provided needed labor in the meat packing plants which opened in 1868, and by 1880, the pop. numbered 3,200. In 1886, Wyandotte and the neighboring towns of Armourdale, Armstrong, KC and Riverview to the S, formed KC. By the turn of the century the pop. numbered 50,000. After 1900, KC started the trend of situating manufacturing plants away from residential zones, and also initiated the first of the state's urban renewal projects during the 1950s. An industrial center, it is the state's second largest city. Today KC leads in livestock marketing, automobile assembly, soap manufacturing and flour milling.

GOVERNMENT. KC has a commission form of govt. consisting of a mayor and two commissioners, all elected at large to four-year terms.

ECONOMY AND INDUSTRY. There are approx. 300 manufacturing firms, employing some 37,000, in KC, which is the major industrial center of E KS. Processed foods lead the area's industrial products, followed by automobiles, fiberglass and soap. The flour mills, livestock markets and grain elevators operating in the city make it a center of agriculture. KC is included the KC met. area, which in June, 1979, had a labor force of 706,700 and an unemployment rate of 3.9%. Avg. income per capita was $4,516.

BANKING. In 1978, total deposits for the 16 banks headquartered in KC were $753,042,000, while assets were $999,196,000. Banks include Commercial Natl., Security Natl., Home State, Brotherhood State, Industrial State, Twin City State and Rosedale State Bank and Trust.

HOSPITALS. There are three gen. hosps. in KC, Bethany Medical Center,

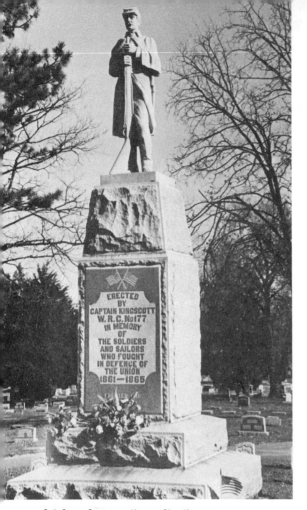

KANSAS CITY
MISSOURI

CITY LOCATION-SIZE-EXTENT. KC, located in W MO at the junction of the MO and KS Rivers near the geog. center of the US, encompasses 316 sq. mi. at 39°17' N lat. and 94°43' W long. Its greater met. area includes Jackson Co. and extends into the counties of Clay to the N, Platte to the NW, Cass to the SW and Ray to the NE and into the KS counties of Johnson and Wyandotte.

TOPOGRAPHY. The terrain of KC, situated in the W Plains Region of MO, varies from flat to gently rolling hills. The MO River runs E-W through the city. The mean elev. is 800'.

CLIMATE. The climate of KC is modified continental, characterized by rapid changes which are unobstructed by any topog. barriers. The avg. annual temp. of 56.8°F ranges from monthly means of 27.1°F in Jan. to 77.5°F in July. The avg. annual rainfall of 38.98" primarily occurs between Apr. and Sept., and the avg. annual snowfall of 20" occurs during the remaining months. The RH ranges from 51% to 87%. The avg. growing season is approx. 200 days. KC is located in the CSTZ and observes DST.

FLORA AND FAUNA. Animals native to KC include the raccoon, whitetail deer and opossum. Typical birds are the sparrow, pheasant, bluebird, cardinal, mockingbird, and meadowlark. Bullfrogs, toads, box

Civic Center Square, Kansas City, Kansas

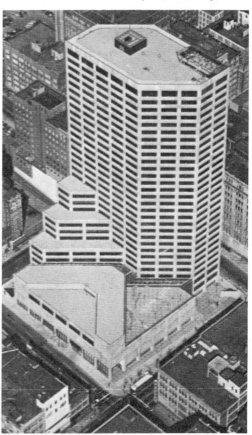

Oak Grove Cemetary, Kansas City, Kansas

Providence-St. Margaret Health Center and the U of KS Medical Center Hosp.

EDUCATION. The U of KS Medical Center, located in KC, originated in 1880 as a "preparatory course" established at the Lawrence Campus of the U of KS. In 1905, the KC Medical Col., the Medico-Chirurgical Col. and the Col. of Physicians and Surgeons were merged to form the final two-year program of a four-year medical course offered by the U of KS. The School of Medicine was consolidated on one campus in 1962. In 1978 the U enrolled approx. 1,800. KC, KS Comm. Jr. Col. established in 1923, awards associate degrees. In 1978, it enrolled approx. 3,000. Other institutions include Donnelly Col. and Central Baptist Theological Seminary. Lib. facilities are available through the KC Pub. Lib.

ENTERTAINMENT. Events, sports and other forms of entertainment are available in neighboring KC, MO.

ACCOMMODATIONS. There are many hotels and motels in KC, including Best Western, Colonial Inn, Holiday Inn-Towers, Penrod Motel and Resort and W Haven Motel.

FACILITIES. There are several parks in KC, including Garden Center-Loose, Hobby Hill Nature Center and Wyandotte Co. Tennis courts can be found at several locations and golf courses are available at five local country clubs.

CULTURAL ACTIVITIES. KC shares cultural activities with its twin city, KC, MO.

LANDMARKS AND SIGHTSEEING SPOTS. The three remaining buildings of the Shawnee Methodist Mission, established in 1830 as a mission and school for Indian children, display original furnishings. Ft. Dodge, now a state home for vets., was an army post constructed in 1865 to protect the Santa Fe Trail from native Americans. Such historic characters as "Wild Bill" Hickock, "Buffalo Bill" Cody and George Custer played important roles in the fort's history. The Huron Indian Cemetery, an Indian burial ground, has been preserved downtown.

turtles, water snakes and the venomous copperhead, rattlesnake, and water moccasin are found in the area. Typical trees are the dogwood, oak, elm and willow. Smaller plants include hawthorn, broomsedge, goat grass and primrose.

POPULATION. According to the US census, the pop. of KC in 1970 was 507,330. In 1978, it was estimated that it had decreased to 485,007.

ETHNIC GROUPS. In 1978, the ethnic distribution of KC was approx. 77.5% Caucasian, 22.1% Black and 2.7% Hispanic (a percentage of the Hispanic total is also included in the Caucasian total).

TRANSPORTATION. Interstate hwys. 29, 70 and 35 and US hwys. 50, 71 and 69 provide major motor access to KC. *Railroads* serving the city include Chicago NW, Kansas City S, St. Louis, San Francisco, IL Central Gulf, Union Pacific, and AMTRAK. *Airlines* serving KC Intl. Airport include ZV, RP, BN, TW, DL, UA, CO, Midway, FL, OZ, NC, RW and MVA. *Bus lines* include Continental Trailways, Greyhound, Jefferson Lines and the local KC Area Transportation Authority. There are 20 docks and terminals available for barge shipping on the MO River, with an annual tonnage of over one million tons.

COMMUNICATIONS. Communications, broadcasting and print media originating in KC are: *AM radio stations*: WDAF 610 (ABC/I Contemp., MOR); WHB 710 (Indep., Pop. Mus., News); KCMO 810 (ABC/E, Adult, Personality); KMBZ 980 (Indep., MOR); KJLA 1190 (Indep., Disco) and KPRT 1590 (Natl., Blk.); *FM radio stations*: KCUR 89.3 (NPR, Clas., Pub. Affairs); KTSR 90.1 (Indep., Relig.); KCEZ 94.9 (Indep., Btfl. Mus.); KWKI 93.3 (ABC/FM, Relig.); KXTR 96.5 (Indep., Clas.); KMBR 99.7 (Indep., Btfl. Mus.); KYYS 102.1 (Indep., Rock) and KPRS 103.3 (Indep., Soul Rock); *television stations*: WDAF Ch. 4 (NBC); KCMO Ch. 5 (CBS); KMBC Ch. 9 (ABC); KCPT Ch. 19 (PBS); KBMA Ch. 41 (ABC); KYFC Ch. 50 (Relig.) and cable; *press*: two major dailies serve the area the *Star*, issued evenings, and the *Times*, issued mornings; KC Kansan, Examiner and Olathe Daily News; other publications include *NE News*, *Livestock Market Digest*, *The Independent*, *Northlander*, *The Call*, *Labor Beacon*,

Central Kansas City, Missouri

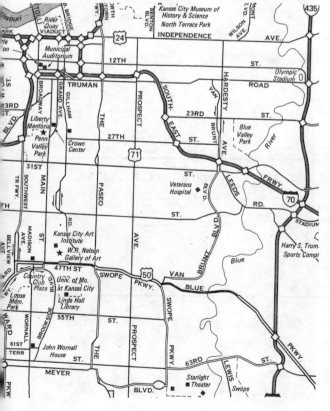

Jewish Chronicle, Liberty Tribune, Grandview Tribune, Lee's Summit Tribune, Clay Co. Sun, Clay Co. Chronicle, Scout Sun and *The Wed. Magazine*, all published weekly. Monthly publications include *Flower and Garden Magazine*, *VFW Magazine*, *Broadcast Engineering*, *MO Beef Cattleman*, *Modern Jeweler*, and *Retail Banking Today*. Other publications are *Gladstone Dispatch*, *Platte Dispatch*, and *Press Dispatch*.

HISTORY. Native Americans of the KS tribe lived at the confluence of the KS and MO rivers until the 1820s, when they left the area in accordance with treaty commitments. The following year Francois Chouteau established a trading post, later known as Chouteau's Landing, which grew into a settlement that attracted employees of the American Fur Co. to the area. Westport, the second settlement, was founded in the early 1830s some four mi. S of Chouteau's Landing. In 1833, John C. McCoy built a log cabin trading post there. Westport served as an important trading center for NM as the Santa Fe Trail passed through Westport. In 1838 a group of investors purchased the Chouteau Landing site and named the settlement the Town of KS after the previous Indian inhabitants. The Town of KS benefited from the overland trade, serving as the river port for Westport and was often referred to as Westport Landing. The town was incorporated in 1850 under the name City of KS with a population of about 2,500. The town's economy was seriously disrupted during the Civil War causing a mass exodus of people and capital. In 1869 the city opened the first RR bridge over the MO River, thereby linking the city with the nation's trans-continental RR system. During the 1870s and 1880s the city developed a market for grain and also became a stockyard center as cattle was shipped in from the W. Meat packing and flour milling plants were also established. In 1889 Westport and the City of KS were officially chartered as KC. The pop. reached 163,752 by the turn of the century. The city continued to prosper after 1900 as a center of commerce and industry. The city's residents numbered 324,410 by 1920. At that time the Democratic Party machine, under Thomas J. Pendergast, gained control of city govt. and did not relinquish it until 1939. Although some civic improvements were made, there was much corruption in city govt., and in 1940 a reform group was voted into office. KC was a center of defense industry during WW II. The city has initiated urban renewal projects, to be completed in the 1980s.

GOVERNMENT. KC is administered by a council-mgr. form of govt. The mayor is a voting member of council. The council is composed of 13 members, seven of whom, including the mayor, are elected at large and six elected by district. All members serve four-year terms. The council appoints a city mgr. who carries out council policies and prepares the annual budget.

ECONOMY AND INDUSTRY. KC is a major manufacturing and distribution center. The met. area's more than 1,700 manufacturing firms together with wholesale, trade and services and fed., state and local govts. are major employers. The most important manufacturing industries are printing and publishing and food processing. KC leads the nation in producing envelopes and greeting cards, distributing farm equipment, storing and distributing frozen foods, marketing hard winter wheat and providing foreign trade zone and underground storage space. It has a stable economy, with a June, 1979, met. labor force of 706,700 and an unemployment rate of 3.9%.

BANKING. There are 43 commercial banks and 12 savings and loan assns. in KC. In 1978, total deposits for the 46 banks headquartered in the city were

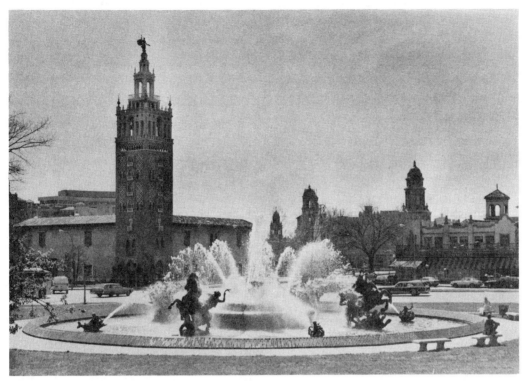

J.C. Nichols Fountain in the Country Club Plaza, Kansas City, Missouri

$3,900,734,00, while assets were $5,194,461,000. Banks include Commerce of KC, First Natl. of KC, United MO of KC, Columbia Union Natl. Bank and Trust and Boatmen's Bank and Trust Co. of KC.

HOSPITALS. There are 22 hosps., 14 clinics and 48 extended care facilities in KC, including Baptist Memorial, St. Joseph's, St. Mary's, Truman Medical Center, W MO Mental Health Center, Trinity Lutheran and St. Lukes.

EDUCATION. The KC branch of the U of MO enrolled its first students in 1933. The U offers grad. and undergrad. instruction and, in 1978, enrolled approx. 11,000. The U MO-Columbia at KC Extension offers professional license training in engineering, in addition to its other programs, and enrolled more than 4,000 in 1978. Rockhurst Col., founded in 1917 by the Society of Jesus and operating under the auspices of the Roman Catholic Church, offers a jr. year abroad. A four-year coed liberal arts col., it enrolled more than 3,500 in 1978. Other institutions include Park Col., Avila Col., Cleveland Chiropractic Col., Penn Valley Comm. Col., Maple Woods Comm. Col., Midwestern Baptist Theological Seminary, MO Institute of Technology, Calvary Bible Col., and Art Institute. Public schools in KC enroll nearly 100,000 students in 129 elementary, 21 sr. high and 21 jr. high schools. There are 48 parochial and three private schools. The city's 23 public libs. include one braille lib. The Linda Hall Lib. is one of the nation's largest privately supported libs. housing references on scientific and technical research.

ENTERTAINMENT. Annual events in KC include the Plaza Christmas lighting ceremony each Thanksgiving night, the Renaissance Festival in fall and the American Royal Livestock and Horse Show and the Future Farmers of America Natl. Convention in Oct. The football Chiefs of the NFL-AFC, the baseball Royals of the AL and the basketball Kings of the NBA offer professional sports. Collegiate sports are offered by the U of MO Kangaroos. Each Mar. the city hosts the NAIA Tournament.

ACCOMMODATIONS. There are numerous hotels and motels in KC, including the Radisson Muehlebach, Marriott, Alameda Plaza, Best Western, TraveLodge, Howard Johnson's, Crown Center Hotel and Sheraton, Hilton, Breckenridge, Holiday and Ramada inns.

FACILITIES. There are approx. 157 parks in KC, including four public golf courses, 15 swimming pools, 101 tennis courts and 146 ball diamonds. The 1,769-acre Swope Park, the largest park in the city, contains the Zoo, a nature center and a braille trail. Fleming Park has a 100-acre lake and offers shelter houses, fishing, nature trails, wildlife exhibits and an historic village. Line Creek Park includes 100 acres with buffalo, elk and deer and contains an archeological site. The 75-acre Loose Park, located on the site of a civil war battle, features a rose garden, lake and horticulture reference lib.

CULTURAL ACTIVITIES. KC is served musically by the Philharmonic Orchestra and the Lyric Opera. Concerts and theater-in-the-park are produced each summer by the Parks and Recreation Dept. Also, the Starlight Theater, a 7,600-seat outdoor amphitheater, hosts summer musical programs. The Nelson Gallery-Atkins Museum is one of the nation's largest art museums and exhibits collections of American and Oriental art. Other museums include the KC RR Museum, Lone Jack Museum and the KC Museum of History and Science.

LANDMARKS AND SIGHTSEEING SPOTS. KC is known as "The City of Fountains" because of its numerous fountains, most evident in the shopping area known as the Plaza, which also contains many art objects imported from Spain. Al Jolson, Fannie Brice and Maude Adams performed and Jack Johnson and Jack Dempsey fought at the neoclassical Standard Theater, which dates from the early 1900s. Adjoined by the Livestock Exchange Building, the stockyards began in 1870 and are still active as a livestock market. Built on the site of the early city hall and courthouse buildings, the City Market has been in operation in the same location since 1840. Preserved 19th-century buildings of interest include the Janssen Place residences, Grace and Holy Trinity Cathedral, the Bunker Bldg., the St. Luke's A.M.E. Church and Parsonage, the August R. Meyer Residence and the Rev. Nathan Scarritt residence. A 22-ft. high sculpture, the Eagle Scout Memorial, reminds citizens that KC has produced more Eagle Scouts than any other council. The Pioneer Mother Memorial stands as a tribute to all pioneer mothers, while the victims of WW I are commemorated by the Liberty Memorial. Overlooking the confluence of the MO and KS Rivers, the

Lewis and Clark Memorial honors the two men who mapped the site in 1806 as a good location for a ft. The Agriculture Hall of Fame is nearby at Bonner Springs.

KNOXVILLE, TENNESSEE

CITY LOCATION-SIZE-EXTENT. Knoxville, the seat of Knox Co. and the third largest city in the state, encompasses 77.1 sq. mi. of land 70 mi. NE of Chattanooga at 35°49' N lat. and 83°59' W long. in E TN. The met. area extends N into Union, W into Anderson, SW into Loudon, S into Blount, SE into Sevier and NE into Jefferson counties.

TOPOGRAPHY. Knoxville lies in the Appalachian Ridge and Valley Region, on the TN River in a broad valley between the Cumberland Mts., which lie NW of the city, and the Great Smokey Mts., which lie SE of the city. The area in the immediate vicinity of the TN River is generally flat, but slopes abruptly upwards into ridges to the E and W of the river approaching the mt. ranges. The mean elev. is 890'.

CLIMATE. The climate of Knoxville is moderate continental and is influenced by the Cumberland Mts. and the Great Smokey Mts. Monthly mean temps. range from 39.2°F during Jan. to 78°F during July, with an annual avg. of 59°F. The annual avg. rainfall is 48", with Sept. and Oct. being the driest months. The annual snowfall avg. 12". The growing season lasts approx. 228 days. The RH ranges from 50% to 92%. Knoxville is in the ESTZ and observes DST.

FLORA AND FAUNA. Animals native to Knoxville include the whitetail deer, raccoon, opossum and fox. Common birds include the cardinal, crow, bluebird, thrasher, oriole and sharp-shinned hawks. Box turtles, toads, salamanders, spring peepers, garter snakes and the venomous timber rattlesnake and copperhead, are found in the area. Typical trees include the pine, oak, elm, hickory, poplar (state tree) and maple. Smaller plants include the iris (state flower), mayapple, meadow rue, tulip, foxglove and violet.

POPULATION. According to the US census, the pop. of Knoxville in 1970 was 174,587. In 1978, it was estimated that it had increased to 187,800.

ETHNIC GROUPS. In 1978, the ethnic distribution of Knoxville was approx. 87% Caucasian, 12.7% Black and 0.3% Hispanic.

Knoxville, Tennessee

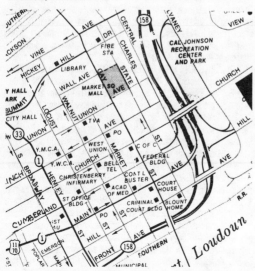

TRANSPORTATION. Interstate hwys. 40, 75 and 640, US hwys. 11, 25, 70, 129 and 441 and state hwys. 1, 9, 33, 34, 61, 62, 71, 73, 131 and 158 provide major motor access to Knoxville. The two *railroads* serving the city are the L & N and Southern. *Airlines* serving McGhee Tyson Municipal Airport, 13 mi. S, are AA, DL, UA, PL and SO. The municipally-operated Downtown Island Airport and two private airfields offer facilities for private and charter flights. The Inter-city Greyhound and Trailways and the local Knoxville Transit *bus lines* serve the city.

COMMUNICATIONS. Communications, broadcasting and print media originating in Knoxville are: *AM radio stations* WRJZ 620 (Indep., Contemp.); WIVK 850 (Indep., Contemp., C&W); WNOX 990 (Indep., Contemp.); WBIR 1240 (CBS, Contemp.); WKGN 1340 (ABC/C, AOR); WJBE 1430 (Indep., R&B, Gospel, Jazz); WKVQ 1490 (Indep., MOR) and WSKT 1580 (MBS, Inspir., News); *FM radio stations* WKCS 91.1 (H.S., Rock); WUOT 91.9 (NPR, Clas.); WEZK 97.5 (Indep., Good Mus.); WBIR 103.5 (ABC/FM, Top 40) and WIVK 107.7 (Indep., Btfl. Mus.); *television stations* WATE Ch. 6 (NBC); WBIR Ch. 10 (CBS); WTVK Ch. 26 (ABC) and cable; *press*: the two major daily publications serving the area are the *Journal*, issued mornings, and *News-Sentinel*, issued evenings; other publications include the *U of T Daily Beacon*, *The Aurora*, *TN Law Review*, *TN Alumnus* and *TN Farm & Home Science*.

HISTORY. Native Americans of the Cherokee tribe first inhabited the site of Knoxville. In 1786, Gen. James White brought his family to the area and built a house called White's Fort. In 1791, Gov. William Blount arrived, having chosen the vicinity of White's Fort as a territorial capital. Several months later he signed a treaty with 41 Cherokee chiefs whereby the Native Americans relinquished all land claims to the Knoxville region. Incorporated in 1791, Knoxville was named in honor of Gen. Henry Knox, Secretary of War in Pres. Washington's Cabinet. Knoxville served as TN's capital from its inception as a state in 1796 until 1812, and again from 1817-1818. In 1837, the first wholesale house—destined to become important to Knoxville's economy—was established. By 1850, Knoxville had a pop. of 2,076. Although during the Civil War Knoxville was initially a Confed. region, its citizens had mixed sympathies. Later, Union forces won an important battle fought at Ft. Sanders on Knoxville's W side. After the Civil War ended, the jobbing business arrived, and improved transportation led to the construction of numerous wholesale houses. Rapid industrialization boosted Knoxville's pop. from 8,682 in 1870 to 32,637 by the turn of the century. City expansion in 1917 further increased the pop. to 77,818 by 1920. TN Valley Authority (TVA) projects in the 1930s furnished new supplies of electric power and contributed to Knoxville's development as a manufacturing center. Industry continued to grow during the 1960s; this period also saw the initiation of urban renewal projects. Today, Knoxville is the business center of the rich E TN Valley, a burly tobacco market and livestock center.

GOVERNMENT. Knoxville has a council-mgr. form of govt. The five council members are elected at large to a four-year term, while the mayor is elected at large to a two-year term. The mayor, though not a member of council, may vote in special cases.

ECONOMY AND INDUSTRY. The TVA and the U of TN are Knoxville's major employers. Manufacturing is represented with more than 400 industrial plants producing heating equipment, clothing, food products, plastic products and metals. The city is also the retail center of E TN. The met. area had a June, 1979, labor force of 209,000 and a rate of unemployment of 4.4%.

BANKING. There are seven commercial banks and eight savings and loan assns. in Knoxville. In 1978, total deposits for the seven banks headquartered in the city were $1,280,221,000, while assets were

$1,524,884,000. Banks include United American, Park Natl., Valley Fidelity and Trust Co., Knoxville, First TN and First American.

HOSPITALS. Knoxville has eight hosps., including U of TN Memorial, E TN Baptist, E TN Children's, Ft. Sanders Presbyterian, Park W, St. Mary's Medical Center, NW Gen. and Lakeshore Mental Health Institute.

EDUCATION. The U of TN at Knoxville, founded in 1794 and state-supported, offers grad. as well as undergrad. instruction. In 1978, it enrolled 30,468 students. The State Technical Institute at Knoxville offers associate's degrees in engineering and science. In 1978, enrollment was 979. Among other teaching and research institutions are Knoxville Col., Knoxville Bus. Col., Draughon Bus. Col., Johnson Bible Col. and the U of TN Memorial Research Center. The city and co. maintain 105 schools with an avg. daily attendance of 58,859. There are 14 private and parochial schools. The Public Lib. System of Knoxville and Knox Co., with 20 branches, contains 1,514,472 volumes. The libs. of the U of TN, Knoxville Col. and the AVA are also available.

ENTERTAINMENT. Knoxville offers dining entertainment at the W Side Dinner Theatre. Annual events include Dogwood Arts Festival in April, a celebration of spring. It features entertainment, art shows and tours. The TVA & I Fair, the largest agricultural fair in E TN, is presented each fall. The White Sox, SL, present professional baseball to the city. Collegiate sports are provided by the U of TN at Knoxville Volunteers.

ACCOMMODATIONS. Knoxville hotels and motels include the Best Western Country Squire Motel, Howard Johnson's, Hyatt Regency, the Quality, Days and several Holiday inns.

FACILITIES. Recreational facilities in Knoxville include 11 swimming pools, 51 athletic and recreation centers, three golf courses, 119 tennis courts and 75 playgrounds. Chilhowee Park contains an amusement park. Knoxville Zoological Park houses over 250 species, including African elephants and Bengal tigers, and has a reptile complex.

CULTURAL ACTIVITIES. Knoxville is served by the Knoxville Symphony Orchestra and the Carousel and Clarence Brown Theatres at U of TN. The TN Artists Gallery displays the original work of local amateur and professional artists. The Dulin Gallery of Art is housed in a neoclassical mansion built by John Russell Pope, architect of the Jefferson Memorial. Indian artifacts and period furnishings from old local homes are among the exhibits displayed at the Frank H. McClung Museum. The Beck Cultural Exchange Center promotes interracial teamwork through the arts and cultural activities as well as preserving Black history. Other museums include the Student's Museum, the American Museum of Science and Energy, the Knoxville Academy of Medicine and Geology & Zoology Museums at the U of TN.

LANDMARKS AND SIGHTSEEING SPOTS. Blount Mansion, a Natl. Historic Landmark built in 1792, was the home of William Blount, a signer of the US Constitution and Gov. of the Territory S of the OH River. Confed. Memorial Hall, an antebellum mansion, houses Civil War and early S life relics, and was the headquarters for Gen. Longstreet during a Confed. siege in the Civil War. Other historic buildings include James White's Ft., the John Sevier Home, the Craig Jackson House (1818), the Crescent Bend-Armstrong House (1830) and the Market House (1897).

Ayres Hall of the University of Tennessee, Knoxville, Tennessee

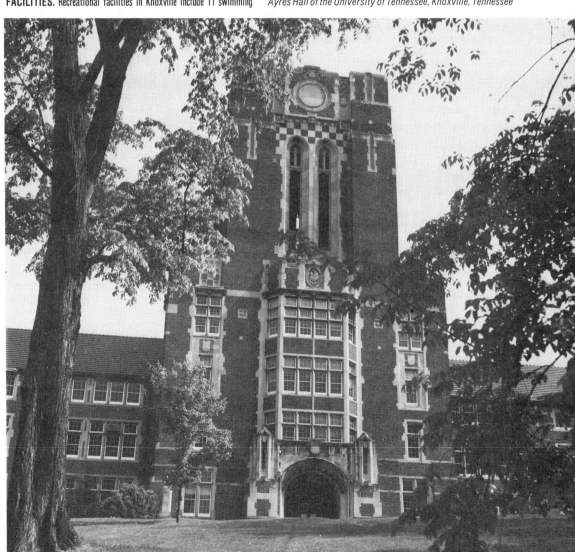

LAKEWOOD
COLORADO

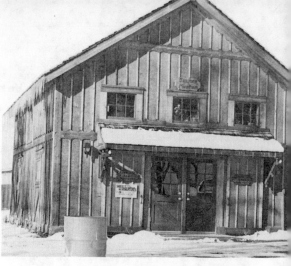

Belmar Museum Lakewood Colorado

CITY LOCATION-SIZE-EXTENT. Lakewood encompasses 18.5 sq. mi. in Jefferson Co., five mi. W of Denver, in N central CO, at 39°44'4" N lat. and 105°4'7" W long. The greater met. area extends into the counties of Clear Creek to the W, Gilpin to the NW and Boulder to the N and is part of the Denver met. area.

TOPOGRAPHY. The topography of Lakewood, which is situated at the foot of the E slope of the Rocky Mts. in the Rocky Mt. region of CO, is characterized by mountainous terrain. The mean elev. is 5,450'.

CLIMATE. The climate of Lakewood is mild, sunny and semi-arid, influenced by the sheltering effect of the Rocky Mts., which moderate prevailing westerlies and enable the city to escape extreme weather conditions. Monthly mean temps. range from 30°F in Jan. to 73°F in July, with an avg. annual temp. of 50°F. Most of the 14" avg. annual rainfall occurs during the warmer months. Snowfall avgs. 59" per year. The RH ranges from 35% to 71%. Lakewood lies in the MSTZ and observes DST.

FLORA AND FAUNA. Animals native to Lakewood include the mule deer, black bear, chipmunk, porcupine and bighorn sheep. Common birds are the golden and lark bunting, mountain bluebird, roadrunner, crow, bald eagle and scrub jay. Garter snakes, horned and fence lizards and the venomous prairie rattlesnake, are found in the area. Typical trees are the spruce, willow, juniper and fir. Smaller plants include the columbine, larkspur, lupine and rabbit brush.

POPULATION. According to the US census, the pop. of Lakewood in 1970 was 92,743. In 1978, it was estimated that it had increased to 131,700.

ETHNIC GROUPS. In 1978, the ethnic distribution of Lakewood was approx. 99.3% Caucasian, 0.1% Black and 4.7% Hispanic. (A percentage of the Hispanic total is also included in the Caucasian total.)

Central Lakewood, Colorado

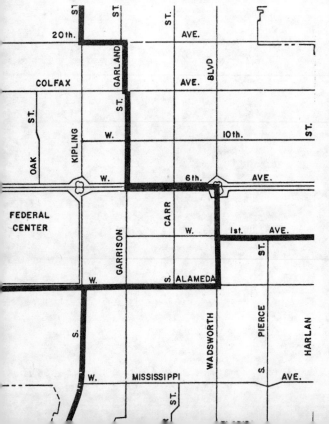

TRANSPORTATION. Interstate hwy. 70, US hwys. 6, 40 and 285 and state hwys. 58, 74 and 119 provide major motor access to Lakewood. *Railroads* and *bus lines* serve the city through Denver. All major *airlines* serve nearby Stapleton Intl. Airport in Denver.

COMMUNICATIONS. Communications, broadcasting and print media originating from Lakewood are: *AM radio station* KLAK 1600 (Indep., C&W); *FM radio station* KPPL 107.5 (Indep., MOR); no *television stations* originate from the city, which receives broadcasting from nearby Denver; *press*: two major weekly publications serve the city, the *E Jefferson Star* and the *S Jefferson Star*.

HISTORY. Gold discoveries in CO in 1859 attracted many settlers who traveled on rtes. which crossed the site of present-day Lakewood. Farms and ranches were established in the area and, in 1889, the name "Lakewood" first entered Jefferson Co. records to designate a proposed subdivision. The Panic of 1893, when the US govt. canceled its silver contracts, crippled the real estate development and it was not until June 29, 1969, that Lakewood was incorporated as a city with the greatest pop. of any US city at the time of incorporation. Today, Lakewood is a satellite city of Denver.

GOVERNMENT. Lakewood has a mayor-council form of govt. Ten council members are elected by district to two-year terms, while the mayor, a member of council, is elected at large to a two-year term. The mayor votes only in a tie.

ECONOMY AND INDUSTRY. There are approx. 66 manufacturing plants in Lakewood. Major products include kidney dialysis machines, organic chemicals, surgical equipment and sheet metal. Printing and boat building are also important industries. The median family income in 1978 was $18,420.

BANKING. In 1978, total deposits for the 11 banks headquartered in Lakewood were $378,018,000, while assets were $451,142,000. Banks include Jefferson Bank and Trust, First Bank of Westland, Govt. Employees' Industrial, United of Lakewood, Lakewood Natl., Jefferson S and Green Mt.

HOSPITALS. Hospitals are available to Lakewood residents in met. Denver.

EDUCATION. The CO School of Trades located in Lakewood is accredited by the Natl. Assn. of Trade and Technical Schools. Enrollment was over 250 in 1978. Libs. include the Jefferson Public Lib. and the Natl. Park Service Lib.

ENTERTAINMENT. Lakewood's proximity to Denver enables its residents to take advantage of that city's dinner theater entertainment, festivals, annual events and sporting activities.

ACCOMMODATIONS. There are several hotels and motels in Lakewood, including the Ramada W, Homestead and Rockin' R motels.

FACILITIES. There are 46 improved and unimproved park areas in Lakewood, encompassing a total of approx. 2,300 acres. Tennis facilities are available at the 27 public and three private tennis courts. The two country clubs in Lakewood offer golfing facilities. Horseback riding is also available in the city.

CULTURAL ACTIVITIES. Lakewood is an integral part of the Denver area and has access to the cultural facilities in that city.

LANDMARKS AND SIGHTSEEING SPOTS. The renovated Hone House, built in Lakewood sometime between 1859 and 1864, is used by many groups under the auspices of the Parks and Recreation Department. The Belmar Museum, a restored calving barn located in Belmar Park, houses items significant to Lakewood history.

LANSING
MICHIGAN

CITY LOCATION-SIZE-EXTENT. Lansing, the capital city of MI and seat of Ingham Co., encompasses 34.37 sq. mi. at the junction of the Grand and Red Cedar rivers in S central MI, 85 mi. NW of Detroit at 42°47' N lat. and 84°36' W long. Its met. area extends into the neighboring cos. of Eaton on the W and Clinton on the N.

TOPOGRAPHY. The terrain of Lansing, which is situated in the Great Lakes Plains Regions of MI, varies from flat to gently rolling, with some high bluffs and hills bordering the river valley. The mean elev. is 860'.

CLIMATE. The climate of Lansing is continental mod-erated at times by the influence of the Great Lakes. The avg. annual temp. of 46.8°F ranges from a Jan. mean of 22°F to a July mean of 71°F. The avg. annual rainfall of 30.77" is distributed evenly throughout the year. The avg. annual snowfall is 49" and the RH ranges from 54% to 90%. The avg. growing season is approx. 154 days. Infrequent tornadoes and occasional floods, along with destructive electrical storms and windstorms, occur in the area. Lansing is located in the ESTZ and observes DST.

FLORA AND FAUNA. Animals native to Lansing include the fox, skunk, opposum, whitetail deer, raccoon and squirrel. Common birds include the robin (the state bird), the cardinal, blue jay, woodcock, green heron and great horned owl. About 150 mi. directly N of Lansing are the only known breeding grounds of the endangered Kirtland's warbler. Salamanders, bullfrogs, skinks, box turtles, E garter and racer snakes, and the venomous E Massasauga (a pygmy rattler), are also found in the area. Typical trees are the white pine (the state tree), the oak, maple and elm. Smaller plants include the blackberry, sunflower, pepperweed, Queen Anne's lace and May apple.

POPULATION. According to the US census, the pop. of Lansing in 1970 was 131,403. In 1978, it was estimated that it had decreased to 129,000.

ETHNIC GROUPS. In 1978, the ethnic distribution of Lansing was

The State Capitol Building, Lansing, Michigan

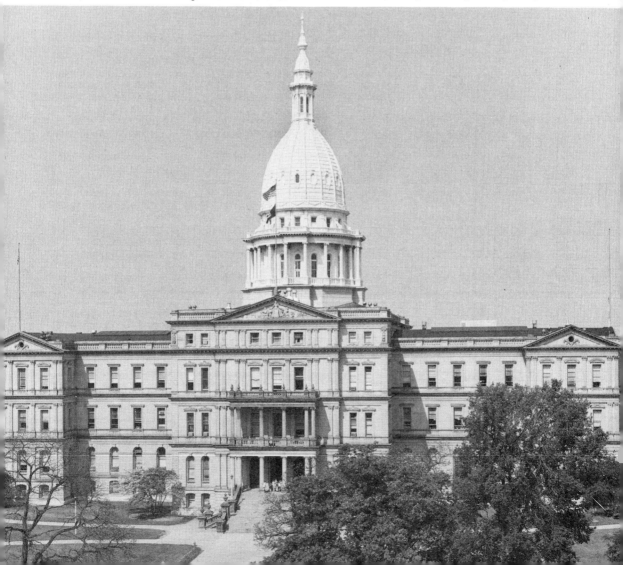

approx. 90.1% Caucasian, 9.3% Black and 3.9% Hispanic. (A percentage of the Hispanic total is also included in the Caucasian total.)

TRANSPORTATION. Interstate hwys. 69, 96 and 496, US hwys. 27 and 127 and state hwys. 43, 78 and 99 provide major motor access to Lansing. *Railroads* serving the city are ConRail, Chessie, Grand Trunk and AMTRAK. *Airlines* serving the Capital City Airport include UA and NC. *Bus lines* serving the city include Greyhound, Indian Trails, N Star Lines and the local Capital Area Transportation Authority.

COMMUNICATIONS. Communications, broadcasting and print media serving Lansing are: *AM radio stations* WITL 1010 (Indep., Ctry. Gold); WJIM 1240 (NBC, MOR) and WILS 1320 (Indep., Top 40); *FM radio stations* WJIM 97.5 (NBC, Btfl. Mus.); WITL 100.7 (Indep., Mod. Ctry.) and WILS 101.7 (Indep., Jazz, Progsv.); *televison stations* WJIM Ch. 6 (CBS) and cable; *press*: one major daily newspaper is published in the city, the evening *State Journal*; other publications include the *Weekly Towne Courier*, *The Catholic Weekly* , *MI Farmer*, *MI Out-of-Doors* and *MI Farm News*.

HISTORY. Lansing was settled in the late 1830s. Two enterprising brothers, whose names nobody remembers, sold lots in a fictitious city called "Biddle" to some citizens of Lansing, NY. When the buyers arrived at the site, they found only forest. Some remained and founded the nearly inaccessible village of Lansing, naming it after the village in NY where they used to live. In 1842, the village was officially designated Lansing Township. During a controversy over the location of a new state capital, in 1847, the MI Legislature voted to move it to Lansing from Detroit. The plank road built from the new capital to Detroit in 1852 made the city accessible for the first time. In 1857, Agricultural Col., now MSU, was founded. Lansing received a city charter in 1859, when its pop. was 4,000. The RRs

Central Lansing, Michigan

reached Lansing in 1871 and industrial expansion followed. Lansing had physical features adaptable to the auto industry. When that industry began to emerge after the turn of the century, the city became a leader in auto manufacturing. Increased job opportunities in the automobile and other industries contributed to Lansing's growth.

GOVERNMENT. Lansing has a mayor council form of govt. The mayor (who is elected at large to a four-year term) and eight council members, four of whom are elected at large and four from wards, serve four-year terms.

ECONOMY AND INDUSTRY. Lansing is a center for the automotive industry. MI State govt. is the city's largest employer. MI State U. is also a significant employer. In June, 1979, the total labor force for the met. area totaled 241,200 and the rate of unemployment was 6.0%.

BANKING. There are nine commercial banks in Lansing. In 1978, total deposits for the four banks headquartered in the city were $1,966,937,000, while assets were $2,327,430,000. Banks include MI Natl., American Bank and Trust, Bank of Lansing, NBD Commerce, E Lansing State, People's State Clinton Natl. and Pacesetter Bank of Lansing.

HOSPITALS. There are five hosps. in Lansing—Ingham Medical, Sparrow, St. Lawrence, Provincial and Lansing General Osteopathic. The MI Cancer Treatment Center is located at Provincial Hosp. and the Rehabilitation Medical Center is at Sparrow Hosp.

EDUCATION. MI State U (MSU) of E Lansing is one of the largest in MI. The first state school to offer agricultural courses for credit, MSU now offers programs leading to bachelor and doctoral degrees. In 1978, enrollment was approx. 47,380. Other institutions include Lansing Comm. Col., Great Lakes Bible Col., Davenport Business Col., Cooley Law School and Edward W. Sparrow Hosp. There are 46 elementary, five intermediate and four high schools in the public school system. Total enrollment in 1978 was approx. 27,600. There are six parochial schools in the area, with an enrollment of approx. 1,800. The MI School for the Blind and the MI Vocational School are also in the city. The Lansing Public, State and the MI Historical Commission libs. provide lib. facilities in the area.

ENTERTAINMENT. Annual events in Lansing include the Easter Seal telethon and Farmer's Week at MSU in Mar. and the Memorial Day Parade. MI Week is observed state-wide from May 19 through 26. Sports teams from Lansing Comm. Col. and the Spartans of MSU participate in collegiate sports in the Big Ten Conference. Other sporting teams include the Lansing Laurels, a women's amateur softball team.

ACCOMMODATIONS. There are a number of hotels and motels in Lansing, including the Ramada, Harley, University, Red Roof, Howard Johnson's, Knight's and Hilton inns, the Plaza Hotel and the Kellogg Center.

FACILITIES. The 45 parks in Lansing include Bancroft, Frances, Moore's, St. Joseph and Riverfront and feature facilities for basketball, football, boccie, tennis, baseball, softball and boating. The Carl G. Fenner Arboretum exhibits prairie animals and features nature trails, including one designed for the visually handicapped. The Potter Park and Zoo offers pony rides, canoe rentals and refreshments in the summer. There are several public golf courses, including Groesbeck and Akers, at MSU.

CULTURAL ACTIVITIES. The Symphony Orchestra in Lansing presents regular performances led by famous guest conductors. The Boar's Head Theater is the only professional theater in MI outside Detroit. Drama is also presented on the campuses of MSU and Lansing Comm. Col. The Arts Information Center, a division of the Met. Lansing Fine Arts Council, sponsors touring art exhibits and theatrical and musical performances. The MI Historical Museum is housed in the James Turner family home on the Lansing Comm. Col. campus, while the Kresge Art Gallery is on the MSU Campus. Other museums and galleries include the MI Historical and R. E. Olds museums, Impression S and the Lansing and Capitol Art Galleries.

LANDMARKS AND SIGHTSEEING SPOTS. The Capitol Building in Lansing was erected in 1873 and is an example of 19th-century architecture. The Abrams Planetarium is on the campus of MSU. The Ledges, 10 mi. W of Lansing, are rock ledges estimated to be over 300 million years old.

LAS VEGAS
NEVADA

CITY LOCATION-SIZE-EXTENT. Las Vegas, the largest city in the state and seat of Clark Co., encompasses 54.3 sq. mi. in SE NV at 36°85' N lat. and 115°10' N. long. More than half the pop. of NV lives in the Las Vegas greater met. area, which includes all of Clark Co., bordered by the neighboring counties of Nye on the W, and Lincoln on the N and the AZ and CA state borders to the E and S respectively.

TOPOGRAPHY. Situated in the Basin and Range Region of NV, Las Vegas is near the center of a broad valley which slopes gradually upwards towards the surrounding mts., the elev. of which ranges from 2,000' to 10,000' above the valley floor. The CO River and Hoover Dam lie 30 mi. to the E. The mean elev. is 2,162'.

CLIMATE. The climate of Las Vegas is continental, characterized by well defined seasons and summers typical of the desert, with max. temps. usually of 100°F or more. Winds are usually downslope toward the center of the valley causing temps. in the lower parts of the city to be 15°F to 25°F cooler than the higher parts. The avg. annual temp. of 66°F ranges from a monthly mean of 44°F in Jan. to 89.7°F in July. The avg. annual rainfall of 4.06" is distributed relatively evenly throughout the year. The lack of moisture is due to the effects of the Sierra NV Mts. of CA and the Spring Mts. W of the Vegas Valley, which act as barriers to storms moving E from the Pacific Ocean. The RH ranges from 11% to 54%. Las Vegas lies in the PSTZ and observes DST.

FLORA AND FAUNA. Animals native to Las Vegas include the fox, bobcat, striped skunk, ringtail and coyote. Common birds include the roadrunner, Gambel's quail, prairie falcon, and cactus wren. Nightsnakes, ground snakes, coachwhip snakes, tree lizards, horned lizards and the venomous rattlesnake and gila monster, are found in the area. Typical trees are the oak, pinyon, juniper and desert willow. Smaller plants include the rabbitbrush, poppy, creosote and filaree.

POPULATION. The 31.6% increase in pop. experienced in Las Vegas between 1970 and 1977 was one of the highest in the US. According to the US census, the pop. of Las Vegas in 1970 was 125,787. In 1978, it was estimated that it had increased to 161,200.

ETHNIC GROUPS. In 1978, the ethnic distribution of Las Vegas was approx. 87.6% Caucasian, 11.2% Black and 4.6% Hispanic (a percentage of the Hispanic total is also included in the Caucasian total).

TRANSPORTATION. Interstate hwy. 15, US hwys. 466, 93, and 95 and state hwy. 6 provide major motor access to Las Vegas. *Railroads* serving the area include AMTRAK and Union Pacific. *Airlines* serving the city through McCarran Intl. Airport include TW, UA, DL, FL, RW, NA, WA, BN, CO, TI, Pacific SW Air, AA and NW Orient. Air facilities are also available at N Las Vegas Airport and Hughes Executive Terminal. *Bus Lines* serving the city include Trailways, Greyhound, LTR Stage Lines and the local Las Vegas Transit System.

COMMUNICATIONS. Communications, broadcasting and print media originating from Las Vegas are: *AM radio stations*: KOWN 720 (MBS, MOR); KORK 920 (NBC, MOR, Personality); KNUU 970 (ABC/I, MBS, All News); KLUC 1140 (Indep., Top 40); KLAV 1230 (CBS, MOR); KRAM 1340 (ABC/E, Mod. Ctry.) and KENO 1460 (ABC/C, Top 40, Rock); *FM radio stations*: KUDO 93.1 (Indep., Btfl. Mus.); KORK 97.1 (Indep., Btfl. Mus.); KLUC 98.5 (Indep., Top 40) and KENO 101.9 (Indep., Top 40); *television stations* KORK Ch. 3 (NBC); KVVU Ch. 5 (Indep.); KLAS Ch. 8 (CBS); KLVX Ch. 10 (PBS); KSHO Ch. 13 (ABC) and cable; *press*: two major dailies serve the city, the morning *Sun* and the evening *Review-Journal*; other publications include *Panorama* and *Israelite*.

HISTORY. Artifacts discovered near Las Vegas indicate that the area was the site of a primitive culture 20,000 years ago. At one time, Native Americans of the Pueblo tribe lived there, and prior to the arrival of white settlers the region was inhabited by Native Americans of the Paiute tribe. In 1855, the Bringhurst Party came from Salt Lake City to teach the Native Americans agriculture and build a ft., which was abandoned in 1858. The town boomed briefly during the silver rush, and revived again with ranching in the late 1800s. Las Vegas was founded in 1905 after the Union Pacific RR announced that the site had been designated a major RR division point and then auctioned off lots. The name Las Vegas which is derived from two Spanish words meaning "the meadows", was chartered as a city in 1911. It was a slowly-developing agricultural area until 1931, when legalized gambling proved a windfall to the desert town. That year the pop. expanded when workers arrived to construct the Boulder (now Hoover) Dam on the nearby CO River. Nevis AFB was established during WW II, and after the war's end, Las Vegas' fame as a resort grew. The first large gambling casino opened in 1946. By the late 1960s, Las Vegas alone drew 15 million tourists annually to NV. Billionaire Howard Hughes moved to Las Vegas in 1966 and bought airports, land, hotels, casinos, and a TV station. Las Vegas continues to grow rapidly, its development generated by the tourist industry, with an estimated

Las Vegas Convention Center, Las Vegas, Nevada

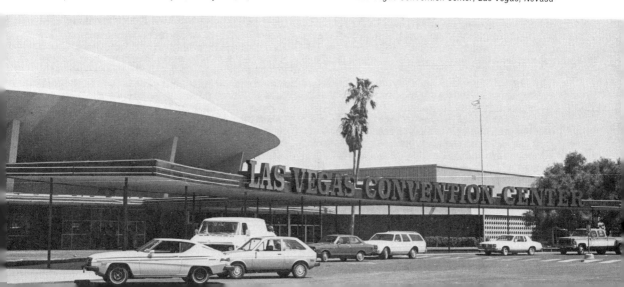

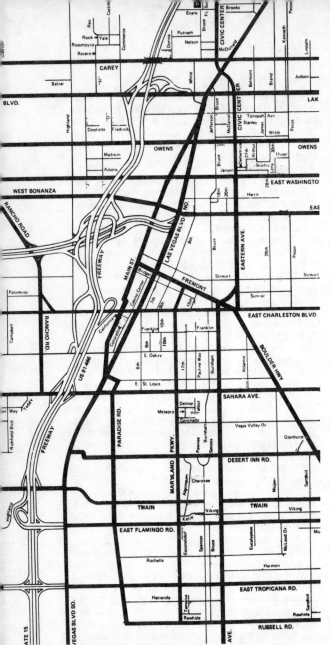

Las Vegas, Nevada, including the Famous "Strip"

350,000 residents now living in the city. Ranked as the 6th fastest-growing city in the nation, Las Vegas is also drawing non-gambling industries, attracted to the area by low construction and operating costs. The city also serves as a distribution point for a large mining and ranching area.

GOVERNMENT. Las Vegas has a council-mgr. form of govt. Four council members are elected by district and the mayor, a voting member of council, is elected at large. All serve four-year terms.

ECONOMY AND INDUSTRY. Tourism and conventions are the major industries in Las Vegas. Legalized gambling, top entertainment and year-round outdoor recreation draws an avg. of 25,000 visitors daily. Development of major industries is a city priority. Three major warehousing operations began in 1978 and the world's largest lithium battery plant is to open in 1980. The city is developing a motion picture and TV production industry. It is also becoming a major retirement

community. The total labor force for the Las Vegas area in June, 1979, was 186,300 and the rate of unemployment was 7.0%. Wages and salaries in 1978 totaled was $1,812,922,054. The 1978 avg. per capita income (measured in 1958 dollars) was $4,644.

BANKING. There are six banks and seven savings and loan assns. in Las Vegas. In 1978, total deposits for the three banks headquartered in the city were $1,016,309,000, while assets were $1,132,509,000. Banks include Valley of NV, NV Bank, and NV State.

HOSPITALS. There are several hosps. in Las Vegas including Sunrise, NV Memorial, Valley, Desert Springs, N. Las Vegas, St. Rose Delima, and Women's. Public health care facilities and agencies include the Clark Co. Health District, which conducts a continuing communicable disease testing program involving all workers employed in the food service areas.

EDUCATION. Located in Las Vegas and founded as a coordinate campus of the U of NV, the UNV at Las Vegas (UNLV) grants grad as well as undergrad degrees. In 1978, approx. 8,700 students enrolled. Other teaching institutions are Clark Co. Comm. Col., Dana McKay Business Col. and Education Dynamics Institute. The Clark Co. public school system consists of 67 elementary, 15 jr., four jr.-sr. and 15 high schools. Lib. facilities are provided by the Las Vegas Public, the Clark Co. and the UNLV libs.

ENTERTAINMENT. Las Vegas claims to be "The Entertainment Capital of the World", where the biggest stars in show business perform nightly along the famous "Strip" and downtown "Casino Center." The Helldorado Rodeo, a four-day celebration in May, features street dances and parades where participants wear Old W costumes. Wayne Newton also hosts a rodeo in the city. Other festivals and annual events include the Intl. Festival, NV State Fair, and Youth Fair. Sports entertainment is offered by the UNLV Running Rebels and the Las Vegas Seagulls, a pro soccer team.

ACCOMMODATIONS. The hotels and motels in Las Vegas, include Caesar's Palace, Del Webb's Sahara, Mint, Horseshoe, Circus Circus, Dunes, El Morroco, Four Queens, Flamingo Hilton, Fremont, Frontier, Golden Nugget, Las Vegas Hilton, MGM Grand, La Concha, Riviera, Sands, the 20th Century and Union Plaza, and Holiday, Docort, Rodeway and Best Western inns.

FACILITIES. There are several parks in Las Vegas including the Floyd R. Lamb State, which contains a zoo; Jaycee; Lions-Sunset; Fountain; Hadland; and Lorenzi, which features a jogging track. Jogging tracks are also provided at Valley, Las Vegas and W high schools and Supreme Court. There is a municipal golf course and additional public courses are available at four privately operated facilities. Public tennis courts are available at four privately operated facilities. Some of the major hotels provide their own tennis courts and golf courses.

CULTURAL ACTIVITIES. Las Vegas is served musically by the Civic Symphony and the U of NV at Las Vegas (UNLV) Music Dept. Concerts are sponsored by the Musician's Union and Young Audience, Inc., while classical music, opera and ballet are presented at Artemus Ham Concert Hall. Both the Reed Whipple Cultural Arts Center and the City of Las Vegas Dept. of Recreation and Leisure Activities (Cultural and Comm. Affairs) offer classes, workshops and activities, in addition to presentations of the performing arts. Cultural and educational programs are also sponsored by the Junior League. Dramatic productions are staged by the Comm. Theater of the Theater Arts Society, Inc., Rainbow Co., Jelly Bean Theater, the UNLV, Judy Bayley Theater, Meadows Theater, and the Aladdin Theater. Dance is performed by the UNLV Contemporary Dance Theater and the Center for Modern Dance. Changing exhibits by local and nationally known artists are displayed by the Las Vegas Art League and Museum. Other museums include the UNLV Art Gallery and Museum, the Museum of Natural History and the S NV Museum and Cultural Center.

LANDMARKS AND SIGHTSEEING SPOTS. Las Vegas' primary attraction lies in its casinos and nightclubs, most of which are located downtown on Fremont Street. One such establishment, Binion's Horseshoe, displays 100 US banknotes worth $10,000 each between sheets of bulletproof glass, suspended from a giant golden horseshoe. The Mint Hotel and Casino, also located downtown, offers behind-the-scenes glimpses of a plush casino. Circus Circus is a tent-shaped hotel casino on The Strip, where most of the casinos not situated on Fremont are located. Other attractions include the Mormon Ft., the Kiel Ranch and the Spring Mt. Ranch.

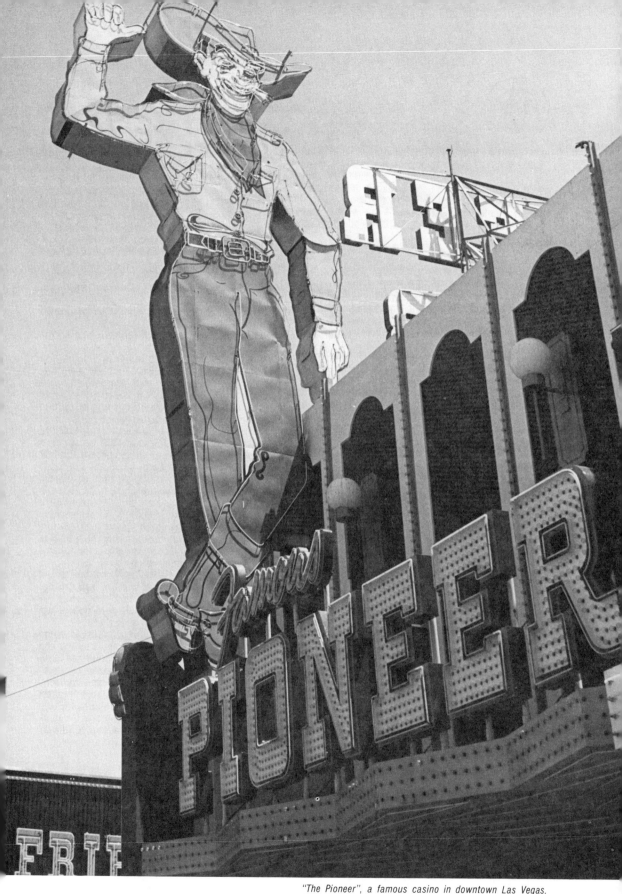

"The Pioneer", a famous casino in downtown Las Vegas, Nevada

LEXINGTON
KENTUCKY

CITY LOCATION-SIZE-EXTENT. Lexington, the seat of Fayette Co., is located in N central KY, 94 mi. E of Louisville and 80 mi. S of Cincinnati, at 38°02' N lat. and 84°36' W long. The Urban Service District of Lexington encompasses 73.4 sq. mi., while the met. area extends into the counties of Jessamine to the SW, Woodford to the NW, Scott to the N, Bourbon to the NE and Clark to the E.

TOPOGRAPHY. The topography of Lexington, which is situated on a plateau in the heart of the Bluegrass region, is characterized by gently rolling terrain which varies in elev. from 90' to 1050', with a mean elev. of 983'.

CLIMATE. Lexington's climate is temperate and continental with a large temp. range. Monthly mean temps. range from 33.3°F in Jan. to 76.2°F in July with an avg. annual temp. of 55.1°F. The avg. annual rainfall of 43.81" is evenly distributed with slightly less occurring in the fall. The avg. annual snowfall of 16.7" occurs primarily from Jan. through Mar. The RH ranges from 54% to 88%. Lexington lies in the ESTZ and observes DST.

FLORA AND FAUNA. Animals native to Lexington include the woodchuck, fox, whitetail deer and raccoon. Common birds include the cardinal, blue jay, thrasher, robin and red-eyed vireo. Tree frogs, toads, box turtles and garter snakes, as well as the venomous copperhead and timber rattlesnake, are found in the area. Typical trees include the KY coffee tree, oak, maple, elm and ash. Smaller plants include the honeysuckle, blackberry, ironweed and corn cockle.

POPULATION. According to the US census, the pop. of Lexington in 1970 was 174,323. In 1978, it was estimated that it had increased to 193,200.

ETHNIC GROUPS. In 1978, the ethnic distribution of Lexington was approx. 87.5% Caucasian, 12.4% Black and 0.5% Hispanic (a percentage of the Hispanic total is also included in the Caucasian total).

TRANSPORTATION. Interstate hwys. 64, 75, 71 and 264, US hwys. 25, 27, 42, 60, 68 and 421 and state hwys. 4, 57, 353, 922, 956, 1681, 1973 and 1974 provide major motor access to Lexington. *Railroads* serving the

Central Lexington, Kentucky

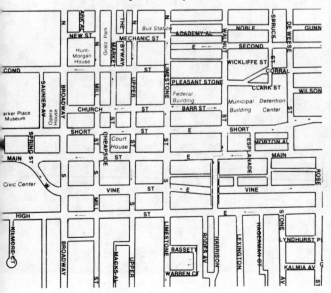

city include Chesapeake & OH, KY Union, KY Central, Louisville & Nashville and Cincinnati S. *Airlines* serving Blue Grass Field Terminal include DL, EA, PI and US Air. *Bus lines* include Greyhound and the local LexTran.

COMMUNICATIONS. Communications, broadcasting and print media originating from Lexington are: *AM radio stations* WVLK 590 (ABC/I, Contemp.); WLAP 630 (CBS, Pop., Contemp.) and WBLG 1300 (NBC, MOR); *FM radio stations* WBKY 91.3 (NPR, Clas., Jazz, Bluegrass); WVLK 92.9 (Indep., Btfl. Mus.); WLAP 94.5 (Indep., Contemp.) and WKQQ 98.1 (Indep., Progsv.); *television stations* WLEX Ch. 18 (NBC); WKYT Ch. 27 (CBS); WKLE Ch. 46 (Educ.); WTVQ Ch. 62 (ABC) and cable; *press*: two major dailies serve the area, the morning *Herald* and the evening *Leader*; other publications include *The Blood-Horse*, *KY Kernel*, *Around the Town*, *State Govt. News*, *Bluegrass Woman*, *KY Turf*, *Horseman and Fair World* and *Leaders Magazine*.

HISTORY. Lexington received its name in 1775, when a group of hunters, including Robert Patterson and Simon Kenton, named their campsite after the Revolutionary War battle of Lexington, MA. The first permanent settlement was established in the spring of 1779, when Robert Patterson returned to the campsite with a small group of settlers. The Block House, Patterson's cabin, was built in April, 1779. Transylvania Col., the first institution of learning established in the W, opened at Lexington in 1780. The town was incorporated by the State of VA in 1782, and later that year KY achieved statehood. The KY Legislature held its first sessions in Lexington. The city's horse racing industry began in its early years, as the first race track was built in 1798 and the Jockey Club was organized in 1809. Secretary of State Henry Clay was one of the organizers and first members of the Jockey Club. Lexington's tobacco industry began in 1825 when hogsheads of tobacco were first sold in the city. The city was chartered in 1832. Horse racing became more popular after the Civil War and the area's thoroughbred horse breeding industry prospered. Lexington's growth in the late 1800s and early 1900s was based on agriculture and the thoroughbred industry. Today, the city is the nation's largest loose-leaf tobacco market.

GOVERNMENT. Lexington has a mayor-council form of govt. The City of Lexington and Fayette Co. govts. merged in 1973 to create the unified Lexington-Fayette Urban Co. Govt. Three of the 15 council members are elected at large and 12 are elected by district. The mayor, elected at large, chairs the council meetings and votes only in case of a tie.

ECONOMY AND INDUSTRY. Govt. is the largest employer in Lexington, followed by trade, manufacturing and services. The chief manufactured products are furniture, automotive parts, tools and machinery, fertilizers, typewriters, electrical parts, house products, apparel, flour, concrete and asphalt, paper products and whiskey. Lexington is the largest Burley tobacco market in the world, and also an important livestock market. The met. area, including Fayette Co., had a labor force of 162,300 in June, 1979, and an unemployment rate of 3.1%.

BANKING. In 1978, total deposits for the seven banks headquartered in Lexington were $1,075,880,000, while assets were $1,250,500,000. Banks include First Security Natl. Bank and Trust, Central Bank and Trust, Citizens' Union Natl., Second Natl. Bank and Trust, Bank of Commerce and Trust, Bank of Lexington and Bank of the Bluegrass.

HOSPITALS. There are a number of hosps. in Lexington, including Cardinal Hill, Central Baptist, Good Samaritan, St. Joseph's, U of KY, Shriner's Hosp. for Crippled Children, E State and two V.A. hosps.

EDUCATION. The U of KY, founded in Lexington in 1865, offers grad and undergrad degrees. In 1978, the U enrolled more than 22,300. Transylvania Col. a privately-supported, liberal arts col., was chartered in 1780 by the VA

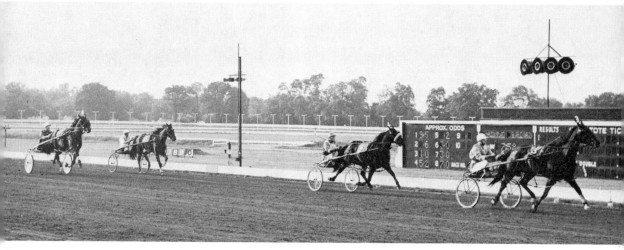

Harness Racing at the Redmile, Lexington, Kentucky

Legislature and has been affiliated with the Christian Church (Disciples of Christ) since 1865. In 1978, enrollment was approx. 780. There are three female seminaries In the city, including Hamilton Female Col. Other institutions include Fugazzi Business Col., KY Business Col., Lexington Technical Institute and St. Joseph's Hosp. Libs. include the Lexington Public Lib. and the lib. of the Lexington Theological Seminary. The Keeneland Lib. is a leading depository of thoroughbred racing material.

ENTERTAINMENT. Lexington's Diner's Playhouse offers dinner theater entertainment. The U of KY Wildcats participate in intercollegiate sports. Horse racing is offered at the Keeneland Race Course and at Red Mile. Racing meets in spring and fall include the Blue Grass Stakes, held in Apr., an important preliminary race for the KY Derby. The Lions Club Blue Grass Fair is held in July, as is the Lexington Jr. League Horse Show.

ACCOMMODATIONS. There are many hotels and motels in Lexington, including the Continental, Lexington Hilton and Sheraton, Hospitality, Holiday, Quality and Ramada inns and Hyatt Regency Hotel.

FACILITIES. The 1032-acre KY Horse Park, near Lexington, contains training facilities and has demonstrations highlighting the region's equine heritage, and also contains camping and picnic facilities. Public golf courses can be found at Lakeside, Meadowbrook, and Tates Creek golf courses.

CULTURAL ACTIVITIES. The Lexington Opera House is the home of the Lexington Philharmonic Orchestra. Approx. 12 events are sponsored annually by the Central KY Concert and Lecture Series. The U of KY School of Music presents many public performances. Exhibits on KY culture are housed in the KY Life Museum. The U of KY Art Gallery has collections of historical and contemporary prints and drawings. Transylvania Col.'s Mitchell Fine Arts Center is the site of the Morland Gallery.

LANDMARKS AND SIGHTSEEING SPOTS. Located in Lexington is Ashland, the home of Henry Clay, which houses Clay family possessions and contains one of the first private racetracks. Hopemont, the home of Confederate Gen. John Hunt Morgan, was erected about 1814 and still stands in the city. Pres. Abraham Lincoln's future wife, Mary Todd, lived in what is now called the Mary Todd Lincoln Home. Bryan Station Memorial honors the pioneer women who risked their lives to bring water to the ft. when it was under assault by Canadians and Indians.

Kentucky Horse Park, Lexington, Kentucky

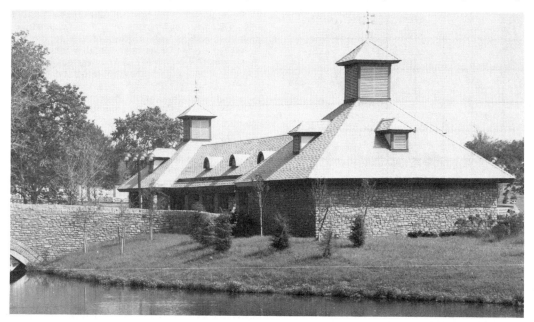

LINCOLN
NEBRASKA

CITY LOCATION-SIZE-EXTENT. Lincoln, the capital of NE and the seat of Lancaster Co., encompasses 58.66 sq. mi. at 40°49' N lat. and 96°42' W long. The second largest city in NE, its met. area extends NE into Cass Co., S into Gage Co., SW into Saline Co., NW into Seward and Butler Counties., N into Saunders Co., SE into Johnson Co. and approaches Otoe Co. on the SE.

TOPOGRAPHY. The terrain of Lincoln lies in the Dissected Till Plains Region and consists of gently rolling prairie. However, the W edge of the city is in the flat basin of Salt Creek. Holmes, Capitol Beach and Oak lakes are all within the city limits. The mean elev. is 1,167'.

CLIMATE. The climate of Lincoln is continental, characterized by cold winters and hot summers. Warm winds from the Rockies, 500 mi. to the W, often produce rapid rises in temp. in the winter. Monthly mean temps. range from 23.4°F in Jan. to 77.9°F in July, with an avg. annual temp. of 51.7°F. The avg. annual rainfall of 27.7" is heavier during the warm season. The avg. annual snowfall is 28.7". The RH ranges between 45% and 86%.

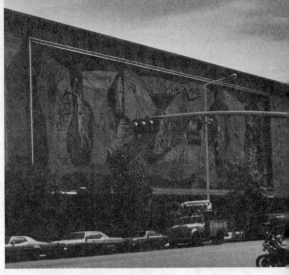

Pershing Municipal Auditorium, Lincoln, Nebraska

approx. 97.7% Caucasian, 1.5% Black and 0.8% others.

TRANSPORTATION. Interstate hwys. 80 and 180, US hwys. 6, 34 and 77 and state hwy. 2 provides major motor access to Lincoln. *Railroads* include Union Pacific, Chicago & N, Burlington N, MO Pacific, Rock Island and AMTRAK. *Airlines* serving Lincoln Municipal Airport include Air WI, FL, UA and Pioneer. *Bus lines* include Greyhound, Trailways and the Lincoln Transit System.

COMMUNICATIONS. Broadcasting, communications and print media originating from Lincoln are: *AM radio stations* KFOR 1240 (ABC/I, MOR); KBRL 1300 (Indep., C&W); KICX 1360 (ABC/C, MOR); KLIN 1400 (MBS, MOR); KLMS 1480 (Indep., Top 40) and KECK 1530 (Indep., C&W); *FM radio stations* KRNU 90.3 (ABC/C, MBS, Clas., MOR); KUCV 91.3 (Indep., Relig., Clas., Educ.); KBHL 95.3 (Indep., Contemp., Relig.); KFMQ 101.9 (Indep., Adult Rock); KFOR 102.7 (Indep., Btfl. Mus.); KHAT 106.3 (Indep., C&W) and KLIN 107.3 (Indep., MOR); *television stations* KOLN Ch. 10 (CBS); KUON Ch. 12 (PBS) and cable; *press*: two major dailies serve the city, the evening *Journal* and the morning *Star*; other publications include the weekly *Lincolnland Sun, The News, The Voice* and *The Wesleyan*; monthly publications include *The Children's Friend, Christian Record, Young and Alive, NE Medical Journal, The NE Newspaper* and *Nebraskaland*.

HISTORY. The site of present-day Lincoln was first inhabited by native Americans of the Sioux tribe, who discovered salt in the basin of Salt Creek. After this discovery, various attempts were made to build a salt industry, and in 1859, a group of salt prospectors formed the city of Lancaster, situated near the salt flats. In 1867, after a bitter quarrel over location of the state capital, Lancaster was selected and renamed Lincoln, in honor of Abraham Lincoln. Within a year the pop. had jumped to over 500. The comm. grew rapidly. With the advent of the Burlington RR in 1870, the pop. continued to increase until, by the turn of the century, 40,000 people lived there. During the early 1900s, the city became an important business and industrial center and a dominant wholesale and retail location. In 1935, the state legislature in Lincoln voted to establish a unicameral system of govt., the only one in the country. The city ranked third nationally in quality of life among cities of its size in a recent indep. survey. Among its list of distinguished citizens are William Jennings Bryan, WW I leader, Gen. John J. Pershing, and author Willa Cather.

GOVERNMENT. Lincoln has a mayor-council form of govt. consisting of seven council members and a mayor. Three council members and the mayor are elected at large and four by district, all to four-year terms. The mayor is not a voting member of the council, but has the right of veto, which may be overridden by a 5/7 majority vote in the council.

ECONOMY AND INDUSTRY. Lincoln has a broad-based

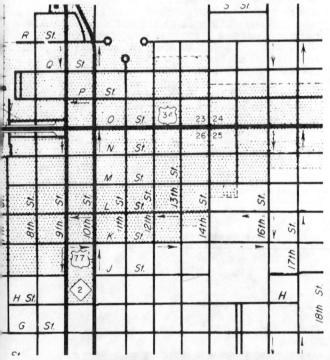

Lincoln, Nebraska

The avg. growing season lasts approx. 183 days. Lincoln is in the CSTZ and observes DST.

FLORA AND FAUNA. Animals native to Lincoln include the red fox, whitetail deer, raccoon and coyote. Typical birds include the pheasant, bobwhite, red-tailed hawk, shrike and swallow. Mud turtles, skinks, American toads, and hognose snakes. Trees include the locust, oak, ash, maple and hackberry. Smaller plants include the musk thistle.

POPULATION. According to the US census, the pop. of Lincoln in 1970 was 149,518. In 1978, it was estimated that it had increased to 168,800.

ETHNIC GROUPS. In 1978, the ethnic distribution of Lincoln was

economy. As the home of local and state govt. and a number of public and private educational institutions, including the main campus of the U of NE, Lincoln has relatively-high levels of employment in govt. and education. Important industries include electronics, research, agriculture, meatpacking and food processing. Major products are motor scooters, rubber belting, electrical and telephone appliances, RR cars, dairy products, meat and flour. The Burlington RR is the city's largest private employer. The total labor force for the area in June, 1979, was 112,750, and the unemployment rate was 3%. Avg. hourly wages for production workers in manufacturing was $6.50.

BANKING. In 1978, total deposits for the 11 banks headquartered in Lincoln were $882,249,000, while assets were $1,178,010,000. Banks include First Natl. and Trust Co. of Lincoln, Natl. of Commerce Trust and Savings Assn., Gateway Bank and Trust Co., Havelock, Citizens' State, Citibank and Trust Co. of Lincoln and Lincoln Bank S Inc.

HOSPITALS. Hosps. in Lincoln include St. Elizabeth's, Bryan and Lincoln Gen., NE Regional Center Psychiatric and the V.A.

EDUCATION. The largest U in Lincoln is the U of NE, Lincoln, whose forerunner was the State U and Agricultural Col., established by the State Legislature in 1869. Offering degrees from associate to doctorate, the U of NE enrolled 22,256 in 1978. NE Wesleyan U is a private institution created in 1887 as the result of the merging of three small Methodist cols. Offering programs leading to bachelor degrees, the U enrolled 1,108 in 1978. Union Col., founded in 1891 by the Seventh Day Adventists, offers courses leading to associate and bachelor degrees. In 1978, this private institution enrolled 923. The SE Comm. Col., a publicly-supported two-year institution, offers courses leading to the associate degree and, in 1978, enrolled 1,199. Lincoln School of Commerce, a private school granting the associate degree, enrolled over 375 in 1978. Other institutions include Bryan Memorial Hosp., St. Elizabeth Comm. Health Center and Lincoln Aviation Institute. There are 33 elementary and 17 secondary schools in the public school system and 13 non-public schools. Lib. facilities include the Bennett Martin Public Lib., with eight branches, and its Heritage Room, housing a collection of Lincoln and NE historical materials; Love Public Lib.; Lincoln Regional Center; NE Lib. Commission and NE State Lib.

ENTERTAINMENT. The Lincolnfest is held in the city each year as well as the U Rodeo. The NE State Fair is held each Sept. Horse racing is also available. The U of NE Plainsmen and Wesleyan teams participate in intercollegiate sports.

ACCOMMODATIONS. Hotels and motels in Lincoln include the Hilton, Villager and Clayton House, and the Congress, Airport, Ramada and Holiday inns.

FACILITIES. Lincoln's city park system covers over 4,496 acres. There are 64 parks, including Holmes, Pioneer, Wilderness, Oak Lake and Antelope. In addition, the parks system features the Chet Ager Nature Center, the Sunken Gardens and the Woods Rose Gardens. There are three zoos, the James Ager Memorial, Pioneers and the Arnott Folsom Children's. Public golf courses are located at Hidden Valley, Holmes, Mahoney, Pine Lake, Pioneers and Ager Memorial Jr. parks. Joggers enjoy the Roberts Park and the Wilderness Park Physical Fitness Course. There are ten outdoor ice skating locations.

CULTURAL ACTIVITIES. Lincoln is served by a symphony orchestra, the Comm. Playhouse, and the music and drama depts. of the U of NE and of NE Wesleyan U. The NE State Historical Society Museum includes displays on native American history and life, period rooms and pioneer exhibits. An extensive collection of modern and fossil elephants is featured at the U of NE State Museum. Lincoln art galleries include the Elder, Sheldon Memorial, Wesleyan and Haymarket.

LANDMARKS AND SIGHTSEEING SPOTS. Historic buildings of interest include the State Capitol building; Fairview, once occupied by the William Jennings Bryan family and now restored with early 1900s period furniture and the Thomas P. Kennard House, built in 1869 and considered the oldest house in Lincoln. The Gov.'s Mansion is also available for tours. Mueller Planetarium is another Lincoln attraction.

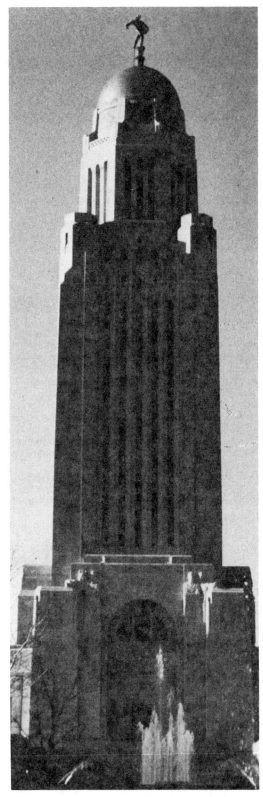

State Capitol Building, Lincoln, Nebraska

LITTLE ROCK
ARKANSAS

CITY LOCATION-SIZE-EXTENT. Little Rock, capital of AR and seat of Pulaski Co., encompasses 56.9 sq. mi. on the S bank of the AR river, at 34°14' N lat. and 92°14' W long. Its met. area includes all of Pulaski Co. and extends N into Faulkner, W into Lonoke and SE into Jefferson counties.

TOPOGRAPHY. The terrain of Little Rock rises slightly from E to W between the flat lowlands of the MS Valley on the E and the Ouachita Mts. to the W. The elev. ranges from 222' to 600'. The mean elev. is 257'.

CLIMATE. Little Rock's continental climate is influenced by all of the N American air masses and, because of its proximity to the Gulf of Mexico, summers are marked by prolonged periods of warm and humid weather. The avg. annual temp. of 62.1°F ranges between a Jan. mean of 41.5°F and a July mean of 81.4°F. The 48.26" avg. annual rainfall is well distributed throughout the year, with the driest period occurring in the late summer and early fall. The RH ranges from 41% to 89%. Snowfall avgs. 5.4" annually. Approx. 62% of the normal rainfall occurs during the growing season, which avgs. 288 days. Little Rock lies in the CSTZ and observes DST.

FLORA AND FAUNA. Animals native to Little Rock include the squirrel, whitetail deer, raccoon and opossum. Common birds include the sharp-shinned hawk, mockingbird, cardinal, great horned owl and bobwhite. Bullfrogs, toads, salamanders, box turtles, king snakes and the venomous copperhead, cottonmouth, coral snake and rattlesnake, are also found here. Typical trees include the pine, oak, elm and sycamore. Smaller plants include honeysuckle, possumhaw, sparkleberry and ironweed.

POPULATION. According to the US census, the pop. of Little Rock in 1970 was 132,483. In 1979, it was estimated that it had increased to 155,000.

ETHNIC GROUPS. In 1978, the ethnic distribution of Little Rock was approx. 74.7% Caucasian, 25% Black and .7% Hispanic (a percentage of the Hispanic total is also included in the Caucasian total).

TRANSPORTATION. Interstate hwys. 30, 40, 430 and 630, US hwys. 65, 67, 70, 167 and 365 and state rtes. 4, 10, 107, 176 and 338 provide major motor access to Little Rock. *Railroads* serving the city include MO

Downtown Little Rock, Arkansas

Pacific, Chicago, Rock Is. & Pacific and St. Louis SW. *Airlines* serving Adams Field include AM, BN, DL, FL, TI, OZ and Skyways. *Bus lines* include Greyhound, Trailways and Central AR Transit. The McClellan-Kerr AR-MS River Navigation System provides a 448-mi. navigation channel to the Verdigris River and includes 17 locks and dams. The Little Rock Port Industrial Park has been designated as a foreign trade zone by the US Dept. of Commerce, allowing storage and processing of duty-free imports.

COMMUNICATIONS. Communications, broadcasting and print media originating from Little Rock are: *AM radio stations* KARN 920 (NBC, Btfl. Mus.); KLRA 1010 (CBS, Easy Ctry.); KSOH 1050 (Indep., Relig.); KAAY 1090 (ABC/C, Top 40) and KITA 1440 (Mut. Blk.); *FM radio stations* KLRE 90.5 (Indep., Clas.); KEZQ 94.1 (ABC/C, Btfl. Mus.); KXXA 95.7 (Indep., All News); KLAZ 98.5 (ABC/FM, Top 40) and KKYK 103.7 (NBC, Rock); *television stations* KETN Ch. 2 (PBS); KARK Ch. 4 (NBC); KATV Ch. 7 (ABC), KTHV Ch. 11 (CBS) and cable; *press*: two major dailies serve the city, the *AR Democrat* and *AR Gazette*. Other publications include *AR Methodist*, *Baptist Trumpet*, *S Mediator Journal* and *AR Cattle Business*.

HISTORY. Quapaw Indians first inhabited the area that is now Little Rock. In 1722, the French explorer Bernard de la Harpe led a party up the AR River to establish trade with the Indians. The name Little Rock, contrary to the popular belief that it was used to describe the smaller of two outcropping rocks along the river bank, evolved from usage and, during the early 1800s, was commonly used to describe the area. Although travelers passed through the area, no one settled until 1814, and then, in 1820, William Russell, a land speculator, established a town there. In 1819, AR became a territory, and in 1820, Little Rock was incorporated as a town. That same year, AR chose Little Rock as the territorial capital although the pop. was less than 20. This, coupled with the town's strategic situation on the AR River, led to its development as a trading center. It was chartered as a city in 1831. During the Civil War, the town served as a supply center for the Confederate Army. In 1863, however, the state govt. was forced to move to Washington, in Hempstead Co., and Union troops, followed by the Union govt. under Isaac Murphy, occupied the town. Trade increased after the war and the city became a significant cotton and lumber market. The city continued to grow. After WW II, the state's industrialization efforts stimulated pop. growth in Little Rock as more factories were established. An increase in govt. employment also brought more people to the city. In 1957, world attention was drawn to the problems of desegregation in Little Rock when the Gov., then Orval E. Faubus, opposed integration of Central High School. As the result of a navigation project on the AR River completed in 1968, Little Rock now has a direct water route to the open sea and barges can go inland into OK via the Inland Waterway.

GOVERNMENT. Little Rock has a city-mgr. form of govt. A seven-member board of directors is elected every two years for four-year terms to determine city policy. The board elects the mayor from its members.

ECONOMY AND INDUSTRY. Agriculture, wholesale and retail trade and manufacturing dominate the economy of met. Little Rock. Over 376 manufacturers in the area produce fabricated metals, chemicals, primary metals, food products, apparel, machinery, textiles and paper products. Little Rock is a chief market for cotton, rice and soybeans. Avg. income per capita, in 1976, was $5,244, while avg. income per household was $15,300. The labor force in the met. area totaled 191,600 in June, 1979, while unemployment was 4.1%.

BANKING. There are 10 banks and six savings and loan assns. in Little Rock. In 1978, total deposits for the six banks headquartered in the city

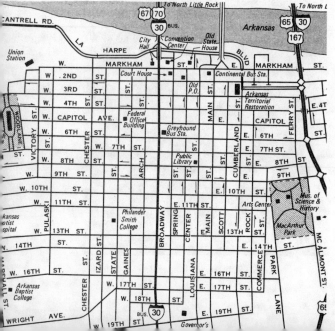

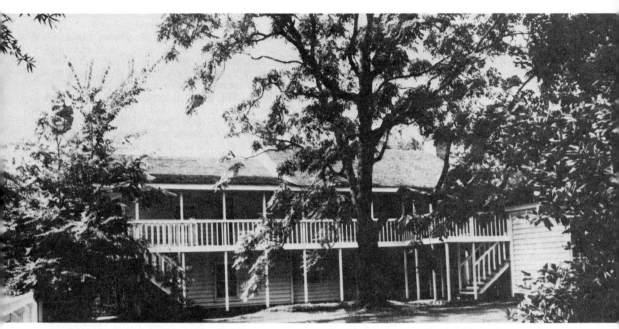

Arkansas Territorial Restoration, Little Rock Arkansas

were $1,240,210,000, while assets were $1,627,586,000. Banks include Worthern Bank and Trust, First Natl., Commercial Natl., Union Natl. Bank, Pulaski Bank and Trust and Met. Natl.

HOSPITALS. Little Rock is the center of medicine in AR and hosps. include, the U of AR Medical Center, an important center of kidney transplant and R&D; the new Baptist Medical Center; St. Vincent Infirmary; Central Baptist; Doctors; Memorial; AR Children's; MO Pacific (for RR employees); V.A.; and State, a leading mental health treatment center.

EDUCATION. The U of AR at Little Rock, which enrolled 10,004 students in 1979, is a state-supported institution offering programs leading to bachelor and master degrees. The Grad Institute of Technology; Grad School of Social Work; and Law School and Medical Center of the U of AR, are also located in the city. The U of AR Medical Sciences Campus enrolled 1,500 in 1979. Other institutions include the AR Baptist Col., Philander Smith Col., Capital City Business Col., United Electronics Institute, Shorter Col. and Draughon School of Business. The Little Rock School District consists of one vocational, 14 primary, 14 intermediate, seven jr. and three sr. high schools. There are 14 parochial and numerous private schools in the area. There are also special schools including the AR School for the Blind and the AR School for the Deaf. Public libs. in the met. area include the AR Lib. Commission, Little Rock Public Lib. and the Pulaski-Perry Regional Lib. and its branches.

ENTERTAINMENT. Each year, Little Rock hosts the AR Livestock Exposition in Oct., the AR State Festival of the Arts in May and the AR State Fair in Sept. The city's pro baseball team, the AR Travelers, is a farm club of the St. Louis Cardinals and plays at Ray Winder Field. Collegiate football is provided by the U of AR's Razorbacks.

ACCOMMODATIONS. Hotels and motels in Little Rock include the Hilton, LaQuinta and Sands and the Americana, Camelot, Coachman's Vagabond, Holiday and Magnolia inns.

FACILITIES. The 15,000-acre Little Rock met. park system includes 43 parks featuring three municipal pools, 28 ball fields, 18 pavillions, a pistol range and tennis facilities including Walker Tennis Center. Public golf courses are available at Pine Valley, Rock Creek, Hindman, Rebsamen and War Memorial parks. The zoo, located in War Memorial Park, includes a tropical rain forest display, aquarium, chimpanzee island, sea lion display, bear dens and flamingo area. Other parks include Overlook, Boyule, Burns and MacArthur. Fishing and boating are available at nearby David D. Terry Lake, which together with Murray Lock and Dam, providing an extra 771 acres to the parks of Greater Little Rock.

CULTURAL ACTIVITIES. The AR Arts Center in Little Rock contains four galleries with exhibits on visual and performing arts and a 400-seat theater. The theater is used by the Little Rock Comm. Theatre, the Little Rock Musical Coterie and the Arts Center's Children's Theatre. The Symphony Orchestra and the Repertory Theatre perform at the Little Rock Convention Center. Other cultural groups include the Orchestra Guild, Chamber Music Society, Comm. Concert Assn., AR Opera Theatre, The Broadway Theatre Series, the U of AR at Little Rock Theatre Group, Youth Orchestra Group and Little Rock Ballet Co. The Museum of Science and Natural History presents lecture tours on ancient cultures, pioneers, native Americans and ecology. The Planetarium and Observatory at U of AR are open to the public.

Quapaw Quarter, Little Rock, Arkansas

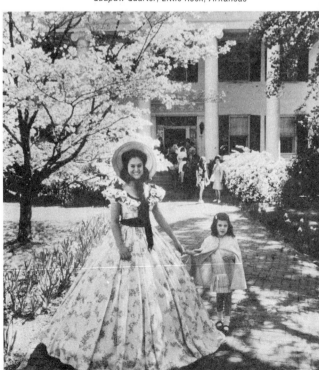

LANDMARKS AND SIGHTSEEING SPOTS. Named for native Americans of the Quapaw tribe, Quapaw Quarter is the oldest residential section of Little Rock. Among the historic houses is Trapnall Hall, built in 1843 in the classic Greek Revival style, as the home for AR's pioneer lawyer, Frederick W. Trapnall. Located on W Markham Street is Old State House, the State Capitol from 1836 to 1911, also in the classic Greek Revival style, originally designed by Gideon Shyrock and restored by the state. Built of hand-hewn logs and clay chinking between 1826 and 1828, the Hinderliter House is believed to be the meeting place of the last Territorial Legislature in 1835. Other historic homes include the Woodruff House and the Noland House. Old Mill, a paper mill built in the 19th century, was the setting for an opening scene in the movie "Gone With the Wind." There is a marker on the bank of the AR river near where Bernard de la Harpe first landed and named the area "La Petite Roche"—in English, Little Rock.

LIVONIA
MICHIGAN

CITY LOCATION-SIZE-EXTENT. Livonia, in SE MI, encompasses 36.1 sq. mi. two mi. W of Detroit in Wayne Co., at 42°23′ N lat. and 83°22′5″ W long. It is a part of the greater Detroit met. area.

TOPOGRAPHY. The terrain of Livonia, which is situated in the Great Lakes plains, varies from gently sloping areas to hilly regions to the NW. The mean elev. is 581′.

CLIMATE. The climate of Livonia is characterized by winter storms bringing periods of snow or rain, summer storms bringing brief showers and occasional thundershowers or damaging winds, and is influenced by the Great Lakes, which moderate most climatic extremes. The avg. annual temp. of 48.5°F ranges from a Jan. mean of 22.5°F to a July mean of 71.7°F. Most of the 31″ avg. annual rainfall occurs during the warmer months. Approx. 50% of the 40″ avg. annual snowfall occurs during Dec. and Jan. The RH ranges from 50% to 88%. The avg. growing season is approx. 180 days. Livonia lies in the ESTZ and observes DST.

FLORA AND FAUNA. Animals native to Livonia include the fox, raccoon and deer. Common birds include the goldfinch, crow, sparrow, robin, blackbird and cowbird. Bullfrogs, salamanders, milk snakes and skinks, as well as the venomous E massasauga (a pygmy rattler), are also found here.

Central Livonia, Michigan

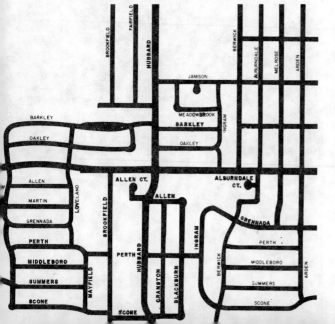

Typical trees are the maple, pine, beech, oak and elm. Smaller plants include the dogwood, rose, blackberry and goldenrod.

POPULATION. According to the US census, the pop. of Livonia in 1970 was 110,109. In 1978, it was estimated that it had increased to 110,800.

ETHNIC GROUPS. In 1978, the ethnic distribution of Livonia was approx. 99.7% Caucasian and 0.8% Hispanic (a percentage of the Hispanic total is also included in the Caucasian total).

TRANSPORTATION. Interstate hwys. 96 and 275 provide major motor access to Livonia. The Chesapeake & OH *Railroad* provides rail service to the city. Detroit Met. Airport, seven mi. S, offers service on all major *airlines. Bus lines* serving the city include Greyhound, Trailways and the local SE MI Transportation Authority (SEMTA).

COMMUNICATIONS. Communications, broadcasting and print media serving Livonia are: no *AM radio stations, FM radio stations*, or *television stations* originate in Livonia, which receives broadcasting and print media from the Detroit met. area; *press*: publications include the bi-weekly *Observer* and the *Ceramic Teaching Projects and Trade News, Ceramic Arts & Crafts*

HISTORY. Native Americans of the Wyandot tribe occupied the region near present-day Livonia before the first white settlers arrived from N.E. and NY. Settlers were first attracted to Livonia by the area's lucrative fur-trapping enterprise, and later by the agricultural promise shown in the rich soil. When the settlement became the Township of Livonia in 1835, the transition from wilderness to farmland was nearly complete. The name, derived from a former province in W Russia, is thought to have been chosen because its uniqueness insured incorporation without delay. When Livonia was chartered as a city in 1950, with a pop. of 17,000, it encompassed the entire township. By 1978, the city's residents numbered 110,800. Livonia's advantageous position on a major RR and a major hwy. has made it a transportation center and created industrial and commercial growth.

GOVERNMENT. Livonia has a mayor-council form of govt. The mayor, not a voting member of the council, is elected at large to a four-year term, while the seven council members are elected at large to two- or four-year terms.

ECONOMY AND INDUSTRY. The combination of a major RR and a major hwy. has made Livonia an industrial corridor, providing transportation to all parts of the met. area. The city's industry grew from 22 plants in 1950 to 255 in 1970, while, during the same period, employment in industrial plants increased from 579 to 27,000. Area manufacturers produce food products, machinery, plastics, automotive parts, furnaces and ovens and welding and electrical apparatus. The economy of Livonia, part of the greater Detroit met. area, is reflected in the economic data of that city.

BANKING. There are eight commercial banks in Livonia. In 1978, total deposits for the three banks headquartered in the city were $248,919,000, while assets were $278,360,000. Banks include MI Natl.-W Met., Detroit-Livonia and Manufacturers' of Livonia.

HOSPITALS. St. Mary's, a gen. hosp., and Ardmore Acres, a private psychiatric hosp., are located in Livonia. Additional health care facilities are available in nearby Detroit.

EDUCATION. There are three institutions of higher learning in Livonia. Schoolcraft Col. is a locally-controlled col. offering associate degrees. Established in 1961, it enrolled more than 10,000 in 1978. Madonna Col., a private, liberal arts col. affiliated with the Felician Sisters of the Roman Catholic Church, awards bachelor degrees. Incorporated as a sr. col. in 1947, the col. enrolled approx. 2,500 in 1978. Dorsey School of Business is also located in the city. The Livonia Public School District maintains approx. 24 elementary, seven jr. high and four high schools. Catholic and Lutheran schools are also located in the city. Lib. facilities are provided through the Livonia Public Lib.

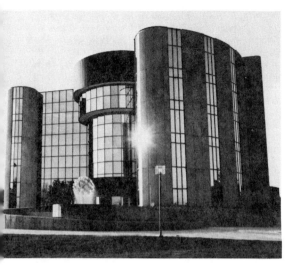

New City Hall, Livonia, Michigan

ENTERTAINMENT. Collegiate sports entertainment is offered by the Schoolcraft Col. Ocelots. Additional entertainment is available in the area.

ACCOMMODATIONS. There is a Holiday Inn in Livonia and other lodging is available nearby .

FACILITIES. Livonia offers several recreational facilities, including two public golf courses and tennis courts at a local racquet club. Skating facilities are also available. Nearby Detroit offers many recreational facilities.

CULTURAL ACTIVITIES. The 90-piece Oakwood Symphony Orchestra is based in Livonia. Other cultural activities are available in the Detroit Met. area.

LANDMARKS AND SIGHTSEEING SPOTS. The Greenmead Farm in Livonia is listed on the Natl. Register of Historic Places. Many other attractions are also available in nearby Detroit.

LONG BEACH
CALIFORNIA

CITY LOCATION-SIZE-EXTENT. Long Beach encompasses 50.1 sq. mi. in LA Co. in central SW CA at 33°49' N lat. and 118°9' W long. It is 100 mi. N of San Diego and 25 mi. S of LA, bordered by Orange Co. to the SE and is part of the LA met. area.

TOPOGRAPHY. Long Beach lies in the LA Ranges region. Its terrain is flat to rolling. The city has one major hill, Signal Hill, with an elev. of 320'. The city has 5.5 mi. of beach along the San Pedro Bay. The San Gabriel Mts. are 30 mi. to the N and the Santa Ana Mts. are 20 mi. to the E. The mean elev. is 35'.

CLIMATE. The climate of Long Beach is coastal marine. The avg. annual temp. of 63°F ranges from a July mean of 72.6°F to a Jan. mean of 54.6°F. The avg. annual rainfall is 10.27", most of which occurs during the winter months. The RH ranges between 50% and 80%. Long Beach lies in the PSTZ and observes DST.

FLORA AND FAUNA. Animals native to Long Beach include the pocket gopher, skunk and opossum. Common birds are the gull, egret, great blue heron, house finch and W kingbird. Tree frogs, bullfrogs, salamanders and toads, are found in the area. Typical trees include the introduced eucalyptus and pine and palm. Smaller plants include chaparral shrubs and bunch grasses.

POPULATION. According to the US census, the pop. of Long Beach in 1970 was 361,427. In 1978, it was estimated that it had decreased to 345,000, and the 1979 estimate ranges between 350,000 and 360,000.

ETHNIC GROUPS. In 1976, the ethnic distribution of Long Beach was approx. 74% Caucasian, 9% Black, 12% Hispanic and 5% other.

TRANSPORTATION. Interstate hwys. 405 and 605 and state rtes. 1, 7, 11 and 19 provide major motor access to Long Beach. *Railroads* include Santa Fe, Pacific and Union Pacific. Long Beach Airport offers intra-state passenger service, freight, commuter and charter service. The only major commercial carrier utilizing the airport is Pacific SW Airlines. All major natl. and intl. *airlines* serve nearby LA Intl. Airport. *Bus lines* include Greyhound, Trailways, S CA Rapid Transit District and Long Beach Transit. The Port of Long Beach has the deepest harbor on the US W coast handling approx. 40 million tons annually.

COMMUNICATIONS. Communications, broadcasting and print media originating from the Long Beach area are: *AM radio stations* KFOX 1280 (Indep., C&W) and KGER 1390 (Indep., Relig., Blk.); *FM radio stations* KLON 88.1 (NPR, Ed.); KSUL 90.1 (Indep., Var); KNOB 97.9 (UPI) and KNAC 105.5 (Indep.); *television stations* Long Beach receives television broadcasting from LA; *press*: two jointly-owned major daily newspapers are published in the city, the morning *Independent* and the evening *Press-Telegram*; other publications include the weekly *Cycle News W, Cycle News E, Marina News, Argus, Pacific News, Signal Hill Tribune, Viking* and the monthly *Apartment Owner/Builder* and *Computer*, the bi-weekly *Biker*, the bi-monthly *Dynamic Years*, the daily *Forty-Niner*, the semi-weekly *Reporter*, and the semi-monthly *Modern Maturity* and *NRTA Journal*.

HISTORY. Native Americans of the Shoshone tribe inhabited the Long Beach area prior to white settlement. The region was first documented by the Spanish explorer Cabrillo, who led an expedition there in 1542. In 1784, it was included in the Spanish land grant to Manuel Nieto, later divided into the Los Cerritos and

Civic Center, Long Beach, California

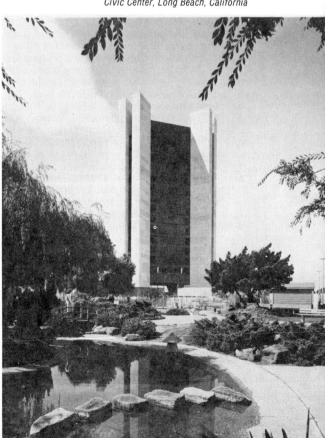

Los Alamitos Ranchos. Following the Mexican War these lands were sold for a low price. In 1870, the English developer William Ervin Willmore first glimpsed the site, and 12 years later he returned with a group of investors and founded the township of Willmore City. When the venture failed two years later, Willmore departed for AZ, but other settlers remained. The city was renamed Long Beach after its fine shoreline and in 1888 was incorporated as a city. In 1897 citizens opposed to liquor prohibition joined forces with those dissatisfied with taxes and voted to disincorporate the town. This state of affairs, however, was shortlived. The development of Long Beach into a resort city was facilitated by its beaches and warm climate. Oil discovered at Signal Hill in 1921 caused the pop. to boom from 55,593 in 1920 to 142,032 in 1930. In 1933 an earthquake in the city killed 52 people and caused extensive damage. In 1936, the larger Wilmington Oil Field was discovered. The outbreak of WW II initiated development of the aircraft industry and the establishment of a Naval Shipyard in Long Beach. Land in the harbor was found to be slowly sinking in the 1940s and threatened to close the Naval Shipyard and damage a larger section of the city. It was determined that this was the result of extensive oil removal, and salt water was pumped back into the ground to restore pressure. The pop. of Long Beach reached 250,767 in 1950, spurred by the growth of industry. During the 1970s the city began construction of a series of civic improvements.

GOVERNMENT. Long Beach, a charter city, has a council-mgr. form of govt. consisting of nine council members including the mayor. The council members are elected every four years by district and the mayor is selected by fellow council members; he is a voting member of the council. The city mgr. is appointed.

ECONOMY AND INDUSTRY. There are over 400 manufacturing firms in Long Beach. Leading manufactured products are transportation equipment, including airframe and shipbuilding; petroleum products; chemicals and allied products; fabricated metal products and food and products. The city has over 400 wholesale establishments, over 3,000 retailing establishments and over 3,000 service-related establishments. The city has rich oil deposits including the large Wilmington Oil Field. As of 1976, the labor force in Long Beach was estimated to be 147,000. Manufacturing was the largest sector (33,000 employees) followed by govt. (30,000) and services (29,000). The unemployment figure in June, 1979, for the area including LA was 5.2%.

BANKING. In 1978, total deposits for the five banks headquartered in Long Beach were $369,002,000, while assets were $446,941,000. Banks include Farmers and Merchants of Long Beach, Coast Bank, Harbor Bank, Natl. of Long Beach, Farmers and Merchants Trust Co., Bank of America, City Natl., Harbor, Lloyds of CA, Security Pacific Natl., The Sumitomo of CA and Union.

Long Beach, California

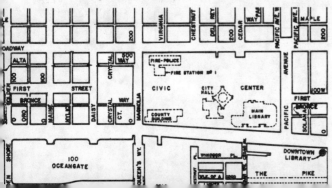

HOSPITALS. Long Beach has eight gen. hosps., including Long Beach, Comm., Long Beach Gen., Los Altos, Memorial, Pacific, Westside Comm. and Woodruff Comm. There are also a V.A. Hosp., and a Navy Hosp.

EDUCATION. CA State U at Long Beach, established in 1949, was the birthplace of the first Intl. Sculpture Symposium held in the US and was the first U in the world to sponsor such an event. The public supported liberal arts coeducational col. grants bachelor degrees and master degrees in over 50 major areas. Enrollment in 1978 was 36,895. Other institutions are Pacific Coast U, Long Beach City Col., Brooks Col., Long Beach Col. of Bus., CA Col. of Commerce and S CA Comm. Bible Col. Long Beach has 56 elementary schools, 15 jr. high schools and eight sr. high schools. Long Beach Lib. serves the city.

ENTERTAINMENT. The Long Beach Grand Prix held annually each Apr. attracts the world's best drivers to compete over a challenging course laid out on downtown city streets. The only collegiate sports team in the city is the CA State U at Long Beach 49ers. Dinner theater, professional and collegiate sports and annual events are accessible to Long Beach residents in nearby LA.

ACCOMMODATIONS. Hotels and motor inns in Long Beach include the Queen Mary Hyatt, Long Beach Hyatt, the Queensway Hilton and the Holiday Inn. The new Hyatt Regency, to be located at the Long Beach Convention Center, is scheduled for completion in 1982.

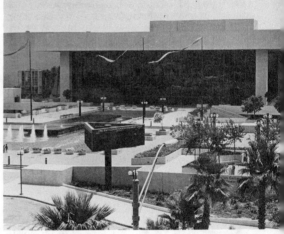

Convention and Entertainment Center, Long Beach, California

FACILITIES. Long Beach is well known for the 5.5 mi. of beach front which initially gave the city its name. The 1,850-slip Long Beach Marina in the E part of the city will be joined in 1982 by a new 1,650-slip downtown marina. Belmont Pier provides a fishing platform and boating facilities. Belmont Olympic Pool, a huge indoor facility on the beach front, offers recreational swimming and has hosted Olympic swimming and diving trials. The city has an extensive park and recreational system, including the regional El Dorado Park. Included in the latter park is the El Dorado Nature Center, an 80-acre semi-wilderness area which contains well-marked nature trails. There are three 18-hole and one nine-hole public golf courses. Tennis court facilities are located in several parks, including the Billie Jean King Tennis Center. Plans are now proceeding for a new Shoreline Aquatic Park on the city's downtown shoreline.

CULTURAL ACTIVITIES. Long Beach is served by a Symphony Orchestra, a Municipal Band and a Civic Light Opera Company. Dramatic productions are staged in the Comm. Playhouse. The Long Beach Arts Museum houses art and sculpture. Rancho Los Cerritos is an historical museum and reference lib.

LANDMARKS AND SIGHTSEEING SPOTS. Ranchos Los Alamitos, constructed in 1884 and one of the oldest adobe structures still in use in CA, is located in Long Beach. The *Queen Mary*, one of the largest passenger liners ever built, is permanently docked at Pier J. It houses a sea marine exhibit designed by Jacques Cousteau.

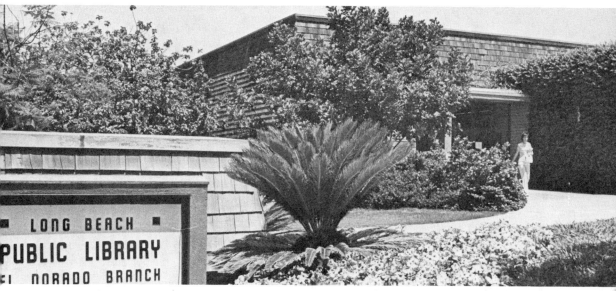

Public Library, Long Beach, California

LOS ANGELES
CALIFORNIA

CITY LOCATION-SIZE-EXTENT. LA, the largest city in the state in both pop. and area, the third largest in pop. in the nation and the seat of LA Co., encompasses 463.9 sq. mi. on the Pacific Ocean coast of SW CA at 34°03' N lat. and 118°14' W long. The second most populous in the nation, the met. area extends into the counties of Orange to the S, San Bernardino to the W, Ventura to the NW and Riverside to the SE and consists of a sprawling complex of intermingling comms., including Burbank, Glendale, Hollywood, Long Beach and many others.

TOPOGRAPHY. The terrain of LA, which is situated in the LA Ranges, varies from beaches and coastal plains on the E to coastal mt. ranges to the W of the city. The Hollywood Hills and Santa Monica Mts. extend E and W in the N section of the city. Several reservoirs, including Chatsworth, Encino and Stone Canyon, lie within the city. The coastal hills attain maximum elevs. of 5,049', while the mean elev. is 287'.

CLIMATE. The climate of LA is maritime, characterized by normally pleasant and mild weather which is maintained throughout the year by the moderating influences of the Pacific Ocean and the S CA coastal mt. ranges. The avg. annual temp. of 62.8°F ranges from a Jan. mean of 55.4°F to an Aug. mean of 70.9°F. Daily temp. variations range from 15°F to 30°F, depending on location. Approx. 85% of the avg. annual rainfall of 13.57" occurs during Nov. through Mar., while summers receive virtually no rainfall. Light fog occurs each month, although heavy fog rarely occurs during the summer. The RH ranges from 45% to 84%. LA lies in the PSTZ and observes DST.

FLORA AND FAUNA. Animals native to LA include the coyote, pocket gopher, opossum and deer mouse. Common birds include the scrub jay, house finch, mourning dove, hummingbird and W kingbird. Bullfrogs, toads, salamanders and pond turtles, as well as the venomous Pacific rattlesnake,

are found in the area. Typical trees include the pine, oak, willow and fir. Smaller plants are the chaparral shrub, poppy and blue blossom.

POPULATION. According to the US census, the pop. of LA in 1970 was 2,811,801. In 1978, it was estimated that it had decreased to 2,795,000.

ETHNIC GROUPS. In 1978, the ethnic distribution of LA was approx. 77.5% Caucasian, 17.9% Black and 18.4% Hispanic (a percentage of the Hispanic total is also included in the Caucasian total).

TRANSPORTATION. Interstate hwys. 5, 10, 210 and 405, US hwy. 101 and state hwys. 1, 11, 27 and 118 provide major motor access to LA. There are 15 *railroads* serving the city, including AMTRAK, Burlington N, ConRail, Consolidated Rail, French Natl., Mexican, Santa Fe, S Pacific and Union Pacific. *Airlines* serving LA Intl. Airport, ranked among the top ten freight airports in the world, include AA, BN, CO, DL, EA, FT, NA, NW, PA, RD, RW, RI, TW, UA and WA. Hollywood-Burbank Airport offers flights on CO, RW and TI. *Bus lines* serving the city include Greyhound, American Pacific Stage Co., Trailways and the local S CA Rapid Transit District (SCRTD).

COMMUNICATIONS. Communications, broadcasting and print media originating from LA are: *AM radio stations* KLAC 570 (Indep., C&W); KFI 640 (ABC/E, MOR); KMPC 710 (Indep., Adult Contemp.); KABC 790 (ABC/I, Talk); KHJ 930 (Indep., Top 40); KFWB 980 (Indep., News); KTNQ 1020 (Indep., Top 40); KNX 1070 (CBS, News); KIIS 1150 (ABC/C, MOR); KKTT 1230 (Indep., Blk.); KFAC 1330 (MBS, Clas.) and KPOL 1540 (CBS, Good Mus.); *FM radio stations* KXLU 88.9 (Indep., Clas.); KPFK 90.7 (Indep., Educ.); KFAC 92.3 (MBS, Clas.); KNX 93.1 (CBS, Good Contemp.); KPOL 93.9 (Indep., Good Mus.); KMET 94.7 (Indep., Progsv.); KLOS 95.5 (ABC/FM, Rock); KFSG 96.3 (Indep., Relig.); KGBS 97.1 (NBC, Clas.); KJOI 98.7 (Indep., Btfl. Mus.); KHOF 99.5 (Indep., Relig.); KIQQ 100.3 (Indep., Top 40); KRTH 101.1 (Indep., Oldies); KIIS 102.7 (Indep., Top 40); KOST 103.5 (Indep., Btfl. Mus.); KBIG 104.3 (Indep., Btfl. Mus.); KBCA 105.1 (Indep., Jazz); KWST 105.9 (Indep., Progsv.) and KLVE 107.5 (Indep., Soft Rock); *television stations* KNXT Ch. 2 (CBS); KNBC Ch. 4 (NBC); KTLA Ch. 5 (Indep.); KABC Ch. 7 (ABC); KHJ Ch. 9 (Indep.); KTTV Ch. 11 (Indep.); KCOP Ch. 9 (Indep.); KWHY Ch. 22 (Indep.); KCET Ch. 28 (PBS); KMEX Ch. 34 (Indep.); KLXA Ch. 40 (Indep.); KBSA Ch. 467 (Metro.); KBSC Ch. 52 (Indep.); KLCS Ch. 58 (PBS) and cable; *press*: two major dailies serve the city, the *Times*, issued mornings, and the *Herald-Examiner*, issued evenings; other daily publications include *LA Opinion, Met. News, Daily Racing Form* and *Daily Trojan;* weekly publications include *LA City News, LA City Press, NW Leader, Central News, SE Wave-Star, Southside Journal, SW Sun, SW News, SW Topics-Wave* and *SW Wave*. Major monthly publications include *Coast Magazine, Motor Trend, Off-Road, Everywoman, Popular Cycling, Guns and*

Ammo, Hot Rod Magazine, Human Behavior and *CA Magazine.* Quarterly publications include *Financial Observer, Ostomy Quarterly, The Personalist* and *Gems & Gemology.*

HISTORY. Native Americans of the Shoshone tribe inhabited a village on the site of present-day LA when a Spanish expedition in search of Monterey visited the site, naming it "Nuestra Senora la Reina de Los Angeles de Porciuncula" or "Our Lady the Queen of the Angels of Porciuncula". The Mission San Gabriel was established nearby in 1771, and, in 1781, Spanish Gov. Felipe de Neve led 11 families to establish a town on the site as part of Spain's efforts to colonize CA. The area, which had been divided into large cattle ranches, came under Mexican rule in 1821, when Mexico won independence from Spain. LA alternated with Monterey as the capital of the territory. Americans made their first appearance in the city when fur trapper Jedediah Smith arrived in 1826 and settlers arrived in 1841. In 1847, LA was the last place to surrender to the US after war erupted between the US and Mexico in 1846. CA became a US territory after the 1848 signing of the Treaty of Guadalupe Hidalgo. In 1850, LA was incorporated as a city and CA gained statehood. The pop. of the city, which in 1850 totaled approx. 1,600, increased slowly until RRs, completed in 1876 and 1886, provided easy access of people into and produce from the city. The pop. doubled during the decade preceding 1900, increasing from 50,000 to 100,000. The early 1900s were years of progress, as oil fields were discovered, the first movie was filmed in the city ("The Count of Monte Cristo", completed in 1907), an artificial harbor was built at San Pedro (completed in 1914) and aircraft factories opened. An economic slump during the Great Depression was followed during WW II by great activity within the war plants and an influx of workers, particularly blacks, which increased the pop. to more than 1.5 milion by 1945. The pop. continued to increase, reaching approx. 2.5 million by 1960. Overcrowding within the city created unemployment, traffic congestion, inadequate public transit and pollution, problems which plagued the city through the 1970s. In 1965, riots in Watts left 34 dead, while 64 died in a 1971 earthquake. Today, LA is a center of tourism, trade and the aerospace and electronic industries.

Los Angeles, California

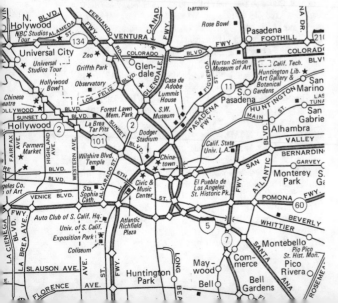

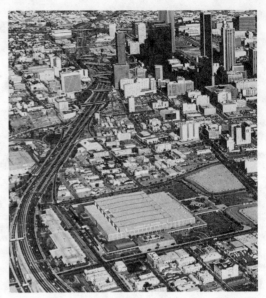

Aerial view of Downtown, Los Angeles, California

GOVERNMENT. LA has a mayor-council form of govt. The mayor, elected at large to a three-year term, is not a voting member of council, but is empowered to appoint the 23 commissioners to direct the 23 city depts. The council meets each weekday and its 15 members are full-time council persons. All members are elected by district to four-year terms.

ECONOMY AND INDUSTRY. The third largest manufacturing center in the US, LA has a highly-diversified industrial base. Approx. one-eighth of the area's manufacturing plants are involved in the aerospace industry. Other major industries include tourism, construction, automobile assembly, machinery and metals fabrication, motion-picture production, agriculture, fishing and publishing. Major products include plastics and instruments, primary metals, electronics, food, apparel, chemicals, rubber, furniture and armaments. The labor force in Mar., 1979, for LA Co. was 3,515,000, while the rate of unemployment was 5.7%. In 1977, the per capita income was $6,922, while the median household effective buying income was $15,452.

BANKING. There are 38 banking institutions in LA. In 1978, total deposits for the 38 banks headquartered in the city were $35,744,555,000, while assets were $43,765,255,000. Banks include Security Pacific Natl., United CA, Union, Lloyds of CA, Manufacturers, Imperial, Mitsubishi of CA, American City and First LA.

HOSPITALS. There are more than 55 hosps. in LA, including Beverly Glen, CA Hosp. and Medical Center, Cedars Sinai Medical Center, Children's of LA, City View, French of LA, Hollywood Presbyterian Medical Center, Hosp. of Good Samaritan, Kaiser, Martin Luther King, Jr. Gen., St. Vincent's, Temple, U CA LA HOSP., LA U of S CA Medical Center and Shriner's for Crippled Children. The two V.A. facilities are Brentwood and Wadsworth.

EDUCATION. The largest public institution in the city is the U of CA at LA, one of the nine branches of the U CA. Academically ranked among the leading universities in the nation, the U began with 250 students in 1919 and enrolled more than 31,700 in 1978. CA State U at LA, established in 1947, is a state-controlled institution with a 1978 enrollment of approx. 26,400. The privately-supported U of S CA, prominent in research, offers bachelor, master and doctoral degrees.It enrolled approx. 28,000 in 1978. LA City Col., a publicly-supported institution, awards associate degrees. In 1978, it enrolled approx. 20,000. Other institutions include Occidental Col., CA School of Professional Psychology, Center for Early Education, Fashion Institute of Design and Merchandising, Immaculate Heart Col., Intl. Col.,

L.I.F.E. Bible Col., LA SW Col., LA Trade-Technical Col., Loyola Marymount U, Mount St. Mary's Col., Otis Art Institute of LA Co., SW U School of Law, U of Judaism, W Coast U and Woodbury U. The LA public school system, the second largest in the US, enrolls more than 750,000 in approx. 600 schools. More than 50,000 attend the nearly 225 private and parochial schools in the city. Libs. include the LA Co. Law Lib., the LA Co. Medical Assistants Lib., the LA Co. Public Lib. System and the Natural Historical Museum of LA Co.

ENTERTAINMENT. Annual events in LA include the Chinese New Year Celebration in Jan. or Feb., the Great W Livestock and Poultry show in Dec., the LA Co. Fair in Sept. and Nisei Week in Aug. The area has many movie theaters, befitting its image as "Film Capital of the World". The Rams of NFL-NFC football, the Dodgers of NL baseball, the Lakers of NBA basketball, the Kings of NHL-POWC hockey, the Monarchs of PHL hockey, the Aztecs of NASL soccer and the Strings of WTT tennis, offer professional sports entertainment, while the UCLA Bruins, the USC Trojans, the U of LA Co. Diablos and the LA City Cubs participate in intercollegiate sports.

ACCOMMODATIONS. There are numerous hotels and motels in LA, including the LA Bonaventure, LA Hilton, New Otani, Hyatt House, Pacifica, Hotel Bel Air, Beverly Ilills Hotel, Beverly Hilton, Beverly Wilshire, Century Plaza, L'Ermitage, Royal Palace, Westwood Marquis, Sportsmen's Lodge, Beverly Hillcrest, Beverly House, Broadway Plaza Hyatt, Marina del Rey, Hotel Bel Air, TraveLodge, Best Western, Howard Johnson's and Holiday, Quality and Ramada inns.

FACILITIES. There are approx 75 mi. of beaches, providing year-round surfing and swimming, and 210 parks and playgrounds in LA. The 4,000-acre Griffith Park, the largest municipal park in the nation, features ballfields, bridlepaths, golf courses, tennis courts and 113-acre LA Zoo. The five continental areas of the LA Zoo provide a natural setting for more than 2,000 mammals, birds and reptiles, while the children's zoo features an animal nursery and petting yard. The city maintains 14 public golf courses. Tennis courts are available at Griffith Park and many other locations.

CULTURAL ACTIVITIES. A major cultural center in LA is the Music Center for the Performing Arts, part of the Civic Center. It consists of 3,250-seat Dorothy Chandler Pavillion, a concert hall, the 2,100-seat Ahmanson Theatre and the 750-seat Mark Taper Forum. Ballet, drama, dance and opera troupes, the LA Philharmonic, the Center Theatre Group, the LA Civic Light Opera, the LA Master Chorale, and the LA Neophonic Orchestra perform in the Mark Taper Forum. Two open-air theaters, the 20,000-seat Hollywood Bowl and the 4,000-seat Greek Theatre, are also in the city. Other theaters and concert halls in LA incude the Century City Playhouse, the Huntington Hartford Theatre, The Ivar Theatre and the Shrine Auditorium. UCLA and USC also present musical and dramatic programs in their campus theaters. The LA Co. Museum of Art, the city's largest, houses exhibits ranging from ancient Egyptian articles to modern art. Other museums include the Henry E. Huntington Lib. and Art Gallery, the LA Municipal Art Gallery and the SW Museum. The LA Co. Museum of Natural History, in Exposition Park, features a collection of pre-historic fossils. The most famous theater in the city is Mann's, formerly Graumann's Chinese Theatre, known for its unusual exterior. Other theaters are the ABC Entertainment Center, Amphitheatre, Mayfair Music Hall, Pantages Theatre, Westwood Playhouse and Schubert Theatre.

LANDMARKS AND SIGHTSEEING SPOTS. Several sections of LA offer shops and cafes of a particular heritage, including Chinatown and Little Tokyo, Heritage Square and Carroll Ave. are reminiscent of the Victorian period, while Olvera Street features a bricked walkway which passes through an authentic-appearing marketplace. The 52-floor Atlantic-Richfield Plaza is one of the largest office complexes in the W. The Watts Towers, three web-like towers constructed on concrete-coated steel rods, shells, tile and glass, represent 33 years of work for the tilesetter Simon Rodia. Casa de Adobe, furnished in the style of the 1880s, is a reconstructed Spanish Colonial hacienda, while the architecture of Frank Lloyd Wright is represented at Hollyhock House. There are many interesting churches and temples in LA, including the First Baptist Church and its rose windows (replicas of those in the cathedral at Chartres, France) and ceiling (a replica of a palace ceiling in Mantova, Italy); the world's largest Mormon Temple, including a 15' statue of the Angel Moroni on its 257' tower; St. John's Church, a replica of an 11th-century church at Toscannella, Italy; St. Sophia

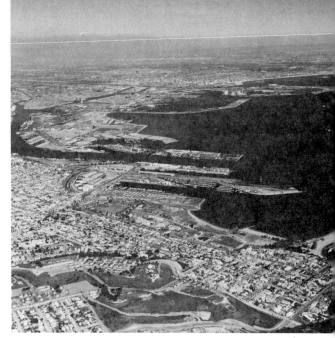

Harbor, Los Angeles, California

Cathedral, housing stained-glass windows, murals and crystal chandeliers; St. Vincent De Paul Church, featuring mosaic tiles from Mexico and Wilshire Boulevard Temple, housing a 135' dome inlaid with mosaic, a huge rose window, Byzantine columns of black Belgian marble and bronze chandeliers. In Griffith Park, atop Mt. Hollywood, is the Griffith Observatory and Planetarium. In nearby Burbank, a studio tour is offered which emphasizes the technical aspects of TV and film production and features the home of Warner Bros. and Columbia Pictures. Constructed in 1893 with wrought iron and marble trappings, ornate elevators and Victorian flourishes, the Bradbury Building is the set for many well-known movies.

LOUISVILLE
KENTUCKY

CITY LOCATION-SIZE-EXTENT. Louisville, located in N central KY on the S bank of the OH River, encompasses 65.2 sq. mi. in Jefferson Co. at 38°11' N lat. and 85°44' W long. The met. area extends S into Bullit, NE into Oldham and NW into Clark and Floyd counties, IN.

TOPOGRAPHY. Louisville lies in the Bluegrass region of KY on the S bank of the OH River in a broad river valley surrounded by a plateau and the knobs of the river valley area. The mean elev. is 465'.

CLIMATE. The climate of Louisville is continental. The annual avg. temp. of 56.8°F ranges from a Jan. mean of 34.4°F to a July mean of 78.3°F. The 42.9" avg. annual rainfall is heaviest in Mar. and lightest in Oct. The avg. annual snowfall of 18.3" occurs from Nov. and Mar. The RH ranges between 53% to 89%. The avg. growing season lasts 28 weeks. Louisville lies in the ESTZ and observes DST.

FLORA AND FAUNA. Animals native to Louisville include the whitetail deer, squirrel, rabbit, opossum and raccoon. Common birds include the cardinal (state bird), robin, thrasher, crow and flycatcher. Box turtles, tree frogs, salamanders, toads, green snakes and the venomous timber rattlesnake and copperhead are common to the area. Typical trees include the elm, oak, pine and maple. Smaller plants include iris, blackberry, dogwood and honeysuckle.

POPULATION. According to the US census, the pop. of Louisville was 361,706 in 1970. It was estimated in 1979 that it had decreased to 318,200.

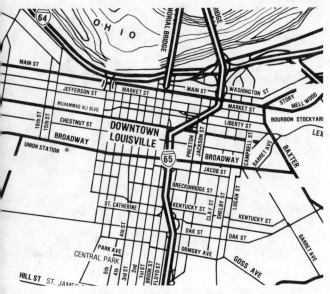

Louisville, Kentucky

ETHNIC GROUPS. In 1978, the ethnic distribution of Louisville was approx. 70.0% Caucasian, 29.5% Black and 0.4% Hispanic. (A percentage of the Hispanic total is included in the Caucasian.)

TRANSPORTATION. Interstate hwys. 64, 65, 71 and 264, US hwys 31E, 31W, 42, 60, 61 and 150 and state hwys. 22, 61, 146, 155 and 864 provide major motor access to Louisville. *Railroad* service is provided by AMTRAK, Baltimore & OH, Burlington N, Chessie System, ConRail, IL Central, KY & IN, The Milwaukee and S Railway. *Airlines* serving Standiford Field include AM, US Air, DL, EA, OZ, PI and TW. *Bus lines* include Greyhound, Trailways and the Transit Authority of River City which provides intra-city service.

COMMUNICATIONS. Communications, broadcasting and print media originating from Louisville are: *AM radio stations* WTMT 620 (Indep., C&W); WAKY 790 (Indep., Contemp.); WHAS 840 (CBS, MOR); WFIA 900 (UPI, Relig.); WAVE 970 (NBC, MOR); WKLO 1080 (ABC/C Top 40); WINN 1240 (ABC/E, C&W); and WLOU 1350 (Natl. Blk.); *FM radio stations* WFPL 89.3 (Indep., Talk); WUOL 90.5 (NPR, Clas.); WFPK 91.9 (NPR, Clas., Educ.); WAMZ 97.5 (MBS, MOR); WLRS 102.3 (ABC/FM, Rock, AOR) and WVEZ 106.9 (Indep., Btfl. Mus.); *television stations* WAVE Ch. 3 (NBC); WHAS Ch. 11 (CBS); WKPC Ch. 15 (PBS); WLKY Ch. 32 (ABC); WDRB Ch. 41 (Indep.) and WKMJ Ch. 68 (Indep.); *press*: two major dailies serve the Louisville area; *Louisville Times*, published evenings and *Courier-Journal*, published mornings and Sunday, weekly publications include *KY Labor News*, *The Record*, *Voice-Jeffersonian*; monthly publications include *Louisville Magazine*, *KY Farm Bureau News*, *Masonic Home Journal*, *Natl. Horseman*, *Retreader's Journal*, *Rural Kentuckian* and *Word and Work*.

HISTORY. Louisville was established in 1778 during the American Revolution by a group of pioneers from PA led by the explorer George Rogers Clark. In gratitude to King Louis XVI for France's role in the Revolution, Clark named the settlement Louisville. Louisville's location on the falls of the OH River made it an important river port immediately. It became the distribution and transshipment point and main artery for settlers moving from the E seaboard states to the W and S. The first ocean-going vessel arrived in 1779. The pop. reached 350 by 1800, and prosperity stimulated the new city's continued growth. The U of Louisville was established in 1798. Among the newcomers to Louisville was the family of Zachary Taylor, the 12th Pres. of the US. A city

charter was granted in 1828. In 1830, the Portland Canal was completed, allowing ships to bypass the falls of the OH River and thereby increasing water transportation. Louisville became one of the top tobacco processing centers in the 1830s, and was a world tobacco center by 1840. The city's residents numbered approx. 43,000 by 1850, and the arrival of the RR the following year further boosted Louisville's growth. During the Civil War the city was used as a supply depot by Union troops, although local sympathies were divided between the N and S. Louisville prospered after the war as S markets were re-established. In 1875 the first KY Derby was held, and since then horse racing has dominated local sports. Between 1870 and 1900 the pop. more than doubled, from 100,000 to 205,000. In 1937, the OH River caused extensive damage when it overflowed and flooded the city, leading to the construction of a floodwall around the city. During WW II the city grew larger when an influx of rural workers arrived seeking factory jobs in the defense industry. In the 1950s and 1960s Louisville public schools and facilities were integrated. Urban renewal and beautification projects were initiated in the 1970s. Today, Louisville is KY's largest city and a major SE manufacturing center.

GOVERNMENT. Louisville has a mayor-council form of govt., with the mayor (who may not succeed himself) and 12 aldermen. The aldermen are elected at large every two years and the mayor is also elected at large every four years. The mayor is not a member and has no vote.

ECONOMY AND INDUSTRY. Products of Louisville's industries include chemicals, electric appliances, paints, varnishes, synthetic rubber, food and beverage (including distilling), lumber and timber products, machinery, motor vehicles and parts, farm equipment, printing and publishing, stone and clay products, textiles and tobacco products. The 1979 labor force for the Louisville met. area was 429,600 workers with an unemployment rate of 5.3%.

BANKING. There are 11 commercial banks in Louisville. In 1978, total deposits for the eight banks headquartered in the city were $2,822,811,000, while total assets were $5,030,460,000. Banks include Bank of Louisville, Citizens Fidelity Bank and Trust, First Natl. Bank and Liberty Natl. Bank and Trust.

HOSPITALS. There are 19 hosps. in Louisville, including Baptist, U of Louisville Gen., Jewish, Kosair Crippled Children's, Norton Children's, Our Lady of Peace, Methodist, Audubon, St. Mary, Elizabeth and SW Jefferson. There are also several psychiatric facilities, and a V.A. hosp.

EDUCATION. Louisville is the home of the Kentuckiana Metroversity, a consortium of six colleges and universities in the met. area. Member academic institutions include Bellarmine Col., Indiana U-SE, Louisville Presbyterian Theological Seminary, S Baptist Theological Seminary, Spalding Col. and the U of Louisville. The U of Louisville is one of the oldest municipal universities in the country. Established in 1798 as Jefferson Seminary, it became known as Louisville Col., in 1846. Approx. 17,398 students attended this institution in 1978, which grants every degree from associate to doctorate. Other institutions here are Jefferson Comm. College and the Simmons U, LOU Bible Col., Col. of the Scriptures, Sullivan Jr. Col. of Bus., Wattersdon Col. and Spencerian Bus. Col. Public school students attend schools of Jefferson Co., with total public school enrollment over 100,000 pupils in 172 schools. Seventy-one Catholic schools in the city and co. educated over 25,000 students. Denominational schools, Montessori schools and a school for the perceptually handicapped are also located in the city. The Louisville Free Public Lib., founded in 1816 as one of the nation's first public lib. systems, has 24 branches.

ENTERTAINMENT. There are several annual festivals in Louisville, including the KY State Fair, held every Aug., the Louisville Salute to the Arts each Sept. and the Derby festival in May. The Derby Festival is held a week

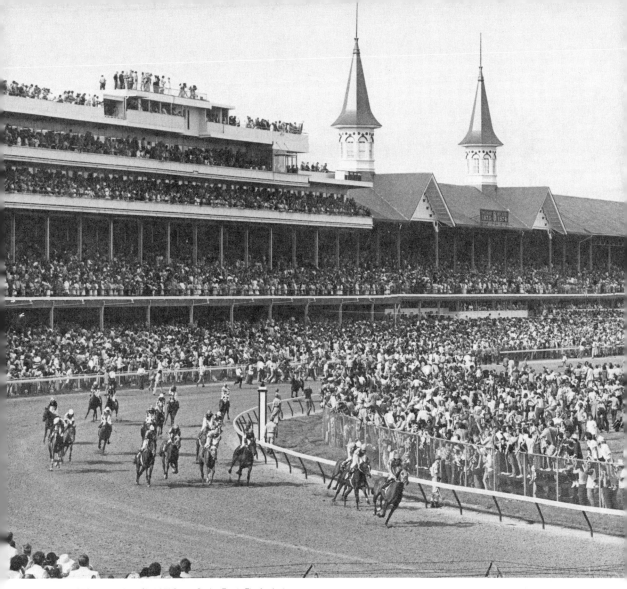

before the KY Derby is held at Churchill Downs Racing Track. The festival features the Pegasus Parade, a balloon race, concerts, a basketball classic, a steamboat race, derby of cycling and fireworks. Heritage Festivals, celebrating different ethnic cultures are held summer weekends. The U of Louisville Cardinals play collegiate basketball. The KY Colonels, a pro basketball team belonging to the American Basketball Assn., have their home in Louisville.

ACCOMMODATIONS. Louisville hotels and motels include the Galt House, the Hyatt Regency, the Lexington Hilton and Stouffer's Louisville, Clarksville-Louisville Marriott, Hilton, Ramada, Holiday, Howard Johnson's and Executive inns.

FACILITIES. There are over 160 parks spread over 7,000 acres of land in Louisville. The larger parks are Shawnee and Seneca Parks. An 1,800-acre forest in Fairdale brings wildlife to the doorstep of the urban area. The Louisville Zoo consists of 58 developed acres containing over 500 animals found in 60 exhibits. The city offers nine public golf courses, over 200 tennis courts, two Exer-21 exercise courses, 15 swimming pools, a skating rink, a riding stable, archery and bowhunter ranges and hiking and bridle paths. Horse racing enthusiasts enjoy Churchill Downs, the racetrack where the KY Derby is held annually. Riding Academies can be found at Aubrey Dude Ranch, Houchin Horse Center and Rock Creek Riding Club.

CULTURAL ACTIVITIES. Since reopening in 1962, the Brown Theatre (now the Macauley Theatre) has been home for the Louisville Orchestra, KY. Opera Assn. and Louisville-Jefferson Co. Youth Orchestra. Actors Theatre of Louisville, a repertory theater, has been designated as the state theater of

Churchill Downs, home of the Kentucky Derby, Louisville, Kentucky

Ky. Dramatic productions are staged by the U of Louisville, Belknap Theatre and Shakespeare-in-the-park, while the Louisville Theatrical Assn. sponsors Broadway shows. The city is also served by a ballet company and the Louisville Dance Council. Paintings by such masters as Rembrandt and Rubens are displayed at the J. B. Speed Art Museum. "Man and the River" is the theme of the Museum of Natural History and Science exhibits. The American Saddle Horse Museum—the only one of its kind in the nation—is housed in a Victorian style structure built in 1884 by the Hart Hardware Company. On the S Baptist Theological Seminary Campus are the Eisenberg Museum of Egyptian and Near E Antiquities and the Nicol Museum of Biblical Archeology, featuring artifacts from Jerusalem and Bethlehem.

LANDMARKS AND SIGHTSEEING SPOTS. Historic buildings of interest include Locust Grove, the home of Louisville's founder, George Rogers Clark, from 1809 until his death in 1818; the Farmington (1810), designed by Thomas Jefferson and encompassing an early 19th-century garden, working blacksmith shop and reconstructed barn; the Hart Hardware Co. Building, now listed on the Natl. Register of Historic Places and the Culbertson Mansion, completed in 1868. Other landmarks include Cave Hill cemetery, gravesite of George Rogers Clark; the Zachary Taylor Natl. Cemetery, and the tree stump on display at the Filson Club, reputedly inscribed by Daniel Boone in 1803. Churchill Downs, home of the KY Derby, is a popular visitor's stop.

LUBBOCK
TEXAS

CITY LOCATION-SIZE-EXTENT. Lubbock, the seat of Lubbock Co., encompasses 83.8 sq. mi. in N TX on the Double Mt. fork of the Brazos River, 110 mi. S of Amarillo, at 33°39' N lat. and 101°49' W long. The greater met. area extends E into Hockley Co. and S into Lynn Co.

TOPOGRAPHY. The terrain of Lubbock, which is situated on a plateau in the S plains, is extremely flat, while the area contains numerous small depressions and valleys carved by small streams. The mean elev. is 3,241'.

CLIMATE. The climate of Lubbock is semi-arid, intermediate between desert conditions to the W and humid conditions to the E and SE. The avg. annual temp. of 60°F ranges from a Jan. mean of 39°F to a July mean of 79.5°F. Most of the 17.7" avg. annual rainfall occurs during May through Sept., when warm moist tropical air from the Gulf of Mexico is carried into the area. The annual 9.7" avg. snowfall usually occurs in light amounts which seldom remain on the ground for more than three days. Late winter and spring low pressure centers bring prolonged winds, with the strongest usually from the W. The RH ranges from 52% to 81%. Lubbock lies in the CSTZ and observes DST.

FLORA AND FAUNA. Animals native to Lubbock include the prairie dog, coyote, jack rabbit and whitetail deer. Typical birds include the scissor-tailed flycatcher, scaled quail, dove, mockingbird (the state bird of TX), prairie chicken and vulture. Toads, horned lizards, leopard frogs, Great Plains skinks, collared lizards and garter snakes, as well as the venomous rattlesnake, are found in the area. Typical trees include the mesquite, hackberry, cottonwood and pecan (the state tree of TX). Smaller plants include the prickly pear cactus, cat's claw, yucca, sagebrush, prairie flower and bluebonnet (the state flower of TX). Residents are encouraged to plant chrysanthemums to support the city's claim as the "Chrysanthemum Capitol of the World."

POPULATION. According to the US census, the pop. of Lubbock in 1970 was 149,101. In 1978, it was estimated that it had increased to 175,250.

ETHNIC GROUPS. In 1978, the ethnic distribution of Lubbock was approx. 71.5% Caucasian, 8.5% Black and 21% Hispanic. (A percentage of the Hispanic total is also included in the Caucasian total.)

Lubbock, Texas

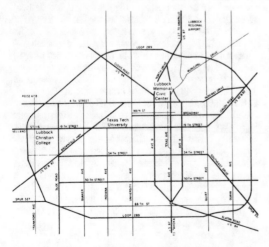

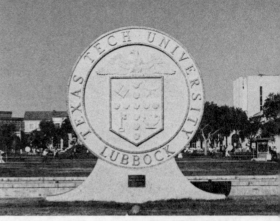

Seal which marks the entrance to Texas Tech University, Lubbock, Texas

TRANSPORTATION. Interstate hwys. 62, 82, 84 and 87, US hwy. 27 and state Hwy. 114 provide major motor access to Lubbock. Two major *railroads* serve the city, the Atchison, Topeka & Santa Fe Co. and Burlington-Northern. *Airlines* serving Lubbock Intl. Airport are BN, CO,TI, SW, ZV, Big Bend and Crown Air. *Bus lines* serving Lubbock are T.N. M.&O Coaches.

COMMUNICATIONS. Communications, broadcasting and print media originating in Lubbock are: *AM radio stations* KRLB 580 (Indep., C&W); KFYO 790 (CBS, MOR); KSEL 950 (Indep., Contemp., Top 40); KLBK 1340 (ABC/C, MOR); KLFB 1420 (Indep., Span.); KLLL 1460 (NBC, C&W) and KEND 1590 (Indep., C&W); *FM radio stations* KOHM 91.1 (Indep., Progsv.); KTXT 91.9 (ABC/FM, Jazz/Progsv.); KSEL 93.7 (Indep., C&W); KLBK 94.5 (ABC/C, Soft Rock); KLLL 96.3 (NBC, 25% AM Simulcast); KWGO 99.5 (Indep., Contemp.) and KTEZ 101.1 (Indep., Btfl. Mus.); *television stations* KTXT Ch. 5 (PBS); KCBD Ch. 11 (NBC); KLBK Ch. 13 (CBS) and KAMC Ch. 28 (ABC); *press*: one major daily serves the city, the *Avalanche-Journal*, published mornings and evenings; other publications include the *U Daily*, *W TX Times*, *Duster*, *Suburban Today*, *Grain Sorghum News*, *Greater Lubbock*, *Wolffort Plainsman* and *Lubbock Digest*.

HISTORY. Before the arrival of the first Quaker settlers, native Americans of the Comanche tribe roamed the area of present-day Lubbock. Lubbock was formed in 1891 by the merger of two small villages—Old Lubbock and Monterey—that had recently sprung up on ranching lands. The city's founders—W. E. Rayner, W. D. Crump and Frank Wheelock—named it in honor of Tom S. Lubbock, a former TX Ranger, signer of TX Declaration of Independence and a Confed. war hero. The area cattle industry expanded rapidly throughout the 1880s due to abundant amount of grass growing there, which led to the establishment of cattle empires on the plains. The brand of the first cattle empire was the IOA. Discovery of water close to the ground's surface and the introduction of cotton at the turn of the century stimulated an influx of people, who arrived to farm this oasis in an otherwise arid region. In 1909, the city of Lubbock was incorporated and that year the first train arrived from Plainview. TX Tech. U was chartered in 1923, and opened in 1925. The Ft. Worth and Denver RR opened for traffic in Lubbock in 1928. In 1941, Lubbock Army Air Field (now Reese AFB) opened. Lubbock became the hub of the vast S central plains of TX as a major transportation center. Large scale irrigation helped assure the city's future, which today is the largest inland cotton market in the world. Lubbock has the largest assembly of cotton mills and produces one-fifth of the nation's sorghum.

GOVERNMENT. The city of Lubbock has a council-mgr. form of govt. The five council members, including the mayor as a voting member, are elected at large. Council members serve four-year terms, while the mayor serves a two-year term.

ECONOMICS AND INDUSTRY. Agriculture is an important sector of the economy of Lubbock. Agricultural products include cotton and cotton by-products, grain, vegetables, livestock, poultry, dairy products and grain sorghum. Through the production of the city's three major cottonseed oil mills, Lubbock has become the "Cottonseed Oil Capitol of the World". Three plants in the city slaughter approx. 250,000 cattle annually. Manufacturing employment has increased 112.7% since 1968. Major manufactured products include canvas products, electronic components, heavy machinery and textiles. In 1979, the met. labor force totaled 101,900, while the rate of unemployment was 4.3%.

BANKING. There are nine banks and savings and loan assns. in Lubbock. In 1978, total deposits for the nine banks headquartered in the city were $1,104,496,000, while assets were $1,293,964,000. Banks include First Natl. and Lubbock Natl.

HOSPITALS. There are seven hosps. in Lubbock, The Health Science Center Hosp., opened in Lubbock in 1978, is the primary testing facility for the TX Tech. U School of Medicine. The hosp. operated by the Lubbock Co. Hosp. District has the only neonatal intensive care unit located between Dallas and Denver. Other hosps. are Comm., Highland Mercy, Methodist, St. Mary's, U and W TX.

EDUCATION. Located in Lubbock is TX Tech. U, the fourth-largest university in the state, which has been designated as one of the four multipurpose universities in TX. The U awards undergrad. degrees in 96 major fields and 101 grad. and postgrad. degrees. In 1978, this institution enrolled more than 22,300. Lubbock Christian Col., established in 1957, is a four-year liberal arts col. offering undergrad. level courses. In 1978, it enrolled approx. 1,200. S Plains Col., a publicly-supported two-year col., enrolled more than 2,000 in 1978. Thirty-five elementary schools, 15 jr. and sr. high schools and three special schools are included in the public school system, which enrolls more than 31,000. There are also two parochial schools and numerous private schools, academies and specialty schools in the city. Libs. include the Lubbock City Lib. and its three branches.

ENTERTAINMENT. The Country Squire Dinner Theater provides dining entertainment in Lubbock. Two annual rodeos are presented in the spring and the annual Pan Handle-S Plains Fair draws more than a quarter-million visitors annually. The TX Tech U Red Raiders participate in intercollegiate sports in the SWC.

ACCOMMODATIONS. There are many hotels and motels in Lubbock, including the Best Westerns-Southpark and Village, La Quinta and the Hilton, Holiday, Lubbock and Ramada inns.

Civic Center, Lubbock, Texas

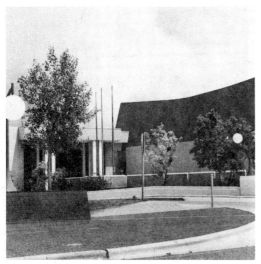

FACILITIES. The 3,137-acre Lubbock park system includes swimming pools, party houses, a golf course, a city tennis center, tennis courts, basketball courts, baseball diamonds and soccer fields. The Yellowhouse Canyon Lakes Project is a series of six lakes running from the NW to the SE corners of the city, which include picnic areas, wilderness trails and bicycle paths. The lakes may be utilized by non-motored boats. Nearby is the MacKenzie State Park, which contains Prairie Dog Town, one of the few remaining colonies of its type in the nation. Buffalo Springs Lake, located five mi. SE of the city, provides opportunities for fishing, boating and skiing. Several public golf courses are available. Tennis courts can be found at the Lubbock Municipal Tennis Center.

CULTURAL ACTIVITIES. Lubbock is served musically by the Lubbock Symphony, Civic Chorale, Music Club, Youth Chamber Orchestra, TX Tech Symphony, Band and Choir and the TX Christian Col. Band. Dramatic Productions are staged by local and TX Tech theater groups, who present ballet and dance as well. Museums include the TX Tech U Museum, where Colonial buildings house American Revolution memorabilia such as a letter written by George Washington. The Lubbock Art, Fine Arts Crafts and Lubbock Art Assns. sponsor local arts events.

LANDMARKS AND SIGHTSEEING SPOTS. Ranching Heritage Center, adjacent to the Museum of TX Tech U, consists of 20 restored buildings recreating the history of ranching in TX. The Moody Planetarium, also part of the Museum, offers programs each weekend. Prairie Dog Town in MacKenzie State Park is the last refuge for the nearly extinct prairie dog. Lubbock Lake Project is an archeological site located on old meander bend of Yellowhouse Draw.

MACON
GEORGIA

CITY LOCATION-SIZE-EXTENT. Macon encompasses 49.5 sq. mi. of Bibb Co. in central GA, just 75 mi. SE of Atlanta, at 32°42' N lat. and 83°39'W long. The met. area extends into the counties of Jones on the N, Houston on the S, Monroe on the NW, Crawford on the SW and Twiggs on the SE.

TOPOGRAPHY. Macon lies in the Piedmont Plateau Region, consisting of terrain that is predominantly flat. The outlying area of the city is swampy with several creeks in the vicinity. To the W of the city a range of hills runs in a general NW-SE direction. The mean elev. is 434'.

CLIMATE. The climate of Macon is a blend of marine and continental. Monthly mean temps. range from a Jan. mean of 47.5°F to a July mean of 80.8°F with an avg. annual temp. of 64.6°F. The 44.71" avg. annual rainfall is heavier during June through Aug. Snowfall is scant, occuring most winters. The RH ranges from 47% to 93%. The avg. growing season is 246 days. Macon is in the ESTZ and observes DST.

FLORA AND FAUNA. Animals native to Macon include the opossum, whitetail deer, raccoon and beaver. Common birds are the oriole, summer tanager, yellow-billed cuckoo, swallow, chuck-will's-widow and mockingbird. Rat snakes, green anoles, turtles, toads and four types of venomous snakes reside here. Typical trees are the pine, and live oak (the state tree), smaller plants are the marigold, boxwood and sassanqua.

POPULATION. According to the US census, the pop. of Macon in 1970 was 122,423. In 1978, it was estimated that it had decreased to 120,300.

ETHNIC GROUPS. In 1978, the ethnic distribution of Macon was approx. 62.6% Caucasian, 37.3% Black, and .3% Hispanic. (A percentage of the Hispanic total is also included in the Caucasian total.)

TRANSPORTATION. Interstate hwys. 16, 75 and 475, U.S. hwys. 23, 41, 80 and 129 and state hwys. 11, 22, 19, 49, 87, 148 and 247 provide major

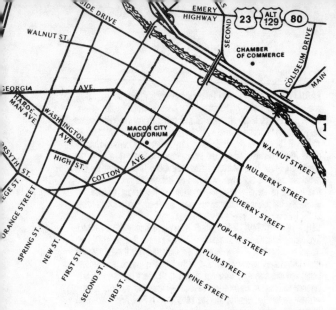

Macon, Georgia

motor access to Macon. *Railroads* include IL Central gulf, St. Louis, Seaboard, Western and the Louisville & Nashville. The Herbert Smart and the Lewis B. Wilson Airports offer *airline* service on DL and Air S (commuter). *Bus lines* serving the city include the local Bibb Transit line, Greyhound and Trailways.

COMMUNICATIONS. Communications, broadcasting and print media originating from Macon are: *AM radio stations* WBML 900 (MBS, Relig.); WMAZ 940 (CBS, MOR); WDDO 1240 (Natl., Blk.); WIBB 1280 (Mut., Blk.); WNEX 1400 (ABC/C, Top 40) and WDEN 1500 (Indep., Mod. Ctry.); *FM radio stations* WMAZ 99.1 (ABC/FM, Top 40); WDEN 105.3 (Indep., Dups AM 15%) and WCRY 107.9 (Indep., Btfl. Mus.); *television stations* WMAZ Ch. 13 (CBS, ABC) and WCWB Ch. 41 (NBC) and cable; *press*: two major dailies serve the area, the morning *Telegraph* and the evening *News*; other publications include the *Herald*, *GA Farm Bureau News*, *Wesleyan College NOW*, *Christian Messenger*, *Livestock Breeder Journal* and *Mercer Cluster*.

HISTORY. As early as 8,000 B.C., Indians were inhabiting the Macon area. Native Americans of the Creek Tribe were settled there when Macon was founded and incorporated in 1823, on the site of Fort Hawkins, which was established by Thomas Jefferson in 1806. In 1826, the final treaty was signed, which divested the Creek Tribe of their lands. The remaining members of the tribe were relocated in the OK Territory. The city was named for Nathaniel Macon, a NC congressman. Macon became the focal point for education and culture in mid-GA. Wesleyan Col. was founded in 1836, the first in the US to grant degrees to women. Mercer U, established in Penfield, GA, in 1833, moved to the town in 1871. Poet Sidney Lanier was born there in 1842. Wealthy planters and businessmen in pre-Civil War days moved to Macon. During the 1840s and 1850s, Macon became a RR center. During the Civil War, Macon was a confederate depository and had several munitions plants in the city. Confederate troops repelled two Union attacks, but the city was eventually occupied in 1865. Macon became the temporary state capital during Gen. Sherman's march to Atlanta. The city has since become a manufacturing and trade center for GA's famous peach region.

GOVERNMENT. The city of Macon has a mayor-council form of govt. consisting of the mayor and 15 council members. The mayor is elected at large every four years; he is not a council member. The council members are elected every four years; 10 are elected by district and five at-large.

ECONOMY AND INDUSTRY. Leading industries in Macon include chemicals, food processing, clothing, lumber, steel and meatpacking. In 1979 the labor force for the

Macon met. area totaled 102,400, with an unemployment rate of 6%. The 1978 medium income was $5,638.

BANKING. There are five commercial banks in Macon. In 1978, total deposits for the five banks headquartered in the city were $287,094,000, while total assets were $341,412,000. Banks include Macon, Central of GA, GA, First Natl., and Citizens & Southern.

HOSPITALS. Macon has four general hosps.—Coliseum Park, College Street, Medical Center of Central GA, Middle GA and Riverside Clinic.

EDUCATION. Macon is the site of Mercer U and Wesleyan Col. Mercer U, a private, liberal arts U is controlled by the S Baptist Convention. Established in 1833, this institution offers programs leading to the bachelor, master and doctorate degrees. In 1978, Mercer U enrolled 2,150 students Wesleyan Col., a private liberal arts col. for women, is controlled by the Methodist Church. Wesleyan obtained the first state charter for granting degrees to women in 1836. Over 500 enrolled in 1978. Macon Jr. Col., a publicly-supported jr. col., offers transfer and vocational programs leading to an associate degree. In 1978, MJC enrolled 2,420 students. Other institutions include Crandall Col., a private college offering programs leading to the associate degree, certificates and diplomas. In 1978, Crandall enrolled over 145 students. The GA Academy for the Blind is also located here. There are 55 public schools with approx. 28,000 enrolled in 1978. Lib. facilities are available through the Middle GA Regional Lib. with 13 branches.

ENTERTAINMENT. Macon hosts the GA State Fair and the SE Arts and Crafts Festival annually. The Mercer U Bears and the Macon Chiefs provide sporting events in the city. Wesleyan Col. participates in intercollegiate sports.

ACCOMMODATIONS. Hotel and motels include the Macon Hilton, Howard Johnson's and the Sheraton, Ramada, Quality and Day's inns.

FACILITIES. There are 32 parks in the Macon park system. The larger ones are Central City, Freedom, Bloomfield, Eastside and Memorial. Nearby is the Piedmont Natl. Wildlife Refuge, which encompasses 32,000 acres.

Mercer University, Macon, Georgia

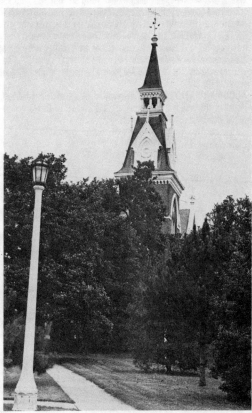

There are two public golf courses in the city. Public tennis courts can be found at the Macon Tennis Center in Tatnall Square Park. Boating facilities can be found at a local boat club.

CULTURAL ACTIVITIES. The Macon Area Comm. Theatre and Macon Little Theatre offer theatrical entertainment in Macon. Musical entertainment is provided by the Middle GA Symphony and the Heart of GA Barbershop Chorus. The Museum of Arts and Sciences houses scientific, historic, nature and art displays, GA's second largest planetarium, and the home of author Harry Stillwell Edwards. Galleries in the city include Soter, Anne Tutt Studio and Ocmulgee Arts.

LANDMARKS AND SIGHTSEEING SPOTS. Macon's Ocmulgee Natl. Monument is the site of an early Indian civilization and includes an Indian museum, burial ground and lodge. Hay House (1855) features period furnishings, antiques and art works. Fort Hawkins (1806), a reconstructed blockhouse, served as a ft. and trading post. The Grand Opera House (1883) was the original home of the old Academy of Music. The renovated building presented the early Ben Hur production, complete with chariot race scene, on its huge stage. Old Cannonball House (1857), a 24-room, Greek revival structure furnished in ante bellum style, was built by Judge Asa Ilolt, and features antique furnishings and art works, including a Waterford chandelier. Other preserved homes include the Raines-Miller-Carmichael House, Hatcher-Groover-Schwartz House, T.C. Burke House, Isaac-Scott-Johnson House, Harrin-Pliny Hall Houses, Dunlap Farm House, Randolph-Whittle-Davis House, Munro-Goolsby House and Green-Poe House. Also located in the city is the Macon Coliseum, a $6 million building with a profile resembling an Indian mound.

MADISON
WISCONSIN

CITY LOCATION-SIZE-EXTENT. Madison, the capital and second largest city in the state and the seat of Dane Co., encompasses 54 sq. mi. along a natural isthmus between two fresh water lakes, the Monona and Mendota, in S central WI, 79 mi. W of Milwaukee and 142 mi. N of Chicago, at 43°08' N lat. and 89°20' W long. The greater met. area extends into the counties of Jefferson to the W, Columbia to the N, Dodge to the NE, Green to the SE, Rock to the SW, Iowa to the E and Sauk to the NW.

TOPOGRAPHY. The terrain of Madison, which is situated in the Great Lakes plains of WI, consists of rolling to hilly areas between two lakes, Mendota and Monona. The city encompasses lakes Waubesa, Kenosha and Wingra. The mean elev. is 845'.

CLIMATE. The climate of Madison is continental, characterized by air masses from the polar regions which produce pleasant summers and moderate extremes in temp. and humidity. Monthly mean temps. range from 17°F in Jan. to 71°F in July, with an annual avg. of 46°F. The annual precip. of 31" occurs mainly during the warmer months. Snowfall avgs. 40.5" per year, occurring mainly during Dec. through Mar. The RH ranges from 54% to 92%. The growing season avgs. 175 days. Madison lies in the CSTZ and observes DST.

FLORA AND FAUNA. Animals native to Madison include the fox, whitetail deer and squirrel. Common birds include the robin, meadowlark, bittern, blackbird and swallow. Bullfrogs, salamanders, painted turtles, and skinks, as well as the venomous E massasauga (a pygmy rattler) and timber rattlesnake, are found in the area. Common trees include the sugar maple, ash, elm and oak. Smaller plants include the sumac, wood violet, saxifrage, bell flower and geranium.

POPULATION. According to the US census, the pop. of Madison in 1970 was 171,769. In 1979, it was estimated that it had increased to 173,051.

ETHNIC GROUPS. In 1978, the ethnic distribution of Madison was approx. 95.5% Caucasian, 2% Black, 1% Hispanic and 1.5% other.

TRANSPORTATION. Interstate hwys. 90 and 94, US hwys. 12, 14, 18, 51 and 151 and state hwys. 30 and 113 provide major motor access to Madison. The three *railroads* serving the city are Chicago & NW, IL Central and the Milwaukee Road. *Airlines* serving Dane Co. Regional Airport include NW, NC Republic and OZ. Twelve *bus lines* serve the city, including Madison Metro, Badger, Greyhound and Commuter Service.

COMMUNICATIONS. Communications, broadcasting and print media originating from Madison are: *AM radio stations* WHA 970 (NPR, Educ.); WTSO 1070 (Indep., C&W); WIBA 1310 (NBC, MOR); WISM 1480 (Indep., Contemp.) and WWQM 1550 (ABC/C, C&W); *FM radio stations* WERN 88.7 (Indep., Educ.); WORT 89.7 (Indep., Jazz, Clas.); WISM 98.1 (Indep., MOR); WIBA 101.5 (CBS Progsv.); WNWC 102.5 (Indep., Relig.) and WZEE 104.1 (Indep., Top 40); *television stations* WISC Ch. 3 (CBS); WMTV Ch. 15 (NBC); WHA Ch. 21 (CBS); WKOW Ch. 27 (ABC) and cable; *press:* two major dailies serve the city, the *Capital Times*, printed evenings, and the *WI State Journal*, issued mornings and Sun. Monthly publications include *Select Magazine*, *US Hockey & Arena Biz*, *Badger Farm Bureau News*, *Municipality* and *Progressive*; quarterly publications include *Social Biology*, *WI Magazine of History*, *WI Press*, *Contemporary Design*, *Land Economics* and *MBAA Technical Quarterly*.

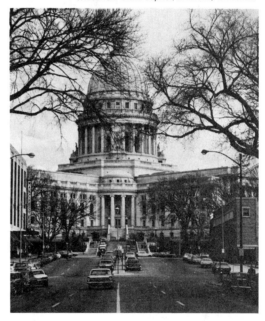

Wisconsin State Capitol, Madison, Wisconsin

HISTORY. Native Americans of the Winnebago tribe originally inhabited the Madison area. James D. Doty, a former fed. judge, and Stevens T. Mason, gov. of the MI territory, first purchased the site. Several years later, in 1836, Madison was created by the first legislature of the WI territorial govt., although the comm. did not actually exist. It was intended to be the state capital and named in honor of James Madison. Known as the "Four Lakes City," Madison's site was chosen because of the lakes in the vicinity, carved out by a glacier centuries ago. The only access to the new capital was by trail. Eben and Rosaline Peck became the region's first white settlers when they arrived in 1837 and erected a tavern and an inn. Madison began functioning as a capital in 1838, with a pop. of 62. When incorporated as a village in 1846, the pop. was 626. In 1854, the first RR reached Madison from Milwaukee. The city

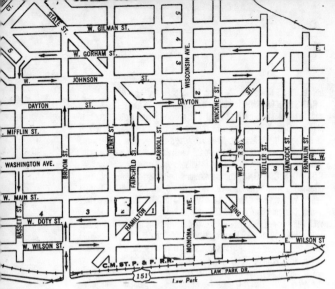

Downtown Madison, Wisconsin

was incorporated in 1856, with a pop. of 7,000. The Chicago & NW RR arrived in 1864, enabling the town to slowly prosper and grow. Madison's growth depended mainly on govt. employment and WI U (created in 1835). During the Civil War many soldiers were quartered at Camp Randall, built on the state fairgrounds. By 1899, 20,000 people lived in Madison. In 1919, Oscar Mayer and Co. opened a meat-packing plant in the city, which made it a major food processing center. During the 1920s, the Progressive Party was based in Madison, led by the LaFollette family. A rapid increase in state and govt. employment during the 1960s led to a sharp rise in Madison's pop. By 1970, the number of residents reached 171,769. Today the city serves as a center of health care and recreation, as well as an important agricultural market.

GOVERNMENT. Madison has a mayor-council form of govt. The mayor, elected at large to a two-year term, is not a member of the council and votes only to break a tie. The 22 council members are elected by district to two-year terms.

ECONOMY AND INDUSTRY. There are more than 260 manufacturing firms, employing approx. 18,000 in the Madison met. area. Processed meats, storage batteries, hosp. equipment, air circulating fixtures and dairy and agricultural equipment are major products. Agriculture is an important economic factor, with approx. one-sixth of all WI dairy farms in the Madison area. Leading agricultural products are corn, alfalfa, tobacco, oats, eggs, cattle, hogs and dairy products. The median household income for 1978 in Madison was

Bradley House, Madison, Wisconsin

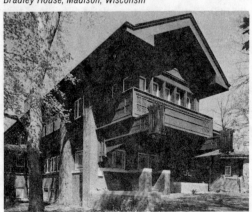

$17,714. The labor force in 1978 totaled 166,200, while the rate of unemployment was approx. 4.6%.

BANKING. In 1978, total deposits for the 12 banks headquartered in Madison were $822,062,000, while assets were $954,068,000. Banks include First WI Natl., Affiliated of Madison, Affiliated of Hilldale, United Bank and Trust and Security Marine.

HOSPITALS. There are seven hosps. in Madison, including Madison Gen., Methodist, St. Mary's, the Mendota Mental Health Institute, U Hosp. and the V.A. facility. Completion of the new $100 million Clinical Health Sciences Center, the largest building in the state, leaves the older complex for expansion of the U of WI-Madison training and research facility.

EDUCATION. The state-supported U of WI-Madison was founded in 1849 and offers courses leading to degrees ranging from associate to doctoral. The U enrolled more than 39,000 in 1978. The U of WI Center System, also located in Madison, offers associate degrees. It enrolled approx. 8,600 in 1978. Edgewood Col., a four-year institution established in 1941, is one of the most recent educational units developed by the Dominican Sisters of Sinsinawa, WI. The col. awards bachelor degrees and, in 1978, it enrolled more than 500. Other institutions include Madison Business Col., WI School of Electronics, Madison Gen. Hosp. and St. Mary's Hosp. Medical Center. The public school system consists of 29 elementary, 10 middle and four high schools. Also provided are several special educational facilities, including two alternative-education high schools, several Montessori preschools and many special education services for those with mental and physical handicaps. Libs. include the Madison Public Lib., WI State Historical Society Lib., WI Legislative Reference Bureau and WI State Law Lib.

ENTERTAINMENT. Wilson St. E Dinner Playhouse provides dining entertainment in Madison. Annually, the city hosts a sidewalk Art Festival, a Dairy Exposition, an Equinox Festival and the Dane Co. Jr. Fair. The U of WI-Madison Badgers participate in intercollegiate sports.

ACCOMMODATIONS. There are several hotels and motels in Madison, including Concourse, Edgewater Motor Hotel, Park, Sheraton Inn, Howard Johnson's and Best Western-Town Campus.

FACILITIES. There are 5,000 acres of parkland, including 70 neighborhood parks, 12 comm. parks and eight conservation parks in Madison. Among the larger parks are Olbrich, Olin, Tenney, Vilas and Warner. The 67-acre Vilas Park Zoo, located near Lake Wingra, contains a wide variety of wild animal species. A children's zoo has also been constructed through the efforts of the Madison Jaycees. The U of WI operates a 1,256 acre arboretum which contains 24 mi. of foot trails through a variety of plant communities, including restored prairies, coniferous forests, oak woods, maple woods and marshlands. The arboretum also includes acres of horticultural collections. The met. area includes 18,000 acres of lake surface, including five lakes within the city itself. The city provides eight golf courses, 50 supervised playgrounds, seven playfields, 14 beaches, 11 boat launching sites, two toboggan runs and 61 ice skating rinks. Public golf courses include Glenway, Yahara Hills and Odana Hills. Tennis courts can be found at several tennis clubs and the U of WI Nielsen Tennis Stadium, the world's largest indoor facility of its kind.

CULTURAL ACTIVITIES. Madison is served musically by the Symphony Orchestra, Civic Chorus and the music dept. of the U of WI. Dramatic productions are staged by the Theatre Guild and Civic Reportory Theatre. A local ballet and the U of WI dance troupe present performances. Drama performances are presented in the Auditorium and the Isthmus Theatre of the new Madison Civic Center. The U of WI Elvehjem Art Center, designed by Chicago architect Harvey Weese, functions both as a teaching center and museum. The Sidewalk Art Fair, held annually, displays the work of 400 carefully selected artists and crafts people from around the country. Madison is also the location of the State Historical Society Museum.

LANDMARK AND SIGHTSEEING SPOTS. Situated on a 13.4 acre park in the heart of the city, the State Capitol features a 200' illuminated dome and a gold and bronze statue called "Miss Forward." The Indian Mounds include one that is the effigy of an Eagle with a 624' wingspan. The Unitarian Meeting House is among the noted buildings designed by Frank Lloyd Wright, while the Bradley House, built in 1909, was designed by Louis Sullivan. Other points of interest include the Tenney Boat Locks.

MEMPHIS
TENNESSEE

CITY LOCATION-SIZE-EXTENT. Memphis, the seat of Shelby co., encompasses 280.89 sq. mi. on the MS River in the SW corner of TN at 35°3' N lat. and 90° W long. The greater met. area extends into the neighboring cos. of Tipton to the N, Crittenden, AR across the MS to the W and De Soto, MS to the S.

TOPOGRAPHY. The terrain of Memphis, which is situated on the MS alluvial plain of TN on high bluffs overlooking the river, is level to slightly rolling. The mean elev. is 258'.

CLIMATE. The climate of Memphis is continental, characterized by frequent variations in the weather. The avg. annual temp. of 62°F varies from a Jan. mean of 41°F to a July mean of 81°F. The avg. annual rainfall of 49" is fairly well-distributed throughout the year. The avg. annual snowfall is 5.5". The RH ranges from 51% to 86% and the avg. growing season is approx. 230 days. Memphis lies in the CSTZ and observes DST.

FLORA AND FAUNA. Animals native to Memphis include the whitetail deer, raccoon, rabbit and opossum. Common birds include the mockingbird (the state bird), bluebird, robin, vireo, egret and barn owl. Water snakes, bullfrogs, salamanders, snapping turtles and toads and the venomous rattlesnake, copperhead and water moccasin are found in the area. Typical trees include the tulip, poplar (the state tree), oak, elm and sycamore. Smaller plants include the honeysuckle, camas, bellflower and iris (the state flower).

POPULATION. According to the US census, the pop. of Memphis in 1970 was 623,988. In 1978, it was estimated that it had increased to approx. 680,000.

ETHNIC GROUPS. In 1978, the ethnic distribution of Memphis was approx. 60.9% Caucasian, 36.9% Black and 0.4% Hispanic and 1.8% other.

TRANSPORTATION. Interstate hwys. 40, 55, 240 and US hwys. 51, 61, 64, 70, 72, 78 and 79 and State hwy. 14 provide major motor access to Memphis. *Railroads* serving the city include the Chicago, Rock Island & Pacific, IL Central Gulf, Louisville & Nashville, MO Pacific, St. Louis-San Francisco, St. Louis-SW and S. Barge lines providing service to the Pt. of Memphis, the second largest inland pt. on the MS River, include American Commercial, Fed., OH, Sioux City & New Orleans, Union Meckling and Valley. *Airlines* serving Memphis Intl. Airport include AA, BN, DL, US Air, Frontier PI, Republic and UA. *Bus lines* serving the city include Trailways, Greyhound and the local Bridge Transit and Memphis Transit Authority.

COMMUNICATIONS. Communications, broadcasting and print media originating from Memphis are: *AM radio stations* WHBQ 560 (UPI Top 40); WREC 600 (CBS, MOR); WMPS 680 (ABC/C, Contemp.); WMC 790 (NBC, Ctry.); KWAM 990 (Indep., Relig., Blk.); WDIA 1070 (MBS, Mut. Blk.); WLOK 1340 (Mut. Blk.); WWEE 1430 (ABC/I, Talk) and WMQM 1480 (Indep., C&W); *FM radio stations* WQOX 88.5 (Indep., Educ.); WLYX 89.3 (ABC/FM, Progsv.); WEVL 90.3 (Indep., Divers.); WKNO 91.1 (NPR, Var.); WSWS 91.7 (ABC top 40); WLVS 94.3 (ABC, Rock); WHRK 97.1 (ABC, Disco); WMC 99.7 (NBC Contemp., Rock); KWAM 101.1 (ABC/E, C&W); WZXR 102.7 (Indep., AOR); WQUD 104.5 (Indep., Good Mus.) and WEZI 105.9 (Indep., Btfl. Mus.); *television stations* WREG Ch. 3 (CBS); WMC Ch. 5 (NBC); WKNO Ch. 10 (PBS); WHBQ Ch. 13 (ABC) WPTY Ch. 24 (Indep.) and cable; *press:* two daily newspapers are published in the city, the morning *Commercial Appeal* and the evening *Press-Scimitar,* other publications include the *Daily News, Helmsman, Memphis Magazine, Bell Tower, Christian Observer, Cotton Farming, Resort Management, Shelter, Whitehaven Press* and the *Whole Truth.*

HISTORY. Native Amerians of the Chickasaw tribe

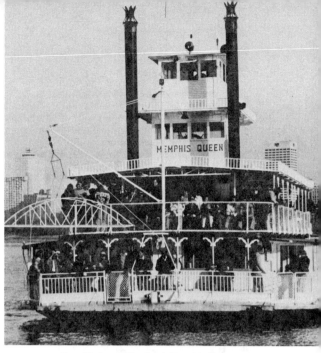

Memphis Queen Riverboat, Memphis, Tennessee

inhabited the area of present-day Memphis when explorer Louis Joliet and missionary Fr. Marquette arrived and traded with them in 1673. Nine years later, LaSalle claimed the area for France. In 1739, the French built Ft. Assumption on the bluffs overlooking the MS River. The region passed to the British and then to the US and, in 1819, the town of Memphis was founded by Gen. Andrew Jackson and two partners, Judge John Overton and Gen. James Winchester, from a fed. land grant. The town, named after the ancient Egyptian capital because of the Nile-like appearance of the MS, quickly became a leading river pt. During the early part of the 19th century, cotton plantations were established in the area and, as slave labor was brought in to work on them, the town became the largest slave market in the central S. Memphis was incorporated as a city in 1849, and, by 1860, its pop. had reached 23,000. For a brief period during the Civil War, the city became the Confed. capital of TN, but, after the sinking of a Confed. fleet near the city by fed. gunboats in 1862, it fell to fed. forces. River trade decreased and many plantations were destroyed by a series of yellow fever epidemics in the 1870s. The worst epidemic, in 1878, killed more than 5,000 people, half of the survivors fled, and, in 1879, the charter of the city was revoked. The town was rebuilt slowly and not without difficulty, but in 1893, it regained its city charter. By the turn of the century, the city began to experience greater growth and prosperity and became the hardware lumber center and busiest cotton pt. of the US. Industry continued to expand throughout the 20th century. During the 1960s, the city experienced a building boom, increased its area by 53% through an active policy of annexation and began a program of racial integration of public schools. In 1968, Martin Luther King, Jr., was assassinated in the city. Subsequent efforts by both white and black leaders, however, helped ease racial tensions, and urban renewal programs were also initiated. Today, the city is an important agri-business center.

GOVERNMENT. Memphis has a mayor-council form of govt. consisting of 13 council members, a mayor and a mayor-appointed chief administrator. The mayor and six council members are elected at large, and seven council members are elected by district to four-year terms.

ECONOMY AND INDUSTRY. More than 40% of the US cotton crop is traded in Memphis, which is the largest spot cotton market in the world as well as the second largest processor of soybeans and third largest meat and food processor in the US. Approx. 850 industrial plants in the met. area manufacture such products as lumber and wood products. The city is also a major producer of hardwood flooring, fabricated metals, non-electrical and electrical machinery, chemicals, clothing and paper products. The city is also a major sales and distribution center to the farm and industry levels of agri-business. In June, 1979. the labor force of the greater met. area totaled approx. 385,000, while the rate of unemployment was 5.4%.

BANKING. There are 31 banks and six savings and loan assns. in Memphis. In 1978, total deposits at the nine banks headquartered in the city were approx. $3,055,499,000, while assets totaled approx. $3,743,653,000. Banks include First TN, Union Planters Natl., Natl. Bank of Commerce, Memphis Bank & Trust, Commercial & Industrial, United American, Commerce Union, City Natl. and Tri State.

HOSPITALS. There are more than 20 gen. hosps. in the Memphis met. area, as well as US Naval and V.A. hosps. The Memphis Medical Center, the largest in the S, consists of 20 short- and long-term care facilities including the largest private hosp. in the US (Baptist Memorial), the 10th largest medical school and specialty clinics. Hosps. include City of Memphis, Crittenden, Doctors, Methodist, Methodist N, Methodist S, St. Joseph's, St. Joseph's E, TN Psychiatric, Le Bonheur Children's, Shelby Co., W TN Chest Disease, St. Jude Children's Research and Oakville Memorial Supplemental services are provided by Memphis and Shelby Co. Health Dept., Memphis Speech & Hearing, Les Passees Rehabilitation and the Mental Health Centers, the W TN Cancer Clinic and the U of TN Center for the Health Sciences.

EDUCATION. Memphis State U (MSU). the largest in the city, was established in 1912 as the W TN State Normal School. It became a sr. col. in 1925 and achieved its present status in 1951, when it was reorganized to include a grad. school. Approx. 21,200 enrolled in 1978. Offering programs leading to degrees in such fields as dentistry, medicine, medical technology, nursing and social work, the U of TN Medical Units enrolled approx. 2,120 in 1978. Christian Brothers Col., a privately-supported institution affiliated with the Catholic U of America, grants bachelor degrees, and, in 1978, enrolled approx. 1,000. LeMoyne-Owen Col., established through the merger of Owen and LeMoyne cols. in 1968, is a privately-supported institution affiliated with the United Church and the TN Baptist Missionary and

Education Convention. In 1978, approx. 1,000 enrolled. Other educational institutions include the Shelby State Comm. Col., Memphis Academy of Arts, S Col. of Optometry, SW at Memphis and the State Technical Institute at Memphis. There are approx. 110 elementary and 50 jr. and sr. high schools in the public school system which enrolls more than 150,000. In addition, more than 14,000 students attend 50 private and parochial schools. The Memphis-Shelby Co. Public Lib. provides lib. facilities.

ENTERTAINMENT. Annual events held in the city include the Memphis in May Intl. Festival; the Cotton Carnival in late May and early June; the Music Heritage Festival on Labor Day Weekend; the Mid-S Fair & Exposition in Sept. and the Oktoberfest. Professional sports entertainment is provided by a SL farm club of the Montreal Expos NL baseball team and the Memphis Rogues, an NASL soccer team. The Memphis State U Tigers play at the Liberty Bowl Memorial Stadium, which is the site of the annual Liberty Bowl Classic. The Danny Thomas Memphis PGA Classic is held annually in late June or early July at one of the golf courses in the city. The World Championship Tennis Racquet Classic, a major tennis competition, is also held in the city.

ACCOMMODATIONS. There are numerous hotels and motels in Memphis, including the TraveLodge, Executive Plaza, Hyatt Regency, Medical Center Plaza, Howard Johnson's, Best Western and the Sheraton, Ramada, Days, Downtown Motor, Pilot House Motor and Holiday inns.

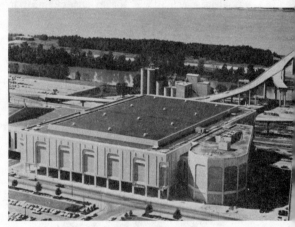

Cook Convention Center, Memphis, Tennessee

FACILITIES. The Memphis Park System consists of 197 public parks encompassing more than 6,200 acres. Among the parks are the 590-acre McKellar featuring four lakes, hiking trails and a boat dock; the 398-acre King-Riverside with facilities for golf, tennis and hiking; the 360-acre Audubon featuring facilities for skiing, boating, swimming and sailing; and the 320-acre Overton, which houses more than 2,000 mammals, reptiles, birds and fish and contains a zoo, a petting zoo for children and an aquarium. Volunteer Park, along Mud Island, which will feature a yacht club, a picnic garden and a man-made lake for row boats, is currently under construction. The kT.O. Fuller State Park offers a swimming pool, golf course and picnicking and camping facilities. The 88-acre Botanic Gardens contains thousands of varieties of flowers and trees. Public tennis courses and golfing courses are provided throughout the park system. The Park Commission also supervises 150 playgrounds during the summer and provides equipment for athletic and recreational sports, sports clinics, day camps, country weekends and 19 mobile units, which feature arts and crafts and science and nature programs. There are 26 comm. centers as well as centers for hobbies, the handicapped and sr. citizens. The nearby 13,500-acre Meeman-Shelby Forest State Park, located along the MS River, contains lakes offering fishing, and provides five hiking trails, a riding stable, campgrounds, a museum and nature center.

CULTURAL ACTIVITIES. The Memphis Arts Council, consisting of approx. 20 member groups, promotes and supports the arts in the comm. Performing arts organizations in the city include the Theatre Memphis,

Downtown Memphis, Tennessee

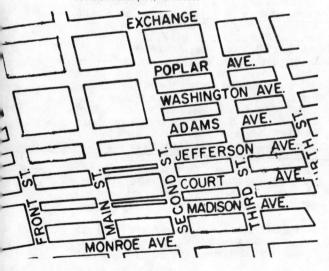

Memphis Ballet Society, Memphis Symphony Orchestra, Opera Theatre and Beethoven Club. The Brooks Memorial Art Gallery exhibits American and European art, including its Kress Collection. The Dixon Gallery and Gardens displays French and American Impressionist art. The Memphis Academy of Arts also features permanent and changing exhibits. The Pink Palace Museum and Planetarium features history and resources of the region.

LANDMARKS AND SIGHTSEEING SPOTS. The Victorian Village Complex, a Natl. Historic District on Adams St. in Memphis, consists of 10 restored homes furnished with period pieces, including the Magerney House, a clapboard cottage built in 1831; the Mallory-Neely House, an Italianate-Victorian mansion built in 1860, and the Fontaine House, a French Victorian mansion housing antiques of the Colonial to Victorian periods. The Beale St. home of W. C. Handy, the "Father of the Blues", has been restored as a center of black culture and entertainment. Graceland, the home of the late Elvis Presley, built in the architectural style of the old S, dominates spacious grounds. The Memphis State U operates the Chucalissa Indian Village Project and Museum, an archaeological site dating from 900 AD, where Choctaw Indians act as guides and demonstrate crafts. Overton Square in the mid-town area features shops, restaurants, sidewalk cafes, art galleries and a cooking school. Tours of the Cotton Exchange and cruises on the MS River are available. Liberty Land, a family theme amusement park, features several rides and other entertainment.

MESA
ARIZONA

CITY LOCATION-SIZE-EXTENT. Mesa encompasses 67 sq. mi. of Maricopa Co., 15 mi. E of Phoenix, in central AZ, at 33°25′ N lat. and 110°52′ W long. The met. area, which is a part of the greater Phoenix met. area, extends into Pinal Co. on the SE.

TOPOGRAPHY. The terrain of Mesa, which is situated in the Salt River Valley, is nearly flat, while mts. virtually surround the city. The mean elev. is 1,240.'

CLIMATE. The climate of Mesa is arid, typical of the surrounding desert. Monthly mean temps. range from 52°F in Jan. to 91°F in July, with an avg. annual temp. of 70°F. Daily extremes occur mostly in winter, when nighttime temps. drop below freezing, while afternoons are sunny and warm. The two annual wet seasons occur during Nov. through Mar., due to storms from the Pacific Ocean, and during July and Aug., due to thunderstorms originating in the Gulf of Mexico and along the Mexican W coast. The avg. annual rainfall is only 7.4". The RH ranges from 12% to 68%. The sun shines 86% of the daylight hours. Mesa lies in the MSTZ and does not observe DST.

FLORA AND FAUNA. Animals native to Mesa include the badger, coyote, skunk and bat. Common birds include the roadrunner, cactus wren, Gambel quail and hummingbird. Many reptiles, including the venomous gila monster, AZ coral snake and several species of rattlesnakes, are found in the area. Desert plants, such as the Saguaro cactus, and the palm and palo verde trees, are among the flora of this area.

POPULATION. According to the US census, the pop. of Mesa in 1970 was 62,990. In 1979, it was estimated that it had increased to 156,000.

ETHNIC GROUPS. In 1978, the ethnic distribution of Mesa was approx. 86% Caucasian, 1.2% Black, 11.7% Hispanic and 1.1% other.

TRANSPORTATION. US hwys. 60, 70, 80 and state hwys. 87 and 93 provide major motor access to Mesa. *Railroads* serving the city include S Pacific and Santa Fe. *Airlines* serving Phoenix Sky Harbor Intl. and Mesa Falcon Field Municipal airports include RW, AM, WA, CO, DL, TW, Cochise and FL lines. *Bus lines* include Greyhound, Trailways and the local Sun Valley and Safeway Suburban Stages.

COMMUNICATIONS. Communications, broadcasting and print media originating from Mesa are: *AM radio stations* KQXE 1310 (Indep., Contemp.) and KDKB 1510 (Indep., Soft Rock); *FM radio stations* KDKB 93.3 (Indep., AOR); and KIOC 104.7 (Indep., Soft Rock); no *television stations* originate from Mesa, which receives television broadcasting from nearby Phoenix; *press:* one major daily serves the city, the evening *Tribune.*

HISTORY. Mesa was established in 1878 by a company of Mormons from Idaho and Utah led by Charles I. Robson, Francis Pomeroy, George W. Sirrine and Charles Crismon. In Feb. 1878 the rest of the group reached Jonesville, present day Lehi, then moved up river to a temporary camp. Work on a new canal to irrigate the land was begun immediately and, along with construction of a town site, this occupied the attention of the company in the early months.

Temple of the Church of Jesus Christ of Latter Day Saint's, Mesa, Arizona

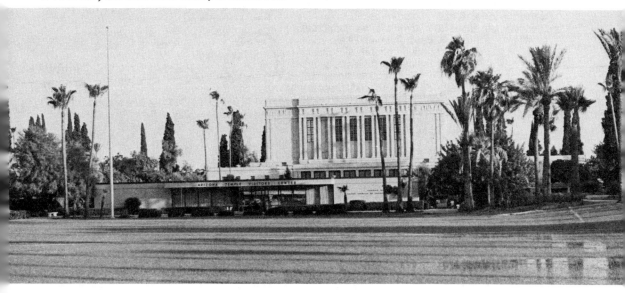

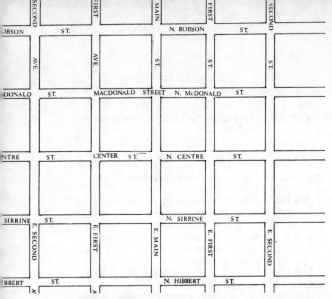

Downtown Mesa, Arizona

Capt. W. A. Hancock and A. M. Jones surveyed and marked corners of 12 sections of land and, by May, 1878, Theodore Sirrine had completed platting of the Mesa townsite. The town's name was derived from the Spanish word "Mesa", meaning table, which the settlers used to describe the bluff on which the new town was situated. on January 17, 1879. Early in 1880, a third party of settlers arrived and established Stringtown, to the west of the Mesa townsite. In 1882, the first adobe building designed specifically as a school was erected. Mesa was incorporated as a village in 1883 with a pop. of 300. Mesa's growth in the early years was slow. The new village government had to contend with an outbreak of smallpox. Mesa remained largely an agricultural comm. till the early 1950s, when a manufacturing plant was built there. The industrial base has now expanded to more than 40 firms. Jonesville, renamed Lehi in 1884, officially became a part of Mesa in 1970. By 1978 Mesa's pop. had grown to 135,000.

GOVERNMENT. The city of Mesa has a council-mgr. form of govt. The six council members are elected in staggered-year elections to four-year terms. The mayor, elected to a two-year term, presides over council meetings and serves as the ceremonial head of govt. He is empowered to make minor decisions when council is not in session and may appoint advisory board members, subject to council approval. The city mgr. is the administrative head of city govt.

ECONOMY AND INDUSTRY. There are more than 40 manufacturing firms in Mesa. Tourism is the chief industry, followed by electronics, aircraft renovation, citrus packing, food processing and the manufacture of apparel. Maricopa Co. ranks fourth among US counties in agricultural production. Principal crops are cotton, alfalfa, cereal grains, citrus fruits, sugar beets, lettuce, onions, potatoes and tomatoes. The median household income in 1978 was $13,226. The unemployment rate in 1978 was 5%.

BANKING. There are six commercial banks and six savings and loan assns. in Mesa. In 1978, total deposits for the one bank headquartered in the city were $16,108,000, while assets were $17,764,000. Banks include Arizona, Continental, Copper State, First Natl. and Valley Natl.

HOSPITALS. There are three hospitals in Mesa—Desert Samaritan, Mesa Lutheran and Mesa Gen. Osteopathic.

EDUCATION. Mesa Comm. Col., located in Mesa, is a branch of the Maricopa Co. Comm. Col. District. It awards the associate degree and, in 1978, it enrolled approx. 12,400. The U of AZ Agricultural Station is also located in the city. There are 27 elementary, seven jr. and four sr. high schools in the district, plus three special schools. Lib. facilities include the Mesa Public Lib. and the genealogical lib. of the Latter-day Saints Church.

ENTERTAINMENT. Annual events in Mesa include a Miniature Parade, Scandinavian Festival and Family Living Conference. Mesa is the spring training camp for the Chicago Cubs baseball team of the NL. The AZ State U Sun Devils and the Mesa Comm. Col. Thunderbirds compete in intercollegiate sports.

ACCOMMODATIONS. There are numerous hotels and motels in Mesa, including the Royal Mesa, Mezona Motor Hotel, Maricopa, Dobson Ranch and Superstition inns.

FACILITIES. There are 19 major parks and playgrounds in Mesa, offering picnic facilities, playground equipment, shuffleboard, tennis, croquet and handball courts and softball fields, most of which are lighted for evening use. Larger parks include Pioneer, Reed, Palo Verde, Hohokam and Fitch, which features a special "Fitness Trail." There are 76 tennis courts in the city, and 14 golf courses, including the municipal Dobson Ranch course.

CULTURAL ACTIVITIES. The Mesa Fine Arts Assn. sponsors local cultural activities, such as the Sun Valley Orchestra and the Tri-City Band. Dramatic productions are staged by the Musical Theatre and the Little Theatre. The Activity Center and Art Barn offer arts and crafts programs. The Museum of Archeology and History features exhibits on the valley's prehistory.

LANDMARKS AND SIGHTSEEING SPOTS. Local points of interest include Montezuma's Canal and other ancient Indian ruins in the area and the AZ Temple of the Church of Jesus Christ of Latter-Day Saints. The Little Adobe Schoolhouse was built in 1976 by Mesa public school students, as a replica of the first adobe building designed specifically as a school which was originally built in 1882.

Centennial Hall, Mesa, Arizona

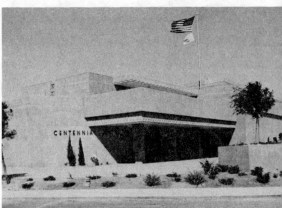

MIAMI
FLORIDA

CITY LOCATION-SIZE-EXTENT. Miami encompasses 34.3 sq. mi. on Biscayne Bay in Dade Co., on the lower E coast of FL, at 25°47' N lat. and 80°11' W long. The greater met. area extends N into Broward Co.

TOPOGRAPHY. The terrain of Miami, which is situated on the Atlantic Coast, is very level and includes sandy beaches along the bay and sparsely wooded areas further inland. It is located at the mouth of the Miami River and is connected to Lake Okeechobee, approx. 90 mi. to the NW, by a man-made canal. The mean elev. is 10'.

CLIMATE. The climate of Miami is subtropical marine, characterized by long, warm and rainy summers and short, mild and dry winters. The area is subject to winds from the E or SE approx. 50% of the time. The avg. annual temp. of 75.5°F varies slightly from a mean

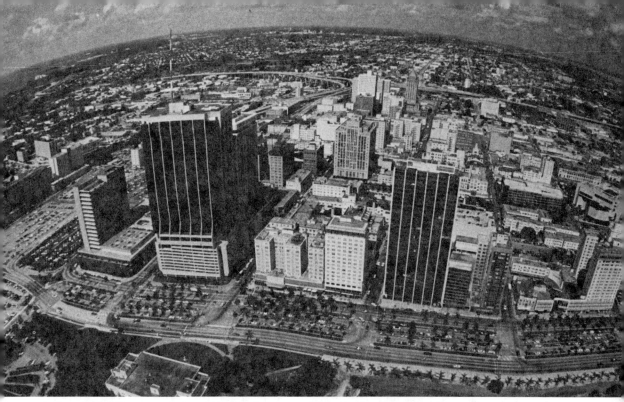

in Jan. of 67.2°F to a mean in Aug. of 82.7°F. Approx. 66% of the annual mean rainfall of 58.93" occurs during the period from late spring to early fall. Tropical hurricanes affect the area, with most occurring during Sept. and Oct. The RH ranges from 54% to 89%. Miami lies in the ESTZ and observes DST.

FLORA AND FAUNA. Animals native to Miami include the whitetail deer, opossum and raccoon. Common birds include the grackle, heron, ibis, egret and gull. Beckos, skinks, sirens, newts, tree frogs and cricket frogs as well as the venomous coral snake, rattlesnake and water moccasin are found in the area. Typical trees include the palm, mangrove, mahogany and cypress. Smaller plants include the palmetto, yucca, bay and holly.

POPULATION. According to the US census, the pop. of Miami in 1970 was 334,859. In 1978, it was estimated that it had increased to 354,000.

ETHNIC GROUPS. In 1978, the ethnic distribution of Miami was approx. 23% Caucasian, 22% Black and 55% Hispanic.

TRANSPORTATION. Interstate hwys. 95 and 195, US hwys. 1, 41, 441 and 27 and state hwys. 9, 25 and 836 provide major motor access to Miami. *Railroads* serving the city include AMTRAK, Auto-Train, ConRail, FL E Coast, French Natl., Seaboard Coast Lines and S. *Airlines* serving Miami Intl. Airport are BN, CO, DL, EA, NA, NW, PA, PI, RD, TW and UA. *Bus lines* serving the city include Greyhound, Trailways and the local Dade Metro Transit Authority.

COMMUNICATIONS. Communications, broadcasting and print media originating from Miami are: *AM radio stations* WQAM 560 (Indep., Contemp.); WIOD 610 (MBS, Divers); WGBS 710 (Indep., MOR); WINZ 940 (CBS, All News); WQBA 1140 (Indep., Spec. Progsv.); WCMQ 1220 (Indep., Latin Contemp.); WWOK 1260 (MBS, C&W) and WOCN 1450 (Indep., Spec. Progsv.); *FM radio stations* WMCV 89.7 (Indep., Educ., Relig.); WLRN 91.3 (NPR, Clas., Jazz, Divers.); WTMI 93.1 (Indep., Clas.); WMJX 96.3 (Indep., Contemp.); WAIA 97.3 (Natl. Blk.); WLYF 101.5 (Indep., Btfl. Mus.) and WIGL 107.5 (Indep., Ctry.); *television stations* WPBT Ch. 2 (PBS); WTVJ Ch. 4 (CBS); WCIX Ch. 6 (NBC); WPLG Ch. 10 (ABC); WLRN Ch. 17 (PBS); WLTV Ch. 23 (Span.); WHFT Ch. 45. (Relig.) and cable; *press:* four major dailies serve the area, the *Herald* and the *Diario de Las Americas*, both issued mornings, *News*, issued evenings; and *Miami Review* a business daily. Weekly publications include *Greater Miami Beach Journal*, *Times*, *Jewish Floridian*, *This Week in Miami Beach* and *The Voice*; monthly publications include *Miami Magazine, FL Sportsman, Go Boating, Golf Industry* and *Welding Journal*.

Wide Angle View of Downtown Miami, Florida

HISTORY. Native Americans of the Tequesta tribe inhabited the Miami area prior to white settlement. In 1567 the first Spanish mission was established when Menendez tried to convert the native Americans, but this effort failed and it wasn't attempted again until 1743 when a Spanish mission was constructed near present-day Coconut Grove. An early FL settler named Julia Tuttle persuaded RR builder Henry Flagler that the region had potential as a fertile agricultural area by sending him some flowers that survived a damaging cold spell. Flagler received land for extending the FL E Coast RR to the area in 1896. Miami received its charter that year with a pop. of 1,500. The first white settlers built homes on Biscayne Bay, which provided a good harbor. The comm.'s name was derived from the Miami River. Aided by the RR, the number of residents reached 5,000 by 1910. Enterprising promoters drained Miami swamps and dredged Biscayne Bay to enlarge Miami Beach at the turn of the century. Fortunes were made and lost in real estate during the land boom of the 1920s. As it began to collapse, a hurricane wreaked havoc on the city in 1926 and again two years later. Still, Miami's pop. rose to 110,000 by 1930. WW II also contributed to the city's development, for thousands of servicemen who lived in Miami while it was a military center returned there after the war. The 1970s brought problems of unemployment and a scarcity of inexpensive housing to Miami. These problems were combatted with job training programs for unskilled workers and urban renewal projects. Today, Miami is the fastest growing city E of the MS River, the second largest city in FL and over 10 million people visit the world famous resort each year.

GOVERNMENT. Miami has a council-mgr. form of govt. Four council members are elected at large to four-year terms. The mayor, a voting member of the council, is elected at large to a two-year term.

ECONOMY AND INDUSTRY. Tourism is the chief industry of the Miami met. area, while the city is developing light, diversified industry and has more than 2,000

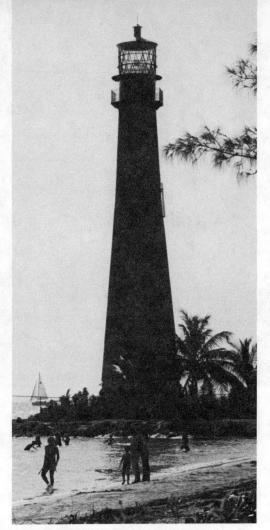

Cape Florida Lighthouse, Miami, Florida

ENTERTAINMENT. Featured each year is Miami's King Orange Jamboree, which culminates with the Orange Bowl football game on New Year's Day. The Miami Dolphins of NFL-AFC football offer pro. sports. Horseracing and Jai Alai are two popular gaming sports. The $50,000 annual LPGA Tourney is the richest tournament on the LPGA circuit and leads off the season. Intercollegiate sports are provided by the Miami Hurricanes and the Florida Intl. U Sunblazers. The city is also the site of the annual N-S Col. All Star Game.

ACCOMMODATIONS. With tourism one of its major industries, Miami has 485 hotels and 366 motels. These include Omni Intl., Key Biscayne and Doral Country Club hotels, Miami Marriott, River House, Coconut Grove, Newport Resort, Pan American, Dupont Plaza, Everglades, Intercontinental, Howard Johnson's, Sonesta, Best Western and Quality, Holiday, Ramada and Sheraton inns.

FACILITIES. There are 4,083 acres of parkland, including 105 parks and playgrounds, in Miami. The major parks are Bicentennial, Cape FL Lighthouse, Peacock, Bayfront and Simpson. Beaches are located at Bill Baggs Cape, FL State Recreation Area, Crandon Park and VA Beach. Adjacent to Miami is Miami Beach, which includes 250 acres of land forming 33 parks. Also located in the area are Miami Seaquarium, Parrot Jungle and the zoo in Crandon Park. Jogging and exercise courses are located at the U of Miami and Bicentennial, Kennedy and Morningside parks. Public courses include Colonial Palms, Briar Bay and Par Three, while public tennis courts are available at Marco Polo-Waikiki's Tennis Center, McDonald Tennis Court and Milander Tennis Court.

CULTURAL ACTIVITIES. The Miami Philharmonic and Miami Opera Guild perform at the Expo Center; programs are also presented at Gusman Philharmonic Hall. Dramatic productions are staged by the Players State Theater at Coconut Grove Playhouse. A variety of presentations are featured at the Miami Beach Theater of the Performing Arts. Paintings, wood sculpture and two of the world's largest tapestries are featured at the Bass Museum. The Museum of Science houses exhibits of science, gem-cutting, early FL cultures and wildlife. Vizcaya, formerly the estate of James Deering, is now the Dade Co. Art Museum. Other city museums include the Historical Museum of S FL, the Cuban Museum of Arts and Culture, the Lowe Art Museum and the Metropolitan Museum and Art Center.

LANDMARKS AND SIGHTSEEING SPOTS. The man who established Miami Beach and deeded many public beaches and parks to Miami is honored by the Carl Fisher Monument. The Miami Wax Museum offers recorded tours of over 40 diaramas with life-sized wax figures portraying historical events of FL and the US. A large collection of parrot-type and other exotic birds are exhibited in the Parrot Jungle. The Miami Seaquarium features a diversified display of marine life in four separate show arenas. An authentic indoor cloud, rainstorm and a captive hurricane are recreated at Planet Ocean, an educational ocean science center which is headquarters for the Intl. Oceanography Foundation. The Space Transit Planetarium is also located in Miami.

manufacturing firms. Clothing is a major product and Miami ranks second only to NYC in its production. Other products include electronics, furniture, metal products, printed matter and automotive equipment. Met. Dade Co. is the city's single largest employer with the more than 136 US and foreign airlines serving Miami Intl. Airport ranking second. Total labor force for the Miami area in Sept., 1979, was 704,500, while the rate of unemployment was 6.1%. The median per capita income in 1977 was $7,755.

BANKING. There are 74 commercial banks, one state savings and loan assn. and 21 fed. savings and loan assns. in Miami. In 1978, total deposits for the 26 banks headquartered in the city were $4,361,858,000, while assets were $5,370,540,000. Banks include SE First Natl., FL Natl., City Natl., Pan American, Barnett and Republic Natl.

HOSPITALS. There are 41 gen. hosps. and two govt. hosps. in Miami, including Jackson Memorial, Cedars of Lebanon, Mount Sinai, Mercy, S Miami and Baptist.

EDUCATION. FL's first Catholic col., Barry Col., is located in Miami. It opened in 1940 and is operated by the Sisters of St. Dominic of Adrian, MI. In 1978, it enrolled approx. 1,800. The largest col. in Miami is the Miami-Dade Comm. Col. It offers associate degrees and, in 1978, it enrolled approx. 39,500. Other institutions include Biscayne Col., FL Memorial Col., Intl. Fine Arts Col., Miami Christian Col., St. John Vianney Col. Seminary and FL Intl. U. The Dade Co. Pub. School System operates approx. 173 elementary and 60 jr.,sr. high and 6 special education schools. Approx. 140 private and church-supported schools serve the area. The area's 29 public libs. include the Miami-Dade Public Lib. System.

Miami, Florida

MILWAUKEE
WISCONSIN

CITY LOCATION-SIZE-EXTENT. Milwaukee, the largest city in WI and seat of Milwaukee Co., encompasses 95 sq. mi. on the W shore of Lake MI in SE WI, at the confluence of the Milwaukee, Menomonee and Kinnichinnic rivers at 42°02' N lat. and 87°54' W long. The greater met. area extends into the neighboring counties of Racine to the S, Waukesha to the SW and WA and Ozaukee to the N.

TOPOGRAPHY. The terrain of Milwaukee, situated on a bluff in the Great Lakes Plains Region, is generally flat and encompasses 10 mi. of sandy beaches along the Lake MI shoreline. There are several lakes in the area, including Muskego, Little Muskego, Wind, Long and Waubeesee, all to the SW. The mean elev. is 635'.

CLIMATE. The climate of Milwaukee is greatly influenced by Lake MI as well as by storms moving E across the Upper OH River Valley and Great Lakes region and the large high pressure systems moving SE out of Canada. Monthly mean temps. range from 20.9°F in Jan. to 70.7°F in July, with an avg. annual temp. of 47°F. About 66% of the annual rainfall of 30" occurs during the growing season, which avgs. 178 days. Annual snowfall avgs. 46", of which 50% falls in Dec. and Jan. The RH ranges from 65% to 81%. Milwaukee lies in the CSTZ and observes DST.

FLORA AND FAUNA. Animals native to Milwaukee include the E chipmunk, gray squirrel, whitetail deer, muskrat, shrew, woodchuck and raccoon. Common birds are the robin (the state bird), blue jay, screech owl, mourning dove, golden eye mallard, rock dove, grackle, oriole, brown thrasher and chickadee. Spring peepers, leopard frogs and garter snakes are common to the area. Typical trees are the oak, hawthorne, tasswood, dogwood, elm and sugar maple (the state tree). Smaller plants include the blue violet (the state flower), marsh marigold and spring beauty.

POPULATION. According to the US census, the pop. of Milwaukee in 1970 was 717,372. In 1978, it was estimated that it had decreased to 620,160.

ETHNIC GROUPS. In 1970, the ethnic distribution of Milwaukee was approx. 84.4% Caucasian, 14.7% Black, 0.5% Native American and 2.2% Hispanic. (A percentage of the Hispanic total is also included in the Caucasian total.)

TRANSPORTATION. Interstate hwys. 43, 94, 794 and 894, US hwys. 18, 41 and 45 and state hwys. 15, 16, 24, 32, 38, 57, 59, 62, 74, 100, 145, 181 and 190 provide major motor access to Milwaukee. *Railroads* serving the city include AMTRAK, Milwaukee Road, Chicago & NW and the Soo Line. *Airlines* serving Gen. Mitchell Field include EA, RP, NW, BN, OZ, UA, RW, and WE. *Bus lines* serving the city include American, Badger, Mid America, Royal, WI and WI-MI coach lines, Greyhound, and the local Milwaukee Co. Transit System. The Port of Milwaukee, on Lake MI, serves 350 cities in 31 states and several foreign markets. Cargo is shipped to the E seaboard via the St. Lawrence Seaway, with more than six million tons of cargo passing through the port annually.

COMMUNICATIONS. Communications, broadcasting and print media originating in Milwaukee are: *AM radio stations* WTMJ 620 (NBC, MOR); WNOV 860 (Indep., Blk.); WOKY 920 (Indep., Contemp.); WISN 1100 (ABC/I, MOR); WEMP 1250 (CBS, C&W); WZUU 1290 (Indep., Top 40); and WBCS 1340 (APR, C&W); *FM radio stations* WYMS 88.4 (Indep., Educ.); WUWM 89.7 (Indep., Divers.); WQFM 93.3 (Indep., Progsv.); WKTI 94.5 (IABC/FM, Progsv.); WZUU 95.7 (Indep., Top 40); WFMR 96.5 (Indep., Clas., Jazz); WLPX 97.3 (Indep., ADR); WNUW 99.1 (Indep., MOR); WAWA 102.1 (Indep., Blk.); WBCS 102.9 (Indep., C&W); and WVCY 107.7 (Indep., Relig.); *television stations* WTMJ Ch. 4 (NBC); WITI Ch. 6 (CBS); WMVS Ch. 10 (PBS); WISN Ch. 12 (ABC); WVTV Ch. 18 (Indep.); 24 (Indep.); WMVT Ch. 36

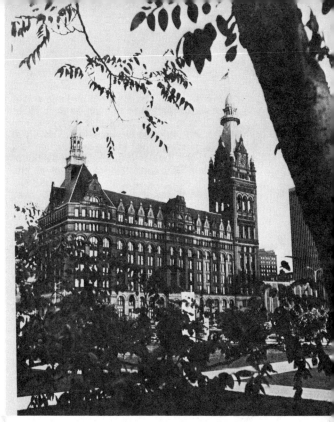

City Hall, Milwaukee, Wisconsin

(PBS) and cable; *press*: two major dailies serve the city, the *Journal*, issued evenings, and the *Sentinel*, issued mornings; other publications include the *Milwaukee Labor Press, Herald, Post, Courier, Deutsche Zeitung, Daily Reporter* and quarterly *Milwaukee Milwaukee.*

HISTORY. Prior to the arrival of white settlers, the site of present-day Milwaukee served as hunting grounds for native Americans of the Fox, Mascouten and Potawatomi tribes who called it Mahn-a-waukee Seepe "gathering place by the river." The French missionary, Jacques Marquette, became the area's first recorded visitor, in 1674. Although the region remained in contact with passing fur traders and missionaries, it was not until 1795 that a fur trader named Jacques Vieau established a trading post in the area. In 1818, Solomon Juneau, Vieau's clerk, settled there, and, 15 years later, established a town on the E bank of the Milwaukee River. The area expanded during the 1830s, with the arrival of settlers from the E and entrepreneurs, such as Byron Kilbourne of CT, who developed the W bank of the Milwaukee River, and George Walker of VA, who developed the land S of the Menomonee River. The Village of Milwaukee was formed in 1839 by the merger of Juneautown, and Kilbourntown as two wards of the town of Milwaukee. In 1845, Walker's Point joined the merger and the three wards were incorporated as the City of Milwaukee in 1846, with Juneau as the first mayor. The city's residents numbered 12,000 in 1847. An influx of German, Polish and Irish immigrants began arriving in the 1840s, and later formed the nuclei of the city's ethnic makeup. The 1850s and 1860s saw Milwaukee's development as a commercial center, and, with the improvement of transportation facilities, an important flour and wheat market as well. In 1867, the first practical typewriter was designed in Milwaukee. With the development of the meatpacking and tanning industries, the city's economic emphasis shifted to manufacturing, after 1870. By 1890, 200,000 persons

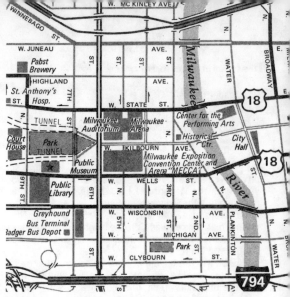

inhabited Milwaukee. The city developed into one of the nation's major brewing centers in the early 1900s. Industrial growth led to socialist political agitation during this time, although this consisted primarily of inhabited organizing labor. Milwaukee had the first Socialist mayor in a major US city, upon the election of Emil Seidel in 1910. With the enlargement of city harbors in the early 1950s, ocean-going vessels could be accommodated, and, when the St. Lawrence Seaway was opened in 1959, Milwaukee's importance as an intl. seaport facilty was established. The pop. had reached 741,324 by 1960, but subsequently declined, as many city residents moved to the suburbs.

Two projects are underway for the 1980s, to revitalize the downtown area. The Menomonee River Valley Project will redevelop an industrial area to employ about 30,000. The WI Ave. Mall Project is under construction.

GOVERNMENT. Milwaukee has a mayor-council form of govt. The 16 aldermen who form the common council are elected, by district, and the mayor is elected at-large, to four-year terms.

ECONOMY AND INDUSTRY. There are 26,758 business establishments in Milwaukee. Major products include textiles, apparel, lumber, furniture, paper, printing and publishing, petroleum and coal products, rubber, plastics, machinery, prime metal and fabricated metal products. Milwaukee produces more beer than any other city and has three of the four largest breweries. In 1979, the total labor force for the city was 680,000, while the rate of unemployment was 3.7%. In 1978, the median family income in the greater met. area before taxes was $13,000.

BANKING. There are over 97 banks in Milwaukee. In 1978, total deposits for the 30 banks headquartered in the city were $4,304,576,000, while total assets were $5,987,804,000. Banks include the First WI Natl., Marshall & Isley, Marine Natl., First Bank and Heritage.

HOSPITALS. The hosps. and health care centers in Milwaukee include Columbia, Mt. Sinai, Deaconess, Lutheran, NW Gen., St. Anthony, St. Francis, St. Joseph's, St. Luke's, St. Mary's Hills, St. Michael, Milwaukee Co. complex and Milwaukee Children's.

EDUCATION. The U of WI Milwaukee, the largest U in the city was

St. Joan of Arc Church, originally built in France, sits on Marquette University Campus, Milwaukee, Wisconsin

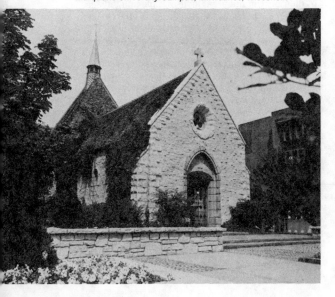

established in 1956 and offers work courses leading to bachelor, master and doctorate degrees. Enrollment was 24,281 in 1978. Marquette U, an institution supported by the Society of Jesus, was founded in 1881 and is one of the largest Catholic institutions in the nation. Offering courses leading to bachelor, master and doctorate degrees; Marquette U enrolled 10,855 in 1978. Alverno Col., a private, liberal arts col. for women, founded in 1936 by the School Sisters of St. Francis, offers programs leading to the bachelor degree. In 1978, Alverno Col. enrolled 1,101. Other institutions include Cardinal Stritch Col., St. Francis de Sales Col., Concordia Col., Mt. Mary Col., WI Conservatory of Music, the Medical Col. of WI, the Milwaukee School of Engineering. The Milwaukee Area Technical Col. is one of the nation's largest vocational/adult education centers. The public school includes 106 elementary, 18 middle, 15 sr. high and 7 special education education schools and enrolls over 92,523 annually. Approx. 29,179 students attend 127 private and parochial schools. The Milwaukee Public Lib. and its 15 branches serve the city.

ENTERTAINMENT. Some of the festivals and events held annually in Milwaukee WI are the WI Festival of Arts (May); Brady Street, Monarch Dance and Lakefront Arts festivals (June); the Marquette Summer Theatre, Alewives Jazz festival and Summerfest (June-July); Kool Jazz Festival (July); Volk Fest and Festa Italiana (July); the WI State Fair (Aug.); Oktoberfest (Oct.) and Holiday Folk Fair (Nov.). The Milwaukee Bucks, an NBA basketball team and the Brewers, an AL baseball team provide pro sports entertainment. The Green Bay Packers football team of the NFL-NFC usually play one game per season in Milwaukee. The Marquette U Warriors and U of WI Panthers participate in collegiate sports.

ACCOMMODATIONS. Hotels and motels in Milwaukee include the Marc Plaza, Milwaukee River Hilton, Pfister Hotel and Tower, the Sheraton Mayfair, two Holiday inns, Marriott, Hyatt Regency, Ramada, Howard Johnson and Best Western.

FACILITIES. The Milwaukee Co. Park System encompasses 14,000 acres in 128 parks and includes six beaches along the lakefront in Bradford, McKinley, Grant, S Shore, Bay View and Doctors' parks. Swimming pools are featured at Carver, Dineen, Gordon, Greenfield, Hales Corners, Hoyt, Jackson, Kosciuszko, Lincoln, Madison, McCarthy, McGovern, Oak Creek, Sheridan, Washington and Wilson, while Holler, Pulaski and Moody have indoor/outdoor pools. A 76 mi. bicycle trail forms a loop throughout Milwaukee Co. utilizing many of the major parks. Ice skating ponds and skiing facilities are also available. Boating facilities are located at McKinley Marina and S Shore Park. Whitnall Park, the largest in the co. has many natural features, including hills, lagoons and nature trails. The Todd Wehr Nature Center offers a wildlife preserve with many trails for hiking and cross-country skiing. Included in Whitnall Park are the Boerner Botanical Gardens—an outdoor formal display of numerous flowering plants, trees and shrubs. There are 134 tennis courts and 15 golf courses in the park system. Over 6,000 animals are featured in barless enclosures and natural habitats at the Milwaukee Co. Zoo. The Mitchell Park Conservatory is composed of three domes, arid, tropical and a changing show dome.

Milwaukee, Wisconsin

CULTURAL ACTIVITIES. The Milwaukee Symphony Orchestra, Repertory Theatre Co., Ballet Co., Bel Canto Chorus, Florentine Opera Co., and Pabst Theater are located in Milwaukee. Musicals are presented at the Temple of Music in WA Park and Melody Top Theater, while the Performing Arts Center and Theatre X stage dramatic productions. Native American, African, Pre-Columbian and European Village exhibitions, as well as displays of the city's history, are housed in the Milwaukee Public Museum. An Italian-style villa built in 1923, Villa Terrace now exhibits decorative arts, with furnishings of periods ranging from 1660 to 1820. The Charles Allis Art Lib. contains a collection of Oriental art objects among other exhibits. Other museums include the Brooks Stevens Automotive, Experimental Aircraft Assn., Milwaukee Co. Historical Center and the Milwaukee Arts Center in the War Memorial complex containing an art collection.

LANDMARKS AND SIGHTSEEING SPOTS. Milwaukee is the site of Frank Lloyd Wright's last major work, the Annunciation Greek Orthodox Church, a saucer-shaped building with a blue dome roof. St. Josaphat Basilica, modeled after St. Peter's in Rome, is one of two Polish basilicas in N America. Large homes dating from the early 19th century are located in the water tower area. Both the Pabst Mansion (1893) and City Hall (1895) are examples of Flemish Renaissance architecture. One of the city's three original settlers, George H. Walker, founded Walker's Point, a surviving 19th century neighborhood that has been nominated as a Natl. Historic District. Other historic buildings are the Kilbourntown House (1844) and Pabst Theatre (1895). Other attractions are the Allen-Bradley clock, featuring a face 40' in diameter; the Bowling Hall of Fame; the John Plankington Arcade, an enclosed mall of shops and offices patterned after European arcades; three breweries, which are designated as historic landmarks and the 42 story First WI Center, with an observation deck on top.

MINNEAPOLIS
MINNESOTA

CITY LOCATION-SIZE-EXTENT. Minneapolis, located in SW MN, encompasses 58.7 sq. mi. in Hennepin Co. at 44°53' N lat and 93°13' W long. Its met. area, which is contiguous with the St. Paul area, extends into Scott and Carver counties on the SW and Sherburne and Wright counties on the NW.

TOPOGRAPHY. Minneapolis is located at the confluence of the MS River and the MN River over the heart of an artesian water basin. The city's flat to gently rolling terrain varies little in elev. The area is dotted with numerous lakes and lakelets which are relatively small and shallow and are ice covered during the winter. The mean elev. is 831'.

CLIMATE. Minneapolis has a typical continental climate characterized by wide variations in temp., including substantial summer rains. Annual snowfall avgs. 46.3". Over 70% of the avg. annual rainfall of 26.64" occurs from Apr. to Sept. Mean temps. range from 12.9°F in Jan. to 73.1°F in July, with an annual avg. of 44.9°F. The RH ranges from 50% to 82%. Minneapolis is in the CSTZ and observes DST.

FLORA AND FAUNA. Animals native to Minneapolis include the deer, raccoon, beaver and muskrat. Common birds are the sparrow, duck, loon (the state bird), bittern, rail, goldfinch and kingfisher. Bullfrogs, leopard frogs, snapping turtles and mudpuppies are found in the area. Typical trees include maple, Norway pine (the state tree), oak, elm and willow. Smaller plants include the lilac, lady-slipper (the state flower), buttercup, hepatica and fireweed.

POPULATION. According to the US census, the pop. of Minneapolis in 1970 was 434,000. In 1978, it was estimated that it had decreased to 375,000.

ETHNIC GROUPS. In 1978, the ethnic distribution of Minneapolis was approx. 89% Caucasian, 7.5% Black, 2.3% American Indian and 1.2% other.

TRANSPORTATION. Interstate hwys. 94, 35 W and 494, US Hwys. 52, 12, 169, 65 and 212 and state hwys. 200 and 36 provide major motor access to Minneapolis. *Railroads* serving Minneapolis are AMTRAK, Burlington N, Chicago-Milwaukee-St. Paul & Pacific, Chicago ConRail, Milwaukee RR, Minneapolis Northfield & S, Santa Fe, Soo Line, S Pacific, S Union Pacific and W Pacific. Eight *airlines* use the Minneapolis/St. Paul Intl. Airport: US AIR, BN, EA, NC, NW, OZ, TW and UA. Inter-city *bus lines* are Suburban, Richfield, Greyhound, Jefferson and Medicine Lake. The Met. Transit Commission provides city bus service.

COMMUNICATIONS. Communications, broadcasting and print media originating from Minneapolis are: *AM radio stations* KDWB 630 (Indep., Contemp.); KTCR 690 (MBS, C&W); KUOM 770 (NPR, Educ.); WCCO 830 (CBS, Var.); KTIS 900 (Indep., Relig.); WAYL 980 (Indep., Btfl. Mus.); WDGY 1130 (Indep., Contemp.); WWTC 1280 (NBC, MBS, UPS, All News); WLOL 1330 (ABC/I, Var.); WDAN 1370 (Indep., MOR); KEEY 1400 (Indep., MOR) and KSTP 1500 (Indep., Educ./Com. Ser.); *FM radio stations* KSJN 91.1 (NPR, Clas., News); WAYL 93.7 (Indep., Var.); KSTP 94.5 (Indep., Bright MOR); KBEM 88.5 (Indep., Educ., Comm. Ser.); KFAI 90.3 (Indep., Var.); KNOF 95.3 (Indep., Gospel); KTCR 97.1 (Indep., Btfl. Mus.); KTIS 98.5 (Indep., Relig.); WLOL 99.5 (Indep., MOR); WCTS 100.3 (Indep., Relig.); KDWB 101.3 (Indep., MOR); KEEY 102.1 (Indep., Btfl. Mus.) and WCCO 120.9 (ABC/C, MOR); *television stations* KTCA Ch. 2 (PBS); WCCO Ch. 4 (CBS); KSTP Ch. 5 (ABC); KMSP Ch. 9 (Indep.) WTCN Ch. 11 (NBC); KTCI Ch. 23 (Indep.) and cable; *press*: the major dailies serving the area are *The Star*, an evening newspaper, the *Daily* and the *Tribune*, published mornings; other publications include the *Labor Reader*, *Skyway News*, the *Spokesman* and the *Twin Cities Reader*, weekly publications include the *Corporative Builder*, *N Hennepin* and *N Minneapolis Posts* and *The Progress Register*, monthly publications include The *MN Chemist*, *MN Press*, *NW Lumberman* and the *Twin Cities Woman*.

Longfellow's Minnehaha Falls in Winter, Minneapolis, Minn.

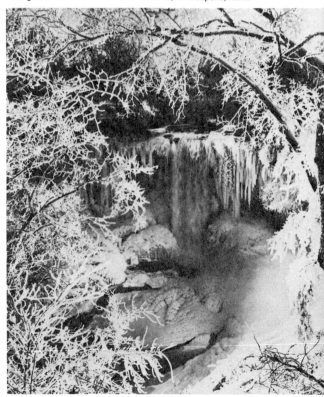

HISTORY. The first inhabitants of the Minneapolis area were native Americans of the Sioux Tribe. Minneapolis was founded as a lumbering village in 1849 and named All Saints. The name was changed in 1852 to Minneapolis, coming from the Indian and Greek words "minne", meaning water, and "polis", meaning city. The city is on the site of the MS River and St. Anthony Falls, which were discovered by Louis Hennepin in 1680. Ft. Snelling was built in the area by American soldiers in the 1820s, and from then until the 1850s the ft. was a trading center. In the mid 1850s, the city's agricultural development was enhanced by the construction of grain elevators for wheat farming. The city was incorporated in 1856. After the Civil War, the power of the St. Anthony Falls was harnessed and, by 1882, Minneapolis was the world's leading flour milling center. It became a transportation center, as did St. Paul, its sister city and MN's state capital. The city's

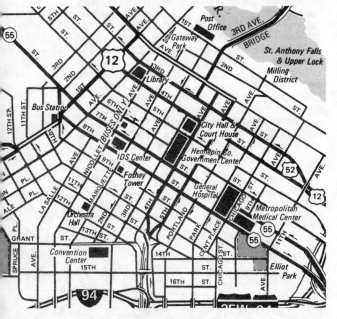

Downtown Minneapolis, Minnesota

industrial growth began to outpace that of St. Paul which was, instead, more involved with river trade and agriculture. By the turn of the century, Minneapolis had become a world center for lumber trade. The lumber industry declined in the early 20th century when overcutting depleted the lumber supply. A 1920s increase in freight rates ended the city's flour mill expansion. After World War II, Minneapolis became a leader in electronic equipment, farm machinery and computer industries. During the 1960s and 70s, a massive privately-funded redevelopment project renewed the city's downtown section.

GOVERNMENT. Minneapolis has a mayor-council form of govt. consisting of a mayor and 13 council members. Council members are elected by district every two years. The mayor is elected at large every two years, but is not a member of the council and has no vote.

ECONOMY AND INDUSTRY. Minneapolis is a major center for industry, trade and finance. There are approx. 3,000 manufacturers in the met. area producing approx. $3 billion worth of goods annually. Leading industries are food processing, chemicals, electronics, research,

meat packing and publishing. The Minneapolis-St. Paul met. area had a total labor force of 1,099,100 in 1979 and an unemployment rate of 3.2%.

BANKING. In 1978, total deposits for the 26 banks headquartered in Minneapolis were $6,196,652,000, while total assets were $8,435,363,000. Banks include Minneapolis Fed. Reserve, Farmers' and Mechanics' Savings, Mid-W Fed., NW Natl., First Minneapolis and First Natl.

HOSPITALS. There are several hospitals in the city including Hennepin Co. Gen., Fairview, Abbot—NW, U of MN, Methodist, N. Memorial, V.A., Gillette Children's and Shriners Hosp. for Crippled Children.

EDUCATION. The U of MN operates its main campus in Minneapolis. Chartered in 1851 as a preparatory school, the U grew to include three additional campuses. The school enrolled 4,629 students in 1979 and offers grad and undergrad courses and degrees. The Minneapolis Col. of Art and Design is a private professional school awarding the baccalaureate degree. Augsburg Col. is a private liberal arts institution supported by the American Lutheran Church, offering course work leading to bachelor degrees. The col. enrolled 1,751 students in 1978. Other cols. include Golden Valley Lutheran, St. Mary's Jr., Minneapolis Bus. and Minneapolis Drafting. The public school system includes approx. 96 elementary and high schools, with a 1979 enrollment of about 53,007 students. There are 36 parochial and private schools in the city. The Minneapolis Public Lib. has 15 branches and houses more than a million books.

ENTERTAINMENT. Annual festivals include the Syttende Mai, a Swedish festival held every May, and in July there is the Aquatennial with canoe races, water ballets, costume balls and a parade. Among the sports teams in Minneapolis are the MN Twins, AL baseball; the Kicks, NASL soccer; The MN Vikings, NFL-NFC football; and the MN Northstars, NHL-POWC hockey. The U of MN Golden Gophers and the Metro Comm. Col. Marauders participate in collegiate leagues.

ACCOMMODATIONS. Hotels and motels in Minneapolis include the Marquette Inn, Sheraton Ritz, Radisson, Howard Johnson's, L'Hotel de France, the Registry, Best Western, Holiday Inn, Concord, Leamington, Normandy, Fair Oaks and Northstar.

FACILITIES. Minneapolis has over 100 parks and playgrounds covering 5,500 acres. In addition, 22 natural lakes in the area provide various water sports. The largest parks are Wirth Park and Minnehaha Park, where the Minnehaha Falls—of Longfellow's "Song of Hiawatha"——are found. Como Park Zoo and the children's zoo are other city attractions. The MN Zoological Gardens cover over 500 acres and house more than 250 species of animals as well as 2,000 varieties of plants. Outdoor sports facilities are also available. There are several public golf courses including, Breamar, Hampton Hill and Silver Springs. Public tennis courts are located at the Minneapolis Tennis Club and at the Nicollet Indoor Tennis and Roller Garden. The Theodore Wirth Ski lift is available for skiers.

CULTURAL ACTIVITIES. Minneapolis is the home of several natl.-known institutions. The Guthrie Theater, featuring a resident repertory co. and performing in Guthrie Hall, offers special performances and concerts throughout the year. The MN Symphony Orchestra performs in Orchestra Hall. The Minneapolis Civic Orchestra, Cricket Theater, Children's Theater Co., MN Opera and Theater in the Round Players also give performances. Minneapolis museums and galleries include the Science Museum, Hennepin Co. Historical Society and Museum, Bell Museum of Natural History, Walker Art Institute, the Minneapolis Institute of Arts—with over 60,000 works, including sculpture, photography, paintings, drawings and prints—and the Swedish Institute, which houses a valuable art collection of pioneer items, Swedish glass and ceramics, textiles and furniture.

LANDMARKS AND SIGHTSEEING SPOTS. The Investors Diversified Services (IDS) Center, comprised of four buildings, contains the tallest structure in Minneapolis, a 57-story tower with an observation platform. The large, glass-enclosed Crystal Court is also a popular spot. Main Street, U.S.A., a miniature replica of an early 1900 street, is made up of II buildings containing over 1,500 miniatures from around the world. Historical Ft. Snelling was established in 1820 as one of the first American military posts W of the MS River. The colorfully lit fountains of Gateway Center, near Hennepin and Washington avenues, may be viewed from dusk to midnight.

MOBILE
ALABAMA

CITY LOCATION-SIZE-EXTENT. Mobile, the seat of Mobile Co., encompasses 141.9 sq. mi. on the W shore of Mobile Bay in SW AL, approx. 30 mi. N of the Gulf of Mexico, at 30°41' N lat. and 88°15' W long. The greater met. area extends into the counties of Baldwin to the E, Washington to the N and Jackson, MS, to the W.

TOPOGRAPHY. The topography of Mobile, which is situated in the Mobile River Delta of the E Gulf Coastal plains, is characterized by low, swampy terrain. Many bayous run through the rolling grasslands, while the area immediately surrounding the bay is covered by sandy beaches. The elev. ranges from 7' to 217', with a mean elev. of 211'.

CLIMATE. The climate of Mobile is marine, characterized by the moderating influences of the Gulf of Mexico. The avg. annual temp. of 67.5°F ranges between monthly means of 51.7°F in Jan. and 81.8°F in July. Extremes in temps. are rare. The 67.5" avg. annual rainfall, among the highest in the US, is fairly evenly distributed throughout the year. The RH ranges from 50% to 90%. The growing season avgs. 274 days. Mobile lies in the CSTZ and observes DST.

FLORA AND FAUNA. Animals native to Mobile include the opossum, racoon and skunk. Common birds include the gallinule, kite, heron, egret, quail, dove and swallow. Sirens, waterdogs, alligators, several species of frogs and salamanders, as well as the venomous copperhead, cottonmouth, coral snake and rattlesnake, are found in the area. Typical trees include the pine, oak, pecan and palm. Smaller plants include the azalea, camellia and marsh grass.

POPULATION. According to the US census, the pop. of Mobile in 1970 was 190,026. In 1978, it was estimated that it had increased to 203,000.

ETHNIC GROUPS. In 1978, the ethnic distribution of Mobile was 64.3% Caucasian, 35.4% Black, 0.9% Hispanic and 0.23% other. (A percentage of the Hispanic total is included in the Caucasian total.)

TRANSPORTATION. Interstate hwys. 10 and 65, US hwys. 31, 43, 45, 90 and 98 and state hwys. 5, 12, 16, 42 and 163 provide major motor access to Mobile. *Railroads* serving the city include IL Central Gulf, St. Louis-San Francisco , the Family Line System (SCL/L&N) and S Railway. *Airlines* serving Mobile Municipal Airport include NA, EA and SO. Air service is also available at Brookley Field in downtown Mobile. *Bus lines* serving the city include Greyhound, Colonial, Trailways, Gulf Transport and the local Mobile Transit Authority. Navigable river systems connecting the city to major market areas are the Tombigbee-Warrior, AL Coosa, Chattahoochee and TN rivers.

COMMUNICATIONS. Broadcasting communications, and print media originating from Mobile are: *AM radio stations* WKRG 710 (CBS, MOR); WMOB 840 (ABC/E, MOR, Talk); WGOK 900 (Mut Rlk); WLIQ 1360 (MBS, C&W); WUNI 1410 (NBC, C&W); WABB 1480 (ABC/C, Top 40) and WMOO 1550 (Indep., Gospel); *FM radio stations* WHIL 91.3 (Indep., Divers.); WBLX 92.9 (Natl. Blk.); WKSJ 94.9 (Indep., C&W); WLPR 96.1 (Indep., MOR); WABB 97.5 (Indep., Contemp. Rock) and WKRG 99.9 (ABC/FM, MOR); *television stations* WEAR Ch. 3 (ABC); WKRG Ch. 5 (CBS); WALA Ch. 10 (NBC); WEIQ Ch. 42 (PBS) and cable; *press.* two major dailies serve in the city, the evening *Mobile*, and the morning *Register*; other publications include *Mobile Beacon, AL Citizen, Chickasaw News Herald, S Shopper, Mobile City News, Elevator World* and *The Masonic Monthly*.

HISTORY. In 1702, the French Canadian explorer Jean Baptiste Le Moyne built a trading post some 27 mi. N of present-day Mobile. He named it Ft. Louis de La Mobile, after native Americans of the Maubila tribe, part of the

Municipal Auditorium, Mobile, Alabama

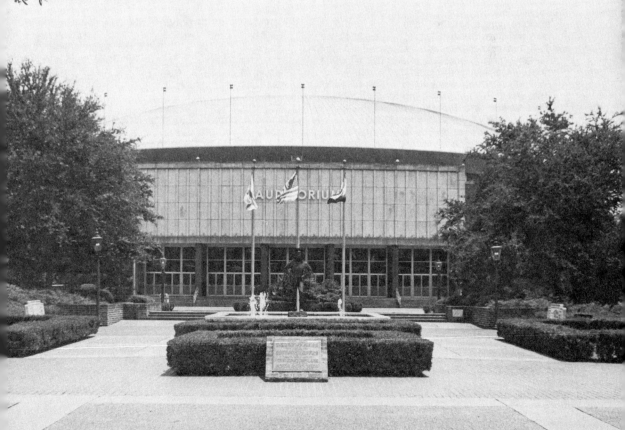

Choctaw Nation, who lived in the area. Mobile became the capital of French Louisiana, and was moved to the present site in 1711, after floods forced the evacuation of the original settlement. In 1763, the French ceded Mobile to Great Britain. Spain later took possession in 1780. After the Louisiana Purchase (1803) Americans began settling in the area although it was under Spanish control. Gen. James Wilkinson seized the city for the US in 1813 and Gen. Andrew Jackson made Mobile his headquarters when campaigning against the British. Municipal govt. was organized in Mobile for the first time in its 150-year history when elections were held in 1814 to choose a mayor and city council. The city was incorporated that year. Mobile remained an important port and cotton center during the early 1800s. When Alabama joined the Confederacy in 1861, Mobile's importance as a port city prompted the Union Army to blockade it. The city fell to the Union Army after the Battle of Mobile. Reconstruction was slow as Mobile's economy gradually strengthened. During WW I and II, the city's port and shipbuilding facilities were utilized for the nation's war effort. Mobile has grown steadily since WW II, as new industries have moved to the area.

GOVERNMENT. Mobile has a commission form of govt., consisting of three commissioners elected at large to four-year terms. Each commissioner serves a 16-month, rotating term as mayor, presiding over meetings. All have an equal vote.

ECONOMY AND INDUSTRY. Manufacturing, state and fed. govt., and shipping are the three largest sectors of Mobile's economy. The city has over 100 factories and the chief industry is the production of lumber and wood pulp for paper, followed by shipbuilding and repairing, cement, aluminum, clothing production, steel fabricating and metal stamping, iron and steel and oil refining. Products include bakery products, chemicals, furniture, pumps, batteries, rayon fibers, roofing, seafood and goods related to the aviation industry. In 1978, avg. per capita income was estimated at $5,444. The labor force in June, 1979, totaled 188,100, while the rate of unemployment was 9.2%.

BANKING. In 1978, total deposits for the six banks headquartered in Mobile were $1,268,816,000, while assets were $1,437,347,000. Banks include Merchants' Natl., First Natl., American Natl. Bank & Trust, Commercial Guaranty, Central and Commonwealth Natl.

HOSPITALS. There are six gen. hosps. and one private mental health hosp. in Mobile including Doctor's, Mobile Infirmary, Providence, Spring Hill, Southland and the U of S AL Medical Center. Searcy Hospital and the Albert P. Brewer Center are also located in Mobile.

EDUCATION. The state-supported U of S AL, located in Mobile, awards

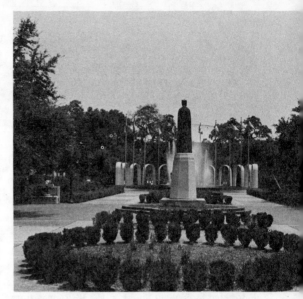

Spanish Plaza, Mobile, Alabama

bachelor, master and doctorate degrees. In 1978, it enrolled approx. 7,000. Spring Hill Col., the oldest institution of higher learning in AL, was founded in 1830, and has been operated by the Society of Jesus since 1847. It became coed in 1952 and, in 1954, it accepted black students. Awarding bachelor degrees, it enrolled approx. 900 in 1978. Other institutions include Mobile Col., S. D. Bishop State Jr. Col., AL Christian Col., Carver State Technical Trade School and SW State Technical School. There are approx. 88 schools in the Mobile Co. School System, enrolling approx. 67,000. More than 16,000 are enrolled in 70 private and parochial schools. Libs. include the Mobile Public Lib. and its five branches.

ENTERTAINMENT. The Entertainer provides dinner theater entertainment in Mobile. Annually, the city hosts the Azalea Trail and America's Jr. Miss Pageant. Mobile has one pro football team, the Mobile Generals. Spring Hill Col. and the U of S AL Jaguars compete in intercollegiate sports. The city is the site of football's nationally-televised, annual Sr. Bowl Game in Jan. Each summer, Pacer and Late Model racing is held at Mobile's Intl. Raceway.

ACCOMMODATIONS. There are many hotels and motels in Mobile including the Sheraton, Hilton, Quality, Ramada, Holiday, Malaya, Day's and Rodeway inns, Howard Johnson's, La Quinta and TraveLodge.

FACILITIES. There are 58 parks in Mobile including the 700-acre Langan (including its 40-acre lake) and Chickasabouge Lake. The park system offers playgrounds, swimming pools, tennis courts, ballfields, basketball courts and fishing. Nearby is Bellingrath Gardens, featuring 75 acres of gardens, which include the camellia, azelea, mt. laurel and dogwood. Public golf courses are located at local golf clubs and Pritchard Municipal Golf Course, while public tennis courts can be found at Mobile and Lyon's Park tennis centers. Greyhound races are held at the Mobile Greyhound Park. Beaches are available at Dauphin Island and Fairhope Municipal Pier.

CULTURAL ACTIVITIES. The Allied Arts Council coordinates programs in performing, visual and graphic arts, including live comm. theater, opera, ballet and symphonic concerts. The Mobile Symphony Pop Orchestra also presents musical performances. Works of art are displayed at the Municipal Art Gallery and Museum and the Patio Art Gallery.

LANDMARKS AND SIGHTSEEING SPOTS. Mobile has four historic districts—Church Street, Tonti Square, Oakleigh and Spring Hill, all listed on the Natl. Register of Historic Places. Together, these historic districts protect some 250 buildings of various architectural designs. The Ft. Conde-Charlotte House, completed in 1735, and restored in 1975-1976, was successively occupied by French, Spanish, British and American troops. The USS *Alabama* stands as a memorial to AL war veterans.

Downtown Mobile, Alabama

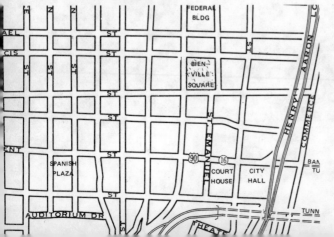

MONTGOMERY
ALABAMA

CITY LOCATION-SIZE-EXTENT. Montgomery, the capital of the state and seat of Montgomery Co.,encompasses 50 sq. mi. in S central AL at 32°18' N lat. and 86°24' W long. Situated on the AL River, the city is 85 mi. SE of Birmingham. The greater met. area extends NE into Elmore Co. and NW into Autanga Co.

TOPOGRAPHY. The terrain of Montgomery, which is located on the E Gulf coastal plain is characterized by gently rolling hills extending SW to the fertile Black Belt area. The terrain to the NE and E is flat as well as gently sloping. The mean elev. is 195'.

CLIMATE. Extremes of either cold or hot temps. in Montgomery are rare. Avg. monthly temps. range from 48.5°F in Jan. to 81.6°F in July, with an annual avg. of 65.6°F. During Dec., Jan. and Feb., there are frequent shifts between mild, moist air from the Gulf of Mexico and dry, cool continental air. Most of the avg. annual rainfall of 50.94" falls during late winter and early spring. The RH ranges from 52% to 90%. Snowfall is negligible. The avg. growing season is 253 days. Montgomery lies in the CSTZ and observes DST.

FLORA AND FAUNA. Animals native to Montgomery include the beaver, whitetail deer, opossum and raccoon. Typical birds are the egret, flicker, cardinal, Carolina wren and blue jay. Bullfrogs, red-eared turtles, watersnakes and toads inhabit the area, as do the venomous copperhead, rattlesnake, water moccasin and coral snake. Common trees are the magnolia, ash, oak, elm and pine. Smaller plants include the hagberry, maclura, mock orange shrub, camellia, honeysuckle, orchid, bluecurl and meadow beauty.

POPULATION. According to the US census, the pop. of Montgomery in 1970 was 167,790. In 1978, it was estimated that it had increased to 195,704.

ETHNIC GROUPS. In 1978, the ethnic distribution of Montgomery was approx. 56% Caucasian, 34.1% Black, .04% Hispanic and 9.86% other.

TRANSPORTATION. Interstate hwys. 65 and 85 and US hwys. 31, 231, 331, 80 and 82 provide major motor access to Montgomery. *Railroads* serving the city include L&N, Seaboard, AMTRAK, Western Railway and Central of GA. *Airlines* serving Dannelly Field include DL, EA and RP. *Bus lines* include Greyhound, Trailways and the local Montgomery Area Transit System.

COMMUNICATIONS. Communications, broadcasting and print media originating in Montgomery are: *AM radio stations* WBAM 740 (Indep., Mod. C&W); WMGY 800 (ABC/I, Relig.); WLSQ 950 (MBS, Top 40), WQTY 1000 (CBS, MOR, Talk); WCOV 1170 (NBC, MOR); WHHY 1440 (ABC/C, Top 40) and WXVI 1600 (Mut., Blk.); *FM radio stations* WLWI 92.3 (ABC/FM, MOR); WFMI 98.9 (Indep., Btfl. Mus.); WHHY 101.9 (Indep., MOR) and WREZ 103.3 (Indep., Var.); *television stations* WSFA Ch. 12 (NBC); WCOV Ch. 20 (CBS); WAIQ Ch. 26 (PBS); WKAB Ch. 32 (ABC) and cable; *press*: two major daily newspapers serve the city, the *Advertiser*, a morning publication, and the *Journal*, issued evenings; other publications include the *Independent, Times, Spectra, AL Conservation, AL Forests, AL News Magazine, AL Trucker, AREA Magazine, Loggin' Times, Neighbors, Pulpwood Production and Timber Harvesting* and *Southern Outdoors.*

HISTORY. Native Americans of the Alibamu and Creek tribes inhabited the site of present-day Montgomery when Spanish explorer Hernando de Soto camped in the area in 1540 and again in 1560. In 1715, Sieur de Bienville, a Frenchman, led an expedition up the AL River and built Ft. Toulouse in the area. In 1817, Andrew Dexter of MA established the town of New Philadelphia

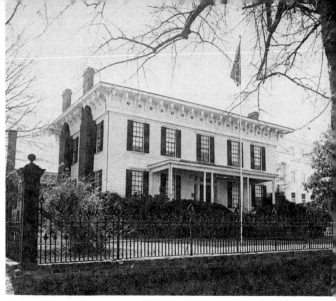

First White House of the Confederacy, Montgomery, Alabama

near what was to become Montgomery. In 1819, the towns of New Philadelphia and nearby AL Town, settled by Gen. John Scott of GA in 1817 and renamed E AL in 1818, merged and formed a new town named Montgomery in honor of Revolutionary War hero Brig. Gen. Richard Montgomery. Incorporated as a city in 1837, it became the capital of AL in 1847. On Feb. 8, 1861, the Confederate States of America was established in the city, which served as the first Confederate capital until May 21 of the same year when Richmond, VA became the capital. Jefferson Davis was inaugurated Pres. of the Confederacy in the city's Capitol, and Montgomery became known as "The Cradle of the Confederacy". The city was an important cotton market prior to the Civil War, during which it suffered destruction and looting while under siege by fed. troops. By the 1880s Montgomery had once again become a thriving cotton center, and its pop. grew steadily. The first cotton mill in AL was established in the city in 1881, and the first electric streetcar in the world began operating there on Apr. 7, 1885. The city also became a center of agricultural trade in the late 1800s, with the largest livestock market and dairy industry in the SE. In the early 1900s, the Wright Brothers' Flight School was established at the present site of Maxwell AFB. In 1956, a fed. court ordered the city to desegregate its public bus system as a result of boycotts led by civil rights leader Martin Luther King, Jr. in 1955 and 1956. Prior to the order, Blacks had been required by law to sit in the rear. In Mar., 1965, King led a five day march from

State Capitol, Montgomery, Alabama

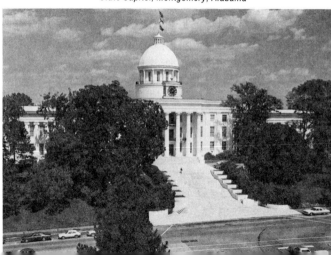

Selma to Montgomery to protest voter registration discrimination, an action which influenced the passage of the Voting Rights Act—enfranchising thousands of AL blacks—by Congress in Aug. of that year.

GOVERNMENT. Montgomery has a mayor-council form of govt. The nine council members, elected by district, select one member to serve as pres. The mayor, not a member of council, is elected at large. All serve four-year terms.

ECONOMY AND INDUSTRY. Major manufactured products in Montgomery include machinery, clothing, glass products, food products and lumber and wood products. The city is also a major S agricultural center. In addition, govt. and trade each employ about 20% of the work force. In June, 1979, the total labor force of the

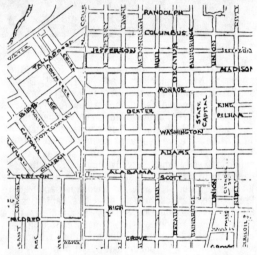

Downtown Mobile, Alabama

greater met. area was approx. 122,000, while the rate of unemployment was 6.7%. In 1978, avg. per capita income was $6,544. Gunther and Maxwell AF bases are major govt. employers.

BANKING. In 1978, total deposits for the six banks headquartered in Montgomery were approx. $940,684,000, while total assets were $1,140,646,000. Banks include First AL, Union Bank and Trust, AL Natl., Central, Exchange Natl. and Southern.

HOSPITALS. There are five gen. hosps. in Montgomery, St. Margaret's, Fairview, Jackson, Baptist Medical Center and Southland. Other facilities include the V.A. hospital, the Air Force Hosp., and the Mental Health Center.

EDUCATION. AL State U at Montgomery, once called the AL Colored People's U, opened in 1887 and first offered grad. degrees in 1940. The U, which offers courses leading to bachelor and master degrees, enrolled more than 4,700 students in 1978. Auburn U at Montgomery, a state-controlled U founded as a private school in 1866 by the Methodist Church, offers bachelor and master degrees and enrolled more than 4,400 students in 1978. Comm. colleges include Trenholm State Technical and John M. Patterson State Technical. Other institutions include Huntingdon Col., Jones Law Institute, Troy State U at Montgomery and AL Christian Col. There are 52 schools with more than 36,200 students in the public school system. Libs. in the city include Montgomery Public Lib. and its five branches, the State Dept. of Archives and History and the AL Supreme Court Lib. A regional library is available for the blind and physically handicapped.

ENTERTAINMENT. Montgomery annually hosts the Festival in the Park, the Blue Grass Festival, Jubilee, the S AL State Fair and the SE Livestock Show and Rodeo. The Lamplighter offers dinner theater. Sports entertainment is offered by the Rebels, a baseball farm club of the Detroit Tigers, which plays in the S League. The AL State U Crimson Tide and the Auburn Tigers participate in collegiate football. The annual Blue-Gray

football classic, played between college seniors from the N and S, is held in Dec. at the Crampton Bowl. Stock car racing, rodeos, horse shows and motocross are other spectator sports activities in the area.

ACCOMMODATIONS. There are several hotels and motels in Montgomery, including the Days, Sheraton, Holiday and Ramada inns, Governor's House, Highway Host and Howard Johnson's.

FACILITIES. There are 38 parks, 25 playgrounds and 19 comm. centers in Montgomery. Lagoon Park is the largest, while a children's zoo is located at Chisholm Park. There are two public golf courses and several tennis courts in the city. Hunting, fishing, water sports and camping facilities are available at 11 area lakes.

CULTURAL ACTIVITIES. The Montgomery Museum of Fine Arts, the oldest in AL, features permanent collections and art shows with historical displays. The 1850 Ordeman-Shaw House and complex, a restored Italianate town house and its servant quarters, features an art collection. The Tumbling Water Museum of Flags features a natl. commemorative collection among its exhibits, while the Archives and History Building, houses a museum depicting life in AL from the time of the native Americans to the present. A municipal orchestra—which presents a comm. concert series—the Montgomery Civic Ballet and the Montgomery Little Theatre— which performs in the 19th-century Junius Bragg Smith Theatre—provide cultural entertainment. Each of the colleges and universities in Montgomery, as well as Maxwell and Gunter AF bases, offer lectures, concerts and plays. The First White House of the Confederacy, a white frame house built in 1852 which served as the presidential home of the Jefferson Davis in the first months of the Confederacy, has been preserved as a Confederate museum.

LANDMARKS AND SIGHTSEEING SPOTS. The AL state capitol building, which closely resembles the natl. capitol in its Greek Revival architectural style, is one of Montgomery's most impressive landmarks. It is located on Capitol Hill, also known as Goat Hill. A self-suspended, double spiral staircase winds from the first to the third floors, and inside the 97' dome is a 13' high mural depicting some of the state's historic events. Other historic points are Ft. Toulouse, the turn of the century Gov.'s Mansion, and the 1855 St. John's Episcopal Church, the oldest Episcopal church in the city. Jasmine Hill, one of the S's most famous gardens, contains camellias, azaleas, cherry trees, pools and fountains. The W.A. Gayle Space Transit Planetarium, the largest in AL and jointly operated by Troy State U and the City of Montgomery, presents a program simulating space travel. The Gen. Richard Montgomery Riverboat, a replica of an original sternwheeler, is docked at Riverfront Park and regularly conducts cruises on the AL River. Other Montgomery landmarks are Oakwood Cemetery, the city's oldest (donated to Montgomery by city founders Andrew Dexter and John Scott); Court Square McMonnie Fountain, designed by the famous sculptor and known as "The Big Basin", and the Curb Market, offering fresh fruits and vegetables and homemade jams and jellies; the AL War Memorial and the Governor's Mansion.

NASHVILLE
TENNESSEE

CITY LOCATION-SIZE-EXTENT. Nashville, the capital of TN, is on the Cumberland River in N central TN at 36°7' N lat. and 86°41' W long. The city covers 532 sq. mi. which includes all of Davidson Co. The greater met. area extends into surrounding counties, Williamson to the S, Cheatham to the W, Robertson to the N, Wilson to the E and Sumner to the NE.

TOPOGRAPHY. Nashville has a varied topography combining the flatlands of W TN with the mts. of the state's E section. The terrain is generally hilly, featuring a number of creeks and valleys. There are several bodies of water nearby, including Old Hickory Lake, Percy Priest Lake and the Cumberland River, all of which are

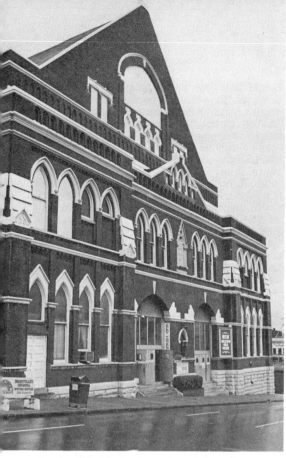

Former Home of 'Grand Ole Opry' Nashville, Tenn.

part of the Cheatham Reservoir. The mean elev. is 590'.

CLIMATE. Nashville's climate is moderate continental. The avg. annual temp. of 60°F varies from a Jan. mean of 39°F to a July mean of 79°F. Most of the avg. annual rainfall of 47" occurs during the winter and early spring. The avg. annual snowfall is 11.2". The RH ranges from 51% to 92% and the avg. growing season lasts 211 days. Nashville is in the CSTZ and observes DST.

FLORA AND FAUNA. Animals native to Nashville include the whitetail deer, raccoon and opossum. Common birds include the quail, night heron, robin, bluejay, thrasher, oriole and catbird. Several species of frogs, turtles and snakes, including the venomous rattlesnake, copperhead and cottonmouth, are found here. Trees include the oak, red bud and dogwood. There is an abundance of wildflowers, including the iris, the state flower.

POPULATION. According to the US census, the pop. of Nashville in 1970 was 444,489. In 1978, it was estimated that it had increased to 451,000.

ETHNIC GROUPS. In 1978, the ethnic distribution of Nashville was 80.1% Caucasian, 19.6% Black and 0.6% Hispanic (a percentage of the Hispanic total is also included in the Caucasian total).

TRANSPORTATION. Interstate hwys. 24, 40, 65 and 265, US hwys. 31, 41, 70 and 431 and state hwys. 100 and 155 provide major motor access to Nashville. *Railroads* include Louisville & Nashville and the IL Central. *Airlines* serving the Met. Nashville Municipal Airport-Berry Field include PI, AA, DL, SO, OZ, BN, TW, AL and EA. The privately operated Cornelia Fort Airport is also available to smaller aircraft. *Bus lines* include Greyhound, Trailways, Trailblazers and the city-owned Metro Transit Authority. Barge lines operate through ports on the Cumberland River.

COMMUNICATIONS. Communications, broadcasting and print media serving Nashville are: *AM radio stations* WSM 650 (NBC, MOR); WSIX 980 (ABC/I, MOR); WAMB 1190 (MBS, Big Band); WKDA 1240 (CBS, C&W); WMAK 1300 (Indep., Contemp.); WNAH 1360 (Indep., Relig.); WLAC 1510 (Indep., Top 40) and WWGM 1560 (Indep., Contemp., Relig.); *FM radio stations* WNAZ 88.9 (ABC/I, Top 40); WPLN 90.3 (NPR, Var.); WRVU 91.1 (Indep., Progsv.); WZEZ 92.9 (Indep., Btfl. Mus.); WSM 95.5 (ABC/FM, Var.); WSIX 97.9 (ABC/E, Metro., Ctry.); WKDF 103.3 (Indep., AOR) and WLAC 10549 (Indep., MOR); *television stations* WGNE Ch. 2 (ABC); WSM Ch. 4 (NBC); WTVE Ch. 5 (CBS); WDCN Ch. 8 (PBS); WZTV Ch. 17 (Indep.) and cable; *press*: two major dailies serve the city area are the evening *Banner*, and the morning *Tennessean*; other publications include the weekly *Suburban News, Donelson Diary, Madison News, Goodlettsville Gazette, Westview, Gospel Advocate, Record* and *TN Register*, the monthly *Kindergartner, Market Bulletin, Music City News, Nashville, Outreach, S Beef Producer, The Sunbelt Dairyman, TN Farmer, TN Magazine* and *TN Teacher*.

HISTORY. Nashville was founded in 1779 by a group of settlers from NC led by James Robertson and John Donelson. They named the settlement Ft. Nashborough in honor of Gen. Francis Nash, a Revolutionary War hero. The area served as hunting grounds for native Americans of the Cherokee, Chickasaw and Shawnee tribes before Ft. Nashborough was built. The first white men to come to the area were French fur traders in the 1710s and later the "long hunters" (so named because they hunted for very long periods of time). In April, 1780, a week after the arrival of the rest of the settlers, they entered into the Cumberland Pact to provide a civic government for themselves. In April, 1781, Ft. Nashborough survived a Cherokee attack. In time, the comm. began to grow. In 1784, its name was changed from Ft. Nashborough to Nashville. Among some of the early Nashville citizens who influenced state, natl. and intl. affairs were Andrew Jackson, seventh Pres. of the US, John Overton, Judge of the Supreme Court of TN, and William Walker, who went on to become the Pres. of Nicaragua—the only American ever to become the pres. of a foreign country. In 1796, TN became the 16th state. Nashville, then a trading center, was one of several temporary capitals of TN. Nashville was chartered as a city in 1806. The first steamboat arrived in the city in 1818. Nashville was selected as the permanent state capital in 1843. By 1860, Nashville was a prosperous city. During the Civil War, Nashville was occupied by Union troops because of its location on the river and because of its RR links with Louisville, Chattanooga and Atlanta. The war left Nashville in shambles. A slow period of growth began during the Reconstruction. This was marked in Nash-

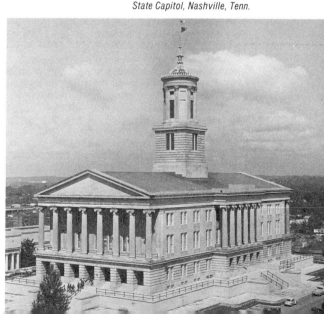

State Capitol, Nashville, Tenn.

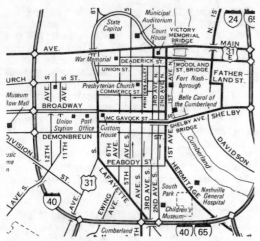

Nashville, Tennessee

ville by expansion of higher education. Fisk U opened in 1866, Vanderbilt U in 1873 and Meharry Medical Col. in 1876. Nashville became an important distribution and wholesale center, in addition to being a printing center. Nashville marked its centenary with an exposition in 1880 that attracted people from all over the country. By 1900, the city's pop. had grown to 80,865. The Old Hickory Powder Plant was built during WW I to manufacture smokeless gunpowder. Nashville is today known as the home of country music. It is also a leading center of higher education, business and manufacturing.

GOVERNMENT. Nashville has a mayor-council form of govt. with the vice mayor presiding over the 40-member council. The council members are elected to four-year terms; six are elected at large and 35 by district. The mayor is elected at large to a four-year term and is not a member of the council.

ECONOMY AND INDUSTRY. There are approx. 650 industrial plants in Nashville. The most important industry is the production of commercial, industrial and agricultural chemicals. Printing and publishing provide major employment. Several religious denominations have publishing headquarters here and it is also a center for publication of school annuals, national magazines and telephone directories. Nashville is second only to NYC as a recording center. Music-related industry contributes an estimated $100 million to its economy annually. Other major areas of employment are education and health care, insurance and banking, and food and clothing production. Seven insurance companies have home offices here with total assets over $3 billion. The govt. is also a major employer. Fifty businesses in the area employ more than 500 persons. The Nashville-Davidson area had a labor force of 406,500 in June, 1979, and an unemployment rate of 4.7%. Avg. hourly earnings for production workers in manufacturing were $5.89. Median per capita income in 1975 was $4,887.

BANKING. There are seven major banks and six savings and loan assns. in Nashville. In 1978, total deposits for the seven banks headquartered in the city were $3,485,147,000, while assets were $4,118,332,000. Banks include Commerce Union, First American Natl., Third Natl. in Nashville, First TN Bank of Nashville and Citizens Savings Bank and Trust Co.

HOSPITALS. Vanderbilt and Meharry Medical Cols. in Nashville offer grad. medical training. Both have major hosps. Vanderbilt and George Hubbard. Other hosps.—include St. Thomas Baptist, Memorial Nashville Gen. and Bordeaux, Madison and Donelson.

EDUCATION. Vanderbilt, an independent private U founded in 1873, by the Methodist Episcopal Church has campuses in France and Spain, and offers grad., professional and undergrad. degrees. In 1978, enrollment was 7,269. Fisk U, founded in 1866 as a school for students of all races, colors and creeds, offers bachelor and master degrees and, in 1978, enrolled 1,124. TN State U, established in 1912, enrolled 5,362 in 1978. Other teaching institutions include George Peabody Col. for Teachers, the U of TN at Nashville, enrolling 5,685 in 1978; Meharry Medical, Belmont, David Lipscomb, Trevacca Nazarene, John A. Yuxton, Free Will Baptist and Draughton cols.; Aquinas Jr. Col.; the YMCA Night Law School and the American Baptist Theological Seminary. There are approx. 120 elementary and 20 high schools in met. Nashville's pub. school system, and approx. 85,000 students are enrolled. Approx. 40 private and parochial schools supplement the public system. The Public Lib. has 14 branches, the largest being the Joint U Lib. belonging to Vanderbilt and George Peabody.

ENTERTAINMENT. The Barn Dinner Theater offers dining entertainment. Festivals and annual events in Nashville include the TN State Fair in Sept., the Steeplechase in May, the Market Street Festival-Courthouse Day in Oct., the Easter Parade and the Franklin Rodeo. Nashville is the home of the Nashville Sounds, an AA Baseball Club in the SL which led the minor league in attendance in 1978 and 1979. The Vanderbilt U Commodores compete in the SE Conference. The Fisk U Bulldogs and TN State U Tigers both participate in major intercollegiate sports.

ACCOMMODATIONS. Nashville hotels and motels include Opryland, Maxwell House, Hyatt Regency, Radisson, Spence Manor and the Sheraton, Airport Hilton, Airport Rodeway and Vanderbilt Holiday inns.

FACILITIES. Nashville's park system consists of 67 parks covering 6,613 acres. The major parks include Centennial, Percy and Edwin Warner, Cedar Hill and Sevier. Children and adults will enjoy the Ellington Agriculture Center and the nearby TN Game Farm Zoo. There are four private and several public golf courses, including McCabe, Shelby Park, Rhodes, Riverview and Two Rivers Park. public tennis courts can be found at Tennis Unlimited. Other facilities are available to the public at Hermitage Landing Recreation area.

CULTURAL ACTIVITIES. Best known for its country and W music heritage, Nashville is the site of the Grand Ole Opry, where leading musicians perform. Orchestras in the city include the Nashville Symphony Orchestra, which performs in the Municipal Auditorium. Live theater is provided year-round by such groups as the Circle Players and the Nashville Children's Theater. The Country Music Hall of Fame & Museum and the Country Music Wax Museum offer exhibits on country music. Other museums in the city are the TN State Historical Museum, Creekwood and the Peabody Art Museum.

LANDMARKS AND SIGHTSEEING SPOTS. Among Nashville's historic homes are the Hermitage (Andrew Jackson's home), Traveller's Rest (the home of Judge John Overton) and Belle Meade Mansion. There is a statue of Gen. Sam Houston (TX War of Independence hero) in front of the capitol, and, on the capitol grounds is buried James K. Polk, the 11th Pres. of the US. A reconstructed version of Ft. Nashborough is in downtown Nashville. Many early settlers, including James Robertson and Capt. William Driver who named the US flag "Old Glory", are buried in the Old Cemetery on Fourth Avenue S. An exact replica of the Parthenon stands in Nashville's Centennial Park.

The "Hermitage" Home of Pres. Jackson, Nashville, Tenn.

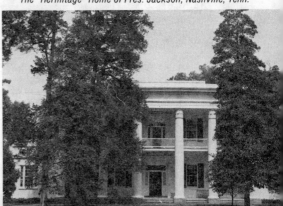

NEWARK
NEW JERSEY

CITY LOCATION-SIZE-EXTENT. Newark, the seat of Essex Co., encompasses 24 sq. mi. in NE NJ, across the Hudson and Newark bays from NYC, at the mouth of the Passaic River, at 40°42' N lat. and 74°10' W long. The greater met. area extends E into Hudson Co. and overlaps the met. area of Elizabeth to the S.

TOPOGRAPHY. The terrain of Newark, which is situated in the Piedmont region, varies from flat to marshy areas, with some high ridges running in a S-SW to N-NE direction. The mean elev. is 146'.

CLIMATE. The climate of Newark is moderate, characterized by the drying effect of downslope westerlies and the ocean influence carried by E winds. The avg. annual temp. of 53.8°F ranges from monthly means of 31.5°F in Jan. to 76.3°F in July. The 42" avg. annual rainfall is fairly evenly distributed throughout the year. Most of the 28" avg. annual snowfall occurs between Dec. and Feb. The RH ranges from 45% to 78%. The avg. growing season is 200 days. Newark lies in the ESTZ and observes DST.

FLORA AND FAUNA. Animals native to Newark include the squirrel, and opossum. Common birds are the blue jay, cardinal, goldfinch, crow and E gold finch (the state bird). Salamanders, frogs, newts and garter snakes, are found in the area. Typical trees are the red oak (the state tree), dogwood, maple, elm and chestnut. Smaller plants include the violet, viburnum, white cockle and purple violet (the state flower).

POPULATION. According to the US census, the pop. of Newark in 1970 was 381,930. In 1978, it was estimated that it had decreased to 320,000.

ETHNIC GROUPS. In 1978, the ethnic distribution of Newark was approx. 44.7% Caucasian, 54.3% Black and 7.2% Hispanic. (A percentage of the Hispanic total is also included in the Caucasian total.)

TRANSPORTATION. Interstate hwys. 78, 80, 95 and 280, US hwys. 1, 9 and 22 and state hwys. 10, 21, 23, 27 and 124 provide major motor access to Newark. *Railroads* serving the city include AMTRAK, ConRail and PATH. Major *airlines* serving Newark Intl. Airport are AA, US Air, BN, DL, EA, NA, NW, NY, PI, TW and UA. *Bus lines* serving the city include Trailways, Greyhound, Irving, Lincoln, Martz and Transport of NJ.

COMMUNICATIONS. Communications, broadcasting and print media originating from Newark are: *AM radio stations* WVNJ 620 (ABC/E, Btfl. Mus.) and WNJR 1430 (Mut. Blk, Rock); *FM radio stations* WBGO 88.3 (Indep., Educ.); WFME 94.7 (Indep., Relig.); WVNJ 100.3 (Indep., Btfl. Mus.) and WHBI 105.9 (Indep., Blk.); *television stations* WNJU Ch. 47 (Indep.) and WWHT Ch. 68 (Indep.) *press:* one major daily serves the city, the *Star Ledger*; other publications include *Information, NJ Afro-American, Italian Tribune, NJ Law Journal* and *Rutgers-Newark Observer.*

HISTORY. The early inhabitants of the present-day Newark area were native Americans of the Delaware tribe. The city was founded in 1666 by 30 Puritan families from the CT colony and named after Newark-on-Trent, England. The city's growth began with iron-making, in the middle of the 18th century, when area mines began operation, while toward the end of the century, the tanning industry began. During the early 1800s the manufacturers of shoes and other leather goods were a major employer. Patent leather was invented in Newark during the early 1800s. In 1831, the Morris Canal linked the city with PA's Lehigh Valley coal mining area. Newark was incorporated in 1836. During the latter half of the 19th century, large numbers of European immigrants arrived to work in industry. During this period the chemical industry was begun. In

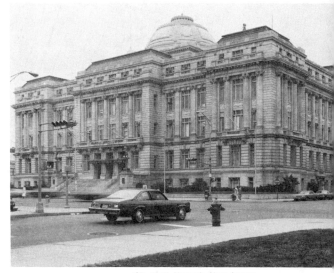

City Hall, Newark, New Jersey

1915, the Port of Newark was opened. The following decade brought industrial expansion, particularly in chemicals. The Great Depression had a tremendous impact on Newark, as hundreds of factories were closed and areas of the city deteriorated. WW II saw an influx of S blacks to work in defense plants increasing the pop. in the poor areas of the city. In the decade following the war, large numbers of more affluent people moved out of the city which, by the 1960s, did not have adequate funds to deal with its problems. A racial riot in 1967 caused 23 deaths. Following the riots, investigators found widespread dishonesty in city govt. and, in 1970, a black mayor, Kenneth A. Gibson, was elected. During the 1970s, Newark leaders have worked to solve the city's employment problems and improve its housing.

GOVERNMENT. Newark has a mayor-council form of govt. The nine council members are elected to four-year terms—four at large and five by district. The mayor, not a voting member of council, serves four years

ECONOMY AND INDUSTRY. Newark is headquarters for Prudential and Mutual Benefit Life Insurance Cos. The diverse industries of Newark produce paint, varnish, electrical machinery, liquors, chemicals, leather products, apparel, motor parts, radio parts, perfume and cosmetics. Meat packing is an important industry. The 1979 labor force for the met. area totaled 977,300, while the rate of unemployment was 6.9%.

BANKING. In 1978, total deposits for the nine banks headquartered in Newark were $6,249,931,000, while total assets were $7,473,036,000. Banks include Howard Savings, Midlantic Natl., US Savings and First Natl.

HOSPITALS. There are six hosps. in Newark, including St. James, St. Michael's, Columbus, Newark Beth Israel, Col. of Med. and Dentistry of NJ and the United Hosp., which includes Children's of Newark, Hosp. for Crippled Children & Adults, Newark Eye and Ear Infimary (Presbyterian); United Hosp. Medical Center and United Hosp. Orthopedic.

EDUCATION. The publicly-supported Col. of Medicine and Dentistry of NJ at Newark is coed and awards professional degrees in medicine and dentistry, as well as the doctorate in biomedical science. The 1978 enrollment was more than 1,300. Rutgers, the State U of NJ-Newark Campus, awards associate, bachelor's, master's and doctoral degrees and includes the Col. of Nursing. The Newark Col. of Arts and Sciences, incorporated into Rutgers U in 1946, offers grad. as well as undergrad. instruction. In 1978,

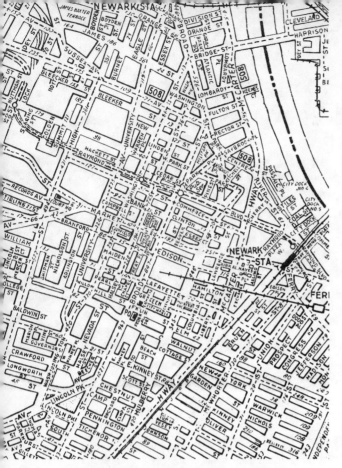

Downtown Newark, New Jersey

the campus enrolled approx. 10,000. Other institutions include the Seton Hall U Law Sch., NJ Institute of Technology, Essex Co. Col., Essex Col. of Business, and Lyons Institute. There are approx. 80 public schools, with an enrollment of approx. 61,400. The Newark Public Lib. includes a main lib. and 10 branches.

ENTERTAINMENT. The Cherry Blossom Display is held each Apr. in Newark. Annual neighborhood and ethnic parades and festivals are held in the summer. Rutgers U Scarlet Raiders and Essex Co. Col. teams participate in intercollegiate sports.

ACCOMMODATIONS. There are many hotels and motels in Newark, including the Hilton Gateway, Holiday Inn and Howard Johnson's.

FACILITIES. There are 10 major parks in Newark. A golf course is located at Weequahic Park, while ice skating facilities can be found at Branch Brook Park.

CULTURAL ACTIVITIES. Performing arts organizations in Newark include the NJ Symphony Orchestra and the NJ State Opera based at Symphony Hall. Rutgers U-Newark sponsors a concert and lecture series, while its Col. of Arts and Sciences presents musical performances. The Newark Museum, established in 1909, features the Schaeffer Collection of ancient glass, Tibetan objects and Indian relics, and includes exhibits of art, science, history and technology. A valuable collection of 10,000 prints is housed at the of Newark Public Lib. NJ portraits, drawings and prints have been collected for preservation by the NJ Historical Society.

LANDMARKS AND SIGHTSEEING SPOTS. The Catholic Cathedral of the Sacred Heart, located in Newark, is comparable in size to Westminster Abbey. Of French Gothic design,it resembles the famed basilica at Rheims. Military Park in downtown Newark features a major outdoor statuary depicting "Wars of America" by Gutzon Borglum of Mt. Rushmore fame. Also at the park is a bust of Pres. Kennedy by Jacques Lipchitz. Other landmarks include Old First Presbyterian dedicated in Jan. 1791 and the Blume House built in 1710 which is still used as a rectory by the House of Prayer Episcopal Church. It was here that Rev. Hannibert Goodwin invented the flexible photographic film in 1887.

NEW BEDFORD
MASSACHUSETTS

CITY LOCATION-SIZE-EXTENT. New Bedford encompasses 18.99 sq. mi. in Bristol Co. in SE MA 33 mi. E of Providence and 56 mi. S of Boston, on the W shore of Buzzards Bay on the Atlantic Ocean, at 41°38' N lat. and 70°56' W long. The met. area extends NE into Plymouth Co. and includes the towns of Acushnet in the NE, Fairhaven in the S, Dartmouth to the W and Freetown to the N.

TOPOGRAPHY. The terrain of New Bedford which is situated in the coastal lowlands region, is generally flat and includes 11.4 mi. of shoreline along the bay. Turner Pond and the Pamanset River are to the W of the city, while the Mattapoisett River is to the NE. The mean elev. is 50'.

CLIMATE. The climate of New Bedford is continental, characterized by mild winters and cool summers produced by the modifying effects of Buzzard's Bay and the Atlantic Ocean. The avg. annual temp. of 50°F ranges from monthly means of 30°F in Jan. and 73°F in July. The avg. annual rainfall of approx. 40" is well distributed throughout the year. More than 50% of the avg. annual snowfall of 39" occurs in Jan. and Feb. The RH ranges from 50% to 88%. New Bedford is in the ESTZ and observes DST.

FLORA AND FAUNA. Animals native to New Bedford include the raccoon, fox and rabbit. Common birds are the chickadee, tern, gull, dove and crow. Salamanders, newts, frogs, garter snakes and venomous timber rattlesnake and copperhead, are also found in the area. Typical trees are the oak, elm, maple, E white swamp cedar and juniper. Smaller plants include the mayflower, dogwood, violet and thistle.

Whaling Museum, New Bedford, Massachusetts

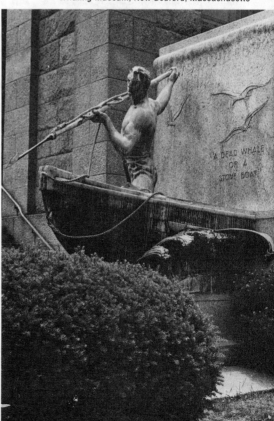

POPULATION. According to the US census, the pop. of New Bedford in 1970 was 101,777. In 1978, it was estimated that it had decreased to 100,075.

ETHNIC GROUPS. In 1978, the ethnic distribution of New Bedford was approx. 86% Caucasian, 3.5% Black, 2% native Americans, 8% Cape Verdeans and 2% Hispanic (a percentage of the Hispanic total is also included in the Caucasian total).

TRANSPORTATION. Interstate hwy. 195, US hwy. 6 and state hwys. 140 and 18 provide major motor access to New Bedford. *Railroad* service to the city is provided by ConRail. *Airlines* serving New Bedford Municipal Airport are NE and NorEast. Seaplane transportation is available through Island Air Service. Ferry service is available from New Bedford to Cuttyhunk and Martha's Vineyard. *Bus lines* serving the city include Brander and the local SE Regional Transit Authority.

COMMUNICATIONS. Communications, broadcasting and print media originating from New Bedford are: *AM radio stations* WNBH 1340 (ABC, MOR) and WBSM 1420 (Indep., MOR, Talk); *FM radio station* WJFD 97.3 (Indep., Portuguese) and WMYS 98.1 (ABC, Adult Contcmp.); *television stations* WTEV Ch. 6 (CBS); *press:* one major newspaper serves the city, the evening *Standard-Times.*

HISTORY. The New Bedford area was first inhabited by native Americans of the Wampanoag tribe. Although Norsemcn had landed in the area in the 11th century and, in 1602, Bartholomew Gasnold had landed on "Smoking Rocks" (the site of present day New Bedford), it was not until 1652 that the region was settled by white men. In that year, 36 dissenters from Plymouth Colony purchased the site of Bedford Village from Massasoit, Chief of the Wampanoags. In 1664, Bedford Village (named in honor of the Duke of Bedford's family) and several other settlements along the river were incorporated as the town of Dartmouth. The early development of Bedford was based on agriculture. However, in the 1760s, whaling became the most important industry and, by 1775, Bedford Village was the second largest whaling port in the world. During the Revolutionary War, Bedford Village served as a refuge and supply center for American privateers and consequently was invaded in 1778 by British forces who destroyed most of the village. Bedford Village, Fairhaven and Acushnet were incorporated as the town of New Bedford in 1787. A temporary setback in its development was caused by the War of 1812, and also by the severance of Fairhaven and Acushnet when they formed the separate town of Fairhaven in the same year. However, by 1830 New Bedford had become the whaling center of the world. Portuguese and other foreign seafaring people were drawn to the area by the whaling industry, which remained important until the discovery of petroleum in PA in 1859. The successful Wamsetta textile mill was started in 1846. The additional growth led to the chartering of New Bedford as a city in 1847. During the Civil War, whalers were used as merchant ships and blockaders and many vessels were sunk by hostile ships. After the war, the decline of the whaling industry proved to be the impetus for the development of textiles, when 26 more mills were built and by the 1880s the city was a leading producer. It led the world in textile production until the Great Depression crippled the industry. Govt. work programs and WW II helped the city hurdle the economic impact of the Depression. Since the war, New Bedford has encouraged the establishment of new industry and further broadened its economic base through the creation of an industrial park. City business has been increased by urban renewal projects and an improved road system. Today, New Bedford has a pop. of 100,345. It serves as a trade and distribution center for SE MA and as an important fishing port; tourism further bolsters the city's economy.

GOVERNMENT. New Bedford has a mayor-council form of govt. The 11 council members are selected in non-partisan elections, six by ward and five at large. The mayor, a member of the council, is elected at large and votes only to break a tie. All serve two-year terms.

ECONOMY AND INDUSTRY. Jobs in manufacturing constitute approx. 55% of the New Bedford total employment with much of it in the textile industry. Other important products include sports equipment, cotton goods, shoes, electrical products, synthetics, rubber and apparel. In the non-manufacturing sector wholesale and retail, the fishing industry and govt. are major employers. Avg. income per family in 1978 was $11,640. The met. labor force in June, 1979, was 87,300, while the unemployment rate was 5.8%.

BANKING. There are eight commercial banks, four savings banks, three cooperative banks and one savings and loan assn. in New Bedford. In 1978, total deposits for the six banks headquartered in the city were $735,341,000, while assets were $847,153,000. Banks include New Bedford Five Cent Savings, First Natl., Baybank Merchants, SE Bank and Trust Co. and Old Stone Banking Co. of Bristol Co.

HOSPITALS. There are several liusps. in New Bedford, including St. Luke's and Union. The New Bedford Area Center for Human Services, active in mental health care and the prevention and treatment of drug and alcohol abuse, is operated in affiliation with Union Hosp.

EDUCATION. Swain School of Design, established in 1881, awards bachelor degrees in fine, applied, graphic and industrial arts. In 1978, it enrolled approx. 209. The public school system includes 26 elementary, three jr. and one sr. high schools. There are several parochial elementary and two high schools. The New Bedford Pub. Lib., the first free public Lib. in the nation, maintains a main lib. and four branches, including a Portuguese-language dept.

Fishing boat, New Bedford, Massachusetts

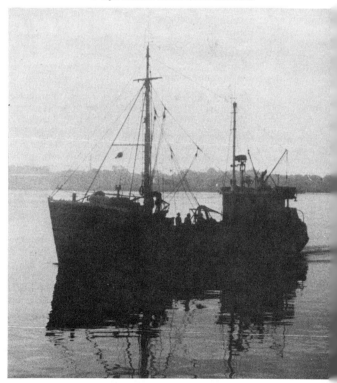

ENTERTAINMENT. Annual events in New Bedford include Rediscover New Bedford Days, Whaling City Festival, Portuguese Feast and the Center Street Festival. State championship competition in softball is held in the city. Buzzard's Bay is a training ground for competition yachts.

ACCOMMODATIONS. There are several hotels and motels in New Bedford, including the Holiday Inn and Skipper Motor Inn.

FACILITIES. Parks in New Bedford include Buttonwood, Brooklawn, Hazelwood, Ashley and Marine. A zoo, including a children's zoo, is located in Buttonwood Park. A public golf course is available at Whaling City Golf Course. Softball fields and basketball and tennis courts are available at the city's parks. Bowling on the green is offered at Hazelwood Park. Bathing facilities can be found at the city's pavillion and beach house on W Rodny French Blvd. and two beaches are available for swimming and sunning. The state maintains an ice-skating rink open 24 hours daily.

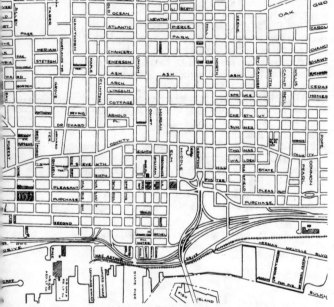

Downtown New Bedford, Massachusetts

CULTURAL ACTIVITIES. New Bedford is served by a symphony orchestra and two comm. theater groups, as well as the Comm. Chorus. Visiting artists perform at the SMU Auditorium. Located in the city's restored historic district, the New Bedford Whaling Museum houses whaling relics, while the Glass Museum includes 1,500 examples of American art and craftsmanship in glass among its silver plate and copperware exhibits. Artwork exhibited at the Crapo Art Gallery reflects the area's maritime influence. The US Coast Guard recently converted the lightship *New Bedford* to a floating maritime museum, with special emphasis on the role the Coast Guard has played in the development of the area. Fire Station Four, a Bi-centennial project, contains fire-fighting artifacts and equipment spanning the history of the industry.

LANDMARKS AND SIGHTSEEING SPOTS. The original buildings in New Bedford's Historic District, a once-shabby commercial district, have been renovated and the area now forms the basis of the tourist industry. Seaman's Bethel, the "whaleman's chapel" in Herman Melville's *Moby Dick*, pre-dates the district's other landmarks. Opened in 1832, it stands at 15 Johnny Cake Hill in commemoration of early religious patriots. Rotch Rodman House is a lavish granite mansion built between 1818 and 1833 by the great-grandson of Joseph Rotch, who purchased the original 10-acre tract in Bedford Village. The former home of a Civil War hero, the St. Carney homestead was built in 1852 and now features handicrafts of the 1800s. Fort Taber, New Bedford's Civil War coastal fortress, was partly designed by Colonel Robert E. Lee when he served as an engineer with the US Army.

NEW HAVEN
CONNECTICUT

CITY LOCATION-SIZE-EXTENT. New Haven, located on Long Island Sound at the mouth of the Quinnipac River in S CT, 75 mi. NE of NYC and 35 mi. SW of Hartford in New Haven Co., encompasses 18.4 sq. mi. at 41°18' N lat. and 72°54' W long. It is bordered by the cities of E Haven to the E, N Haven and Hamden to the N, and Woodbridge, Orange, and W Haven to the W.

TOPOGRAPHY. The terrain of New Haven, situated in the coastal lowlands region, is rolling, with hills to the E and W. There are several lakes in the area, including Lake Saltonstall to the E and Maltby Lakes to the W. The W River empties into New Haven Harbor S of the city. The mean elev. is 25'.

CLIMATE. The climate of New Haven is intermediate continental, characterized by temps. which vary by several degrees from inland to coastal areas, which are cooler during summer and warmer during winter. The avg. annual temp. of 51°F ranges from a Jan. mean of 28°F to a July mean of 73°F. The avg. annual rainfall of 44" is evenly distributed. Snowfall avgs. 28" annual-ly, with more than 50% occurring during Jan. and Feb. The RH ranges from 52% to 84%. New Haven lies in the ESTZ and observes DST.

FLORA AND FAUNA. Animals native to New Haven include the shrew, mole, raccoon, bat, woodchuck, white-footed mouse and muskrat. Common birds include the gull, tern, robin and blue jay. Salamanders, frogs, newts and milk snakes as well as the venomous copperhead and timber rattlesnake, are also found in the area. Typical trees are the dogwood, oak, pine, beech, elm birch and maple. Smaller plants include mt. laurel, vibernum, violet, thistle and hemlock.

POPULATION. According to the US census, the pop. of New Haven in 1970 was 137,721. In 1978, it was estimated that it had decreased to approx. 133,000.

ETHNIC GROUPS. In 1978, the ethnic distribution of New Haven was approx. 72.9% Caucasian, 26.3% Black and 3.6% Hispanic (a percentage of the Hispanic total is also included in the Caucasian total).

TRANSPORTATION. Interstate hwys. 84, 91 and 95, US hwys 1 and 5 and state hwys 10, 15, 17, 34 and 80 provide major motor access to New Haven. *Railroads* serving the city include AMTRAK, Penn Central, Central VT and ConRail. *Airlines* serving Tweed New Haven Airport include Ransome, US Air, Pilgrim and New Haven Airways. *Bus lines* serving the city include Greyhound, Trailways and the local New Haven Bus Service Inc. The Port of New Haven, served by a 35' deep ocean channel, is headquarters for the US Coast Guard in LI Sound.

COMMUNICATIONS. Communications, broadcasting and print media originating from New Haven are: *AM radio station* WELI 960 (Indep., MOR); WAVZ 1300 (Indep., Top 40) and WNHC 1340 (MBS, MOR, News, Talk); *FM radio stations* WYBC 94.3 (ABC/FM, Blk., Jazz) and WPLR 99.1 (Indep., AOR); *television stations* WTNH Ch. 8 (ABC); WTVU Ch. 59 (Indep.); WEDY Ch. 65 (PBS) and cable; *press:* two major dailies serve the city, the *Journal-Courier*, issued mornings, and the *Register*, issued evenings; other publications include *Yale Daily News*, *Advocate* and *Information*.

HISTORY. In 1638 New Haven was founded as a trading comm. by a group of Puritans led by Rev. John Davenport and Theophilus Eaton. Known first as Quinnipiac after the Indian village which once occupied the site, the settlement was renamed New Haven two years later. Within a few years about 800 people lived there, and the little colony expanded rapidly. However, two initial commercial ventures—private shipping to England and fur trading in Delaware Bay—failed, and by 1660, the comm. was so poor it was unable to send an emissary to England to apply for a new charter. New Haven was absorbed by the CT Colony in 1665. In 1716 the "Collegiate School," later known as Yale U, was persuaded to relocate in the little town. During the 1700s, New Haven developed a thriving trade industry with Boston, NY and the W Indies, facilitated by its natural harbor. Pop. soared from 1,400 in 1748 to 8,000 in 1774. British troops invaded New Haven and burned E shore homes during the Revolutionary War in 1779. Intended to divert Washington's army in NY state, the raid was unsuccessful. In 1784, New Haven was incorporated as a city with a pop. of 3,500. The advent of industrialization and immigration during the 19th century changed New Haven from a small commercial town to a large industrial city, further boosted by Eli Whitney's manufacturing system of interchangeable parts. The first influx of immigrants occurred in the 1830s and continued through the 1850s. By 1861, New Haven's residents numbered approx. 40,000. In 1864 a hardware manufacturing plant was established in the city, and a firearms factory in 1870. Breweries, retail stores and additional factories followed. A second wave of immigrants began arriving during the 1880s and peaked in 1896. The city had some 108,000 inhabitants at the turn of the century. In the late 19th and early 20th century, New Haven was a major oystering center. WWI provided economic impetus for further industrial expansion. In 1927, a dredging project was initiated to accommodate New Haven's harbor to ocean-going vessels, reclaiming its importance as a major port. The pop. reached 163,000 by 1938. Following WW II and the exodus of many residents to the suburbs, an urban renewal project was begun in 1950 to combat urban blight. Today New Haven is CT's third largest city and an important N.E. wholesale and education center.

GOVERNMENT. New Haven has a mayor-council form of govt. The 27 council members are elected by ward to two-year terms. The mayor, elected at large to a two-year term, is not a member of council.

ECONOMY AND INDUSTRY. There are approx. 1,400 manufacturing firms in New Haven. Major products include chemicals and petrochemicals, electronics, fabricated metals, machinery, transportation equipment, rubber, plastics, primary metals, apparel and textiles. Printing and publishing are significant to the city's economy, as is research. Yale U is New Haven's largest employer. The city has experienced high rates of unemployment in recent years. In 1978, the total labor force of the greater met. area was approx. 62,479, while the rate of unemployment was 9.8%.

BANKING. There are 12 banks in New Haven. In 1978, total deposits for the five banks headquartered in the city were $2,747,591,000, while assets were $3,135,660,000. Banks include Union Trust, New Haven Savings, CT Savings, First Natl. Savings, Colonial, First Fed. Savings and CT Bank & Trust.

HOSPITALS. There are two major hospitals in New Haven, Yale-New Haven, which contains the Yale School of Medicine and St. Raphael's. Other hosps. include the V.A. Hosp., CT Mental Health Center, C-Med and Comprehensive Cancer Center for CT.

EDUCATION. Yale U, founded in 1701, is the nation's second oldest collegiate institution and was the first to award doctorate degrees. The privately-supported school became coed. in 1969 and enrolled over 9,600 students in 1978. Other teaching and research institutions include Albertus Magnus Col., Berkeley Divinity School, S CT State Col., S Central Comm. Col.,

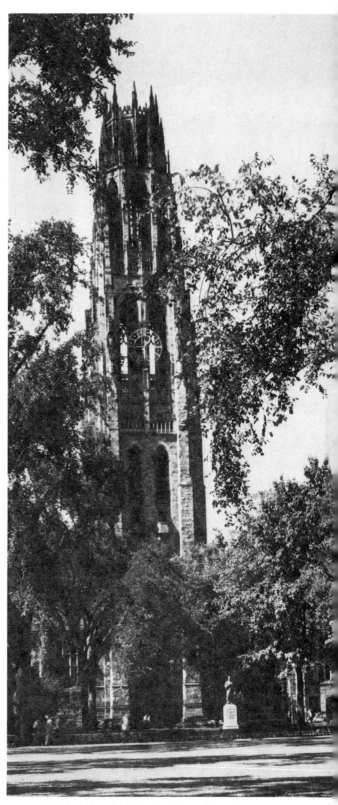

Harkness Memorial Tower, New Haven, Connecticut

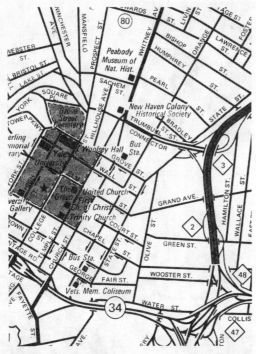

Downtown New Haven, Conn.

a professional group also performs. Dramatic productions are staged by the Long Wharf Theatre, and visiting theatrical companies perform in Shubert Theater. Dance is offered by the pro CT Ballet, Inc., the New Haven Ballet, Intl. Folk Dancers and the Royal Scottish Country Dance Society. The Victorian John Slade Ely House, a cultural center for the visual and performing arts, offers instruction in arts and handcrafts, as does the Creative Arts Workshop. Museums and galleries at Yale include the U Art Gallery, founded in 1832 and housing works of art by Picasso, Matisse, Renoir and Cezanne; the Yale Center for British Art, containing an extensive collection of 18th-century art; the Peabody Museum of Natural History and the Beinecke Rare Book and Manuscript Lib. Other museums in the city include the New Haven Colony, the CT Afro-American Historical Societies' and the Children's Museums.

LANDMARKS AND SIGHTSEEING SPOTS. When New Haven was planned in 1638, the Green was laid out in nine squares and designated as the marketplace and public square. Four blocks from the Green, Wooster Square, named for revolutionary war hero, David Wooster contains several homes from the 1840s and 1850s and is listed in the Natl. Registry of Historic Places. Located on the E side are Ft. Nathan Hale and Black Rock Ft., the site of a major defense during the Revolutionary War. Three churches, each of special architectural interest, were built between 1812 and 1814. Many prominent colonial figures, including traitor Benedict Arnold's mother, are buried in the Colonial Burial Ground. A plaque commemorating Benedict Arnold's leadership of the New Haven militia to Lexington in 1775 is located on the New Haven City Hall, a Victorian gothic building. The Pardee-Morris House, built around 1680, and the oldest house in New Haven, has been restored to 18th-century appearance. Three of Cromwell's officers who carried out the death warrant of Charles I took refuge from British troops in Judge's Cave, now located in a state park on the outskirts of the city.

Stone School of Business. CT School of Electronics, Yale-New Haven Hosp. and Hosp. of St. Raphael. New Haven's public school system enrolls approx. 21,000. There are also six private schools, including the Hopkins-Day Prospect Hill School, the nation's oldest. Libs. include the New Haven Public Lib. with nine branches, Yale U's Sterling Memorial and the Beinecke Rare Book and Manuscript Lib.

ENTERTAINMENT. Each year New Haven hosts the New Haven 20 Km. Road Race Marathon. The annual Mary Magdalene Festival features foods, music and displays. Every fourth of July, the city's cultural resources are celebrated in the Festival-on-the-Green. Pro sports teams include the Nighthawks (AHL, Hockey) and baseball's N.E. Pilgrims. Yale U's Bulldogs participate in intercollegiate sports.

ACCOMMODATIONS. There are numerous hotels and motels in New Haven, including the Holiday Inn, Sheraton Park Plaza, Hotel Duncan, Three Judges and Howard Johnson's.

FACILITIES. There are 15 parks in New Haven, including E Rock, Edgewood, Nathan Hale, Edgerton and Ft. Wooster. W Rock Park features a 400' cliff, "Judges Cave", a 40-acre nature center and a zoo with native animals. Public tennis courts are available at Edgewood and Clinton Avenue Parks, while Lighthouse Point Park has public beaches.

CULTURAL ACTIVITIES. New Haven has a Symphony Orchestra, Chorale, Civic Opera and stages the Woolsey Hall Concert Series. An annual three-day jazz festival is held at Quinnipiac Col. Yale U's Repertory Theatre, *Woolsey Hall, New Haven, Conn.*

NEW ORLEANS
LOUISIANA

CITY LOCATION-SIZE-EXTENT. New Orleans, in Orleans Parish of SE LA, encompasses 197.1 sq. mi. at 29°54' N lat. and 90°15' W long. The met. area extends to the surrounding parishes—W into St. Charles, S into Jefferson, S into Plaquemines, SE into St. Bernard and N into St. Tammany.

TOPOGRAPHY. New Orleans lies on the Mississippi Delta, which consists of swamps and bayous. The main portion of the city is virtually surrounded by water. Lake Pontchartrain borders the city on the N and is connected to the Gulf of Mexico through Lake Borgne, which borders the city on the E. The MS River is in the S section of the city—it curves as it passes through the city, inspiring the city nickname "Crescent City". Lake St. Catherine borders the city on the NE. The mean elev. is 5'.

CLIMATE. The climate of New Orleans is humid and subtropical, with the surrounding waters of the Gulf of Mexico, Lake Pontchartrain and the MS Delta modifying temp. extremes. The monthly mean temp. ranges from 53.8°F. in Jan. to 82.3°F. in July, with an avg. annual temp. of 68.9°F. Rainfall occurs throughout the year, with an annual avg. of 59.35". Snowfall is negligible. Waterspouts are observed quite often on nearby lakes. Three hurricanes have hit the area since 1900. The RH ranges from 59% to 91%. New Orleans is in the CSTZ and observes DST.

FLORA AND FAUNA. Animals native to New Orleans include the

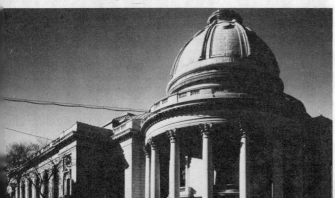

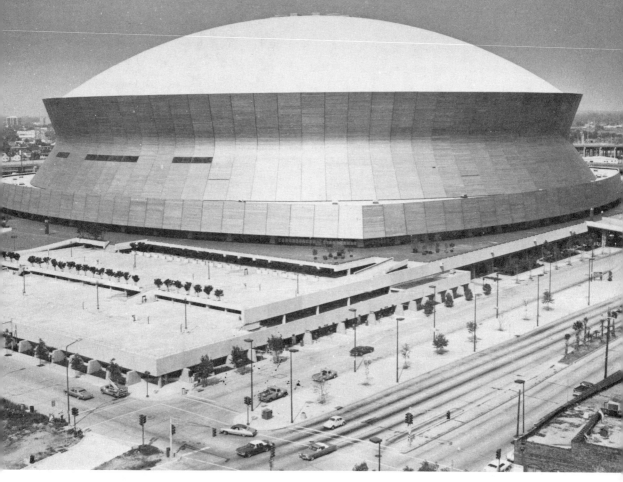

Superdome, New Orleans, Louisiana

opossum, armadillo, muskrat and raccoon. Common birds are the mockingbird, cardinal, egret, heron, gull and tern. Alligators, water snakes green anole lizards, toads, frogs and the venomous copperhead, cottonmouth, coral snake and rattlesnake are common to the area. Typical trees include the magnolia (the state flower of LA), oak, sweetgum and elm. Smaller plants include the gardenia, Spanish moss and mallow and marsh grass.

POPULATION. According to the US census, the pop. of New Orleans in 1970 was 593,471. In 1978, it was estimated that it had decreased to 555,000.

ETHNIC GROUPS. In 1978, the ethnic distribution of New Orleans was approx. 54.6% Caucasian, 45.0% Black and 4.4% Hispanic. (A percentage of the Hispanic total is included in the Caucasian total.)

TRANSPORTATION. Interstate hwy. 10 , US hwys. 11, 61 and 90 and state hwys. 39 and 45 provide major motor access to New Orleans. *Railroads* serving the city include AMTRAK, Illinois Central, Louisville Nashville, Southern Pacific, Southern Railway System, Union Pacific, Burlington Northern, Missouri Pacific and Santa Fe. *Airlines* serving New Orleans Intl. Airport include BN, CO, DL, EA, NA, NW, SO, TI and UA. Additional airports in the area include New Orleans Lakefront and Alvin Callender Naval Air Station. *Bus lines* serving the city include Greyhound and Trailways. Local service is provided by New Orleans Public Service, which operats a trolley line. The Port of New Orleans ranks as the nation's second largest in total water-borne commerce. In 1978, more than 163 million tons of cargo were handled. The port operates the only seaport-related foreign trade zone on the Gulf Coast permitting foreign and domestic goods to be stored, processed and exported without being subject to US customs and regulations. Additional transportation facilities are offered by the MS River, the Intracoastal Waterway and the connecting Interharbor Navigation Canal and the MS River-Gulf Outlet.

COMMUNICATIONS. Communications, broadcasting and print media originating from New Orleans are: *AM radio stations* WVOG 600 (Indep., Relig.); WTIX 690 (Indep., Top 40); WSHO 800 (MBS, C&W); WWL 870 (CBS, Var.); WYLD 940 (Indep., Blk.); WNNR 990 (MBS, Nostalgic, Rock); WNDE 1060 (Indep. Contemp, Top 40); WBOK 1230 (Natl., Blk.); WGSO 1280 (ABC/I, Var.); WSMB 1350 (ABC/E, WWNO 89.9 (NPR, Clas., Jazz); WWOZ 90.7 (Indep., Clas.); WTUL 91.5 (UPI, Prog. Jazz); WQUE 93.3 (ABC/I Top 40); WRNO 99.5 (ABC/FM, AOR); WBYU 95.7 (Indep., Btfl. Mus.); WEZB 97.1 (Indep., Btfl. Mus.); WYLD 98.5 (Indep., Jazz, Prog.); WRNO 99.5 (ABC/FM, ADR); WNDE 101.0 (Indep., AOR) and WWL 101.9 (Indep., Prog.); *television stations* WWL Ch. 4 (CBS); WDSU Ch. 6 (NBC); WVUE Ch. 8 (ABC); WYES Ch. 12 (PBS); WGNO Ch. 26 (ABC) and cable; *press:* two major dailies serve the area, the *States-Item*, issued evenings, and the *Times-Picayune*, issued mornings; other publications include the weekly *Orleans Guide, LA Weekly, Clarion-Herald, Jefferson Democrat, Loyola Maroon;* the monthly *Coin Industry Play Meter, Sugar Journal* and *Xavier Herald;* and the quarterly *LA Conservatist, The Second Line* and *Tulanian.*

HISTORY. New Orleans was founded in 1718 by Jean Baptiste Le Moyne Sieur de Bienville, gov. of the French colony of LA. In 1721, Adrien de Pauger, assistant to the Royal Engineer, drew up plans of the city, marking out a square where important public buildings were to be located. This Place d'Armes (renamed Jackson Square in 1849) was the beginning of the area known today as the French Quarter or Vieux Carre. New Orleans became the capital of the LA colony in 1722. In 1750, the city's limits were marked out and a surrounding moat and wall built. In 1762, Louis XV ceded LA to Charles III of Spain. The Spanish gov. did not arrive in the town until 1766. A revolution by the French settlers was put down in 1769. It was during the period of Spanish rule that the sugar industry developed on nearby plantations and granulated sugar was perfected. Much of the city was rebuilt after a fire in 1788, resulting in the combined French and Spanish architecture seen today in the French Quarter. LA was returned to France by a treaty negotiated in 1801, and which was formalized in New Orleans in Nov., 1803. France sold LA to the US in Apr., 1803, and the formal transfer took place in Dec. of that year. For the first 85 years, New Orleans had been an agrarian-based comm. sustained by the MS River. The coming of the Americans brought a faster rate of change. In 1805, New Orleans was incorporated as a city. LA became a state of the Union in 1812. The War of 1812 destroyed the ill feeling between Creoles and Americans who united under Andrew Jackson to defeat the British in the Battle of New Orleans at Chalmette in 1815. Unrestricted trade with the other states, especially in cotton and sugarcane, brought prosperity. The city grew to a pop. of 102,000 in 1840, making it the fourth largest city in the US. New Orleans was firmly established as a major trade center, but was also known for its Creole-style of life and gaiety. The first Mardi Gras parade was held in 1857. In the Civil War the port of New Orleans was taken by Admiral Farragut and Gen. B.F. Butler. The capital moved from New Orleans to Donaldsonville and to Baton Rouge after the Civil War. Reconstruction after the war was not successful until the 1870s, when the Fed. troops left. More settlers came, and the MS channel was deepened to allow ocean-going vessels to reach New Orleans. After the turn of the century, the water control programs began in the 1870s and 1880s were completed, to help eliminate the danger of flooding from the river. The Port of New Orleans regained its position as a major port. WW II brought shipbuilding industries to the area and these, in conjunction with the petroleum and petrochemical industries boom and a developing tourist industry, contributed to the city's growth. By 1960, the pop. had reached 627,000. During the 1960s, the Natl. Aeronautics and Space Administration began fabrication in New Orleans of the first stages of the Saturn B and the Saturn V launch vehicles, giving the city a supporting role in America's space exploration program. **GOVERNMENT.** New Orleans has a mayor-council form of govt. The mayor is the chief executive officer and does not have a vote in council, but

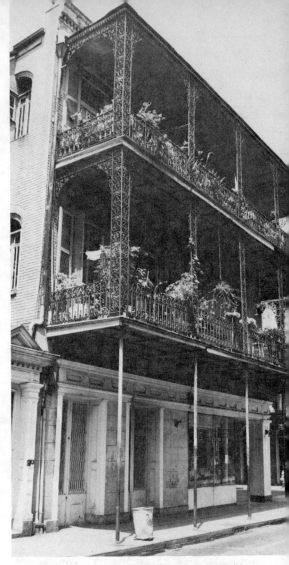

French Quarter, New Orleans, Louisiana

retains veto power. He is elected for a four-year term and may not serve more than two consecutive terms. The city council consists of seven members elected to a four-year term—five are elected by district and two at large. The council has the power to override a mayoral veto by a two-thirds majority vote.

ECONOMY AND INDUSTRY. Port activity is the largest industry in New Orleans. The port generates approx. 72,000 jobs, with payrolls totaling $600 million annually. Tourism is the second major industry. Approx. 5.8 million tourists visited the area in 1976 and accounted for 10% of the city's retail sales. Industrial activity is highlighted by shipbuilding and repair, oil/gas exploration, refining and petrochemical activity, food processing, primary metal production, and metal fabrication. There are approx. 1,000 manufacturing and processing plants in the met. area, including the nation's second largest primary aluminum plant, a major new nickel and copper refining plant and a giant petrochemical complex. Approx. 750 mining firms are engaged in the extraction of oil, natural gas and sulphur operate in the area. Retail sales reached $3.9 billion in 1977, an increase of 113% since 1970. Govt. is a major employer. The avg. per capita income in New Orleans in 1978 was $5,608. The met. area had a labor force of 473,500 in June, 1979, and an unemployment rate of 6.5%. Total personal income in 1978 was approx.

Central New Orleans, Louisiana

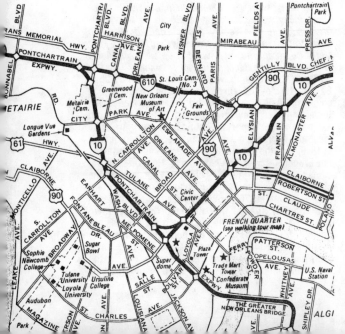

$3,882,000,000. Total effective buying power in 1977 was approx. $7 billion, a 109% increase since 1970.

BANKING. New Orleans is the financial center of the Gulf South. Located in the area are a branch bank of the Sixth Fed. Reserve District, 1 Fed. Land Bank, 39 commercial banks and more than 40 savings and loan assns. In 1978, total deposits for the ten banks headquartered in the city were $3,540,727,000, while assets were $4,510,665,000. Banks include Whitney Natl. of New Orleans, First Natl. Commerce, Hibernia Natl., Natl. American and Bank of New Orleans and Trust Co.

HOSPITALS. New Orleans is considered an intl. center of medicine, having 22 hosps. and more than three-fourths of the region's hosp. beds. Near the central business district is one of the largest complexes of medical treatment and training facilities in the US. The complex consists of the state-operated Charity Hosp., the US V.A. Hosp., and the medical schools of both Tulane and LSU. Ochsner Foundation Hosp. is known world-wide for its work in tropical medicine and open-heart surgery. Other hosps. include Children's, Eye, Ear Nose and Throat, Flint Goodridge of Dillard U, Hotel Dieu, Jo Ellen Smith Memorial, Mercy, Methodist, St. Charles Gen., St. Claude Gen. and Southern Baptist.

EDUCATION. The U of New Orleans, a branch of the LA State U System, offers grad. and undergrad. degrees. In 1978, this institution enrolled over 14,161 students. Tulane U, a private, nonsectarian U, also offers courses leading to grad. and undergrad. degrees. The U has a sister col., Newcomb Col., which admits only women to its programs. The school is known for its programs in medicine and law. In 1978, it enrolled 9,463 students. Dillard U, established in 1869, is one of the oldest, predominantly black institutions in the country. It was formed by the merger of Straight Col. (Congregational) and New Orleans U (Methodist). Other privately-endowed institutions include Loyola U, Our Lady of the Holy Cross Col., St. Mary's Dominican Col., New Orleans Baptist Theological Seminary., Notre Dame Seminary and Delgado Col. Publicly-supported campuses include LA State U Medical Center, and S U in New Orleans. The Orleans parish pub. school system enrolls more than 93,000 students in its schools. There are 65 parochial and 53 private schools in the city. LA's first pub. subscription lib. was founded in the city in 1805 and the New Orleans Public Lib. was established in 1896.

ENTERTAINMENT. While much of the entertainment action is in the French Quarter, other areas of New Orleans, such as Fat City, also offer top entertainment. The France-LA Festival each July, New Orleans Food Festival in July or Aug., New Orleans Jazz and Heritage Festival in Apr. and the Spring Festival in Apr. or May are among the city's annual festivals. The "world's biggest party" is the Mardi Gras held in either Feb. or Mar. each year. Parades, balls, parties and festivities abound. Professional sports include the Saints (NFL, football), and N.O. Pride (Women's Pro. Basketball). Collegiate sports are offered by the Tulane U Green Wave, LA State U Black Knight, U of New Orleans Privateers and Dillard U Blue Devils. Major sporting events are presented in New Orleans' Superdome, including New Year Eve's classic football competition, the Sugar Bowl Tournament.

ACCOMMODATIONS. Hotels and motels in downtown New Orleans include the Hyatt Regency, Grand Hotel, Le Richeleiu, Le Pavillion, Maison Dupuy, Marriott, Monteleone, Hilton, Marie Antoinette, Bienville House, Place d'Aremes, Royal Orleans, Royal Sonesta, St. Ann French Quarter Inn and the Saint Louis. Holiday, Quality, Best Western, Travelodge, Day's inns, and Howard Johnson's have facilities throughout the city.

FACILITIES. New Orleans' parks include Audubon, City, Lakefront and Pontchartrain Beach Amusement. Audubon Park was once part of the Etienne de Bore Plantation. It contains tree-shaded lagoons, gardens, bridle paths, golf courses and a swimming pool. The park houses the Audubon Zoo and Odenheimer Aquarium. City Park, one of the country's larger municipal parks, covers 1,500 acres of a former plantation and offers picnic sites, lagoons for boating, golf courses, bicycle rentals, tennis court, houses, carnival rides, and a children's storyland. Lakefront Park has picnic tables, shelters, benches and a seawall located along Lake Pontchartrain. Pontchartrain Beach Amusement Park, with more than 100 rides and attractions, is situated on the shores of Lake Pontchartrain. The Longue Vue Gardens consist of an eight-acre private estate garden now open to the pub. The gardens offer a combination of fountains, flowers and manicured greenery. The park system has many golf courses, including five courses in

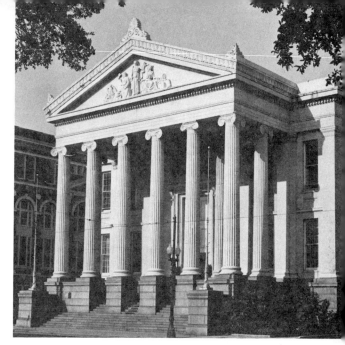

Gallier Hall, New Orleans, LA

City Park, one each in Audubon Park, Brechtel Park and Pontchartrain Park. Other pub. golf courses can be found at 12 locations throughout the city. Tennis courts are available at various locations. Lake Pontchartrain, many bayous and the Gulf of Mexico provide opportunity for boating and fishing. Bicycle rentals are available at City and Audubon Park and in the Vieux Carre. Horseback riding is permitted in the two major parks and horses may be rented at two local stables. Horse racing is presented at the Fairgrounds Racetrack.

CULTURAL ACTIVITIES. New Orleans is the home of jazz, which is everywhere evident, from the many clubs on Bourbon St. to funeral processions. The Jazz Club presents concerts. The Philharmonic Symphony Orchestra performs at the Theatre for the Performing Arts. The Summer Pops presents a summer series at the Municipal Auditorium. Chamber Music recitals are presented by the Friends of Music. The Opera House Assn. presents six operas annually. The Opera

Jackson Square & St. Louis Cathedral, New Orleans, Louisiana

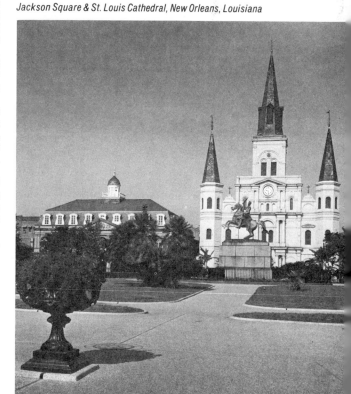

Guild sponsors a variety of productions by world famous orchestras, dance companies, singers and ballet troupes. The Comm. Concert Assn. sponsors a range of performances, including instrumental and choral groups. There are several theaters in the city. The Theater for the Performing Arts is part of a cultural complex that includes a theater-in-the-round. The Beverly Dinner Playhouse offers Broadway productions. Children's Corner Le Petit Theatre du Vieux Carre houses a comm. theater group which presents musicals for children. The Gallery Circle Theater, a theater-in-the-round, presents three musicals and three dramas each season. Performances at the Nord Theater are sponsored by the New Orleans Recreation Dept. The Dashiki Project Theatre is a black comm. theater performing plays of black experience. The Free Southern Theatre is the oldest black art institution in the South. The Historic New Orleans Museum of Art features several complete collections, including pre-Columbian masterworks from Mexico and the Samuel Kress Collection of masterpieces of Renaissance Italy. The museum also has an educational program for children, a lecture series, a film series, concerts and programs. Other galleries and museums are the Confed. Memorial Museum, LA State Wildlife Museum, Historic New Orleans Collection, the Jazz Museum, Lampe Gallery of Fine Art, Middle American Research Institute, the New Orleans Pub. Lib., U of New Orleans Gallery, Ursuline Museum, LA Maritime Museum, LA State Museum and Tulane Gallery.

LANDMARKS AND SIGHTSEEING SPOTS. New Orleans' French Quarter offers 70 blocks of well-preserved historical buildings, straight, narrow streets, Franco-Spanish architecture, "iron-lace" balconies, and fan windows, patios and courtyards. Established in 1721, Jackson Square is named for the hero of the Battle of New Orleans, Andrew Jackson. St. Louis Cathedral is the oldest cathedral in the US. The third church structure on the site, it was completed in 1794, after the fire of 1788. Other structures dating from the eighteenth century include Lafitte's Blacksmith Shop, the House of Jean Pascal (which some researchers say is the oldest building in the MS Valley), Merieult House, Maison de Flechier, the Presbytere, the Cabildo and the Casa de Comercio. Dating from the 19th century are these structures— Old Bank of LA, Old Absinthe House, The Hermann House, Old Bank of the US, Maison Seignouret, LeMonnier House, Old LA State Bank, Casa Faurie, Court of Two Lions, Maison LeMonnier (a three-story building that is said to be the "first skyscraper"), Orleans Ballroom, 1850 House, the Pontalbe buildings, LeCarpentier House, Soniat House, Thierry House, Clay House, LaLaurie House, Gallier House and Miltenberger House. Other points of interest in the city include the Cabrini Doll Museum and Art Center, presenting a worldwide collection of dolls; the Loom Room, offering demonstrations and exhibits of weaving; Musee Conti Wax Museum, featuring historical wax figures and the Haunted Dungeon; the Pharmacy Museum, dating back to 1820 and displaying old apothecary items and Voodoo potions; Pontalba Historical Puppetorium, in which automated marionettes portray the life of Jean Lafitte, the pirate; The Women's Opera Guild House, a pre-Civil War mansion of Greek Revival Style and Italian architecture; the LA Superdome; old cemeteries throughout the city where tombs of solid masonry 100 or more feet long lie above ground; the Nicholas D. Burke Siesmographical Observatory; and the Lake Pontchartrain Causeway, the longest, overwater highway bridge in the world.

NEWPORT NEWS
VIRGINIA

CITY LOCATION-SIZE-EXTENT. Newport News, an independent city, encompasses 69.1 sq. mi. on the James River in SE VA in the Tidewater Region at 36°58' N lat. and 76°25' W long. The greater met. area extends into the counties of S Hampton and York to the W and James City to the N. The cities of Hampton and Norfolk lie to the SE.

TOPOGRAPHY. The terrain of Newport News, which is situated in the lower VA peninsula of the coastal plain,

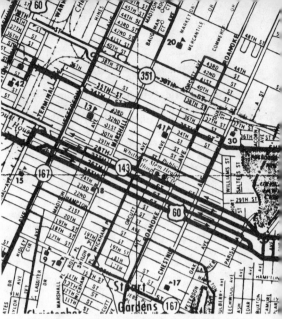

Central Newport News, Virginia

is characterized by level lowlands. The city has several lakes and creeks, while Chesapeake Bay lies to the NE, James River lies to the SW and Hampton Roads Estuary lies to the W and S. The mean elev. is 25'.

CLIMATE. The climate of Newport News is modified marine, due to the effects of the surrounding waters of Chesapeake Bay and Hampton Roads. The avg. annual temp. of 60°F ranges from a Jan. mean of 41°F to a July mean of 79°F. The warmer months receive most of the avg. annual rainfall of 44.4''. Most of the annual snowfall of 7.2'' occurs during Jan. and Feb. The RH ranges from 55% to 90%. The growing season avgs. 240 days. Newport News lies in the ESTZ and observes DST.

FLORA AND FAUNA. Animals native to Newport News include the Southern flying squirrel, raccoon, opossum and striped skunk. Common birds include the cardinal, bluebird, tree swallow, gull, tern and willit. Blue crab and oysters are also found in the area, as are bullfrogs, toads, painted turtles, water snakes and the venomous rattlesnake, copperhead and cottonmouth. Typical trees are the loblolly pine, yellow poplar, oak, dogwood and sweetgum. Smaller plants include the honeysuckle, water lily and cattail.

POPULATION. According to the US census the pop. of Newport News in 1970 was 138,177. In 1978, it was estimated that it had increased to 164,637.

ETHNIC GROUPS. In 1978, the ethnic distribution in Newport News was approx. 70.8% Caucasian, 28.4% Black and 1.5% Hispanic (a percentage of the Hispanic total is also included in the Caucasian total).

TRANSPORTATION. Interstate hwy. 64, US hwys. 60 and 17 and state hwys. 143, 167, 168, 173 and 351 provide major motor access to Newport News. *Railroads* serving the city include Chesapeake & OH and AMTRAK. *Airlines* serving Patrick Henry Intl. Airport are UA, US Air and Wheeler. *Buslines* serving the city include Greyhound and the local Pentran. The Port of Newport News handles more than 885,000 tons annually and is one of the world's largest facilities for the export of coal.

COMMUNICATIONS. Broadcasting, communications and print media originating from Newport News: *AM radio station* WOKT 1270 (MBS, C&W, Relig.) and WGH 1310 (APR., Top 40); *FM radio stations* WGH 97.3 (Apr. Clas..) and WQRK 104.5 (MBS, Top 40). (Indep.,) no *television stations* originate in Newport News, which receives broadcasting from nearby Norfolk and Portsmouth; *press*: two major dailies serve the area, the *Daily Press*, issued mornings, and *Times-Herald*, issued evenings; among bi-weekly newspapers is *The Wheel*.

HISTORY. Jamestown settlers used the site of present-day Newport News as a point from which to await news of the return of Capt. Christopher Newport from Eng-

day Newport News as a point from which to await news of the return of Capt. Christopher Newport from England, hence giving the site the name Newportes News. The name first appeared in English records in 1619, making it the oldest English location name of any city in the US. The first settlement at the site was established when Daniel Gookin led 50 men to the location in 1621 to establish a plantation. One of the area's finest plantations, Denbigh Plantation, was established in 1629 by Capt. Samuel Mathews. Newport News was part of the Corporation of Kecoughtan from 1617 until 1634, when it became part of Warwick River Shire, later renamed Warwick Co. In June, 1667, the Dutch, angered by the closing of colonial ports to Dutch ships, burned many of the 20 tobacco ships moored in Newport Harbor. The peace and prosperity of the wheat and tobacco farmers, which prevailed during the 1700s, was marred only by a brief battle during Cornwallis' Peninsula campaign in 1781, which ended in a British retreat. During the War of 1812, British warships occupied Hampton Roads, blockading the settlement's port. Newport News remained sparsely settled during the following years, with Warwick Co. maintaining a nearly constant pop. of approx. 1,600 between 1790 and 1870. In May, 1861, Union troops occupied and established fortifications at Newport News, which served as a staging area for Union troops until the end of the war. In March, 1862, the iron-clad confed. ship, the *Merrimack*, destroyed two Union ships. The following day the Union iron-clad ship, the *Monitor*, met the *Merrimack* and the resulting battle ended with both ships retreating and claiming victory. The city served as a union prisoner-of-war camp for several months at the end of the Civil War. By 1880, CN merchant Collis Potter Huntington had purchased land for a RR right-of-way, ushering in a new phase in the growth of the city as a center of transportation and industry. The city's pop. increased rapidly until construction of the RR began to slacken. In the late 1880s Huntington established a shipbuilding yard, initially to service the ships which were transporting RR commerce. Newport News served as the county seat between 1888 and 1896, when it was incorporated as a city. A temporary exodus from the city occurred when yellow fever struck in 1898. Early in

Victory Arch, Newport News, Virginia

1916, the Curtiss Flying School was established nearby as a training center for airmen involved in WW I. The pop. grew steadily and by war's end totaled 100,000. Black singers Pearl Bailey and Ella Fitzgerald were born in the city in 1918. A depression occurred in 1921 when an Intl. Disarmament Conf. was held in Washington, D.C. and, to demonstrate its sincerity, the US canceled $70,000,000 in shipyard contracts at Newport News. The economic slump continued through the Great Depression, and was reversed only when WWII placed shipbuilding demands on the city. In 1958, Newport News and Warwick Co. were merged to become the greater Newport News. Today the city remains a major shipbuilding center.

Shipbuilding Yard, Newport News, Virginia

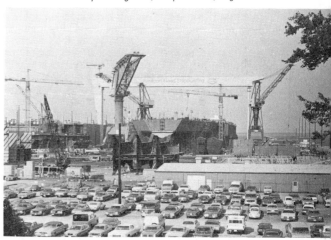

GOVERNMENT. Newport News has a council-mgr. form of govt. The seven council members, including the mayor, are elected at large to four-year terms. The council selects a mayor and vice-mayor by majority vote from within the council. Both are voting members of the council and serve two-year terms.

ECONOMY AND INDUSTRY. Shipbuilding and repair is the largest industry in Newport News. The world's largest private shipyard, employing more than 25,500, is located in the city. Other important industries include port activities, fishing, tourism, R&D and the manufacture of apparel and electronics. In June, 1979, the Newport News-Hampton met. area labor force totaled 163,700, while the rate of unemployment was 5.7%. The avg. per capita income in 1978 was $6,548.

BANKING. In 1978, total deposits for the three banks headquartered in Newport News were $185,487,00, while assets were $207,189,000. Banks include VA Natl., Bank of VA, United VA, Dominion Natl., Fidelity American and First City.

HOSPITALS. There are four hosps. in Newport News, including Riverside, Whittaker, Mary Immaculate and Patrick Henry. Riverside, the largest, offers the broadest range of services on the peninsula. Riverside Hosp. contains the Peninsula Mental Health Clinic, while the Newport News Public Health Dept. provides outpatient services.

EDUCATION. The publicly-supported Christopher Newport Col., located in Newport News, awards bachelor degrees. In 1978, it enrolled more than 3,700. Other educational services include the VA Associated Research Campus, which provides research and grad. study through the cooperative efforts of the Col. of William and Mary and Old Dominion U. The public school system includes 29 elementary, four intermediate and four high schools and enrolls approx. 24,000. There are many private and parochial schools in the area, offering classes ranging from nursery through the

12th grade. Other institutions include the Vocational/Technical Center, a shipbuilding apprentice school and NASA's apprentice technician program. Lib. facilities include seven municipal branch libraries and the Schuylen Technical Lib.

ENTERTAINMENT. More than 100 traditional craftspeople, musicians and dancers participate in the annual Newport News Festival of Folklife. Other annual events include Spring Thing, Arts in the Parks and the July Fourth celebration. The Peninsula Pilots offer Class A baseball, while Christopher Newport Col. participates in intercollegiate sports.

ACCOMMODATIONS. There are 24 hotels and motels in Newport News, including the Hotel Warwick, Colonial Courts, King James Motor Hotel. Holiday, Ramada, Traveler's and Old London inns.

FACILITIES. The 13 municipal parks in Newport News encompass 8,682 acres and contain swimming pools, three lakes, a salt water beach, tennis courts, picnic grounds and more than 200 campsites. Parks include Mariners Museum, Newport News, Christopher Newport and Deer. The Peninsula Nature and Science Center/Planetarium, located at Deer Park, features a live animal room, aquarium, observatory and nature trail. A 36-hole municipal golf course is available, while a local country club maintains a private course. There are 42 free and 10 admission public tennis courts in the city. Two parks contain jogging tracks. The surrounding waters provide opportunities for fishing, boating, swimming and water skiing.

CULTURAL ACTIVITIES. Performing organizations in Newport News include a Symphony Orchestra, a 100-voice Choral Society, a Civic Opera, a Ballet Co. and a dance co. Mariners Museum contains one of the most extensive collections of maritime artifacts in the world. War Memorial Museum, also in Newport News, features more than 18,000 exhibits representing American conflicts, including the world's largest collection of wartime posters. Art galleries include the Peninsula Fine Arts Center and Sherman Galleries.

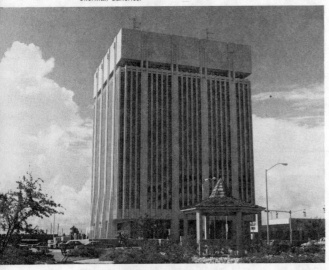

City Hall, Newport News, Virginia

LANDMARKS AND SIGHTSEEING SPOTS. The Victory Arch was erected in 1919 to receive the returning troops after WW I. The temporary wood and plaster structure was replaced with a permanent arch in 1962. Ships from every nation harbor at the C&O Port Terminal, one of the world's largest tobacco ports. Tours of the city include a Harbor Cruise, which visits the shipyards and the site of the battle between the *Monitor* and the *Merrimack*. Newport News is also the home of Ft. Eustis, a US Army Transportation Center which features a port area, the Memorial Chapel of the Transportation Corps and the Transportation Corps Museum. Five sites in the city are designated in the Natl. Register of Historic Places, including the Hilton Village Historic District, Lee Hall Mansion, the Matthew Jones House (built in 1660 and located at Ft. Eustis), Ft. Crafford and Denbigh Plantation Site.

NEW YORK CITY
NEW YORK

CITY LOCATION-SIZE-EXTENT. NYC, the largest city in the US, encompasses 314 sq. mi. at the mouth of the Hudson River and borders LI Sound and the Atlantic Ocean, at 40°47' N lat. and 73°58' W long. The city encompasses five counties, Bronx, Kings, NY, Queens and Richmond and is composed of five boroughs, Brooklyn, Manhattan, Queens, Staten Island and The Bronx (primarily a residential area). The Bronx is the only borough attached to the mainland. The met. area extends into the NY counties of Rockland on the NW, Westchester on the N and Nassau on the E, as well as into the NJ counties of Bergen and Hudson on the W and Middlesex on the SW.

TOPOGRAPHY. The terrain of NYC, which is situated on the Atlantic Coastal range, varies from hills to the W, N and NW to low lying areas of the coastal plain and traverse the area and all of the boroughs, but one, are situated on islands. The elev. varies from less than 50' to 800'.

CLIMATE. The climate of NYC is predominantly continental, due to the storm and frontal systems which approach the city from the W, although a marine influence moderates summer temps. The avg. annual temp of 54°F varies between monthly means of 32°F in Jan. to 76°F in July. The annual avg. rainfall of 43" occurs fairly evenly throughout the year. Most of the avg. snowfall of approx. 25" occurs during Dec. through Mar. The RH ranges from 48% to 80%. The growing season avgs. 200 days. NYC lies in the ESTZ and observes DST.

FLORA AND FAUNA. Animals native to NYC include the raccoon, and squirrel. Common birds include the starling, sparrow, pigeon, bluejay and gull. Salamanders, frogs, milk snakes and box turtles, as well as the venomous timber rattlesnake and copperhead, are also found in the area. Common trees include the oak, maple, elm and pine. Smaller plants include the rose, vibernium, violet, honeysuckle and cattail.

POPULATION. Between 1970 and 1977, the NYC met. area pop., the largest in the nation, declined by approx. 4.8%. According to the US census, the pop. of NYC in 1970 was 7,895,563. In 1978, it was estimated that it had decreased to 7,414,800.

ETHNIC GROUPS. In 1978, the ethnic distribution of NYC was approx. 77.2% Caucasian, 21.1% Black and 10.3% Hispanic (a percentage of the Hispanic total is included in the Caucasian total).

TRANSPORTATION. Interstate hwys. 78, 80, 87, 95, 278, 280, 495, 678 and 895, US hwys. 1, 9, 22, 45 and 46 and state hwys. 21, 24, 25, 27, 35, 58 and 82 provide major motor access to NYC. *Railroads* serving the city include AMTRAK, Burlington N, Canadian Natl., ConRail, FL E Coast, French Natl. Metroliner, Santa Fe, S Pacific and Union Pacific. *Airlines* serving John F. Kennedy Intl. Airport, which handles more intl. flights than any other airport (approx. 220 daily), are AA, US Air, BN, DL, WA, FL, NA, NW, NY, PA, RD, SB, TW and UA. LaGuardia and Newark Airports also serve the area. *Bus lines* serving the city include Atlantic City, Lincoln Transit, Bonanza, Gray Line, Greyhound and Trailways. The city's subways, the world's busiest, cover 237 mi. and handle 4.5 million passengers daily. The Port of NYC clears more than 26,000 vessels annually, shipping 40% of the entire foreign trade of the US.

COMMUNICATIONS. Communications, broadcasting and print media originating from NYC are: *AM radio stations* WMAC 570 (MBS, Talk); WNBC 660 (NBC, Contemp.); WOR 710 (Indep., Talk); WABC 770 (ABC/C, Mass Appeal); WCBS 880 (CBS, All News); WINS 1010 (Indep., News); WNEW 1130 (Indep., MOR); WLIB 1190 (Indep., Blk.); WADO 1280 (Indep., Spec. Prog.);

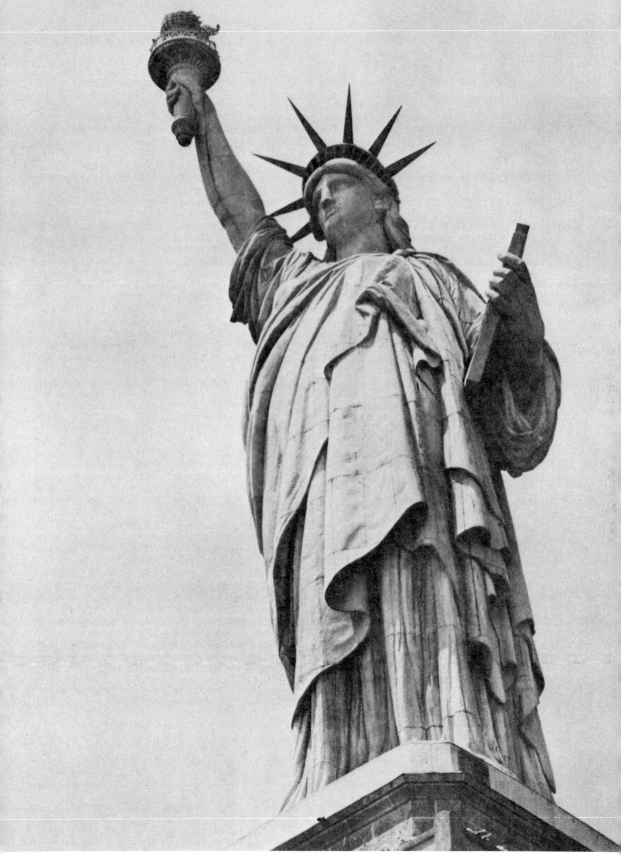

Statue of Liberty, New York, New York

WPOW 1330 (Indep., Var.); WBNX 1380 (Indep., Spec. Prog.); WJIT 1480 (Indep., Spec. Prog.); WQXR 1560 (Indep., Clas.) and WWRL 1600 (Indep., Blk.) *FM radio stations* WKCR 89.9 (Indep., Clas., Jazz); WNYU 89.1 (Indep., Divers.); WFUV 90.7 (ABC/E, Clas., Educ., Contemp.); WNYE 91.5 (Indep., Educ.); WKTU 92.3 (Indep., Mellow); WNYC 93.9 (Indep., Talk, Clas.); WPLJ 95.5 (ABC/FM, Mass Appeal); WQXR 96.3 (Indep., Clas.); WYNY 97.1 (Indep., Rock); WEUD 97.9 (Indep., Divers.); WXLO 98.7 (Indep., Talk); WBAI 99.5 (Indep., Divers.); WCBS 101.1 (CBS, Rock); WPIX 101.9 (Indep., AOR); WNEW 102.7 (Indep., Progsv.); WNCN 104.3 (Indep., Clas.); WRFM 105.1 (Indep., Btfl. Mus.); WRVR 106.7 (Indep., Jazz) and WBLS 107.5 (MBS, Blk.); *television stations* WCBS Ch. 2 (CBS); WNBC Ch. 4 (NBC); WNEW Ch. 5 (Indep.); WABC Ch. 7 (NBC); WOR Ch. 9 (Indep.); WPIX Ch. 11 (Indep.); WNET Ch. 13 (PBS); WYNE Ch. 25 (PBS); WNYC Ch. 31 (PBS) and cable; *press:* three major dailies serve the area, the *Daily News* and *Times*, both issued mornings, and *Post*, issued evenings; other daily publications include *The China Post, Natl. Herald* and *Wall Street Journal*; weekly publications include *Amsterdam News, Cue, E Side Herald, Editor and Publisher, Gramercy Herald, Newsweek, The New Yorker, NY Magazine, Parade, Publishers Weekly* and *Time*; monthly publications include *Humpty Dumpty's Magazine, Cosmopolitan, Esquire, Gallery Magazine, Glamour, Good Housekeeping, High Times, Ladies Home Journal, Mademoiselle, McCall's Magazine, Modern Photography, Money, Natl. Lampoon, Vogue, Penthouse* and *People*; quarterly publications include the *Curator, The Hudson Review, Political Science Quarterly* and the *Ukrainian Quarterly*.

HISTORY. The first white men to explore the area of present-day NYC were Italian navigator Giovanni da Verrazano in 1524 and English explorer Henry Hudson in 1609. Hudson, sailing for the Dutch E India Co., is responsible for the name of the NYC borough Staten Island, derived from his naming of the island as "Staaten Eyelandt". In 1613, four trading houses were erected and, in 1614, a permanent settlement was established in the area. Dutch colonists began the construction of a ft. on Manhattan Island in 1625, naming the resulting comm. New Amsterdam. The following year the island was purchased from the Native Americans by Dutch Gov. Peter Minuit for $24 worth of trinkets. The first church was built in 1633, and eventually the original ft. was replaced by Ft. Amsterdam. By 1653, the new ft. had a pop. of 800. The Duke of York seized the area from the Dutch in a nonviolent 1664 takeover. The British renamed the city after the Duke of York, and it was chartered on Apr. 27, 1686. During the Revolutionary War, Washington was defeated in the Battle of LI by Sir William Howe's British

View of Lower Manhattan as seen from Brooklyn Heights Mall, New York, New York

troops and NYC was under British control until 1783. Between 1785 and 1790, Congress convened in NYC, also the site of Pres. Washington's inauguration. The stream of European immigration into the city began in the late 1700s, increasing NYC's pop. to 60,000 by 1800. A city expansion plan was established in 1811, and, in 1825, waterway transportation to Buffalo was made possible by the opening of the Erie Canal. The 1800s brought the arrival of a nearly constant flow of immigrants from Germany, Ireland and other European countries resulting in poor living conditions and political corruption. Tammany Hall, the Democratic Party machine, traded advice and favors to the immigrants for votes for the party and maintained a stronghold on city govt. In 1871, the Tammany boss Tweed's Ring was broken up, but the machine soon regained control of the city. The 1883 completion of the Brooklyn Bridge led to greater dependence between the area's cities, and in 1898, Brooklyn, the Bronx, Queens and Staten Island were joined with Manhattan to become Greater NYC. Manhattan then had 2/3 of the city's three million people, but improved transportation allowed the pop. to spread to the other boroughs. In 1900, the city's pop. was more than seven million. Fiorello LaGuardia, a popular mayor who served between 1934 and 1945, was able to permanently destroy Tammany Hall. NYC, long a manufacturing and financial center, was boosted in its industry by WW I and WW II. Its position as a cultural center was furthered when it was selected in 1946 as the home of the United Nations. Attention was focused on the city during its hosting of World Fairs in 1939 and 1964. Although the city has always had problems with crowding, these problems have increased in recent years. A 1966 strike by sanitation workers and a 1971 police strike demonstrated unrest among public servants. In 1975, the city was unable to meet its budget. Both the State legislature and the US Congress established a loan guarantee program administered by the Municipal Assistance Corp. NYC was able to borrow enough funds from the corp. to see it through the financial crisis. Today, NYC is the major financial, industrial and cultural center in the US.

GOVERNMENT. NYC has a mayor-council form of govt. consisting of a mayor and 43 council members. Each borough of the city (including the Bronx, Queens, Manhattan, Staten Island and Brooklyn) elects two members at large and 33 are elected by district. The pres. of the council is elected at large. The mayor is not a member of the council and thus has no vote. The mayor's chief strength lies in his or her appointive powers, including the naming of the deputy mayors and heads of city departments. Each borough also elects a borough pres., whose responsibility it is to advise the mayor on matters of importance to his or her specific borough.

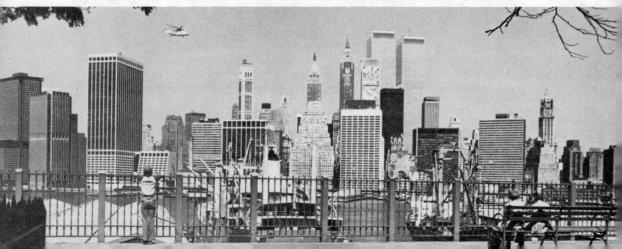

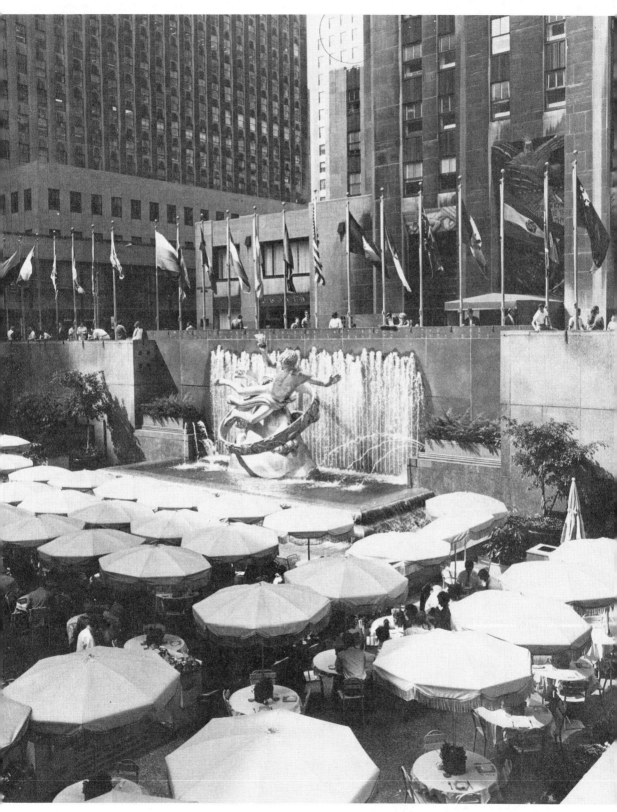

Rockefeller Center, New York, New York

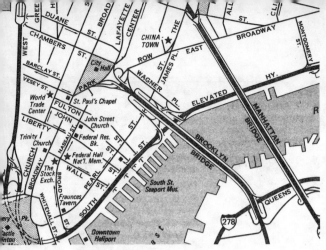

New York City, New York

ECONOMY AND INDUSTRY.
Major industries in NYC include finance, printing and publishing, insurance, tourism and the manufacture of apparel, machinery, food products and metal products. Several oil companies are headquartered in the city. Three quarters of the nation's books and more than 100 magazines are published in NYC. In 1978, approx. 17,000,000 tourists spent $1.8 billion in the five boroughs, while approx. 875 conventions were hosted in the city. The 1979 labor force in NYC was 3,084,000, while the rate of unemployment was 10%.

BANKING.
There are 250 banking institutions serving NYC. In 1978, total deposits for the 137 banks headquartered in the city were $303,102,824,000, while total assets were $394,876,327,000. Among the many banks serving the area are Bank of America, Bank of NY, Banker's Trust, Citibank, Chase Manhattan, Emigrant Savings, NY Bank for Savings, Bowery Savings Bank and Barclays Intl.

HOSPITALS.
There are more than 130 hosps. and health care institutions in NYC, including Montefiore with the Albert Einstein School of Medicine, Misericordia, NY Eye & Ear, Bellevue, Beth Israel, N Central Bronx, Parkchester Gen., Queens, Presbyterian, Prospect, Richmond Memorial Roosevelt, St. Clares, St. Johns Episcopal, St. Lukes, St. Vincents, State U, Staten Island, St. Barnabas, NYU Medical Center, Brookdale, NY Medical Col., Hosp. for Special Surgery, Cabrini, Bronx Lebanon, Brooklyn, Coney Island, Lenox Hill, King's Co., LI Col., Met. Hosp. Center, Methodist Brooklyn, Harlem, Bronx Psychiatric and Memorial Cancer. NYC has many research facilities, including Sloan-Kettering Cancer Research Institute. The V.A. maintains two facilities.

EDUCATION.
The oldest educational center in NYC, Columbia U, was founded in 1754 as King's Col. In 1897, after several moves, the col. located at its present address and was recognized as a U by the State of NY in 1912. Currently one of the top 10 research U's in the US, Columbia offers grad. and undergrad. programs. In 1978, it enrolled more than 17,000. Its affiliate Barnard Col., a private liberal arts col. for women, offers bachelor degrees. In 1978, 2,250 enrolled. The city's largest U is NYU, a private U founded in 1831. Offering 34 degree programs recognized by professional and accrediting agencies, NYU enrolled 31,197 in 1978. Other institutions are the New School for Social Research, which emphasizes adult education; Rockefeller U, specializing in scientific and medical research; Pratt Institute, focusing on fine arts and Cooper Union, dealing with engineering, architecture and the arts. The City U of NY has branches scattered throughout the five boroughs. Other institutes include the Bank Street Col. of Education, Kingsborough Comm. Col., Hebrew Union Col.-Jewish Institute of Religion, Jewish Theological Seminary of America, Fordham U, Juilliard School, St. John's U, Pace U and Yeshiva U. NYC has the largest school system of any urban center in the world. The public school system consists of about 900 schools enrolling half a million children. Lib. facilities are provided by the American Museum of Natural History, the Engineering Society Lib., the Fed. Reserve Bank of NY Lib., the Gen. Society of Mechanics and Tradesmen Lib., the Grolier Club Lib., the Mercantile Lib. Assn., the Met. Museum of Art Lib., the Municipal Reference and Research Center, the NY Academy of Medicine, the NYC Lawyers Assn., the NY Historical Society Lib., the NY Law Institute Lib., the NY Public Lib., Time Inc. Lib. and Yivo Institute for Jewish Research Lib.

ENTERTAINMENT.
There are several annual events in NYC. Old Home Day in Oct. is held in Staten Island, The Atlantic Antic Street Festival is held in Oct., St. Jude's Feast in October in Brooklyn, the fall flower shows at the Queens Botanical Gardens, Newport Jazz Festival, Natl. Horse Show and New Years Eve in Times Square. Parades include Pulaski Day, Columbus Day, United Hispanic American Day, Ragamuffin Parade in Brooklyn and the Massing of the Colors are all held in Oct. and Macy's Thanksgiving Day Parade. Two pro-baseball teams, the Yankees (AL) and the Mets (NL) compete in NYC. The city is home of the the Giants (NFL-NFC) and the Jets (NFL-AFC) football teams. The Knickerbockers (NBA) play basketball, while the Cosmos play soccer and the Islanders and the NY Rangers of the NHL play hockey. The NYC Apples play in the World Team Tennis League. Collegiate sports are highlighted by the NYC Violets, the Columbia U Lions, the Fordham U Rams, Hunter Col. Hawks, the City of NY Bees and the Kingsborough Comm. Col. Lions. The city is the home of the US Soccer Federation Hall of Fame. The annual horse race, the Belmont Stakes, is held in NYC.

ACCOMMODATIONS.
NYC hotels and motels include the Hilton, Marriott's Essex, Park Land, St. Moritz On-the-Park, Barbizon Plaza, Sheraton, Carlyle, Drake, Loew's Summit, Hotel Pierre, Regency,

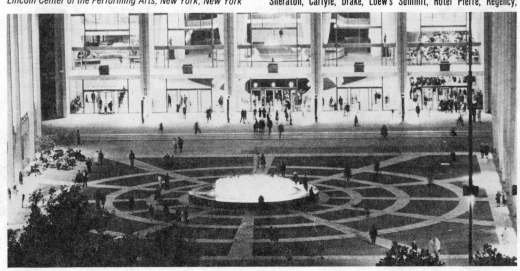

Lincoln Center of the Performing Arts, New York, New York

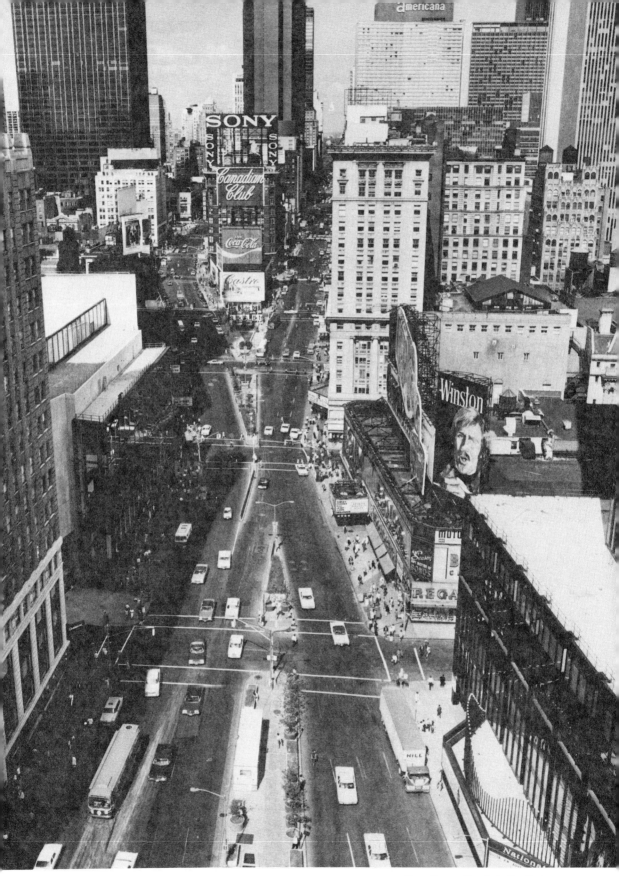

Times Square, New York, New York

St. Regis Sheraton, Sherry Netherland, United Nations Plaza, Waldorf-Astoria, Westbury, Warwick, Windsor, Statler Hilton, Sheraton Russell, Algonquin, Americana of NY, Howard Johnson's, Travelodge, Holiday, Sheraton, Ramada, Rodeway and Quality inns.

FACILITIES. There are 1,100 parks in the city park system covering nearly 27,000 acres, including Central, Van Corlandt, Prospect, Flushing Meadows-Corona and Bronx parks. Central Park contains 840 acres of wooded and landscaped grounds, lakes, two outdoor skating rinks, a swimming pool, a merry-go-round, and a children's zoo. Biking is popular in the park and horseback riding trails are available. Prospect Park contains a zoo, Quaker graveyard, gardens, trails, and boating facilities on its 526 acres. Flushing Meadows-Corona Park was the site of NYC's World Fairs in 1939-40 and 1964-65. Featured are bicycle paths, a boat lake, carousel, fresh water fishing facilities and pitch and putt golf, and an indoor ice-skating rink. In addition, there are picnic grounds, a marina, pony rides, an outdoor swimming pool, baseball, cricket, football and softball fields and boccie and tennis courts. NY Zoological Park houses the Bronx Zoo and botanical gardens. Brooklyn has botanic gardens and another zoo can be found on Staten Island. There are several beaches available, including Coney Island, Manhattan Beach, Rockaway Beach and S Beach. Also, there is the Gateway Natl. Recreation area, a 26,172 acre park along the Hudson River. There are 107 tennis courts in nine locations in Manhattan. There are no golf courses in Manhattan, although 12 18-hole public courses are available in other parts of NYC.

CULTURAL ACTIVITIES. With more than 120 museums, 400 art galleries and 35 Broadway theaters. NYC is an undisputed cultural center. The performing arts are well represented at the $185 million Lincoln Center for the Performing Arts. The 14-acre site contains many educational and artistic institutions, including Alice Tully Hall, home of the Chamber Music Society of Lincoln Center; Avery Fisher Hall, housing the NY Philharmonic Orchestra; Juilliard School, a world-famous music school; the NY Public Lib. at Lincoln Center, housing material on performing arts and a small auditorium; NY State Theatre, home of the NYC Ballet and the NYC Opera; and the Vivian Beaumont Theatre and the Mitzi E. Newhouse Theatre, maintained by the NY Shakespeare Festival at the Lincoln Center. During the 1978-79 season some 9.8 million people attended Broadway theaters. Local theaters include the Brooklyn Academy of Music, Chelsea Theatre, Opera House and Music Hall. Many of the most prominent theatrical companies have performed at the Brooklyn Academy of Music including the Royal Shakespeare Co. Cherry Lane Theatre, the oldest in NY, is located in Greenwich Village. A well-known "off-Broadway" theater, it presents a variety of shows. Other theaters include Joseph Papp's Public Theatre in the E Village, the Manhattan Theatre Club, the Gramercy Arts Institute, the Sullivan Street Playhouse and the Village Gate. The Theater Development fund operates "TKTS" booths in Duffy Square, where half-price same-day-of-performance tickets may be purchased. Free theater is offered by the Delacorte Theatre with Shakespearean performances in Central Park and Theatre-in-the-Black at the Brooklyn Museum. The Met. Museum, one of the largest in the world, houses extensive collections on Near East, Egyptian, Greek, Roman, European and American arts. The Solomon R. Guggenheim Museum, designed by Frank Lloyd Wright, features exhibits of lesser-known artists, in addition to its permanent displays. The Museum of Modern Art houses collections of sculpture, design, drawing, prints, photography and films. The Whitney Museum of American Art features contemporary American sculpture, paintings and watercolors. The American Museum of Natural History has an extensive display on the origin of man. Museums specializing in ethnic art include the African-American Institute; the Asia House Gallery, featuring four exhibitions of Asian art annually; Japan House; Museum of American Folk Art; the Jewish Museum, featuring relics from the early Middle Ages and Jacques Marchais Center of Tibetan Art, housing Tibetan Buddhist art. An indoor-outdoor museum, S St. Seaport, includes several blocks on the E River waterfront which are being restored to their appearance during the early port days. It contains historic ships, a printing shop, a market and a lighthouse. The Frick Collection contains paintings, antiques and furnishings of Henry Clay Frick. The Brooklyn Museum houses an Egyptian collection and an outdoor sculpture garden. Other museums located in the Bronx include the Bronx Museum of the Arts,

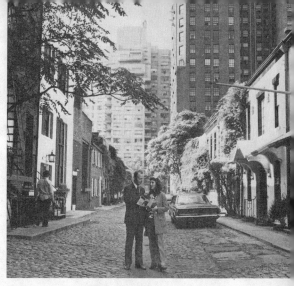

Greenwich Village, New York, New York

City Island Historical Nautical Museum, Museum of Bronx History and Museum of Migrating People. Midtown museums include Kodak Gallery and Photo Info Center and the Museum of Broadcasting. The Cloisters located at Washington Heights, is devoted to medieval art. Staten Island Museums include Staten Island Institute of Arts and Sciences, Garibaldi Meucci Museum, Snug Harbor Cultural Center and Staten Island Children's Museum. The Hall of Science, Jamaica Arts Center, Queens Museum and Storefront Museum/Paul Roberson Theatre are located in Queens.

LANDMARKS AND SIGHTSEEING SPOTS. Among the numerous sightseeing spots in NYC is the City Hall, in Lower Manhattan, which has been the seat of NYC municipal govt. since 1811. It is near the site where, on presence of Gen. Washington. Fed. Hall Natl. Memorial on the site of the presence of Gen. Washington. Fed. Hall Natl. Memorial is on the site of the first US Capitol, contains George Washington memorabilia and includes the site where Washington was inaugurated. The first American War Dept. was housed in Fraunces Tavern, a neo-Georgian structure built in 1719. George Washington and Gov. George Clinton had personal pews at St. Paul's Chapel, which was dedicated in 1766. Commemorating the alliance of France and the US during the American Revolution, France presented the Statue of Liberty to the US in 1884. The Statue of Liberty Natl. Monument measures 152' high and stands on a 150' pedestal, making it the tallest statue of modern times. Ellis Island was the first stop for over 12 million European immigrants during a wave of European immigration between 1892 and 1924. The Theodore Roosevelt Birthplace Natl. Historic Site contains many relics relating to the only Pres. born in NYC. Alexander Hamilton and Robert Fulton are buried at Trinity Church. Although it was originally built in 1697, the current edifice was completed in 1846. Trinity Church was the original location of King's Col., now Columbia U. Lower Manhattan is also the location of WA Square, containing designer Stanford White's WA Arch. A 13th-century Gothic-style structure, St. Patrick's cathedral is one of the largest churches in the US and the seat of the Roman Catholic Archdiocese in NY. The largest synagogue in the world, Temple Emanu-el, was built in 1845. Built in 1783, Dyckman House is the only remaining Dutch farmhouse on Manhattan Island. The Gen. Grant Natl. Memorial houses the graves of Pres. Ulysses S. Grant and his wife. Built in 1765, the historical Morris-Jumel Mansion served as Army headquarters for Washington in 1776. The Riverside Church is home to a 74-bell Laura Spelman Rockefeller Carillon. The Bronx is home to Poe Cottage, the home of Edgar Allen Poe from 1846 until his death in 1849. It is furnished from Poe's time and contains some of his possessions. In the Brooklyn area, the Lefferts Homestead contains relics of colonial and Revolutionary America. Abolitionist Henry Ward Beecher pastored Plymouth Church of the Pilgrims. Its windows depict the history of Puritanism. The Staten Island Conference House (1680) was the location where Benjamin Franklin, John Adams and Edward Rutledge met with Gen. Howe to discuss peace before the Revolutionary War. One can find Delacorte geyser in the E River, which expells purified water 400' in the air. The Hayden Planetarium features presentations and lectures on astronomy. NY Aquarium houses marine life in indoor and outdoor pools near the Coney Island Amusement Park. Known as the city's Bohemian center, Greenwich

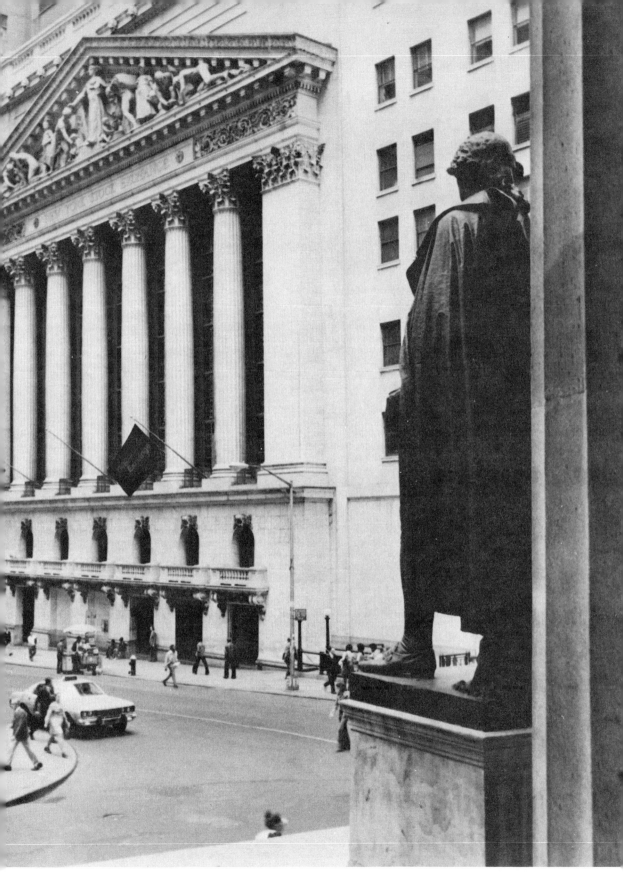

Stock Exchange, New York, New York

Village is famous for its old houses, landmarks, shows, shops and restaurants. The twin towers (110 stories) of the World Trade Center are the second tallest buildings in the world. The famous Empire State Building is one of the world's largest office buildings. Now more than 40 years old, it soars 1,472' upward. The Rockefeller Center includes the Plaza, the RCA Building (with a 70th floor observation deck), a theater and NBC studios. The United Nations Headquarters contains several buildings, a conference building and the Hammarskjold Lib. The public may attend the official meetings of the United Nations.

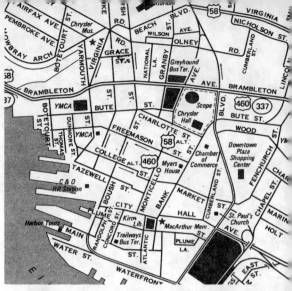

Norfolk, Virginia

NORFOLK
VIRGINIA

CITY LOCATION-SIZE-EXTENT. Norfolk, an indep. city and the largest city in the state encompasses 64 sq. mi., including 12 sq. mi. of waterways in SE VA 150 mi. S of Washington, D.C., it is at 36°51'N lat. and 26°17'W long. Norfolk, Portsmouth to the SW and VA Beach to the SE comprise a met. area. Chesapeake is S of the city, which is bordered on the W by the mouth of the Elizabeth River, on the NW by Hampton Roads, an arm of Chesapeake Bay, on the N by Chesapeake Bay and on the E by the Atlantic Ocean.

TOPOGRAPHY. The terrain of Norfolk, which is located in the VA tidewater region of the Atlantic Coastal Plain, and almost completely surrounded by water, is generally low and flat. There are several rivers in the area, including the James, Lafayette and Nonsemone. The mean elev. is 12'.

CLIMATE. The climate of Norfolk, due to its flat terrain, is modified marine, characterized by mild winters, long, warm summers and pleasant spring and fall. The avg. annual temp. of 60°F ranges from a Jan. mean of 41°F to a July mean of 78.6°F. Rainfall is heaviest during the summer and avgs. 45" annually. Most of the avg. annual snowfall of 7.2" occurs in Jan. and Feb. The city is located S of the usual path of N storms. The RH ranges from 50% to 80% and the growing season avgs. 244 days. Norfolk is in the ESTZ and observes DST.

FLORA AND FAUNA. Animals native to Norfolk include the whitetail deer, squirrel, raccoon and opossum. Common birds include the warbler, vireo, gull, tern and egret. Bullfrogs, tree frogs, diamond-back terrapins, toads, and salamanders, as well as venomous water moccasins, canebreak rattlesnakes and copperheads are found in the area. Typical trees are the oak, elm and sweetbay. Smaller plants include the arrowhead, dogwood (the state flower), blue-eyed grass, rose gentian and vervain.

POPULATION. According to the US census, the pop. of Norfolk in 1970 was 307,951. In 1978, it was estimated that it had decreased to approx. 286,000.

ETHNIC GROUPS. In 1978, the ethnic distribution of Norfolk was approx. 69.9% Caucasian, 28.3% Black, 1.6% Hispanic and .2% other.

TRANSPORTATION. Interstate hwys. 64 and 564, US hwys. 60, 58 and state hwys. 165, 44, 168 and 170 provide major motor access to Norfolk. *Railroads* serving the city are AMTRAK, the Chessie System, Fruit Growers Express, Norfolk & Portsmouth, Norfolk & Western, Seaboard Coast, Southern and the VA & MD. *Airlines* serving Norfolk Intl. Airport include NA, US Air, PI, UA, PA, TW, EA, NW and Skyline. The Port of Norfolk, with a 45' deep channel serves 35 steamship companies with 12 gen. cargo warehouses.

COMMUNICATIONS. Communications, broadcasting and print media originating from Norfolk are: *AM radio stations* WTAR 790 (CBS, MOR); WRAP 850 (Natl. Blk., Contemp.); WCMS 1050 (Indep., C&W); WZAM 1110 (Indep., Progsv. Ctry.) and WNOR 1230 (ABC/C, MBS, Contemp.); *FM radio stations* WTGM 89.5 (NPR, Clas., C&W); WKEZ 95.7 (Indep., Btfl.

Mus.); WNOR 98.7 (ABC/C, MBS, AOR); WYFI 99.7 (Indep., Relig.); WECMS 100.5 (Indep., C&W); WOWI 102.9 (Mut. Blk., Jazz, Top 40,) and WORK 104.5 (Indep., Top 40); *television stations* WTAR Ch. 3 (CBS); WAVY Ch. 10 (NBC); WVEC Ch. 13 (ABC); WHRO Ch. 15 (PBS) and cable; *press* two major daily publications serve the city the *Ledger-Star*, issued evenings, and the *VA Pilot*, issued mornings; other publications include the *Mace and Crown, Metro, Magazine of SE VA, Journal and Guide Tidewater Motorists, Tidewater VA* and *VA Ports*.

HISTORY. Native Americans of the Pouhatan tribe inhabited the area of present day Norfolk before the first white settlers arrived. In 1680, upon orders from England, Norfolk was established by the VA Gen. Assembly as a port to serve ships from England and the W Indies. Two years later, the colonial govt. purchased the parcel from Nicholas Wise, a planter, for $400 worth of tobacco (five tons). By the early 1700s marine trade and commerce with area plantations flourished. In 1736, Norfolk was chartered as a borough by King George II, and a local govt. was establised. Gov. of VA ordered his ships to bombard the borough after British control was repudiated. Although much of Norfolk was destroyed by the citizens themselves to prevent it from falling in the hands of the British it gradually recovered, aided by the establishment of a shipyard at Gosport (now the Norfolk Naval Shipyard). A British blockade of the city again resulted in economic hardship. Norfolk was incorporated as a city in 1845. By 1855, the pop. of the city had reached 15,000, and a yellow fever epidemic forced 10,000 to evacuate for several months, while more than 1,500 of those remaining died. As an important shipping and naval base, Norfolk was an object of contention during the Civil War. In 1862, the Confed. ironclad *Virginia* (formerly, the *Merrimac*), which was built at the shipyard, fought the *Monitor* in Hampton Roads. Post-war reconstruction initiated slow economic development. During WW I, a Naval Base constructed in the area in stimulated the city's economy and created thousands of new jobs. During WW II, more people came to the city to work at the Naval Shipyard and the expanded base. From 1940 to 1950, the pop. of the city grew from 144,300 to more than 213,500. In 1951, the city undertook an urban renewal project, which included replacing slums.

GOVERNMENT. The city of Norfolk has a council-mgr. form of govt. Seven councillors, who elect one of their number to serve a two-year term as mayor, are elected at large to four-year terms. A mgr. is appointed to administer city govt.

ECONOMY AND INDUSTRY. Services and wholesale and retail trade each employ approx. 25% of the total work force of the greater Norfolk met. area, followed by manufacturing (approx. 15%). The Norfolk Naval Base, headquarters for the Atlantic Command of the N Atlantic Treaty Organization (NATO), is the largest naval installation in the US. More than 300 manufacturing plants produce chemicals, metal, electrical, building and food products among others. In June 1979, the labor force of the Norfolk-VA Beach-Portsmouth met. area was approx. 326,300, while the rate of unemployment was 6.3%.

BANKING. There are 11 banks and eight savings and loan assns. in Norfolk. In 1978, total deposits for the eight banks headquartered in the city were approx. $2,907,735,000, while total assets were $3,419,035,000. Among the banks serving the city are VA Natl., United VA, Seaboard Natl., Fidelity American, First VA of Tidewater, Commonwealth and Heritage Bank and Trust.

HOSPITALS. There are several gen. care hosps. in Norfolk, including De Paul Leigh Memorial, Medical Center and Norfolk Gen.

EDUCATION. Norfolk State U, a state-supported institution granting associate, bachelor and master degrees was founded in 1935 as a division of VA Union Col. More than 7,200 students enrolled in 1978. Old Dominion U, a state-supported institution established in 1930 as a branch of the Col. of William and Mary, offers associate, bachelor and master degree programs. In 1978, nearly 14,200 enrolled VA Wesleyan Col., chartered in 1961 and affiliated with the Methodist Church, offers liberal arts programs leading to bachelor degrees. In 1978, approx. 750 enrolled. Other institutions include E VA Medical School the newest in the State, Keels Business Col. and Tidewater Broadcasting School. There are approx. 55 elementary, 10 jr. high and five sr. high schools in the public school system. Lib. facilities include the Norfolk Public Lib.

ENTERTAINMENT. Among the annual events held in Norfolk are the Azalea Festival, the Harborfest, which takes place in June and the VA Festival of Performing Arts, held in July. Professional sports entertainment is provided, the Tidewater Tides, a farm club of the NY Mets baseball organization, which plays in the IL, collegiate sports entertainment is provided by the Norfolk State U Spartans. The Tidewater Dinner Theater also offers entertainment.

ACCOMMODATIONS. There are several hotels and motels in Norfolk,

Adam Thoroughgood House, built 1636 Norfolk, Virginia

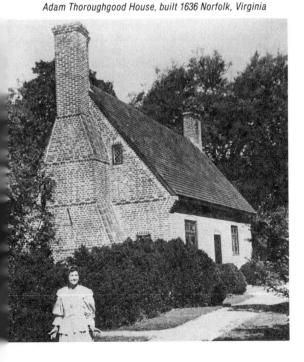

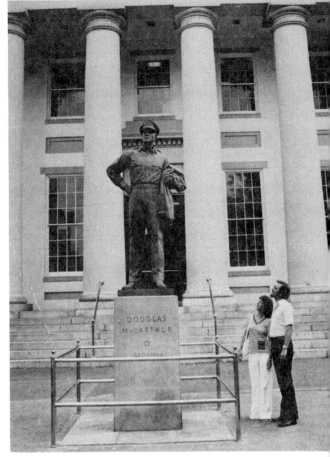

Douglas MacArthur Memorial, Norfolk, Virginia

including the Omni Intl., Lafayette, Bel Air, VA Reel and the Holiday, Quality, Ramada and Sheraton inns.

FACILITIES. The park system in Norfolk consists of four parks and three playgrounds and includes one outdoor, and three indoor swimming pools, five public golf courses, including the 105-acre Ocean View, and 150 tennis courts. The 55-acre Lafayette Zoological Park houses more than 350 animals including a pair of rare S white rhinos in natural settings. Norfolk Gardens by-the-sea, located on a 175-acre site, offers 12 mi. of boating, hiking and trackless train as well as picnic areas. There are several beaches for swimming and sunning, including Ocean View, Sarah Constant, Comm. and City.

CULTURAL ACTIVITIES. Performances of the Norfolk Symphony, as well as Broadway shows and ballet and other musical productions, are held at Chrysler Hall, part of SCOPE, the city's new cultural and convention complex. The Chrysler Museum contains a vast comprehensive collection of art which includes treasures from every period in civilization. The Hermitage Foundation Museum, located in a mansion on the banks of the Lafayette River and surrounded by 12 wooded and landscaped acres, houses collections of oriental and W art.

LANDMARKS AND SIGHTSEEING SPOTS. Gen. Douglas MacArthur, the youngest gen. in WW I, is honored by a memorial encompassing an entire city block in Norfolk. It contains many of his medals, war souvenirs, mementos, personal papers and grave. The Moses Meyers House, built in 1729 by one of the first American millionaires, and visited by such historical figures as James Monroe, Daniel Webster and the Marquis de Lafayette, contains more than half of the original furnishings. The Adam Thoroughgood House, built in 1636, is the oldest brick home in the US. St. Paul's Church (1739), the only one that survived the bombardment and subsequent destruction of the city on Jan. 1, 1776, features a cannonball fired by Lord Dunmore during that battle.

OAKLAND
CALIFORNIA

CITY LOCATION-SIZE-EXTENT. Oakland, the seat of Alameda Co., encompasses 53.4 sq. mi. (including 27 mi. of bay coastline) on the E shore of the San Francisco Bay in W central CA at 37°44' N lat. and122°12' W long. Connected to San Francisco, across the bay, by the San Francisco-Oakland Bay Bridge, the city is part of the San Francisco-Oakland met. area. Oakland is separated from Alameda on the W by the Oakland Inner Harbor, while San Leandro lies to the S and Berkeley lies to the N.

TOPOGRAPHY. Oakland is situated in a crescent-shaped section of a broad valley between the San Francisco Bay on the W and the Pacific coastal hills on the N and E. The largest urban salt water lake in the country, Lake Merritt, is located in the city. The elev. of the area ranges from 0' at the shoreline to 1900' in the San Leandro Hills E of Oakland. The mean elev. is 6'.

CLIMATE. The climate of Oakland is marine, influenced by the prevailing W winds from the Pacific Ocean and characterized by mild and moderately wet winters and cool, dry summers. Monthly mean temps. range from 48.1°F in Jan. to 64.4°F in July, with an annual avg. of 57.1°F. There is only slight temp. variation from month to month and daily temps. above 90°F are rare. Approx. 90% of the avg. annual rainfall of 17.75" occurs from Nov. through Apr. The RH ranges from 63% to 84%. Oakland lies in the PSTZ and observes DST.

FLORA AND FAUNA. Animals native to Oakland include the pocket gopher, deer, skunk, coyote and opossum. Common birds include the gull, egret, great blue heron, housefinch and mourning dove. Gopher snakes, alligator lizards, pond turtles, red-legged frogs and the venomous Pacific rattlesnake are also found in the area. Typical trees include the oak, hickory, eucalyptus and pine. Smaller plants include the chaparral shrub, manzanita, bunch grass, brodeia, creamcup and poppy (the state flower).

POPULATION. According to the US census, the pop. of Oakland in 1970

Oakland, California

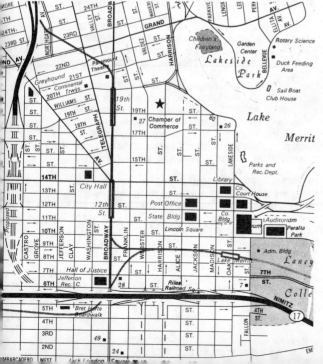

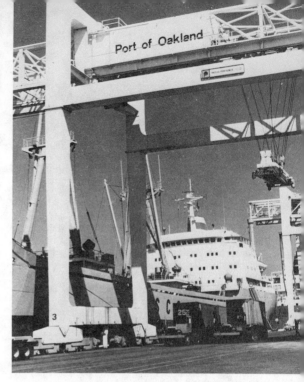

Port of Oakland, California

was 361,561. In 1978, it was estimated that it had decreased to 333,055.

ETHNIC GROUPS. In 1978, the ethnic distribution of Oakland was approx. 46.1% Caucasian, 44.7% Black, 2.2% Hispanic and 7.0% Asian.

TRANSPORTATION. Interstate hwys. 80 and 580 and state hwys 13, 17, 24, 61, 123 and 185 provide major motor access to Oakland. *Railroads* serving the city include AMTRAK, S Pacific and Santa Fe. *Airlines* serving Oakland Intl. Airport include Pacific SW, AA, DL, RW, TW, UA and WA. *Bus lines* serving the city include Greyhound, Trailways, Peerless Stages, AC Transit, Golden West and the San Francisco Bay Area Rapid Transit (BART), which is headquartered in Oakland. The Port of Oakland is one of the world's largest container ports.

COMMUNICATIONS. Communications, broadcasting and print media originating from Oakland are: *AM radio stations* KNEW 910 (ABC/E, MBS, C&W); KABL 960 (Indep., Btfl. Mus.) and KDIA 1310 (Indep., Blk.); no *FM*; *television stations* KTVU Ch. 2 (Indep.); *press*: one major daily serves Oakland, the *Tribune*, issued evenings; other publications include *Montclarion, Oakland Post, CA Voice, Rural American, Piedmont/Oakland Bulletin, Walnut Kernel, Oakland Post Enquirer, Oakland Times Journal, El Mundo* and *Oakland Magazine*.

HISTORY. Native Americans of the Costanoan tribe inhabited the area of present-day Oakland when Spanish explorers arrived during the 1770s. The city was founded in the late 1840s, during the CA gold rush, when prospectors settled in an area which had once been part of an 1820 Spanish land grant to Luis Maria Peralta. The city was incorporated in 1852 and in 1869, a RR from the E arrived, producing a pop. increase. After the 1906 earthquake in San Francisco, some 65,000 fled that city and settled in Oakland. The Bay Bridge opened in 1936, linking San Francisco and Oakland. During WW II, Oakland became an important port and two shipbuilding industries were established. In 1972, the Bay Area Rapid Transit System began operations from Oakland, while a route from the city to San Francisco was established in 1974.

GOVERNMENT. Oakland has a council-mgr. form of govt. The nine council members, including the mayor as a voting member, are elected at large to four-year terms.

ECONOMY AND INDUSTRY. Traditionally a center of manufacturing, distribution, retail trade and medical care, Oakland is a rapidly developing port and ship-building point. Govt. and service are major employers. Processed foods are the major manufactured products, followed by fabricated metals, transportation equipment, non-electrical machinery, apparel and printed materials. The labor force for the Oakland met. area totaled 176,800 in 1978, while the rate of unemployment was 8%.

BANKING. There are 17 banking institutions in Oakland. In 1978, total deposits for the two banks headquartered in the city were $500,132,000, while assets were $555,293,000. Banks include Central, First Enterprise, Crocker, Barclay and Union.

HOSPITALS. There are several hosps. in Oakland, including Children's, Merritt, Highland, Alta Bates and Peralta.

EDUCATION. The Peralta Comm. Col. District has two cols. in Oakland, Merritt and Laney. The publicly-supported cols. award associate degrees. In 1978, Laney Col. enrolled more than 12,000, while Merritt Col. enrolled more than 9,000. Mills Col., a private liberal arts col. which enrolls only women in its undergrad. programs, was founded in 1852 and moved to its present site in 1871. In 1978, the col. enrolled approx. 1,000. Other educational institutions include Vista Col., Holy Names Col., E Bay Skills Col. and Law School of Marine Engineering. There are 60 elementary, 14 jr. high and eight sr. high schools in the public school system. Libs. include the Oakland Public Lib. and the Asian Comm. and Latin American libs.

ENTERTAINMENT. Annual events in Oakland include the Children's Easter Egg Roll in the City Hall Plaza and the Oakland Flower Show, the Greek Festival and the Art Auction and Sale in May. Professional sports entertainment is offered by the Raiders of NFL-AFC football, the A's of AL baseball, the Golden State Warriors of basketball and the Golden Gators of WTT tennis, while the Laney Col. Eagles and the Merritt Col. Thunderbirds participate in intercollegiate sports.

ACCOMMODATIONS. There are several hotels and motels in Oakland, including the Oakland Airport Hilton, Oakland Hyatt, Holiday Inn and the Best Western Thunderbird Lodge.

FACILITIES. There are 64 parks in the 45,000-acre Oakland park system, including E Bay Regional, Joaquin Miller, Lakeside and Knowland. The Oakland Zoo at Knowland Park features a zoo-fari, an aerial tram and a children's zoo. Flowers are exhibited at the Morcum Amphitheatre of Roses. Lake Merritt, in the heart of Oakland, is a 155-acre body of salt water which offers tree-shaded paths and the Lakeside Park Garden Center. Golf courses can be found at Galbraith, Montclair, Oak Port and Lake Chabot Municipal golf courses, while tennis courts are available at the Davie Tennis Stadium. A jogging track is provided at Lake Merritt.

CULTURAL ACTIVITIES. The Paramount Theatre of the Performing Arts hosts many of Oakland's cultural offerings. Among the city's cultural organizations are the Oakland Symphony Orchestra, Oakland Ballet Co., Met. Ballet, Oakland Ensemble Theatre, Oakland City Theatre, The Actors' Society Intl. and the Oakland Youth Chorus. Museums in the city include the Rogues Gallery, CA Col. of Arts, the E. B. Negro Historical Society, Patti McClain's Museum of Vintage Fashions, Art Gallery (on Mills Col. campus)

Mills College, Oakland, California

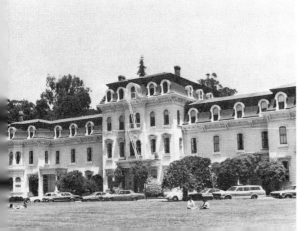

and Kaiser Center. The Oakland Museum houses displays on CA art and history.

LANDMARKS AND SIGHTSEEING SPOTS. Jack London, a popular turn-of-the-century writer who lived in Oakland, has a square named for him. Located at Jack London Square are restored shops and houses, including Heinold's First and Last Chance Saloon, the author's favorite hangout. Similarly honored is author Bret Harte, another native of Oakland. A row of Victorian homes housing shops and restaurants stand on Bret Harte Boardwalk. Another Oakland landmark is the Mormon Temple, atop a hill with beautifully landscaped grounds.

OKLAHOMA CITY
OKLAHOMA

CITY LOCATION-SIZE-EXTENT. OK City, the capital of the state and the seat of OK Co., encompasses 621.4 sq. mi. (ranking among the three largest cities in the nation in area) along the N Canadian River near the geographical center of OK at 35°24' N lat. and 97°37' W long. The greater met. area extends into the counties of Logan to the N, Kingfisher to the NW, Canadian to the W, Grady to the SW, McClain to the S, Cleveland and Pottawatomie to the SE and Lincoln to the NE.

TOPOGRAPHY. The terrain of OK City, which is situated in

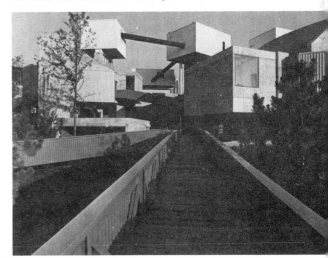

Oklahoma Theater Center, Oklahoma City, Oklahoma

the Red Beds plains, is gently rolling, while the nearest hills or low mts. lie 80 mi. to the S. There are numerous lakes in the area, including Hefner, Overholser, Thunderbird and Stanley Draper. The mean elev. is 1,207'.

CLIMATE. The climate of OK City is continental, characterized by short, mild winters and long, usually hot summers. Monthly mean temps. vary from 37°F in Jan. to 81°F in July and Aug., with an annual avg. of 60°F. Most of the annual avg. rainfall of 31.5" occurs during late spring, summer and early fall. The snowfall avgs. 9.2" annually. The RH ranges from 46% to 85%. The growing season avgs. 220 days. OK City lies in the CSTZ and observes DST.

FLORA AND FAUNA. Animals native to OK City include the armadillo, rabbits, squirrels, opossum, raccoon, skunk, beaver and coyote. Common birds include the scissor-tailed flycatcher (the state bird), bluebird, mockingbird and cardinal. Horned lizards, collared lizards, mud turtles and

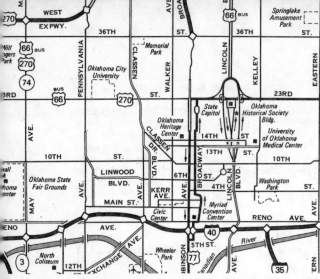

Oklahoma City, Oklahoma

king snakes, as well as the venomous rattlesnake and copperhead, are found in the area. Located on the W edge of the Cross Timber Region, the area's trees include the cottonwood, sycamore, oak, pine, elm, redbud (the state tree) and dogwood trees. Smaller plants include the bluestem, sunflower and mistletoe (the state flower).

POPULATION. According to the US census, the pop. of OK City in 1970 was 368,164. In 1978, it was estimated that it had increased to 379,800.

ETHNIC GROUPS. In 1978, the ethnic distribution of OK City was approx. 83.45% Caucasian, 14.0% Black, 2.19% Indian and 0.36% other.

TRANSPORTATION. Interstate hwys. 35, 40 and 240, US hwys. 62, 66, 77 and 270 and state hwys. 3 and 74 provide major motor acces to OK City. *Railroads* serving the city include Santa Fe, Frisco, Katy and Rock Island. *Airlines* serving Will Rogers World Airport include AA, BN, TI, CO, FL and TW. *Bus lines* serving the city include Greyhound, Trailways, MK & O, Mid-Continent and the OK Transportation Co.

COMMUNICATIONS. Communications, broadcasting and print media originating from OK City are: *AM radio stations* KQVC 800 (Indep., Relig.); KBYE 890 (APR., Relig.); WKY 930 (Indep., Progsv.); KTOK 1000 (ABC/I, MOR); KATT 1140 (Indep., AOR); KOCY 1340 (CBS, C&W) and KOMA 1520 (Indep., Contemp.); *FM radio stations* KKNG 92.5 (Indep., Btfl. Mus.); KEBC 94.7 (ABC/E, C&W); KXXY 96.1 (Indep., Contemp.); KTLS 98.9 (Indep., Blk.); KATT 100.5 (Indep., AOR); KFNB 101.9 (Indep., Btfl. Mus.); KZUE 102.7 (Indep., MOR); KOFM 104.1 (Indep., Adult Rock) and KAEZ 107.7 (Indep., Btfl. Mus.); *television stations* KTVY Ch. 4 (NBC); KOCO Ch. 5 (ABC); KWTV Ch. 9 (CBS); KETA Ch. 13 (PBS); KGMC Ch. 34 (Indep.); KOKH Ch. 25 (Indep.) and cable; *press*: three major dailies serve the city, the *OK Journal* and the *Oklahoman*, issued mornings and the *Times*, issued evenings; other publications include *Capitol Hill Beacon, N Star Advertiser, Friday, OK Union Farmer, Outdoor OK, Persimmon Hill, Black Dispatch, OK Sports, OK Business, OK Monthly* and *OK Living*.

HISTORY. Native Americans of the Cherokee, Chickasaw, Choctaw, Creek and Seminole tribes inhabited the area of present-day OK City before white settlers arrived. When Pres. Benjamin Harrison opened up the area to the famous Land Run on April 22, 1889, a tent city of nearly 10,000 was established at the site in a single day, and 10 days later an unofficial township organization had been established. The city was incorporated in 1890. The first municipal water well was completed shortly after 1900 to ease water scarcity in the rapidly expanding city. By 1910, OK City was the largest city in the state, with a pop. of more than 64,000, and had replaced Guthrie as the OK state capital. Four RR companies served the city during this time. In 1919, the Lake Overholser Reservoir was completed and by 1920 the pop. stood at more than 91,000. The Post Office officially adopted the name OK City in 1923. In 1928, an economic boom began with the discovery of oil in the

city, which became a center of the petroleum industry, as many oil firms erected refineries in the area. Tinker AFB, the largest aircraft supply and repair depot in the world, was constructed during WW II. During the post-war years, iron, steel, electronic and aviation industries were established in the city. Through annexation of surrounding areas, OK City expanded from approx. 310 sq. mi. in the early 1960s to approx. 635 sq. mi. in 1970. In 1965, internationally known architect I. M. Pei presented a plan for redevelopment of the central business district and work on this project continued into the 1970s. In 1979, a major automotive manufacturing plant was established in the city.

GOVERNMENT. OK City has a council-mgr. form of govt. The eight council members are elected by district to a four-year term. The mayor, elected at large to a four-year term, is a voting member of council.

ECONOMY AND INDUSTRY. Petroleum is the major industry in OK City, with more than 2,000 wells adjoining or within city limits. Other major industries include agriculture, the manufacture of fabricated metal products, electronics, meatpacking, food processing and distribution. Tinker AFB is the largest employer in the city, while the Fed. Aviation Administration at Will Rogers World Airport is another major employer. Approx. 27% of the city labor is employed by fed. and state govt. In 1978, the avg. household income was $15,694. The total labor force for the met. area in June, 1978, was 405,800, while the rate of unemployment was 3.2%.

Buffalo Bill Monument, Oklahoma City, Oklahoma

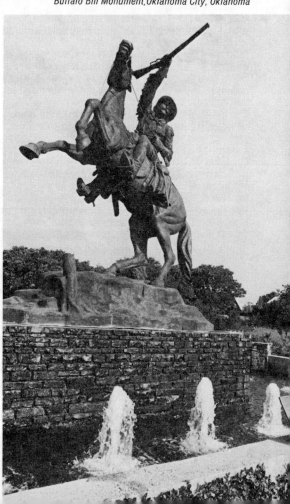

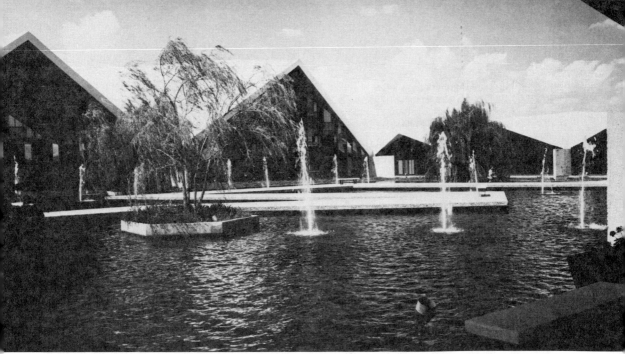

National Cowboy Hall of Fame, Oklahoma City, Oklahoma

BANKING. In 1978, total deposits for the 30 banks headquartered in OK City were $3,648,284,000, while assets were $4,534,543,000. Banks include First Natl. Bank & Trust, Liberty Natl. Bank & Trust, Fidelity, Citizens Natl. Bank & Trust, Union Bank & Trust, United OK, Penn Square, Central Natl., Guaranty Bank & Trust and Central Natl.

HOSPITALS. There are several hosps. in OK City, including St. Anthony, Presbyterian, University, Deaconess, Mercy Health Center, Baptist Medical Center, the V.A. Hosp., Children's Memorial and S Comm. Hosp.

EDUCATION. The U of OK Health Center, established at Norman in 1900 and merged with Epworth Medical Col. in OK City in 1910, awards grad. degrees in medical science, public health, nursing and pharmacy at the OK City HSC campus. In 1978, it enrolled approx. 2,500. The OK State U Technical Institute at OK City enrolled more than 2,000 in 1978. Other educational institutions include OK Christian Col., OK City U, S OK City Jr. Col., SW Col. and Midwest Christian Col. Teaching and research institutions include OK Medical Research Foundation, St. Anthony's Hosp., Children's Hosp., OK U Health Sciences Center and Dean McGee Eye Institute. There are approx. 105 public schools and 15 private and parochial schools in OK City. Libs. include the OK Met. System, OK State, U of OK and OK Historical Society Archives.

ENTERTAINMENT. Among the dinner theaters in the city are Star Supper Club and Gaslight Dinner Theatre. Annual events in OK City include the Festival of Arts, Fall Festival, OK State Fair and Exposition in Sept. and Natl. Finals Rodeo (the "World Series of Rodeo") in Dec. The Stars of CHL hockey and the 89ers of AA baseball provide professional sports entertainment, while the OK U Sooners, the OK State U Cowboys and the OK City U Chiefs participate in intercollegiate sports.

ACCOMMODATIONS. There are numerous hotels and motels in OK City, including Sheraton Century Center, Skirvin Plaza and Holiday, Ramada, Best Western, Southgate and Lincoln Plaza inns.

FACILITIES. There are approx. 128 parks in OK City, covering 3,500 acres. Among the larger parks are Will Rogers, Trosper, Martin Park Nature Center, Lincoln and Myriad Gardens. The 632-acre Lincoln Park, the largest, houses the OK City Zoo. The zoo contains more than 400 animal species, a survival center for rare, hoofed animals, a children's zoo with baby animals and a herpetarium with reptile displays. Lakes Hefner, Overholser and Stanley Draper offer fishing and boating. Lincoln Park also contains a lake. Golf courses can be found at Lincoln, Earlywine, Hefner and Trosper Lake, while a jogging track is provided at Memorial Park. The downtown revitalization plan will include a riverfront park.

CULTURAL ACTIVITIES. In the heart of the city is the six-block-long Civic Center, the home of the OK City Symphony and the Lyric Theatre of OK City U. The Church of Tomorrow maintains a theatre-in-the-round. On display at the W Heritage Center are paintings and sculptures depicting the American W. Exhibits in the OK Historical Society Building and Museum trace the history of the state. The Kirkpatrick Planetarium is part of the OK Science and Arts Foundation. Other museums include the OK Art Center, OK State Firefighters' Museum and the Omniplex, a science museum.

LANDMARKS AND SIGHTSEEING SPOTS. The OK Heritage Center, located in OK City, was once the home of Judge R. A. Hefner. Among other antiques, the structure houses a Louis XVI salon table. At the S entrance of the State Capitol, an adaptation of Roman Corinthian architecture, stands the "Statue of a Cowboy" by Constance Warren. The Natl. Cowboy Hall of Fame, also located in the city, honors the cowboy and his contribution to the development of the W. The hall features recreations of Indian and pioneer villages, mining and trapping scenes and the James Fraser sculpture, "The End of the Trail".

OMAHA
NEBRASKA

CITY LOCATION-SIZE-EXTENT. Omaha, the state's largest city, encompasses 83 sq. mi. in Douglas Co. at 41°18' N lat. and 95°54' W long. The met. area extends N into Washington Co., S into Sarpy Co. and E across the MO River to Council Bluff, IA in Pottawattamie Co.

TOPOGRAPHY. Omaha is situated on rolling hills in the Till Plains region of E NE on the W bank of the MO River. The area is cut by many streams and glacial residues are exposed. The mean elev. is 1,040'.

CLIMATE. The climate of Omaha is continental. The avg. annual temp of 50°F ranges from a Jan. mean of 20°F to a July mean of 76.5°F. Approx. 75% of the annual avg. rainfall of 29" occurs during Apr. through Sept. Snowfall avgs. 29" per year. The RH ranges from 49% to 87%. The avg. growing season lasts 188 days. Omaha lies in the CSTZ and observes DST.

FLORA AND FAUNA. Animals native to Omaha are the whitetail deer, raccoon, muskrat, rabbit and squirrel. Typical birds include the meadowlark, swallow, pheasant and night hawk. Reptiles and amphibians include the bull frog, skink, salamander, painted turtle, and the venomous copperhead and E massasauga (a pygmy rattler) are common to the area. Typical trees include the cottonwood, oak and elm. Smaller plants include the buttercup, bluebell, ironweed and blue sedge.

POPULATION. According to the US census, the pop. of Omaha in 1970 was 358,452. In 1978, it was estimated that it had increased to 375,400.

ETHNIC GROUPS. In 1978, the ethnic distribution of Omaha was approx. 89.3% Caucasian, 9.6% Black and 3.6% Hispanic (a percentage of the Hispanic total is also included in the Caucasian total).

TRANSPORTATION. Interstate hwys. 29, 80, 480 and 680, US hwys. 34, 75 and 275 and state hwys. 36, 92, 183 and 191 provide major motor access to Omaha. *Railroads* serving the city include AMTRAK, Burlington N, Chicago and NW, IL Central Gulf, KC S, LA & AR, MO Pacific, Rock Island and Union Pacific lines. *Airlines* serving Eppley Airfield are AA, BN, EA, FL, NC, OZ, UA TW, Pioneer and Air Nebraska. *Bus lines* include the local Metro Area Transit and the inter-city Stage, Greyhound and Trailways.

COMMUNICATIONS. Communications, broadcasting and print media originating from Omaha are: *AM radio stations* WOW 590 (ABC/C, MOR); KOWH 660 (ABC/E, Relig.); KFAB 1110 (NBC, Progsv.); KOIL 1290 (Indep., Top 40); KOOO 1420 (CBS, UPI, Talk) and KYNN 1490 (MBS & C&W); *FM radio stations* KVNO 90.7 (MBS, Fine Arts); KEZO 92.3 (Indep., MOR); KOWH 94.1 (ABC/E, Blk.); KEFM 96.1 (Indep., C&W); KGOR 99.9 (Indep., Var.); KGBI 100.7 (Indep., Relig.) and KOOO 104.5 (CBS, UPI., MOR); *television stations* KMTV Ch. 3 (NBC); WOWT Ch. 6 (CBS); KETV Ch. 7 (ABC) and KYNE Ch. 26 (PBS); *press:* one major daily serves the area, *World-Herald*, published mornings and afternoons; other publications include *Daily Record, The Catholic Voice, Everybody, Omaha Profile, Midlands Busn. Journal, German Tribune, Omaha Magazine, Star, Spectacle Magazine* and *The Sun.*

HISTORY. The first inhabitants of the Omaha area included the Otoe and the Omaha native Americans. Following a treaty between the US govt. and the Omaha tribe, Omaha was founded in 1854 by a land development co. The site had served as winter quarters for the Mormons during 1846-47. Pushing W to UT, they fell victim to the bitter cold and 600 died there. Several years after Omaha's founding, Pres. Lincoln designated it as the point from which the transcontinental RR should start W. The Union Pacific began its construction in 1863. Omaha was selected capital of the NE Territory in 1855. (Lincoln later became state capital.) The city was incorporated in 1857. The discovery of gold in CO gave an impetus to Omaha's growth as it was a supply center for people heading W. The development of the meat processing industry and the building of the Union stockyards in 1884 further increased the pop. After the turn of the century, a number of small factories opened. In 1948, the city was

Father Flanagan Statue in front of Boystown, Omaha, Nebraska.

selected as headquarters for the Strategic Air Command. Today, Omaha ranks as the world's largest cattle market and serves as a trading center.

GOVERNMENT. Omaha has a mayor-council form of govt. The mayor and seven council members are elected to four-year terms. The mayor is not a member of the council and votes only to break a tie.

ECONOMY AND INDUSTRY. Among US cities, Omaha is ranked first in meat processing, second in the production of frozen foods, fourth in RR activity and first in reservation services. The city has nearly 670 manufacturing concerns and its principal activities are meat packing, food processing and telephone communications. Services, retail trade and manufacturing employ nearly 59.6% of the total labor force. In June, 1979, the met. labor force was 279,000, while unemployment was 4.9%.

BANKING. In 1978, total deposits for the 20 banks headquartered in Omaha were $1,924,959,000, while assets were $2,371,721,000. Banks include Omaha Natl., First Natl. of Omaha, NW Natl., Center and Packers Natl. in Omaha.

HOSPITALS. Omaha has many medical facilities, including Archbishop Bergen Mercy, Clarkson Memorial, Douglas Co., NE Methodist, St. Joseph, U of NE Medical Center, Lutheran Medical Center, NE Psychiatric Institute, Childrens Memorial and Immanuel Medical Center. The Boys Town Institute for Communication Disorders in Children is also located here.

EDUCATION. Eight cols. and universities are located in Omaha. Among them is the U NE at Omaha. Founded in 1908 as Omaha U, this institution became part of the state U system in 1968. Granting degrees from associate's to master's, the U enrolled 14,696 students in 1978. The U NE Medical Center includes the Col. of Med., Nursing and Pharmacy and Grad. Col., as well as the School of Allied Health Professions. The 1978 enrollment was 1,896. Creighton U, a coed. facility operated by the Jesuits, offers programs leading to degrees from bachelor's to doctoral. In 1978, enrollment was 4,979. The Col. of St. Mary, a private independent liberal arts school for women, was founded by the Sisters of Mercy in 1923 and offers both the associate and bachelor's degrees. In 1978, this col. enrolled 540 students. Other institutions include Grace Col. of the Bible, Bellevue Col., Met. Technical Comm. Col., NE Col. of Business, Omaha Col. of Health Careers, and Universal Technical Institute. Omaha public schools serve approx. 50,000 students in eight high, 13 jr. high and 73 elementary schools. The Omaha Public Lib., with its nine branches and several bookmobiles, serve the city.

ENTERTAINMENT. Entertainment in Omaha includes the Midtown Upstairs Supper Theater and the Firehouse Dinner Theater. Annually, the city hosts the Omaha Marathon and two other 26-mile runs. In Sept. the

Omaha, Nebraska

AK-Sar-Ben Rodeo and Livestock show takes place. Omaha is the home of the Royals, the AAA farm club of the KC Royals baseball team. The U of NE and the Creigton U Blue Jays compete in intercollegiate sports. The Col. World Series in baseball is held every June at Rosenblatt Stadium.

ACCOMMODATIONS. Omaha has numerous hotels and motels, including the Granada Royale Hometel, Omaha Hilton, Howard Johnson's, Tower, Holiday, Sheraton and Ramada inns.

FACILITIES. There are 120 parks covering 6,000 acres in Omaha. The largest parks include Levi Carter, Dodge, Marina and Benson. The park system provides 140 tennis courts, a public indoor tennis center, 20 outdoor swimming pools and two indoor swimming pools, two ice arenas, nine fulltime recreation centers, nine golf courses, 100 ball fields, three marinas, a stadium, a trap and skeet range and numerous bike and jogging trails. The 100-acre Henry Doorly Zoo includes some 500 mammals and a rare cat collection. Neale Woods is owned by Fontenelle Forest Nature Center and provides hiking trails for weekend outings. The Peony Amusement Park has a pool, a half-mile of sandy beach, an artesian well, an outdoor pavillion, an indoor ballroom, banquet and party facilities, a games gallery and dozens of amusement rides. The MO River, Carter Lake and Lake Manawa are a few of the areas available for boating and sailing recreation during the summer months.

CULTURAL ACTIVITIES. The Omaha Musicians Assn. sponsors summertime concerts in parks and downtown areas. Opera Omaha, the Symphonic Chorus and the NE Wind Symphony all present regular performances. The Joslyn Art Museum presents its chamber music series in the Witherspoon Concert Hall at the museum, and also presents a dance series. Other dance performers include the Omaha Ballet, Dance Theatre '76 and Creighton U's A Company of Dancers. Major performances are held in the Ak-Sar-Ben Coliseum, the City Auditorium and Music Hall and the Orpheum Theater. Theaters in the city include the Chanticleer Comm. Theater, Eppley Little Theater, NE Theater Caravan, Offutt Theater Guild, Comm. Playhouse the Omaha Jr., Magic, U and Rudyard Norton theaters. The Joslyn Art Museum houses a permanent visual arts collection encompassing 50 centuries of art. Other galleries include the Artists' Cooperative, Gallery '72, Creighton, the U of NE at Omaha and the Old Market Craftsmen's Guild. The Great Plains Black Museum features Black history exhibits. The Puppet Theater Museum also offers classes in puppetry. Other museums include the Strategic Aerospace, Union Pacific RR Historical and W Heritage museums.

LANDMARKS AND SIGHTSEEING SPOTS. Serving as a natl. landmark for Omaha is Boys Town. Here hundreds of underprivileged and homeless boys run a comm. govt., a Boys Town lib., farm, and dairy. Ft. Omaha, built in 1868, is a natl. landmark. Other landmarks designated in the Natl. Register of Historic Places include the Burlington Building. City Natl. Bank, Orpheum Theater, Omaha Building, Astro-Riviera Theater, Union Depot, Burlington Station, Grace Bible Institute, Aquila Court, Fontenelle Bank, Old Log Cabin, Hamilton House, Burlington Depot, Gen. Crook House, Bank of Florence, G. Barton House, Gottlieb Horz House and Joslyn Castle. Other interesting landmarks include Douglas Co. Courthouse, Pioneer Mormon Cemetery, Florence Mill, Waterworks, Mercer Mansion, Cecilia's Cathedral and the Gerald Ford Birthsite.

Courtyard in Joslyn Art Museum, Omaha, Nebraska.

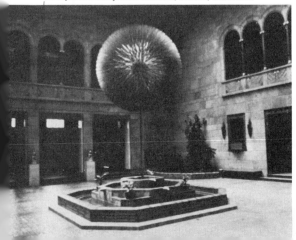

ORLANDO
FLORIDA

CITY LOCATION-SIZE-EXTENT. Orlando, the seat of Orange Co., encompasses 42.87 sq. mi. (including 51.99 mi. of shoreline) at the heart of the "Sunshine State" in central FL at 28°32' N lat. and 81°22' W long. The greater met. area includes Walt Disney World and extends into the counties of Osceola to the S and Seminole to the N.

TOPOGRAPHY. The terrain of Orlando, which is situated in the central section of the FL peninsula, is gently rolling. The city encompasses 69 lakes, including Lakes Orlando, Turkey and Underhill. The mean. elev. is 109'.

CLIMATE. The climate of Orlando is subtropical marine, characterized by a high RH year round. The avg. annual

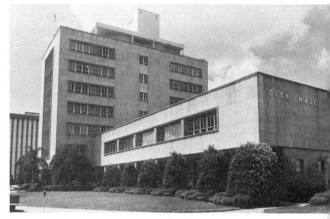

City Hall, Orlando, Florida

temp. of 72.5°F varies from a monthly mean of 60.7°F in Jan. to 82.4°F in Aug. The avg. annual rainfall of 50.26" occurs mainly during the summer months, with July being the wettest month and Nov. the driest. The RH ranges from 45% to 92%. Orlando lies in the ESTZ and observes DST.

FLORA AND FAUNA. Animals native to Orlando include the shrew, opossum and skunk. Common birds are the bluejay, grackle, tern, gull and egret. Frogs, toads, newts, sirens and terrapins, as well as the venomous coral snake, rattlesnake and water mocassin, are found in the area. Typical trees include the oak and cypress. Smaller plants include the yucca, palmetto and mangrove.

POPULATION. According to the US census, the pop. of Orlando in 1970 was 99,006. In 1978, it was estimated that it had increased to 122,090.

ETHNIC GROUPS. In 1978, the ethnic distribution of Orlando was approx. 70.2% Caucasian, 29.5% Black and 0.3% other.

TRANSPORTATION. Interstate hwy. 4, US hwys. 17, 92 and 441 and state hwys. 50 and 436 provide major motor access to Orlando. *Railroads* serving the city include Seaboard Coastline, AMTRAK and Auto-Train. *Airlines* serving Orlando Intl. Airport include DL, EA, SO, NA and RD. Herndon Airport, a 1,000-acre facility near downtown Orlando, services private and corporate planes. *Bus lines* serving the city include Greyhound, Trailways and the local Orange-Seminole-Osceola Transit Authority.

COMMUNICATIONS. Communications, broadcasting and print media originating from Orlando are: *AM radio stations* WDBO 580 (CBS, MOR); WKIS 740 (Indep., MOR); WLOF 950 (Indep., Top 40); WHOO 990

(ABC/I, Mod. Ctry.) and WMJK 1220 (Indep., Span.); *FM radio stations* WDBO 92.3 (Indep., Btfl. Mus.); WHOO 96.5 (NBC, Contemp., Btfl. Mus.); WDIZ 100.3 (ABC/C, Top 40) and WBJW 105.1 (Indep., Btfl. Mus.); *television stations* WESH Ch. 2 (NBC); WDBO Ch. 6 (CBS); WFTV Ch. 9 (ABC); WMFE, Ch. 24 (PBS) and WSWB Ch. 35 (Indep.); *press:* one major daily serves the city, the *Sentinel Star*, printed mornings; other publications include *Times, The FL Catholic, Central FL Scene, Avi-ation Journal, FL Aviation News, Orlando-Land, SE Dairy Review* and *Walt Disney World News.*

HISTORY. During the Seminole Wars (1835-1842), US soldiers camped near the site of present-day Orlando on the shores of Lake Cherokee. There during the night, according to legend, a young sentry named Orlando Reeves fired a warning shot to alert his sleeping comrades. Reeves was killed by the Seminoles, but the army successfully defended the camp and later buried Orlando under an oak tree on the S bank of Lake Eola. Among the earliest settlers to arrive at the end of the wars was Aaron Jernigan, who arrived in 1842. By 1850, a post office had been established under the name Jernigan near Ft. Gatlin. In 1857, B. F. Caldwell deeded the land known as Orlando's Grave to Orange Co. to establish a village and the town was named

Central Orlando, Florida

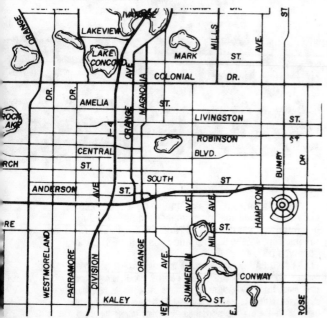

Orlando. The first courthouse opened in 1863 under a confed. flag and the city was incorporated in 1875. The citrus industry accounted for Orlando's first economic boom, with the first citrus nursery and the first commerical grove planted in the same year. A RR link with Sanford provided an outlet to N markets in 1880. A fire destroyed portions of the business district in 1884. On Feb. 4, 1885, Orlando received a city charter. The citrus boom was brought to a halt by the Great Freeze of 1895 and the farmers who remained grew other crops. Orlando experienced another upturn in its economy during the land speculation rush of the 1920 s, but the economy declined during the Great Depression. An economic revival and a pop. increase resulted from the 1950s opening of a space center (currently called Kennedy Space Center). Between 1950 and 1960 the

pop. of Orlando increased 124%. The 1971 opening of Disney World made the city a major tourist center.

GOVERNMENT. Orlando has a mayor-council form of govt. The six council members are elected by district to four-year terms. The mayor, elected at large to a four-year term, is a voting member of council.

ECONOMY AND INDUSTRY. Walt Disney World is the major employer in the area, which also has a massive agric. industry, including crop production, chemical, container and fertilizer manufacturing, marketing, distribution and other agribusiness industries. Since 1970, more than 300 manufacturing companies have opened or expanded in the area, while more than 150 electronics firms are located in the city. The city is also one of the SE's major insurance centers. The met. area labor force totaled 319,500 in June, 1979, while the rate of unemployment was 5.9%. The city ranked 39th of 40 large met. areas in cost of living in 1978.

BANKING. There are 35 commercial banks in Orlando. In 1978, total deposits for the 11 banks headquartered in the city were $1,023,227,000, while assets were $1,227,826,000. Banks include Sun First Natl., SE Natl., Pan Am, FL Natl., Atlantic and Landmark.

HOSPITALS. There are several hosps. in Orlando, including Orlando Gen., Mercy, Orlando Regional Medical Center, FL, Lucerne, Winter Park Memorial and Parkland Health Center.

EDUCATION. The state-controlled U of Central FL, located in Orlando, awards associate, bachelor and master degrees. It was established in 1963 and, in 1978, it enrolled more than 10,000. Valencia Comm. Col. awards associate degrees and, in 1978, it enrolled approx. 9,000. Other institutions include Central FL Bible Col., Charron Williams Col., Jones Col., Mid-FL Technical Institute and Data Processing Institute S Col. The Orlando public school system enrolls approx. 127,000. There are 14 parochial and 22 private schools in the area. Libs. include the Orlando Public Lib. and the Law Lib. in the County Courthouse.

ENTERTAINMENT. Once Upon a Stage Dinner Theatre offers dining entertainment in Orlando. The city annually hosts the PGA Citrus Open Golf Tournament and, in Dec., the football Tangerine Bowl. Spring training camps for baseball's AL MN Twins and Soccer's NAHL N.E. Tea Men are located in the city. The U of Central FL Knights participate in intercollegiate sports.

ACCOMMODATIONS. The opening of Disney World spawned unprecedented growth in the accommodations of Orlando, which is now sixth in the world in the number of hotel-motel rooms with 31,000 rooms. Included are the Orland Marriott, Red Carpet, Howard Johnson's, TraveLodge, Hotel Royal Plaza, Best Western, Econo-Inn, Days Lodge, Rodeway and Sheraton, Gold Key, Quality, Holiday, Knight, Dutch, Day's, 1776 Resort and Ramada inns.

FACILITIES. There are several city parks in Orlando, including Audubon, Turkey Lake, Moss, Azalea, Delaney, George Barker and Mathews. Flowers and other botanical specimens are on view at the Harry P. Leu Botanical Gardens. Lake Eola Park, located in the central city, offers landscaped acres and a lake. Rented paddle boats are available. A private golf course is available at a local country club and public golf course locations include a golf club and Fairways and Dubsdread golf courses. Private tennis courts can be found at several locations and public tennis courts are available at a local golf and tennis club.

Municipal Auditorium, Orlando, Florida

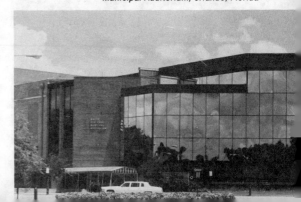

CULTURAL ACTIVITIES The Mayor Bob Carr Auditorium hosts Broadway shows and ballet performances. It is also used by the FL Symphony for concerts. Church Street Station is a block long entertainment complex in Orlando featuring Dixieland jazz, singing bartenders and dancing waiters. The Loch Haven Art Center and Maitland Art Center feature art exhibits. Specialized museums reflect Orlando's economic bases in tourism, entertainment and industry. Among these are the Cartoon Museum, the Six Flags Star Hall of Fame, the Tupperware Food Container Museum and the Shell Museum. Located near the Orlando Intl. Airport, an aviation and automotive museum, Wings and Wheels, opened in 1979.

LANDMARKS AND SIGHTSEEING SPORTS. Circus World, located in Orlando, is a Ringling Bros. and Barnum & Baily entertainment center which features more than 50 human and animal performers. Sea World, the world's largest and most elaborate marine park, includes Japanese and Hawaiian villages and performing sea animals. Orlando also offers the Seminole Harness Raceway, Ben White Raceway, a harness racing training facility and the Orlando-Seminole Jai-Alai Fronton. Walt Disney World is approx. 16 mi. SW of Orlando.

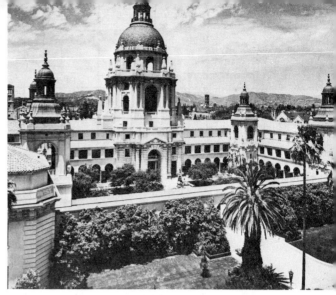

City Hall, Pasadena, California

PASADENA
CALIFORNIA

CITY LOCATION-SIZE-EXTENT. Pasadena encompasses 35.85 sq. mi. in LA Co., 10 mi. NE of LA, in W central CA at 34°8' N lat. and 98°5' W long. The city is part of the LA met. area and neighboring cities include Glendale to the W, S Pasadena to the S and Arcadia to the E.

TOPOGRAPHY. The terrain of Pasadena, which is situated in the LA ranges, consists of a slightly hilly area in the foothills of the San Gabriel Mts., overlooking the San Gabriel Valley. The mean elev. is 864'.

CLIMATE. The climate of Pasadena is marine, influenced primarily by prevailing westerlies. The avg. annual temp. of 64°F ranges from monthly means of 56°F in Jan. to 72°F in July. Daily temps. may vary as much as 30°F, producing warm to hot afternoons and cool to cold evenings. Nearly 85% of the annual avg. of 20" of rainfall occurs during the winter months. The RH ranges from 45% to 84%. Pasadena lies in the PSTZ and observes DST.

FLORA AND FAUNA. Animals native to Pasadena include the coyote, pocket gopher, opossum and the skunk. Common birds include the W kingbird, lesser goldfinch, scrubjay, housefinch and hummingbird. Garter snakes, alligator lizards, skinks, horned lizards and the venomous Pacific rattlesnake are found in the area. Typical trees include the fir, oak and pine. Smaller plants include the CA golden poppy, chaparral shrub, bunch grass and geranium.

POPULATION. According to the US census, the pop. of Pasadena in 1970 was 113,000. In 1978, it was estimated that it had decreased to 106,700.

ETHNIC GROUPS. In 1978, the ethnic distribution of Pasadena was approx. 60% Caucasian, 19% Black, 17% Hispanic and 4% other.

TRANSPORTATION. Interstate hwys. 210 (Foothill Frw.) and state hwys. 134 (Ventura Frw.), 11 (Pasadena Frw.) and 7 (Long Beach Frw.) provide major motor access to Pasadena. *Railroad* service is provided by AMTRAK. All major *airlines* serve the airports in the area, including Burbank-Glendale-Pasadena, LA Intl. and Ontario Intl. *Bus lines* serving the city include Trailways and Greyhound.

COMMUNICATIONS. Communications, broadcasting and print media originating from Pasadena are: *AM radio stations* KRLA 1100 (Indep., Contemp.); KPPC 1240 (Indep., Relig., Ethnic) and KWKW 1300 (Indep., Span., Var.); *FM radio stations* KPCS 89.3 (NPR, Var.) and KROQ 106.7 (Indep., AOR); no *television stations* originate from Pasadena, which receives broadcasting from the LA met. area; *press*: one major daily serves the area, the *Star-News*, issued mornings and evenings; other publications include the *Chronicle*, *Gazette* and *Plain Truth*.

HISTORY. In 1771, Spanish priests established the San Gabriel Mission on the site of present-day Pasadena. In 1874, the Indiana Colony headed by Thomas Elliott, purchased land which was once part of the mission and called the new community the IN Colony. The name was changed in 1875 to Pasadena, a Chippewa word meaning "crown of the valley". Incorporated in 1886, Pasadena received its city charter in 1901. The Tournament of Roses Parade was first held in 1890, and the following year, Throop U (now the CA Institute of Technology) was established. Today, Pasadena is the home of the Rose Bowl and the suburban retail center for the San Gabriel Valley.

GOVERNMENT. Pasadena has a council-mgr. form of govt. The seven council members are elected by district to four-year terms. The mayor, a voting member of council, is elected by the council from within its membership and serves a one-year term.

ECONOMY AND INDUSTRY. Aerospace is the major industry in Pasadena. Major manufactured products include cameras, precision instruments, ceramics, optical instruments, chemicals, electronics, pharmaceuticals, apparel, printed materials and cosmetics. The Sept., 1978, Pasadena labor force was estimated at 58,853, while the rate of unemployment was 4.6%.

BANKING. There are nine commericial banks and 17 savings and loan assns. in Pasadena. In 1978, total deposits for the only bank headquartered

Public Library, Pasadena, California

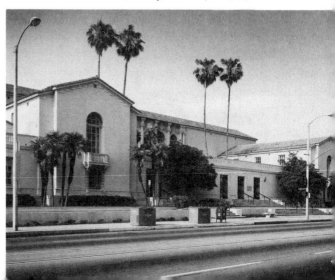

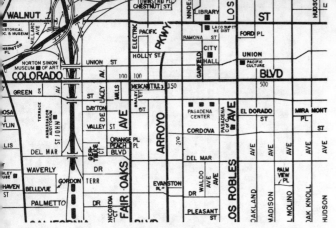

Pasadena, California

PASADENA
TEXAS

in Pasadena were $21,66,000, while assets were $24,579,000. The bank is Citizens Commercial Trust and Savings.

HOSPITALS. There are three gen. hosps. in Pasadena including, St. Lukes, Huntington Memorial and Pasadena Comm.

EDUCATION. The CA Institute of Technology, located in Pasadena, is ranked among the top 10 research institutes in the nation. Founded in 1891 as a school of arts and crafts, it currently offers grad. and undergrad. degrees. Six alumni of the institute have received Nobel prizes. In 1978, the institute enrolled more than 1,600. Pasadena City Col., awarding associate degrees, enrolled more than 18,800 in 1978. Other institutions include Pacific Oaks Col., American Academy of Dramatic Arts-W, Art Center Col. of Design, Pasadena Col. of Chiropractic and Fuller Theological Seminary. There are 17 public elementary schools, five public high schools and 28 parochial schools in the city. Libs. include the public lib. and its eight branches.

ENTERTAINMENT. The most famous annual event in Pasadena is the Tournament of Roses, which features a nationally-televised parade with flower-decorated floats, and the Rose Bowl football game, a New Year's Day competition between col. teams of the Big 10 and the PAC 10. The CA Institute of Technology Beavers participate in intercollegiate sports.

ACCOMMODATIONS. There are three hotels and 11 motels in Pasadena, including the Hi-Way Host Motel, Holiday Inn, Huntington-Sheraton, Pasadena Hilton and Vagabond Motor Hotel.

FACILITIES. There are 24 parks and 33 playgrounds in Pasadena. Public golf courses are located at Brookside and Eaton Canyon, while public tennis courts are available at many of the parks and campuses. Riding facilities can be found at a local stable. Lower Arroyo Park offers a nature trail and archery ranges.

CULTURAL ACTIVITIES. The Norton Simon Museum of Art, located in Pasadena, exhibits tapestries, sculpture and paintings dating from the 15th century. The Pacific Culture Asia Museum houses historical, cultural and art exhibits of the Far E and Pacific. Exhibits are also housed at the Huntington Lib. Art Gallery.

LANDMARKS AND SIGHTSEEING SPOTS. Constructed in Pasadena in 1908, Gamble House is a bungalow-style home with sculptured woodwork, hand-shaped beams and projecting rafters. The Tournament House, a mansion once owned by William Wrigley, Jr., features memorabilia of notable Rose Bowl events.

Gamble House, Pasadena, California

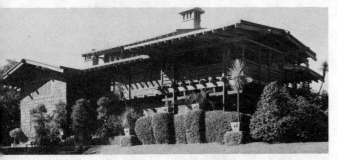

CITY LOCATION-SIZE-EXTENT. Pasadena encompasses 55 sq. mi. of Harris Co. in SE TX, bordering Houston and the Houston Ship Channel, at 29°42' N lat. and 95°12' W Long. It is part of the greater Houston met. area.

TOPOGRAPHY. The terrain of Pasadena, which is situated in the SE Gulf Coastal Plain, is low and flat. Nearby bodies of water include Pasadena, Clear and Taylor lakes and Galveston Bay. The mean elev. is 32'.

CLIMATE. The climate of Pasadena is predominantly marine, characterized by the mild winters, cool summer nights and plentiful rainfall produced by SE and S prevailing winds. Monthly mean temps. range from 50°F in Jan. to 82°F in July, with an avg. annual temp. of 68°F. The avg. annual rainfall of 50" is evenly distributed throughout the year. Thundersqualls and tropical storms occasionally pass through the city. Air pollution is a climatic factor, but is usually swept away by prevailing winds, Light fog occurs approx. 62 days each year. The RH ranges from 57% to 94%. Pasadena lies in the CSTZ and observes DST.

FLORA AND FAUNA. Animals native to Pasadena include the opossum, armadillo, raccoon and the swamp rabbit. Common birds are the cardinal, mockingbird (the state bird of TX), egret, nighthawk and purple martin. The venomous copperhead, water moccasin, coral snake and rattlesnake are also found in the area. Typical trees are the mulberry, live oak, palm, pine, pecan (the state tree of TX), hickory, elm and tallow. Smaller plants include the bluebonnet (the TX state flower), Indian paintbrush, black-eyed Susan, dewberry, blackberry, amaryllis and azalea.

POPULATION. According to the US census, the pop. of Pasadena in 1970 was 89,277. In 1978, it was estimated that it had increased to 118,000.

ETHNIC GROUPS. In 1978, the ethnic distribution of Pasadena was approx. 86.9% Caucasian, 0.1% Black, 12.6% Hispanic, 0.1% Asian and .3% other.

TRANSPORTATION. Interstate hwy. 610 and state hwys. 8, 146 and 225, 246, E Beltway 8 and Spencer Hwy. provide major motor access to Pasadena. *Railroads* serving the city include Port Terminal RR, S Pacific and Santa Fe. All major *airlines* serve the area through the Houston Intercontinental and Hobby airports. *Bus lines* include TX and Greyhound.

COMMUNICATIONS. Communications, broadcasting and print media originating from Pasadena are: *AM radio station* KLVL (Indep., Span.); *FM radio stations* KYND 92.5 (Indep. Btfl. Mus.) and KIKK 95.7 (Indep., C&W); although no *television stations* originate from Pasadena, broadcasting is received from Houston; *press*: one major daily serves the area, the *News Citizen*, issued mornings; the *Pasadena Press* is published weekly.

HISTORY. Pasadena was founded in 1895 by Col. J. H. Burnett. The city was incorporated in 1928. Within the city limits of Pasadena is the site of the Battle of San Jacinto. On this site outnumbered Texans, under Gen. Sam Houston, defeated Gen. Santa Ana's Mexican regular army on Apr. 21, 1836. The defeated army returned to Mexico and the new Republic of TX was born. Today, Pasadena is a major center of the petrochemical industry.

GOVERNMENT. Pasadena is a Home-Rule Charter city with a mayor-council form of govt. The mayor, is elected to a four-year term, while the six councilmen, two of whom are elected at large and four by district, serve two-year terms.

ECONOMY AND INDUSTRY. Pasadena is a major center of the petrochemical industry. Tire production, research, electronics and food processing are also important

industries. In 1978, the avg. per capita income of
Pasadena was $21,000, the highest in the nation. The
total labor force of the greater met. area was 60,593,
while the rate of unemployment was approx. 3.4%.

BANKING. In 1978, total deposits for the four banks headquartered in
Pasadena were $320,669,00, while assets were $356,802,000. Banks include
First Pasadena State, San Jacinto State, Pasadena Natl. and TX
Independence.

HOSPITALS. There are five hospitals in Pasadena, Southmore, Bayshore,
Strawberry Clinic, Pasadena Gen. and Memorial.

EDUCATION. The U of Houston, a publicly supported institution,
maintains a campus in Pasadena. San Jacinto Jr. Col. is a publicly supported
two-year institution offering associate degrees. Enrollment in 1978 was
approx. 9,900. TX Chiropractic Col., established in 1908, offers professional
degrees and enrolled approx. 300 in 1978. There are 40 public schools in the
city including 4 sr. high, 9 intermediate and 27 elementary schools which
enrolled approx. 38,000 in 1978. There are approx. 10 to 15 private schools
in the city. Libs. include the Pasadena Public Lib. and San Jacinto Lib.

ENTERTAINMENT. Festivals and annual events in Pasadena include the
Pasadena Youth Rodeo, Pasadena Annual Rodeo, Strawberry Festival, Silver
Slipper Revue and the Special Olympics. Another main attraction is the
world-famous Gilley's Club—the largest country and W nightclub as noted
in the *Guiness World Book Of Records.*

ACCOMMODATIONS. There are several motels and inns in Pasadena,
including the Ramada and Rodeway inns and the Tropicana Motel.

FACILITIES. There are five comm. parks in Pasadena, including
Strawberry, Memorial, Red Bluff, Sunset and Armand Bayou. Three
ecological zones are represented at Armand Bayou Park—the piney woods,
the Gulf Coast prairie and the salt marsh. A municipal golf course is located
N of Ellington AFB. Jogging tracks are located in Memorial Park, Pasadena
Auxiliary Stadium and Deepwater School.

CULTURAL ACTIVITIES. The Pasadena Little Theater stages dramatic
productions, while the Pasadena Municipal Band presents musical and
dramatic performances throughout the year. The Pasadena Art Assn.
sponsors exhibits. Other museums include the Parks House and Historical
museums.

LANDMARKS AND SIGHTSEEING SPOTS. The San Jacinto
Monument commemorates the famed battle between Mexican forces
directed by Gen. Santa Anna and the TX army under Gen. Sam Houston,
which led to TX independence. The Pasadena Freedom Trail contains 37

Central Pasadena, Texas

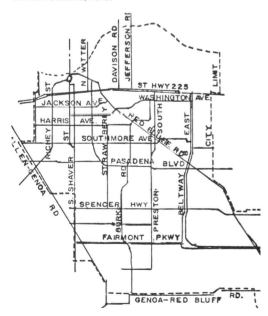

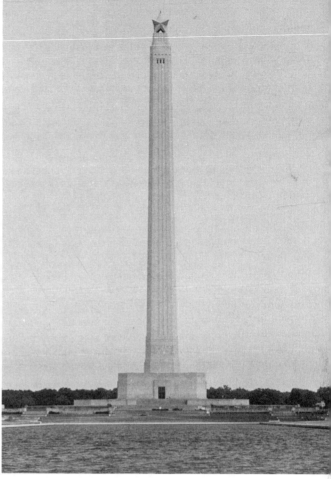

San Jacinto Monument, Pasadena, Texas

historical markers designating significant moments in TX history. A
survivor of two WWs and many campaigns, the battleship *Texas* was
presented to TX by the US Navy and brought to Pasadena by the nickels and
dimes of TX school children. The Port of Houston on Pasadena's N boundary
also includes large industrial plants and is a popular sightseeing spot.

PATERSON
NEW JERSEY

CITY LOCATION-SIZE-EXTENT. Paterson, the seat of Passaic Co., is located at the falls of the Passaic River,
encompassing 8.4 sq. mi. at 40°55' N lat and 74°10' W
long. The city is 12 mi. N of Newark and 12 mi. NW of
NYC. Its met. area includes Clifton to the S and
Fairlawn to the NE.

TOPOGRAPHY. Paterson is located in the Piedmont area
of NJ. This area is characterized by low hills and rolling
terrain. The mean elev. is 100'.

CLIMATE. The climate of Paterson is continental, characterized by marine influences. Monthly mean temps.
range from 32°F during Jan. to 76°F during July, with
an avg. annual of 54°F. The avg. annual rainfall is 43".
Most of the avg. annual snowfall of 29" occurs during
Dec. through Mar. The RH ranges from 48% to 80%. The
avg. growing season is approx. 200 days. Paterson is in
the ESTZ and observes DST.

FLORA AND FAUNA. Animals native to Paterson include the raccoon,
squirrel and rabbit. Common birds include the robin, goldfinch (the state
bird), starling and cardinal. Salamanders, frogs rat snakes, garter snakes

and the venomous timber rattlesnake and copperhead, are also found here. Typical trees include the oak, pine, elm and maple. Smaller plants include the violet, Queen-Anne's lace, rhododendron and rose.

POPULATION. According to the US census, the pop. of Paterson in 1970 was 144,824. In 1978 it was estimated that it had increased to 154,256.

ETHNIC GROUPS. In 1978, the ethnic distribution of Paterson was approx. 72.5% Caucasian, 26.9% Black, and 8.2% Hispanic. (A percentage of the Hispanic total is also included in the Caucasian total.)

TRANSPORTATION. Interstate hwy. 80, US hwy. 46, and state hwy. 23 and Garden State Parkway provide major motor access to Paterson. *Railroads* serving the city include *AMTRAK, ConRail* and *Morris Central.* All major *airlines* serve the nearby NYC airports. Approx. 20 *bus lines* serve the area, including All Jersey, Arrow, Manhattan Lines, Transport of NJ and Greyhound.

COMMUNICATIONS. Communications, broadcasting and print media originating in Paterson are *AM radio station* WPAT 930 (Indep., Btfl. Mus.); and *FM radio station* WPAT 93.1 (Indep., Var.); NYC; *television station* WXPTV Ch. 41 (Span.); *press*: one major daily newspaper serves the city, the morning *News*; the weekly *La Voce Italiana* is also published in the city.

HISTORY. Paterson was founded in 1791 by Alexander Hamilton, who, seeing the potential for power production of the Great Falls, formed the "Society for the Establishment of Usefull Manufactures" (SUM) and, given power to control the falls by NJ, laid the basis for America's first planned industrial city. The city was named after the NJ Gov., William Paterson, who supported Hamilton's plans. The harnessing of the water for industry was begun by Pierre L'Enfant who had designed Washington, DC, and completed by SUM under the direction of Peter Colt. Mills were constructed and operated by SUM which remained a power developer for more than 150 years. By the early 1800s, industrialists had invested in the area and brought large-scale immigration. The first industry was cotton. By 1825, 3 million yards of fabric were being produced annually and by 1831 Paterson mills were making all the sails for the American navy. In 1836, Samuel Colt invented his revolver and began manufacturing in 1842. The next 20 years saw the development of the silk and locomotive industries. In the 1840s, George Murray and John Ryle founded the Pioneer Silk Co. and by the 1880s, Paterson was the "Silk City of the New World" with annual revenues exceeding $30 million. Secondary industries such as dyeing, braiding and machinery

Central Paterson, New Jersey

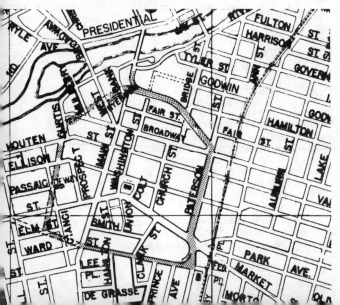

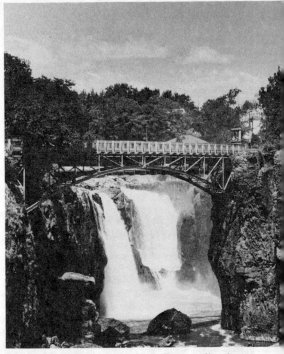

Great Falls, Paterson, New Jersey

production followed. Thomas Rogers' firm began production of steam locomotives in 1835 and with such engines as the *Sandusky 119,* and the *General* that beat the *TX (also built in Paterson by Cooke Locomotive)* in the Great Civil War Locomotive Chase of 1862, became America's major locomotive producer. Paterson was incorporated as a city in 1851 and by 1900 was the 15th largest city in the nation. The Panic of 1912 and subsequent strikes (25,000 silk workers struck in 1913), the discovery of rayon, changes in industrial technology and the industrial exodus to the S, caused a decline in the milling industries. Restoration of historic industrial buildings in the 1960s and 1970s under the auspices of the Great Falls Historic District, has brought revitalization to Paterson.

GOVERNMENT. Paterson's mayor-council form of govt. was established in 1974 under Plan D of NJ's Faulkner Act. It consists of nine council members, six elected by district and three at large, in staggered-year elections, while the mayor is elected every four years.

ECONOMY AND INDUSTRY. The Paterson met. area, which includes Clifton and Passaic had a labor force of 221,200 in June, 1979, and an unemployment rate of 9.0%. Silk and rayon production make up about 30% of Paterson's manufacturing industries. Other manufactured products include apparel, chemicals, textiles and electrical products.

BANKING. There are ten commercial banks in Paterson. In 1978, total deposits for the two banks headquartered in Paterson were $192,406,000, while assets were $221,414,000. Banks include Broadway Bank and Trust and Franklin.

HOSPITALS. Paterson is served by St. Joseph's, Greater Paterson Gen. and Barnert Memorial hosps.

EDUCATION. Passaic Comm. Col., a publicly-supported two-year col. offering associate degrees, enrolled 1,458 students in 1978. William Paterson Col. in nearby Wayne offers Bachelor and Master degrees and in 1978 enrolled 12,000. Lyons Institute is a privately-supported trade and technical school. The city's pub. schools enroll 27,000 students in 34 facilities. Lib. facilities include the Passaic Co. Local History Center and the Danforth Memorial, the Haledon Pub. and the Paterson Pub. libs.

ENTERTAINMENT. Paterson annually hosts the Great Falls Festival on Labor Day.

ACCOMMODATIONS. Hotels and motels in Paterson include Best Western, Holiday Inn, Regency House and Sheraton Heights Hotel.

FACILITIES. Paterson's major parks are Westside, Eastside and Great Falls. Westside Park, featuring boating and swimming facilities, is located on the Passaic River and includes the original Holland submarine and the 1800s brownstone Van Houten House. Eastside Park features Victorian landscaping created in the 1890s. Garrett Mt. Reservation is also located in the city. Riverside Oval, Putnam Oval, The Commons, Titus Field, Vreeland Avenue mini-parks, Dean McNulty Playground, Upper Raceway, Pennington and Brades Oval, offer softball fields, playgrounds, swimming pools, picnic areas, a pavillion, tennis courts and a running track. A six-mi. bikeway connects 10 parks with the downtown area and the Great Falls Historic District.

CULTURAL ACTIVITIES. Orchestral concerts and band recitals are held in Paterson at Hinchliffe Stadium. Operas are also sponsored in the city. Dramatic productions are staged by the Genesis Theater Company. The Learning Theater teaches high school students dramatic arts and the Inner City Ensemble gives lessons to teenagers in dance, acting, arts and crafts. The Paterson Museum houses a collection of Paterson and American Artifacts and also features Indian, mineralogy, archeological, geological and zoological exhibits. A new section devoted to American industrial history is being developed.

LANDMARKS AND SIGHTSEEING SPOTS. Lambert Castle, constructed in 1891 in the Garret Mt. Reservation overlooking Paterson, was built by the wealthy silk manufacturer, Catholina Lambert. It contains the Passaic Co. Historical Society Museum, whose collections include the McKinley-Hobart documents. The Great Falls Historic District is listed on both the NJ and Natl. Registers of Historic Places. Highlights include the Great Falls, a waterfall 77' high and 280' wide; the SUM hydroelectric plant; Middle Raceway, the first section of the three-tiered water raceway system begun in 1793; the Question Mark Bar, known as "Nag's Head" bar during the silk strikes of 1911 to 1913 and Dublin Spring and Spring's "No More" Monument, sculpted in bronze by Gaetano Federici. Other buildings of interest include the Ivanhoe Papermill Wheelhouse, constructed in 1865 and the only remaining building of the Ivanhoe Papermill Complex; Barbour Linen and Flax Complex (1879); Rogers Locomotive Erecting Shop; the John Ryle House (1840), Daniel Thompson House (1835); the Colt Gun Mill (1836); and Phoenix (1816) and Hamil Mills. Elm St. is the most nearly intact streetscape featuring workmen's homes built between 1840 and 1880. The Old German Church, built in 1840, is also located in the area. City Hall, a Beaux Arts structure designed by Carrerre and Hastings and built between 1894 and 1896, was rebuilt after the Great Fire of 1902.

PEORIA
ILLINOIS

CITY LOCATION-SIZE-EXTENT. Peoria, the seat of Peoria Co., encompasses 38.2 sq. mi. on the W shore of the IL River in central IL, midway between Chicago and St. Louis, at 40°40' N lat. and 89°41' W long. The greater met. area extends into the counties of Woodford to the NE and Tazewell to the SE.

TOPOGRAPHY. The topography of Peoria, which is situated in the Till plains, is characterized by gently-rolling, well-drained terrain, slightly removed from the flood plain of the IL River. The mean elev. is 652'.

CLIMATE. The climate of Peoria is continental, characterized by changeable weather and a wide range of temp. extremes. The avg. annual temp. of 51°F ranges between monthly means of 24°F in Jan. to 75°F in July.

The avg. annual rainfall is 35.06". The annual snowfall avgs. 24.6" with approx. 50% falling during Dec. and Jan. The RH ranges from 55% to 88%. The growing season avgs. 189 days. Peoria lies in the CSTZ and observes DST.

FLORA AND FAUNA. Animals native to Peoria include the muskrat, beaver, raccoon and opossum. Common birds include the cardinal, blue jay, redwinged blackbird and woodpecker. The bullfrog, salamander, toad, soft-shelled turtle and skink, as well as the venomous copperhead, timber rattlesnake and E massasauga (a pygmy rattler), are also found in the area. Trees include the oak, pine, elm and maple. Smaller plants include the violet, rose and honeysuckle.

POPULATION. According to the US census, the pop. of Peoria in 1970 was 126,963. In 1978, it was estimated that it had increased to 135,400.

ETHNIC GROUPS. In 1978, the ethnic distribution of Peoria was approx. 88.1% Caucasian, 16.5% Black and 0.9% Hispanic. (A percentage of the Hispanic total is also included in the Caucasian total.)

TRANSPORTATION. Interstate hwys. 74 and 474, US hwys. 24 and 150 and state hwys. 8, 9, 29, 87, 88, 91, 98, 116, 121, 122, 172 and 174 provide major motor access to Peoria. *Railroads* serving the city include Burlington Northern, Chicago & NW, ConRail, IL Central Gulf, IL Terminal Norfolk & W, Penn Central Peoria & E, Peoria & Pekin Union, Rock Island, Santa Fe & Toledo and Peoria & W. *Airlines* serving the Greater Peoria Airport include OZ, CO, Fed. Express and Emery Air Freight. Area gen. aviation airports are Mt. Hawley, Pekin and Waddell. *Bus lines* serving the city include Trailways and the local Greater Peoria Mass Transit District and Crown Transit. Barge transportation is available. The IL River has a nine-foot channel operational year round.

COMMUNICATIONS. Communications, broadcasting and print media originating from Peoria are: *AM radio stations* WPEO 1020 (MBS, Relig.); WIRL 1290 (Indep., Contemp.); WXCL 1350 (ABC/I, C&W) and WMBD 1470 (CBS, MOR); *FM radio stations* WCBU 89.9 (ABC/E, NPR, Clas.);

Civil War Monument, Peoria, Illinois

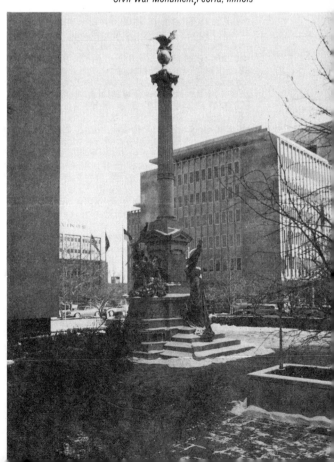

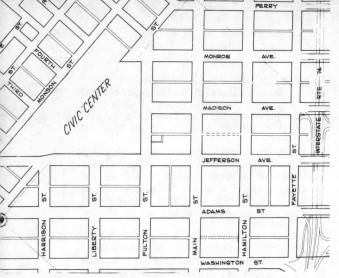

Downtown Peoria, Illinois

WKZW 93.3 (Indep., Top 40); WWCT 105.7 (ABC/C, Rock) and WSWT 106.9 (Indep., Good Mus.); *television stations* WRAU Ch. 19 (ABC); WEEK Ch. 25 (NBC); WMBD Ch. 31 (CBS) and WTVP Ch. 47 (PBS); *press*: one major daily serves the city, the morning and evening *Journal Star*; other publications include *Catholic Post*, *Observer*, *The Prairie Sun*, *Peoria Today*, *Shooting Times*, *Duroc News*, *Labor News* and *Heights Herald*.

HISTORY. Native Americans inhabited the area of present-day Peoria until the late 1600s, when they were joined by French settlers. Frenchmen and Indians of mixed blood coexisted in the area until 1812, when an American militia razed their village, believing them to be sympathetic to hostile Indians. Ft. Clark was constructed on the site in 1813, and a permanent settlement was established in 1819. Becoming the seat of Peoria Co. in 1825, Peoria was incorporated as a town in 1835, and, in 1845, the city was chartered. Today, Peoria has a pop. of 126,963 and ranks third in size among cities in IL. It is noted for the production of beer and whiskey.

GOVERNMENT. Peoria has a council-mgr. form of govt. consisting of nine members including the mayor. The mayor and three council members are elected at large, and the remaining five by district, to four year terms.

ECONOMY AND INDUSTRY. There are 372 manufacturing firms in the Peoria area. Major products include earthmoving equipment, steel, wire, beer, distilled spirits, off-highway trucks, and electrical equipment. There are large jobbing and wholesale businesses in the city, while a number of coal-producing mines are located nearby. The Peoria met. area had a labor force of 178,800 in June, 1979, while the rate of unemployment was 5.3%. The 1976 per capita income in Peoria Co. was $7,706. The household income for the met. area in 1977 was $18,346.

BANKING. There are 21 banks and six savings and loan assns. in Peoria. In 1978, total deposits for the 10 banks headquartered in the city were $824,875,000, while assets were $1,036,496,000. Banks include Commercial Natl., Jefferson Trust & Savings, S Side Trust & Savings, Prospect Natl., U Natl., Madison Park, NW and Pioneer State.

HOSPITALS. There are four hosps. in Peoria—Methodist Medical Center, St. Francis, Proctor Comm. and Shrine. The Institute of Physical Medicine and Rehabilitation, the Peoria Municipal T.B. Sanitarium and the Geo. Zeller Mental Health Center are also located in the city.

EDUCATION. Bradley U, a private university founded in Peoria in 1897 by Mrs. Lydia Moss Bradley, grants both grad. and undergrad. degrees. In 1978, it enrolled more than 5,000. IL Central Col., a publicly-supported institution awarding associate degrees, enrolled more than 5,000 in 1978. Other educational institutions include U IL Peoria School of Medicine and Midstate Col. The Research Laboratory of the US Dept. of Agriculture is also

located in the city. There are 37 public schools in Peoria, with a 1978 total enrollment of more than 21,000. Nine parochial schools enrolled more than 4,000 in 1978. Libs. include Peoria Public Lib. and its 12 branches, IL Valley Lib. System and the Peoria Co. Law Lib.

ENTERTAINMENT. The Heart of IL Fair is held in Peoria each July. The Peoria Bradley U Braves participate in inter-collegiate sports.

ACCOMMODATIONS. There are many hotels and motels in Peoria, including the Day's, Holiday and Best inns, Howard Johnson Motor Lodge, Peoria Hilton and Continental Regency.

FACILITIES. There are several parks in Peoria, including Trewyn, Bradley, Leisure Oaks, Glen Oak and Forest. Forest Park includes 800 acres of woodlands maintained as a wildlife refuge and nature education center. Five mi. of nature trails and a nature museum with displays of animals, birds and plants are maintained at the park. The 100-acre Glen Oak Park contains a zoo, a conservatory, gardens, floral displays, picnic areas ad tennis courts. The zoo houses displays of birds, large cats, monkeys, reptiles and fish, while the botanical gardens consist of four acres of gardens, trees and a conservatory and features the Formal Rose Garden, Annual Flower Gardens, All Season's Garden, a herb garden and a perennial flower garden. There are seven golf courses, while tennis courts can be found at two private centers and at Bradley Park. Year round swimming is offered at the Central Park pool and seasonal swimming pools are provided at Carver, Glen Oak and Lakeview parks and Proctor Center.

CULTURAL ACTIVITIES. The Lakeview Museum for Art and Sciences, located in Peoria, features changing art exhibits and natural science displays and a planetarium. The Peoria Historical Society maintains a museum in the oldest home in Peoria, built in 1837 by John Flanagan. Art galleries in the city include the Bradley U Gallery, IL Comm. Col. Gallery, Peoria Art Guild, Peoria Heights Lib., Peoria Public Lib., Tower Park Gallery and Asia Gallery.

LANDMARKS AND SIGHTSEEING SPOTS. One of the pioneer educational institutions in Peoria is the Jubilee Col. and Historical Site. Completed in 1839 by Bishop Philander Chase, the chapel and main building are made of native limestone. Bishop Chase is buried in the church yard. The Museum of Central IL Agriculture features replicas of a country home, general store and barn. Tours are available of the largest bourbon distiller in the world, located in Peoria.

PHILADELPHIA
PENNSYLVANIA.

CITY LOCATION-SIZE-EXTENT. Philadelphia, the largest city in PA, is located at the junction of the Delaware and Schuylkill rivers near the NJ and DL borders and encompasses 127.9 sq. mi. at 39°53' N lat. and 75°15' W long. The greater met. area includes all of Philadelphia Co. and extends into the surrounding cos. of Bucks to the N, Chester to the SW, Montgomery to the NW and across the DL River into Camden Co., NJ to the E.

TOPOGRAPHY. The terrain of Philadelphia, which lies on the Atlantic coastal plain, is generally flat, although it becomes more hilly in the W, near the Appalachian Piedmont region. The mean elev. is 45'.

CLIMATE. The climate of Philadelphia is moderate, influenced by its position between the Appalachian Mts. to the W and the Atlantic Ocean to the E. During the summer, maritime air engulfs the area, resulting in high humidity. SW winds prevail in summer, while NW winds dominate in winter. The avg. annual temp. of 54.6°F varies from monthly means of 33°F in Jan. to 76.6°F in July. The annual avg. rainfall of 41" is distributed evenly throughout the year. More than 50% of the annual 21" of snowfall occurs during Jan. and Feb. The RH ranges from 47% to 83%. Philadelphia lies in the ESTZ and observes DST.

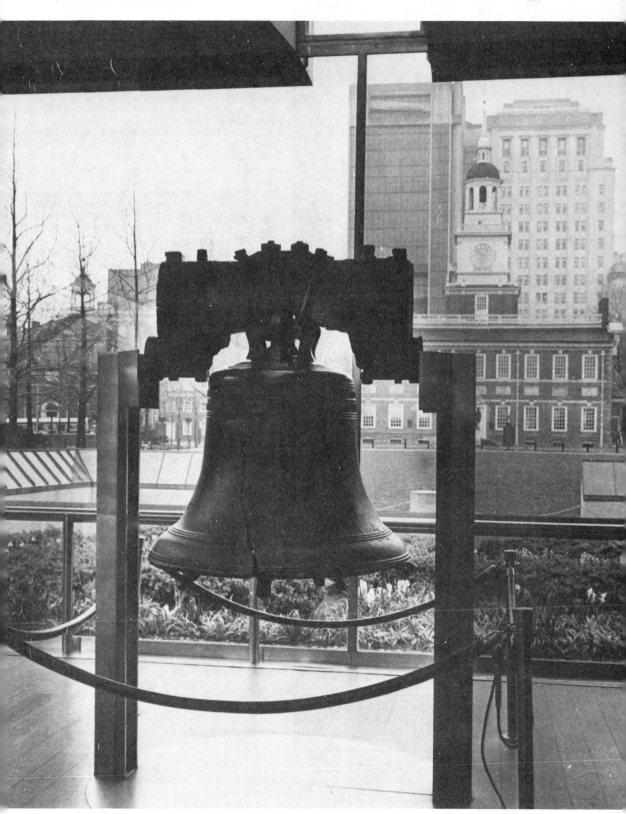

The Liberty Bell, symbol of the nation's independence, Philadelphia, Pennsylvania

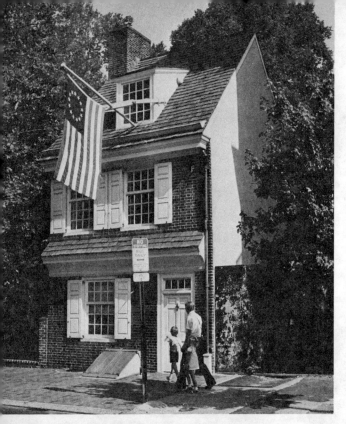

Betsy Ross House, Philadelphia, Pennsylvania

FLORA AND FAUNA. Animals native to Philadelphia include the opossum, raccoon and fox. Common birds are the goldfinch, robin, bluejay and crow. Frogs, salamanders, toads and milk snakes, as well as the venomous copperhead and timber rattlesnake are found in the area. Typical trees are the oak, elm, maple and hemlock. Smaller plants include the rose, rhododendron and goldenrod.

POPULATION. According to the US census, the pop. of Philadelphia in 1970 was 1,949,996. In 1978, it was estimated that it had decreased to 1,765,000.

ETHNIC GROUPS. In 1978, the ethnic distribution of Philadelphia was approx. 65.8% Caucasian, 33.5% Black and 1.4% Hispanic (a percentage of the Hispanic total is also included in the Caucasian total).

TRANSPORTATION. Interstate hwys. 76 and 95, US hwys. 1, 13, 30 and 422 and state hwys. 291, 73, 611 and 309 provide major motor access to Philadelphia. *Railroads* serving the city include PA-Central, Reading and

Philadelphia, Pennsylvania

AMTRAK. The SE PA Transportation Authority and the Pt. Authority Transit Corp. offer rail service to NJ. *Airlines* serving Philadelphia Intl. Airport include AA, US Air, DL, EA, FT, NA, NW, OZ, PA, TW and UA. *Bus lines* serving the city include Greyhound, Trailways and the local Transport of NJ. The Pt. of Philadelphia, the world's largest freshwater harbor, serves one-third of the US pop. and trades with 300 pts. in 100 countries.

COMMUNICATIONS. Communications, broadcasting and print media originating from Philadelphia are: *AM radio stations* WFIL 560 (Indep., MOR); WIP 610 (Indep., Contemp., MOR); WTEL 860 (Indep., Relig.); WFLN 900 (NBC, Clas.); WPEN 950 (ABC/E, MBS, MOR); KYW 1060 (ABC/I, All News); WCAU 1210 (CBS, News); WHAT 1340 (Mut. Blk., Blk., R&B). WDAS 1480 (Natl. Blk.) and WRCP 1540 (ABC/E, C&W); *FM radio stations* WXPN 88.9 (Indep., Var. Spec. Prog.); WRTI 90.1 (ABC/I, Jazz, Ethnic); WUHY 90.9 (NPR, Var.); WPWT 91.7 (Indep., diver.); WKDU 91.7 (Indep., Prog. Blk.) WIFI 92.5 (Indep., Btfl. Mus.); WMMR 93.3 (Indep., Progsv., Rock); WYSP 94.1 (Indep., AOR); WFLN 95.7 (NBC, Clas.); WWDB 96.5 (Indep., Talk); WCAU 98.1 (Indep., Disco, Jazz); WIOQ 102.1 (ABC/FM, AOR); WMGK 102.9 (Indep., Soft Mus.); WSNI 104.5 (Indep., Btfl. Mus., C&W); WDAS 105.3 (Indep., Blk.) and WWSH 106.1 (Indep., Btfl. Mus.); *television stations* KYW Ch. 3 (NBC); WPVI Ch 6 (ABC); WCAU Ch. 10 (CBS); WPHL Ch. 17 (Indep.); WTAF Ch. 29 (Indep.) and WKBS Ch. 48 (Indep.); *press:* three major dailies serve the city, the *Bulletin* and the *News*, both issued evenings, and the *Inquirer*, issued mornings; weekly publications include the *Carrier Pidgeon*, *Germantown Center* and the *NE Times*; other publications include the monthly *Philadelphia Gazette*, *Philadelphia Magazine*, *Playbill* and *Successful Meetings*.

HISTORY. Philadelphia was founded as a haven for religious dissenters by William Penn in 1682 on land granted to him by King Charles II of England. He named the city Philadelphia, which means "city of brotherly love" in Greek. The first European settlers on the present site of Philadelphia were the Swedes and Dutch, who arrived in the 1630s and 1640s. But by 1674, the British had won control over the area. Penn maintained friendly relations with native Americans of the DL tribe, who lived in the area, and signed a treaty with them at Shackamaxon. From the beginning, Penn's Colony of PA and its capital town, Philadelphia, attracted numerous religious dissidents from Europe. In 1683, the first German settlers, led by Francis Pastorius, arrived and founded Germantown, now a part of Philadelphia. By 1700 the city's pop. stood at 4,500 and in 1701 it was incorporated. The early 1700s marked a period of industrial growth resulting in further pop. expansion. By 1710, Philadelphia was the largest city in the colonies. In 1723, a 17-year-old apprentice printer named Benjamin Franklin moved from Boston to Philadelphia. The newspaper that he founded and the almanac he published spurred the city's development as a publishing center. The city's leadership role in commerce, industry and education in the 18th century is exemplified by the many "firsts" dating from that period. The first hospital, lib., university, medical school, law school, paper mill, theater, bank, insurance company, stock exchange, street lighting, baloon ascension, navy yard, US mint, fire company, botanic garden, magazine and learned society were established in Philadelphia. The city became the center of colonial protest during and after the Revolutionary period. The Continental Congress met in Carpenters Hall in 1774 and again in 1775. The Declaration of Independence was adopted at the PA State House (now Independence Hall) in 1776. The British attacked and occupied the city in 1777, withdrawing in 1778 for fear of being trapped there after the French sent a fleet to aid the revolutionaries. In 1787, the US

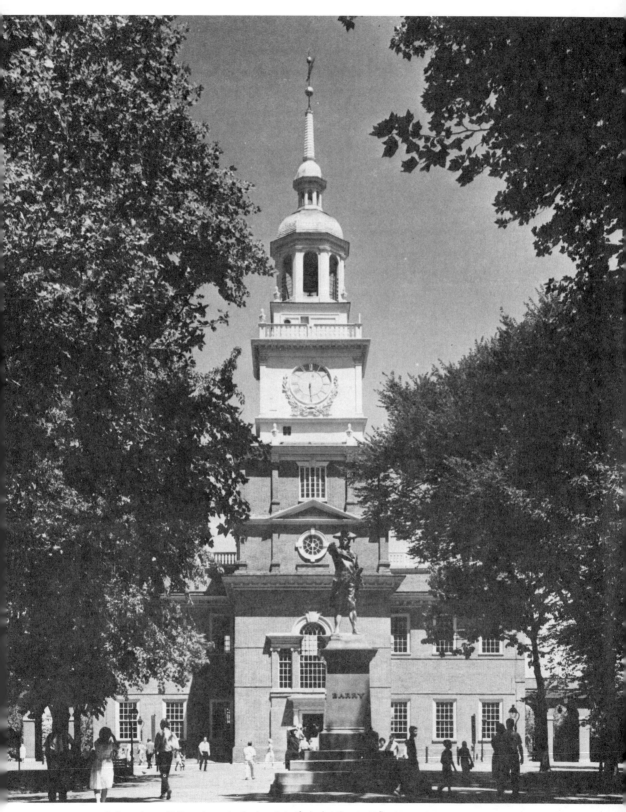

Independence Hall , where the Declaration of Independence was signed in 1776, Philadelphia, Pennsylvania

Constitution was adopted in the city. Philadelphia served as the capital of the US from 1790 to 1800. Lancaster replaced Philadelphia as state capital in 1799. The early part of the 19th century was marked by continued economic growth. Construction of canals and RRs increased trade with the Midwest. As the center of the iron, textile, locomotive and shipbuilding industries, the city attracted immigrants from Ireland and rural whites and blacks to its workforce. Tensions mounted and, in 1844, riots between native-born Protestants and Irish Catholics resulted in some 30 deaths. Philadelphia was merged with 11 nearby towns in 1854. By 1860, the pop. stood at 565,529. In the mid 1800s, the city became a center of the anti-slavery movement and was the home of abolitionists such as Lucretia C. Mott, James Forten and Robert Purvis. In the ensuing Civil War, Jay Cooke, a Philadelphia banker, was the Union's chief financial agent. During the War, Philadelphia's economy was geared toward producing war material. In 1876, Philadelphia hosted the Centennial Expo, the first world fair held in the US, to mark the nation's first century. With the advent of electric trolleys in the 1890s, Philadelphians could live further away from the center of the city, where they worked. The city's expansion continued into the 1920s. After WW II, the city launched a vast urban renewal program to restore the downtown area. Rev. Leon H. Sullivan, a black minister, began to develop self-help projects to train unemployed black inner-city youths. In 1964 he founded Opportunities Industrialization Center (OIC), which operates today on a nationwide basis. Philadelphia's rebuilding efforts are continuing into the 1980s.

GOVERNMENT. Philadelphia has a mayor-council form of govt. The mayor, elected at-large to a four-year term, has no council vote but is empowered to veto legislation, plan budgets and appoint administrative officials. The 17 council members serve four-year terms. Ten are elected by district and seven at-large. The chief legislative body, the council can override a mayoral veto by a two-third's majority vote.

ECONOMY AND INDUSTRY. The approx. 3,000 manufacturing plants in Philadelphia produce $6.5 billion in goods annually. There are also 18,764 retail and 3,904 wholesale establishments. The most important manufacturing industries are apparel and processed food. Other products include pharmaceuticals, chemicals, electronics and metal products. Printing and publishing and insurance are important to the area's

City Hall Tower in Downtown Philadelphia, Pennsylvania

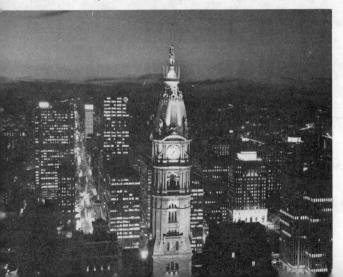

economy and the city is a major US banking center as well. Approx. 57% of the area's labor force is employed in trades and services. In June, 1979, the total labor force of the greater met. area was 2,126,300, while the rate of unemployment was 7.5%.

BANKING. In 1978, total deposits for the five banks headquartered in Philadelphia were $1,483,731,000, while assets were $1,588,119,000. Banks include Beneficial Mutual Savings, Frankford Trust Co., Marian, Glemede Trust Co. and Bank of Leumi-Le-Israel.

HOSPITALS. There are 74 gen. and special hosps. in Philadelphia, including the Albert Einstein Medical Center, J.F.K. Memorial, American Onocologic, Philadelphia Psychiatric and V.A.

EDUCATION. The U of PA, a private coeducational institution founded in 1740, offers courses leading from bachelor to doctorate degrees. Its Wharton School of Finance and Commerce was the first business school in the US to offer college level courses. In 1978, enrollment was 22,078. Temple U, Philadelphia's largest institution of higher education, was founded in 1894 and became a state-related institution in 1965. In 1978, Temple enrolled 36,339 students. Other institutions include the Moore Col. of Art, the nation's oldest art school for women; the Med. Col. of PA, founded in 1850 and the first medical school in the US for women only; Thomas Jefferson U; St. Joseph's Col. and the PA Col. of Optometry. There are more than 250 public schools in Philadelphia with an enrollment of 286,907. The approx. 145 private schools enroll 115,937 students. Libs. include the Free Public Lib. of Philadelphia, the Lib. for the Blind and Physically Handicapped, the Films Dept. Lib. Loan Service, the Athenaeum of Philadelphia, the Lib. Col. of PA and the Philadelphia Museum of Art Lib.

ENTERTAINMENT. The New Year's Day Mummers Parade features costumed celebrations. Other annual events include the Sportsmen's Show in Feb., the PA Relay Carnival in Apr., the Artist's Masked Ball in May, a Flag Day celebration, a pageant at Gloria Dei Church and Freedom Week in June. Dining entertainment is offered at the Riverfront Dinner Theater. Philadelphia is the home of the Phillies (NL, baseball), the Eagles (NFL-NFC, football), the 76ers (NBA, basketball), the Fury (NASL, soccer), the Firebirds (AHL, hockey) and the Flyers (NHL, hockey). The U of PA's Quakers and Temple U's Owls participate in intercollegiate sports and each Nov. the city hosts the Army-Navy football game.

ACCOMMODATIONS. There are numerous hotels and motels in Philadelphia, including the Barclay, Benjamin Franklin, Philadelphia Sheraton and the Hilton and several Holiday inns. Other accommodations in the area include the Philadelphia Marriott, George Washington Motor Lodge and Warwick.

FACILITIES. The Philadelphia met. park system includes 325 parks and playgrounds. Fairmount Park, the largest, encompasses 8,579 acres which extend along both sides of the Schuylkill River and includes miles of scenic drives, walks, a bicycle rte. and bridle trails. It also offers facilities for tennis, golf, archery, lawn bowling, boating and fishing. The Morris Arboretum is comprised of 100 acres of domestic and exotic trees and shrubs, while the Schuylkill Valley Nature Center includes woodlands, wildlife and several nature trails. More than 1,600 mammals, birds and reptiles are housed at the Philadelphia Zoo, which also contains a children's zoo. Ice skating facilities are available at Penn Center.

CULTURAL ACTIVITIES. The Philadelphia Orchestra performs at the Academy of Music, the oldest US opera house still in use, which is also the home for the Philadelphia Opera Co. and PA Ballet. Outdoor performances are presented by the Rittenhouse Opera Society. Dramatic productions are staged by Playhouse in the Park and Society Hill Playhouse, while Shubert Theatre hosts musicals. Over 200 works by the French sculptor Auguste Rodin are exhibited at the Rodin Museum. Hundreds of statues, reliefs and other sculptures designed by Alexander M. Calder are part of the overall City Hall structure. The PA Academy of Fine Arts Museum is the oldest art museum in the US. Other museums include the Balch Institute, Maritime Museum, Afro-American Historical Center, Please Touch Museum for children and the Franklin Institute.

LANDMARKS AND SIGHTSEEING SPOTS. Independence Hall Park in Philadelphia relates the story of the nation's and city's birth. Situated in the park are Independence Hall, Congress Hall, Carpenters' Hall and City

Tavern—all symbols of the American Revolution—as well as Graff House, where Thomas Jefferson drafted the Declaration of Independence. Benjamin Franklin and six other signers of the Declaration of Independence are buried in the cemetery of Christ Church. Also located on park grounds is Philadelphia's Old City Hall. Other historic houses in the park are the Bishop White House, the Todd House (where Dolly Madison grew up), the Free Quaker Meeting House and St. Joseph's Church. Wealthy Philadelphians have restored and now occupy hundreds of the 200-year-old houses in Society Hill, another historic neighborhood. Some of the city's oldest churches are located here, including St. Mary Church (1763), Old Pine Presbyterian Church (1768), and Mother Bethel A M E Zion Church (1818). Southwark, Philadelphia's oldest section, was first settled by Swedish immigrants in the early 1600s and is the site of PA's oldest church, Gloria Dei (Old Swedes Church). City Hall, a French Renaissance structure completed in 1901, is crowned with a massive statue of city and state founder William Penn on its tower. Other city landmarks include St. John Neumann Shrine (tomb of a Philadelphian bishop cannonized by Pope Paul VI), Penn Station, Penn's Landing and the Betsy Ross House.

PHOENIX
ARIZONA

CITY LOCATION-SIZE-EXTENT. Phoenix, the state capital, seat of Maricopa Co. and largest city in the state, encompasses 325.2 sq. mi. in the Salt River Valley in central AZ at 33°26' N lat. and 112°01' W long. The greater met. area extends S and SE into Pinal Co. and includes the cities of Glendale, Mesa, Scottsdale and Tempe in the region known as "Paradise Valley".

TOPOGRAPHY. Situated in the Basin and Range Region of AZ, Phoenix lies in a broad, oval-shaped, nearly flat plain in the center of the usually dry Salt River Valley. The city is surrounded by mt. ranges which reach elevs. of 4,500', including the Salt River Mts. to the S, the Phoenix Mts. to the N, the Sierra Estrella to the SW and the White Fox Mts. to the NW. The mean elev. is 1,100'.

CLIMATE. The climate of Phoenix is arid continental, characterized by extreme ranges in daily temps., especially during the winter, and little rainfall. The annual avg. temp of 70.4°F ranges from monthly means of 51.7°F in Jan. to 91°F in July. Most of the avg. annual rainfall of 7.44" occurs from Nov. through Mar. (resulting from storms originating in the Pacific Ocean), and during July and Aug. (from thunderstorms originating in the Gulf of Mexico and along the W coast of Mexico). Snowfall has not been registered during the last 50 years. The growing season is year-round. The RH ranges from 12% to 68%, with an avg. RH of approx. 30%. The sun shines approx. 86% of the time. Phoenix lies in the MSTZ and does not observe DST.

FLORA AND FAUNA. Animals native to Phoenix include the bobcat, spotted skunk, ringtail and kangaroo rat. Common birds include the hummingbird, roadrunner, cactus wren (the state bird) and turkey vulture. Coachwhip snakes, horned chuckawallas, whiptail lizards, and geckos, as well as the venomous gila monster, coral snake and rattlesnake, are found in the area. Typical trees include the redbud, pinion and juniper. Smaller plants are the creosote bush, saguaro cactus and acacia.

POPULATION. According to the US census, the pop. of Phoenix in 1970 was 589,016. In 1979, it was estimated that it had increased to approx. 762,300.

ETHNIC GROUPS. In 1978, the ethnic distribution of Phoenix was approx. 93.5% Caucasian, 4.7% Black and 14% Hispanic (a percentage of the Hispanic total is also included in the Caucasian total).

TRANSPORTATION. Interstate hwys. 10 and 17, US hwys. 60, 80 and 89 and state hwys. 85, 88 and 93 provide major motor access to Phoenix. *Railroads* serving the area include AMTRAK, Burlington N, ConRail, MO Pacific, Pacific Fruit Express, Rock Island, Santa Fe, S Pacific and Union Pacific. *Airlines* serving Phoenix Sky Harbor Intl. Airport include CO, DL, FL, RW, BN, US Air, EA, TW, NW Orient, AA, WA and several regional carriers. *Bus lines* serving the city include Greyhound, Trailways, AZ, Las Vegas-Tonopah-Reno State, Sun Valley and the local Phoenix Transit System.

COMMUNICATIONS. Communications, broadcasting and print media originating from Phoenix are: *AM Radio stations* KOY 550 (Indep., MOR); KTAR 620 (ABC/I, MBS, News, Sports); KMEO 740 (Indep., Btfl. Mus.); KIFN 860 (Indep., Span.); KJJJ 910 (ABC/E, C&W); KARZ 960 (CBS, MOR, Personality, News); KXEG 1010 (Indep., Relig.); KHEP 1280 (Indep., Relig.); KVIX 1400 (NBC, MOR, Personality, Talk); KPHX 1480 (Indep., Span.); KASA 1540 (Indep., Relig.) and KNIX 1580 (Indep., C&W); *FM radio stations* KMCR 91.5 (NPR, Divers.); KDKB 93.3 (Indep., AOR); KOOL 94.5 (Indep., Contemp.) KQYT 95.5 (Indep., Btfl. Mus.); KMEO 96.0 (Indep. Btfl. Mus.); KBBC 98.7 (ABC/C, AOR); KHEP 101.5 (Indep., Clas.) and KNIX 102.5 (Indep., C&W);

Downtown Phoenix, Arizona

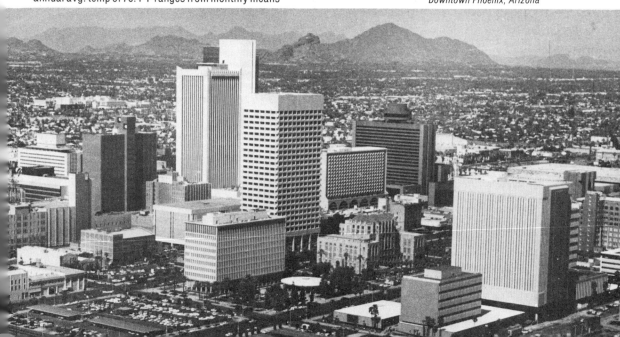

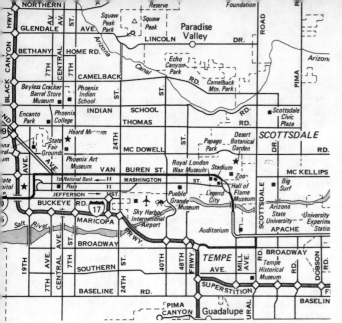

Phoenix, Arizona

television stations KTVK Ch. 3 (ABC); KPHO Ch. 5 (Indep.); KAET Ch. 8 (PBS); KOOL Ch. 10 (CBS); KPNX Ch. 12 (NBC); KNXV Ch. 15 (Indep.); KPAZ Ch. 21 (Indep.) and KTVW Ch. 33 (Indep.); *press*: one major daily newspaper is published in the city, the morning *AZ Republic*; weekly publications include the *AZ Weekly Gazette, Maryvale Star, New Times Weekly, Today, AZ Mobile Citizen, AZ Weekly, Phoenix, Press Weekly* and *Paradise Valley News-Progress*; monthly publications include the *AZ Farm Bureau News, AZ Highways, AZ Farmer Ranchman, Phoenix Magazine, American Patriot* and *Outdoor AZ*.

HISTORY. Native Americans of the Hohokam tribe inhabited the Salt River Valley and the area of present-day Phoenix until about 1450 AD, when they disappeared for unknown reasons. When white trader Y. T. Smith arrived in 1865, the region was occupied by native Americans of the Pima and Maricopa tribes. In 1867, the first settlers arrived, and named the comm. after the legendary Egyptian bird which burned itself every 500 to 600 years and then returned to life from its own ashes. Irrigation canals were soon constructed, and within a year (1868) the first crops were harvested. About 1,500 people lived in the settlement. In 1879, the town became a supply center for mines in the N AZ Territory. The stagecoaches, and with them lawless elements, arrived in the comm., and, by the end of the 19th century, two public hangings were staged in an attempt to regain some law and order. Incorporated as a city in 1881, Phoenix became the capital of the territory in 1889, and in 1912 of the state. In 1977, Roosevelt Dam on the Salt River, which provided additional irrigation and power for industry, was completed. Between 1900 and 1920, the pop. of the city rose from approx. 5,000 to more than 29,000. In 1926, the arrival of the S Pacific RR in the area provided a link to the E and many people, including retirees attracted by the dry climate, came to visit and live in the city. During WW II, the US military conducted desert warfare and aviation training in the area. The development of air conditioning in the post-war years resulted in additional industrial expansion and the arrival of more retired people and veterans in the city. By 1960, the pop. of the city reached nearly 439,200. In the late 1960s, the US Congress authorized the construction of the Central AZ Project, scheduled for completion in the mid-1980s to transport water, a factor in the continual growth of the city, from the CO River to Phoenix. An important resort area and industrial and agricultural center, the city pursued an active policy of annexation in the 1970s which resulted in a 20% increase in its area and growth in its pop.

GOVERNMENT. Phoenix has a council-mgr. form of govt. The seven council members, including the mayor as a voting member, are elected at large to two-year terms. The city mgr. is appointed by the council and serves as the chief administrator.

ECONOMY AND INDUSTRY. Major products of the manufacturing plants located in Phoenix, which is both an agricultural and industrial center, are electronic components, electrical products, computers, cosmetics, chemicals, aerospace technology, military armaments, fertilizers and processed foods. Agricultural products grown in the area include cotton, citrus fruit, olives, dates and other subtropical fruits and vegetables. Tourism and two military installations, Luke and Williams AFBs, are also important to the economy of the area. The labor force of the greater met. area totaled approx. 629,800 in June, 1979, while the rate of unemployment was 5.2%.

BANKING. There are 14 banking institutions in Phoenix. In 1978, total deposits at the 11 banks headquartered in the city were approx. $8,646,338,000, while assets totaled $9,931,871,000. Banks include Valley Natl. of AZ, First Natl., of AZ, AZ, United of AZ, Great W Bank & Trust, Continental, Thunderbird, American Bank of Commerce and Bank of Paradise Valley.

HOSPITALS. There are several hospitals in the city, including Gen., Baptist Gen., St. Joseph's, St. Luke's, Desert Samaritan, Good Samaritan, Lincoln, Maryvale Samaritan, AZ Children's, Barrow Neurological, Camelback Psychiatric, County, V.A., AZ State and US Public Health Service Indian Medical Center.

EDUCATION. Grand Canyon Col. is a private liberal arts and teachers col. in Phoenix sponsored by the AZ Baptist Convention. Awarding bachelor degrees, it enrolled more than 1,100 in 1978. Maricopa Technical Comm. Col. (which enrolled approx. 5,200 in 1978) and Phoenix Col. (more than 14,000) are two-year publicly-supported institutions of the Maricopa Co. Comm. Col. District that award associate degrees. There are more than 250 public elementary and high schools and 45 private and parochial schools in the city. Lib. facilities include the Phoenix Public, Maricopa Co. and AZ State libs.

ENTERTAINMENT. Among the dinner theaters in Phoenix is the Windmill. Annual events include the Natl. Livestock Show, held in Jan., and the AZ State Fair, held in late Oct. and early Nov. Pro sports entertainment is provided by the Phoenix Suns, an NBA basketball team, the Roadrunners, a PHL hockey team and a minor league PCL baseball team of the San Francisco Giants of the NL. The Antelopes of Grand Canyon Col. participate in collegiate sports. Horse and greyhound racing are held at Turf Paradise during the winter months.

ACCOMMODATIONS. There are several hotels and motels in Phoenix, including the Pointe, Hyatt Regency, Del Webb's Townehouse, AZ Biltmore, Adams Hotel, Granada Royale, Registry, Wigwam, Mt. Shadows and Caravan, Camelwalk, Sheraton and Ramada, Holiday and Rodeway inns.

FACILITIES. There are several parks in Phoenix, including Thunderbird, Papago and Encanto. Encanto features facilities for golf, swimming, boating, tennis and shuffleboard, as well as a lagoon and islands which serve as a waterfowl refuge and contain unusual trees and shrubs. Papago Park houses the Desert Botanical Garden and the Phoenix Zoo, which features an AZ exhibit, a children's zoo and a herd of rare Arabian Oryx. The Tropic Gardens Zoo houses monkeys, birds, mini-kangaroos, deer and flamingos in a shaded tropical setting. The Japanese Flower Gardens feature brilliantly-colored flora. There are numerous golf courses and tennis courts in the city, which also maintains S Mt. Park, the largest municipal park in the US. Other nearby parks are Estrella, Mt. Regional, Lake Pleasant Regional and N Mt. Parks, featuring lakes and desert wildlife.

CULTURAL ACTIVITIES. The Phoenix Symphony, the Theatre Phoenix and the Phoenix Little Theatre present regular performances in the city.

Primitive native American art and anthropology are exhibited at the Heard Museum. The Hall of Flame contains the largest collection of fire engines in the US. The Phoenix Museum of History features exhibits relating to early state history, while an ancient Hohokam dwelling is featured at the Pueblo Grande Museum and ruins. Displays of paintings, sculpture and graphics ranging from Renaissance to contemporary are housed in the Phoenix Art Museum. The AZ History Room features exhibits which reflect the lives and cultures of native Americans, Spaniards, Mexicans and pioneer Americans. Other museums are the AZ Mineral Museum and the AZ Museum.

LANDMARKS AND SIGHTSEEING SPOTS. Built of tufa stone from the Kirkland Junction and granite from the Salt River Mts., the State capitol in Phoenix features a mural of Estevanico, the black guide of the leader of a Spanish expedition into AZ in 1539, Fray Marcos de Niza. Included in the Royal London Wax Museum are scenes of the old W and statutes of pioneers, pres. and performers. The Bayless Cracker Barrel Museum recreates a gen. store of the 1890s.

PITTSBURGH
PENNSYLVANIA

CITY LOCATION-SIZE-EXTENT. Pittsburgh, the seat of Allegheny Co., encompasses 55.5 sq. mi. in SW PA at 4°27' N lat. and 80° W long. The Allegheny and Monongahela rivers join within the city to form the OH River and the triangular section of land produced within the boundaries of the rivers gives the business

53°F varies from a Jan. mean of 30.3°F to a July mean of 74.4°F. The avg. annual rainfall of 36" is well distributed throughout the year. More than 87% of the 40" avg. annual snowfall occurs from Dec. through Mar. The RH ranges from 50% to 86%. The growing season is approx. 180 days. Pittsburgh lies in the ESTZ and observes DST.

FLORA AND FAUNA. Animals native to Pittsburgh include the raccoon, rabbit, weasel, opossum and whitetail deer. Common birds include the ruffed grouse (the state bird), warbler, song sparrow, bluebird, purple martin and sparrow hawk. Salamanders, frogs, box turtles, milk snakes and the venomous copperhead, timber rattlesnake and E massasauga (a pygmy rattler), are also found here. Typical trees include the hemlock (the state tree), elm, oak and maple. Smaller plants include the mountain laurel (the state flower), rhododendron, bunch berry and bugbane.

POPULATION. According to the US census, the pop. of Pittsburgh in 1970 was 520,089. In 1978, it was estimated that it had decreased to 421,000.

ETHNIC GROUPS. In 1978, the ethnic distribution of Pittsburgh was approx. 79.3% Caucasian, 20.2% Black and 0.5% other.

TRANSPORTATION. Interstate hwys. 279 and 376, US hwys. 19, 22 and 30 and state hwys. 28, 51 and 837 provide major motor access to Pittsburgh. *Railroads* serving the city include Bessemer & Lake Erie, Chessie System, McKeesport, Monongahela, Norfolk & W, Pittsburgh Chartiers & Youghiegheny, Pittsburgh & Lake Erie and Union. *Airlines* serving Greater Pittsburgh Intl. Airport are AA, US Air, EA, NW, TW and UA. Allegheny Co. Airport offers private plane facilities. *Bus lines* include Trailways, Greyhound and the local Port Authority (PAT).

Point Fountain at Point State Park, Pittsburgh, Pennsylvania

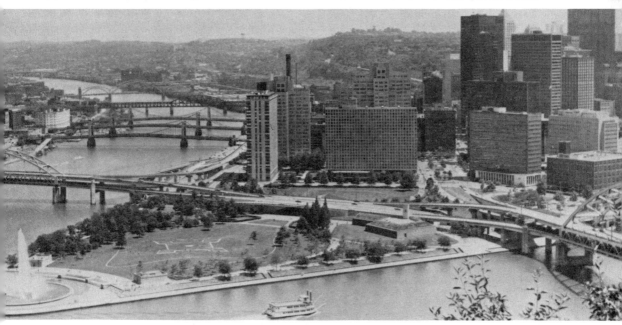

district its title, "The Golden Triangle." The met. area extends into the neighboring counties of Beaver on the NW, WA on the SW, Westmoreland on the E and Butler on the N.

TOPOGRAPHY. The topography of Pittsburgh, which is situated in the Appalachian Plateau region of PA, is characterized by a rolling terrain with many broken hills and wooded slopes. The mean elev. is 760'.

CLIMATE. The climate of Pittsburgh is humid and continental, modified only slightly by the Atlantic Ocean and the Great Lakes. The avg. annual temp. of

COMMUNICATIONS. Communications, broadcasting and print media originating from Pittsburgh are: *AM radio stations* WPIT 730 (Indep., Relig.); WWSW 970 (ABC/I, MOR); KDKA 1020 (Indep., MOR, Top 40); WEEP 1080 (MBS, C&W); WTAE 1250 (ABC/E, Adult Contemp.); WKTQ 1320 (Indep., Top 40) and KQV 1410 (Indep., All News); *FM radio stations* WRCT 88.3 (Indep., Educ.); WQED 89.3 (NPR, Fine Arts); WDUQ 90.5 (NPR, C&W); WYEP 91.5 (NPR, Divers.); KDKA 92.9 (Indep., MOR); WJOL 93.7 (Indep., Btfl. Mus.); WPEZ 94.5 (ABC/C, Top 40); WXKX 96.1 (Indep., Contemp.); WSHH 99.7 (Indep., Btfl. Mus.); WPIT 101.5 (Indep., Dups. AM 20%); WDVE 102.5 (Indep., AOR); WYDD 104.7 (Indep., Progsv.) and WEEP 107.9 (Indep., Dups. AM 50%); *television stations* KDKA Ch. 2 (CBS); WTAE Ch. 4 (ABC); WIIC Ch. 11

(NBC); WQED Ch. 13 (PBS); WQEX Ch. 16 (Indep.); WPCB Ch. 22 (Indep.) and WGPH Ch. 53 (Indep.); *press*: two major dailies serve the city, the morning *Post Gazette* and the evening *Press*; other publications include the weekly *Brookline Journal, Catholic Observer, Jewish Chronicle, Liberty Ledger, Mt. WA News, New Pittsburgh Courier* and *Reporter*, and the monthly *Carnegie Magazine, Country Music News, Iron and Steel Engineer, Pittsburgh Magazine, W PA Motorist* and *Winged Head*.

HISTORY. The Pittsburgh area was first inhabited by native Americans of the Iroquois Nation. Pittsburgh's founding goes back to the 1750s and the struggle between the French and the British to control the area. In 1758, Gen. John Forbes defeated the French and their Indian allies, destroyed the French-held Ft. Duquesne, and built a new ft. at the junction of the Monongahela, Allegheny and OH rivers. The settlement that grew up around the ft. was named Pittsborough in honor of the British statesman, William Pitt. After the Revolution, Pittsborough, by then called Pittsburgh, grew as a trading and industrial center. The first flat boats left Pittsburgh for New Orleans in 1782, beginning the heavy river traffic to the Gulf port. Pittsburgh became the seat of Allegheny Co. in 1788. Coal mining began in the nearby hills. The first glassworks were opened, and in 1792, the Anschutz blast furnace was built. This foreshadowed the iron industry, born locally in 1805 with the construction of a foundry. In 1811, the first steamboat was launched in Pittsburgh on the OH and MS rivers. Pittsburgh was incorporated in 1816. The PA Canal System, linking Pittsburgh and Philadelphia, opened in 1834. The first RR came to the town in 1851. Industry expanded rapidly during the first half of the 19th century. Pittsburgh's many iron and steel plants gave Pittsburgh the nickname "The Iron City." The city was a major supplier of armaments for the Union Army during the Civil War. After the war, industry continued to expand, with steel tycoons Andrew Carnegie and Henry Frick playing major roles. In 1888, the world's first aluminum plant was constructed in Pittsburgh. Industrial development continued throughout the first decades of the 20th century, bringing large numbers of immigrant workers from Europe and the S. Pittsburgh acquired the name of "Smoky City", as increasing numbers of industrial smoke stacks were built. In 1936, the St. Patrick's Day Flood of the two major rivers resulted in 45 deaths and millions of dollars in damage. But the city bounced back and completed a massive flood control program. During WW II, Pittsburgh was a

major steel producer. Following the war, the city initiated an ambitious anti-smoke program that eventually made the air cleaner than that of most major US cities. During the 1950s, there was a decrease in pop. as more people moved to the suburbs. However, during the 1960s and 1970s the downtown area underwent a redevelopment program and skyscrapers began to rise again as a number of large corps. moved their headquarters to Pittsburgh.

GOVERNMENT. Pittsburgh has a mayor-council form of govt. The nine council members and the mayor are elected at large to four-year terms. The mayor is not a council member and has no vote.

ECONOMY AND INDUSTRY. Pittsburgh is one of the leading industrial cities in the US, due primarily to the area's supply of crude ores. The city produces much of the nation's steel, iron and coke. More than 2,500 manufacturing plants in the city produce food products, chemicals, petroleum and coal products, fabricated metals, machinery and electronic equipment. Manufacturing employs approx. 33% of the area's labor force. In June, 1979, the met. area had a labor force of 1,020,000 and an unemployment rate of 6.3%.

BANKING. There are 43 commercial banks (with over 290 branches) in greater Pittsburgh. In 1978, total deposits for the nine banks headquartered in the city were $12,731,596,000, while assets were $16,341,835,000. Banks include Mellon, Equity, Dollar Savings, Union Natl., N Side Deposit and Iron and Glass.

HOSPITALS. Among the numerous hosps. in Pittsburgh are the U of Pittsburgh's Medical Center which has schools of Dentistry, Medicine, Nursing, Pharmacy and Public Health, and also operates the Falk Clinic, W Psychiatric Institute and the Sara Mellon Scaife Cyclotron. Other hosps. include, Children's, Allegheney Gen., Magee Women's, Mercy, Montefiore, Divine Providence, Eye and Ear Hosp., Presbyterian U, St. John's Gen., St. Margaret's, Shadyside and W Penn.

EDUCATION. The U of Pittsburgh, one of the state's largest centers of higher education, was founded in 1787 as a private U and became a state-related U in 1966. Offering degrees from associate to doctorate, the U enrolled approx. 29,700 in 1978. Carnegie-Mellon U, a private U created through the merger of Carnegie Institute of Technology and the Mellon Institute of Research awards degrees from bachelor to doctorate, and enrolled approx. 5,300 in 1978. Duquesne U; La Roche; Robert Morris; Point Park and Carlow cols.; the Comm. Col. of Allegheny; Pittsburgh Theological Seminary; Columbia Health Center and the Art Institute of Pittsburgh, are all located in the city. The city's 115 public schools enrolled approx. 70,000 in 1978, while enrollment in the approx. 100 parochial and private schools was 40,000. Lib. facilities are provided by the Carnegie Central Lib. and its 18 branches, and the Hunt Institute for Botanical Documentation.

ENTERTAINMENT. Annual events in Pittsburgh include the Glass Manufacturers' Show in Jan., the Three Rivers Art Festival in May and the Intl. Exhibition of Paintings at the Museum of Art of the Carnegie Institute in Oct. Pro sports entertainment is offered by the Pirates (NL, baseball), the Steelers (NFL-NFC, football), the Penguins (NHL-POWC, hockey) and the Spirits (soccer). Collegiate sports teams include the U of Pittsburgh Panthers, the Duquesne Dukes, the Robert Morris Colonials, the Allegheny Comm. Col. Cougars, the Point Park Col. Pioneers, and the Carnegie-Mellon U. Tarters.

ACCOMMODATIONS. There are numerous hotels and motels in the city including the Pittsburgh Hilton, William Penn, Hyatt House, Carlton House, Marriott, Howard Johnson's and the Sheraton, Hilton Airport, Red Roof and Holiday inns.

FACILITIES. The 2,500-acre Pittsburgh park system includes the 499-acre Frick, 456.1-acre Schenley, and the Riverview, Highland, W and E parks. Schenley Park features a lake, playground, picnic areas,tennis courts, baseball fields, fishing, bike trails, a miniature golf course, a regulation golf course and an ice skating rink. Frick Park, while providing picnic areas and tennis courts, remains largely undeveloped, with nature trails winding through ravines and hills. Highland Park houses the Pittsburgh Zoo, which

Central Pittsburgh, Pennsylvania

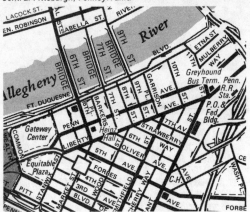

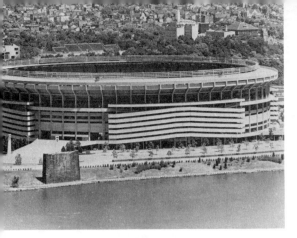

Three-River Stadium, Pittsburgh, Pennsylvania

contains approx. 2,000 animals and includes the Aquazoo and the Twilight zoo which is a 300' tunnel containing 16 exhibits of rare, nocturnal animals. The Pittsburgh Conservatory-Aviary, exhibiting birds in naturalistic, planted environments, includes three walk-through exhibits and eight ecological displays featuring birds from various regions of the world. Phipps Conservatory displays 53,000 permanent plants, including 6,000 species, and houses water gardens and an herbaceous garden. Public golf courses are available through the city park system. Public tennis courts are located at Natl. WA Plaza. Skating facilities are available at the Greater Pittsburgh Coliseum and Park arena.

CULTURAL ACTIVITIES. Andre Previn conducts the Pittsburgh Symphony Orchestra, which performs during the regular season at Heinz Hall. Duquesne U's Tamburitzans is a folk ensemble that emphasizes music of the Balkans. Also performing in Pittsburgh are the Civic Light Opera and the Carnegie-Mellon U Drama Dept. The Frick Art Museum exhibits Italian, French and Flemish paintings from early Renaissance through the 18th century. Regional historical exhibits are on display at the Historical Society of W PA. A new convention and exposition center is scheduled to open in the fall of 1980.

LANDMARKS AND SIGHTSEEING SPOTS. Ft. Pitt Blockhouse, built in 1764, is the oldest surviving building in Pittsburgh. Ft. Ligonier (1758), built by Gen. John Forbes, contains a museum featuring the living room of Gen. Arthur St. Clair, the Pres. of the Continental Congress. One of Frank Lloyd Wright's unique residential designs, Fallingwater, which actually bridges Bear Run Creek, was completed in the 1930s as a home for the Edgar J. Kaufmann family. Old Economy, a small 19th-century village, was founded by the Harmony Society as an experiment in communal living. Heinz Memorial Chapel is modeled after the 13th-century Gothic chapel, Sainte Chapelle, in France. The Inclines (passenger cable cars), which date back to the 1850s, were once a major means of transportation along the steep hillsides of Pittsburgh.

PORTLAND
OREGON

CITY LOCATION-SIZE-EXTENT. Portland, located in NW OR on the Willamette River near the junction of the Columbia River is the seat of Multnomah Co. and encompasses 93.5 sq. mi., including 6 sq. mi. of inland water, at 45°36' N lat. and 122°36' W long. An important W coast port city, Portland is situated 65 mi. inland from the Pacific Ocean. Its greater met. area extends into the counties of Columbia to the NW, WA to the W, Yarnhill to the SW and Clackamas to the SE.

TOPOGRAPHY. Situated in the Willamette Lowland region in the fertile Willamette Valley, the terrain of Portland is gently rolling farm and forest land. The city is midway between the Coastal Mt. Range on the W and the Cascade Range on the E. The mean elev. is 77'.

CLIMATE. The climate of Portland is relatively mild,

influenced by the Coastal Mt. Range, which shields the city from the Pacific Ocean, and the Cascade Range, which acts as a barrier to continental air masses and moderates the annual rainfall. The avg. annual mean temp. of 52.5°F ranges from monthly means of 38.6°F in Jan. to 66°F in July. Nearly 47% of the avg. annual rainfall of 37.5" occurs in Nov. through Jan. Fog is most frequent during fall and early winter. Portland has a year round growing season. RH ranges between 45% and 90%. Portland lies in the PSTZ and observes DST.

FLORA AND FAUNA. Animals native to Portland include the deer, elk, mountain lion, porcupine and chipmunk. Common birds are the gray jay, raven, blue spruce grouse, red crossbill and finch. Alligator lizards, rubber boas and gopher snakes as well as the venomous Pacific rattlesnake are found in the area. Typical trees include the Douglas fir and spruce. Smaller plants include the OR grape, tarweed, camas, geranium and godetia.

POPULATION. According to the US census, the pop. of Portland in 1970 was 382,352. In 1978, it was estimated that it had decreased to 368,000.

ETHNIC GROUPS. In 1978, the ethnic distribution of Portland was approx. 92.3% Caucasian, 5.6% Black, 1.7% Hispanic and .4% other.

TRANSPORTATION. Interstate hwys. 5, 80, 205 and 405, US hwys. 26 and 30 and state hwys. 8, 10, 99 and 213 provide major motor access to Portland. *Railroads* serving the city include AMTRAK, ConRail, Burlington N, Union-Pacific and W Pacific. *Airlines* serving the Portland Airport include Air Canada, Air W, BN, CO, EA, NW Orient, UA and WA. *Bus lines* serving the city include Pacific, Trailways and the local Tri-Met.

COMMUNICATIONS. Communications, broadcasting and print media originating from Portland are: *AM radio stations* KGW 620 (NBC, Contemp.); KXL 750 (ABC/I, MOR); KPDQ 800 (Indep., Relig.); KOLN 970 (Indep., Top 40); KWJJ 1080 (ABC, C&W); KKEY 1150 (MBS, Talk); KEX 1190 (ABC/I, MOR); KLIQ 1290 (Indep., Top 40); KUPL 1330 (Indep., Btfl. Mus.); KPAM 1410 (ABC/C, Top 40); KBPS 1450 (NPR, Spec. Progsv.); *FM radio stations* KRRC 89.3 (Indep., Var.); KBOO 90.7 (NPR, Clas., Jazz); KOAP 90.7 (NPR, MOR); KGON 92.3 (Indep., AOR); KPDQ 93.7 (Indep., Btfl. Mus.); KPAM 97.1 (Indep., Contemp., Top 40); KUPL 98.5 (Indep., Btfl. Mus.); KJIB 99.5 (Indep., Btfl. Mus.); KQFM 100.3 (Indep., MOR); KINK 101.9 (Indep., Progsv.); *television stations* KATU Ch. 2 (ABC); KOIN Ch. 6 (CBS); KGW Ch. 8 (NBC); KOAP Ch. 10 (PBS) and KPTV Ch. 12 (Indep.); *press*: two major dailies serve the city, the *Oregonian*, issued mornings, and the *OR Journal*, issued evenings; other publications include the *Daily Journal of Commerce*, *The Bridge*, *The Buyer's Guide*, *Catholic Sentinel*, *Arab Student Bulletin*, *Chain Saw Age*, *OR Labor Press* and the *Portland Magazine*.

HISTORY. The site of present-day Portland was originally inhabited by native Americans of the Chinook tribe. In 1829 the French-Canadian trapper Etienne Lucier built a log cabin in the area, becoming its earliest white settler. In 1844 Portland was founded by Asa Lovejoy and Francis Pettygrove, N.E. land developers who

Pittock Mansion, Portland, Oregon

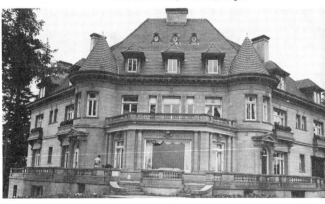

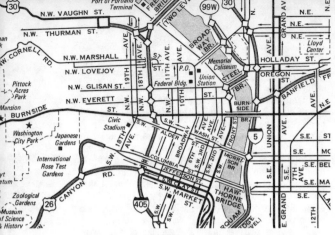

Downtown Portland, Oregon

believed that someday a port would be needed at the confluence of the Columbia and Willamette rivers. Named after Portland, ME, the city was the largest in the Pacific NW when incorporated in 1851. The area was settled by farmers and Portland became a commercial center for the marketing of fur, grain, lumber and wool. Manufacturing industries were boosted by the completion of a RR line, in 1883, which provided access to the E. Portland's position as a supply center during the Klondike gold rush of the late 1800s stimulated city commerce. During the first decade of the 1900s, Portland's pop. more than doubled, exceeding 200,000. In 1905, the city hosted the Lewis and Clarke Expedition Exposition, which drew three million tourists. For many years, lumbering was the primary industry and major source of employment. However, in 1933 a fire destroyed area forests and the lack of lumber forced many sawmills to close. Various industries dependent upon electricity moved into the city during the 1930s, when power-generating dams were built on the principal rivers. During WW II, shipbuilding and defense industries attracted tens of thousands of new workers to Portland, many of whom stayed. During the early 1970s, the city renovated existing roads and planned alternate rtes. Today, Portland is a major port and the state's largest city.

GOVERNMENT. Portland has a commission form of govt. consisting of five commission members, including the mayor, who are elected at large to four-year terms. The mayor is a voting member of the commission.

ECONOMY AND INDUSTRY. Manufactured goods produced by leading industries include metal products, electronics, chemicals and lumber. Portland is one of the leading cities in the country in wheat and lumber products for export. Portland's freshwater harbor ranks third in ocean-borne shipping on the Pacific coast. In 1979, the total labor force of the greater met. area was approx. 587,200, while the rate of unemployment ,was 5.4%.

BANKING. There are 14 banks in Portland. In 1978, total deposits for the nine banks headquartered in the city were $7,785,876,000 while total assets were $9,671,337,000. Banks include First Natl. of OR, US Natl. of OR, First State Bank of OR, and The OR Bank.

Skidmore Fountain, Portland, Oregon

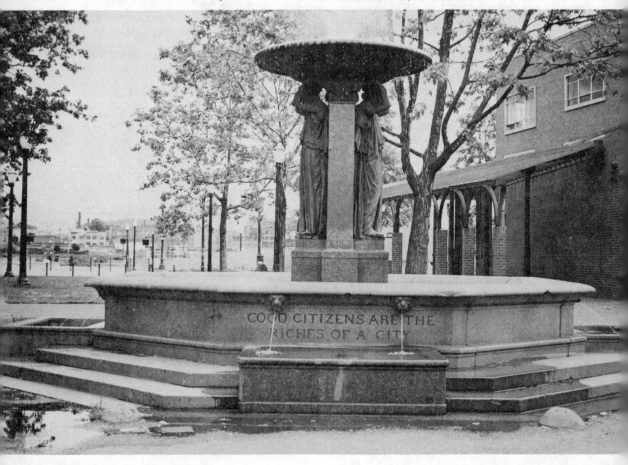

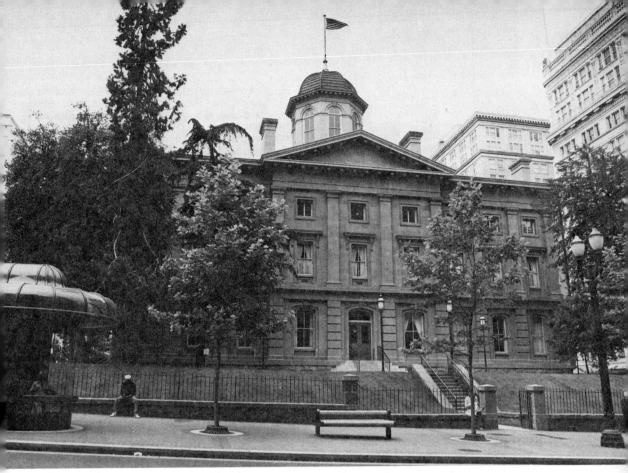

Pioneer Courthouse, Portland, Oregon

HOSPITALS. There are several hosps. in Portland, including Good Samaritan Emanuel, Medical Center, Eastmoreland Gen. and St. Vincent's. The U of OR Health Science Center is located in Portland as are the U's medical and dental schools.

EDUCATION. Portland State U was established in 1946 as Vanport Extension Center in order to assimilate the overflow of student veterans after WW II. Awarding bachelor and master degrees, PSU enrolled 15,888 in 1978. The U of Portland, a privately supported U founded in 1901 by the Congregation of the Holy Cross, awards grad. and undergrad. degrees and enrolled 2,540 in 1978. Lewis and Clarke Col., a private liberal arts col. established in 1867, is affiliated with the United Presbyterian Church in the US and enrolled 3,150 in 1978. Other institutions include the Museum Art School, Warner Pac. Col., W Conservative Baptist Seminary, Concordia Col., Judson Baptist Col., Portland Comm. Col. and the dental and medical schools of the U of OR. Almost 100 elementary and sr. high schools serve Portland. Libs. include the main building and 18 branches of the Multnomah Co. Lib. and special libs. at the OR Historical Society, the Portland Art Museum and the OR State Lib.

ENTERTAINMENT. Annual events in Portland include the Wintering-in Harvest Festival (Sept.), Pacific Intl. Livestock Exposition (Oct.), OR Herb Society Show and Sale (May), WA Park Summer Festival (July) and the Multnomah Co. Fair (July). The most popular festival is the Annual Portland Rose Festival (in Dec.). The Rose festival features the coronation of a festival queen, Starlight Parade, Jr. Parade, Rose Show, Festival of Bands, Rose Cup Sports Car Races and the grand Floral Parade. Portland is the home of the NBA Trailblazers and the NASL Timbers. The Winterhawks are a resident pro hockey team belonging to the WHL. In baseball, the Beavers compete in the PCL. The U of Portland Pilots and the Portland State U Vikings participate in intercollegiate sports.

ACCOMMODATIONS. There are numerous hotels and motels in Portland, including the Benson, Hilton, Marriott, Red Lion Riverside W, Best Western, Thunderbird Motor, Sheraton, Portland Airport inns and Portland Hotel and Travelodge.

FACILITIES. The 5,000 acre Portland met. park system encompasses six parks and stretches nine mi. across the W hills. At one end is WA Park with intl. rose test and Japanese gardens, while Forest Park at the other end consists of tangled wilderness. The area in-between features many trails. Other parks include Mt. Tabor, Tyron Creek Street, Eastmoreland and Waterfront. WA Park Zoo houses over 400 exotic and domestic animals and a children's zoo. Hoyt Arboretum occupies 213 acres and contains 650 varieties of trees, while the Sunken Rose Garden in Peninsula Park features more than 700 varieties of roses. Several public golf courses and tennis courts are available throughout the park system. Jogging tracks can be found in Duniway and Tyrone Creek Park.

CULTURAL ACTIVITIES. Musical performances are presented by the OR Symphony, and Portland Jr. Symphony an opera company. Dramatic productions are staged by the civic theater troupe, Storefront Actors, Portland Black Repertory Theatre, and the Matrix Theatre. Diverse acts can be seen at the Paramont Theatre and Civic Auditorium, Memorial Coliseum and Multnomah Co. Exposition Center. Museums in the city include the Portland Black Repertory Theatre, and the Matrix Theatre. Diverse plays can be seen at the Paramount Theatre and Civic Auditorium, Memorial Coliseum human body, and a planetarium. Other museums include the OR Historical Society, Museum of Police History and the W Forest Center. The Fountain Gallery of Art features contemporary work of NW artists.

LANDMARKS AND SIGHTSEEING SPOTS. The former residence of *Daily Oregonian* founder Henry L. P. Hock, the Pittock Manion is located in Pittock Acres Park. The French Renaissance structure, completed in 1914, contains many ultramodern features, including a central vacuum cleaning system, elevators and a telephone system between rooms. Old Town is an historic section of the city. A fine example of "carpenter Gothic," the Old Church is the city's oldest surviving church building. Built in 1856, the Bybee Howell House has been restored to reflect its 19th-century origin. Erected by Servite fathers, the Natl. Sanctuary of Our Sorrowful Mother contains a cave in a 10-story cliff on the 60-acre plot. The Lloyd Center, one of the nation's largest shopping centers, occupies 50 acres near downtown and includes a large outdoor ice skating rink.

PORTSMOUTH
VIRGINIA

CITY LOCATION-SIZE-EXTENT. Portsmouth is an independent city located in SE VA, next to the Elizabeth River near Hampton Roads, encompassing 45.5 sq. mi. at 36°44' N lat. and 76°32' W long. Its greater met. area extends into the surrounding cities of Newport News to the N, Norfolk and VA Beach to the E and Chesapeake to the S.

TOPOGRAPHY. The terrain of Portsmouth, situated in the VA Tidewater region, is mostly level, with some slight sloping toward the mts. to the W. The mean elev. is 5'.

CLIMATE. The climate of Portsmouth is modified marine, influenced by Hampton Roads to the N and the Atlantic Ocean to the E. The avg. annual temp of 60°F ranges from a Jan. mean of 41°F to a July mean of 79°F. Most of the 45" avg. annual rainfall occurs during the summer. Most of the 7.2" avg. annual snowfall occurs in Jan. and Feb. The RH ranges from 50% to 86% and the growing season avgs. 244 days. Portsmouth lies in the ESTZ and observes DST.

FLORA AND FAUNA. Animals native to Portsmouth include the raccoon, striped skunk and muskrat. Common birds are the cardinal, bluejay, wren, swallow and gull. Bullfrogs, salamanders, box turtles and king snakes, as well as the venomous rattlesnake, cottonmouth and copperhead, are found in the area. Typical trees are the oak, pine, redbud and dogwood. Smaller plants include marsh grass.

POPULATION. According to the US census, the pop. of Portsmouth in 1970 was 110,963. In 1978, it was estimated that it had decreased to approx. 108,400.

ETHNIC GROUPS. In 1970, the ethnic distribution of Portsmouth was approx. 59.4% Caucasian, 39.9% Black and 0.7% Hispanic.

TRANSPORTATION. Interstate hwys. 264 and 464, US hwys. 17, 58 and 460 and state hwys. 125 and 135 provide major motor access to Portsmouth. *Railroads* serving the city are Norfolk & Portsmouth Beltline, Norfolk & W, Penn Central, Seaboard Coastline & S Railway. *Airlines* serving the Norfolk Intl. Airport include US Air, PI, EA, NA and UA. *Bus lines* serving the city include Trailways and Greyhound.

COMMUNICATIONS. Communications, broadcasting and print media originating from Portsmouth are: *AM radio stations* WPMH 1010 (Indep., Relig.); WHNE 1350 (ABC/E, C&W) and WPCE 1400 (Mut. Blk., Blk.); *FM radio stations* WNHS 88.7 (Indep., Educ. Top 40); WAVY Ch. 10 and

Downtown, Portsmouth, Virginia

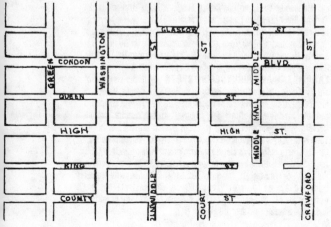

television stations WYAH Ch. 27 (Indep.); *press*: two major dailies serve the city, the *Ledger Star* and *Virginian-Pilot*; other publications include the local *Metro* and *Tidewater VA* magazines.

HISTORY. Due to its favorable location, Portsmouth began as a shipbuilding facility. English settlers arrived in the area as early as 1607, and in 1620, John Wood was granted 400 acres for a shipbuilding yard. In 1752, the town of Portsmouth was founded by William Crawford and incorporated; its name derived from the English seaport city. A few years after it was founded, the shipbuilding and repairing center of Gosport Shipyard was built. Strategically important, Portsmouth was repeatedly occupied and Gosport burned during the Revolutionary War. However, the town was quickly rebuilt and Gosport became the first shipyard of the new US Navy. In 1794 the frigate *Chesapeake* was constructed in Gosport Yard. Portsmouth was again attacked during the War of 1812, but the British were rebuffed. The city was chartered in 1858. Ships were built at Gosport Shipyard until the Civil War, when it was burned by the retreating Union Army. The Confederates, however, built a base on the site. The pop. remained at only a few thousand during the 1800s. At the end of the century, the economy of Portsmouth revolved around shipbuilding. The city boomed during WWs I and II, spurred by the increased demand for war vessels. During WW II, the yard, now the Norfolk Naval Shipyard, turned out 101 new ships and repaired or converted many more for the war effort. Today the city is part of the Hampton Roads port complex and home of the Norfolk Naval Shipyard and naval hospital. Portsmouth is combatting social and economic problems with urban renewal, historic preservation, and industrial expansion.

GOVERNMENT. Portsmouth has a council-mgr. form of govt. which consists of seven council members, including the mayor. The council members and the mayor (a voting member) are elected at large for four-year terms.

ECONOMY AND INDUSTRY. Portsmouth's major employer is the Naval Shipyard, with electronics and food processing also significant to the city's economy. Major products include clothing and chemicals. The avg. income per capita in 1977 was $4,550. In 1979, the total labor force for the greater met. area was approx. 326,300 workers, with a rate of unemployment of 6.3%.

BANKING. There are six banks in Portsmouth. In 1978, total deposits for the one bank headquartered in the city were $71,538,000, while assets were $79,775,000. Among the banks serving the city are VA Natl., Dominion Natl., Bank of VA, United VA, Fidelity American and Citizens' Trust.

HOSPITALS. There are three hospitals in Portsmouth, Maryview, Portsmouth and Portsmouth Psychiatric. The nation's oldest USN medical center, Portsmouth Naval Hosp., is also located there.

EDUCATION. Tidewater Comm. Col., a publicly-supported school, offers associate degrees in a variety of programs. Enrollment was 13,033 in 1978. There are 34 schools in the Portsmouth public school system, with a 1979 enrollment of 20,000. Libs. include the Portsmouth Public, William Collins Hill, Multi-Ethnic and Memorial Horticultural.

ENTERTAINMENT. Hunting and Fishing Day and the Seawall Art Show are held annually in Portsmouth. The Tidewater Mets (IL) play baseball in the Portsmouth-Norfolk area.

ACCOMMODATIONS. There are several hotels and motels in Portsmouth, including the Imperial 400 and Sunset Manor Motels and the Holiday and Quality inns.

FACILITIES. There are three parks in Portsmouth including, Portsmouth City and Sleepy Hole which both have golf courses, and Churchland.

CULTURAL ACTIVITIES. Musical performances are presented by the Comm. Concert Series, and Portsmouth is also served by the Comm. Art

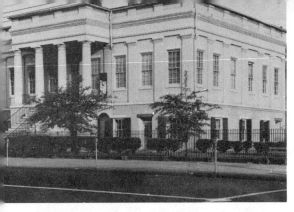

1846 Courthouse, Portsmouth, Virginia

Center. The Norfolk Naval Shipyard Museum features a collection of model ships from all eras and displays illustrations of the shipyard's history. A 70-year-old ship, the *Lightship Museum*, is now stationed inland and exhibits Coast Guard memorabilia.

LANDMARKS AND SIGHTSEEING SPOTS. The historic Old Towne section of Portsmouth is a restored residential district. Virginians who made their mark in sports are commemorated in the VA Sports Hall of Fame, which exhibits photographs and mementos of the athletes. Other historic buildings include the Courthouse, constructed in a Roman classic style; the Trinity Church (1762); St. John's Church (1898); the Grice-Neely House; the Murdaugh Residence (1812); the Watts House (1799); and the Ball-Nivison House (1784).

PROVIDENCE
RHODE ISLAND

CITY LOCATION-SIZE-EXTENT. Providence, the capital of RI and the seat of Providence Co., is located at the head of Narragansett Bay on the Providence River and encompasses 20 sq. mi. at 40°44' N lat. and 71°26' W long. Its greater met. area includes the cities of N Providence to the NW, E Providence, to the SE, Pawtucket to the NE, and Cranston to the S, and extends throughout Providence Co. and into Kent Co. to the S.

TOPOGRAPHY. Providence is partially situated in the coastal lowlands near the Atlantic Coast. The terrain rises slightly to the W and NW to the sloping hill areas of the N.E. uplands. The mean elev. is 51'.

CLIMATE. The climate of Providence is influenced by its position near Narragansett Bay and the Atlantic Ocean, which temper cold air masses moving into the area, producing mild winters and cool summers. The avg. annual temp. of 50.5°F ranges from monthly means of 29°F during Jan. to 73°F during July. The avg. annual rainfall of 41" is distributed throughout the year. More than 50% of the annual 39" of snowfall occurs in Jan. and Feb. The growing season avgs. 195 days. The RH ranges from 46% to 84%. Providence lies in the ESTZ and observes DST.

FLORA AND FAUNA. Animals native to Providence include the opossum, fox and squirrel. Common birds are the goldfinch, gull, tern, chickadee and woodpecker. Frogs, salamanders and milksnakes, as well as the venomous timber rattlesnake and copperhead, are found in the area. Typical trees are the maple, elm, oak and cedar. Smaller plants include the violet, rose, mayflower, field daisy and meadowrue.

POPULATION. According to the US census, the pop. of Providence in 1970 was 179,116. In 1978, it was estimated that it had decreased to 167,729. Approx. 20% of RI's pop. resides in Providence.

ETHNIC GROUPS. In 1978, the ethnic distribution of Providence was approx. 90.1% Caucasian, 8.9% Black, 0.8% Hispanic and 0.2% other.

TRANSPORTATION. Interstate hwys. 95 and 195, US hwys 1, 6 and 44 and state rtes. 2, 7, 14, 46 and 95 provide major motor access to Providence. *Railroads* include AMTRAK, Auto-Train, ConRail and the Providence & Worcester Co. *Airlines* serving Theodore Francis Greene Airport are US Air, EA, NE, TWA and UA. *Bus lines* are Greyhound, Bonanza, ABC, Tauton Interstate Coach and the local RI Public Transit Authority.

COMMUNICATIONS. Communications, broadcasting and print media originating from Providence are: *AM radio stations* WPRO 630 (Indep., Contemp.); WEAN 790 (MBS, All News); WJAR 920 (NBC, MOR, Personality); WLKW 990 (ABC/I, Btfl. Mus.); WHIM 1110 (ABC/E, C&W); WRIB 1220 (Indep., Relig., Spec. Prog.) and WICE 1290 (Indep., Contemp.); *FM radio stations* WDOM 91.3 (MBS, Educ., Progsv.); WPRO 92.3 (Indep., Top 40); WHJY 94.1 (ABC/E); WBRU 95.5 (ABC/FM, Progsv. Rock); WLKW 101.5 (Indep., Top 40) and WPJB 105.1 (Indep., Top 40); *television stations* WTEV Ch. 6 (CBS); WJAR Ch. 10 (NBC); WPRI Ch. 12 (ABC); WSBE Ch. 36 (PBS); New TV Ch. 64 (Indep.) and cable; *press:* two major dailies serve the city, the *Evening Bulletin*, issued evenings, and *Journal*, issued mornings; other publications include *The Italian Echo, Visitor, Brown Daily Herald, Anchor, The Cowl, Eastside-Westside, RI Labor News, RI Medical Journal* and *Bulletin of the American Mathematical Society*.

HISTORY. Native Americans of the Narragansett tribe originally inhabited the Providence area. The first white comm. in RI, Providence was founded in 1636 by Roger Williams, after he was banished from MA for his religious convictions. Williams purchased the land from the Narragansetts and named the comm. "Providence Plantations" in gratitude for reaching the location. By 1647, there were 200 settlers in the comm. The region's early inhabitants were primarily planters, but by the late 1600s the economic emphasis shifted from agriculture to small business and commerce. Maritime

Financial district and world's widest bridge, Providence, Rhode Island.

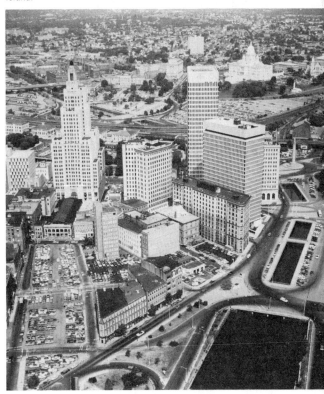

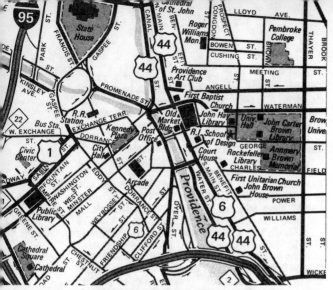

Central Providence, Rhode Island

commerce between RI, the W Indies and the other colonies was flourishing by 1700. Some 4,300 persons lived in Providence in 1775. During the Revolutionary War Providence served as RI's defensive stronghold and was strategically important due to its position near Boston. The city prospered from the war industries and lucrative privateering—legalized piracy—and emerged as RI's major urban center after the war. A thriving trade in spices, silks and porcelain was initiated in 1787 by a merchant named John Brown, who sent the first RI ship to Canton. In 1786, the first hand-powered machine for spinning cotton was built in Providence. Better technology and the simultaneous decline of the shipping industry in the 1800s led to the town's development into one of the leading US textile centers. In 1794, the silversmith Nehemiah Dodge started the first local jewelry business after discovering a process whereby cheap metals could be covered by more expensive ones. Jewelry making was to become an important industry in RI. Providence was incorporated as a city in 1832. Increased industrialization attracted an influx of immigrants to Providence factories during the 1840s and the pop. reached 104,857 by 1880. One of several RI capitals since 1663, Providence became the sole capital of the state in 1900. Production of military supplies proved to be profitable during WWs I and II. However, following each war many industries sought to defray expenses by relocating to the S, and the pop. declined from a high of 248,674 in 1950 to 179,116 in 1970. An urban renewal project was initiated in the 1960s. Today, the city serves as a major NE commercial industrial and educational center as well as an important seaport. Home to one-fifth of RI's pop., Providence is the state's largest city.

GOVERNMENT. Providence has a mayor-council form of govt. The mayor, who is not a member of the council, serves a four-year term, while the 26 council members are elected by district to four-year terms.

ECONOMY AND INDUSTRY. Manufacturing is the predominant sector of the Providence area economy, followed by services and trade. Major products include jewelry, textiles, precision machinery and metals. In 1976, the labor force for the met. area was 125,400. The rate of unemployment was 7.1% in 1979.

BANKING. There are 12 banks in Providence. In 1978, total deposits for the 10 banks headquartered in the city were $5,087,311,000, while assets were $6,292,757,000. Banks include Industrial Natl., Hosp. Trust, Old Stone, Citizens Savings and Peoples Savings.

HOSPITALS. There are seven major hosps. in Providence, including Miriam, RI, Roger Williams General, St. Joseph, Butler, V.A. and Women and Infants. Several specialized medical care centers, emergency care services and several smaller hosps. are also located in the city.

EDUCATION. Brown U, chartered in 1764, moved to the city from Warren in 1770. One of the nation's first colleges, Brown U, is a privately-supported institution offering course work leading to bachelor, master and doctorate degrees. Enrollment in 1978 was more than 6,700. RI School of Design, founded in 1877, is a privately-supported institution offering instruction in all forms of art. Bachelor degrees, Architecture and Landscape Architecture degrees, as well as master degrees in teaching and art education are granted. More than 1,400 enrolled there in 1978. Other institutions include RI Col., Providence Col., Johnson and Wales Col., U RI Extension N.E. Institute of Technology and Roger Williams Col.-Providence Branch. Libs. include the Providence Public Lib., largest in the state, with nine branches; the RI state Lib., the RI Historical Society Lib. and the Providence City Archives, located in City Hall.

ENTERTAINMENT. The Providence Col. Friars and Brown U Bruins participate in intercollegiate sports.

ACCOMMODATIONS. There are numerous hotels and motels in the Providence area including the Biltmore Plaza, Marriott, Ramada, Holiday Inn, Howard Johnson's and the Sheraton Islander.

FACILITIES. Roger Williams Park features a zoo and recreational facilities. Public golf courses and tennis courts are available in the area.

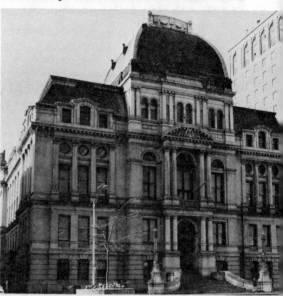

Built 1878, City Hall, Providence, Rhode Island

CULTURAL ACTIVITIES. The Trinity Square Repertory Co. stages productions in Lederer Theater, while the RI Philharmonic Orchestra performs at the newly renovated Ocean State Theater in downtown Providence. The new Civic Center hosts concerts. Located in the RI School of Design, the Museum of Art features masterpieces from ancient Greece and Rome, 20 centuries of Oriental art, a noted selection of French art and the Pendleton House collection of American furniture and decorative arts. Among the 14 art galleries and museums in Providence are the Wheeler Gallery and the List Art Gallery at Brown U. The Providence Art Club occupies two houses dating from 1786 and 1791. Shows are presented by the Cormack Planetarium in the Roger Williams Park Museum of Natural History. The John Brown House is the home of the RI Historical Society, while the Museum of RI History is housed in the Aldrich House.

LANDMARKS AND SIGHTSEEING SPOTS. Built in pre-revolutionary days, the First Baptist Meeting House is one of the oldest buildings in the city. Providence founder Roger Williams belonged to this congregation. The First Unitarian Church of Providence (1816) has the largest bell cast in the foundry of Paul Revere. Tablets on the Old Market Building, completed in 1774, commemorating the 1775 Providence Tea Party and the Great Gale of 1815. The State House contains the original parchment charter of 1663, granted by King Charles II, as well as many relics and notable paintings. Other historic buildings of interest include the John Brown House, constructed in 1786 for Providence's wealthiest merchant, the Gov. Stephen Hopkins House (1707-1743) and the Betsy Williams Cottage, built in 1773. Roger Williams is buried at the base of the Roger Williams monument. The College Hill Historic District is a Natl. Historic Landmark which perserves many old houses and buildings.

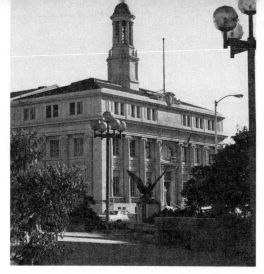

City Hall, Pueblo, Colorado

PUEBLO
COLORADO

LOCATION-SIZE-EXTENT. Pueblo, the seat of Pueblo Co., is located at the junction of the AR and Fountain rivers, approx. 50 mi. S of CO Springs in S Central CO and encompasses 33.5 sq. mi. at 38°15' N lat. and 104°37' long.

TOPOGRAPHY. The terrain of Pueblo, which lies in the Great Plains region, part of the Interior Plain of N America, slopes gradually from E to W toward the base of the Rocky Mts. and consists of rolling plains broken by shallow, usually dry ditches. The mts. extend to within 25 mi. of the city to the SW and 35 mi. to the NW. The mean elev. is 4,700'.

CLIMATE. The climate of Pueblo is semi-arid with wide daily temp. variations. During the summer, the temp. ranges from 90°F to 57°F. In the winter, daytime temps. reach 50°F while nighttime temps drop to freezing. The avg. annual temp. of 52.2°F ranges from a Jan. mean of 30.7°F to a July mean of 75.4°F. The avg. annual rainfall of 11.91" occurs mainly during the spring and summer months. Most of the avg. annual snowfall of 29.3" occurs in Mar. The growing season avgs. 149 days. The RH ranges from 48% to 82%. Pueblo is in the MSTZ and observes DST.

FLORA AND FAUNA. Animals native to Pueblo include the mule deer, coyote, prairie dog, cottontail rabbit, jackrabbit and pronghorn antelope. Common birds are the roadrunner, scaled quail, mt. bluebird, woodpecker and bittern. Chorus frogs, fence lizards and green snakes as well as the venomous prairie rattlesnake, are found in the area. Typical trees are the pine, cottonwood, juniper, pinyon and aspen. Smaller plants include the groundsel, lupine, penstemon, columbine, grama, kochia and buffalo grass.

POPULATION. According to the US census, the pop. of Pueblo in 1970 was 97,453. In 1978, it was estimated that it had increased to 110,668.

ETHNIC GROUPS. In 1978 the ethnic distribution of Pueblo was approx. 62.5% Caucasian, 1.9% Black, 35% Hispanic and .6% other.

TRANSPORTATION. Interstate Hwy. 25, US hwys. 50, 85 and 87 and state hwys. 76 and 96 provide major motor access to Pueblo. *Railroads* serving the city are Burlington N, MO Pacific Lines, Denver & Rio Grande, W and Santa Fe. *Airlines* serving Pueblo Memorial Airport include FL and Rocky Mt. Airways. *Bus lines* serving the city include Greyhound and Trailways.

COMMUNICATIONS. Communications, broadcasting and print media originating from Pueblo are *AM radio stations* KCSJ 590 (MBS,MOR); KAPI 690 (Indep., Span.); KFEL 970 (Indep., Mus., Relig.); KDZA 1230 (ABC/E, Top 40); KIDN 1350 (Indep., C&W) and KPUB (ABC/I, C&W); *FM Radio stations* KYCC 98 (Indep., CHO); KPLV 98.9 (Indep., Btfl.Mus.); KYNR 99.9 (Indep., Bftl. Mus.) and KZLO 100.7 (Indep., MOR); *television stations* KOAA Ch. 5 (NBC); KTSC Ch. 8 (PBS) and cable; *press:* two major dailies serve the city, the *Chieftan*, issued mornings, and *Star-Journal*, issued evenings.

HISTORY. The settlement of Ft. Pueblo was established in 1840, but was razed 14 years later by native Americans of the Ute tribe. In 1854, Fountain City was founded on

its site by entrepreneurs searching for gold. In 1860, Fountain City was renamed Pueblo (which is Spanish for village) after the original comm. and townsite were laid out. Incorporated as a town in 1870, Pueblo received its city charter in 1873. Today Pueblo is a major industrial center and the third largest city in CO.

GOVERNMENT. Pueblo has a council-mgr. form of govt. The seven council members are elected to four-year terms, three at large and four by district. The council president is selected from among the ranks of the council; a voting member, he serves a one-year term.

ECONOMY AND INDUSTRY. Pueblo's major industry is steel manufacturing. Other industries include clothing, auto parts, construction and building blocks, meat processing, retail and wholesale trade, aluminum pistons, insulation and soft drink bottling. In 1979, the city's total labor force was approx. 49,870 with an unemployment rate of 5.9%.

BANKING. There are 16 banks in Pueblo. In 1978 total deposits for the 11 banks headquartered in the city were $302,807,000, while assets were $351,441,000. Banks include First Natl., Pueblo Bank and Trust, Minnequa, United, Republic Natl. and Midtown Natl.

HOSPITALS. There are two gen. hosps. in Pueblo, Parkview Episcopal and St. Mary Corwin. The CO State Hosp. and Pueblo Neighborhood Health Center are also located in the city. The Spanish Peaks Mental Health Center offers specialized medical treatment.

EDUCATION. The U of S CO., a state-supported liberal arts and technological institution established in 1933, offers course work leading to associate, bachelor and master degrees. The U enrolled 5,659 in 1978. The private Midwest Business Col. enrolled nearly 150 in 1978. The newly created Pueblo Vocational Comm. Col. offers two-year technical programs. The Pueblo Regional Lib. and the U of S CO Lib. serve the area.

ENTERTAINMENT. The CO State Fair, held annually in late Aug. and

Mineral Lake, Pueblo, Colorado

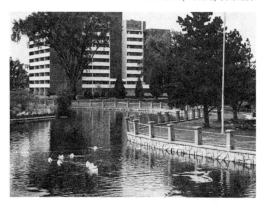

early Sept. features rodeos, pari-mutuel horse racing, exhibits, and a midway. There is Greyhound racing during the summer months. Semi-pro sports are offered by the Olympia Brewers baseball team and the Pueblo Peps hockey team. U of CO's Indians participate in collegiate sports.

ACCOMMODATIONS. There are several hotels and motels in Pueblo including the Claymar, Holiday and Ramada inns, the Town House Motel and Travelodge.

FACILITIES. The pueblo met. park system encompasses five parks, the City, Minnequa, Mitchell, Mineral Palace and Pueblo Mt. Public golf courses are located at the City Park and Pueblo W. River Trails feature a jogging trail and 16 mi. for biking and horseback riding.

CULTURAL ACTIVITIES. Musical organizations serving Pueblo include a civic symphony, jr. symphony and civic ballet co. The Symphony Orchestra and Chorale perform at the Sangre de Cristo Arts Conf. Center. The Center also hosts Broadway plays. Dramatic productions are also staged by

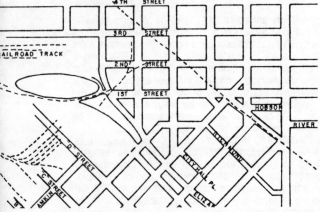

Pueblo, Colorado

the Impossible Playhouse. The El Pueblo Museum features a full-size reproduction of Ft. Pueblo and an exhibition depicting the evolution of iron and steel. The Pueblo Met. Museum, situated on the former Thatcher Estate, displays artifacts from the late 1800's. A Geological Museum is located at the U of S CO.

LANDMARKS AND SIGHTSEEING SPOTS. Pike's Stockade is a replica of the stockade Lt. Pike built in Pueblo when he was in the area in Nov. of 1806 to map the AR River and the LA purchase. Other landmarks include the Goodnight Barn, the last remaining building of the Charles Goodnight cattle empire. Union Depot, one time hub of the S CO RR system and the old Co. Courthouse with its ornate dome which still houses the co. govt.

RALEIGH
NORTH CAROLINA.

CITY LOCATION-SIZE-EXTENT. Raleigh, the capital of NC and seat of Wake Co., encompasses 49.46 sq. mi. in central NC at 35°52' N lat. and 78°47' W long. Raleigh and the city of Durham form a met. area that extends SE into Johnston, SW into Harnett, NW into Durham, W into Chatham, N into Granville and NE into Franklin.

TOPOGRAPHY. Raleigh is located in the transition zone between the Coastal Plain and the Piedmont Plateau where the surrounding terrain is generally rolling, rising slightly towards the Blue Ridge Mts. in the W. The mean elev. is 434'.

CLIMATE. The climate of Raleigh is continental. The avg. annual temp of 59.9°F ranges from a mean of 41.5°F during Jan. to a mean of 78.2° F during July. The annual

avg. rainfall of 45" is well distributed with the greatest amount falling in July and the least in Nov. The annual avg. snowfall is a scant 7.1". The RH ranges from 48% to 93%. The avg. growing season lasts approx. 210 days. Raleigh is located in the ESTZ and observes DST.

FLORA AND FAUNA. Animals native to Raleigh include the whitetail deer, opossum, raccoon, beaver, fox and chipmunk. Common birds include the warbler, vireo, mockingbird, bluejay and cardinal (the state bird). Bullfrogs, water snakes, toads, salamanders and box turtles as well as the venomous cottonmouth, copperhead, coral snakes and rattlesnake are found here. Trees include beech, oak, maple, elm, crepe myrtle, sycamore, sweetgum and pine (the state tree). Smaller plants include dogwood (the state flower), mt. laurel, honeysuckle and azalea.

POPULATION. According to the US census, the pop. of Raleigh in 1970 was 122,830. In 1978, it was estimated that it had increased to 156,256.

ETHNIC GROUPS. In 1978, the ethnic distribution of Raleigh was approx. 76.7% Caucasian, 22.6% Black, and 0.7% other.

TRANSPORTATION. Interstate hwy. 40, US hwys. 1, 64, 70 and 401 and state rtes. 50 and 54 provide major motor access to Raleigh. *Railroads* include AMTRAK, Seaboard Coast Line and S Railway. *Airlines* serving the city through the Raleigh-Durham Regional Airport include EA, DL, UA and PI. *Bus lines* include Carolina Trailways, Greyhound, S Coach Co. and Carolina Coach Co. and the local Capital Area Transit (CAT).

COMMUNICATIONS. Communications, broadcasting and print media originating from Raleigh are: *AM radio stations* WLLE 570 (Mut. Blk.); WPTF 680 (NBC, MOR); WKIX 850 (Indep., Contemp.); WPJL 1240 (MBS, Relig.) and WYNA 1550 (ABC/E, CUW); *FM radio stations* WKNC 88.1 (ABC/I, Educ., Top 40); WSHA 88.9 (Indep. Blk., Educ., Jazz); WCPE 89.7 (Indep., Educ.); WQDR 94.7 (Indep., AOR); WYYD 96.1 (Indep., Btfl. Mus.) and WRAL 101.5 (Indep., Contemp.); *television stations* WRAL Ch. 5 (ABC); WTVD Ch. 11 (CBS) and WRDU Ch. 28 (NBC); *press:* two major dailies serve the city, the morning *News & Observer* and the *Times*; other publications include *Biblical Recorder Technician, Carolina Co-operation, Carolina Country, NC Education, NC Farm Bureau News, NC Legion News, The State, Tarheel Wheels, We The People of NC, Newsweekly, The Carolinian, The Spectator* and the *Triangle Leader.*

HISTORY. Raleigh was founded in 1792 as the "unalterable seat of govt." for NC by the State's General Assembly. The city was named for Sir Walter Raleigh, who established the first English colony in America in the 16th century. The site chosen by the Assembly was purchased from a plantation owner, Joel Lane. A city engineer was appointed to design a city plan within 10

Leglislature Building, Raleigh, North Carolina

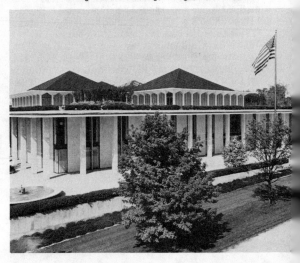

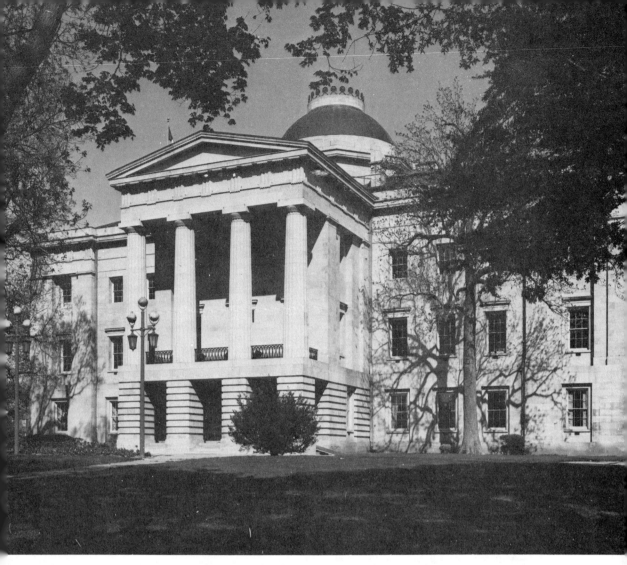

State Capitol, Raleigh, North Carolina

mi. of Hunter's Tavern. Andrew Johnson, the 17th President of the US, was born in Raleigh in 1808. Construction of state offices occupied the early part of the 19th century. The present capitol building was completed in 1840. That same year, the Raleigh & Gaston RR opened for business and brought growth to the city. The city's growth was halted only by the Civil War. While Raleigh escaped much of the destruction associated with Gen. Sherman's march to the sea, the Gov.'s Mansion had to be rebuilt after the war because it lay in ruins. Raleigh has continued to grow and it is now a center of scientific industrial research, a leading tobacco growing and curing market and home of several institutions of higher learning.

GOVERNMENT. Raleigh has a council-mgr. form of govt. consisting of eight members including the mayor, who is a voting member. The mayor and two council members are elected at large and five are elected by district, all for two-year terms. The council employs the city mgr.

ECONOMY AND INDUSTRY. The economy of Raleigh is greatly influenced by state govt. It is also the location of six public and private institutions of higher learning. Raleigh is a wholesale, retail trade and light manufacturing center. The establishment of Research Triangle Park has attracted research institutions to the area and there are currently 25 such agencies there, including business machines, the US Environmental Protection Agency and the Natl. Institute of Health. The service sector is the largest employer, followed by trade and manufacturing. Manufactured products include measuring and timing devices, data processing and electronic equipment, batteries, steel fabricators and dairy products. Retail sales in 1978 were $1,896,886,799. Avg. per capita income for the city in 1977 was $5,464. The total labor force for the Raleigh-Durham area in June, 1979, was 282,500 and the unemployment rate was 3.6%.

BANKING. There are 19 banking institutions in Raleigh. In 1978, total deposits for the three banks headquartered in the city were $1,172,366,000, while assets were $1,344,810,00. Banks include State Bank of Raleigh, Capitol Natl., First Citizens Bank & Trust Co., Bank of NC and Peoples Bank and Trust Co.

HOSPITALS. Wake Co. Medical Center in Raleigh is a full-service facility sharing its extensive diagnostic and therapeutic services with four suburban hosps., Wake, W Wake, E Wake and N Wake. The Dorothea Dix State Mental Hosp., Rex, Raleigh Comm. and Holly Hills hosps. are located here. Other medical services include the Wake Co. Mental Helath Center and the Inner City Mental Health Center.

EDUCATION. Raleigh, a U city, has NC State U (NCSU), one of the nation's larger and older public universities. First chartered in 1889, after its founding in 1887 as a land-grant institution and named NC Col. of Agriculture and Mechanic Arts, NCSU expanded rapidly to provide programs leading to every degree from associate to doctorate. Enrollment in 1978 was 17,809. Meredith Col, a private four-year col. for women founded in 1891 by the NC Baptist Convention, offers programs leading to the bachelor degree. Its engineering program is cooperatively arranged with NCSU, leading to a dual degree granted by both schools. In 1978, 1,378 students enrolled. St. Augustine's Col. is a four-year liberal arts col. founded by the Freemen's Commission of the Protestant Episcopal Church and members of the Episcopal Diocese of NC. Although nonracial in its admission policies, St. Augustine serves mainly the black pop. of the region. Peace Col., a two-year Presbyterian col., St. Mary's Jr. Co., offering the associate degree, and the Wake Technical Institute are other institutions in the city. All of these institutions are members of Cooperating Raleigh Colleges, a consortium whereby undergraduate students may enroll in any course not offered at his or her school, receiving credit upon completion. In 1979, over 25,864 enrolled in the consortium. Use of libs. and participation in cultural affairs and social events is included in this sharing arrangement. In 1976, Raleigh and Wake Co. public school systems merged and the system enrolled 55,000 students in 77 schools, from elementary to sr. high. The Wake Co. Public Lib. with branches throughout the co. is the largest and most widely used lib. in the area. Other libs. are the NC Museum of Fine Arts lib. and the law, medical, transportation and other specialized libs. of the state govt. are available for public use.

ENTERTAINMENT. The State Fair is held each Oct. in Raleigh. The NCSU's Wolfpack competes in intercollegiate football, basketball, and women's basketball. Shaw U Bears compete in basketball and Peace Col. has an all-women tennis team and the Green Giants basketball team.

ACCOMMODATIONS. Raleigh hotel and motel facilities include the Royal Villa Hotel, Velvet Cloak, Hilton, Holiday, Sheraton-Crabtree Motor and Plantation inns and Howard Johnson's.

FACILITIES. There are more than 25,000 acres of land and water available in the Raleigh area. There are 120 park sites with 34 major parks and 300 acres (6.7 miles of Greenway). Some of the major parks are Chavis, Sanderford Road, Pullen, Eastgate, Lake Johnson Nature, Lake Wheeler, Shelley Lake and Umstead State. Seventy-two-acre Pullen Park contains Howell Lake where pedal boats are available to the public. Lake Wheeler has 540 acres of water and 60 acres of land, offering facilities for boating, fishing, skiing, and picnicing. Umstead State Park covers 5,200 acres and offers a variety of recreational activities including organized group camping, picnicking, rowboats, fishing and nature trails. There is a 38-mi. bikeway system in the city consisting of 3.8 mi. of bike paths and 34.2 mi. of bike rtes. Public golf courses can be found at Cheviot Hills, Raleigh Golf Assn., and Wilmar Golf. Public tennis courts are available through the city park system and the Millbrook Tennis Center. Skating facilities and riding academies are also available.

Raleigh, North Carolina

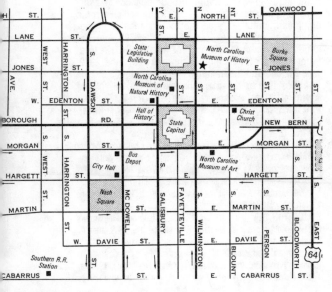

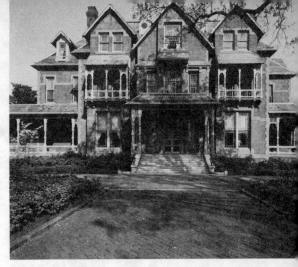

Governor's Mansion, Raleigh, North Carolina

CULTURAL ACTIVITIES. The NC Symphony, a state-sponsored organization, performs at the Memorial Auditorium. NC State U has its own student faculty symphonic ensemble performing on campus and giving public concerts. Raleigh Little Theater & Rose Garden, Theatre-in-the-Park and Stewart Theater present annual programs of musical and nonmusical works for the stage. The Raleigh Civic Ballet includes nonpro and pro choreographers and musicians in their performances. The NC Museum of Art contains works by Rembrandt, Rubens, Goyer, Monet, Wyeth and other W masters. It also sponsors an art appreciation program for the blind at the Mary Duke Biddle Gallery for the Blind. The Art Museum's Samuel H. Kress collection of Renaissance and Baroque art is among the largest in the country. There is a Museum of Natural History.

LANDMARKS AND SIGHTSEEING SPOTS. Raleigh is the birthplace of Andrew Johnson, the 17th President of the US, and the tiny house in which he was born is now located in Mordecai Historic Park. Among the historic homes in Raleigh are the Joel Lane House (1760) and the Charles Lee Smith House (1850). The Henry Clay Oak still marks the site where the statesman wrote his "Texas Question" letter which most likely cost him the US Presidency. Christ Episcopal Church, constructed about 1840, is one of the foremost examples of Gothic Revival buildings in the S. The State Capitol, built between 1833 and 1840, is a neo classical structure that has been restored to its 1840-1860 appearance. Located on a 5,200 acre site is Research Triangle Park, a center for research activities of private industry and govt. agencies.

RICHMOND
VIRGINIA

CITY LOCATION-SIZE-EXTENT. Richmond, the capital of VA, is an independent city located in the E central part of the state at 37°30' N lat. and 77°20' W long. Encompassing 62.5 sq. mi., including 3 sq. mi. of waterways, it lies at the head of the James River navigation system. It is bordered on the N and E by Henrico Co. and on the S and W by Chesterfield Co. Chesapeake Bay is 60 mi. to the E.

TOPOGRAPHY. Richmond is situated in an area between the Coastal Plain and the Piedmont Plateau regions. Its terrain is characterized by gently rolling hills. The mean elev. is 84".

CLIMATE. Richmond's climate is continental, and is considerably influenced by the mts. to the W that temper cold air masses moving into the area. Chesapeake Bay and the Atlantic Ocean contribute to humid summers and mild winters. The 58°F avg. annual temp. ranges between monthly means of 38°F in Jan. to 78°F in July. Almost a fourth of the 44' avg. annual rainfall occurs in July and Aug. The avg. growing season is 216

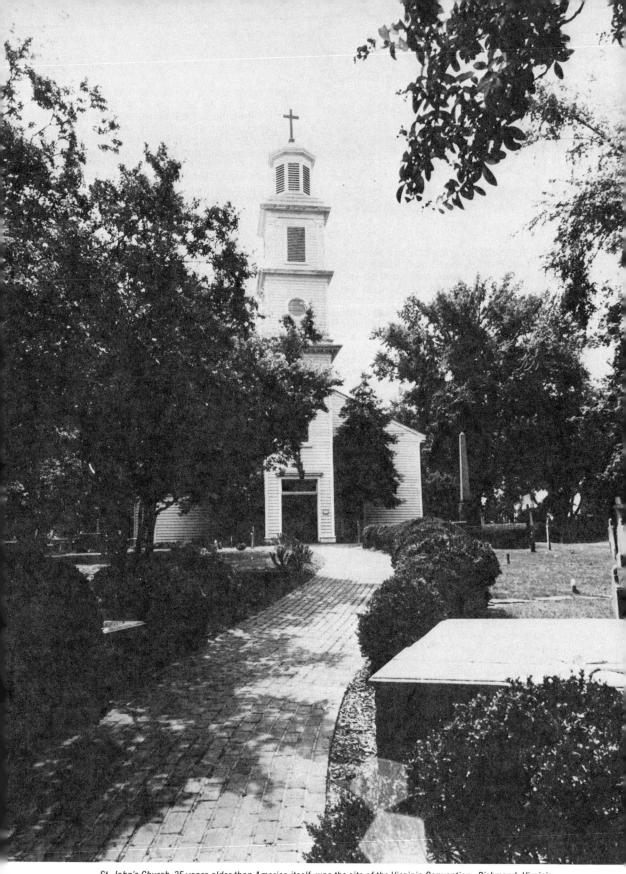

St. John's Church, 35 years older than America itself, was the site of the Virginia Convention , Richmond, Virginia.

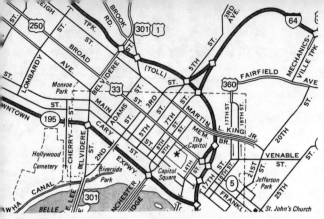

Central Richmond, Virginia

days. Richmond lies in the ESTZ and observes DST.

FLORA AND FAUNA. Animals native to Richmond include the opossum, gray and fox squirrels, cottontail rabbit, ground hog, and chipmunk. Common birds are the robin, blue jay, cardinal, wren and brown thrasher. Waterfowl and shorebirds winter on nearby Chesapeake Bay. Several species of reptiles, including the venomous rattlesnake, copperhead and cottonmouth, are found in the area. Typical trees are the maple, elm, oak, pine, ash and sweetgum. Flowering plants include the water lily, azalea, cattail and dogwood.

POPULATION. According to the US census, the pop. of Richmond in 1970 was 249,431. In 1978, it was estimated that it had decreased to 216,300.

ETHNIC GROUPS. In 1978, the ethnic distribution of Richmond was approx. 57.6% Caucasian, 42% Black and 0.4% other races.

TRANSPORTATION. Interstate hwys. 64, 95 and 195, US hwys. 1, 33, 60, 301 and 360 and state hwys. 6, 147 and 197 provide major motor access to Richmond. *Railroads* serving the area include AMTRAK, Chesapeake & OH, Chessie System, ConRail, MO Pacific, Norfolk & W, Richmond, Fredricksburg & Potomac, Rock Island, Seaboard Coast and S. *Airlines* serving Richard E. Byrd Intl. Airport are EA, PI and UA. *Bus lines* include Greyhound, Trailways and the local Greater Richmond Transit Co.

COMMUNICATIONS. Communications, broadcasting and print media originating from Richmond are: *AM radio stations* WRNL 910 (ABC/I, Contemp.); WXGI 950 (Indep., C&W); WANT 990 (Natl. Blk.); WRVA 1140 (NBC, MOR); WEET 1320 (ABC/E, Contemp. Ctry.); WTVR 1380 (CBS, Btfl. Mus.); WBBL 1480 (Indep., Contemp.); WLEE 1480 (ABC/C, Contemp.); WKIE 1540 (MBS, APR., MOR) and WGOE 1590 (Indep., Progsv.); *FM radio stations* WRVQ 94.5 (Indep., Top 40); WTVR 98.1 (Indep., Btfl. Mus.); WRXL 102.1 (Indep., AOR); WEZS 103.7 (Indep., Easy List.) and WRFK 106.5 (NPR, Clas., Jazz, Relig.); *television stations* WTVR Ch. 6 (CBS); WXEX Ch. 8 (ABC); WWBT Ch. 12 (NBC); WCVE Ch. 23 (PBS) and WCVW Ch. 57 (Indep.); *press:* two dailies serve the city, the *News Leader,* issued evenings and the *Times-Dispatch,* issued mornings; other publications include the *Afro-American and Planet, Catholic Virginian, Commonwealth Times, VA Churchman* and *Lifestyle Magazine.*

HISTORY. Native Americans of the Powhatan tribe lived in what is now Richmond. Richmond's first white visitors were Capts. John Smith and Christopher Newport who sailed up the James River within days after their historic 1607 landing in Jamestown. They were stopped by the Fall Line which is now the site of the city. Two years later, in 1609, Capt. Francis West built a ft. in the area. The ft. was abandoned due to attacks by native Americans. The site was resettled by Thomas Stegg in 1637, but it was Col. Wm. Byrd II who developed the settlement into a commercial center and planned a town on the site. It was laid out in 1737. Byrd named the settlement Richmond after Richmond-on-the-Thames, an English borough with a similar appearance. Richmond was incorporated as a town in 1742. It was the site of the second and third VA conventions of the Revolution in 1775 and became the state capital in 1779. It was captured in 1781 by British troops under Benedict Arnold, then in the British service, and rescued by Lafayette in 1782. The town's industry grew

and it manufactured the first American iron and brick, mined coal for the first time in the New World and started the nation's tobacco industry. Richmond was incorporated as a city in 1842. Between the 1830s and the Civil War, the city was a major slave market. As an industrial center, Richmond attracted many freed black males who were able to maintain themselves as wage earners. In 1861, Richmond became the capital of the Confederacy. Many battles occurred near the city during the Civil War. In 1865, when Confed. defenses in the area collapsed, parts of the city were burned during its evacuation to prevent its being captured undamaged by Union troops. After a difficult reconstruction period, Richmond became an industrial, financial, education and commercial center. Diverse industries were established in the city in the early 1900s, causing the pop. to grow to 230,310 by 1950. Richmond is one of the major S cities in which integration of schools and public facilities did not lead to racial riots or social dislocation in the 1950s and 60s. A 1970 annexation led to a suit against the city by a civil rights leader charging that the annexation would dilute the black vote. But the annexation was upheld by a 1976 ruling.

GOVERNMENT. Richmond has a council-mgr. form of govt. whose nine members are elected by district for two-year terms. The mayor is selected by the council.

Robert E. Lee Monument, Richmond, Virginia

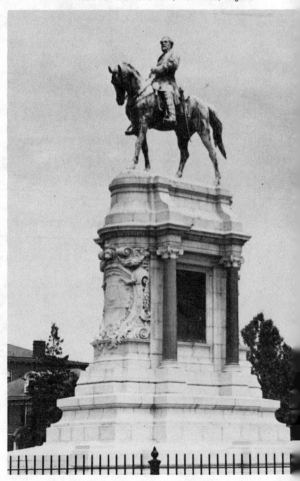

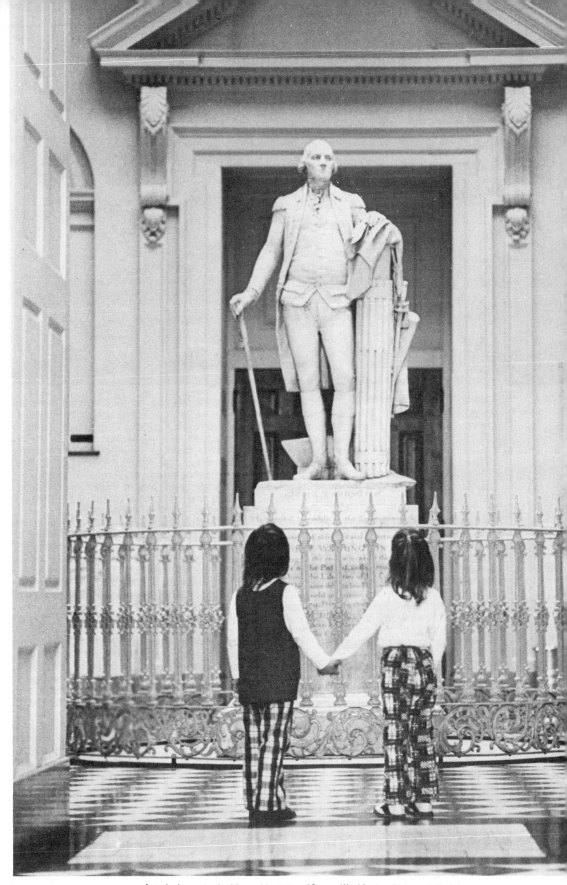

America's most valuable marble statue of George Washington, Richmond, Virginia

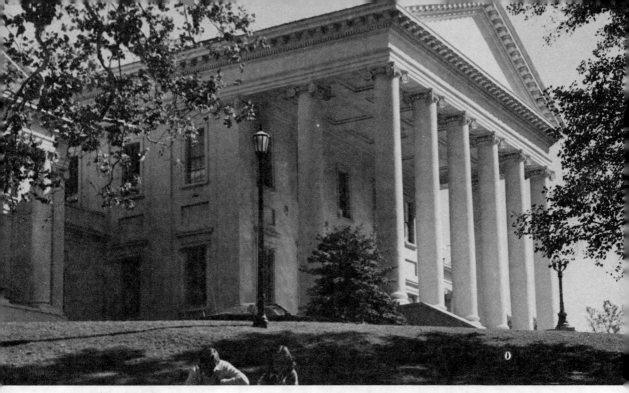

State Capitol, Richmond, Virginia

ECONOMY AND INDUSTRY. Known as the "Tobacco Capital of the World", Richmond produces more than 25% of the nation's cigarettes. Major manufactured products include chemicals, aluminum, paper, pharmaceuticals, paints, fertilizers, food, metal products, clothing and heavy sewn textiles. In June 1979, the met. labor force was 326,900 and the unemployment rate was 3.6%. The avg. income per capita in 1975 was $5.192.

BANKING. There are 12 banks and 77 other banking offices in Richmond. In 1978, total deposits for the 11 banks headquartered in the city were $4,687,547,000, while assets were $5,817,747,000. Banks include First and Merchant's Natl., Bank of VA, United VA, Central Natl. and S. The city is headquarters for the Fifth District Fed. Reserve Bank.

HOSPITALS. The AMA has designated Richmond a prime medical center, a rating given only to those cities which provide every type of care and surgery. There are 17 hosps. in Richmond including Chippenham, Grace, Johnston-Willis Richmond Memorial, St. Luke's, St. Elizabeth, St. Mary's Stuart Circle, The Medical Col. of VA Hosp. (the city's largest), Richmond Eye, Henrico Doctors', Commonwealth Psychiatric, Westbrook and Crippled Children's.

EDUCATION. The state-supported VA Commonwealth U and its medical sciences division, The Medical Col. of VA, offers degrees from associate to doctorate. Total enrollment in 1978 was 19,100, the city's largest. The J. Sargeant Reynolds Comm. Col., which enrolled approx. 8,700 in 1978, serves the area with a downtown campus and a campus in Henrico Co. Church-related institutions include the U of Richmond, VA Union, Union Theological Seminary and the Presbyterian School of Christian Education. The public school system maintains five high, nine middle and 29 elementary schools as well as seven special education centers and a technical center, with a total enrollment of approx. 32,577. Fifteen private schools are also located in the city.

ENTERTAINMENT. Theater entertainment and dining are offered at the Barn Dinner Theater, Swift Creek Mill Playhouse, Barksdale Theater, W End Dinner Theater and the Haymarket Dinner Theater. Annual events include the June Jubilee, the summer Festival of the Arts, the State Fair of VA held in Sept. and the Oct. Tobacco Bowl Festival. The city is the home of the Richmond Braves, an IL baseball team and the Rifles, an EHL hockey team. The U of Richmond Spiders, the VA Commonwealth U Rams and VA Union Panthers are intercollegiate sports teams.

ACCOMMODATIONS. Richmond's hotels and motels include the Jefferson, John Marshall and Hyatt hotels and the Best Western, Howard Johnson's, Ramada, Sheraton Motor, Scottish and Holiday inns.

FACILITIES. Richmond's 25-unit park system includes the Bryan, Byrd, Chimborazo, James River and Maymount parks. Among the unique features of the Maymount park are its Parson's Nature Center, which features the area's natural inhabitants, native VA wildlife habitats and the herb, Italian and Japanese gardens. There are numerous public golf courses, several skating rinks, jogging tracks and swimming pools. Nearby is the Wintergreen skiing center and resort.

CULTURAL ACTIVITIES. The VA Museum Theater, the VA Chamber Music Society and the VA Dance Society provide programs at the VA Museum of Fine Arts. The Richmond Orchestra offers performances at a municipal theater. Battle Abbey, the Confed. Memorial Institute, houses materials on VA history, including many manuscripts on Confed. VA. The Confed. Museum, once the home of Confed. Pres. Jefferson Davis, exhibits relics of the Confederacy. The VA Museum of Fine Arts contains one of the world's finest collections of Fabrege eggs. The Valentine Museum, designed by Robert Mills, was built in 1812 and houses exhibits and relics of local history.

LANDMARKS AND SIGHTSEEING SPOTS. The VA Capitol, which was designed by Thomas Jefferson, is a replica of a Roman temple in Nimes, France. A statue of George Washington, done from a life mask by Antoine Hudon, stands in the rotunda. An equestrian statue of Washington stands in the Sq. A statue of Bill "Bo Jangles" Robinson is located in the Jackson Ward area. St. John's Church, also located in the city, was the site of Patrick Henry's famous "Give me liberty or give me death" speech. Many leading Virginians, including Pres. John Tyler and James Monroe, and Jefferson Davis and Gen. Fitzhugh Lee, are buried in Hollywood Cemetery. The cemetery also contains a granite memorial to 18,000 Confed. soldiers buried there. Historical houses open to the public include, Lee House, John Marshall House, Agecroft Hall, VA House and Wilton House. The VA WWII, Korea and Vietnam Memorial Shrine contains relics of major land and naval battles. The Richmond Natl. Battlefield Park features permanent exhibits and an audio-visual program which demonstrates the Civil War battles fought near the city. It covers 57 mi. of battle lines, including the outer Richmond defenses. The $26 million Coliseum, opened in 1971, hosted the first indoor US-USSR track meet. Many Victorian townhomes are being restored in the Fan District. The Natl. Park Service is restoring the home of Maggie Walker, the country's first woman bank pres. and a prominent black Virginian and Richmond native. Confed. statues line the hand-paved Monument Ave.

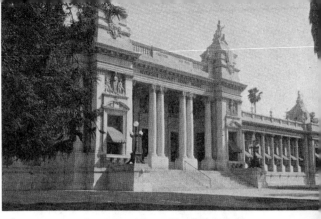

County Court House, Riverside, California

RIVERSIDE
CALIFORNIA

CITY LOCATION-SIZE-EXTENT. Riverside, the seat and largest city of Riverside Co., encompasses 71.3 sq. mi. on the N branch of the Santa Ana River in S CA, approx. 10 mi. S of San Bernadino and 53 mi. E of LA, at 33°58' N lat. and 117°21' W long. The greater met. area includes the cities of Highgrove to the NE, Edgemont to the E, San Bernadino to the NE and Ontario to the NW and extends into San Bernadino Co. on the S and N and Orange Co. on the SW.

TOPOGRAPHY. The terrain of Riverside consists of hilly to mt. areas at the foothills of the San Bernadino Mts., while to the E the land slopes downward into a basin area. The mean elev. is 858'.

CLIMATE. The climate of Riverside is marine, characterized by the prevailing W winds of the Pacific Ocean which, combined with other factors, produce pleasant and mild weather. The avg. annual temp. of 60°F ranges from an Aug. mean of approx. 70°F to a Jan. mean of approx. 50°F. Daily temps. may vary 30°F between afternoon and evening. The 13" of avg. annual rainfall occurs mainly during the winter. The RH ranges from 40% to 80%. Riverside lies in the PSTZ and observes DST.

FLORA AND FAUNA. Animals native to Riverside include the coyote, pocket gopher, ground squirrel, skunk and opossum. Common birds include the scrub jay, CA quail, W kingbird and hummingbird. Alligator lizards, gopher snakes, coachwhip snakes, pond turtles and tree frogs as well as the venomous Pacific rattlesnake, are found in the area. Typical trees are the oak, pine and fir. Smaller plants include the CA golden poppy (the state flower), chaparral shrub and creamcup.

POPULATION. According to the US census, the pop. of Riverside in 1970 was 140,089. In 1978, it was estimated that it had increased to 161,000.

TRANSPORTATION. Interstate Hwy. 15 and state hwys. 60 and 91 provide major motor access to Riverside. *Railroads* serving the city include Union Pacific, Santa Fe and S Pacific. All major *airlines* serve Ontario Intl. Airport, 18 mi. NW of the city. Riverside Municipal Airport offers regular commuter service to LA and Ontario, in addition to private and charter flight facilities. *Bus lines* serving the city include Greyhound, Trailways, Southern CA Rapid Transit District and the local Riverside Transit Agency.

ETHNIC GROUPS. In 1978, the ethnic distribution of Riverside was approx. 93.3% Caucasian, 5.2% Black and 12.7% Hispanic. (A percentage of the Hispanic total is also included in the Caucasian total.)

COMMUNICATIONS. Communications, broadcasting and print media originating from Riverside are: *AM radio stations* KPRO 1440 (CBS, Btfl. Mus.) and KHNY 1570 (MBS, Adult Contemp.); *FM radio stations* KUCR 88.1 (Indep., Var., Educ.); KLLU 89.7 (ABC/I, Relig.); KHNY 92.7 (Indep., Btfl. Mus.); KDUO 97.5 (Indep., MOR) and KBBL 99.1 (Indep., Relig.); no *television* stations originate from Riverside, which receive broadcasting from the nearby LA met. area; *press*: two major dailies serve the city, the *Enterprise*, issued mornings, and the *Press*, issued evenings; other publications include *The Beacon, Highlander, Riverside Arlington Times, Render, Globetrotter* and *Riverside Co. Farm & Agricultural Business News.*

HISTORY. The first inhabitants of the Riverside area, in the Santa Ana River Valley, were native Americans of the Cahuilla and Serrano tribes. In 1774, Captain Juan Bautista de Anza, with a company of Spanish soldiers, camped near the site of Riverside. In 1776, he returned, bringing 242 colonists, to increase CA's Spanish pop.

During the early 19th century the river valley lands were used for sheep grazing, but the herds were destroyed by the flood of 1862 and the droughts of 1863 and 1864. The lands of the Rubidoux Rancho were owned briefly by Louis Prevost and his CA Silk Center Assn. and then bought for development in 1870 by John North and the S CA Colony Assn. The town's name, initially Jurupa, was changed to Riverside in 1871. In 1873, L. C. and Eliza Tibbets planted the first Washington navel orange trees near Riverside. The variety led to the development of the citrus industry in CA and, 1879, the first Citrus Fair was held in the city. Riverside was incorporated in 1883. In 1892, the first marketing cooperative was established in the city, leading to the founding of the CA Fruit Growers' Exchange. The Citrus Research Center at the U of CA at Riverside was established in 1907 and is still active today. During WW I, March Field was constructed nearby to train Army fliers. After the war, industry began to develop among the area's citrus groves. During WW II, March Field was expanded and Camps Haan and Anza were built, greatly increasing local employment. Today, Riverside is a major center of agriculture and industry.

GOVERNMENT. Riverside has a council-mgr. form of govt. consisting of seven councilmen and a mayor. Council members are elected by district to four-year terms. The mayor, elected at large to a four-year term is not a member of council and votes only to break a tie.

ECONOMY AND INDUSTRY. There are more than 200 manufacturing firms in the Riverside area. Leading products are mobile homes, recreational vehicles, electronic components, aircraft and rocket motor assemblies. The Co. of Riverside and the U of CA at Riverside are the major non-manufacturing employers. In June, 1979, the greater met. area, including San Bernardino, had a labor force of 569,900, while the rate of unemployment was 6.5%.

BANKING. In 1978, total deposits for the only bank headquartered in the city, Riverside Natl., were $40,768,000, while assets were $44,850,000.

HOSPITALS. There are three gen. hosps. in Riverside, Riverside Comm., Riverside Gen., UMC and Parkview Comm.

EDUCATION. The U of CA at Riverside was founded in 1947 as an experimental station for research on the control of citrus tree diseases and pests. Offering degrees at both the grad. and undergrad. levels, the U enrolled more than 4,900 in 1978. Riverside City Col., the oldest col. in the city, was established in 1916. The publicly-supported col. awards associate degrees and, in 1978, it enrolled more than 14,100. Other institutions include CA Baptist Col. and the La Sierra Campus of Loma Linda U. Specialized schools located in the city include the CA School for the Deaf and Sherman Indian High School. There are 31 elementary, seven jr. high and six sr. high schools in the public school system, while 18 parochial schools are available. Libs. include the Riverside Main Lib.

ENTERTAINMENT. The Mission Inn in Riverside provides dinner theater for the area. Collegiate sports are provided by the U of CA at Riverside Highlanders, the Riverside City Col. Tigers and the CA Baptist Col. Lancers.

ACCOMMODATIONS. There are several hotels and motels in Riverside,

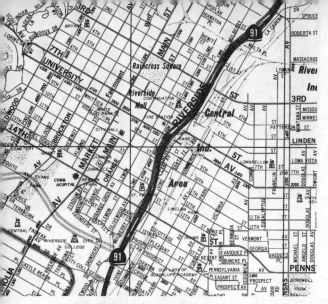

Riverside, California

including the American MotelLodge, Howard Johnson's, Mission, Holiday and Ramada inns.

FACILITIES. There are 23 public parks in Riverside. The largest, Fairmont Park, contains a rose garden, an amusement park, picnic grounds, a playground, a golf course, tennis courts, a lawn-bowling green and a recreation center. It also offers boating and fishing on Lake Evans and horse trails, hiking trails and a nature study area in its wilderness area. Mt. Rubidoux Park rises above the Santa Ana River at the city's W edge and offers hiking. A public golf course is available at Fairmont Park. Public tennis courts are available through the city park system.

CULTURAL ACTIVITIES. Riverside dates the cultural growth of the city back to its earliest existence, when John North sent a circular to the new colony insisting on cultural pursuits. The first addition to cultural life was the Loring Opera House. The early Art Assn. expanded to form the Riverside Opera Assn. Other groups include the Riverside Symphony, the Civic Ballet, the Riverside Chorale, the Arlington Art Guild, the Fine Arts Guild, Riverside Comm. Players and the Children's Theatre. Members of these groups comprise the Riverside Arts Council. The Riverside Museum, built in Italian Renaissance style, contains many exhibits of natural history. The Riverside Art Assn. maintains the Riverside Art Center and Museum.

LANDMARKS AND SIGHTSEEING SPOTS. Mission Inn, an historic mission-style hotel in Riverside, features a 200-year-old altar from Guanajuato, Mexico. The Parent Navel Orange Tree, first planted in 1873 by Luther and Eliza Tibbets, can be seen in the city. There are many 19th-century styled buildings in Riverside, including the Unitarian-Universalist Church, the Bettner-McDavid House (Heritage House), Benedict Castle, the S. C. Evans Home, Sherman Indian Museum, the Riverside Co. Courthouse and the United Magnolia Presbyterian Church, the oldest existing church in Riverside.

ROANOKE
VIRGINIA

CITY LOCATION-SIZE-EXTENT. Roanoke, an independent city, encompasses 43 sq. mi. of SW VA at 37°19' N lat. and 79°58' W long. in the Roanoke River Valley between the Alleghenies to the W and Blue Ridge Mts. to the E. The greater met. area extends into Botetourt Co. to the NE, Bedford Co. to the E, Franklin Co. to the S, Montgomery Co. to the SW, the town of Vinten to the SE, Craig Co. and the city of Salem to the NW.

TOPOGRAPHY. The terrain of Roanoke is characterized by a narrow ridge to the NE that rises sharply from the lower land E and W of it with the ridge broadening to the

S into a plateau. S of the region are VA's highest mt. peaks, Mt. Rogers and Whitetop Mt. Mill Mt., within the city, rises to 2,000'. The mean elev. is 945'.

CLIMATE. The climate in Roanoke, which is mild continental, is moderated by the Roanoke River Valley. Extreme temps. in summer or winter are rare and summer nights are usually cool. The 56.3°F avg. annual temp. ranges between monthly means of 36°F in Jan. to 76°F in July. The 40'' avg. annual rainfall is well distributed throughout the year. Most of the 25'' avg. annual snowfall occurs in Jan. and Feb. The RH ranges from 45% to 77%. The avg. growing season is 190 days. Roanoke lies in the ESTZ and observes DST.

FLORA AND FAUNA. Animals native to Roanoke include the opossum, fox, groundhog, bear, whitetail deer, turkey, squirrel and rabbit. Common birds include the robin, barn swallow, cardinal, wren and brown thrasher. Bullfrogs, salamanders, lizards, turtles and several species of snakes, including the venomous rattlesnake and copperhead, inhabit the area. Typical trees are the pine, poplar, locust, maple, oak and dogwood. Flowering plants include the rhododendron, azalea and mt. laurel.

POPULATION. According to the US census, the pop. of Roanoke in 1970 was 92,115. In 1978, it was estimated that it had increased to 105,500.

ETHNIC GROUPS. In 1978, the ethnic distribution of Roanoke was approx. 81% Caucasian, 18% Black and 1% other.

Central Roanoke, Virginia

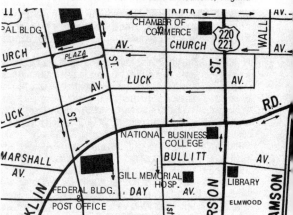

TRANSPORTATION. Interstate hwy. 81, US hwys. 11, 220, 221 and 460 and state hwys. 24 and 311 provide major motor access to Roanoke. The city is also served by one *railroad*, the Norfolk & W. *Airlines* serving Woodrum Municipal Airport include PI and Air VA. *Bus lines* include Greyhound, Trailways and the local Valley Metro.

COMMUNICATIONS. Communications, broadcasting and print media originating from Roanoke are: *AM radio stations* WSLC 610 (NBC, C&W); WTOY 910 (Mut. Blk.); WFIR 960 (CBS, MBS, MOR); WROV 1240 (ABC/C, MOR, Top 40); WRIS 1410 (MBS, MOR) and WKBA 1550 (Indep., C&W, Gospel); *FM radio stations* WWWR 89.1 (NPR, Educ., Info., Cultural); WLRG 92.3 (ABC/E, contemp.); WPVR 94.9 (Indep., MOR) and WSLQ 1550 (Indep., Rock); *television stations* WDBJ Ch. 7 (CBS); WSLS Ch. 10 (NBC) and WBRA Ch. 15 (PBS); *press:* one major daily serves the city, the *Times & World News*, issued both mornings and evenings; other publications include the *Tribune, Norfolk and W Magazine, The Roanoker, Shenadoah Valley Magazine* and *Ski S*.

HISTORY. The town of Big Lick, forerunner of modern day Roanoke, was chartered in 1874. In 1882, the meeting of two major RRs, the Shenandoah Valley RR and the Norfolk & Western RR, at Big Lick gave rise to a new town, renamed Roanoke after the country and the river on whose banks it was situated. The name comes

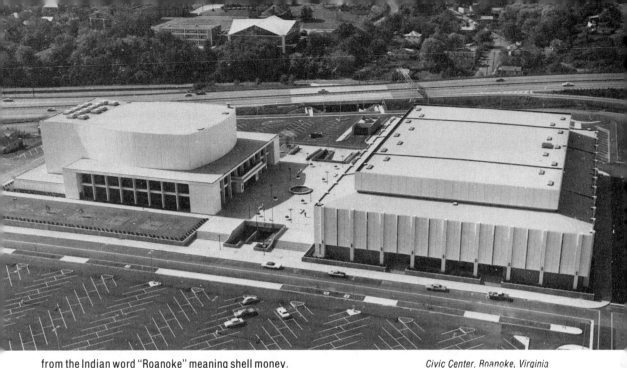

from the Indian word "Roanoke" meaning shell money. The town grew quickly and by 1884 had been chartered as a city. The city's location on the RR lines made it prosper in the 19th century as a major transportation center. Today, the city serves as a manufacturing, commercial and transportation center for the SW part of VA.

GOVERNMENT. Roanoke has a council-mgr. form of govt. consisting of seven council members, including the mayor as a voting member. All are elected at large to staggered four-year terms.

ECONOMY AND INDUSTRY. Wholesale and retailing form the largest industry in Roanoke, with more than 2,486 retail outlets. Electrical equipment, lumber, apparel, plastics, furniture, flour, processed foods, fabricated metal products and machinery are predominant manufactures. The labor force in the met. area totalled 110,700 in 1978, while unemployment was 5.5%. The avg. income per capita for 1978 was $5,572.

BANKING. There are 10 commercial banks and six savings and loan assns. in Roanoke. In 1978, deposits at the two banks headquartered in the city were $893,391,000, while assets totaled $1,060,694,000. Among banks serving the city are First Natl. Exchange Bank, Colonial American Natl. Bank, Bank of VA and First VA Bank of Roanoke.

HOSPITALS. There are several gen. and specialized hosps. in the city including Roanoke Memorial, Comm., Lewis-Gale, White Cross, an alcoholic treatment center and Catawba State, which specializes in geriatrics, TB and mental health.

EDUCATION. The U of VA Extension campus in Roanoke offers both undergrad. and grad. courses, and, in 1978, enrolled approx. 3,800. VA W Comm. Col., established in 1966, offers programs leading to the associate degree, and, in 1978, enrolled approx. 5,303. Roanoke Col., located in nearby Salem, is a private, liberal arts col. that awards bachelor degrees. There are 21 elementary, six intermediate and two high schools with a student enrollment of 18,800; private and parochial schools enroll an additional 1,450. Libs. include the City of Roanoke Public Lib. and the Roanoke Co. Public Lib.

ENTERTAINMENT. The Barn offers dinner theater entertainment in Roanoke. The Festival in the Park is an annual springtime event during which area artists and craftsmen exhibit their work. Each April, beautiful private homes and gardens are open to the public during Historic Garden Week. Other annual events include the Miss VA pageant, City Market Harvest Festival and the Indoor Horse Show. The Salem Pirates baseball club provides pro baseball in Spring. Roanoke Col. participates in collegiate sports.

ACCOMMODATIONS. There are several hotels and motels in Roanoke,

including the Hotel Roanoke, Howard Johnson's, Patrick Henry, TraveLodge, Colony House and the Holiday, Sheraton, Ramada and Day's inns.

FACILITIES. Roanoke's municipal system of 33 parks feature miniature golf courses, driving ranges and roller and ice skating rinks. Atop the 2,000' Mill Mt. is a park with a children's zoo that houses bear cubs, ocelots, giant tortoises, coatimundis and snakes. Other parks include Fallon, Fishburn, Wasena and Washington. Jogging tracks, 176 tennis courts and public swimming pools are also available in the city.

CULTURAL ACTIVITIES. Concerts are presented by the Roanoke Symphony and the Roanoke Jr. Symphony. The Mill Mt. Playhouse, the Showtimers and the Vinton Players offer live theater in the city. The Transportation Museum features exhibits of modern and antique automobiles (including one of the longest model trains in the world). Other museums include the Historical Society, the Science Museum and the Fine Arts Center. There are several art galleries in the city.

LANDMARKS AND SIGHTSEEING SPOTS. Both Firehouse One, built in 1906, and St. Andrew's Catholic Church are listed in the Natl. Register of Historic Places. St. John's Episcopal Church was built in 1892, although its congregation dates back to 1831. The Whitescarver Engineering Building (in which the first bank in Big Lick was housed), the R. H. Angell Building, Flickwir House, the Freight Depot and the Asberry Building (erected in 1890) are other historical buildings in the city. Buried in the Old City Cemetery are members of some of the families prominent in the early days of the city. Legend maintains that those who drink from Dog-Mouth Fountain will some day return to Roanoke.

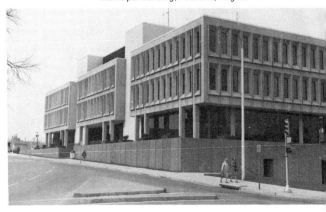

ROCHESTER
NEW YORK

CITY LOCATION-SIZE-EXTENT. Rochester, the seat of Monroe Co. and the third largest city in NY, is a port city in W NY encompassing 36.7 sq. mi. at 43°07' N lat. and 77°40' W long. The met. area borders Lake Ontario on the N and the St. Lawrence Seaway connects the city to the Atlantic Ocean. The met. area includes the cities of Greece to the NW and Irondequoit to the NE and it extends into Wayne Co. to the E, Ontario Co. to the SE, Livingston Co. to the S and Genesee and Orleans Cos. to the W.

TOPOGRAPHY. Rochester is part of the Erie-Ontario Lowland region. Its terrain varies from level to moderately rolling, inclining slightly toward Lake Ontario. The city is divided by the Genesee River, which flows into Lake Ontario. Irondequoit Bay is to the NE and the NY State Barge Canal crosses the city on the SW. The mean elev. is 515'.

CLIMATE. The climate of Rochester is continental and is influenced by Lake Ontario, which extends the winter and summer seasons. The avg. annual temp. of 47.8°F ranges from a Jan. mean of 24.7°F to a July mean of 71.3°F. The 32.6" avg. annual rainfall is evenly distributed throughout the year. Most of the 88.4" avg. annual snowfall occurs from Dec. to Mar. The RH ranges from 53% to 88%. The growing season is approx. 180 days. Rochester is located in the ESTZ and observes DST.

FLORA & FAUNA. Animals native to Rochester include the opossum, raccoon, fox and squirrel. Typical birds include the loon, osprey, bluebird, thrush and goldfinch. Bullfrogs, water snakes, snapping turtles, soft-shell turtles, spring peepers, salamanders and the venomous timber rattlesnake and E massasauga (a pygmy rattlesnake), are common to the area. Typical trees include the oak, willow, maple and elm. Smaller plants include the rose, lilac, rhododendron, blackberry and bull thistle.

POPULATION. According to the US census, the pop. of Rochester in 1970 was 296,233. In 1977, it was estimated that it had decreased to approx. 256,283.

ETHNIC GROUPS. In 1978, the ethnic distribution of Rochester was approx. 79.4% Caucasian, 16.7% Black, 3.0% Hispanic and .9% other races.

TRANSPORTATION. Interstate hwys. 390 and 490, US hwys. 15, 15A

Central Rochester, New York

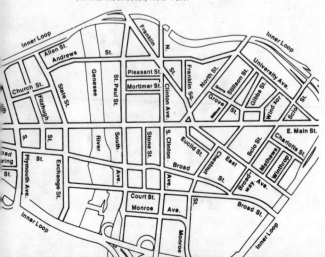

and 104 and state hwys. 47, 15, 31 and 104 provide major motor access to Rochester. *Railroads* serving the city are the Chessie System, ConRail, MO Pacific, S Railway and AMTRAK. *Airlines* serving the Rochester-Monroe Co. Airport include US Air, AA and UA. *Buslines* include Greyhound, Trailways, and the local Regional Transit Service. The Port of Rochester and the Barge Canal Waterway provide water transporation.

COMMUNICATIONS. Communications, broadcasting and print media originating from Rochester are: *AM radio stations* WNYR 680 (ABC/D, C&W); WBBF 950 (ABC/C, Contemp.); WHAM 1180 (ABC/I, MOR); WPXN 1280 (Indep., All News); WSAY 1370 (Indep., C&W); WWWG 1460 (ABC/C, Christian); *FM radio stations:* WRUR 88.5 (ABC/FM, Jazz, Clas.); WITR 89.7 (RII, Progsv.); WIRQ 90.9 (ABC/FM, Var.); WXXI 91.5 (NPR, Clas.); WMJQ 92.5 (Indep., Clas.); WMJQ 92.5 (Indep., Clas.); WCMF 96.5 (Indep., Progsv.); WPX& 97.9 (Indep., Btfl. Mus.); WHFM 98.9 (ABC/C, Rock); WVOR 100.5 (ABC/FM, MOR, Oldies); WEZO 101.3 (Indep., Btfl. Mus.); and WDKX 103.9 (Natl., Blk.); *television stations* WROC Ch. 8 (NBC); WHEC Ch. 10 (CBS); WOKR, Ch. 13 (ABC) and WXXI Ch. 21 (PBS); *press:* two major dailies serve the area, the *Democrat & Chronicle,* issued morning, and the *Times-Union,* issued evenings; other publications include the *Courier-Journal, Eastsider, Gates-Chili News, American Turner Topics, Automatic Machining, NE Tribune, City Newspaper, 10th Ward Courier/Vicinity Post* and *About Time.*

HISTORY. The Algonquins, the original inhabitants of the Rochester area, were followed by the Senecas and the League of the Iroquois. Later, farmers settled the surrounding area, establishing many small towns. In 1812, Colonel Nathaniel Rochester of Maryland and two associates bought tracts of land on both banks of the Genesee River, with the intention of using the Genesee Falls as a power source for a flour mill. A bridge was built across the falls and a comm. began to grow at the site. In 1817, it was chartered as the village of Rochesterville. Rochester was called "the nation's first boom town" when its section of the Erie Canal was opened in 1823, causing its pop. to rapidly increase. The city's many flour mills gave it the nickname "Flour City." Other industries, including the 1880 establishment of a photographic equipment manufacturer, contributed to the steady growth of the city. A railroad reached the city in 1833 and a steam engine arrived in 1836. Rochester had become a major distribution center when it was incorporated as a city in 1834. The harbor was improved in the early 1900s and in 1959 the completion of the St. Lawrence Seaway made Rochester an ocean port. Continued expansion and the construction of major redevelopment projects and civic buildings were pursued in the 1970s. Today the city is the third largest city in NY.

GOVERNMENT. Rochester has a council-mgr. form of govt. There are nine council members, including the mayor—five members are elected at-large and four members are elected by district. All members serve four-year terms. The mayor is appointed from within the council and is a voting member. The council appoints a city mgr.

ECONOMY AND INDUSTRY. Rochester's industries produce photographic material, xerographic equipment, optical instruments and lenses, opthalmic goods, dental equipment, thermometers, and gear-cutting machines. Other important industries are printing and publishing, food processing, petrochemicals, men's apparel, and office equipment. Eastman Kodak is the city's chief employer. The city is also an important distribution center. The 1979 met. area labor force was approx. 479,300 with an unemployment rate of 4.4%.

BANKING. In 1978, total deposits for the seven banks headquartered in Rochester were $4,197,245,000, while assets were $5,077,914,000. Banks include Lincoln First, Comm. Savings, Rochester Savings, Second Trust Co., Monroe Savings, Central Trust Co. and First Natl.

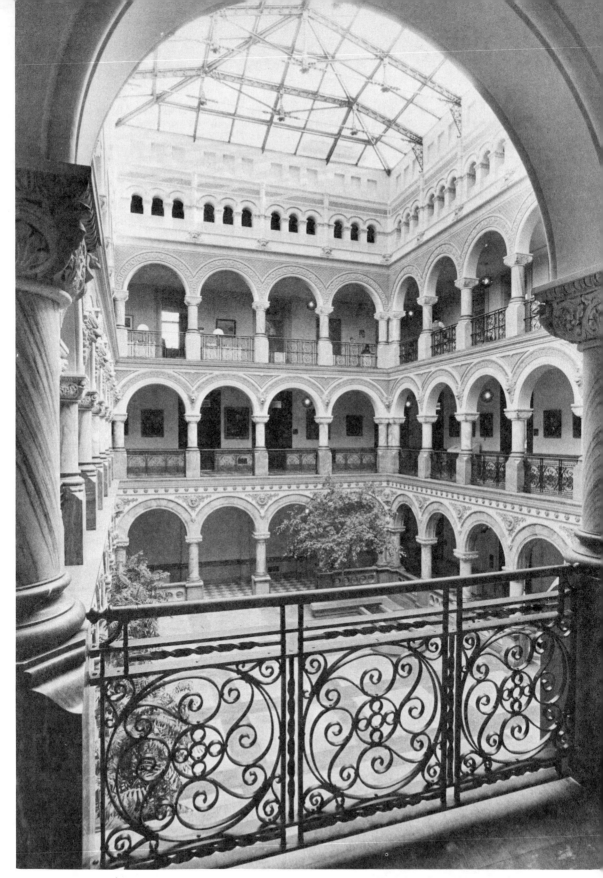

City Hall Atrium, Rochester, New York

HOSPITALS. There are several hosps. in the city, including Strong Memorial of the U of Rochester, Genesee, Lakeside, Rochester General, St. Mary's and Pare Ridge Highland. Strong Memorial specializes in psychiatry, burns, poison control and atomic and space medicine.

EDUCATION. The privately-supported, coeducational U of Rochester, founded in 1850, is one of the nation's smallest leading universities. In 1978, its enrollment was more than 8,750. Its Eastman School of Music has won intl. acclaim. Rochester Institute of Technology, a private, coeducational school founded in 1829, was a pioneer in career-oriented and cooperative work/study education. In 1978, it enrolled more than 12,500. The Institute also established the Natl. Technical Institute for the Deaf, the nation's only post-secondary technical col. for the deaf. Other institutions include Monroe Comm. Col., which enrolled more than 10,000 in 1978, Nazareth Col. of Rochester, St. John Fisher Col., Colgate Rochester Divinity School/Crozerr Theological Seminary, Roberts Wesleyan Col., Rochester Bus. Institute and St. Bernard's Seminary. The public school system includes over 60 elementary and high schools. The Rochester Public Lib. consists of a main lib. with 12 branches. Other lib. include the Pioneer Public Lib. System and the NY State Judicial Dept. Lib.

ENTERTAINMENT. Caesar's Dinner Theater in Rochester provides dining entertainment. Festivals and annual events include Lilac Time, Cornhill Art Festival, Curbstone Craft Festival, La Italiana, Puerto Rico Festival, Pan African Cultural Expo and Oktoberfest. Pro sports are offered by the Americans (AHL, hockey), the Monarchs (NYPMHL, hockey), the Red Wings (IL, baseball) and the Lancers (NASL, hockey). The Rochester Institute of Technology Tigers and the U of Rochester Yellow Jackets provide intercollegiate sports.

ACCOMMODATIONS. Rochester hotels include the Americana, Midtown Tower, TraveLodge, Marriott, One Eleven E Avenue and Hilton, Genesee Plaza/Holiday, Ramada, Sheraton, Gatehouse and Colony E inns.

FACILITIES. There are 16 parks in Rochester's 10,300-acre park system, including Highland, Durand, Eastman, Maplewood and Seneca parks. Highland contains the Botanic Gardens, a conservatory, and a large lilac exhibit. Maplewood contains one of the nation's largest municipal rose gardens. Sailing is a popular sport, with active yacht clubs on Lake Ontario and Irondequoit Bay. Several public golf courses are available.

CULTURAL ACTIVITIES. Opera Under the Stars and the performance of a ballet company are offered in Rochester. The Civic Music Assn. supports the Rochester Philharmonic Orchestra, which presents approx. 200 concerts annually, and an annual Artist Series, featuring nationally prominent musical groups. The Eastman School of Music gives many public performances. A collection of photography and cinematography at the George Eastman House includes cameras, lenses, photographs, motion pictures and other photographic equipment. The museum also houses the

Downtown, Rochester, New York

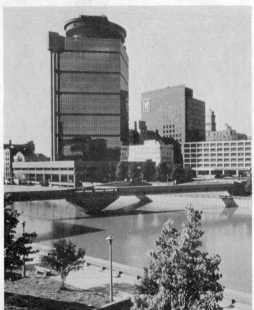

Dryden Theater, which shows classic films to the public. The Rochester Museum of Arts and Sciences is one of the few museums in the nation containing only displays indicative of its geographical location. It features a display of Seneca and Iroquois Indian arts and crafts. The Memorial Art Gallery contains exhibits of art from a variety of periods and offers lectures, films and classes. The Oxford Gallery contains the city's largest collection of paintings, sculpture, graphics ethnic and tribal art. The Shoestring Gallery displays the work of approx. 50 area artists and craftsmen.

LANDMARKS AND SIGHTSEEING SPOTS. The Campbell-Whittlesey House, in Rochester, is a fine example of Greek Revival architecture. It was built in 1835 and has been restored to its original period furnishings. The Stone Tolan House, built in 1792, is believed to be the oldest remaining house in Monroe Co. It contains furnishings appropriate to a pioneer farm site. The residence of suffrage leader Susan B. Anthony is also open to the public. She lived in the house from 1866 to 1906. The Strasenburgh Planetarium offers audiovisual presentations simulating the movement of the Planets. Many local manufacturing plants offer tours of their facilities.

ROCKFORD
ILLINOIS

CITY LOCATION-SIZE-EXTENT. Rockford, second largest city in IL and seat of Winnebago Co., encompasses 36.1 sq. mi. on both banks of the Rock River, midway between Chicago and the MS River, 17 mi. S of the WI border, at 42°12' N lat. and 89°6' W long. Its met. area covers Winnebago Co. and extends into Boone Co. to the E, De Kalb Co. to the SE, Ogle Co. to the S, Stephenson Co. to the W and across the border into WI to the N.

TOPOGRAPHY. Rockford is located in the interior lowlands region of N America. The terrain of Rockford varies from flat to gently rolling farmland and wooded areas. The mean elev. is 721'.

CLIMATE. Climate in Rockford is characterized by hot summers and cold winters. Avg. monthly temps. range from 20.8°F during Jan. to 73.8°F during July, with an avg. annual temp. of 48.6°F. The 35.37" avg. annual rainfall occurs mainly during spring and summer. Nearly 50% of the 34.6" avg. annual snowfall occurs during Dec. and Jan. The RH ranges from 55% to 90% and the avg. growing season is 164 days. Rockford lies in the CSTZ and observes DST.

FLORA AND FAUNA. Animals native to rockford include the raccoon, chipmunk, fox and deer. Common birds are the cardinal, bluejay and mockingbird. Bullfrogs, salamanders, painted turtles and snakes, including the venomous milk snake, E massasauga and timber rattlesnake, inhabit the area. Typical trees are the oak, maple, elm and pine. Smaller plants include the honeysuckle, blackberry, violet, rose and goldenrod.

POPULATION. According to the US census, the pop. of Rockford in 1970 was 147,370. In 1977, it was estimated to have decreased to 128,101.

ETHNIC GROUPS. In 1978, the ethnic distribution of Rockford was approx. 91.4% Caucasian, 8.3% Black and 1.5% Hispanic. (A percentage of the Hispanic total is also included in the Caucasian total.)

TRANSPORTATION. (Interstate) Hwy. 90 and the NW Tollway, US hwys. 20 and 51 and state rtes. 2, 70 and 173 provide major motor access to Rockford. *Railroads* serving the city include, AMTRAK, Burlington N, Chicago, Milwaukee, St. Paul & Pacific, Chicago & NW and IL Central Gulf. The *airline* serving the Greater Rockford Airport is OZ. There is also a private airport serving the city. *Bus lines* are the Rockford Mass Transit District, Loves Park Transit, Greyhound and WI Coach Lines.

COMMUNICATIONS. Communications, broadcasting and print media serving Rockford are: *AM radio stations* WKKN 1150 (MBS, C&W); WHBF 1270 (CBS, C&W); WRRR 1330 (ABC/I, MOR, Talk) and WROK 1440 (ABC/C, Contemp.); *FM radio stations* WZOK 97.5 (Indep., Btfl. Mus.); WHBF 98.9 (Indep., Btfl. Mus.) and WQFL 100.9 (ABC/E, Relig.); *television stations* WREX Ch. 12 (ABC); WTVO Ch. 17 (NBC); WIFR Ch. 23 (CBS); WQRF Ch. 39, (Indep.) and cable; *press:* one major newspaper serves the city, the *Register-Star*, issued mornings; other publications include *Mid-W Observer*, *Labor News*, *Fabricator*, *Chronicle*, *Panorama Magazine*, *Journal*, *Weighing & Measurement* and *Metal Fabricating News*.

HISTORY. The area of Rockford was first inhabited by native Americans of the Blackhawk tribe and was the scene of the Blackhawk War of 1832. Rockford was founded in 1834 by Germanicus Kent and Thatcher Blake and named for the Rock River Fording midway on the stage rte. between Chicago and the booming lead mines at Galena. The early pioneers came from the N.E. states. Two settlements were established on each side of the river. These merged and were incorporated as a town in 1839 with a pop. of 235. The town grew as more settlers arrived, encouraged by the abundant supply of wood, water and excellent farmland. In 1852, Rockford became a city. From its earliest days water power helped make Rockford a manufacturing center. Pumps, harnesses and farming implements were made there. In 1853, John Manny invented and began the manufacture of a combination reaper and mower in the city. Knitting mills and furniture factories were among the earliest industries in Rockford. In 1868, two brothers, W. F. and John Barnes, started the city's machine tool industry. In the second half of the 19th century, the expansion of industry brought more settlers, at first from NY and the NE, and then from Ireland, Sweden, Italy and other European countries. By 1882, there were eight furniture factories in the city, all manned by Swedes. Rockford became one of the largest furniture producing centers in the world. In the 20th century, as industry has expanded, so the city has grown and today Rockford is the second largest city in IL and the producer of more than 6,000 diversified manufactured goods.

GOVERNMENT. Rockford has a mayor-council form of govt. The mayor, who is a member of the council, is elected at large to a four-year term. The council members, who are elected by district, also serve four-year terms.

ECONOMY AND INDUSTRY. Rockford, the metal fastener capital of the world, is also the second largest machine tool center in the country. Other major products include hardware, scales, containers, automobile parts, hand tools, tin cans, electric motors, precision machinery, pet foods, governors, pumps, household appliances, wire goods, paints, plastics, chewing gum, seeds, toys, packaging machinery, textile machinery, aviation instruments, boilers, hosiery, clutches, forgings and barbecue equipment. Agriculture is an important factor in the area's economy, generating about $50 million in income annually. The labor force of the met. area totaled 140,800 in June, 1979, while unemployment was 5.6%. The avg. wage per hour for production workers was $7.00 in April, 1979.

BANKING. There are 15 commercial banks and six savings and loan assns. in Rockford. In 1978, total deposits of the 13 banks headquartered in the city were $881,287,000, while assets were $1,029,981,000. Among the banks serving the city are First Natl. Bank & Trust, United of IL, American Natl., IL Natl., City Natl., Colonial, NW, North Towne Natl. and Alpine State.

HOSPITALS. There are three gen. hosps. in Rockford, Rockford Memorial, St. Anthony, Swedish-American, and the Singer H. Douglas Zone Center for Mental Health. Two hosps. have accredited nursing schools that cooperate

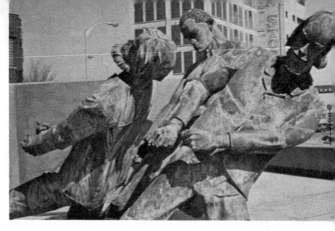

Founder's Memorial, Rockford, Illinois

with the U of IL medical school complex in Rockford.

EDUCATION. Rockford Col., an independent private coed. institution, offers programs leading to bachelor and master degrees. Established in 1847, there were 1,055 students enrolled in 1978. Rockford School of Medicine and Rockford Regional Academic Center are both extensions of the U of IL. Rock Valley Comm. Col. offers courses leading to associate degrees. There are 55 elementary, eight middle, five sr. and four special schools in the Rockford school district. The school district encompasses Cherry Valley and New Milford and enrollment totaled 39,000 in 1978. There are 14 parochial and nine private schools in the area. The public lib. has six branches.

ENTERTAINMENT. Annual festivals include the Rockford Art Assn.'s Greenwich Village Art Fair, Midsummer Festival, Swedish Celebration, Oktoberfest and Riverfront Festival. Rockford Col.'s Regents participate in intercollegiate sports.

ACCOMMODATIONS. There are several hotels and motels in Rockford, including the Albert Pick, Howard Johnson's, the Holiday, Clock Tower inns and the Sweden House Lodge.

FACILITIES. The 2,800-acre Rockford Met. Park System includes 130 parks, featuring a children's zoo and playgrounds. Among the parks are Aldeen, Anna R. Page Forest and Searls parks. Children's Farm features a buffalo, lambs, calves and piglets, with Clydesdale and Belgian horses pulling wagons. The Bicentennial Bike Path is a 3.8 mi. paved bikeway along the E bank of the Rock River. There are three boat launch facilities, located in Riverview Park, Veterans' Park and Martin Park. Local fishing sites include Pierce Lake and Rock River. There are 79 outdoor and 24 indoor tennis courts and six public golf courses in the city. Skating facilities are also available at four centers.

CULTURAL ACTIVITIES. Rockford has a Civic Symphony, Chamber, Youth Symphony and Concert orchestras and the Rockford Concert Band. The Comm. Concert Association sponsors appearances by internationally known artists. Music groups in the city include the Mendelssohn Club, founded in 1884, the Svea Soner Swedish Men's Chorus, founded in 1890, and the Lyran Society, also a men's musical group. Rockford is the home of the 38 voice Kantorei, Singing Boys of Rockford. The Phantom Regiment Drum and Bugle Corps gives regular performances. There are six legitimate theaters in the city, including the New American and Civic theaters and the Red Barn and the Shady Lane playhouses. The Burpee Art Museum features changing exhibits and includes multi-media presentations in its permanent

Tinker Swiss Cottage, built 1865; Rockford, Illinois

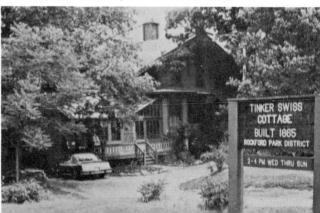

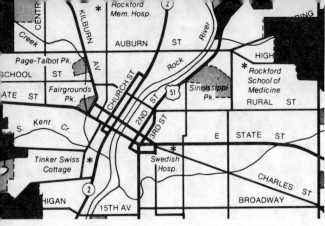

Rockford, Illinois

collection. Other museums include the Burpee Natural History Museum; the Rockford Museum Center, featuring Rockford-crafted furniture, clocks, 19th-century clothing and artifacts; and the unusual Time Museum, which displays antique timepieces from throughout the world.

LANDMARKS AND SIGHTSEEING SPOTS. Memorial Hall houses relics of the Spanish-American and Civil wars and WW I. World traveler Robert Tinker built the Tinker Chalet in 1865 and filled it with antiques and artwork he collected on his travels. The Erlander Home, built in 1871 by John Erlander, was the first brick home built in Rockford. One of three museums of its kind in the US, it features contributions made by the Swedish people in Rockford since 1852 and also contains artifacts of early Rockford.

SACRAMENTO
CALIFORNIA

CITY LOCATION-SIZE-EXTENT. Sacramento, the seat of Sacramento Co. and capital of CA, is located in the Sacramento Valley (part of the Great Central Valley of CA) and encompasses 93.9 sq. mi. at 33°13' N lat. and 121°30' W long. Situated at the junction of the Sacramento and American rivers at the geographical center of the valleys, Sacramento's met. area encompasses the cities of Fair Oaks, Rancho Cordova and Folsom to the E and Citrus Heights, Carmichael and Roseville to the NE, Elk Grove to the S and W Sacramento to the W and includes all of Sacramento Co., extending to the counties of El Dorado and Amador to the E, Yolo to the W, Placer to the NE, Nevada to the N and Sutter to the NW.

TOPOGRAPHY. The terrain of Sacramento, situated in the Sacramento Valley region, is flat. Mts. surround the valley to the W, N and E, providing the area with a plentiful water supply. The mean elev. is 25'.

CLIMATE. The climate of Sacramento is mild, characterized by an abundance of sunshine most of the year. The shielding influence of the surrounding high mts. modifies winter storms, and prevailing winds are S every month except Nov., when they are N. The avg. annual temp. of 60.5°F varies from monthly means of 45.1°F in Jan. to 75.3°F in July. During the summer, prevailing winds from the Pacific Ocean provide cool night breezes. The avg. annual rainfall is 17.05", 75% of which occurs during the winter months of Nov. through Mar. Torrential rains and heavy snows which frequently fall on the W slopes of the surrounding mts. occasionally cause flood conditions along the Sacramento River, but excessive rainfall and damaging windstorms are rare in the valley itself. The RH ranges from 28% to 89%. The avg. growing season is 280 days. Sacramento lies in the PSTZ and observes DST.

FLORA AND FAUNA. Animals native to Sacramento include the mule deer, coyote, skunk, raccoon and ground squirrel. Typical birds are the scrubjay, CA quail, wrentit, lesser goldfinch and mourning dove. Coachwhip snakes, whiptail lizards, Pacific tree frogs and the venomous Pacific rattlesnake, are found in the area. Common trees are the oak, pine and willow. Smaller plants include the chaparral shrub, CA golden poppy (the state flower), bluecurl, wild mustard, monkey flower and blue lupine.

POPULATION. According to the US census, the pop. of Sacramento in 1970 was 257,105. In 1978, it was estimated that it had increased to 260,000.

ETHNIC GROUPS. In 1978, the ethnic distribution of Sacramento was approx. 82% Caucasian, 10.6% Black and 13% Hispanic. (A percentage of the Hispanic total is also included in the Caucasian total.)

TRANSPORTATION. Interstate hwys. 5, 80 and 880, US hwys. 50 and 99, and state hwys. 16, 70 and 160 provide major motor access to Sacramento. *Railroads* serving the city are AMTRAK, Burlington Northern, Sacramento N Railway, S Pacific, Santa Fe, Union Pacific and W Pacific. *Airlines* serving Sacramento Met. Airport include FL, OC PS, RW, UA and WA. *Bus lines* include Greyhound, Trailways and the local Sacramento Regional Transit.

COMMUNICATIONS. Communications, broadcasting and print media originating from Sacramento are: *AM radio stations* KRAK 1140 (Indep., C&W); KCRA 1320 (NBC, ABC/I/E, MOR, News); KNDE 1470 (Indep., Top 40; KFBN 1530 (CBS, All News); *FM radio stations* KFBK 92.5 (Indep., Clas.); KCTC 96.1 (ABC/I, MOR); KROI 96.9 (Indep., Progsv., Top 40); KZAP 98.5 (Indep., Contemp.); KEBR 100.5 (Indep., Relig.); KSFM 102.5 (Indep., Progsv.); KEWT 105.1 (Indep., Btfl. Mus.); KWOD 106.5 (Indep., Adult Contemp.) and KXOA 107.9 (ABC/FM, Soft Rock); *television stations* KCRA Ch. 3 (NBC); KVIE Ch. 6 (PBS); KXTV Ch. 10 (Indep.,); KOVR Ch. 13 (ABC); KMUV Ch. 31 (Indep.) and KTXL Ch. 40 (Indep.); *press:* two major dailies serve the area, the *Bee*, issued evenings, and the *Union*, issued mornings; other publications include *Observer, Report, Valley Union Labor Bulletin, CA Fireman, CA Grange News, CA Highway Patrolman, CA Journal, The CA State Employee, Mainstream* and *Sacramento Magazine.*

HISTORY. Sacramento was founded in 1849 by John A. Sutter, Jr. Ten years earlier, his father, John A. Sutter, Sr., had established near the site the first white settlement in interior CA by pledging allegiance to Mexico. During the 1840s, Sutter's Ft. (located in the downtown area) was the W point for arriving overland settlers. The discovery of gold at Sutter's Mill in 1848 started the great CA goldrush, attracting thousands of prospectors. Named Sacramento after the Sacramento River, the city was incorporated in 1850. That same year a flood leveled most of the city, and an outbreak of cholera caused hundreds of people to flee. In 1850, CA was admitted to the Union and Sacramento was designated the state capital four years later. In 1860,

Downtown Sacramento, California

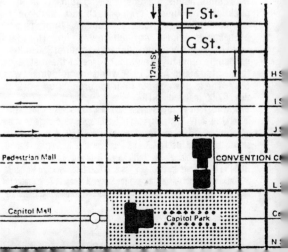

the Pony Express was inaugurated, with Sacramento serving as the W terminal. Construction of the Central Pacific link of the first transcontinental RR began in the city in 1863. The RR was completed in 1869 and provided access to the E. During the late 1800s, area farmers began growing cotton and truck vegetables, making the town an agricultural and trade center. During the early 1900s, canning and food processing became the chief industries. After WW II, a number of new industries located in Sacramento, including the aerospace industry.

GOVERNMENT. Sacramento has a council-mgr. form of govt. consisting of nine members, including the mayor. The council members are elected by districts to four-year terms. The mayor, elected at large to a four-year term, is a voting member of the council.

ECONOMY AND INDUSTRY. Fed., state and local govts. are major Sacramento industries, employing approx. 33% of the area's labor force. The state of CA employs the majority in govt. The military is also a major area employer, as McClellan and Mather AFBS are located in the city. The city's nearly 300 plants produce aerospace products, processed foods, chemicals and wood products. More than 50% of CA's produce is processed in the city, which has the nation's largest almond processing plant. In June, 1979, the total labor force for the greater met. area was 459,600, while the rate of unemployment was 6.8%.

BANKING. There are 23 banks in Sacramento. In 1978, total deposits for the four banks headquartered in the city were $163,418,000, while assets were $184,794,000. Banks include River City, Capitol Bank of Commerce, Merchants Natl. and First Indep. Trust, Wells Fargo, Bank of America and Crocker Citizens.

Pony Express Monument, Sacramento, California

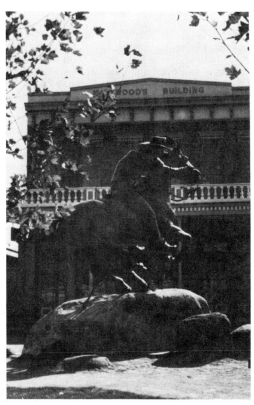

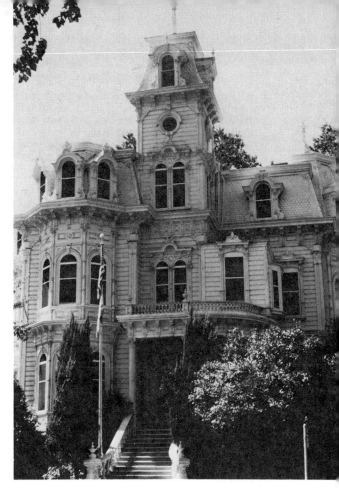

Governor's Mansion, Sacramento, California

HOSPITALS. There are eight gen. hosps. in Sacramento, including Sutter Comm. Hosp. of Sacramento (whose system includes Sutter Gen. and Sutter Memorial), Methodist, Mercy, Comm., Kaiser Foundation, and Sacramento Medical Center.

EDUCATION. CA State U, Sacramento, a publicly-supported institution offering bachelor and master degrees in liberal arts and other areas, enrolled more than 20,000 in 1978. The Los Rios Comm. Col. system maintains three separate campuses of two-year, publicly-supported cols. which offer associate degrees. These include Sacramento City Col., with more than 14,500 enrolled in 1978; American River Col., which enrolled over 23,000 in 1978; and Cosumnes River Col., with an enrollment of more than 5,600 in 1978. Also located in the city is the McGeorge Col. of Law, part of the U of the Pacific in Stockton, CA. The approx. 75 public schools, including seven high schools, enroll some 50,000. Approx. 20 private schools are available. Sacramento City and Co. Public Lib. has a central facility and five branches.

ENTERTAINMENT. Sacramento hosts the annual CA State Fair during the last week of Aug. and the first week of Sept. Other annual events include the Camelia Festival in Mar., the Dixieland Jazz Festival on Memorial Day weekend, Music Circus held May thru Sept., the 20-30 Rodeo in Sept. and the Murieta Music Festival in Oct. The Icecapades present a season of performances in Sacramento each year. Hughes Stadium is the site of football's annual Camelia Bowl on Thanksgiving Day and the annual Pig Bowl each Jan., a football game between the city police and co. sheriffs. CA State U's Hornets participate in intercollegiate sports.

ACCOMMODATIONS. There are numerous hotels and motels in Sacramento, including Best Western, Caravan Inn, Ponderosa, Sandman Motel, the Holiday Inns N and S, Maleville's Coral Reef Lodge, Red Lion Motor, Vagabond Motor Hotel and Sacramento Inn.

FACILITIES. The Sacramento met. park system includes William Land Park, the largest in the city, which occupies land donated by William Land, an early settler in Sacramento. It features the Sacramento Zoo, Fairy Land

and an amusement park. Several large ponds located in the city are the site of children's fishing derby contests.

CULTURAL ACTIVITIES. Sacramento Comm. Center Theatre features symphony, opera and musicals throughout the year. The Bacchus Theatre Playhouse, Gaslight Theatre and Sacramento Civic Theatre stage dramatic productions. The E. B. Crocker Art Gallery, the oldest Museum in the W, features sculpture, paintings, graphic arts, furnishings and tapestries. The CA State Archives house historical documents, including CA's original constitutions of 1849 and 1879. The Indian Museum displays Native American art and artifacts. Silver Wings Aviation Museum depicts the history of aviation in CA.

LANDMARKS AND SIGHTSEEING SPOTS. Old Sacramento is a restoration project that covers 28 acres of old buildings with different architectural designs. Among these are the B. F. Hastings Museum Bldg., which served as quarters for the CA Supreme Court and terminal for the Pony Express; the Old Eagle Theatre; the Pony Express Monument; a one-room schoolhouse and the Central Pacific Passenger Station, which housed rolling stock. The State Capitol (1860-1874), with its gold-leaf dome, and the Gov.'s Mansion (1877-1878) are Victorian-Gothic in design. Sutter's Ft., the first settlement in Sacramento, has been restored to its 1839 design and contains the State Indian Museum housing many exhibits and Native American artifacts, including one of the finest basket collections in existence. Displays include ancient as well as present day life and culture of CA native Americans. The William B. Ide Adobe State Historic Park contains the restored home of the only Pres. of the CA Republic. The Chinese Center features an authentic Chinese comm. complete with restaurants, shops, a bank and a cultural center.

SAINT LOUIS
MISSOURI

CITY LOCATION-SIZE-EXTENT. St. Louis, an independent city, located 10 mi. S of the confluence of the MO and MS rivers, encompasses 61.2 sq. mi. near the geographical center of the US in E central MO, at 38°45' N lat. and 90°22' W long. The met. area includes all of St. Louis Co., and extends into the counties of Jefferson to the S, St. Charles to the NW and Franklin to the SW, as well as the IL counties of St. Clair and Clinton to the E, Madison to the NE and Monroe to the SE. The city is bordered on the E by the MS River and the state of IL.

TOPOGRAPHY. St. Louis is situated on flat to gently rolling terrain. The mean elev. is 470'.

CLIMATE. The climate of St. Louis is continental. The 56.1°F annual temp. ranges between monthly means of 31.4°F in Jan. to 79.3°F in July. The 36.64" of avg. annual rainfall occurs mostly between April and June. The avg. annual snowfall is 19.1". The RH ranges between 54% and 91% and the avg. growing season is about 190 days. St. Louis is in the CSTZ and observes DST.

FLORA AND FAUNA. Animals native to St. Louis include the raccoon,

Central Saint Louis, Missouri

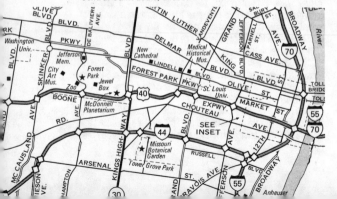

opossum, rabbit, squirrel, skunk and deer. Typical birds include the robin, cardinal, bluejay, wren and swallow. Bull frogs, soft-shelled turtles, salamanders, toads and water snakes, as well as the venomous rattlesnake, copperhead and water moccasin, are found in the area. Typical trees are the willow, elm, oak and dogwood. Smaller plants include the hawthorne, honeysuckle, blackberry, violet and primrose.

POPULATION. According to the US census, the pop. of St. Louis in 1970 was approx. 622,000. In 1978, it was estimated that it had decreased to approx. 489,000.

ETHNIC GROUPS. In 1978, the ethnic distribution of St. Louis was approx. 58.8% Caucasian, 40.9% Black and 1% Hispanic. (A percentage of the Hispanic total is included in the Caucasian total.)

TRANSPORTATION. Interstate hwys. 44, 55, 70 and 270, US hwys. 40, 50, 61 and 67 and state hwys. 21, 30, 100, 180 and 340 provide major motor access to St. Louis. *Railroads* serving the city include AMTRAK, Alton & S, Boston & ME, Burlington N, Chicago Rock Island and Pacific & ConRail. *Airlines* serving Lambert-St. Louis Intl. Airport include AA, US Air, BN, DL, EA, FL, OZ, SO and TW. *Bus Lines* include Great Southern, Greyhound and trailways.

COMMUNICATIONS. Communications, broadcasting and print media originating from St. Louis are: *AM radio stations* KSD 550 (NBC, MOR); KXOR 630 (Indep., Contemp.); KSTL 690 (Indep., C&W); WEW 770 (ABC, Mus.); KXEN 1010 (Indep., Relig.); KMOX 1120 (CBS, Var.); KADI 1320 (Indep., AOR); WIL 1430 (ABC/I, Mod. Ctry.); KIRL 1460 (ABC/C, Adult Contemp.) and KATZ 1600 (MBS, Blk.); *FM radio stations* KLSR 89.7 (Indep., Top 40); KBDY 89.9 (Indep., Var.); KWMU 90.7 (NPR, Educ. News); KSLH 91.5 (Indep., Educ.) KCFM 93.7 (Indep., Btfl. Mus.); KADI 96.3 (ABC/FM, AOR); KSLQ 98.1 (Indep., Top 40); KEZK 102.5 (Indep., Btfl. Mus.); KFOX 103.3 (Indep., MOR); KKSS 107.7 (ABC/C, Blk.); *television stations* KTVI Ch. 2 (ABC); KMOX Ch. 4 (CBS); KSDK Ch. 5 (NBC); KETC Ch. 9 (Indep.); KPLR Ch. 11 (Indep.) and KDNL Ch. 30 (Indep.); *press:* two major dailies serve the area, the *St. Louis Globe-Democrat*, issued mornings, and the *St. Louis Post-Dispatch*, issued evenings; other publications include *Affirmative Action, Labor Tribune* and *MO Teamster*.

HISTORY. The first inhabitants of the St. Louis area were native Americans of the Missouri and Osage Tribes. St. Louis was established as a French trading post in 1764 by Pierre Laclede Liguest. Located at the confluence of the MO and MS rivers, it became the gateway to the W for many explorers and settlers. Lewis and Clark launched their expedition to explore the Pacific NW from there, as did Zebulon Pike. St. Louis was incorporated as a town in 1809 and chartered as a city in 1822, with a pop. of 5,000. In 1837, Army engineer Lt. Robert E. Lee supervised installation of pilings to assure St. Louis' place as a river port. Steamboat traffic up and down the MS River created ties between St. Louis and the S towns of Memphis, Vicksburg and New Orleans. The city had to be rebuilt in the 1840s when it was nearly leveled by flood, cholera and fire. The RR arrived in 1857, and immigrants from Ireland, Germany and other European countries followed. During the Civil War, St. Louis was W headquarters for the Union Army. By 1870, it had become the third largest city in the US after NY and Philadelphia. In 1874, the completion of the Eads Bridge spanning the MS River made the IL coal fields more accessible. Consequently, St. Louis became an important manufacturing center by the end of the century. The 1904 World's Fair, also called the LA Purchase Exposition, at which ice cream, iced tea and hot-dogs were first introduced, was held in the Forest Park area. City businessmen financed Charles Lindbergh's "Spirit of St. Louis" flight over the Atlantic in 1927. During World War II, St. Louis factories played a significant role in the production of munitions. The St. Louis skyline took on a new look in the 1960s with completion of the famed Gateway Arch, part of

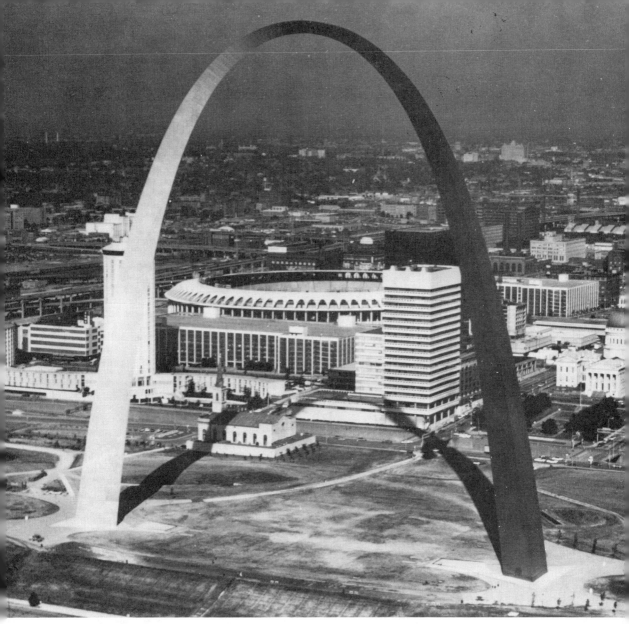

630 foot Gateway Arch, St. Louis, Missouri

one of the largest urban renewal programs in the country. St. Louis is now a major industrial commercial center.

GOVERNMENT. St. Louis has a mayor-council form of govt. Twenty-eight of the 29-member Board of Aldermen are elected by district except the Pres. of the Board who is elected at large. All are elected to four-year terms. The Board is the chief legislative body and selects the city manager, who is the chief administrative officer. The mayor, elected at large to a four-year term, is not a member of council and has no vote.

ECONOMY AND INDUSTRY. There are approx. 3,000 manufacturing plants in St. Louis, a major US transportation and industrial center. Transportation equipment is the chief manufactured product, and the city is a leading producer of automobiles, barges, railroads and tugboats. Other major products include beer, fabricated metal products, chemicals, food products, automobile and aircraft parts and non-electrical machinery. Printing and publishing are also important industries. In 1979, the total labor force for the greater met. area was approx. 1,112,500, while the rate of unemployment was 5.1%. In 1978, the median household income was $18,600.

BANKING. In 1978, total deposits for the 14 banks headquartered in St. Louis were $1,235,170,000, while total assets were $1,442,595,000. Banks include American Natl, Bank of St. Louis, First Natl. of St. Louis and Mercantile.

HOSPITALS. There are several hospitals in St. Louis, including Bethesda, Cardinal Glennon Memorial for Children, St. Louis City, St. Louis Co. and St. Louis State.

EDUCATION. St. Louis U, a private, independent institution founded in 1818 under the auspices of the Society of Jesus, currently offers degree programs in liberal arts, engineering, law, medicine, psychology and social work. Enrollment in 1978 was 10,393. Washington U, established in 1853 as Eliot Seminary, enrolled over 11,147 in 1978. Other institutions of higher learning include Webster Col., a Catholic liberal arts institution established in 1915; Harris Teachers' Col.; the St. Louis campus of the U of MO; Cardinal Glennon Col.; Covenant Theological Seminary; Kenrick Seminary; Maryville Col.; the St. Louis Col. of Pharmacy; Eden Theological Seminary and Fontonne Col. The Jr. Col. District of St. Louis is composed of campus sites at Florissant VBalley, Forest Park and Kirkwood. The public school system includes approx. 150 elementary schools and 13 high schools enrolling over 110,000. An additional 25,000 attend approx. 70 Catholic, 15 Lutheran and

15 other private schools. The St. Louis Public Lib. has 20 branches offering more than one million volumes to its patrons. Also available are the lib. facilities of the MO Botanical Gardens and MO Province Society of Jesus.

ENTERTAINMENT. Dinner theater entertainment in St. Louis is offered by the American Theatre, Loreho-Hilton and Goldenrod Showboat. Annual events include the Valley of Flowers Festival, featuring tours of historic homes and a parade (May); World's Fair Day, a nostalgic observance of the 1904 Fair (May); Intl. Festival, featuring dancing, food and crafts of 35 nations (May); Strassenfest, featuring German food and song (July); Fenton Festival, featuring arts, crafts, horse shows and a carnival (Aug.); Gentry Fair, featuring arts, crafts and antiques (Sept.) and the Oktoberfest, featuring German food, dancing, arts and bands (Oct.). Pro Sports teams include the Cardinals of NFL football, the Cardinals of NL baseball and the Blues of NHL hockey. The Washington U's Billkens participate in collegiate sports.

ACCOMMODATIONS. Downtown St. Louis's hotels and motels include the Bel Air Hilton, the Breckenridge Pavillion, the Chase Park Plaza, the Mayfair, the Sheraton-St. Louis and Stouffer's Riverfront Towers. Others in the area include the Stratford House, the Inn St. Louis, the Drury Inn, and Howard Johnson's.

FACILITIES. St. Louis' park system has approx. 70 parks, including Forest, A.P. Greensfelder, Edgar M. Queeny, and Lone Elk. Lone Elk Park covers 405 acres and bison, elk, white-tailed deer, fallon deer and barbados sheep roam free in the park. Edgar M. Queeny Park's 569 acres offers fishing for children, ice skating indoors-outdoors, tennis courts, swimming pool, nature trails, picnic areas, and a creative play center. A. P. Greensfelder Park features nature trails, saddle horses, an equestrian area with a mustang shelter, rental horses and boarding stables. There are also hayrides, tent or primitive camping areas, picnic areas and a visitors' center. The 14,000-acre Forest Park has 30 mi. of drives and 35 acres of lakes and ponds. Forest Park houses the McDonnell Planetarium, the Jewel Box Floral Conservatory, Zoological Park and the Steinberg Skating Rink. The zoo encompasses 83 acres, with more than 2,000 animals in naturalistic exhibits set in bluffs, woods, pampas lakes, and glades. There is also the Charles Yalem children's zoo, a 3.5 acre miniature world of nature, with a nursery for hand-reared young animals. Also of interest is the MO Botanical Garden including 79 acres of gardens, featuring the Climatron (a geodesic dome greenhouse), a lily pool, Hawaiian garden, an Amazonian jungle, coffee, tea and rubber plantations, Mediterranean and desert plants, a scented garden for the blind and a Japanese garden. There are over 20 public golf courses, including

McDonnell Planetarium, Saint Louis, Missouri

Berry Hill, Glenwood and St. Ann. There are many public tennis courts including Dorsett Racquet Club, Tower Grove Park, and the Butch Buchholz Town and Tennis Club.

CULTURAL ACTIVITIES. Cultural activities in St. Louis include jazz and dinner on riverboats and the second oldest symphony in the U.S., the century-old St. Louis Symphony Orchestra, which performs in Powell Hall. Other performing musical groups are the St. Louis Municipal Opera, the St. Louis Co. Pops, the Baroque Orchestra, the St. Louis Little Symphony and the Philharmonic. The "Gateway to the West" is an arch beneath which is the Museum of Westward Expansion featuring history of the W. The St. Louis Art Museum is important for its 40 galleries and Oriental art exhibits. Other museums include the Laumeier Sculpture Garden, Museum of Science and Natural History, the National Museum of Transporation, the Sports Hall of Fame, the St. Louis Medicine Museum, and the Old Cathedral and Museum. Dramatic presentations can be seen at the American Theatre and the Municipal Open-Air Theatre.

LANDMARKS AND SIGHTSEEING SPOTS. The *Admiral, Delta Queen, MS Queen, Huck Finn, Samuel Clemens, Tom Sawyer* and *Goldenroad,* which are river boats, are available for tours, dining or musical entertainment. The Black Madonna Shrine in the foothills of the Ozarks is a shrine of multi-colored rock grottos built over a period of 22 years by Brother Bronislaus Luscze, a Franciscan monk. The Cathedral of St. Louis, an example of modified Byzantine architecture, contains one of the world's largest organs, along with a Jerusalem, jeweled Resurrection Cross; gold, Eucharistic Chapel and solid marble interiors. The First State Capitol Building is a 19th-century landmark. The Gateway Arch serves as a reminder that St. Louis was the gateway to the W. The 630-foot arch is the nation's tallest and most elegant memorial. Grant's Farm is a 281-acre tract which includes a cabin framed and built by the 18th President, Gen. Ulysses S. Grant. St. Louis's earliest church, Old Cathedral, was restored in 1831 and is still in daily use. Old Courthouse features exhibit rooms of the Louisiana Purchase, Indians and the W and relics relating to Westward Expansion. The Old St. Ferdinand's Shrine is the oldest Catholic church building between the MS River and the Rocky Mts. Soldier's Memorial commemorates the war dead of St. Louis, from the Civil War to the present. McDonnell Planetarium presents lectures on the universe and astronomy. There are several historical restored homes in St. Louis, including the Taille Denoyer Home (1790), the Sappington House (1808), the John B. Myers House (1870), the Hanley House (1894), and the Cupples House (1890). At the N leg of the Gateway Arch, on the MS River, is the USS *Inaugural,* a veteran minesweeper which served in the Battle of Okinawa.

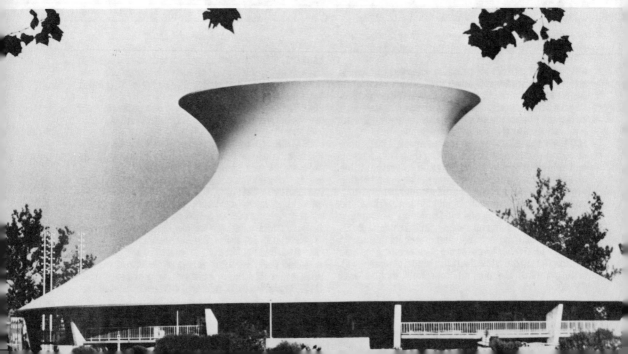

SAINT PAUL
MINNESOTA

CITY LOCATION-SIZE-EXTENT. St. Paul, the seat of Ramsey Co. and capital of MN, is located in E MN on the banks of the MS River, 15 mi. W of the WI border at 44°53' N lat. and 93°13' W long. Minneapolis lies to the W. St. Paul encompasses 55.44 sq. mi. and the met. area overlaps that of Minneapolis, in Hennepin Co., and extends into portions of neighboring Anoka Co. to the N, WA Co. to the E, and Dakota Co. to the S.

TOPOGRAPHY. St. Paul is situated on high bluffs overlooking the MS River. The terrain consists of flat land on terraces. There are many lakes in the area, including Phalen, Como, Pigs Eye and Pickeral. The MN River meets the MS River to the SW. The mean elev. is 834'.

CLIMATE. The climate of St. Paul is continental, characterized by wide variations in temp. and ample summer rainfall. The avg. annual temp. of 44.9°F ranges from a Jan. mean of 19.9°F to a July mean of 73.1°F. Approx. 72% of the 27" avg. annual rainfall occurs from Apr. through Sept. The avg. annual snowfall is 46.3". The RH ranges from 50% to 82%. The growing season avgs. 166 days. An avg. of once in every eight years, St. Paul experiences flooding due to spring snow melt, excessive rainfall, or a combination of both. St. Paul lies in the CSTZ and observes DST.

FLORA AND FAUNA. Animals native to St. Paul include the otter, whitetail deer, fox, beaver, raccoon, skunk and mink. Common birds include the goldfinch, loon, heron, crane, whippoorwill and bittern. Frogs, salamanders, green snakes and snapping turtles are also found here. Trees include the pine, the basswood, oak, elm, walnut, sugar maple, and spruce. Smaller plants include the lady's slipper (the MN state flower), violet, chicory, wood anemone and goldenrod.

POPULATION. According to the US census, the pop. of St. Paul in 1970 was 309,866. In 1978, it was estimated that it had decreased to approx. 277,952.

ETHNIC GROUPS. In 1978, the ethnic distribution of St. Paul was approx. 89.4% Caucasian, 4.7% Black, 3.8% Hispanic, .8% Asian, 1% Native American and .3% other.

TRANSPORTATION. Interstate hwys. 35 and 94, US hwys. 8, 10, 12, 52, 61, 169 and state hwys. 5, 7, 36, 45, 110, 212 and 280 provide major motor access to St. Paul *Railroads* serving the city include AMTRAK, Burlington Northern, Chicago-NW, Milwaukee and Soo Line. *Airlines* serving Minneapolis-St. Paul Intl. Airport are RP, NW Orient, NW, US Air, EA, NC, BN, WA, OZ, SO, TW and UA. There are two intermediate airports—St. Paul Downtown Airport and Anoka Co., and four minor airports—Flying Cloud, Lake Elmo, Crystal and South St. Paul Municipal—all providing commuter, charter, and helicopter services. *Bus lines* include Greyhound, Jefferson, Zephyr, the local Met. Transit Commission and St. Paul & Suburban Bus Co. Four river carriers serve the city on the MS, MN and St. Croix rivers with barge, towing and fleet service.

COMMUNICATIONS. Communications, broadcasting and print media serving St. Paul are: *AM radio stations* KDWB 630 (Indep., Contemp.); KTCR 690 (MBS, C&W); KUOM 770 (NPR, Educ. Progsv.); WCCO 830 (CBS, Var.); KTIS 900 (Indep., Relig.); WAYL 980 (Indep., Btfl. Mus.); WDGY 1130 (NBC, Contemp.); WWTC 1280 (Indep., Contemp.); WLOL 1330 (ABC/I, New Ctry.) KDAN 1370 (Indep., Progsv.); KEEY 1400 (Indep., MOR); and KSTP 1500 (Indep., Contemp.); *FM radio stations* KSJN 19.1 (NPR, Clas., News); WAYL 93.7 (Indep., Btfl. Mus.); KSTP 94.5 (Indep., Bright, MOR); KTCR 97.1 (Indep., Progsv.); KTIS 98.5 (Indep., Inspir. Mus.); WLOL 99.5 (Indep., Btfl. Mus.); KBEM 100.1 (Indep., AM Simulcast); WCTS 100.3 (Indep., Relig.); KDWB 101.3 (Indep., Clas.); KEEY 102.1 (Indep., Btfl. Mus.); WCCO 102.9 (ABC/C, MOR); *television stations* KTCA Ch.2 (PBS); WCCO Ch. 4 (CBS); KSTP Ch. 5 (NBC); KMSP Ch. 9 (ABC); WTCN Ch. 11 (Indep); KTCI Ch. 17 (PBS) and

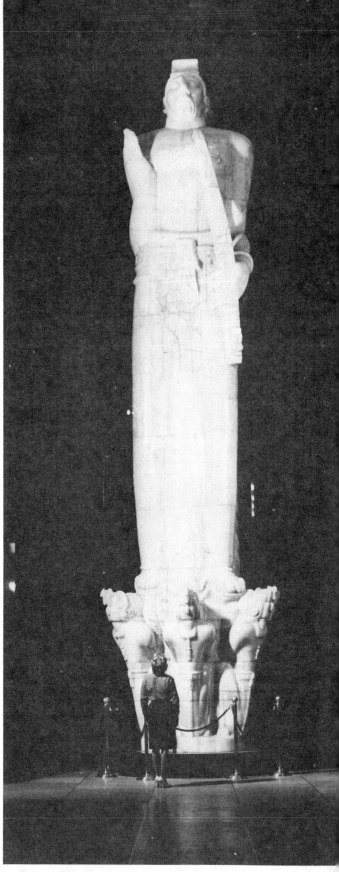

"Indian God of Peace" Statue, Saint Paul, Minnesota

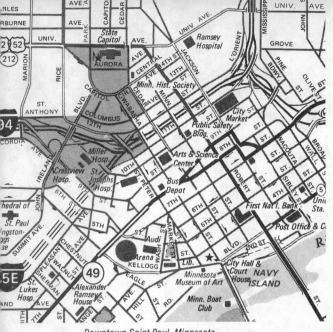

Downtown Saint Paul, Minnesota

arrived. Rich farmlands, iron ore mines and lumbering in the area attracted immigrants from Europe. During the 1880s, the economic interests of St. Paul and its sister city, Minneapolis, began to go in opposite directions, with the latter outpacing St. Paul in pop. because of its large industrial base. The capital continued to prosper through trade and transportation activities. Toward the end of the century, the RR built the Union Stockyards and a cattle market developed. The St. Paul economy suffered during the 1920s and 1930s. By 1940 the downtown area was in need of reclamation. Between 1964 and 1972, urban renewal projects planned during the 50s and 60s were completed, including the building of new apartments, office buildings and stores in the inner city. A new construction boom began in 1976 and is transforming the downtown area. St. Paul continues to serve as the distribution and transportation center for the large midwestern farm area.

GOVERNMENT. St. Paul has a mayor-council form of govt. The seven council members and the mayor are elected at large to two-year terms. The mayor is not a member of the council, but he does have veto power.

ECONOMY AND INDUSTRY. Manufacturing employs approx. 33% of St. Paul's labor force. Major industries are research, electronics, transportation, general insurance, publishing and automobiles. The city is a large collection and distribution center with barge transportation on the MS River making a significant contribution. The city's total labor force in 1978 was 142,871, while the rate of unemployment was 3.9%. Wages and salaries in 1978 totaled $2,582,300,000.

BANKING. There are 27 banks and 9 savings and loan assns. in St. Paul. In 1978, total deposits for the 24 banks headquartered in the city were $2,810,071,000, while assets were $3,827,859,000. Banks include First Natl. American Natl. Bank & Trust, NW Natl., Midway Natl., Commercial State, First State, NW State, First Grand Avenue State, First Security Savings, First Merchants', Liberty State and Midwest Fed.

HOSPITALS. There are 38 hospitals and health care centers in the St. Paul met. area, including Bethesda Lutheran, Midway, St. John's, St. Joseph's, St. Paul's, Ramsey and United.

EDUCATION. Hamline U, established in 1854 and affiliated with the United Methodist Church, offers liberal arts and general programs and had a 1978 enrollment of approx. 1,700. The Col. of St. Catherine, a Roman Catholic-affiliated col., offers bachelor degrees and enrolled more than

KTMA Ch. 23 (Indep.); *press*: two major dailies serve the area, the *Dispatch*, issued evenings, and the *Pioneer Press*, issued mornings; other publications include *MN Legionaire, Catholic Digest, Family Handyman, The Farmer, Farm Industry News, Irrigation Age, ME Advocate, MN Farm Bureau News, Natl. Hog Farmer, Passage, Snow Goer,* and *TWA Ambassador.*

HISTORY. Before white settlers arrived, native Americans of the Sioux tribe inhabited the present day area of St. Paul. In 1805, Lt. Zebulon Pike purchased land from the Sioux. During the 1920s Ft. Snelling was built. Five Swiss refugee families and French-Canadian trader, Pierre "Pig's Eye" Parrant, settled on the ft.'s land and, in 1840, they were ordered off the reservation. The settlers chose a landing on the MS River to form their comm., calling it Pig's Eye, after the trader. In 1841, Father Lucian Galtier built a log cabin chapel in the town, dedicating it to St. Paul, and the comm. adopted the name St. Paul. In 1849, the American Fur Co. made the city its headquarters. The same year, St. Paul was made the territorial capital. It was incorporated as a city in 1854. By the early 1860s the city had become an important trade center and two RRs had

Skyline, Saint Paul, Minnesota

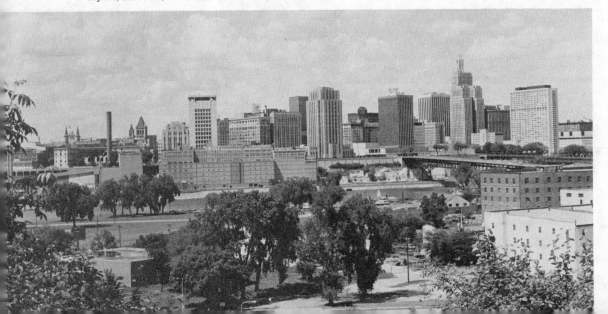

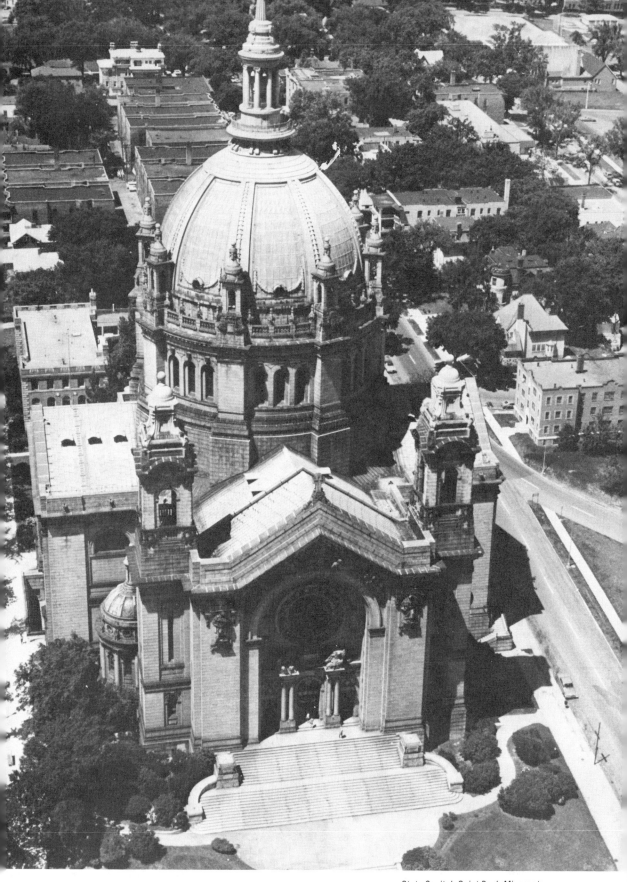

State Capitol, Saint Paul, Minnesota

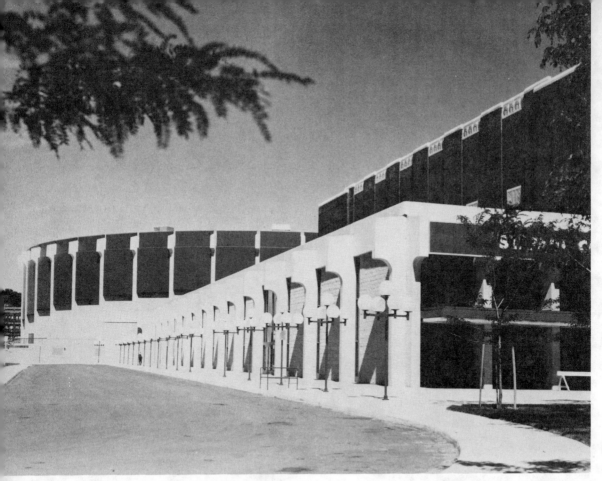

Chamber of Commerce, St. Paul, Minnesota

2,100 in 1978. The Col. of St. Thomas, a liberal arts col., grants bachelor and master degrees and enrolled more than 4,100 in 1978. The publicly-supported state U, the U of MN, maintains campuses in St. Paul and in Minneapolis. The colleges of Agriculture, Forestry, Home Economics, Biological Sciences and Veterinary Medicine are on the St. Paul Campus. Other educational institutions include Bethel, Concordia and Macalester colleges, Globe Col. of Business, Rasmussen School of Business, St. Paul Seminary and Bible Col., the William Mitchell Col. of Law, St. Mary's Jr. Col., the St. Paul Area Vocational-Technical School and three comm. colleges, Lakewood, Anoka-Ramsey and Inver Hills. Approx. 33,729 are enrolled in the city's 46 elementary, 10 jr. high and seven high schools. Approx. 2,000 are enrolled in the 56 special education programs for handicapped children and youth. There are 31 parochial schools with a total enrollment exceeding 14,000. There are seven private schools in the area. Lib. facilities include St. Paul Public Lib., James J. Hill Reference, U of MN, MN State and O'Shaughnessy at the Col. of St. Thomas.

ENTERTAINMENT. The 10-day St. Paul Winter Carnival is held in late Jan. and early Feb. The MN State Fair is held in Aug. The MN Renaissance Festival, recreating a 16th century European marketplace on harvest holiday, is held 25 mi. SW of the city in late Aug. and early Sept. Other annual events include the Harvest Festival of Christmas and Grand Old Days. The Fillies of women's basketball, the Vikings of NFL-NFC football, the N Stars of NHL hockey, the Kicks of NASL soccer and the Norsemen softball team provide professional sports to the Minneapolis-St. Paul area

ACCOMMODATIONS. Hotels and motels in St. Paul include the Radisson-St. Paul, Capp Towers and Golden Steer motor hotels, the Best Western and the TraveLodge motels, McGuire's of Arden Hills, Ramada and Holiday inns.

FACILITIES. The approx. 2,500-acre St. Paul park system includes Phalen, Como, Highland, Crosby and Hidden Falls parks. The zoological gardens in Como Park cover approx. 100 city blocks. The zoo contains ponds, a wooded area, a MN Wildlife exhibit, and a children's zoo/nursery.

The state fairgrounds offer an amusement park. Jogging tracks are available in Como and Phalen parks and MS Bluffs. Boating and fishing are available at the numerous lakes surrounding St. Paul. There are 61 major marinas and 148 swimming beaches and pools. Public golf courses are located at Como, Highland, Phalen and Gross Municipal Parks. Public tennis courts can be found at the Wooddale Recreation Center. Ice skating is permitted in most city parks. Ski lifts can be found in nearby Afton Alps and Buck Hills.

CULTURAL ACTIVITIES. The Council of Arts and Sciences is the center of culture in St. Paul and maintains several cultural organizations, including the Chamber Orchestra, Schubert Club and COMPAS, a comm. arts agency. Other musial groups performing in St. Paul are the Met Youth Orchestra and the MN Opera Assn. There are several theaters in the city, including the Chimera Theatre Co. and Park Sq. Theater. More than 150 musical and theatrical events are presented annually at O'Shaughnessy Hall. Museums and galleries in the city include the Schubert Club's Musical Instrument collection, Gibb's Farm Museum and the Buckley, Col. of St. Catherine, Suzanne Kohn, Kramer and Osbourne galleries, the MN Museum of Art and St. Paul Gallery and Art School.

LANDMARKS AND SIGHTSEEING SPOTS. The State Capitol in St. Paul, designed by Cass Gilbert, the architect of the US Supreme Court Building, and completed in 1904, is constructed of several types of MN stone and 20 varieties of imported marble and features the largest, unsupported, marble dome in the world. St. Paul Cathedral, featuring a copper dome illuminated at dusk, was built in 1905-1907 in classic renaissance style and is akin to Notre Dame in Paris. The Alexander Ramsey house, home of the first gov. of the MN Territory, is maintained in late Victorian style. Other historical sites in the city include the James Hill Mansion, the University Club (of which F. Scott Fitzgerald was a member). The Burbank-Livingstone-Griggs Mansion row house (where F. Scott Fitzgerald lived as a young man) and the Sibley House Museum, the home of the state's first gov. Ft. Snelling, built in 1819, is also of historic interest. A statue by Carl Milles, "Indian God of Peace," may be seen in the lobby of the City Hall-Courthouse.

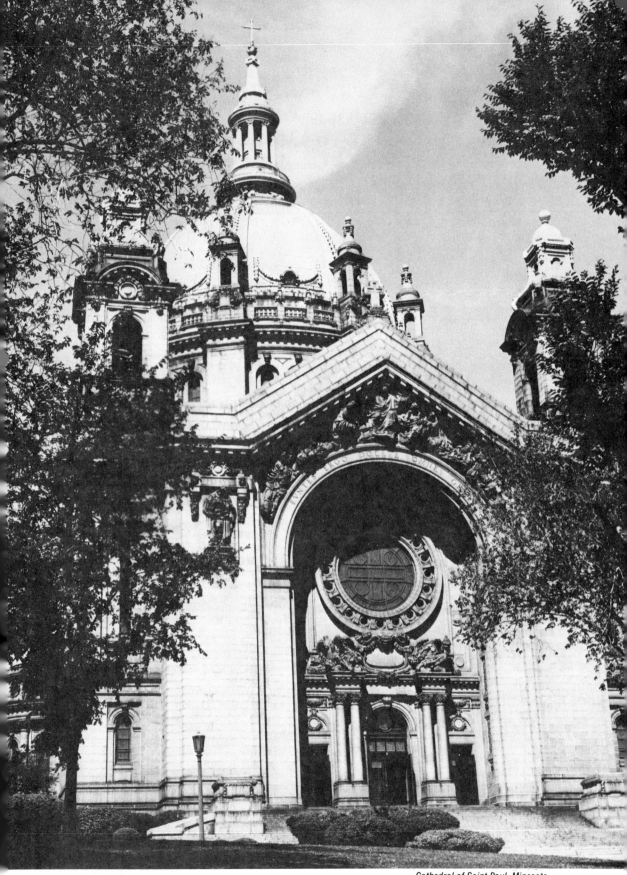

Cathedral of Saint Paul, Minnesota

SAINT PETERSBURG
FLORIDA

CITY LOCATION-SIZE-EXTENT. St. Petersburg encompasses 56.2 sq. mi. in Pinellas Co. on the S end of Pinellas peninsula in central W FL on the W coast of Tampa Bay at 27°46' N lat. and 82°38' W long. The met. area is contiguous with that of Tampa to the NE and also extends N along the FL Gulf Coast into Paseo Co.

TOPOGRAPHY. St. Petersburg lies in the Gulf Coast plain region, and is characterized by level flat terrain. Tampa Bay is to the E of the city, the Gulf of Mexico is to the W and Boca Ciega Bay is to the SW. There are several small lakes, including Maggiore, Mirror and Crescent lakes. The mean elev. is 10'.

CLIMATE. The climate of St. Petersburg is a modified marine type with summer thundershowers and night ground fogs during winter. Monthly mean temps. range from 61°F during Jan. to 82°F in Aug. with an avg. annual temp. of 72°F. Most of the 49" avg. annual rainfall occurs during the summer. The RH ranges from 50% to 93%. Hurricanes occur mainly between June and Oct. St. Petersburg is in the ESTZ and observes DST.

FLORA AND FAUNA. Animals native to St. Petersburg include the raccoon, squirrel, rabbit and opossum. Common birds are the gull, tern, black skimmer pelican, darlin, sandpiper and cormorant. Bullfrogs, mud turtles, toads, lizards and snakes and four types of venomous snakes are common to the area. Typical trees are the palm, slash pine, oak and mangrove. Smaller plants include the palmetto, bayberry, bermuda and dayflower.

POPULATION. According to the US census, the pop. of St. Petersburg in 1970 was 216,159. In 1978, it was estimated that it had increased to 238,450.

ETHNIC GROUPS. In 1978, the ethnic distribution of St. Petersburg was approx. 84% Caucasian, 16% Black, 1.1% Hispanic, and .1% Asian. (A percentage of the Hispanic total is also included in the Caucasian total.)

TRANSPORTATION. Interstate hwy. 275 and US hwys. 19 and 92 and state hwys. 60, 584, 686, 693 and 699 provide major motor access to St. Petersburg. Three airports, Albert Whitted, Tampa Intl. and St. Petersburg and Clearwater Intl. accommodate nearly all major *airlines. Railroads* include Seaboard Coastline and AMTRAK. *Bus lines* include Gray Line, Greyhound, Trailways and Gulf Coast Motor. Dart Handicapped Transportation supplies the handicapped with transportation. St. Petersburn is a close neighbor of Tampa and is developing its own Port of St. Petersburg to handle larger ships than it already does. The current depth is 24'.

Saint Petersburg, Florida

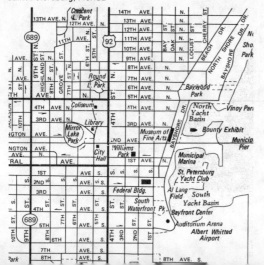

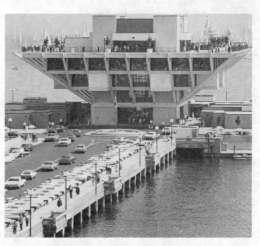

Inverted pyramid structure, Pier Place, St. Petersburg, Florida

COMMUNICATIONS. Communications, broadcasting and print media originating from St. Petersburg are: *AM radio stations* WSUN 620 (ABC/E, Mod. Ctry.); WWBA 680 (Indep., Btfl. Mus.) and WLCY 1380 (ABC/C, Contemp.); *FM radio stations* WLCY 94.9 (Indep., Var.); WQRK 99.5 (MBS, C&W); WKES 101.5 (Indep., Btfl. Mus.) and WWBA 107.3 (Indep., Progsv.); *television stations* WEDU Ch. 3 (PBS); WFLA Ch. 8 (NBC); WLCY Ch. 10 (ABC); WTVT Ch. 13 (CBS); WUSF Ch. 16 (PBS); WTOG Ch. 44 (Indep.) and cable; *press:* two dailies serve the area, the *Times*, issued mornings, and the *Evening Independent*, issued evenings; other publications are *Guide Magazine, The Churchman, Come Unity, Pinellas Review* and *Prizewinner*.

HISTORY. Native Americans had inhabited the present-day St. Petersburg area for nearly 7,000 years before white settlers arrived. Those of the Timucuan tribe were there when explorers de Narvarez and de Soto visited the area during the 1500s. In 1843, Seminole War veteran Antonio Maximo established a "fish ranch" on a land grant, but an 1848 hurricane forced him and his partner to abandon their land. Other settlers followed and in 1856, farmer James R. Hay built the area's first house. During the Civil War, fed. troops raided the settlement and many of its inhabitants were driven from it. In 1875, Gen. John C. Williams purchased land in the area and later, after farming proved unsuccessful, he and Peter Demens decided to extend the Orange Belt RR to the site and establish a city. The RR arrived in 1888 and a town was born. It is believed the two men drew straws to name the new city. Demens won and called it St. Petersburg, after his birthplace in Russia. During the big freeze of 1894-95, the city's citrus groves escaped harm. Less fortunate growers from other parts of the state were attracted to the city, and this played an important role in St. Petersburg's development. The city, incorporated in 1903, realized a tourist boom during the early part of the 1900s, attracting the retired and convalescent. Ramps were installed over curbs, and rows of green benches were placed in parks, establishing the city's natl. reputation as a retirement center. In 1914, the world's first commercial airline began operations from the city. During the 1920s, another land boom took place. In 1922, Gandy Bridge, linking St. Petersburg and Tampa, opened. Other bridges were constructed and helped accelerate the city's growth. St. Petersburg remains a natl. resort city and retirement center.

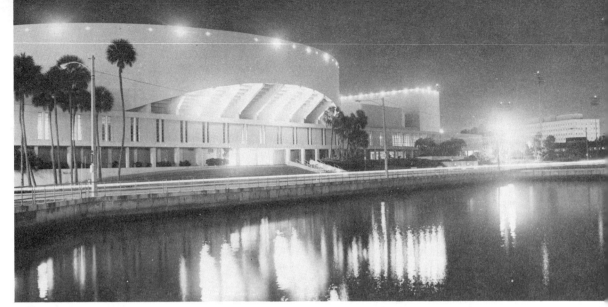

Bayfront Center on Tampa Bay, St. Petersburg, Florida.

GOVERNMENT. St. Petersburg has a council-mgr. form of govt. consisting of seven council members, including the mayor. Six council members are elected by district for four-year terms and one council member (the mayor) is elected at large for a two-year term. The mayor, a voting member of the council, presides at all of the meetings and represents the city on ceremonial occasions. The city mgr., appointed by the council, is in charge of administration, and has no specific term. He serves as long as the council is satisfied with his work.

ECONOMY AND INDUSTRY. Leading industries include tourism, electronics, optical products, research, clothing, fishing, steel, exports, lumber, chemicals, petrochemicals, publishing, food processing and meat packing. The 1979 labor force for the St. Petersburg-Tampa met. area was 590,500, with an unemployment rate of 5.1%. The avg. per capita income in 1977 was $6,966.

BANKING. St. Petersburg has 21 commercial banks and six savings and loan assns. In 1978, total deposits for the 14 banks headquartered in the city were $1,235,170,000, while total assets were $1,442,595,000. Banks include Landmark Union Trust, Century First Natl., St. Petersburg Bank & Trust, FL Natl. Bank and Flagship Bank.

HOSPITALS. Before the turn of the century, a doctors' convention declared St. Petersburg the healthiest spot in the world. There are five hosps. located here, Bayfront Medical Center, Edward H. White II, Memorial, Apollo Medical Center, St. Anthony's and Palm's of Pasadena are total-care facilities, and All Children's specializes in children and young adults up to 21.

EDUCATION. The U of S FL St. Petersburg Campus, a branch of the state-supported institution that opened in 1960, offers grad. and undergrad. programs. The U enrolls approx. 18,000 per quarter. The Stetson U Col. of Law (SUCL), a privately-supported institution supported by the Baptist Convention, offers grad. programs only. SUCL enrolled a portion of the 2,600 total enrolling at the main as well as the branch campus. St. Petersburg Jr. Col., a publicly supported two-year institute, offers programs leading to associate degrees. Eckerd Col., a privately supported liberal arts col. affiliated with the Presbyterian Church, offers programs leading to the bachelor degree. In 1978, there were 881 enrolled. Other research institutions are the U of S FL Marine Science Center of Excellence and the FL Dept. of Natural Resources Marine Research Laboratory. About 120 public schools enroll over 95,000 and over 10,000 attend 51 private and parochial schools. Three adult/vocational educational centers are in St. Petersburg and the Pinellas Vocational/Technical Inst. is nearby. The City Center for Learning serves the needs of students as well as the new and existing industries. Lib. facilities include the public lib. and its branches and mobile lib. service.

ENTERTAINMENT. The Country Dinner Playhouse and the Showboat Dinner Theatre offer dining entertainment. Each year St. Petersburg hosts the Main-Sail Art Festival, S Ocean Racing Conf. and the Festival of States.

Al Lang Stadium in St. Petersburg is the spring training home of the NY Mets and the St. Louis Cardinals of the NL. The city has its own pro baseball team, the Class A Cardinals. The city hosts the Southland Sweepstakes Regatta for power boats and sailing's S Ocean Racing Conf. It also sponsors the annual Big Sun Basketball Tournament which pits four of the nation's finest teams against each other in a two-night tourney.

ACCOMMODATIONS. St. Petersburg has many fine hotels and motels, including the Bayfront Concourse, the Princess Martha Hotel, Howard Johnson's, the Belmar Beach Resort, Breckenridge Resort, the Best Western and Don Ce Sar, and Ramada, Holiday, Sheraton and Suncoast Village Motor inns.

Tampa Bay, Saint Petersburg, Florida

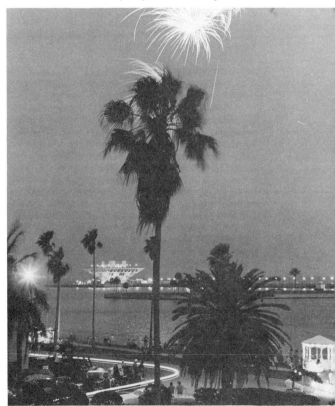

FACILITIES. More than 2,200 acres are devoted to parkland and because two-thirds of St. Petersburg's boundary is water, most of this park land adjoins the water. Some of the parks are Abercrombie, Lake Maggiore, Maximo, Demen's Landing and Williams. Boyd Hill Nature Park, a natural preserve, has 721 acres of lowland hammock, a catwalk that takes visitors above the damp floor of the swampy hammock and numerous nature trails. St. Petersburg maintains five public beaches, Shore, Bay, Spa, Maximo Park and St. Petersburg Municipal. Also of interest are the Sunken Gardens of St. Petersburg which include seven acres of gardens containing over 7,000 varieties, representing native FL plants as well as flora from every tropical country. The city operates 10 swimming pools with instructors. Activities include lessons in swimming, diving and water polo, synchro swimming and master's swimming. Public golf courses can be found at Twin Brooks Municipal Golf. Public tennis courts are available through the city park system and at St. Petersburg Tennis Center.

CULTURAL ACTIVITIES. The FL Gulf Coast Symphony, Comm. Concerts Assn. and Symphony Guild are St. Petersburg's musical organizations. Area cols. maintain theatrical troupes. Performances are presented at Bayfront Center, Palisades Theatre and Little Theatre. The Museum of Fine Arts, exhibits paintings by Monet, Renoir and Rodin. The St. Petersburg Historic Museum features local history exhibits put in culture. Haas Museum is a re-creation of an early village. The St. Petersburg Jr. Col. maintains a planetarium and observatory. Art Galleries include Art Center and those at the local cols.

LANDMARKS AND SIGHTSEEING. Berthed at the downtown waterfront area is MGM's authentic reproduction of Captain Bligh's *Bounty*. An aviation memorial commemorates the "Birthplace of Scheduled Air Transportation". Another memorial, the First European Expedition Monument, commemorates the landing of de Narvarez on FL's beaches. A plaque at Indian Shell Mound is dedicated to Princess Herrihigua, an Indian maiden who rescued explorer Juan Ortiz from her father's death sentence.

SALT LAKE CITY
UTAH

CITY LOCATION-SIZE-EXTENT. Salt Lake City, capital of UT and seat of Salt Lake Co., encompasses 69.5 sq. mi. at 40°46' N lat. and 111°58' W long. The state's largest city, it lies on the Jordan River in N UT, 15 mi. SE of the Great Salt Lake. The greater met. area includes the city of Ogden to the N and extends N into Davis, E into Morgan and Summit, SE into Wasatch, S into Utah and W into Tooele Counties

TOPOGRAPHY. Located in a flat valley, Salt Lake's terrain rises in the E to the slopes of the Wasatch Mts. The Oquirrh Range borders the valley on its W side. The mean elev. is 4,221'.

CLIMATE. The climate of Salt Lake Cty is semi-arid continental. Monthly mean temps. range from a Jan. mean of 28°F to a July mean of 77°F, with an avg. annual temp. of 51.7°F. Rainfall avgs. 15.7" annually, with most occurring in spring. Snowfall avgs. 58.5" annually, with approx. 43% occurring during Dec. and Jan. The RH ranges from 20% to 78%. The avg. growing season is more than five months. Salt Lake City lies in the MSTZ and observes DST.

FLORA AND FAUNA. Animals native to Salt Lake City include the antelope, elk, coyote, bobcat and skunk. Common birds include the pelican, CA gull, sage grouse, rock wren and magpie. Whiptail lizards, sagebrush lizards, gopher snakes, toads, tiger salamanders and the venomous great basin rattlesnake and midget faded rattlesnake, are common to the area. Typical trees are the fir, pinyon, juniper and willow. Smaller plants include sagebrush, sego lilies, pasque flowers, fireweeds and painted cups.

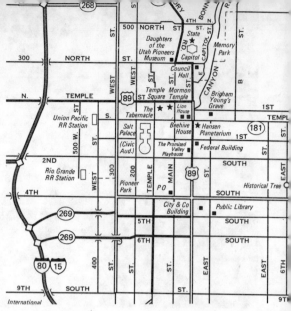

Salt Lake City, Utah.

POPULATION. According to the US census, the pop. of Salt Lake City in 1970 was 175,885. In 1977, it was estimated that it had increased to 180,000.

ETHNIC GROUPS. In 1978, the ethnic distribution of Salt Lake City was approx. 96.8% Caucasian, 1.2% Black, and 6.4% Hispanic. (A percentage of the Hispanic total is included in the Caucasian total.)

TRANSPORTATION. Interstate hwys. 15, 80 and 215, US Hwy. 89 and state hwys. 68, 186 and 201 provide major motor access to Salt Lake City. *Railroads* serving the city include AMTRAK, Burlington N, Rio Grande, Santa Fe, S Pacific, Union Pacific and W Pacific. *Airlines* serving Salt Lake City Intl. Airport are AA, FL, RW, TI, UA and WA. *Bus lines* include Greyhound, Trailways and the local UT Transit Authority.

COMMUNICATIONS. Communications, broadcasting and print media originating from Salt Lake City are: *AM radio stations* KLUB 570 (Indep., Good Mus.); KSXX 630 (NBC, Talk); KWHO 860 (Indep., Clas.); KALL 910 (ABC, MOR); KRSP 1060 (Indep., Contemp., Top 40); KSL 1160 (CBS, MOR); KWMS 1280 (Mut. Blk., All News); KCPX 1320 (Indep., MOR); KSOP 1370 (Indep., C&W) and KRGO 1550 (ABC/E, C&W); *FM radio stations* KUER 90.1 (NPR, Var.); KWHO 93.3 (Indep., Top 40, Oldies); KALL 94.1 (Indep., Var.); KLUB 97.1 (Indep., Btfl. Mus.); KCPX 98.7 (Indep., Top 40); KSL 100.3 (Indep., Btfl. Mus.) and KRSP 103.5 (Indep., Btfl. Mus.); *television stations* KUTV Ch. 2 (NBC); KTVX Ch. 4 (ABC); KSL Ch. 5 (CBS) and KUED Ch. 7 (PBS); *press:* two major dailies serve the area, the *Desert News*, issued evenings, and the *Tribune*, issued mornings; other publications include *UT Chronicle*, *Intermountain Catholic Register*, *Mining Engineering*, *UT Farmer-Stockman*, *UT Cattleman* and *Salt Lake Times*.

HISTORY. The Salt Lake Valley was first inhabited by native Americans of the Paiute, Shoshoni and Ute tribes. Although fur trappers visited the area in 1824, Salt Lake City was not founded until 1847, when a group of Mormons led by Brigham Young reached the Great Salt Lake. The Mormon pioneers immediately laid out the town, started irrigation, planted crops, built forts and homes and began to explore and colonize a large region of the W. Rockies. Salt Lake City served as a seat of govt. of the Provisional State of Deseret, from 1849-1859, and for the Provisional Utah Territory for the remainder of most of the period until 1896. By 1850 there were 5,000 Mormons living in the comm. Great Salt Lake City was incorporated in 1851. After discovery of lead and silver in Brigham Canyon in 1863, the city became a mining center. The city was renamed in 1868, becoming Salt Lake City. In 1869, the country's first transcontinental RR was completed at nearby Promontory Point, providing new markets for the area's agriculture and mining products. During the late 1880s, copper, lead and silver mining boomed. After the turn of the century, large smelters were built and the city expanded rapidly. The city's pop. soared from 53,531 at the turn of the century to over 140,000 in 1930. WW II increased demand for metals, which greatly boosted the development of industry in Salt Lake City. By 1960, the pop. of Salt Lake City reached 189,454, spurred by continued industrial expansion. However, the 60s saw the pop. decline, as many residents migrated to the suburbs. Salt Lake City serves the Rocky Mt. area as a center for finance, industry, transportation and culture. UT's largest city, it is also headquarters of the Church of Jesus Christ of Latter-day Saints, whose members comprise about two-thirds of the city's pop.

GOVERNMENT. Salt Lake City has a commission form of govt., composed of a mayor and four commissioners. The mayor and the commissioners are elected at large to four-year terms.

ECONOMY AND INDUSTRY. Salt Lake City is a major manufacturing center. Mining, oil and ore refining are other major industries, with many natural resources located in the area. Trade is the major area employer, with govt. ranking second. Major products manufactured in the city include refined ores, oil, electrical components and chemicals. The total labor force for the Salt Lake City-Ogden met. area was 387,400 in 1979, with an unemployment rate of 3.9%. Disposable personal income per household for 1977 was $15,600.

BANKING. In 1978, total deposits for the 11 banks headquartered in Salt Lake City were $2,112,932,000, while assets were $2,474,608,000. Banks include Zion's First Natl., Walker Bank and Trust Co., Continental Bank and Trust, Tracy Collins Bank and Trust and First Security State.

HOSPITALS. Nine major hosp. facilities are located in Salt Lake City, including Cottonwood, Holy Cross, Latter-day Saints', Primary Children's Medical Center, St. Mark's Shriners' U. Valley W and the V.A. Hosp.

EDUCATION. Salt Lake City is the site of several institutions of higher education. The U of UT, founded in 1850 as the U of Deseret, is the oldest state university W of the MO River. Renamed in 1892, and now a state-controlled, coeducational U, this institution offers grad. and undergrad. programs. In 1978, over 21,800 students were enrolled. Westminster Col., a private, liberal arts institution established in 1875, is affiliated with the United Presbyterian, United Methodist and United Church of Christ denominations. The col. grants the bachelor degree and enrolled more than 1,400. UT Technical Col., a public two-year institution, awards associate's degrees in vocational/technical programs and enrolled more than 6,400 students in 1978. The Latter-day Saints Bus. Col. offers associate degrees in business-related programs and enrolled nearly 1,000 students in 1978. The city has 45 elementary and high schools, as well as two private and 10 church-supported schools. Lib. facilities are provided by the Intergalactic Lib., the Salt Lake City Public Lib. System, the Salt Lake Co. Public Lib. System and the UT State Lib. Commission.

ENTERTAINMENT. Annual events in Salt Lake City include Statehood Day Celebration on Jan. 4 and the performance of "The Messiah" the Sunday before Christmas. Pro sports are offered by the Golden Eagles (CHL, hockey), the Jazz (NBA, basketball) and the Angels (PCL, baseball). The U of UT Utes provide collegiate sports.

ACCOMMODATIONS. Hotels and motels in Salt Lake City include the Little American Hotel, Salt Lake Hilton, Temple Square, Hotel Utah, the

Famous skyline setting, Salt Lake City, Utah

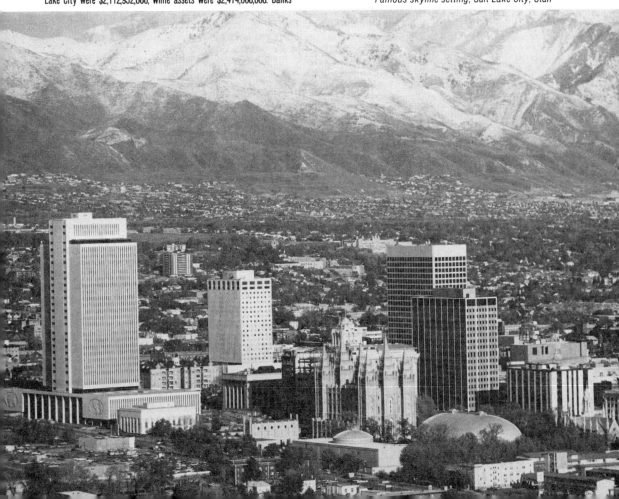

World Motor Hotel and Ramada, Quality and Rinn's Royal Executive inns.
FACILITIES. Salt Lake City has more than 7,000 acres of public parks, playgrounds and municipal golf courses. There are 27 parks, 17 playgrounds, more than 60 baseball and softball diamonds and three municipal swimming pools. The Wasatch Natl. Forest is located adjacent to Salt Lake City on the E and provides some 800 mi. of hiking trails. The Great Salt Lake provides opportunities for sailing, speedboating, water skiing, fishing and jet boating. The Hogel Zoological Gardens, near the entrance to Emigration Canyon, contains a large collection of birds and animals in natural settings. The Intl. Peace Gardens include 14 natl. regions. The garden of each nation represented reflects the nation's heritage and culture. Liberty Park is an 80-acre recreational center with swimming pools, conservatories, a small zoo, an aviary, an amusement park and picnic grounds. Swimming, sailing and freshwater showers are available at the S State Park beaches along the Great Salt Lake State Park on Antelope Island. Approx. 22 public and private golf courses and 273 public and private tennis courts are available.

CULTURAL ACTIVITIES. The Mormon Tabernacle Choir is located in Salt Lake City, which is also the home of the UT Symphony. The city is served by the Ririe-Woodbury Dance Co., the UT Repertory Dance Theatre and Ballet W. The Pioneer Memorial Theater is located on the U of UT and the Promised Valley Playhouse is a replica of the Old Salt Lake Theater, one of the first permanent structures in Salt Lake City. Museums include the UT Museum of Fine Arts, the U of UT Museum and the UT Museum of Natural History. The UT State Historical Society and the Daughters of UT Pioneers' Museum, the Salt Lake City Art Center and the UT State Institute of Fine Arts are also located in Salt Lake City. Pioneer Craft House is both a museum of unique crafts and an art school.

LANDMARKS AND SIGHTSEEING SPOTS. Built without using any nails, Temple Square is the symbolic center of Mormonism and contains the Tabernacle organ, while Trolley Square is a complex of shops and restaurants. The Great Salt Lake is an inland sea so briny that only algae can survive and persons floating in it are unsinkable. Brigham Young is buried, along with three wives and several children in the Brigham Young Cemetery, while the city's founder is also commemorated by a statue. Beehive House, once the official home of Brigham Young, contains most of its original furnishings. Salt Lake City's most distinctive avenue, S Temple, is lined with historic homes and noted buildings as Cathedral of the Madeleine, the Masonic Temple and the Gov.'s mansion. The Hansen Planetarium offers cosmic entertainment. Fort Douglas, built in 1862, once monitored both native Americans and Mormons. A monument in Pioneer Trail State Park commemorates the 100th anniversary of the arrival of the Mormon pioneers in 1847.

Park West ski area, Salt Lake City, Utah

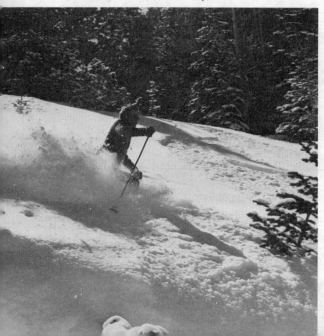

SAN ANTONIO
TEXAS.

CITY LOCATION-SIZE-EXTENT. San Antonio, the seat of Bexar Co., third largest city in the state and tenth largest in the US, encompasses 263.5 sq. mi. on the San Antonio River in S Central TX. approx. 140 mi. NW of the Gulf of Mexico and 190 mi. W of Houston, at 29°32' N lat. and 98°28' W long. Its greater met. area extends throughout Bexar Co.

TOPOGRAPHY. The terrain of San Antonio, which is situated on the wedge of the Gulf coastal plain, slopes upward in the NW towards the Edwards Plateau region of TX and, in the SE, slopes downward towards the Gulf coastal plain. The mean elev. is 701'.

CLIMATE. The climate of San Antonio is continental and subtropical, characterized by dry, mild winters and hot, humid summers. The avg. annual temp. of 69°F ranges from a Jan. mean of 52°F to a July and Aug. mean of 84°F. Most of the avg. annual rainfall of 28" occurs from Apr. through Oct. The avg. annual snowfall is 0.5". Tropical storms in the Gulf of Mexico occasionally result in strong winds and heavy rains in the city. The RH ranges from 45% to 88%. San Antonio lies in the CSTZ and observes DST.

FLORA AND FAUNA. Animals native to San Antonio include the armadillo, whitetail deer, raccoon and opossum. Common birds are the Inca dove, cardinal, mockingbird (the state bird) scissor-tailed flycatcher and chimney swift. TX alligator lizards, TX tortoises and the venomous coral snake, rattlesnake, cottonmouth and copperhead are found in the area. Typical trees are the TX oak, live oak, cedar, elm, juniper and pecan (the state tree). Smaller plants include the mesquite, hackberry, bluebonnet (the state flower) and Indian paintbrush.

POPULATION. According to the US census, the pop. of San Antonio in 1970 was 708,582. In 1978, it was estimated that it had increased to approx. 803,000. The city is one of the fastest growing in the U.S.

ETHNIC GROUPS. In 1978, the ethnic distribution in San Antonio was approx. 91.7% Caucasian, 7.1% Black and 9.1% Hispanic (a percentage of the Hispanic total is also included in the Caucasian total).

TRANSPORTATION. Interstate hwys. 10, 35, 37 and 410, US hwys. 87, 90. 181 and 281 and state hwy 16, provide major motor access to San Antonio. *Railroads* serving the city include AMTRAK, Burlington N, Frisco, MO-KS-TX, Santa Fe, Pacific and MO Pacific. *Airlines* serving San Antonio Intl. Airport are AA, Alamo, BN, CO, DL, EA, TI, Mexicana, SW, Tejas and Amistad. *Bus lines* serving the city include Greyhound, Kerrville, Trailways and the local VIA Met. Transit Authority.

COMMUNICATIONS. Communications, broadcasting and print media originating from San Antonio are: *AM radio stations* KTSA 550 (Indep., Contemp.); KMAC 630 (Indep., Progsv., C&W, Relig.); KKYX 680 (Indep., C&W); KONO 860 (MBS, Contemp.); KQAM 1150 (ABC/C, Top 40); WOAI 1200 (NBC, CBS, Talk, News, Farm); KUKA 1250 (Indep., Span.); KBUC 1310 (ABC/I, C&W); KCOR 1350 (Indep., Span.); KAPE 1480 (ABC/C, Blk.) and KEDA 1540 (Indep., C&W, Spec.); *FM radio stations* KSYM 90.3 (ABC/C, Contemp.); KRTU 91.7 (Indep., Divers.); KITY 92.9 (Indep., Adult Contemp.); KMFM 96.1 (Indep., Clas.); WOAI 97.3 (Indep., Btfl. Mus.); KISS 99.5 (Indep., Progsv.); KZZY 100.3 (ABC/FM, Top 40); KQXT 101.9 (Indep., Btfl. Mus.); KTFM 102.7 (Indep., AOR); KVAR (Span.) and KBUC 107.5 (Indep., Btfl. Mus.); *television stations* KMOL Ch. 4 (NBC); KENS Ch. 5 (CBS); KLRN Ch. 9 (PBS); KSAT Ch. 12 (ABC); KWEX Ch. 41 (Indep.) and cable; *press*: three major daily newspapers serve the city, the *Express*, issued mornings, and the *News* and *Light*, issued evenings. Other publications include *TX Farm and Ranch News*, *Today's Catholic*, *Dental Lab News*, *San Antonio Magazine*, *Seedman's Digest*, *TX Flyer* and *Skeet Shooting Review*.

HISTORY. Native Americans of the Coahuiltee tribe

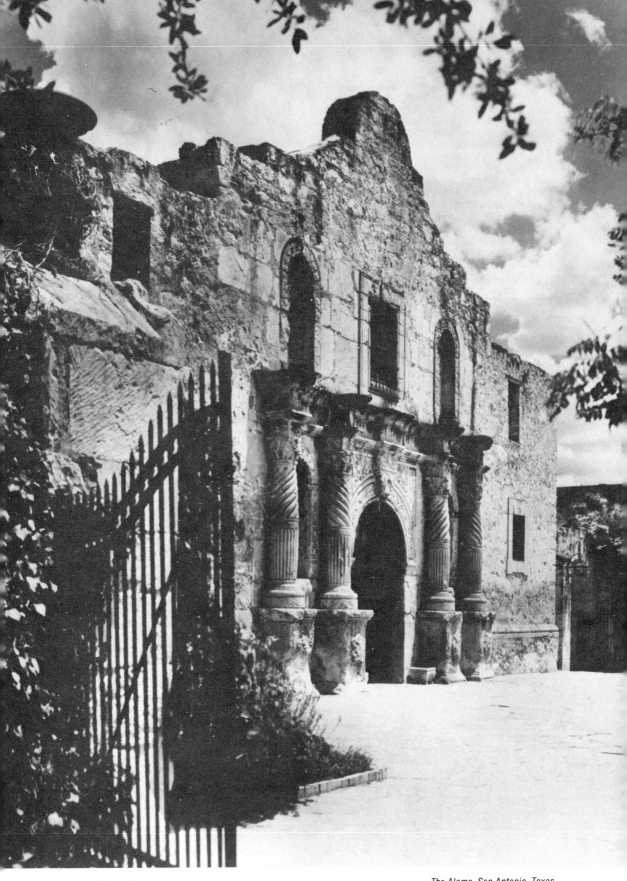

The Alamo, San Antonio, Texas

inhabited the area of present-day San Antonio before the first white settlers, the Spanish, arrived in 1718. The Spaniards established a military post, Ft. San Antonio de Bexar (which later became known as the Alamo), halfway between their missions in E TX and a "presidio" or military settlement, in N Mexico. It also served to protect Mission San Antonio De Valero, established the same year by Fr. Antonio Oliveras, against attacks by native Americans. After it gained independence from Spain in 1821, Mexico controlled the San Antonio area. Hundreds of Americans immigrated to the area between 1821 and 1835, as part of a colonization movement initiated by Stephen F. Austin, the "Father of TX". Resentment against the Mexican govt. grew, however, and in 1835, a small TX army captured San Antonio. The following year, Gen. Santa Ana arrived with a Mexican army of 5,000 soldiers and defeated the courageous TX force of 187 men after a 13-day siege at the Alamo, in which nearly every one of the defenders was killed. Santa Ana was defeated, however, a month later at San Jacinto by troops led by Gen Sam Houston, whose cry was "Remember the Alamo!" The area became part of the Republic of TX. San Antonio was incorporated as a city by the Republic the same year, and became part of the US in 1845, when TX joined the Union. The city grew rapidly thereafter as a point on the cattle drive trail to KS. Business in leather goods began, and in 1877, a RR arrived. Construction was begun on what is now Ft. Sam Houston in 1879, and the city subsequently became established as an important military center. During the early 20th century, oil was discovered near the city. During WW I, the pop. of the city soared because of increased military activity. In the 1930s the rate of growth decreased, but, during WW II, boomed again. The area of the city was doubled during the 1950s when an active policy of annexation was pursued. An urban renewal program was initiated in the 1960s and dilapidated housing was replaced with new structures. In 1968, HemisFair, a world exposition, was held

Central San Antonio, Texas

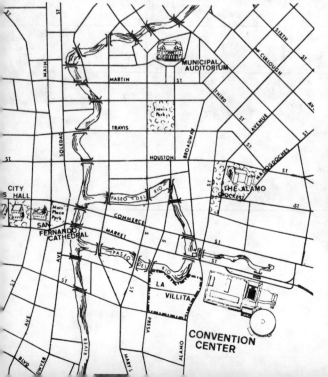

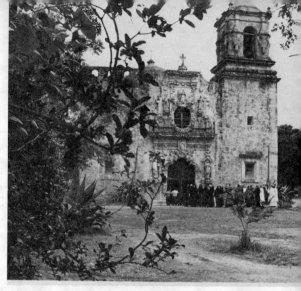

Mission San Jose, built 1720, San Antonio, Texas

in the city. In 1979, the city again attracted world-wide attention when the deposed Shah of Iran was housed at Lackland AFB for several days en route to Panama.

GOVERNMENT. San Antonio has a council-mgr. form of govt., consisting of 11 council members, including the mayor as a voting member, who hires a city mgr., the chief administrator. Ten council members are elected by district, and the mayor at-large, to two-year terms.

ECONOMY AND INDUSTRY. San Antonio is the chief US manufacturing and wholesale and retail market for Mexico. There are nearly 800 manufacturing plants in the met. area. The five military installations in the city, Ft. Sam Houston, Brook, Kelly, Lackland and Randolf AFBs, are significant factors in the economy. Agriculture, including ranching, research and tourism are also major industries. In June, 1979, the labor force of the met. are totaled approx. 413,800, while the rate of unemployment was 6.7%.

BANKING. In 1978, the total deposits at the 42 banks headquartered in San Antonio were approx. $3,362,849,000, while assets totaled approx. $3,957,245,000. Banks include First Natl., Natl. Bank of Commerce, Alamo Natl., Natl. Bank of Ft. Sam Houston, Bexar Co. Natl. and Broadway Natl.

HOSPITALS. There are 15 hosps. in San Antonio, including Santa Rosa Gen. and Children's, Nix, Met. Gen., Baptist, Lutheran, St. Benedict's V.A. three Dept. of Defense hosps., including Wilford Hall USAF at Lackland AFB (the largest in the AF) and three state hosps. Other facilities include The Villa Rose Psychiatric and Rehabilitation Center and S TX Medical Center, which includes a number of hosps. and teaching institutions. The School of Aerospace Medicine at Brook AFB, including Brook Gen. Hosp., offers medical education, research and consultation services.

EDUCATION. The U of TX at San Antonio, a publicly-supported institution established in 1973, offers programs leading to bachelor degrees and enrolled approx. 7,850 in 1978. The U of TX Health Science Center at San Antonio, including medical, dental and nursing schools is a publicly-supported institution which enrolled more than 1,600 in 1978. Other institutions in the city include Trinity U (approx. 3,550), Incarnate Word Col. (1,500), St. Mary's U (approx. 3,200), Our Lady of the Lake U (approx. 1,800), San Antonio Col. (approx. 21,250), St. Phillip's Col. (approx. 7,000), the SW Research Institute and the USAF School of Aerospace Medicine. The San Antonio Independent School District provides public education, and private schools include San Antonio Academy and TX Military Institute. Lib. facilities include the San Antonio Public Lib., which maintains nine branches, and the Lib. of the Daughters of the Republic of TX.

ENTERTAINMENT. Dinner theaters in San Antonio include the Church Theater and the Fiesta Playhouse. The annual Fiesta San Antonio, featuring food, dancing, music and celebrating in the style of old Mexico fiestas, is held in La Villita, or "little town", the earliest settlement within the city. The annual Battle of Flowers Parade is a favorite event. The city also anually hosts the Fiestas Navidenas Starving Artist Show, River Art Show,

TX Folklife Festival and the San Antonio Stock Show and Rodeo. The San Antonio Spurs, a TXL Farm Club team owned by the LA Dodgers, an NL baseball team, offer professional sports entertainment, while the Trinity Tigers and St. Mary's Rattlers participate in intercollegiate sports.

ACCOMMODATIONS. There are numerous hotels and motels in San Antonio, including the St Anthony, Gunther, Menger, Hilton Palacio del Rio, La Mansion del Rio, TraveLodge, Four Seasons, Marriott, Albert Pick, La Mansion del Norte, Town and Country, Oak Hill Motel and Roadway, Passport, Holiday, Sheraton and La Quinta inns.

FACILITIES. There are several parks in San Antonio, including McAllister, San Pedro, S Side Lions, Acequia, Espada and the 363-acre Brackenridge on the San Antonio River, which contains the Sunken Gardens. A former quarry now containing goldfish-filled pools crossed by planted bridges, also includes playgrounds, paddleboats, stables, a mi.-long miniature train, public golf courses, jogging track and zoo. Jogging tracks are also available at Blossom S Side Lions and McAllister parks, and public golf courses and tennis courts are maintained throughout the park system. The San Antonio Natl. Recreation Trail offers a five-mi. hiking/bicycling trail along the river. The Zoological Gardens house more than 3,500 specimens, representing 800 species, in natural settings, and the San Antonio Botanical Center also maintains gardens. Some 2.5 mi. of the Riverwalk is available for paddle boat rides and walking. The San Antonio Zoo features animals, including several rare species in barless pits, designed to simulate their natural environments, and also includes Monkey Island and a tropical aviary.

CULTURAL ACTIVITIES. Among the performing arts organizations in the city are the San Antonio Symphony and its Grand Opera, which perform at the Theater for the Performing Arts. Pops concerts are heard at the Convention Center Banquet Hall. The San Antonio Little Theater offers weekend performances. Comedy farces are presented at the Melodrama Theater and a history program is offered at the Remember the Alamo Theatre and Museum, while other performances are staged at the San Antonio Theater Center and Laurie Auditorium. The audience is separated from the stage at the Arneson River Theater, located on both banks of the San Antonio River. The San Antonio Ballet Co. and San Antonio Choral Society also present regular performances. The Institute of Texan Cultures, maintained by U of TX at San Antonio, contains displays of the cultures of 26 ethnic groups. Witte Museum houses wildlife, historical and artistic exhibits, while the Museum of Transportation displays antique carriages and classic cars. Historical scenes are depicted at the Lone Star Hall of TX History. Other art displays are exhibited at the SW Craft Center Gallery, St. Mary's U Art Center, the McKay Art Institute (a private museum), and the San Antonio Art Institute. Other galleries include San Antonio Museum of Modern Art, Sol del Rio Gallery, Artisan's Alley, Carver and Gallery.

LANDMARKS AND SIGHTSEEING SPOTS. The Alamo, an historic mission in San Antonio, was the scene of the famous battle between the forces of Santa Ana's army and the Texans and is the "Shrine of TX Freedom". Other missions in the city, built by the Franciscans in the 1700s and now restored, include Mission Concepcion (still used as a church), Mission San Jose, (featuring the Rose Window with carved stonework), Mission San Francisco de la Espada (featuring a mi.-long aqueduct built in 1720 to carry water to the mission) and Mission San Juan Capistrano. The old Ursuline Convent is another religious structure of interest. The restored Navarro House, a state historic site, was the home of an early TX patriot, while the monorail and skyride are among the amusements featured. The Spanish Gov. Palace, home of early Spanish settlers, has been restored and furnished with period pieces. HemisFair Plaza, with its futuristic 750' Tower of the Americas, is an interesting contrast to the older structures nearby. El Mercado, a market place, La Villita, an early restored settlement featuring craft shops and boutiques, and River Square on the Paseo del Rio, featuring a variety of shops and restaurants, are interesting sections of the city. Buckhorn Hall of Horns, Fins and Feathers contains more than 3,500 game trophies. More than 20,000 relics of circus life are housed in the Hertzburg Circus Collection. The King William area, one of the oldest neighborhoods in the city, was once one of the most dilapidated. Now almost completely restored, it is one of the most beautiful residential areas in the city, with some homes open for tours.

Famous river walk, San Antonio, Texas

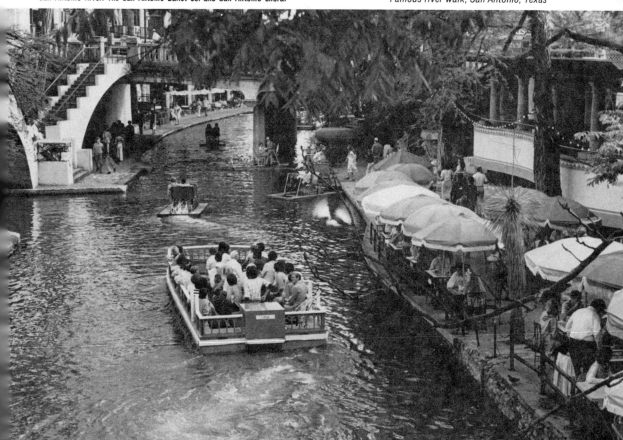

SAN BERNARDINO
CALIFORNIA

CITY LOCATION-SIZE-EXTENT. San Bernardino, the seat of San Bernardino Co. (the largest co. in the US), encompasses 53.22 sq. mi. in S central CA at the foot of the San Bernardino Mts. at 36°06' N lat. and 117°18' W long. Its met. area includes Redlands to the SE and extends S into Riverside Co., which is situated in a valley of the LA Ranges region.

TOPOGRAPHY. The topography of San Bernardino is characterized by flat areas in the E section of the city and hilly to mountainous areas in the W part approaching the San Bernardino Mts. The mean elev. is 1,049'.

CLIMATE. The normally pleasant and mild climate of San Bernardino is influenced primarily by prevailing westerly winds from the Pacific Ocean. Monthly mean temps. range from 50°F in Jan. to 70°F in Aug., with an avg. annual temp. of 60°F. Afternoon and evening temps. vary by as much as 30°F. Most of the 13" avg. annual rainfall occurs during the winter, with little occurring during the summer.

Central San Bernadino, California

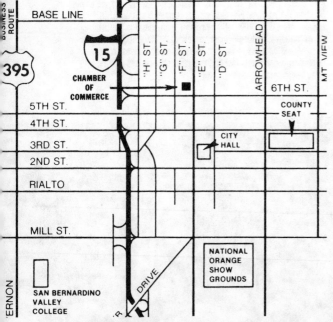

FLORA AND FAUNA. Animals native to San Bernardino include the mule deer, coyote, jackrabbit, ground squirrel, badger and pocket gopher. Common birds include the swallow, hummingbird, white-tail kite, kingbird, quail, scrub jay, golden eagle and woodpecker. Gopher snakes, tree frogs, pond turtles, salamanders and the venomous rattlesnake, are found in the area. Common trees include the pinion, juniper, sycamore, pine and oak. Smaller plants include the manzanita, chaparral shrub, whipple yucca, Indian paintbrush, nemophila, prickly phlox and CA poppy (the state flower).

POPULATION. According to the US census, the pop. of San Bernardino in 1970 was 109,203. In 1978, it was estimated that it had decreased to approx. 107,000.

ETHNIC GROUPS. In 1978, the ethnic distribution of San Bernardino was approx. 60.9% Caucasian, 14.5 Black, 21.3% Hispanic, 1.2% Native American and 2.1% Oriental. (A percentage of the Hispanic total is also included in the Caucasian total.)

TRANSPORTATION. Interstate hwys. 10 and 15, US hwys. 66 and 395 and state hwys. 18, 30, 206 and 330 provide major motor access to San Bernardino. *Railroads* include AMTRAK, Santa Fe, Union Pacific and S Pacific. *Airlines* serving nearby Ontario Intl. Airport include AA, CO, RW, TW, UA and WA. Several other nearby airports offer private and commuter aircraft facilities. *Bus lines* include Greyhound, Trailways, the inter-city Omnitrans System and the local Rapid Transit District.

COMMUNICATIONS. Communications, broadcasting and print media originating from San Bernardino are: *AM radio stations* KFXM 590 (Indep., Top 40); KDIG 1240 (ABC/E, NBC, Btfl. Mus.); KMEN 1290 (ABC/C, Top 40) and KCKC 1350 (CBS, C&W); *FM radio stations* KVCR 91.9 (NPR, Clas.); KQLH 95.1 (ARR., MOR) and KOLA 99.9 (ABC, Top 40); *television stations* KSCI Ch. 18 (Indep.); KVCR Ch. 24 (Indep.) and KHOF Ch. 30 (Indep.); *press*: one major daily serves the city, the *Sun Telegram*, issued both mornings and evenings; other publications include the *Precinct Reporter*, *American*, *Aerospace Safety Magazine* and *El Chicano*.

HISTORY. Native Americans of the Coahilla tribe inhabited the valley in which present-day San Bernardino is located. The first white settlers arrived in 1810. Franciscan Father Francisco Dumetz was sent from Mission San Gabriel to establish an inland mission in the area, which was named San Bernardino in honor of the feast day of St. Bernardino of Sienna. In 1843 Rancho San Bernardino, covering most of the central valley, was granted to Antonio Maria Lugo and his three sons. In 1851, 500 Mormon immigrants from Salt Lake City, led by Capt. Jefferson Hunt, chose the present site of the city as their permanent settlement, purchasing the land from the Lugo and Sepulveda families. The first American settlement in CA, it was incorporated as a town in 1854. In 1858, however, the Mormons left the town after establishing two schoolhouses, a govt. building, three stores, a flour mill, several lumber mills and an irrigation canal to return to Salt Lake City, UT. During the Civil War, the remaining settlers held off Dan Showalter's Irregulars at the Improvised Ft., which was part of the Roman Catholic Mission. In 1862, a flood destroyed part of the city, and in Mar. 1863, the incorporation of the city was rescinded. Thereafter, the town grew steadily, its economy based on trade and agriculture. The S Pacific and Santa Fe RRs arrived in the 1870s and 1880s, and, on Aug. 10, 1886, the city was reincorporated. By 1900, the pop. of the city had reached 6,000. The center of the surrounding agriculture region, the city continued to grow until the 1940s, when its pop. reached approx. 43,650. Between 1940 and 1960, however, the economy began to decline, but it pop. grew nearly 100%, to approx. 87,000, by 1960.

GOVERNMENT. San Bernardino has a mayor-council form of govt. The seven council members are elected by ward to four-year terms. The mayor, elected at large to a four-year term, is not a council member and votes only in a tie. The mayor also has veto power over the council.

ECONOMY AND INDUSTRY. The major employer in San Bernardino is govt., followed by trade, services (including education and health) and manufacturing. Industries include printing and publishing and the manufacture of steel products, furniture, electrical vehicles and apparel. In June, 1979, the total labor force of the Ontario-San Bernardino-Riverside met. area was approx. 569,900, while the rate of unemployment was 6.5%.

BANKING. In 1978, total deposits at the one bank headquartered in San Bernardino were approx. $10,226,000, while assets totaled $11,434,000. Banks include American Security, Bank of CA, Security Pacific Natl. and United CA.

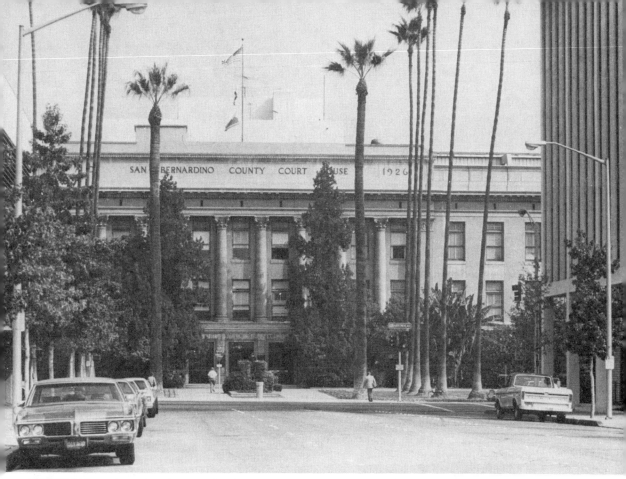

County Courthouse, San Bernardino, California

HOSPITALS. There are three gen. hosps. in the city—St. Bernardine, San Bernardino Comm. and San Bernardino Co., as well as the Patton State Hosp.

EDUCATION. CA State Col. at San Bernardino, a public, liberal arts institution, is one of the largest in the state system. Awarding bachelor and master degrees, it enrolled approx. 5,350 in 1978. San Bernardino Valley Comm. Col., which is also a publicly-supported institution, offers associate degree programs. In 1978, approx. 15,150 were enrolled. There are 37 elementary, six jr. high and seven sr. high schools in the public system, while 16 parochial schools provide private education. Five public libs. are available.

ENTERTAINMENT. The Natl. Orange Show is held each year during Feb. in San Bernardino. The Int'l Council presents a heritage festival in May. The Valley Col. Coyotes participate in intercollegiate sports.

ACCOMMODATIONS. There are several hotels and motels in San Bernardino, including the Hilton, Holiday and Desert inns, Travelodge, and Sands Motel.

FACILITIES. There are 20 parks and playgrounds and six recreation centers in San Bernardino. To the N of the city is the 383-acre San Bernardino Natl. Forest, which contains the highest mts. in S CA, including the 11,502' San Gorgonio Mt. Within the forest, the 65,038 acres set aside as the Cucamonga, San Gorgonio and San Jacinto wilderness areas offer opportunities for walking and driving tours. In addition to the resort centers of Lake Arrowhead and Big Bear Lake, there are campgrounds, picnic areas and seven winter sports areas in the forest. Among the public golf courses in the city is the San Bernardino Golf Course.

CULTURAL ACTIVITIES. The San Bernardino Arts Assn., Civic Light Opera, San Bernardino Symphony Orchestra, Valley Concert Assn., Jr. U Children's Musical Theater and Traditional Arts Assn., all under the auspices of the Arrowhead Allied Arts Council, contribute to the cultural life of the city. Cultural facilities include the CA Theatre of the Performing Arts and the Cultural Arts Center. In addition, San Bernardino Valley Comm. Col. and CA State Col. of San Bernardino present art, dramatic and musical productions.

LANDMARKS AND SIGHTSEEING SPOTS. Attractions in San Bernardino include the site of the first Natl. Orange Show, held at the showgrounds; the Atwood Adobe, which, until its relocation in 1975, was the only remaining structure to withstand the 1862 flood; the Santa Fe RR Depot and the City Clock, which was erected in 1875. Adjacent to the San Bernardino Valley, N of the city, is Arrowhead Mt., on which an unusual separation of soil types and vegetation has produced an arrow-shaped, lightened area on its SW slope. The mt. was named by the Coahilla tribe after, legend maintains, they were driven from their lands and guided to their new home by a flaming arrow on the mt. provided by their god.

City Hall, San Bernardino, California

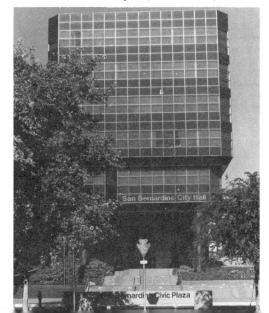

SAN DIEGO
CALIFORNIA

CITY LOCATION-SIZE-EXTENT. San Diego, the seat of San Diego Co., second largest city in the state and ninth largest in the US, encompasses 319.5 sq. mi. E of San Diego Bay in extreme SW CA at 32°44' N lat. and 117°10' W long. The met. area, bounded by Mexico on the S and the Pacific Ocean on the W, extends E into Imperial Co., N into Orange Co. and NE into Riverside Co.

TOPOGRAPHY. The terrain of San Diego, which is located on the Pacific Coastal Plain, varies from flat coast line area in the W part of the city to hilly to mountainous areas in the E approaching the W slope of the San Diego Mts. of the Pacific Coastal Range. The elev. ranges from SL to 822', while the mean elev. is 42'.

CLIMATE. The climate of San Diego is Pacific marine and semi-arid, characterized by cooler summers and warmer winters than other places situated in the same lat. The avg. annual temp. of 62°F ranges from means of 55.2°F in Jan. to 69.8°F in Aug. During Sept. and Oct., dry winds from the E, which often blow for several days in succession, result in temps. in the 90°F and 100°F range. Most of the annual 9.78" avg rainfall occurs from Nov. through Mar., resulting in the need for extensive irrigation. The RH generally ranges between 54% and 81%, but drops below 20% for the duration of the hot, dry winds . San Diego lies in the PSTZ and observes DST.

FLORA AND FAUNA. Animals native to San Diego include the ground squirrel, bobcat, weasel and ringtail. Common birds include the house finch, great blue heron, sea gull, kildeer, hummingbird and woodpecker. Several species of reptiles, including the CA lyre snake, granite night lizard, leaf-toed gecko and the venomous rattlesnake are found in the area. Typical trees include the palm, oak and pine. Smaller plants include the CA golden poppy (the state flower), scotch broom and blue lupine.

POPULATION. According to the US census, the pop. of San Diego in 1970 was 697,027. In 1978, it was estimated that it had increased nearly 20% to approx. 830,000. The city ranks among the 20 fastest-growing in the US.

ETHNIC GROUPS. In 1978, the ethnic distribution of San Diego was approx. 89.2% Caucasian, 7.5% Black and 12.7% Hispanic (a percentage of the Hispanic total is also included in the Caucasian total).

TRANSPORTATION. Interstate hwys. 5, 8, 15 and 805 and state hwys. 67, 75, 78, 94 and 163 provide major motor access to San Diego. *Railroads* serving the city include San Diego & AZ E, AMTRAK, Santa Fe and S Pacific. The Port of San Diego is the base of the Pacific Coast fishing fleet. *Airlines* serving San Diego Intl. Airport include AA, CO, DL, RW, NA, UA, WA and Pacific SW. *Bus lines* serving the city include Greyhound, Trailways, Mexicoach and the local San Diego Transit.

COMMUNICATIONS. Communications, broadcasting and print media originating from San Diego are: *AM radio stations* KOGO 600 (NBC, MOR, Pers.); KFMB 760 (ABC/E, Contemp., MOR); KSDO 1130 (CBS, MBS, News); KCBQ 1170 (Indep., Top 40); KSON 1240 (ABC/I, C&W) and KGB 1360 (Indep., Contemp., Btfl. Mus.); *FM radio stations* KPBS 89.5 (NPR, Public Affairs); KFSD 94.1 (Indep., Clas., Jazz); KLRO 94.9 (Indep., Inspir., Talk); KYXY 96.5 (Indep., Btfl. Mus.); KSON 97.3 (Indep., Easy Ctry.); KIFM 98.1 (Indep., Mellow Mus.); KFMB 100.7 (Indep., Top 40); KGB 101.5 (Indep., Progsv. Rock, News); KEZL 102.9 (Indep., Btfl. Mus.); KOZN 103.7 (Indep. Btfl. Mus.); KITT 105.3 (Indep., MOR) and KPRI 106.5 (Indep., Contemp., Rock); *television stations* KETV Ch. 6 (Indep.,); KFMB Ch. 8 (CBS); KGTV Ch. 10 (ABC); KEWT Ch. 12 (Indep.); KPBS (Ch. 15 (PBS); KCST Ch. 39 (NBC) and KJOG Ch. 51 (Indep.); *press*: two dailies serve the city, the morning *Union* and the evening *Tribune*, other publications include *San Diego Magazine*, *American Handgunner*, *Applause*, *Gun Magazine*, *Sr. World*, *Zoonooz* and *Today in San Diego*.

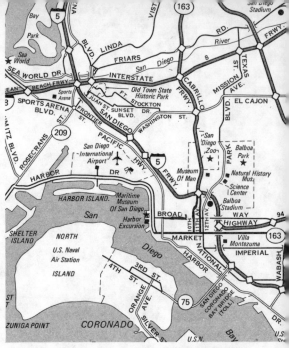

San Diego, California

HISTORY. Native Americans of the Diegueno tribe inhabited the area of present-day San Diego before the first white settlers arrived. In 1542, Portuguese explorer Juan Rodriguez Cabrillo sailed into the bay, which he named in honor of St. Didacus, but colonization did not begin until 1769, when Padre Junipero Serra founded the first CA Mission, San Diego de Alcala, in what is now known as the city's "Old Town." The same year, the first Spanish presidio (military outpost, or fortified settlement) in CA was established in the area as part of Spain's plan to colonize the region. During the early 1800s, the chief industry of the settlement was the trading of cattle hides. San Diego gained pueblo, or village status, in 1835 and remained under Mexican rule until CA became a US territory in 1848. In 1850 (the year CA achieved statehood), San Diego was incorporated

California Tower, San Diego, California

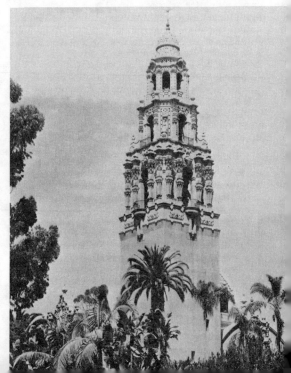

as a city, and, in 1867, businessmen bought vacant land S of the presidio in what is now downtown San Diego, and started a new settlement called "New Town". When the first RR reached the city in 1885, a land boom resulted. Shortly before the turn of the century, the pop. declined. The decline was reversed when the tuna fishing industry boomed and large canneries were built. In 1915, the city hosted the Panama-CA exposition and during World War I, became a major naval center. In 1922, the city was selected as the site for the headquarters of the 11th Naval District. During the 1930s, the aircraft industry became the largest civilian employer in the city and, during WW II, thousands of workers arrived after armed forces bases were built. After the war, many servicemen remained in San Diego. During the 1950s, increased competition from foreign tuna canneries and a slump in the aircraft industry inhibited the growth of the economy of the city, although increased production in the shipbuilding industry offset the losses somewhat. Although the aerospace industry experienced a slump in the 1960s, the development of a large industrial park later helped attract several new industries to the area. The city has continued to grow as a military industrial and educational center and is a popular retirement comm.

GOVERNMENT. San Diego has a council-mgr. form of govt. consisting of nine council members including the mayor as a voting member. The council members and mayor are elected at large to four-year terms, while the city mgr., the administrative head of govt., is appointed.

ECONOMY AND INDUSTRY. There are more than 1,000 manufacturing plants in the San Diego area. Major industries are aerospace, machinery, electronics, R&D, tourism, food processing, printing and publishing, shipbuilding and surfboards. The San Diego Naval Base, which includes the N Island Air Station, is located in the city, which is home for one of the largest complements of armed forces in the US. Fed., state and local govt. employ approx. 25% of the total labor force of the greater met. area, which in June, 1979 was approx. 715,200, while the rate of unemployment was 5.7%.

BANKING. There are 34 banks and 28 savings and loan assns. in San Diego. In 1978, total deposits at the nine banks headquartered in the city were approx. $588,198,000 while assets totaled $646,793,000. Banks include San Diego Trust & Savings, Peninsula, Bank of Commerce, Citizens Western, Mexican American Natl., CA Heritage, CA Coastal, Pacific Coast and Home Fed. Trust.

HOSPITALS. There are 28 gen. hosp. in San Diego, as well as a V.A. Hosp. and two military hosps. Among these are Center City, Mercy, Grossmont, Scripps Memorial, Kaiser, U and Doctors hosps.

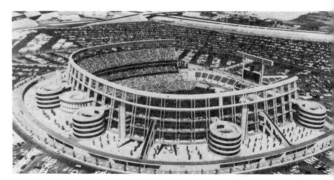

50,000 seat stadium, San Diego, California

EDUCATION. San Diego State U, a publicly-supported liberal arts institution offering programs leading to bachelor, master and doctorate degrees, enrolled nearly 2,400 in 1978. The U of San Diego, a private Roman Catholic institution founded in 1949, is one of 12 diocesan institutes of higher education in the US. More than 3,600 enrolled in 1978. The U of CA at San Diego, established in 1912, enrolled nearly 10,400 in 1978. Other institutions are Point Loma, San Diego City, San Diego Evening and San Diego Mesa cols. and Scripps Institute of Oceanography. There are approx. 150 elementary and high schools in the public school system, with a total enrollment of nearly 154,200. The San Diego Public Lib. system consists of the main lib. and more than 20 branches.

ENTERTAINMENT. Portugal, Mexico, Spain, the US and HI join together for San Diego's annual Cabrillo Festival, a week-long celebration held in Sept. beginning with a flag-raising ceremony and ending with a re-enactment of Cabrillo's landing in San Diego Bay. Commemorating the achievements of Portuguese explorer and navigator Juan Rodriguez Cabrillo, the festival features a band concert, costumed dancers, a banquet, historical seminar, the Cabrillo Art Classic, and a regatta. The Natl. Shakespeare Festival is held annually from June to Sept. at the Old Globe Theatre in Balboa Park. Other festivals include Canadian Maple Leaf Days, America's Finest City Week, Festival de la Primivera and the Carnation Festival in Aug. Pro sports entertainment is provided by the San Diego Chargers an NFL-AFC football team, the San Diego Clippers, an NBA basketball team, the San Diego Padres, a NL baseball team, the Hawks, a minor league, PHL hockey team, and the Friars, a WTT tennis team. The U of San Diego Aztecs and the teams of San Diego State U which participate in the PAC-10 Conf., provide collegiate sports entertainment.

ACCOMMODATIONS. There are several hotels and motels in San Diego, including the Hotel del Coronado, Plaza Intl., Town and Country, Little America Westgate, Sheraton-Harbor Island, Hanales and Bahia Motor hotels, US Grant, TraveLodge Tower, Islandia Hyatt, San Diego Hilton, Vacation Village Motel and the Pickwick, Holiday and Quality inns.

Harbor and skyline of San Diego, California

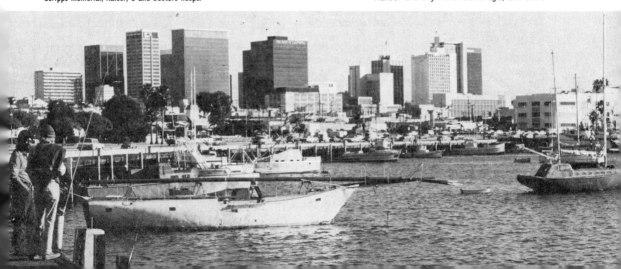

FACILITIES. The 400-acre Balboa Park, located in the heart of San Diego, offers facilities for picnicking, tennis, swimming, archery, badminton, basketball, lawn bowling, square dancing, horseshoe and shuffleboard and contains the San Diego Zoo, famous worldwide for its numerous species of animals. The 4,250-acre Mission Bay Park, an aquatic playground, includes the 50-acre Sea World oceanarium, which displays a killer whale, dolphins, sea lions and walruses. Other city recreational facilities include a 17.5 mi. Pacific Ocean shoreline, with various beaches offering accommodations for water skiing, fishing, sailing, boating, skin diving, surfing, picnicking and swimming. There are numerous public golf courses in the area, including those at Balboa Park, Colina Park, River Valley and Mission Bay.

CULTURAL ACTIVITIES. The San Diego Opera Co. and the San Diego Symphony Orchestra perform at the Civic Center Plays sponsored by the Broadway Theater League are also staged at the center. The Old Globe theatre is a replica of the English playhouse where the plays of William Shakespear were performed. It was destroyed by fire in 1978, is currently being rebuilt and will soon again host Shakespearian plays. There are several art galleries in the city, including The Timken Gallery, which features a large collection of Russian religious painting, the Fine Arts Gallery and The Society for Creative Anachronism maintains medieval pavillions and costumes at the Barony of Calafia. There are several museums in the city, including the San Diego Aerospace Museum in Balboa Park, which commemorates the history of man's attempt to fly and the exploration of outer space; the Sierra Museum in Presidio Park, which features the history of the area; the Fleet Space Theater and Science Center and the Museum of Man, which are located in Balboa Park. The Hall of Champions is an all-sports museum honoring San Diego athletes. The *Star of India*, the oldest iron boat still afloat, is part of the ship collection at the Maritime Museum in San Diego Bay.

LANDMARKS AND SIGHTSEEING SPOTS. Old Town State Historical Park, located in the Old Town section of San Diego, the site of the first settlement in CA, contains many old homes, as well as shops, restaurants and museums of the 1850-1880 period. Among the other structures are the Machado-Stenert Adobe and the Machado-Silvas Adobe. Casa de Estudillo (1827) is a one-story adobe townhouse maintained with period furnishings by the Natl. Society of Colonial Dames. The first parish church in Old Town, the Old Adobe Chapel, was built in 1850. The Mason Street School, which opened in 1865, still serves as a classroom for history and archaeology lectures. Other landmarks are the Plaza San Diego Viejo, Steeley Stable, the Whaley and Pendleton houses, the Old Town Drug Store and the Cabrillo Monument, a statue honoring the Spanish Explorer who landed in the area in 1542. An historic lighthouse, erected in 1855, has been restored with period furnishings.

SAN FRANCISCO
CALIFORNIA

CITY LOCATION-SIZE-EXTENT. San Francisco, the seat of San Francisco Co., encompasses 46.6 sq. mi. on the N tip of a narrow 32 mi.long hilly peninsula between San Francisco Bay on the E and the Pacific Ocean on the W at 37°47' N lat. and 122°25' W long. The city is bounded on the N by the Golden Gate Strait, the only SL entrance through the Coastal Mts. into the Great Valley of CA. The greater met. area extends into the neighboring counties of Marin to the N, San Mateo to the S and, across San Francisco Bay, Contra Costa to the NE and Alameda (including the city of Oakland) to the E.

TOPOGRAPHY. The terrain of San Francisco, which is located near the seismically-active San Andreas Fault in the Coastal Range region of CA, is hilly. The "City of Seven Hills" actually includes more than 40, some reaching heights of nearly 938'. The principal hills are Nob, Russian, Telegraph, Twin Peaks, Mt. Davidson, Rincon and Lone Mt. There are four islands in San Francisco Bay, Alcatraz, Angel, Yerba Buena and Treasure. The Bay forms one of the world's largest land-locked harbors. The freshwater Lake Merced is located in the SW part of the city. The mean elev. is 52'.

CLIMATE. The climate of San Francisco is Pacific marine, characterized by little variation in monthly temp. means or pronounced wet and dry seasons. The 56.4°F avg. annual temp. ranges from 49.2°F in Jan. to 62.4°F in Sept. Some 80% of the avg. annual rainfall of 20" falls from Nov. through Mar. The RH ranges from 59% to 93%. San Francisco lies in the PSTZ and observes DST.

FLORA AND FAUNA. Animals native to San Francisco include the raccoon, pocket gopher and opossum. Common birds are the house finch, starling, swallow and mourning dove. Gopher snakes, tree frogs, salamanders, pond turtles and the venomous Pacific rattlesnake, are also found in the area. Typical trees are the redwood, pine, fir and willow. Smaller plants include the CA golden poppy (the state flower), chaparral shrub, filaree and creamcup.

POPULATION. According to the US census, the pop. of San Francisco in 1970 was 715,674. In 1978, it was estimated that it had decreased to approx. 657,000.

ETHNIC GROUPS. In 1978, the racial distribution of San Francisco was approx. 71.7% Caucasian, 13.4% Black, 14.2% Hispanic and 0.2% other.

TRANSPORTATION. Interstate hwys. 80, 280, 580 and 680, US hwys. 1, 101, 280 and 480 and state routes 9, 17, 35, 82, 84 and 92 provide major motor access to San Francisco. *Railroads* serving the city include Pacific, W Pacific, Union Pacific, Santa Fe and AMTRAK. *Airlines* serving San Francisco Intl. Airport include Air CA, Air Canada, AA, BN, BA, China Airlines, CO, CP/Air, DL, EA, RW, Japan Airlines, Mexicana, NA, NW, PA Philippine, Qantas, Stol Air Commuter, Trans Intl., TW, UA, WA, World

San Francisco, California

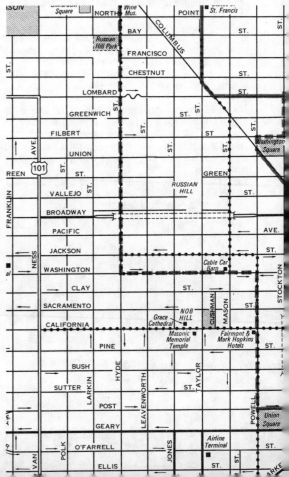

Airways, Lufthansa, Singapore and Yosemite Airlines. *Bus lines* include Greyhound, Trailways, the local A/C Transit, Sam Trans and Golden Gate Transit. Local and commuter transportation is also provided by the Bay Area Rapid Transit system (BART), which links eight city subway stations with 23 E Bay met. area terminals and the San Francisco Municipal Railway system (MUNI) consisting of cable cars, streetcars and buses. The Port of San Francisco is served by gen. cargo, containerized and barge services and handles 1.7 million tons of cargo annually. Both port-to-port and cruise services are available through several trans-Pacific and coastal steamship lines, including the Royal Viking, which offers service to Mexico, Central America, the S Seas, the Carribbean, the Orient and Europe. Ferry service is provided by the Golden Gate (Golden Gate Transit) and Tiburon (Harbor Carriers) ferries.

COMMUNICATIONS. Communications, broadcasting and print media originating from San Francisco are: *AM radio stations* KFRC 610 (Indep., Top 40); KSFO 560 (Indep., MOR): KNBR 680 (NBC, MOR); KCBS 740 (CBS, Adult Contemp.); KGO 810 (ABC); KIQI 960 (Indep., Btfl. Mus.); KIQL 1010 (ABC/C, Adult Contemp.); KFAX 1100 (Indep., Relig.); KYA 1260 (Indep., Top 40); KDIA 1310 (Indep., Blk.); KEST 1450 (Indep., Relig., Ethnic); KALI 1480 (Indep., Span.) and KKHI 1550 (Indep., Clas.); *FM radio stations* KQED 88.5 (Indep., Clas.); KPOO 89.5 (Indep., Var.); KUSF 90.3 (Indep., Educ.); KALW 91.7 (Indep., Educ.); EYA 93.3 (Indep., Progsv.); KSAN 94.9 (Indep., Progsv. Rock); KKHI 95.5 (Indep., Clas.); KOIT 96.5 (Indep., Btfl Mus.); KCBS 97.3 (CBS, Adult Contemp.); KMPX 98.9 (Indep., Swing); KYUU 99.7 (Indep., MOR); KIOI 101.3 (ABC/C., Adult Contemp.); KDFC 102.1 (Indep., Clas.); KFOG 104.5 (Indep. Btfl. Mus.); KBRG 105.3 (Indep., Span.); KMEI 106.1 (Indep., Span.); KMEL 106.1 (Indep., Rock) and KEAR 106.9 (Indep., Relig.) and *television stations* KTVU Ch. 2 (Indep.); KRON Ch. 4 (NBC); KPIX Ch. 5 (CBS); KGO Ch. 7 (ABC); KQED Ch. 9 (PBS); KEMO Ch. 20 (Indep.); KTSF Ch. 26 (Indep.); KQEC Ch. 32 (PBS); KVOF Ch. 38 (Indep.); KBHK Ch. 44 (Indep.); KDTV Ch. 60 (Indep.) and cable; *press*: two major dailies serve the city, the *Chronicle*, issued mornings, and the *Examiner*, issued evenings. Other publications include the weekly *San Francisco Observer*, *This Week in San Francisco* and the *Asian Student*, as well as *The Farmer*, *Sierra*, *San Francisco Magazine*, *Agrichemical Age*, *San Francisco Progress*, *Forest Industries*, *Mother Jones*, *Motorland*, *San Francisco Territorial News* and *This Month in San Francisco and Los Angeles*.

HISTORY. The first permanent white settlements in the area of present-day San Francisco were a presidio or military outpost, and the Franciscan Mission, San Francisco de Asis (later named Mission Dolores), both constructed in 1776. After CA became part of Mexico in the 1820s, the Mexican Gov. appointed an English captain, William Richardson, who camped midway between the Presidio and the Mission, to oversee activities in the Bay area. Other families soon arrived, and, by 1835, a village called Yerba Buena had developed around Richardson's encampment. Trader Jacob Lesse became the first American citizen to settle at Yerba Buena, in 1836. In 1846, the USN and Army troops occupied the area for the duration of the Mexican War, and Lt. Washington A. Bartlett was appointed the first alcalde, or mayor, under American rule. In 1847, the name of the settlement was changed to San Francisco. When gold was discovered in CA in 1848, thousands of prospectors began to arrive in the town—in 1849 alone, more than 40,000 came. A supply center for the miners, San Francisco incorporated as a city on Apr. 15, 1850. A city of many tents and shacks, San Francisco's law enforcement resources were unable to adequately serve the booming pop., and the aid of vigilante groups was required to bring the city's crime wave (especially in the "Barbary Coast" area) under control. Construction of the transcontinental RR attracted thousands of Chinese laborers to the city, which became the "Gateway to the Pacific" when the RR was completed in 1869.

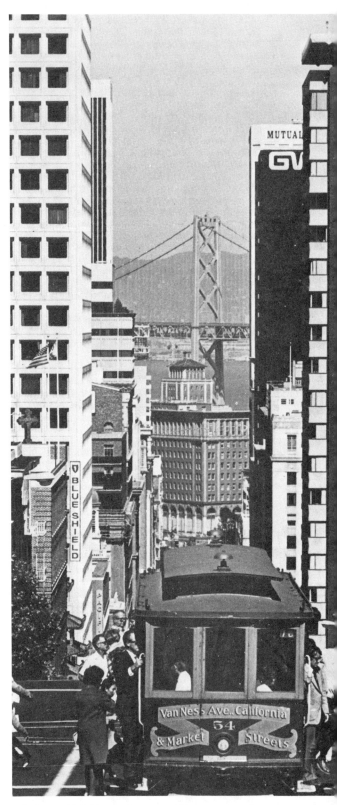

Cablecar with Goldengate Bridge, San Francisco, California

In 1873, the first cable cars in the city began operating. By the turn of the century, the pop. had reached 342,000. In 1906, a powerful earthquake shook the city. An ensuing fire raged out of control and destroyed the entire business district and numerous homes, and more than 700 people were killed. The city was quickly rebuilt, however, and in 1915, hosted the Panama-Pacific Intl. Exposition. The opening of the Panama canal soon after resulted in additional port activity and expansion in the local shipbuilding industry. The city continued to grow during the 1920s and 1930s. In 1936, the San Francisco-Oakland Bay Bridge was opened, while the Golden Gate Bridge was completed the next year. During WW II, the city became the largest shipbuilding center in the world, and thousands of military personnel were based in the Bay area. In 1945, delegates from several nations convened in the city to draft the charter of the UN, which was founded later that year. Throughout the 1950s and 1960s, the pop. of the city, in which the "counterculture" developed, continued to grow. In 1972, the Bay Area Rapid Transit System (BART), opened. In 1978, demonstrations by members of the city's large gay pop. and others followed the killings of George Moscone, the mayor, and Harvey Milk, the first avowed homosexual supervisor in city govt. A city characterized by tolerance since its inception, San Francisco is today the home of diverse ethnic, social and political groups, and one of the most cosmopolitan cities in the US.

GOVERNMENT. The city and co. of San Francisco has a consolidated mayor-council form of govt. The mayor, who is not a council member, is elected to a four-year term. The council, which is the chief legislative body, consists of 11 members, called supervisors, who are elected by district to four-year terms.

ECONOMY AND INDUSTRY. San Francisco is the financial capital of the W, the administrative center for many leading US corporations and the W coast communications center, as well as operation headquarters for several fed. agencies. Service industries, fed., state and local govt., wholesale and retail trade, and real estate, banking and insurance play important roles in the economy of the city. Among the major products manufactured in the city are paper goods, chemicals, pharmaceuticals, food and dairy products, apparel, lumber, forest products, building and hardware products and petroleum products. Tourism is the largest

Chinatown, San Francisco, California

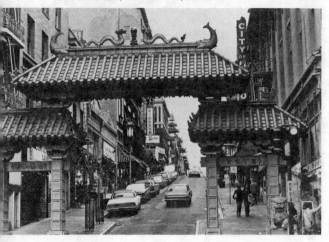

single business in the city, with tourists spending more than one billion dollars annually. Other major fields of employment are shipping, engineering and heavy construction, trucking, transportation, power and communications. In June, 1979, the labor force of the greater met. area (including Oakland) totaled approx. 1,592,400, while the rate of unemployment was 5.2%. In 1978, total taxable retail sales were $2.5 billion, up 10.5% from 1977. In 1977, median per capita income for the San Francisco-Oakland met. area was $7,459 and the median family income was $19,917.

BANKING. There are 40 banks and 25 savings and loan assns. in San Francisco. The headquarters of the largest bank in the world, the Bank of America; four of the largest banks in the US; and agencies for 30 foreign banks, are located in the city. In 1978, total deposits at the 26 banks headquartered in the city were approx. $112,431,863,000 while assets totaled $136,238,480,000. Banks include the Bank of America, Wells Fargo, Crocker Natl., Bank of CA, CA First, Sumitomo of CA, Barclay's of CA, Golden State Sanwa, Union, CA Canadian, Redwood and French of CA.

HOSPITALS. Among the many hosps. in San Francisco are Kaiser, Mt. Zion, Pacific Medical Center, San Francisco Medical Center of the U of CA, SF Gen., St. Joseph's, St. Mary's, Children's, St. Luke's, Marshal Hale, Shriner's, US Public Health Service, Ralph K. Davies, Garden Sullivan, St. Francis, Pacific Medical Center, Chinese, French, Letterman Army and V.A. hosps.

EDUCATION. San Francisco State U, a state-supported institution, was established in 1899 to train elementary school teachers, began to award bachelor degrees in 1923 and master degrees in 1949. In 1978, more than 26,100 enrolled. The City Col. of San Francisco, a two-year institution established in 1935, offers associate degrees. Enrollment in 1978 was approx. 25,350. The San Francisco Comm. Center System, a publicly-supported, two-year institution awarding associate degrees, enrolled approx. 35,950. Golden Gate U, a private pro school established in 1901, offers grad. and undergrad. programs and, in 1978, enrolled nearly 9,100. The U of San Francisco, a Roman Catholic institution operated under the auspices of the Society of Jesus, awards degrees ranging from bachelor to doctorate. Other institutions in the city include San Francisco Conservatory of Music, San Francisco Medical Center of the U of CA, San Francisco Theological Seminary, CA Col. of Podiatric Medicine, San Francisco Law School, San Francisco Art Institute and Simpson Col. There are 97 elementary, 17 jr. and 11 sr. high schools in the city and co. public school system. In 1977, approx. 65,350 enrolled. In addition, some 50 private and parochial schools enrolled approx. 30,000. The San Francisco Public Lib. maintains 25 branches, and there are seven city-co. libs. Other libs. include those at the CA Academy of Sciences and the CA Historical Society.

ENTERTAINMENT. More than 100 festivals and special events are held in San Francisco each year. Among them are the Sports and Boat Show and the E-W Shriner's Football Classic in Jan.; the nine-day Chinese New Year Celebration in late Jan. or early Feb.; the St. Patrick's Day Parade in Mar.; the Nihonmachi (Japantown) Cherry Blossom Festival and the Opening Day Yachting Parade in Apr.; the Bay to Breakers foot race and Master Mariner's Regatta in May; the San Francisco Birthday Celebration in June; the Blessing of the Fishing Fleet held in Sept.; the Columbus Day Celebration and Parade in Oct. and the Grand Natl. Livestock Exposition, Rodeo and Horse Show in late Oct. and early Nov. Professional sports entertainment is provided by the SF 49ers, an NFL-NFC football team, the SF Giants, an NL baseball team the Golden Gaters, a WTT tennis team; and the Shamrocks, a PHL minor league hockey team. The SF State U Dons participate in sports at the collegiate level.

ACCOMMODATIONS. Hotels and motels in San Francisco include the Mark Hopkins, Fairmont, St. Francis, Sir Francis Drake, SF Hilton, Stanford Court, Clift, Sheraton-Palace, Beresford, Sheraton at Fisherman's Wharf, the Carlton, Hyatt Regency, the Miyako and several Best Western motor hotels and Holiday inns.

FACILITIES. There are numerous parks in San Francisco, including Alcatraz Island, Angel Island State Park, Golden Gate Park and Lincoln Park. The 1,017-acre Golden Gate Park includes a conservatory with 5,000 varieties of plants; paddock fields and buffalo; lakes for rowing and model

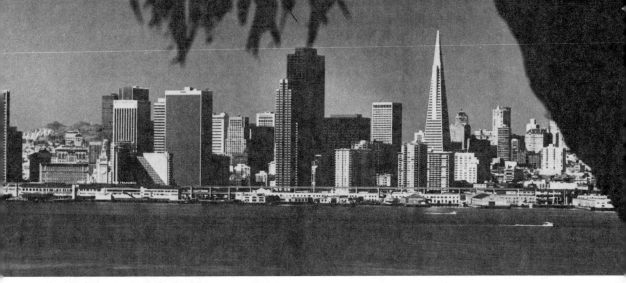

boat sailing; bridle paths; playing fields which accommodate many sports; the San Francisco Zoo, with more than 1,000 animals and birds, and the children's zoo, with its giant, ridable tortoises, and the Japanese Tea Garden, which consists of a tea-house, pagoda, several statues of Buddha, torii gates and several small pools, streams and bridges, including the Moon Bridge. Alcatraz ("Pelican" in Spanish) Island, the site of the first lighthouse built on the Pacific Coast, was once infamous as a fed. prison for such notorious criminals as Al Capone. Tours of the island are conducted by the Natl. Park Service. The 740-acre Angel Island (the largest in the Bay) State Park is a preserve for 200 deer, while facilities are also provided for cyclists, hikers and picnickers. An elephant train tour is also available. The Golden Natl. Recreation Area, a fed. preserve adminstered by the Natl. Park Service, encompasses the shoreline from Fisherman's Wharf to Ft. Funston on the Pacific Ocean, Alcatraz and Angel islands and a 20-mi. stretch of the Marin Co. coast (including beaches, ranchlands and redwoods) N of the Golden Gate Bridge. Adjacent to the San Francisco Zoo is the five-acre Lake Merced, which was an ocean lagoon before it was separated by sand dunes that developed in the area. Now, fed by freshwater springs, it offers boating and the only trout fishing available in the city. The 270-acre Lincoln Park, located on the headlands of Point Lobos, provides a view of the Golden Gate Bridge to the NW, and contains 200' cliffs and a municipal golf course. The Marina Green, a broad, waterfront lawn on the Bay, also provides a view of the Golden Gate Bridge and of boats sailing from the Yacht Harbor. There are several city beaches available to the public, including Ocean Beach, loacted in the W part of the city, which features Seal Rocks—small, stony islands just offshore that are usually inhabited by a colony of Steller Sea Lions. Boating facilities are available at many marinas in the Bay area. Several public golf courses and tennis courts are maintained by the city park system.

CULTURAL ACTIVITIES. Among the performing arts organizations in the city are the San Francisco Symphony Orchestra, which performs at the Opera House, and also presents pop concerts during the summer; the San Francisco Ballet, which annually devotes one of its Dec. performances to the "Nutcracker Suite"; the Curran, Golden Gate and Orpheum theaters, which present major touring Broadway shows; the American Conservatory Theatre, a resident repertory theater; the San Francisco Opera; the W Opera Theatre and the Civic Light Opera. Concert artists, orchestras and dance companies on tour perform at the Opera House and the Masonic Memorial Auditorium. Among the museums and centers, featuring ethnic and historical exhibits, are the Chinese Cultural Center and Wax Museum, the Mexican Museum of San Franciso (the only one of its kind in the US), the San Francisco African Historical and Cultural Center (featuring a Civil War collection), the Asian Art Museum and the Avery Brundage Collection of Oriental Art. The M. H. de Young Memorial Museum features historical items and art treasures from ancient Egypt, Rome and Medieval Europe. Other museums are the San Francisco Museum of Modern Art, the Carlisle Car Barn, the Wine Museum, Morrison Planetarium, the Maritime Museum, the Presidio Army Museum, the Palace of the Legion of Honor and the World of the Unexplained and Ripley's "Believe It or Not" Museum.

LANDMARKS AND SIGHTSEEING SPORTS. The San Francisco cable

As seen from Treasure Island, the skyline of San Francisco, California

car system is the only Natl. Historic Landmark on wheels. Among other historic landmarks are the 1,500-acre Presidio, which is now the headquarters of the 6th US Army, and Mission Dolores (formerly Mission San Francisco de Asis), both of which were built in 1776. The Haas-Lilienthal House, built in 1886, is a Victorian mansion that has been preserved with its period furnishings. The 16 sq.-block Chinatown and Japantown are popular tourist sites. The Whittier Mansion, erected in 1896, is the N headquarters of the CA Historical Society. Nob Hill reflects the cultural diversity of the city. The Old US Mint has been restored and contains presses, gold bullion and numismatic displays. The Wells Fargo History Room, located in the main Wells Fargo Bank, houses a stagecoach, relics of the Gold Rush, and gold nuggets and artifacts dating from 1848 to the earthquake and fire of 1906. "The Brotherhood of Man" is a mural commemorating the signing of the UN charter in the city on June 26, 1945. The Golden Gate Bridge, one of the longest, single-span suspension bridges in the US, built in 1936, spans San Francisco Bay for more than 1.7 mi. and links the city with Marin Co. to the North. Fisherman's Wharf and the nearby Ghirardelli Square, a shopping-eating-entertainment complex, are popular city attractions. Lombard St., comprised of a series of steep, S-shaped curves, is referred to as the "Crookedest Street in the World".

SAN JOSE
CALIFORNIA

CITY LOCATION-SIZE-EXTENT. San Jose, the seat of Santa Clara Co., is located in the central W part of the state and is 48 mi. S of San Francisco encompassing 152 sq. mi. at 37°20′ N lat. and 11°55′ W long. It is the largest city in the Santa Clara Valley and the fourth largest city in CA. Its met. area includes the cities of Santa Clara, Sunnyvale, Mt. View and most of Santa Clara Co., and extends N into Alameda, S into Monterey, SW into San Mateo and SW into Santa Cruz.

TOPOGRAPHY. The terrain of San Jose is basically flat, sloping slightly toward the N. The soil in the area makes it some of the finest farmland in the Santa Clara Valley. The Santa Cruz Mt. and the Diablo Mts. rim the valley. There are several lakes, including Anderson, Coyote and Vasona in the met. area. The city's mean elev. is 67′.

CLIMATE. San Jose's climate is considerably affected by westerlies from the Pacific Ocean. The annual avg. of 56°F ranges from a Jan. mean of 49°F to a Sept. mean of 62°F. Most of the 20′ annual rainfall occurs in the winter months. Snowfall is very rare. The RH ranges

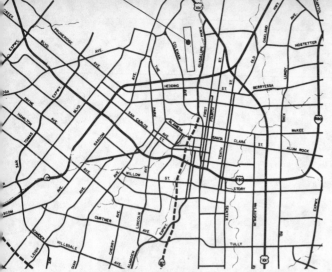

Central San Jose, California

from 56% to 90%. San Jose lies in the PSTZ and observes DST.

FLORA AND FAUNA. Animals native to San Jose include the mule deer, coyote, jackrabbit, desert cottontail and several species of bats. Common birds are the scrub jay, housefinch, great blue heron, Caspian tern and CA quail. The venomous N Pacific rattlesnake inhabits the area. Typical trees include the redwood and pine. Smaller plants include the chaparral bush.

POPULATION. According to the US census, the pop. of San Jose in 1970 was 447,025. In 1978, it was estimated that it had increased to 578,600.

ETHNIC GROUPS. In 1978, the ethnic distribution of San Jose was approx. 72% Caucasian, 3.5% Black, 15.2% Hispanic, 3.3% Asian and 6% other races.

TRANSPORTATION. Interstate hwys. 280 and 680, US hwy. 101 and state hwys. 9, 17 and 82 provide major motor access to San Jose. *Railroads* serving the city include S Pacific, W Pacific and AMTRAK. *Airlines* serving San Jose Municipal Airport are AA, CO, DL, NA, RW, TW, UA and WA. *Bus lines* are Greyhound, Peerless Stage and Santa Clara Transit District. The city is also served by three bay area ports, Oakland, San Francisco and Redwood City.

COMMUNICATIONS. Communications, broadcasting and print media originating from San Jose are: *AM radio stations* KLOK 1170 (UPI, MOR, Personality); KEEN 1370 (UPI, C&W); KNTA 1430 (Indep., Span.); KXRX 1500 (MBS, UPI, Talk) and KLIV 1590 (Indep., Top 40); *FM radio stations* KLEL 89.3 (Indep., Top 40); KSJS 90.7 (Indep., Top 40); KXJO 92.3 (UPI, Progsv.); KOME 98.5 (Indep., Progsv.); KBAY 100.3 (UPI, Btfl. Mus.) and KEZR 106.5 (Indep., Easy Rock); *television stations* KNTV Ch. 11 (ABC); KGSC Ch. 36 (Indep.); KQWT Ch. 48 (Indep.) and KTEH Ch. 54 (PBS); *press*: two major dailies serve the city, the *Mercury*, issued mornings, and the *News*, issued evenings; other daily publications include the *Post Records* and the collegiate *Spartan Daily*; magazines include the *CA School Employee* and *N CA Retailer.*

HISTORY. San Jose, the oldest city in CA, was founded by the Spanish in 1777. It was named Pueblo de San Jose de Guadalupe in honor of St. Joseph. The town grew slowly until American settlers arrived from the E in the 1840s to join the Spanish colonists. San Jose served as the state's first capital from 1849 to 1851. The city was incorporated in 1850. That same year, the first stage coach arrived from San Francisco. By 1864, the pop. was 3,000. The arrival of the RR created a land boom in the area, boosting the pop. to over 9,000 in 1870. San Jose U, the state's first col., was opened in 1871. During the late 1800s and early 20th century, San Jose developed into an important agriculture and wine producing area, and by 1950 was especially noted for prune production. Major growth in the city did not begin until the 1950s, when the aerospace and electronics industries built large facilities changing the region's economy from agricultural to industrial. The influx of people during that period increased the city's pop. to

200,000 by 1960. An urban renewal project was initiated in the late 1960s and early 1970s. During the 1970s the city was faced with problems in housing, pollution, education and public transportation. Today, San Jose is the state's fourth largest city.

GOVERNMENT. San Jose has a council-mgr. form of govt. The mayor, who is a member of the council and the seven members of the council are elected at large to four-year terms.

ECONOMY AND INDUSTRY. The met. area has the highest concentration of high-technology industries in the world. One of every three workers in the met. area is employed in manufacturing. The met. area ranks second in CA and ninth in the nation in value of shipments. In recent years the city's electronics industry has diversified into consumer products, medical instrumentation, and pollution control applications. Aerospace manufacturing is also a leading industry, producing missiles and space vehicles. Other major products include electrical machinery, processed foods, fabricated metals, machinery, chemicals, automobile assembly, and stone and clay. Printing and publishing are a major industries. Avg. income per family in San Jose in 1978 was $24,000. The labor force for the greater met. area totaled 686,200 in 1979, while unemployment was 5.3%. Total wages and salaries in 1978 were approx. $11.9 billion. The 1975 median per capita income was $5,340.

BANKING. There are 22 banking institutions in San Jose. In 1978, total deposits for the four banks headquartered in the city were $606,893,000, while assets were $675,871,000. Banks serving the city are First Natl., Comm., Pacific Valley and CA Security.

HOSPITALS. There are six gen. hosps. in San Jose, including San Jose, Alexian Brothers, Good Samaritan, O'Connor, Santa Teresa Medical Center and Santa Clara Valley Medical. The Agnew State Hosp. is also located in the city.

EDUCATION. San Jose State U, established in 1857 as Minn's Evening School, now offers bachelor and master degrees. Enrollment in 1978 was 28,300. Also serving the area are two comm. colleges Evergreen Valley and San Jose City . There are approx. 154 elementary and 27 high schools in the public school system and more than 20 private schools in the city.Lib. facilities include the San Jose Public Lib. and its 20 branches and the Santa Clara Co. Free Lib.

ENTERTAINMENT. Annual festivals featuring ethnic handicrafts, food and cultural displays include Cinco de Mayo and Tapestry in Talent, held the first weekend in July. The Tapestry in Talent draws 500,000 people to a 16-block area in downtown San Jose to view unique handmade items and sample ethnic foods. San Jose is the home of many sports teams, including the Earthquakes of the NASL, the Missions of the PCL and the Sunbirds of the Women's Pro Softball League. Collegiate sports activities center on the San Jose State U Spartans.

ACCOMMODATIONS. There are many hotels and motels in San Jose, including Motel St. Claire, Hyatt House, Howard Johnson's, Red Lion, Versailles, LeBaron, Petter Tree, TraveLodge and San Jose, Holiday and Ramada inns.

FACILITIES. The 27,000-acre park system includes 137 neighborhood, city and district parks. Alum Rock Park has a jr. museum, riding and hiking trails and picnic areas. Kelley Regional Park features the Happy Hollow Children's Park and Baby Zoo, the Japanese Friendship Garden and Leninger Comm. Center. Golf, archery, rifle and pistol ranges are provided at Santa Teresa Park. Vasona Park, near Los Gatos, offers sailing, fishing and picnicking by a 176-acre lake. The Coyote River, Uvas Canyon and Stevens Creek Parks offer fishing, picnicking, hiking, riding and bicycling. The Municipal Rose Gardens exhibit over 5,000 plants. There are three public golf courses in the city. Jogging tracks can be found at San Jose State U, San Jose City Col. and Evergreen Valley Col.

CULTURAL ACTIVITIES. San Jose is served by a symphony, a city chorus, the Civic Light Opera Co., and the music depts. of Evergreen, San

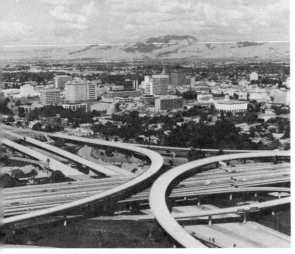

Aerial view of San Jose, California

Jose State and San Jose City Colleges. Among theatrical groups that perform in the city are the Actors Repertory and the San Jose State Art theaters. The San Jose Theatre Guild also sponsors events. The historic Museum of Art building now houses varied art exhibits and presents musical events. Among the exhibits at the Rosicrucian Egyptian Museum, Art Gallery and Planetarium are authentic artifacts and replicas of ancient Egypt. The New Almaden Mercury Mining Museum displays pictures of old mining machinery and Indian artifacts.

LANDMARKS AND SIGHTSEEING SPOTS. The Peralta Adobe, San Jose's only pre-1800 building, has been carefully restored to preserve its original character. Other historic buildings include the Co. Courthouse (1866), St. Joseph's Church (1877) and the Art Museum (1892). Historic San Jose charts Indian, Spanish, Mexican and American influences in early area history and maintains shops, a reconstructed livery and a restored home on its grounds. The Winchester Mystery House is a 160-room house designed by Sarah Winchester, eccentric heiress to the Winchester arms fortune. Paseo de San Antonio features pools, fountains, sculpture, play and picnic areas.

SANTA ANA
CALIFORNIA

CITY LOCATION-SIZE-EXTENT. Santa Ana, located in Orange Co. approx. 33 mi. SE of LA and 90 mi. N of San Diego, encompasses 27.2 sq. mi. at 33°45' N lat. and 117°51' W long. The southernmost city of a triad including Garden Grove and Anaheim, Santa Ana's greater met. area overlaps that of Garden Grove to the NW and Anaheim to the N.

TOPOGRAPHY. Santa Ana is situated in the flat S CA coastal plain which is bordered on the W by the Pacific Ocean and on the E by the Santa Ana Mts. The mean elev. is 133'.

CLIMATE. The climate of Santa Ana is moderate, influenced by prevailing W winds from the Pacific Ocean. The avg. annual temp. of 63°F ranges from a Jan. mean of 55°F to a July mean of 71°F, with temps. varying as much as 25°F from afternoon to night. Nearly 85% of the annual rainfall of 14" occurs during the winter. The RH ranges from 45% to 85%. Santa Ana is in the PSTZ and observes DST.

FLORA AND FAUNA. Animals native to Santa Ana include the coyote, ground squirrel and pocket gopher. Common birds include the egret, scrub jay, house finch and mourning dove. Pond turtles, salamanders, tree frogs and gopher snakes also inhabit the area. Typical trees are pinyon, juniper, pine and willow. Smaller plants include the poppy, chaparral shrub, creamcup and bunch grass.

POPULATION. The Anaheim-Santa Ana-Garden Grove met. area is one of the fastest growing in the nation. Between 1970 and 1977 its pop. increased

28.6%. According to the US census, the pop. of Santa Ana in 1970 was 155,320. In 1978, it was estimated that it had increased to 183,900.

ETHNIC GROUPS. In 1978, the ethnic distribution of Santa Ana was approx. 93.4% Caucasian, 4.3% Black and 25.8% Hispanic (a percentage of the Hispanic total is also included in the Caucasian total).

TRANSPORTATION. Interstate hwys. 5 and 405 and state hwys. 55, 58, 91 and 57 provide major motor access to Santa Ana. *Railroads* serving the city include Santa Fe, S Pacific and AMTRAK. All major *airlines* serve LA Intl. Airport, approx. 37 mi. NW of Santa Ana. Orange Co. Airport, approx. five mi. away, is served by RW. *Bus lines* include Greyhound, RTD and the local Orange Co. Rapid Transit.

COMMUNICATIONS. Communications, broadcasting and print media originating from Santa Ana are: *AM radio station* KWIZ 1480 (Indep., Oldies, MOR); *FM radio stations* KWIZ 96.7 (Indep., MOR); KYMS 106.3 (Indep., Contemp., Relig. Mus.); no *television stations* originate from Santa Ana, which receives broadcasting from nearby LA; *press:* one major daily serving the city is the *Register*, issued both morning and evening; other publications include the monthly *Toastmaster* and *W Landscaping News.*

HISTORY. In 1769, Franciscan Fathers led by Don Gasper Portola celebrated St. Anne's Feast Day with a Mass in a valley they named Santa Ana in her honor. The area was used for cattle grazing in 1810 by Antonio Yorba and Juan Peralta, who had received it in a Spanish land grant. Stretching from the Santa Ana foothills to the ocean, the tract became the Rancho Santiago de Santa Ana. Yorba's heirs sold approx. 70 acres in 1869 to William H. Spurgeon, who laid out the townsite eventually known as Santa Ana after the old rancho and the Santa Ana River. Centrally located in a rich farming area, Santa Ana's development as an agricultural market was aided by the arrival of the S Pacific RR in 1877. Incorporated as a city in 1886, Santa Ana became the Orange Co. seat in 1889. At the turn of the century, Santa Ana's residents numbered 49,333. After WW II, the growth of industry led to further expansion and the town's pop. was 183,900 by 1978. In 1952, Santa Ana was chartered as a city. It is now the financial and governmental center of Orange Co.

GOVERNMENT. Santa Ana has a council-mgr. form of govt. The seven council members are elected at large to four-year terms. The mayor, a voting member of the council, is selected by and from the council and serves a two-year term.

Bowers Museum, Santa Ana, California

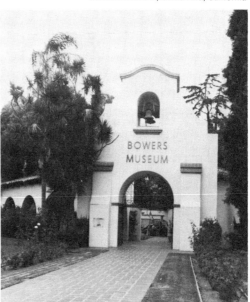

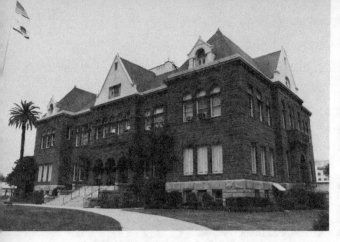

Orange County Courthouse, Santa Ana, California

ECONOMY AND INDUSTRY. There are approx. 180 industrial plants in Santa Ana. Major products include sporting goods, electronic components, fabricated metals, plastics, pharmaceuticals, medical devices and aerospace products. In the non-manufacturing sector, govt. is the largest employer, followed by publishing and insurance companies. In June, 1979, the total labor force of the greater met. area was approx. 1,069,700, while the rate of unemployment was 4.4%.

BANKING. There are six banking institutions in Santa Ana. In 1978, total deposits for the three banks headquartered in the city were $115,234,000, while assets were $124,857,000. Banks include Westlands, Santa Ana State and First American Trust.

HOSPITALS. There are four hosps. in Santa Ana, including Doctors, Mercy Gen., Riverview, Tustin and Psychiatric Hosp. offers specialized medical treatment.

EDUCATION. Santa Ana Col., a public two-year institution offering course work leading to the associate degree, enrolled more than 13,700 in 1978. The Orange School of Law, established in 1964, is a privately-supported coed. col. offering J.D. degrees. Santa Ana's public school system consists of 18 elementary, four jr. high and four sr. high schools. Three schools for the handicapped are also located in the city. The Santa Ana Public Lib. and the Orange Co. Law Lib. serve the city.

ENTERTAINMENT. Harlequin Dinner Playhouse provides theater and dining entertainment in Santa Ana. Santa Ana Col.'s Dons participate in intercollegiate sports.

ACCOMMODATIONS. There are several hotels and motels in Santa Ana, including the Orange Tree, Sandman, El Cortez, TraveLodge and the Saddleback and Ramada inns.

Santa Ana, California

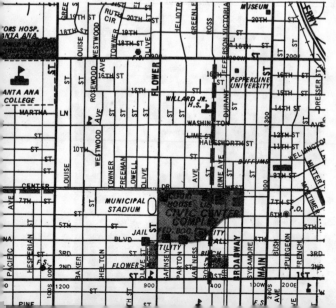

FACILITIES. There are 27 parks in the Santa Ana met. park system, including Adams, Birch, Centennial, Delhi, Edna, Grant, Jerome, Memorial and Santiago parks. A municipal zoo is located at Prentice Park.

CULTURAL ACTIVITIES. Dramatic productions are staged by two local little theater groups. The Bowers Museum exhibits relics pertaining to early CA history. Santa Ana also has access to cultural opportunities in LA and other surrounding met. areas.

LANDMARKS AND SIGHTSEEING SPOTS. One of the nation's largest collections of antique aircrafts, Movieland-of-the-Air, is located at the Orange Co. Airport. The Orange Co. Courthouse, built in 1900, is a state landmark constructed in "Modified Richardson's Romanesque" style. Santa Ana's oldest place of public assembly, the Episcopal Church of the Messiah, was built in 1888 and is also the city's oldest building.

SAVANNAH
GEORGIA

CITY LOCATION-SIZE-EXTENT. Savannah, seat of Chatham Co., encompasses 61.2 sq. mi. of area at 32°8' N lat. and 81°2' W long. The city is located in SE GA at the mouth of the Savannah River, 17 mi. from the Atlantic Ocean. The city's met. area extends N into Effingham Co., W and S into Bryan Co. and NE into Jasper Co.

TOPOGRAPHY. Savannah is surrounded by flat terrain, low and marshy to the N and E, rising to above SL to the W and S. About half the land to the W and S is cleared and the other half in wooded swamp-land. The mean elev. is 41'.

CLIMATE. The climate of Savannah is temperate marine. The avg. annual temp. of 66.8°F ranges from a Jan. mean of 51.6°F to a July mean of 81.4°F. The annual rainfall of 48.34" occurs mostly during the thunderstorm season from June 15 through Sept. 15. The RH ranges from 46% to 91%. The growing season avgs. 273 days. Savannah is in the ESTZ and observes DST.

FLORA AND FAUNA. Animals native to Savannah include the raccoon, whitetail deer, fox, opossum and squirrel. Typical birds are the cardinal, bluejay, wren, heron, gull and sandpiper. Alligators, bullfrogs, tree frogs, snapping turtles and four types of venomous snakes are common to the area. Plants include azaleas, marsh grass and jasmine.

POPULATION. According to the US census, the pop. of Savannah in 1970 was 118,349. In 1978, it was estimated that it had increased to 148,000.

ETHNIC GROUPS. In 1978, the ethnic distribution of Savannah was approx. 57.2% Caucasian, 42% Black, and 0.8% Hispanic.

TRANSPORTATION. Interstate hwys. 16, 95, US hwys. 17, 17A, 80, and 280 and State Hwys. 25 and 26 provide major motor access to Savannah. *Railroads* include Seaboard Coast Line and S Railway, AMTRAK and Central of GA. *Airlines* serving the Savannah Municipal Airport are EA, DL and NA. *Bus lines* include Greyhound, Trailways and the Savannah Transit Authority which operates 60 buses for intra-city service. The port of Savannah is served by 97 steamship lines and 36 deepwater terminals.

COMMUNICATIONS. Communications, broadcasting and news media serving the Savannah area are: *AM radio stations* WKBX 630 (NBC MOR); WEAS 900 (Indep., Relig.); WSOK 1230 (Mut. Blk. Divers.); WWSA 1290 (CBS top 40); WSGA 1400 (ABC/C, Contemp.); WQQT 1450 (Indep. C&W); *FM radio stations* WHCJ 88.5 (Indep., Ed., Jazz); WEAS 93.1 (Indep. Blk.); WWSA 94.1 (Indep., C&W); WSGF 95.5 (Indep., Top 40); WJCL 96.5 (Indep., Btfl. Mus.); WXLM 97.3 (Indep. Btfl. Mus.) and WZAT 102.1 (Indep. Top 40); *television stations* WSAV Ch. 3 (NBC); WVAN Ch. 9 (PBS); WTOC Ch. 11 (CBS) and WJCL Ch. 22 (ABC); *press* two major daily publications serve the area, *Savannah Morning News*, and *Savannah Evening Press*; other print media serving the area include *Herald, Savannah Jewish News*, Tribune, and Georgia Gazette.

HISTORY. Savannah was founded by James Edward Oglethorpe and a group of 120 English settlers in 1733. Designed by Gen. Oglethorpe, it became GA's first colonial city and one of the first planned comm. in the US. The pop. increased with the arrival of Portuguese, Spanish, German, English and Scottish immigrants. The nation's oldest orphanage, Bethesda, opened there in 1740. The city was the capital of the GA colony until the Revolutionary War. During the Revolutionary War, 900 men were garrisoned in the city under Gen. Howe. The city was captured by the British in 1778 and a French and American attempt to retake it in 1779 failed. The British finally left in 1782. Savannah was incorporated in 1789. In 1793, Eli Whitney invented the cotton gin near Savannah. The city became a major cotton seaport. The *S.S. Savannah* was the first steamship to cross the ocean, from Savannah to Liverpool, England, in 1819. The first commercially successful iron steamship, the *S.S. John Randolph* was launched there in 1834. During the Civil War, Savannah served as a Confed. navy yard and supply point until 1862, when Ft. Pulaski was taken by Union forces. In 1864, Gen. Sherman in his march to the sea, entered the city which had been evacuated by Gen. Hardee to prevent its bombardment. In the early 1900s, Savannah constructed one of the finest systems of docks and warehouses in the world. A program for the restoration of historic buldings in the city was undertaken in the 1950s as part of a plan to revitalize the inner city. In 1962, the world's first nuclear-powered merchant ship the *N.S. Savannah*, docked in its home port. The city is one of the chief US ports, a trading center for a large farming area, home of the US Army Flight Training Center for helicopter pilots and a naval stores center. A large pulp and paper center, the city has experienced recent rapid industrial growth.

GOVERNMENT. Savannah has a council-mgr. form of govt. The members of the council are elected for a four-year term; two are elected at large and six are elected by district. The mayor is elected at large to a four-year term and is a voting member of the council.

ECONOMY AND INDUSTRY. There are 181 manufacturers in Savannah. The largest firms produce paper, gulfstream jets, sugar, titanium dioxide and trailers. Other products include food, fiber, building supplies, petrochemicals and assembly. The Hunter-Stewart Military Complex is a major employer and source of income. Savannah has the tenth largest port in the US and is the SE's leading foreign trade port between Baltimore and New Orleans. The port's net tonnage was 11,488,255 in 1977. The avg. per capita income for 1978 was $6,500. The 1979 labor force in the Savannah met. area totaled 91,900 workers with an unemployment rate of 6.1%.

BANKING. There are 12 banks and five savings and loan Assns. in Savannah. In 1978 total deposits for the seven banks headquartered in the city were $2,707,768,000 while total assets were $3,953,287,000. Banks include Citizens & S, Savannah Bank, Trust Co., First Bank of Savannah, and Carver State.

HOSPITALS. Savannah is the medical center for the Coastal Empire area having several gen. hosps including Memorial, Candler, Candler General, Candler-Telfair and St. Joseph's. In addition, there are 12 nursing homes and a new State Regional Mental Hosp. GA Infirmary is a day rehabilitation clinic, for stroke victims and those with other physical impairments.

EDUCATION. Founded in 1935 as a jr. col and offering four-year programs beginning in 1965, Armstrong State Col is a publicly controlled liberal arts col. in Savannah. Preprofessional programs in forestry, veterinary medicine, dentistry, law, medicine and optometry are available,

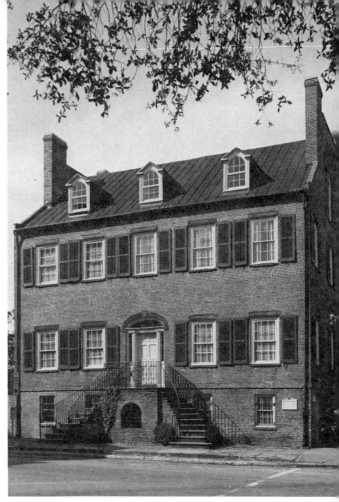

Davenport House, Savannah, Georgia

as well as associate degree programs in nursing and allied medical health fields. The col. enrolled over 3,154 in 1978. Savannah State Col. offers bachelor and master degrees and enrolled 2,824 in 1978. Other institutions include Memorial Medical Center, John Marshall Law School, Savannah Vocational Technical School, Skidway Oceanographic Institute and Oakland Island Technical Center. Savannah has 54 public schools and 22 private schools, which enrolled over 45,000 students in 1978. Lib. include Chatham-Effingham-Liberty Lib. system with 13 branches and the GA Historical Society lib.

ENTERTAINMENT. There are several annual events in Savannah including GA Week Festivities (Feb 12-18), St. Patrick's Day Parade (March 17), Tour of Homes and Gardens (March 25-28), A Night in Old Savannah (April 26-28), A Garden Tour (April 27-28), Savannah Scottish Games (May 5) and a Arts Festival (May 11-13). Pirates and Savannah State Tigers compete in area wide intercollegiate sports activities. The city has a rugby club and a running club known as the Savannah Striders.

ACCOMMODATIONS. Hotels and motels in Savannah include the De Soto Hilton, the John Wesley, the Savannah Inn & Country Club, Howard Johnson's, the Hyatt and Holiday and Ramada inns. Of particular interest are homes such as the historic "Eliza Thompson House", and "17 hundred 90" which have been converted into small hotels.

FACILITIES. There are 42 parks and squares in the Savannah park system, including Forsyth and Bacon parks. Also nearby is Skidaway Island State Park. There are several golf courses in the city including Skidaway Island, Savannah Golf Club, Mury Calder and a municipal golf course in Bacon Park. Public tennis courts can be found in the municipal tennis complex in Bacon Park. Skidaway Island also offers camping, hiking and swimming. The Savannah Beach and numerous waterways offer swimming, fishing, camping, water skiing and sailing facilities. The Oatland Island Zoo is available to the public. Deep sea charter boats are available as are public boat ramps.

Savannah, Georgia

CULTURAL ACTIVITIES. The Telfair Academy of Arts and Sciences, the oldest public art museum in the S, founded in 1875, has exhibits of 18th and 19th century decorative arts and permanent collections of 18th and 19th century American impressionists. The Telfair Academy also maintains the Owens-Thomas House, built in English Regency style and housing a collection of decorative arts. Other galleries and museums include the Science, Ships of the Sea, GA Historical Society, Skidaway Oceanographic and Gallery 209. There are several performing arts groups in Savannah, including Symphony Orch., Concert Assn., Youth Orch., Art Assn. Guild, two ballet guilds, two poetry clubs and a Little Theatre.

LANDMARKS AND SIGHTSEEING SPOTS. Savannah's downtown historic district has been registered as a Natl. Historic Landmark. Historic homes include the William Scarborough House (1818-1819), built by William Jay in Regency style, which houses the Historic Savannah Foundation's headquarters, the Davenport House (1815-1820) features a Davenport china collection, Juliette Gordon Low House, birthplace of the founder of the Girl Scouts; Andrew Low House (1847) and the Gothic-style Green-Meldrim House. On display at City Hall is a model of the steamship *Savannah* and a plaque commemorating the launching of the *S.S. John Randolph*. Factors' Walk is a row of buildings along the riverside on Bay St., a 19th-century meeting place of cotton merchants. Historic churches include Cathedral of St. John the Baptist, Christ church, Evangical Lutheran Church of the Ascension, Independent Presbyterian Church and Wesley Monumental Methodist Church. Forts Jackson, Screven, McCallister and Pulaski are in the vicinity of Savannah.

SEATTLE
WASHINGTON

CITY LOCATION-SIZE-EXTENT. Seattle, the seat of King Co. and the largest city in the state is on an isthumus between Puget Sound on the W and Lake WA on the E in W central WA and encompasses 91.6 sq. at 47°39′ N lat. and 122°18′ W long. It is surrounded by water areas including Elliott Bay to the W. Duwamish Waterway and River to the S, Lake WA Ship Canal which divides Seattle, Lake Union in the center, Green Lake to the N. Portage Bay and Salmon Bay. The greater met. area extends throughout King Co. and into the neighboring counties of Snohomish to the NE and Pierce to the S.

TOPOGRAPHY. The terrain of Seattle consists of rolling hills, which rise abruptly from the Lake WA and Puget Sound shorelines and reach elev. of over 300′ in the central sections and 500′ in the extreme N and SW sections. The city is roughly paralleled by the Cascade

Mts. to the E and the Olympic Mts. on the W and NW. The mean elev. is 125′.

CLIMATE. The climate of Seattle is mild and moderately moist, characterized by warm winters and cool summers and influenced by prevailing westerly air currents from the Pacific Ocean and a steady influx of marine air. Precip. is moderate due to its location on the E side of the Olympic Mts. The avg. annual temp. of 52°F ranges from a Jan. mean of 40°F to a July and Aug. mean of 65°F. Nearly 46% of the annual avg. rainfall of 37.5″ occurs from Nov. to Jan. Snowfall avgs 8″ annually. The RH ranges from 49% to 86%. The growing season avgs. 248 days. Seattle lies in the PSTZ and observes DST.

FLORA AND FAUNA. Animals native to Seattle include the black bear, mule deer, otter, weasel and bat. Common birds are the Canada jay, raven, gull, sandpiper and duck. Frogs, salamanders, and the venomous N Pacific rattlesnake are found in the area. Typical trees are the alder, maple, Douglas fir and W red cedar. Smaller plants include the rhododendron and Brakken fern.

POPULATION. According to the US census, the pop. of Seattle in 1970 was 530,831. In 1978 it was estimated that it had decreased to approx. 470,000.

ETHNIC GROUPS. In 1978 the racial distribution of Seattle was approx. 87.4% Caucasian, 7.1% Black and 2.0% Hispanic and 3.5% other races.

TRANSPORTATION. Interstate hwys 5, 90 and 405 and state hwys. 99, 104, 167, 520 and 522 provide major motor access to Seattle. *Railroads* serving the city include AMTRAK, Burlington-N, Union Pacific and Milwaukee. *Airlines* serving Sea Tac Intl. and Boeing Field are UA, SAS, AS, WE, AA, PA, CO, TW, EA and NW. *Bus lines* include Greyhound, Evergreen, Trailways and the local Metro Transit. The inland Port of Seattle serves the Pacific NW and the Far East and handles some 14 million metric tons of cargo annually.

COMMUNICATIONS. Communications, broadcasting and print media originating in Seattle are: *AM radio stations* KIRO 710 (CBS, MBS, MOR); KVI 570 (Indep., Clas.); KIXI 910 (NBC, Btfl. Mus., News); KBLE 1050 (Indep., Contemp., Top 40); KING 1090 (Indep., MOR); KAYO 1150 (ABC/E, C&W); KJR 950 (ABC/C, Top 40); KMPS 1300 (Indep., C&W); KOMO 1000 (ABC/I, MOR); KYAC 1250 (Indep., AOR) and KZOK 159 (Indep., Btfl. Mus.); *FM radio stations* KNHC 89.5 (Indep., Divers.); KBLE 93.3 (Indep., MOR); KEUT 94.I (Indep., Btfl. Mus) KUOW 94.9 (NPR, Clas.); KIXI 95.7 (Indep., Dups. AM 50%); TYYX 96.5 (MBS, Blk.); KEZX 98.9 (Indep., Btfl. Mus.); KISW 99.9 (ABC/FM, Progsv. Rock); KSEA 100.7 (Indep., Btfl. Mus.); KVDI 101.5 (ABC/C, Top 40); KZOK 102.5 (Indep., AOR); KBIC 105.3 (Indep., Btfl. Mus) and KRAB 107.7 (NPR, Ed.); *television stations* KOMO Ch. 4 (ABC); KING Ch. 5 (NBC); KIRO Ch. 7 (CBS); KCTS Ch. 9 (PBS); KSTW Ch. 11 (Indep.); KCPQ. Ch. 13 (PBS) and cable; *press*: two major dailies serve the area, the *Seattle Post-Intelligence*, issued mornings, and the *Seattle Times*, issued evenings; other publications include the *Ballard Voice*, *Catholic Northwest Progress*, *Fishing and Hunting News*, *The Puget Sounder*, *W Seattle Herald*, *White Center News*, *Planets Alive*, *WA Grange News*, *WA Motorist*, *WEA Action* and *W Farmer*.

HISTORY. Native Americans of the Duwamish, Ino-homish and the Squamish tribes first inhabited the site of present-day Seattle. In 1850 John C. Holgate became the first white man to choose to settle in the area, when he selected a timber claim in the Duwamish Valley (now a section of Seattle). In 1851 a party from IL led by A. A. Denny established a settlement at Alki Point, but the site was ill-chosen and the settlers moved to their own claims the following year. Attracted by Puget Sound's harbor and lumber source, the pioneers settled in the area and named their village for a friendly Indian chief, Sealth. A saw mill was constructed in 1853 and lumber became Seattle's chief industry. Seattle thrived upon development of the coal mining industry in the 1860s and was incorporated as a town in 1865. In 1869, the city was chartered, and by the following year some 1,000 persons lived there. The city was linked to San Francisco by steamship in 1875. When the N Pacific RR reached Seattle in 1884, new markets opened up and the pop. boomed from 3,533 in 1880 to 42,000 10 yrs. later. Despite a fire that destroyed the business section in 1889, the comm. thrived. By 1893, the first transcontinental RR had been extended to Seattle and its shipping industry provided access to the Far E. In 1897, prospectors poured through the city en route to the Klondike gold fields in the Canadian Yukon and AK. The development of AK in turn stimulated Seattle's growth, and its pop. was boosted from 80,000 at the turn of the century to 237,000 in 1910. The city was connected with Atlantic ports upon the opening of the Panama Canal in 1914. Boeing Aircraft, later Seattle's largest company, was established in 1916. Many workers who arrived in Seattle during WW I to work in the defense industries lost their jobs after the war ended and, in 1919, they called the country's first general strike. WW II again stimulated the city's economy, and the increasing industrialization drew many blacks to Seattle. The pop. rose from 368,000 in 1940 to 467,000 in 1950, but dropped during the 1950s and 1960s when many Seattle residents moved to the suburbs. Seattle's economy slumped during the late 1960s and early 1970s when aircraft sales declined. Today, the city ranks as WA's largest and the industrial, commercial, and transportation center of the Pacific NW.

GOVERNMENT. Seattle has a mayor-council form of govt. The mayor, elected at large to a four-year term, is not a member of council, has no vote, but does have veto power. The nine council members are elected at large and serve four-year terms.

ECONOMY AND INDUSTRY. The manufacture of transportation equipment is the primary industry in the Seattle area. Other major products include paper products, primary metals, food products, chemicals, machinery, furniture and fixtures. In 1979 the total labor force for the Seattle-Everett greater met. area was approx. 181,100, while the rate of unemployment was 5.5%.

BANKING. There are 28 banks in Seattle. In 1978, total deposits for the 22 banks headquartered in the city were $13,734,856,000, while assets were $18,321,663,000. Banks include Sea-First Natl., Rainier Natl., People's Natl., Puget Sound Mutual, Pacific and Old Natl.

HOSPITALS. There are more than 20 hospitals in Seattle, including University, Cabrini, Group Health, Harborview, Providence, Seattle Gen., Swedish and Virginia Mason.

EDUCATION. The U of WA, Seattle's largest U, a state-supported institution founded in 1861 moved to its present site in 1895 and awards grad and undergrad degrees. The 1978 enrollment was approx. 37,100. Seattle U., affiliated with the Society of Jesus, offers grad. and undergrad. programs and enrolled more than 3,600 in 1978. Seattle Pacific Col., a privately-supported, liberal arts col. affiliated with the Free Methodist Church of N America, awards bachelor and master degrees and enrolled approx. 2,200 in 1978. Comm. colleges include N Seattle, Seattle Shoreline and S Seattle. Other institutions include Auerswald Business U, Electronic Computer Programming Institute, Griffin Business Col., ITT Peterson School of Business, Ron Bailie School of Broadcast and WA Technical Institute. The public school system enrolls approx. 85,000 in over 110 elementary and high schools. More than 20,000 attend 80 private schools. Lib. facilities are available through the King Co. Lib. System, the Seattle Public Lib. and the Gen. Services Administration Lib.

ENTERTAINMENT. The Seafair, featuring parades, water carnivals, and boat races, is held annually in Seattle during late July and early Aug. Other

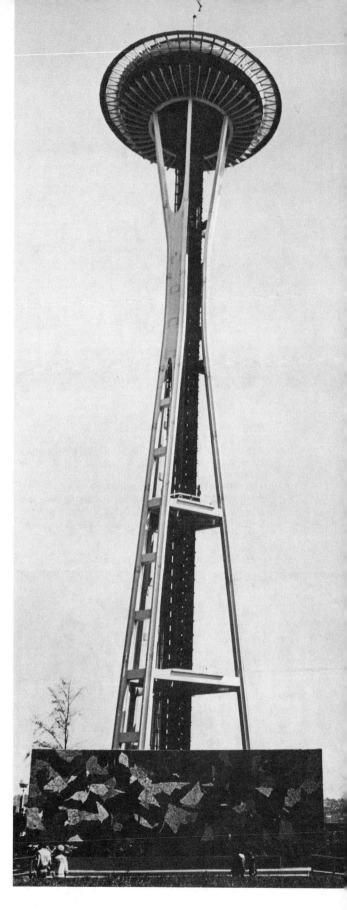

At right: 600 foot space needle with revolving restaurant and observation deck, Seattle, Washington

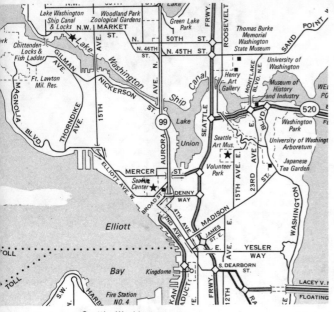

Seattle, Washington

FACILITIES. There are 140 parks and playground in Seattle, encompassing 3,800 acres. The 188-acre Woodland Park contains a zoo housing more than 1,800 animals, an amusement area and gardens. An arboretum is located in WA Park. Puget Sound Alki beach and nearby lakes offer facilities for boating, fishing and skiing. Public golf courses are available at Foster Golf Links, Jackson Park, Jefferson Park, Puetz Evergreen and Tree Valley. Jogging tracks are available at Green Lake, Discovery Park, Lake WA Blvd., and Burke-Gilman Trail.

CULTURAL ACTIVITIES. Seattle is served musically by the Seattle Symphony, Youth Symphony, the Seattle Opera Assn., and the NW Chamber Assn. performs concerts.Theaters in Seattle include the Seattle Repertory Theater and A Contemporary Theater (ACT). Others are presented at Cirque, Skid Road, Intiman, and Bathouse Theaters. The Seattle Art Museum houses an extensive collection of oriental art and one of the two Tupolo ceilings in America. The Henry Art Gallery on the WA U campus specializes in modern arts. Other museums include the Museum of History and Industry, the WA State Fire Service Historical Museum, Inc., the Thomas Burke Memorial WA State Museum, the US Coast Guard Museum and C&E Frye Museum. Space age displays and a reconstructed NW Indian house are among exhibits displayed at the Pacific Science Center.

LANDMARKS & SIGHTSEEING SPOTS. Space Needle provides panoramic views from the topmost platform. Among the 44 scenes in the Pioneer Square Wax Museum are many depicting the early history of Seattle. The Seattle Aquarium features an underwater dome with a view of the sea life of Puget Sound. Some of the world's largest fire boats are housed at Fire Station No.4. The restored Pioneer Square retains much of the city's 19th century charm; with its art galleries, antique shops, boutiques and sidewalk cafes.

events include the King Co. Fair, Fat Tuesday, Trade Fair and Exhibition of NW Art. The Breakers of WH2 hockey, the Supersonics of NBA basketball, the Mariners of AL baseball and the Seahawks of NFL-NFC football provide pro sports entertainment, while Seattle U and the U of WA Huskies participate in intercollegiate sports.

ACCOMMODATIONS. There are numerous hotels in Seattle, including the Olympic, Hotel Seattle, Hilton, Washington Plaza, Mayflower Park, Edgewater, Sea-Tac, Red Lion, Hyatt, Travelodge, America West, Best Western, Thunderbird and the Sherwood, Ramada, Doubletree, Vance Airport and Holiday inns.

Arches of Pacific Science Center, Seattle, Washington

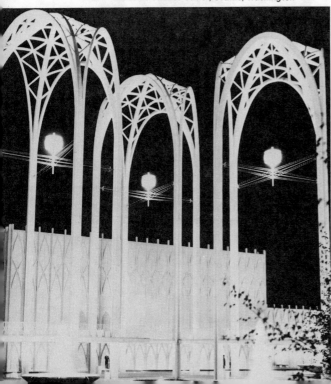

SHREVEPORT
LOUISIANA

CITY LOCATION-SIZE-EXTENT. Shreveport, the seat of Caddo Parish, encompasses 90 sq. mi. on the W bank of the Red River in NW LA, near the AR and TX borders, at 32°30'5'' N lat. and 93°49' W long. The greater met. area extends into the LA parishes of Bossier to the NE and Desoto to the S and into Harrison Co., TX, to the W and includes Bossier City, which lies on the E bank of the Red River.

TOPOGRAPHY. The terrain of Shreveport, which is situated in the W Gulf coastal plain, varies from flat areas in the Red River bottom lands to gently rolling hills beginning one mi. W of the river. Area lakes include Caddo to the NW, Cypress Black Bayou to the NE, Cross to the W, Wallace to the S and Bistineau to the E. The mean elev. is 254'.

CLIMATE. The climate of Shreveport is intermediate between humid sub-tropical and continental. Monthly mean temps. range from 47.3°F in Jan. to 83.1°F in July, with an annual avg. of 66°F. The annual mean rainfall of 44.51'' is fairly evenly distributed throughout the year. Snowfall avgs. 1.7'' annually, with measurable amounts occuring on an avg. of once every two years. The RH ranges from 53% to 90%. The growing season avgs. 254 days. Shreveport lies in the CSTZ and observes DST.

FLORA AND FAUNA. Animals native to Shreveport include the raccoon, opossum, deer and armadillo. Common birds include the cardinal, mourning dove, blackbird, blue jay and mockingbird. Red-eared turtles, bull frogs, box turtles, green anole lizards and toads, as well as the venomous copperhead, cottonmouth and coral snake are also found in the area. Typical trees include the magnolia, oak, pine and willow. Smaller plants include the honeysuckle, bayberry, blackberry and orchid.

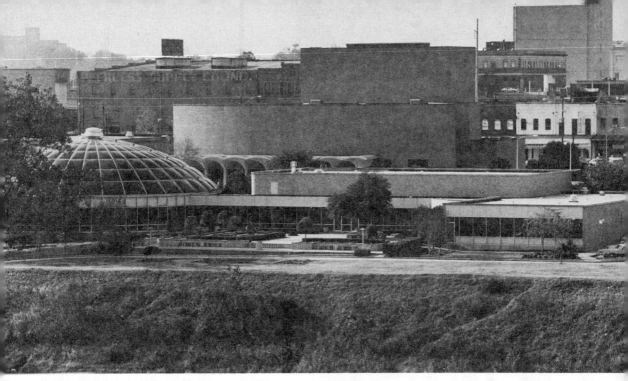

Barnwell Garden and Art Center, Shreveport, Louisiana

POPULATION. According to the US census, the pop. of Shreveport in 1970 was 182,064. In 1978, it was estimated that it had increased to 220,000.

ETHNIC GROUPS. In 1978, the ethnic distribution of Shreveport was approx. 66.3% Caucasian, 34.1% Black and 1.0% Hispanic (a percentage of the Hispanic total is also included in the Caucasian total).

TRANSPORTATION. Interstate hwy. 20, US hwys. 71, 79 and 171 and state hwys. 1, 3, 169 and 175 provide major motor access to Shreveport. *Railroads* serving the city include Cotton Belt, Frisco, IL Central Gulf, KC S, MO & Pacific, S Pacific, S Railway and TX & Pacific. *Airlines* serving the Greater Shreveport Municipal Airport include Royale, FL, DL and TI. *Bus lines* serving the city include Trailways and the local Sportran (the Transit System). Navigation on the Red River is being developed and, by the 1980s, barge traffic will open the river S to the MS River and the Gulf of Mexico.

COMMUNICATIONS. Communications, broadcasting and print media originating from Shreveport are: *AM radio stations* KEEL 710 (ABC/I, Contemp.); KCIJ 980 (Indep., Relig.); KWKH 1130 (MBS, C&W); KBCL 1220 (Indep., MOR); KFLO 1300 (MBS, C&W); KRMD 1340 (NBC, C&W); KJOE 1480 (MBS, News) and KOKA 1550 (ABC/C, Natl. Blk.); *FM radio stations* KMBQ 93.7 (Indep., AOR); KROK 94.5 (Indep., Top 40); KEPT 96.5 (Indep., Relig.); KCOZ 100.1 (Indep., Btfl. Mus.) and KRMD 101.1 (Indep., Dups. AM 50%); *television stations* KTBS Ch. 3 (ABC); KTAL Ch. 6 (NBC); KSLA Ch. 12 (CBS); KLTS Ch. 24 (Indep.) and cable; *press:* two major dailies serve the area, the *Journal*, issued evenings, and the *Times*, issued mornings; other publications include the weekly *Sun* and the monthly *American Rose Magazine*, *S Towne Courier*, *Shreveport Magazine* and *Chain Saw Industry and Power Equipment Dealer*.

HISTORY. Native Americans of the Caddo tribe were the inhabitants of the present-day Shreveport area when Capt. Henry Miller Shreve arrived to clear a massive log jam stretching 165 mi. along the Red River and open the river to navigation. Fed. Indian Agent Jehial Brooks influenced the Indians to sell their lands, and, in 1835, they gave 640 acres to interpreter Larkin Edwards, who sold the land to Angus McNeil and his Shreve Town Co. The comm. established on the site was named for Capt. Shreve, a stockholder in the company, and was incorporated in 1839. With its economy based on trade and shipping, the city expanded rapidly to become the largest in N LA. Due to the isolation of the city, Shreveport served as the state capital from 1863 until the end of the Civil War in 1865. The city continued to prosper as a trading center with the growth of the RRs. Agriculture, lumbering and the oil and gas industry have contributed to the healthy economy of the city, while the importance of the river pt. has waned.

GOVERNMENT. Shreveport has a mayor-council form of govt. The seven council members are elected by district to four-year terms, while the mayor, not a voting member of council, is elected at large to a four-year term.

ECONOMY AND INDUSTRY. The production of oil and gas is the major industry in Shreveport, while agriculture and lumbering are also important to the economy. One of the largest gas transmission company in the nation is headquartered in Shreveport. Recent industrial expansion has brought electrical and automotive plants to the city. Barksdale AFB is located in nearby Bossier City. In June, 1979, the met. area labor force totaled 153,700, while the rate of unemployment was 6%.

BANKING. There are eight banking institutions in Shreveport. In 1978, total deposits for the eight banks headquartered in the city were $1,434,368,000, while assets were $1,722,343,000. Banks are First Natl., Commercial Natl., LA Bank & Trust, Pioneer Bank & Trust, The Bank of Commerce, Shreveport Bank & Trust, United Mercantile and American Bank and Trust.

HOSPITALS. Hosps. in Shreveport include Doctor's, Physicians and Surgeons, Highland, Schumpert Medical Center and Willis-Knighton Memorial. Other medical facilities located in the city include the LSU Medical Center School of Medicine, Shriners Hosp. for Crippled Children, Brentwood Neuro Psychiatric Hosp. and the US Govt. hosp.

EDUCATION. A branch of LA State U was established in Shreveport in 1967 and awards grad. and undergrad. degrees. In 1978, it enrolled more than 3,000. Centenary Col. awards bachelor degrees, and, in 1978, it enrolled approx. 900. Southern U established a branch in the city in 1964 and, in 1979, it enrolled approx. 900. A Medical School of LA State U was established in the city in 1969. The Shreve Memorial Lib. features a petroleum dept., genealogy room and fed., state and parish records.

ENTERTAINMENT. Annual events in Shreveport include the LA State Fair in Oct., the Red River Revel Arts Festival, the Holiday in Dixie Festival and a spring festival commemorating the signing of the LA Purchase in 1803. A farm team of the CA Angels participate in TX League baseball.

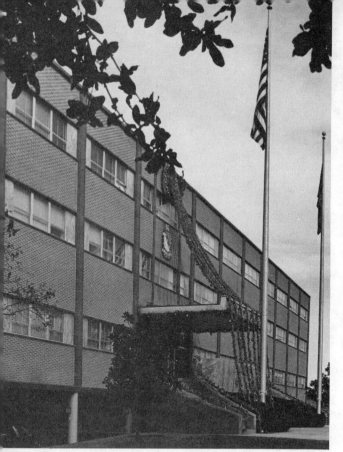

City Hall, Shreveport, Louisiana

Shreveport. The Meadows Museum of Art, on the campus of Centenary Col., houses the Despujol Collection of paintings and drawings of Indochina. Barnwell Memorial Garden & Art Center is one of very few garden/art gallery combinations in the nation. Apart from art exhibits, the S wing contains a glass domed conservatory featuring seasonal planting displays. Norton Art Gallery has one of the leading collections of American Western art. All cultural activities are coordinated by the Shreveport Regional Arts Council.

LANDMARKS AND SIGHTSEEING SPOTS. Restoration projects in Shreveport include the renovation of Shreve Square, named for Capt. Shreve (one of the city founders), and several Victorian warehouses. A statue honoring the Confederate soldiers stands in front of Caddo Parish Courthouse. The American Rose Center, sponsored by the American Rose Society, is one of the largest parks in the US devoted to the cultivation and display of roses. A collection of preserved wild animals is displayed at the Coca-Cola Trophy Room. Ft. Hambug, a Confed. site, is located on Red River, while the Caspiana House is located at the LA State U campus.

Thoroughbred racing is held at LA Downs from July through Nov., while the Independence game is played in the city annually.

ACCOMMODATIONS. There are several hotels and motels in Shreveport, including the Castle, Regency Motor Hotel, Caddo, Chateau Motor and Chez Vous Best Western hotels, and the Sheraton Shreveporter, Quality, Ramada, Hilton, Days and Holiday inns.

FACILITIES. Cross Lake, a Shreveport reservoir, is circled by a drive lined with thousands of redbud trees and offers fishing and boating. Public golf courses are available at Huntington Park and Querbes golf courses, while public tennis courts are provided at S Hills Tennis Center, Querbus Park and Airport Park.

CULTURAL ACTIVITIES. Opera, drama, concerts and symphonies are offered each month in the Convention Hall and Civic Theatre Complex in

Shreveport, Louisiana

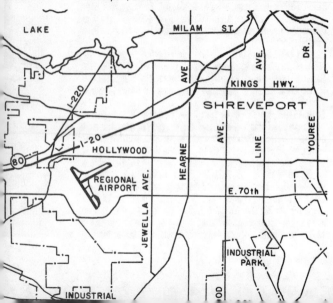

SOUTH BEND
INDIANA

CITY LOCATION-SIZE-EXTENT. South Bend, the seat of St. Joseph Co., is located in N central IN on the bend of the St. Joseph River 20 mi. SE of Lake MI and five mi. S of the MI border and encompasses 30.1 sq. mi. at 41°42' N lat and 86°19' W long. Its greater met. area extends to the city of Mishawaka to the E.

TOPOGRAPHY. The terrain of South Bend, situated in the Plains Region, is predominantly level prairie interspersed with hills. The region also has several small natural lakes. The mean elev. is 710'.

CLIMATE. The climate of South Bend is continental, influenced by the city's location near Lake MI, which moderates temps. during the winter but also produces considerable cloudiness and greater snowfall when NW winds pass over the lake. The avg. annual temp. of 49.5°F ranges from monthly means of 24.4°F in Jan to 73.1°F in July. The annual rainfall of 35.9'' is evenly distributed, while snowfall avgs. 70.4'' annually. The RH ranges from 54% to 89%. The growing season avgs. 165 days. South Bend lies in the ESTZ and observes DST.

FLORA AND FAUNA. Animals native to South Bend include the whitetail deer, chipmunk and fox. Common birds include the cardinal, blue jay, swallow and crow. Bullfrogs, salamanders, tree frogs, American toads, box turtles and the venomous E Massasauga (a pygmy rattler) are found in the area. Typical trees are the poplar, maple, elm and oak. Smaller plants include the peony, goldenrod and thistle.

POPULATION. According to the US census, the pop. in 1970 was 125,580. In 1978, it was estimated that it had decreased to 114,000.

ETHNIC GROUPS. In 1978, the ethnic distribution of South Bend was approx. 85.5% Caucasian, 13.9% Black, and 1.0% Hispanic. (A percentage of the Hispanic total is included in the Caucasian total.)

TRANSPORTATION. Interstate hwys. 80 and 90, US hwys. 20, 31 and 33 and state hwys. 2, 23 and 33 provide major motor access to South Bend. *Railroads* include AMTRAK, ConRail, S Shore, Grand Trunk W, Norfolk & W and the NJ, W & IL. *Airlines* serving Michiana Regional Aiport include NC, VA and Skystream Commuter. *Bus lines* serving the city include Greyhound, Trailways and the local Municipal Busline (TRANSPO). The Port of Indiana, Burns Waterway Harbor, served by a 27' public terminal located at the S end of Lake MI, provides direct access to all the Great Lakes.

COMMUNICATIONS. Communications, broadcasting and print media originating from South Bend are: *AM radio stations* WSBT 960 (CBS, MOR, Contemp.): WNDU 1490 (ABC/1) and WIVA 1580 (MJVA 1580 MBS, C&W): *FM radio stations* WETL 91.7 (Indep., Ed.): WNDU

92.9 (Indep., Hit Parade); WWJY 101.5 (Indep., Btfl. Mus.); WHME 103.1 (Indep., Relig.) and WRBR 103.9 (Indep., Top 40); *television stations* WNDU Ch. 16 (NBC); WSBT Ch. 22 (CBS); WSJV Ch. 28 (ABC); WNIT Ch. 34 (PBS); WHME Ch. 46 (Indep.) and cable; *press*: one major daily serves the area, the *Tribune*, issued evenings; the other publication is the weekly *Tri-County News*.

HISTORY. Rene Cavalier Seiur de la Salle first passed through the South Bend region in 1679. In 1820, Pierre Navarre established a fur trading post and settled in the area. Three yrs. later, Alexis Coquillard arrived, and together with Lathrop Miner Taylor, founded the village of Southold in 1831. Southold's location between Chicago and Ft. Wayne made the town the crossroads of the W. Originally called Big St. Joseph Station, the settlement was later renamed for the southernmost point of the Indiana bend of the St. Joseph River. Following completion of the first dam and millrace in 1844, pulp and grain mills were rapidly constructed, using nearby raw materials. Incorporated as a village in 1835, South Bend became a city in 1865. Until the City Water Works were constructed, periodic fires were a problem, with the worst occurring in 1883 during a blizzard; seven manufacturing plants were destroyed and four others partially ruined. Today, South Bend is a manufacturing center, noted for the production of farm machinery, auto and airplane brake equipment.

GOVERNMENT. South Bend has a mayor-council form of govt. The nine council members are elected to four-year terms, three at large and six by district. The mayor is elected at large to a four-year term; he is not a voting member of council.

ECONOMY AND INDUSTRY. An industrial center, South Bend's major manufactured products are primary metals, prefabricated metals, non-electrical and electrical machinery, transportation equipment, food products, apparel, and printing and publishing equipment. Avg. income per capita in 1977 was $5,931. In June, 1979, the total labor force of the greater met. area was 144,700 while the rate of unemployment was 6.0%

BANKING. There are four banks and five savings and loan assns. in South Bend. In 1978, total deposits for the five banks headquartered in the city were $937,283,00 while assets were $1,085,305,000., Banks include First Bank and Trust, St. Joseph Bank and Trust Co., Natl. Bank and Trust, American Natl. Bank and Trust and W State.

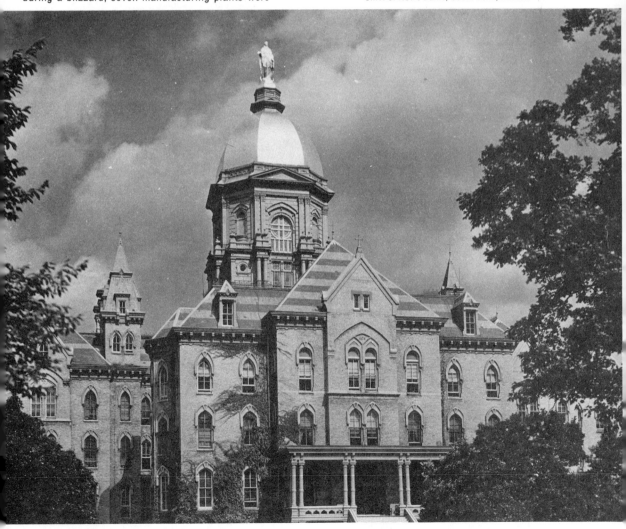

Univ. of Notre Dame, South Bend, Indiana

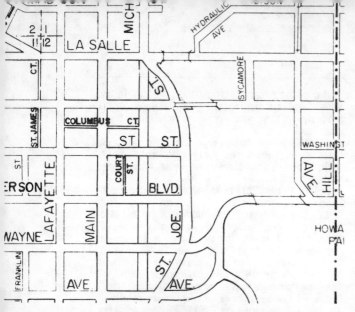

Central South Bend, Indiana

HOSPITALS. There are six hosps. in South Bend, including Memorial, St. Joseph's, N IN State and Developmental Disabilities Center, Healthwin and Osteopathic.

EDUCATION. Adjoining South Bend is the U of Notre Dame founded in 1842 and a privately supported university with a 1978 enrollment of over 8,500 students. The U, under the direction of the Congregation of the Holy Cross, offers grad. and undergrad. programs, students Sophomore Year Abroad, precollege and Freshman programs for educationally disadvantaged, cooperative study in engineering and an extensive intercollegiate sports program. Other teaching institutions are IN U at South Bend (the third largest in the IU system), Holy Cross Jr. Col., Acme Inst. of Technology, IN Vocational Technical Col., South Bend Med. Foundation, Michiana Col. of Commerce and St. Mary's Col. enrolled in the city's 28 elementary and jr. high schools are 21,000 pupils. Six high schools enroll over 7,000 students. Education in 15 private and parochial schools is offered to over 3,500 students. Lib. facilities are provided by the South Bend Pub. Lib.

ENTERTAINMENT. South Bend hosts a variety of annual festivals, including the Union Station Festival and the annual Ethnic Festival. IU and Notre Dame's Fighting Irish participate in intercollegiate sports.

ACCOMMODATIONS. There are several hotels and motels in South Bend, including the Drake, Howard Johnson's, Randall's New Century, and Ramada, Pick Motor, Day's and Holiday Inns.

FACILITIES. The South Bend met. park system encompasses 58 parks, and 15 lakes are located nearby. The 195-acre Bendix Woods Co. Park provides picnic areas, shelters and a nature study center. Facilities for winter sports are available, as well as 5.5 mi. of nature trails, many of which are accessible to the handicapped. Rum Village Park and Nature Trails covers 160 acres, including 55 acres of natural woodland, a children's zoo and small amusement park. A variety of animals are housed at Potawatomi Park Zoo. Four municipal golf courses are located in South Bend.

CULTURAL ACTIVITES. South Bend is served by both a symphony and a chamber orchestra. The Broadway Theatre League of South Bend stages dramatic productions. The Southold Dance Theatre is comprised of local talent. The new Century Center downtown features a 735 seat theater for the performing arts, a recital hall, a museum of industry and a comm. art center in addition to convention facilities. The Studebaker Vehicle collection is housed in the Discovery Hall Museum, which also depicts the the area's industrial history. Early toys, an 1830's pioneer cabin, primitive art works and historical military items are among exhibits displayed at the N IN Historical Society Museum. Studio programs and classes are offered at the Art Center. The Muessel-Ellison-Clark Gallery is located in the Art Center.

LANDMARKS AND SIGHTSEEING SPOTS. South Bend's first settler, Pierre Navarre, lived in the 1820 cabin and fur trading post which now bears his name. Other noted buildings include two Frank Lloyd Wright homes; the Chapin House and Tippecanoe Place and the 1889 mansion of the former Studebaker Co. President, Clement Studebaker.

SPOKANE
WASHINGTON

CITY LOCATION-SIZE-EXTENT. Spokane, seat of Spokane Co. and the largest city between Seattle and Minneapolis, encompasses 52.42 sq. mi. on the Spokane River in E WA, 18 Mi. W of ID and 110 Mi. S of Canada, at 47°38' N lat. and 117°32' W long. The greater met. area encompasses 1,758 sq. mi., in the Inland Empire region and extends into the counties of Whitman to the S, Lincoln to the W, Stevens to the NW, Pend Oreille to the N and Kootenai, ID to the E.

TOPOGRAPHY. Spokane lies in the E part of the Columbia plateau where the gradual upward slope from the Columbia River to the W of the city meets the edge of the more rapid rise of the Rocky Mts. in ID to the E. The Cascade Mts. are W of the Columbia River. The Latah and Little Spokane rivers join the Spokane River NW of the city. The mean elev. is 2,356.'

CLIMATE. The climate of Spokane is characterized by arid continental conditions. Most of the moisture from the air masses reaching the city, primarily brought in by prevailing westerly and southwesterly winds from the Pacific Ocean, is depleted by the Cascade Range to the W. The avg. annual temp. of 48°F ranges from a Jan. mean of 27°F to a July mean of 70°F. Almost 40% of the 16" avg. annual rainfall occurs from Nov. through Jan. More than 60% of the 53.3" avg. annual snowfall occurs during Dec. and Jan. The RH ranges from 25% to 86%. The avg. growing season is approx. 180 days. Spokane lies in the PSTZ and observes DST.

FLORA AND FAUNA. Animals native to Spokane include the fox, bat, rabbit, mule deer and weasel. Common birds are the red crossbill, sparrow, hawk, magpie and gray jay. Leopard frogs, tiger salamanders, painted turtles, W toads and the venomous Pacific rattlesnake are also found in the area. Typical trees are the pine, fir, spruce and oak. Smaller plants include the sagebrush, camas, columbine and trillium.

Downtown Spokane, Washington

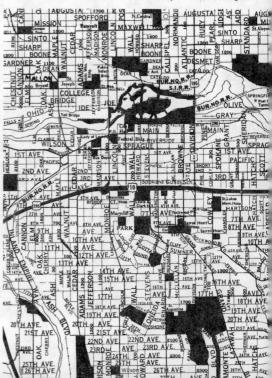

POPULATION. According to the US census, the pop. of Spokane in 1970 was 170,516. In 1978, it was estimated that it had increased to 176,700.
ETHNIC GROUPS. In 1978, the ethnic distribution of Spokane was approx. 97.3% Caucasian, 1.3% Black, 1.1% Hispanic and .3% other.
TRANSPORTATION. Interstate Hwy. 90, US hwys. 2, 195 and 395 and state hwys. 27, 290, 902 and 904 provide major motor access to Spokane. *Railroads* include Burlington N, Milwaukee and Union Pacific. *Airlines* serving Spokane Intl. Airport include NW, UA, FL, RW, Cascade, Columbia Pacific and Flight Craft. Commuter lines and private aircraft serve Felts Field, a city-owned airport. *Bus lines* serving the city include Greyhound and the municipal system.
COMMUNICATIONS. Communications, broadcasting and print media

Falls. Glover became known as the "Father of Spokane". When the Pacific RR reached the comm. in 1881, its area encompassed two sq. mi. and its pop. numbered 1,000. It was chartered as a city that same year, and by 1887, its pop. had reached 15,000. Although a large part of the downtown area was destroyed by fire in 1889, the city was rebuilt and its name changed to Spokane the following year, after WA achieved statehood. By the end of the 19th century, the city had become the largest RR center W of Omaha and a major trade center as well. Additional lead and silver mines opened, and during the early 1900s large numbers of

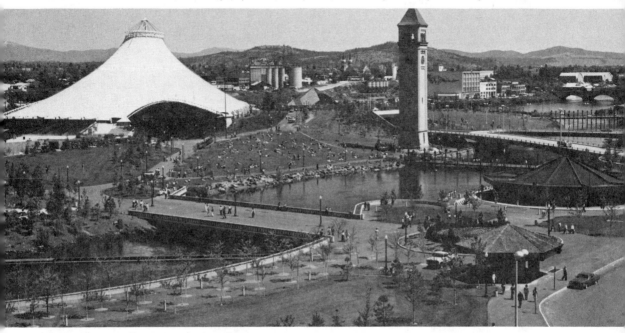

100 acre Riverfront Park, Spokane, Washington

originating from Spokane are: *AM radio stations* KHQ 590 (NBC, MOR); KJRB 790 (Indep., Contemp.); KXLY 920 (CBS, MOR); KREM 970 (Indep., Contemp., Top 40); KSPO 1230 (Indep., All News); KUDY 1280 (Indep., Relig.); KMBI 1330 (Indep., MOR); KEZE 1380 (MBS, Easy List.); KXXR 1440 (ABC/E, C&W) and KGA 1510 (ABC/I, C&W); *FM radio stations* KSFC 91.9 (Indep., Contemp.); KREM 92.9 (Indep., Progsv.); KXXR 93.7 (Indep., Btfl. Mus.); KHQ 98.1 (Indep., Contemp.); KICN 98.9 (Indep., Contemp.); KXLY 99.9 (Indep., Btfl. Mus.); KEZE 105.7 (Indep., Easy List.) and KMBI 107.9 (Indep., Progsv.); *television stations* KREM Ch. 2 (CBS); KXLY Ch. 4 (ABC); KHQ Ch. 6 (NBC); KSPS Ch. 7 (PBS) and cable; *press*: two major dailies serve the city, the *Spokesman-Review*, issued mornings, and the *Chronicle*, issued evenings; other publications include the *Comm. Press*, *Inland Register*, the weekly *Valley Herald* and *Falls*, and the monthly *Spokane Magazine* and *Farmer-Stockman*.
HISTORY. Native Americans of the Spokane (meaning "Sun People" or "Children of the Sun") tribe inhabited the area of present-day Spokane before the first white settlers arrived. In 1807, David Thompson arrived and established a trading post called Spokane House in the area. In 1838, Protestant missionaries also established outposts in the area, but abandoned them in 1847. Completion of wagon roads and the discovery of gold and silver in the region in the 1860s led to interest in establishing a town. The James N. Glover family, attracted by the falls on the Spokane River as a possible power source, settled at the site in 1871 built a house and sawmill and named the comm. Spokane.

Immigrants from Europe arrived. Spokane also became the business and financial hub of the Inland Empire region, whose basic industries were mining and agriculture. Later, the city also became a banking and education center. During WW II, Spokane served as a pilot training center. After the Grand Coulee Dam was constructed, the aluminum industry manufactured various products. Between 1950 and 1960, its pop. grew from approx. 161,700 to more than 181,600. Spokane initiated redevelopment projects in the downtown area during the 1970s, when it hosted the Expo '74 world's fair.
GOVERNMENT. Spokane has a mayor-council-mgr. form of govt. consisting of six council members and the mayor, who are elected at large to staggered four-year terms. A city mgr. is appointed.
ECONOMY AND INDUSTRY. Spokane is the economic hub of the region composed of E WA, NE OR, N ID and W MT, known as the "Inland Empire". Trade, services, govt. and manufacturing are major employers in the area. There are approx. 462 manufacturing plants in Spokane. Major products include primary metals, fabricated metals/machinery, food and kindred products and lumber and wood products. Medical and health related services employ more of the work force than any other area industry, while conventions and tourism

have also become important industries. In June, 1979, the total labor force of the greater met. area was approx. 148,700, while the rate of unemployment was 6.6%. Per capita effective buying income in the area in 1977 was $7,054 and household effective buying income was $14,127.

BANKING. There are nine commercial and three mutual savings banks as well as five savings and loan assns. in Spokane. In 1978, total deposits at the seven banks headquartered in the city were approx. $2,191,209,000, while assets totalled $2,542,005,000. Banks include Old Natl. of WA, Fidelity Mutual Savings, Lincoln Mutual Savings, WA Trust, First Natl., American Commercial and Bank of Spokane.

HOSPITALS. There are six major hosps. in Spokane Co., including Sacred Heart Medical Center, St. Luke's Memorial, Spokane Valley Gen. and V.A. In addition, there are eight specialized hosps., including Edgecliff, E WA State, Interlake, Raleigh Hills, Shriners, Paulsen Medical and Dental, Tri-County and Fairchild AFB Hosp.

EDUCATION. There are two cols., one university and two comm. cols. in Spokane. Ft. Wright Col., a Catholic liberal arts col. for women founded in 1939, enrolled 520 students in 1978. Gonzaga U, an independent Catholic institution, enrolled approx. 3,250 in 1978. Whitworth Col., a private liberal arts institution founded in 1890 and associated with the WA-AK Synod of the United Presbyterian Church. Awarding bachelor and master degrees, it enrolled more than 1,600 in 1978. Other institutions are the publicly-supported, two-year Spokane Comm. Col. and Spokane Falls Comm. Col. The city's school system consists of 35 elementary, one continuation high, seven jr. high, five high and 13 special schools, with a total enrollment of more than 30,300. There are 20 private schools in the city. The Spokane Public Lib. system maintains nine branches and one bookmobile.

ENTERTAINMENT. The greater Spokane Music and Allied Arts Festival and the Lilac Festival are held each year in the city. Spokane is the home of both the Flyers, a pro PHL hockey team, and the Indians, a minor PCL baseball team of the Milwaukee Brewers organization. The Gonzaga U Bulldogs and the Spokane Comm. Col. Sasquath participate in intercollegiate sports. The Spokane Polo Team also provides sports entertainment.

ACCOMMODATIONS. There are approx. 60 hotels and motels in Spokane, including the Davenport, Red Lion, Gateway, Jefferson House, Trade Winds, TraveLodge, Ridpath and, the Holiday, Ramada and Sheraton inns.

FACILITIES. There are 94 parks encompassing more than 7,000 acres in Spokane, providing golf courses, 55 tennis courts and ice skating rinks. Riverfront Park, one of the largest and the former site of Expo '74, has been developed into a multi-faceted cultural, recreational and environmental city park. The John H. Finch Arboretum, the Walk in the Wild Zoo and the Playfair Race Horse Track are also located in the city. Within a 50-mi. radius of Spokane, 76 mt. lakes offer the facilities for fishing, swimming, hunting, boating and sailing. Camping and skiing facilities are also available nearby as are 10 natl. parks and 15 natl. forests.

CULTURAL ACTIVITIES. The Spokane Symphony, which presents 12 major concerts annually, the Riverpark Concert Bank, a 30-piece wind ensemble, the Chorale Society and the Spokane Comm. Concerts Assn. provide musical entertainment in the city. The Spokane Civic Theatre stages dramatic productions, as do troupes from area cols. and universities. Various cultural organizations perform in the Opera House at Riverpark Center, as well as the Coliseum. The Cheney Cowles Memorial Museum and Grace Campbell House display exhibits of the area's early history, while the Museum of Native American Cultures houses an extensive collection of native American art. Other museums are St. John's Cathedral Gallery, Spokane Valley Pioneer Museum, Ft. Wright Historical Museum and the Pacific and NW Indian Center.

LANDMARKS AND SIGHTSEEING SPOTS. Riverfront Park, dedicated by Pres. Jimmy Carter, includes the site of Expo '74, the Japanese Gardens, amphitheaters, an Opera House and Convention Center and the IMAX Theater. A turn-of-the-century carousel, a gondola ride over the falls and the Spokane Story Dioramic Exhibit are other attractions. Crosby Lib., located at Gonzaga U, houses recordings and memorabilia of Bing Crosby. English Gothic architecture is featured at the Cathedral of St. John.

SPRINGFIELD
MASSACHUSETTS

CITY LOCATION-SIZE-EXTENT. Springfield, the seat of Hampden Co. in SW MA, encompasses 31.7 sq. mi. of area at 42°06' N lat. and 72°35' W long. The greater met. area extends N into Hampshire Co. and S into Hartford Co., CT and includes the cities of Chicopee and Holyoke to the N.

TOPOGRAPHY. Springfield lies on the CT River in the S CT River Valley. The terrain is gently rolling with Berkshire Hills to the W. The mean elev. is 200'.

CLIMATE. The climate of Springfield is continental and is influenced by the Berkshire Hills and the Atlantic Ocean, which accounts for the variable climate of cold, dry weather during the winter and warm, maritime temps. during summer. Monthly mean temps. range from 25°F during Jan. to 70°F in July, with an avg. annual temp. of approx. 50°F. The 45" avg. annual rainfall is evenly distributed throughout the year. Nearly 90% of the avg. annual 60" snowfall occurs between Dec. and Mar. The RH ranges between 45% and 85%. The growing season avg. 150 days. Springfield is in the ESTZ and observes DST.

FLORA AND FAUNA. Animals native to Springfield include the opossum, raccoon, fox, squirrel and rabbit. Common birds are the bluejay, goldfinch, robin, crow and hawk. Frogs, salamanders, painted turtles, box turtles and milk snakes, as well as the venomous copperhead and timber rattlesnake, are common to the area. Typical trees are the maple, pine, oak and elm. Smaller plants include the mayflower, buttercup, rhododendron and meadowrue.

POPULATION. According to the US census, the pop. of Springfield in 1970 was 163,905. In 1978, it was estimated that it had increased to 167,500.

ETHNIC GROUPS. In 1978, the ethnic distribution of Springfield was estimated to be 87.2% Caucasian, 12.5% Black and 3.3% Hispanic (a percentage of the Hispanic total is also included in the Caucasian total).

TRANSPORTATION. Interstate hwys. 90, 91 and 291, US hwys. 5, 20 and 202 and state hwys. 21, 57, 83, 116, 141, 147 and 159 provide motor access to Springfield. *Railroads* serving the city include ConRail and AMTRAK. *Airlines* serving Bradley Intl. Airport, 18 mi., from the city are US Air, AA, DL, EA, UA, Altair and Pilgrim. Barnes Airport, 13 mi. from the city, specializes in charter and air taxi services. Merrimac Air System, 8 mi. N of the city, offers commuter service to NYC. *Bus lines* include Greyhound, Trailways, Peter Pan and VT Transit Line.

Central Springfield, Massachusetts

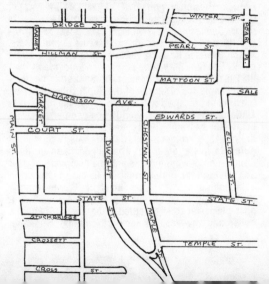

COMMUNICATIONS. Communications, broadcasting and print media originating in Springfield are: *AM radio stations* WGGB 560 (Indep., Contemp.); WSPR 1270 (Indep., MOR); WMAS 1450 (ABC/E, MOR); *FM radio stations* WTRZ 89.1 (Indep., Progsv.); WSCB 89.9 (Mut. Blk., Jazz); WTCC 90.7 (MBS, Progsv.); WAIC 91.9 (ABC/FM, Progsv., Blk.); WHYN 93.1 (Indep., Easy Lis.); WMAS 94.7 (ABC/E, MOR) and WAQY 102.1 (ABC/C, Top 40); *television stations* WFSB Ch. 3 (CBS); WWLP Ch. 22 (NBC); WGGB Ch. 40 (ABC) and WGBY Ch. 57 (PBS); *press*: the two major dailies serving the city are the *News*, issued evenings, and the *Union*, issued mornings; other publications include the *Catholic-Observer, Jewish Weekly News, Republican, Springfield & Four Co. W, New Unity, Press, Yellow Jacket* and *W MA Commercial News.*

HISTORY. The first settlers in the Springfield area arrived in 1636, when a group of Puritans led by pioneer William Pynchon left Roxbury, MA (near Boston) to settle on a tract of land owned by Pynchon. The first settlement, known as Agaswam, was on the W bank of the CT River. The settlers later moved across the river to the present site of the city. The town was named, in 1640, after Springfield, England. A decade later, James Stewart arrived to set up a blacksmithing business. This launched Springfield's great metalworking tradition, which, in turn, led to its weapons industry. During King Philip's War (1675-76), the village was burned by Indians, but was later rebuilt. By the time of the American Revolution, Springfield was the colonial center of the metal trades and a manufacturer of firearms. The Springfield arsenal was the target of an unsuccessful siege by unhappy settlers during Shay's Rebellion in 1786. During the 1800s several Springfield citizens lent their genius to both inventive and social endeavors. Thomas Blanchard invented a lathe to run and finish gun barrels in one process. His *Dexter* steamboat, launched in 1831, was the first that was stern-propelled. John Brown, a leader of the Abolitionist movement, harbored hundreds of runaway slaves in Springfield's Underground RR between 1846 and 1849. After the Civil War, labor began to organize and strong unions appeared in the city. In 1893, the first gasoline auto, built by Charles E. and J. Frank Duryea, made its trial run in Springfield. The Duryea Motor Wagon Co. of Springfield was established in 1895. After the turn of the century, the Springfield and the M-1 rifles of WW I were developed in the city. Among other Springfield firsts are the RR sleeping car, manufactured by George

Mills/Stebbins Villa, Springfield, Massachusetts

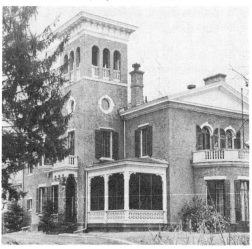

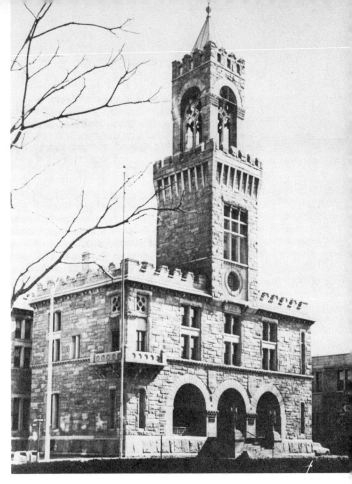

County Courthouse, Springfield, Massachusetts

Pullman, in 1850, and friction matches, invented by Alonzo Phillips in 1836. Also, the game of basketball was created by Springfield's Dr. James Naismith in 1891.

GOVERNMENT. Springfield has a mayor-council form of govt. consisting of nine council members and a mayor, all elected at large to two-year terms. The mayor is not a member of the council and has no vote.

ECONOMY AND INDUSTRY. There are approx. 227 manufacturing firms in Springfield. Many are involved in metal fabrication and allied activities. Other industries are paper, machinery, rubber, plastic and food products, firearms, sports equipment, cosmetics and printing and publishing equipment. Insurance and banking are important non-manufacturing industries. In June, 1979, the met. area had a labor force of 289,500 and an unemployment rate of 4.3%.

BANKING. In 1978, total deposits for the six banks headquartered in Springfield were $1,461,398,000, while assets were $1,699,481,000. Among the banks serving the city are the Institute for Savings, Third Natl. Bank of Hampden City, Valley Bank and Trust, Shawmut First Bank and Trust Co., Hampden Savings and Security Natl.

HOSPITALS. Springfield, the center of health care in W MA, has six gen. and specialized hosps., including the Medical Center of W MA, Baystate, Mercy, Shriners' and Providence.

EDUCATION. Springfield Col., founded in 1885 as the Intl. YMCA Training School and renamed in 1933, offers grad. and undergrad. degrees. In 1978, it enrolled 2,747 students. W N.E. Col., a branch of NE U, was established in 1919. Offering courses at the bachelor, master and professional degrees. In 1978, enrollment was approx. 4,519. American Intl. Col., an independent school, and Springfield Technical Comm. Col. are also located in the city. More than 28,000 students enrolled in the public schools, 30 elementary, six jr. and four sr. high schools in 1978. Approx. 7,000 students are enrolled in 28 private and parochial schools. Libs. include the City Lib., with its eight branches and a bookmobile and the W Regional Lib. System.

ENTERTAINMENT. In early autumn Springfield presents the annual Mattoon Street Arts Festival. Other festivals include Glendi, the annual Fall Greek cultural fair and Big "E." Pro sports are offered by the Indians of the AHL. The Springfield Col. Chiefs compete in intercollegiate sports. It was at Springfield Col., in 1891, that Dr. James A. Naismith invented the game of basketball. The Natl. Basketball Hall of Fame is located in the city.

ACCOMMODATIONS. Hotels and motels in Springfield, are the Marriott, Stonehaven, Highpoint and Best Western and the Ramada, Sheraton, Yankee Pedlar, Holiday and Northhampton Hilton inns.

FACILITIES. Springfield's 735-unit park system features playgrounds, trails, a zoo and clay tennis courts. Forest Park, with 800 acres, is the city's largest and has a kiddieland zoo and a winter ice skating pond. The CT River provides motor boating, sailing, swimming and fishing. Public golf courses are at Veterans Memorial and Franconia. Two amusement parks, Mt. Park and Riverside Park, are also located in the area. Blunt Park also has a winter skating pond.

CULTURAL ACTIVITIES. The Springfield Symphony Orchestra performs at Symphony Hall and encompasses smaller musical groups. Stage is a repertory company which presents classic and experimental plays. The Storrowtown Music Tent provides summer stock theater. Located in the city's Quadrangle are four museums: the George W. V. Smith, the Fine Arts, the Science and the CT Valley Historical. Mini-museums are housed in banks and other buildings.

LANDMARKS AND SIGHTSEEING SPOTS. Springfield's Old Storrowton Village is a restored early N.E. village that includes a restored blacksmith shop, a schoolhouse and a church. The Springfield Armory, which was established by James Stewart in the 1700s and which manufactured arms during the Revolutionary War, is now a museum tracing the history of firearms. Old First Church's congregation was organized in 1637. Atop the present church, built in 1819, is a rooster weathervane which arrived from England in 1749. The Old Day House is filled with antique furnishings. Many other Victorian homes are located on Mattoon St., an historic district. Dr. James Naismith's game is commemorated at the Natl. Basketball Hall of Fame, with exhibits of memorabilia of the game.

SPRINGFIELD
MISSOURI

CITY LOCATION-SIZE-EXTENT. Springfield, the seat of Greene Co. and MO's third largest city, encompasses

Central Springfield, Missouri

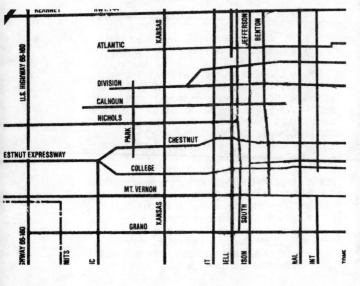

63.2 sq. mi. in the Ozark Mt. resort area at 37°14" N lat. and 93°23' W. It is 220 mi. SW of St. Louis and 176 mi. SE of KC. Its met. area includes most of Greene Co. and extends S into portions of Christian Co.

TOPOGRAPHY. The terrain of Springfield is relatively flat with gently rolling tableland on the crest of the MO Ozark Mt. Plateau. The James and Little Sac rivers are nearby and Lake Springfield is located in the SE portion of the city. The mean elev. is 1,300'.

CLIMATE. Springfield has a "plateau climate", due to its location on the MO Ozark Mt. plateau. Its lat. produces mild winter temps. and its alt. produces cool summer temps. The avg. annual temp. of 55.9°F ranges from a Jan. mean of 32.9°F to a July mean of 77.4°F. The annual rainfall of 40.89" occurs mainly during late spring, summer and early fall. The drier winter months receive an annual snowfall of 15.7". The RH ranges from 53% to 88%. The growing season is approx. 200 days. Springfield is located in the CSTZ and observes DST.

FLORA AND FAUNA. Animals native to Springfield include the squirrel, opossum, fox, deer and raccoon. Common birds are the bluejay, thrasher, bobwhite quail, robin and hawk. Bullfrogs, box turtles, hognose snakes, salamanders and snakes, including venomous cottonmouths, copperheads and rattlesnakes inhabit the area. Typical trees are the oak, pine, elm and hickory. Flowering plants include the honeysuckle, blackberry, ironweed and evening primrose.

POPULATION. According to the US census, the pop. of Springfield in 1970 was 120,096. In 1978, it was estimated to have increased to 134,000.

ETHNIC GROUPS. In 1978, the ethnic distribution of Springfield was estimated to be 97.7% Caucasian, 2% Black, and 0.6% Hispanic. (A percentage of the Hispanic total is included in the Caucasian total.)

TRANSPORTATION. Interstate hwy. 44, US hwys. 60, 65 and 160 and state hwy. 13 provide major motor access to Springfield. The city is also served by two *railroads*, the St. Louis-San Francisco and MO Pacific. The *airline* serving Springfield Municipal Airport is OZ. *Bus lines* are Trailways, Greyhound, Sunnyland Stages and the local City Utilities System.

COMMUNICATIONS. Communications, broadcasting and print media serving Springfield are: *AM radio stations* KBUG 1060 (Indep., MOR); KGBX 1260 (NBC, MOR); KICK 1340 (Indep., Top 40); KTTS 1400 (Indep., C&W) and KLFJ 1550 (Indep., Relig.); *FM radio stations* KSMU 91.1 (NPR, Fine Arts & Info.); KTTS 94.7 (Indep., Ctry.); KWFC 97.3 (ABC/FM, Relig.); KWTO 98.7 (Indep., Rock) and KTXR 101.5 (ABC/E; Easy List.); *television stations* KYTV Ch. 3 (NBC); KOLR, Ch. 10 (CBS); KOZK Ch. 21 (PBS) and KMTC Ch. 27 (ABC); *press*: two major newspapers published in the city are *Leader & Press*, issued evenings, and *Daily News*, issued mornings; other publications serving the area include *Daily Events, The Lance, Pennypower Shopping News, SW Standard, Union Labor Record*, and *Assemblies of God Gospel Group.*

HISTORY. The Kickapoo Indians were the early inhabitants of the present-day Springfield area. The city was founded in 1829 by TN farmer John Polk Campbell, who also contributed 50 acres for the town sq. and co. seat. It was incorporated in 1847 and in 1858 the Butterfield Overland Mail Stagecoach line from St. Louis to San Francisco established a depot in the city. During the Civil War the area was the object of bitter struggles between the N and the S. The Battle of Springfield was fought within the city. The Battle of Wilson Creek, fought 12 mi. SW, ended in a Union retreat to Springfield, but the heavy Confederate casualties suffered in the battle enabled Union troops to take control of the MS River. Pres. Lincoln ranked the battle second only to Gettysburg in its contribution to a Union victory in the Civil War. The city received its first RR in 1870. It maintained a steady growth based on agriculture and light industry and has become one of the fastest growing cities in the midwest. Springfield more than doubled its size between the early 1950s and the late 1970s.

GOVERNMENT. Springfield has a council-mgr. form of govt. The mayor, who is a member of the council and selected at large, serves a two-year term, while the council members, four of whom are elected by residential district, four at large, serve four-year terms.

ECONOMY AND INDUSTRY. Agribusiness, light manufacturing, tourism and education dominate Springfield's economy. Manufacturing employs 18% of the work force and major products include lumber, electronic equipment, durable goods, machinery, processed foods and transportation equipment. Trade, services and transportation comprise a large percentage of the labor force and approx. 953 retail firms and 356 wholesale firms are located in the city. Springfield's livestock and dairy business accounts for approx. $250 million annually. The labor force totalled 104,100 in June, 1978, while unemployment was 3.2%. Avg. income per capita in 1978 was $4,526. In the first quarter of 1978 the city's cost of living index was 22.1% below the natl. avg. and was the lowest index on the survey of 193 US cities.

BANKING. There are eight commercial banks and seven savings and loans assns. in Springfield. In 1978, total deposits for the eight banks headquartered in the city were $681,758,000, while assets were $808,398,000. Among the banks serving the city are Boatmen's Union-Natl., Commerce, Empire, Merchantile, American Natl., Bank of Springfield, Boatmen's Springfield Natl. and United MO of Springfield.

HOSPITALS. There are four hosps. in Springfield, E. Cox Medical Center, St. John's, Springfield Park Central, and Springfield Gen. Osteopathic. There are also eight nursing homes and the US Govt. Medical Center for Fed. Prisoners. More than 320 physicians and 110 dentists serve Springfield.

EDUCATION. SW MO State U, a state-supported U, was founded in 1906 for the training of teachers. It now grants associate, bachelor and master degrees with 13,207 enrolled in 1978. Drury Col., a private liberal arts col., was founded by congregationalists in 1873, and now affiliated with the Disciples of Christ, offers bachelor and master degrees. Its enrollment in 1978 was approx. 2,250. Other institutions in the city include Baptist Bible Col., Assemblies of God Graduate School, Central Bible Col., Evangel and Draughn Business School. There are 43 elementary, eight jr. and five sr. high schools in the public school system. More than 1,500 students attend private schools. Libs. include the Public Lib. of Springfield and Greene Co., the libraries of the city's universities and colleges.

ENTERTAINMENT. Annual events in Springfield include a Fireworks Display on July 4, the Ozark Empire Fair in Aug. and a Christmas Parade in late Nov. Both the SW MO State U Bears and the Drury Panthers participate in intercollegiate sports.

ACCOMMODATIONS. There are several hotels and motels in Springfield, including the Hilton of the Ozarks, Howard Johnson's, the Sheraton, Holiday, Coach House and Drury inns.

FACILITIES. The city's 56-park system features lighted softball and baseball fields and tennis courts. Swimming pools are located at Doling, Westport, Grant Beach, Meador, Fassnight and Silver Springs parks. Phelps Grove Park has a wading pool. The park system conducts baseball, football and basketball leagues. Public golf courses can be found at Grandview Municipal, Horton Smith Municipal and Siler's Shady Acres. A jogging and exercise trail is located at Phelps Grove Park. Dickinson Park has a zoo. Lake Springfield, located within the city, provides a pavillion, picnic facilities, a playground and fishing opportunities. More than 75% of the water in MO (158,000 acres) is within 90 minutes driving time of Springfield, offering a multitude of water sports.

CULTURAL ACTIVITIES. The oldest continuously performing drama group in the Midwest, The Little Theatre, is in Springfield. The Springfield Symphony Assn. has won state-wide acclaim for its musical productions. Theatric entertainment is offered by the SW MO State U Theatre and Drury

Lane Troupers. The Springfield Civic Ballet performs in the city. The Springfield Art Museum annually hosts the nationally famous "Watercolor, U.S.A." show and also features an art education program and continuous programs of exhibits. Area colleges sponsor many other cultural events during the year. An historic museum, containing exhibits of the area's history is located on the Drury Col. campus.

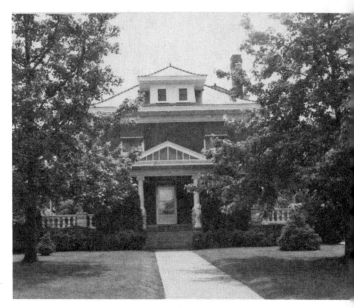

Truman residence, Springfield, Missouri

LANDMARK AND SIGHTSEEING SPOTS. Springfield Natl. Cemetery is one of the few locations in the US where Union and Confederate soldiers are buried side by side. It opened in 1867 and veterans of every US war since 1861 and one veteran of a 1781 battle are buried in the cemetery. It contains many granite and bronze monuments to the Civil War dead. Wilson Creek Natl. Battlefield, 12 mi. SW of Springfield was the location of the most important Civil War battle W of the MS River. It was the second major battle of the war and the first in which Indians fought and regiments from the same state fought each other. More than 2,500 were killed or wounded. Springfield has a recently renovated mall. The square has long been a center of activity and in early Springfield, frontier marshall Wild Bill Hickok was said to have been involved in a shoot-out in front of one of the square's stores.

STAMFORD
CONNECTICUT

CITY LOCATION-SIZE-EXTENT. Stamford encompasses 38.1 sq. mi. in Fairfield Co. in SW CT, 35 mi. NE of NYC, at the mouth of the Rippowam River on LI Sound at 41°03' N lat. and 73°32' W long. The met. area extends throughout the SW section of Fairfield Co., into Westchester Co. on the NW and across the NY border. It overlaps the met. area of Norwalk to the E.

TOPOGRAPHY. Located in the Atlantic Coastal Plain region, Stamford is situated on relatively flat terrain. The mean elev. is 10'.

CLIMATE. The climate of Stamford is both continental and coastal, characterized by temps. which vary from inland temps by being a few degrees warmer in winter

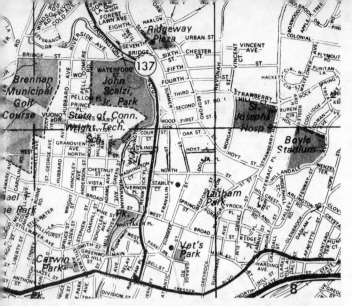

Downtown Stamford, Connecticut

and a few degrees cooler in summer. The avg. annual temp. of 51°F ranges from monthly means of 28°F in Jan. to 73°F in July. The avg. annual rainfall of 44" is well distributed throughout the year. More than half of the avg. annual snowfall of 28" occurs in Jan. and Feb. The RH ranges from 53% to 85%. Stamford lies in the ESTZ and observes DST.

FLORA AND FAUNA. Animals native to Stamford include the whitetail deer, skunk, raccoon, weasel, opossum, otter, muskrat, and fox. Common birds include the gull, tern, crow, blue jay and chickadee. Frogs, salamanders, green snakes and skinks, as well as the venomous copperhead and timber rattlesnake, are found in the area. Typical trees include the oak, pine, beech, maple, hickory and elm. Smaller plants include the field daisy, wood aster, spice bush and shad bush.

POPULATION. According to the US census, the pop. of Stamford in 1970 was 108,798. In 1978, it was estimated that it had decreased to 103,300.

ETHNIC GROUPS. In 1978, the ethnic distribution of Stamford was approx. 87.2% Caucasian, 12.3% Black, and 3.8% Hispanic. (A percentage of the Hispanic total is also included in the Caucasian total).

TRANSPORTATION. Interstate Hwy. 95, US hwys. 1 and 7 and state hwys. 15, 104, 106, 124 and 137 provide major motor access to Stamford. *Railroads* serving the city include AMTRAK and ConRail. Major *airlines* serve nearby Westchester Airport at Purchase, NY. *Bus lines* serving Stamford include Greyhound, Trailways, and the local CT Transit.

COMMUNICATIONS. Communications, broadcasting and print media originating from Stamford are: *AM radio stations* WSTC 1400 (ABC/I, E & FM, MOR); *FM radio stations* WYRS 96.7 (Indep., Btfl. Mus.); no *television stations* originate from Stamford, which receives broadcasting from nearby NYC; *press:* one daily serves the city, the evening *Advocate*, other publications include *The Office, La Voz, Stamford Shopper, Progressive Architecture* and *Teacher.*

HISTORY. Settled in 1641 by members of the Congregational Church, Stamford was incorporated as a village in 1685. It was originally a small agrarian comm. producing subsistence crops and practicing small crafts and trades. The city grew steadily, and by the time of the Revolutionary War, some 3,500 people lived in Stamford. In 1848, the RR arrived, bringing with it a flood of immigrants to work in new mills resulting from the American Industrial Revolution. Stamford's growth into the 20th century paralleled that of N.E.'s, with new, local industries emerging. After WW II, the city's economy jumped sharply upward as research laboratories opened. In 1949, Stamford was merged with surrounding villages and incorporated as a city. Many of its citizens were commuting daily to work in NYC

until during the 1960's, a large number of corporate headquarters began locating in the city and today more workers now commute into Stamford than commute out. Stamford is currently considered the second largest corporate headquarters city in the US, while farming is virtually non-existent.

GOVERNMENT. Stamford has a mayor-council form of govt., consisting of 40 legislators, six finance board members and the mayor. Two members from each of the 20 districts are elected for two-year terms to the 40-member legislature, called the Board of Representatives. The Board of Finance members and the mayor are elected at large and serve four-year and two-year terms respectively.

ECONOMY AND INDUSTRY. Stamford is the headquarters for approx. 21 of the nation's largest industrial firms. It has a sizable industrial base with more than 200 manufacturing firms producing pharmaceuticals, electrical equipment, hair care products, plastics and bearings. The labor force for the Stamford met. area totaled 125,100 in June 1979, while the unemployment rate was 4.1%.

BANKING. There are 11 banking institutions in Stamford. In 1978, total deposits for the four banks headquartered in the city were $518,457,000, while assets were $571,864,000. Banks include Stamford Savings, Citizens Savings, Fidelity Trust, First Stamford Bank and Trust, CT Natl. and Union Trust.

HOSPITALS. There are two general hosps. in Stamford, St. Joseph's and Stamford. There are also several psychiatric facilities as well as the Dubois Day Treatment Center and a regional rehabilitation center.

EDUCATION. St. Basil's Col., founded at Stamford in 1939, is a private seminary-col. for candidates to the Catholic priesthood in the Byzantine Rite. Special courses in Ukrainian language, literature, history and music are offered and the bachelor degree is granted. Enrollment in 1978 was 11. Residents of Stamford are within a 35 mi. commuting distance of NYC and its higher education opportunities. Lib. facilities are provided by the Stamford Public Lib.

ENTERTAINMENT. The Darien Dinner Theatre is in Stamford. Other forms of entertainment may be found in nearby NYC.

ACCOMMODATIONS. Hotels and motels in Stamford include the Executive Hotel, Howard Johnson's, Marriott, Stamford Motor Lodge and Ramada Inn.

FACILITIES. The Stamford Museum and Nature Center features a dairy farm and a zoo. Two golf courses are available, while public tennis courts may be found at five local tennis clubs and many public parks.

Landmark Tower, Stamford, Connecticut

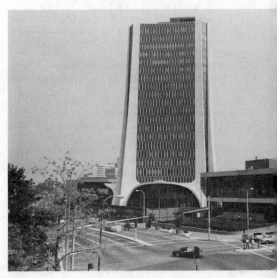

CULTURAL ACTIVITIES. The Stamford Music Society, a symphony, the State Opera and several choral groups offer musical programs throughout the year. Theaters include the Hartman Repertory Theater and a city operated little theater—the Ethel Kweskin Barn. A natural history museum, the Stamford Museum and Nature Center, features an art gallery. Stamford also shares in the cultural activities of the NYC met. area.

LANDMARKS AND SIGHTSEEING SPOTS. The city of Stamford is an historic landmark comm., as it is listed on the Natl. Register of Historic Places. Of special interest are the Landmark Building and Square, Old Town Hall, Veterans Park and the restored Ft. Stamford. The First Presbyterian Church of Stamford features a walk containing more than 100 stones depicting the history of Christianity.

STOCKTON
CALIFORNIA

CITY LOCATION-SIZE-EXTENT. Stockton, the seat of San Joaquin Co., encompasses 40.12 sq. mi., including much of the San Joaquin delta waterway, on the SW portion of the broad delta formed by the confluence of the San Joaquin and Sacramento rivers at 37°54' N lat. and 121°15' W long. One of two inland seaports in CA, it is connected to San Francisco Bay by a 75 mi. long channel. The greater met. area extends into the counties. of Alameda to the SW, Contra Costa to the W, Solano to the NW, Sacramento to the N, Calaveras to the E and Stanislaus to the SE. Stockton is 50 mi. SE of Sacramento.

TOPOGRAPHY. The terrain of Stockton, which is situated in the Great Central Valley region of CA, consists of flat irrigated farm and orchard land with rivers and canals of the delta controlled by a system of levees. The foothills of the Sierra Nevadas Mts. lie approx. 25 mi. to the E and NE, while the CA Coastal Range Mts. lie to the W and SW. The mean elev. is 22'.

CLIMATE. The climate of Stockton is intermediate between marine and continental, as marine influences from the Pacific Ocean periodically pass through the barrier formed by the Coastal Range. The weather is characterized in summer by warm temps., light rains and frequent heavy fogs. The avg. annual temp. of 60.9°F ranges from monthly means of 44.9°F in Jan. to 76.8°F in July. Temps. exceeding 100°F occur on an avg. of six days in July and 15 days in the entire summer. Approx. 90% of the avg. annual rainfall of 13.85" occurs during Nov. through Apr. Snowfall is rare. The RH ranges from 26% to 90%. The growing season avgs. 285 days annually. Stockton lies in the PSTZ and observes DST.

FLORA AND FAUNA. Animals native to Stockton include the coyote, mule deer, pocket gopher, opossum and bobcat. Common birds include the mourning dove, scrub jay, CA quail and house finch. Pacific treefrogs, pond turtles, fence lizards and skinks as well as the venomous Pacific rattlesnake, are also found here. Typical trees include the pine, oak, and willow. Smaller plants include the CA poppy (the state flower), marsh grass, blue lupine, chaparral shrub and mayweed.

POPULATION. According to the US census, the pop. of Stockton in 1970 was 109,963. In 1978, it was estimated that it had increased to 131,100.

ETHNIC GROUPS. In 1978, the ethnic distribution of Stockton was approx. 58.3% Caucasian, 11.0% Black, 21.2% Hispanic and 9.5% other.

TRANSPORTATION. Interstate hwys. 5 and 80, US hwys. 50 and 99 and state hwys. 4, 12, 26, 80, 99 and 120 provide major motor access to Stockton. *Railroads* serving the city include AMTRAK, the Atchison, Topeka & Santa Fe, S Pacific, W Pacific, Central CA Traction, Stockton Terminal and Tidewater S. *Airlines* serving Stockton Municipal Airport

University of the Pacific, Stockton, California

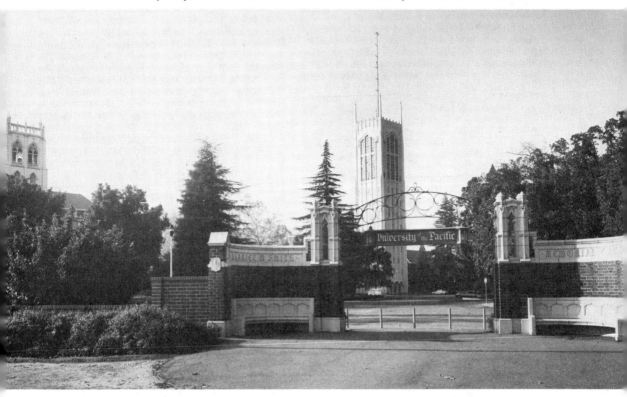

include UA, RW and Pacific SW. *Bus lines* include Trailways, Greyhound and the local Stockton Met. Transit District. The Port of Stockton, CA's largest inland deepwater seaport, serves outgoing vessels through the 30' Stockton Deepwater Channel and the San Joaquin River.

COMMUNICATIONS. Communications, broadcasting and print media originating in Stockton are: *AM radio stations* KWG 1230 (MBS, MOR, C&W); KJOY 1280 (ABC/E, MOR) and KSTN 1420 (ABC/C, Contemp.); *FM radio stations* KSJC 89.5 (MBS, Var.); KCJH 90.5 (Indep., Relig.); KUOP 91.3 (NPR, Clas., Educ., Jazz); KJAX 99.3 (ABC/FM, Btfl. Mus.) and KSTN 107.3 (Indep., C&W); no *television stations* originate from Stockton, however, KOVR Ch. 13 (ABC), Sacramento-Stockton (which originates in Sacramento) has a relay station in Stockton and the city receives additional TV broadcasting from Sacramento and cable; *press:* one major daily serves the city, the *Record*, issued evenings; other publications include the *Advertiser*, *Impact*, *Diamond Walnut News*, *Observer* and *San Joaquin Co. Farm Bureau News*.

HISTORY. Stockton, one of the first two settlements in the San Joaquin Valley, was founded in 1849 by Capt. Charles Weber on land granted to him by Gov. Micheltornea in 1845. The earliest attempt to settle on the site failed when Native Americans of the Yachicumnes tribe, who lived in the area, burned down all 7 houses and killed the stock. Another effort to form a settlement in 1848 was interrupted by the Mexican War. At the end of the war, a successful settlement was established and named Tileburg. The discovery of gold in CA resulted in a large influx of people into the valley. During the gold rush, the settlement became the chief port of departure for area gold mines. In 1850, the town was incorporated and its name officially changed to Stockton, in honor of Capt. Weber's friend, Commodore Robert F. Stockton. The following year an outbreak of fire at the Branch Hotel nearly wiped out the town. However, in 1852, there were over 300 farms in the valley and land prices in Stockton soared. In 1883, Benjamin Holt moved into Stockton and with his brother formed the Holt Manufacturing Co. where he developed and made commercially feasible the caterpillar-type tractor. Construction of a RR to Stockton in the 1880s expanded the market for area crops. In 1933, a 75-mi. deep water channel, with the capacity to berth

Central Stockton, California

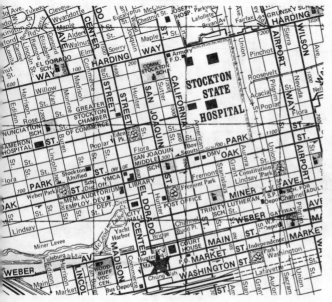

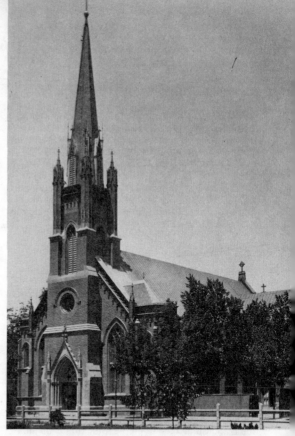

St. Mary's Church, built 1861, Stockton, California

the largest US maritime vessels, linked Stockton to San Francisco. Today, Stockton serves as the main distribution center for products from the San Joaquin Valley.

GOVERNMENT. Stockton has a council-mgr. form of govt. The nine council members are elected by district to four-year terms. The mayor, a voting member of council, is elected at large to a two-year term.

ECONOMY AND INDUSTRY. Agriculture, the largest industry in Stockton, produces milk, grapes, tomatoes, almonds, eggs, hay and corn. The 285 manufacturing firms in the Stockton area produce laminated glass, machinery, paper products, asbestos, cement pipe, wood products, fabricated steel, processed foods, ships and pleasure crafts. Trade, the Port of Stockton and the Sharpe Army Depot and Gen. Services Admin. are also major employers. In June, 1979, the met. area labor force was 167,700, while the rate of unemployment was 8.3%. Unemployment rates fluctuate widely throughout the year because of agriculture.

BANKING. There are 13 banks and seven savings and loan assns. in Stockton. In 1978, total deposits for the three banks headquartered in the city were $360,241,000, while assets were $397,244,000. Banks include Bank of Stockton, Union Safe Deposit, Bank of Agriculture and Commerce, Crocker and Wells Fargo.

HOSPITALS. There are four gen. hosps. in Stockton including, St. Joseph's, Dameron, Oak Park Comm. and San Joaquin Co. Gen.

EDUCATION. The U of the Pacific, located in Stockton, developed the cluster col. concept, in which distinct semi-autonomous units operate within a single U. The privately-supported coed U awards bachelor, master and doctorate degrees. Enrollment in 1978 was approx. 6,000. Other institutions include Humphreys Col. and San Joaquin Delta Col., both jr. colleges. The Stockton Unified School District enrolls more than 30,000. There are 17 private and parochial schools in the area. Libs. include the Stockton Central Lib., the Cooperative Lib. System and the Stockton-San Joaquin Public Lib.

ENTERTAINMENT. Melodrama dinner theater is offered in Stockton at the Pollardville Palace; the Mariners, a minor league baseball team, offers pro sports in Stockton, while the U of the Pacific Tigers participate in intercollegiate sports.

ACCOMMODATIONS. There are numerous hotels and motels in Stockton including the Vagabond Motor Hotel and Hilton, Stockton and Holiday inns.

FACILITIES. There are 43 multi-purpose municipal parks, occupying more than 475 acres in Stockton. Oak Park, one of the largest, features picnic grounds, baseball and softball diamonds, tennis courts, a swimming pool and an ice arena. Both Buckley Cove and Louis parks provide marinas. Pixie Woods, in the Louis Park complex, features an amusement park with a paddle wheel boat, castle, merry-go-round, lagoon, 19th-century mine train and other attractions. Nearby is the delta, providing 1,000 mi. of waterways. Public golf courses are located at Swenson and Van Buskirk parks, while public tennis courts are also provided by the city park system.

CULTURAL ACTIVITIES. The Comm. Concerts Assn. presents musical performances in Stockton. The Opera Co. also performs in the city. European and American paintings and local historic relics are on view at Pioneer Museum and Haggin Gallery, while the life and times in the CA foothills prior to 1940 is depicted in the W Side Collection.

LANDMARKS AND SIGHTSEEING SPOTS. The Pollardville Ghost Town, located in Stockton, recreates a segment of the Old W, featuring 25 old buildings. Erected in 1873, the Weber School is the oldest brick building still standing in Stockton and is listed in the Natl. Register of Historic Places. Other attractions include the Weber Home (built in 1850), the Wong Mansion and St. Mary's Catholic Church.

SUNNYVALE
CALIFORNIA

CITY LOCATION-SIZE-EXTENT. Sunnyvale, located 10 mi. NW of San Jose and 40 mi. S of San Francisco in Santa Clara Co. on the San Francisco Bay peninsula, encompasses 22.95 sq. mi. at 37°22' N lat. and 122°02' W long. and has been developed as a planned comm. Its met. area extends into the surrounding counties of San Jose and Santa Clara to the S and San Mateo to the W.

TOPOGRAPHY. The terrain of Sunnyvale, situated in the broad, flat Santa Clara Valley (part of the fertile Central Valley region in CA) slopes slightly towards the N approaching San Francisco Bay. It lies between the Santa Cruz Mts. on the W and the Diablo range on the E. The mean elev. is 95'.

CLIMATE. The climate of Sunnyvale is mild, influenced by prevailing Pacific Ocean westerlies. The avg. annual temp. of 56°F ranges from monthly means of 49°F in Jan. to 68°F in July. Most of the avg. annual rainfall of 13" occurs from Nov. through Mar. Snowfall is extremely rare. The RH ranges from 60% to 85%. Sunnyvale is in the PSTZ and observes DST.

FLORA AND FAUNA. Animals native to Sunnyvale include the muledeer, pocket gopher, coyote, jackrabbit and bat. Common birds are the scrub jay, mockingbird, swallow, wrentit, Bewick's wren and various gulls and terns. The venomous N Pacific rattlesnake is found in the area. Typical trees are the redwood, live oak, chaparral, walnut, almond, pine and juniper. Smaller plants include the CA golden poppy (the state flower).

POPULATION. According to the US census, the pop. of Sunnyvale in 1970 was 95,408. In 1978, it was estimated that it had increased to 106,050.

ETHNIC GROUPS. In 1978, the ethnic distribution of Sunnyvale was approx. 83.3% Caucasian, 1.9% Black, 6.9% Hispanic, 5.0% Asian and 3.2% other.

TRANSPORTATION. Interstate Hwy. 280 (Junipero Serra Frw.), US Hwy. 101 (Bayshore Frw.) and state hwys. 17, 82, 85 and 237 provide major motor access to Sunnyvale. *Railroads* serving the city include the S Pacific. San Francisco Intl. Airport, less than 30 mi., and San Jose Municipal Airport,

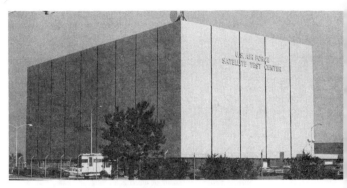

U.S. Air Force Satelite Test Center, Sunnyvale, California

less than 10 mi., from the city, are served by all major *airlines*. *Buslines* serving the city include Greyhound, Trailways and the local Santa Clara Co. Transit System.

COMMUNICATIONS. Communications, broadcasting and print media serving Sunnyvale are: no *AM radio stations, FM radio stations* or *television stations* originate from the city, which receives broadcasting from the nearby San Francisco Met. Bay area; press: two publications serve the city, the *Valley Journal* and the *Scribe* issued weekly on Wed.

HISTORY. Sunnyvale was founded in 1864. Originally called Murphy's Station after landowner Martin Murphy, Jr., it was a flag stop on the S Pacific RR. During the late 1800s, the early settlers called it Encinal. The name Sunnyvale was adopted in 1901 because both Murphy and Encinal were already taken by other CA towns. The city was incorporated in 1912 with a pop. of 2,000. By 1930, the city was an agricultural town with 3,000 people. During the 1950s, the aerospace industries arrived to set the stage for today's development. Sunnyvale is a residential and industrial city that has become a center for both guided missile research and satellite tracking operations.

GOVERNMENT. Sunnyvale has a council-mgr. form of govt. consisting of seven members including the mayor. All members are elected at large to a four-year term. The mayor is selected by the council from the membership; he serves a one-year term and is a voting member of the council.

Picturesque area, Sunnyvale, California

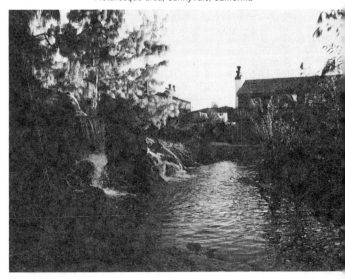

ECONOMY AND INDUSTRY. There are approx. 645 manufacturing plants in Sunnyvale. Aerospace is the most important industry. Major products include computer, communications and electronic systems; electronic video games; chemicals and electronic and missile equipment. The city has a significant number of food processing and research firms. The avg. household income in 1978 was $21,545. In 1978, the total labor force of the greater met. area was approx. 63,189, while the rate of unemployment was 5.5%.

BANKING. There are 18 banks and 10 savings and loan assns. in Sunnyvale. In 1978, total deposits for the one bank headquartered in the city were $10,833,000, while total assets were $11,788,000. Banks include Crocker Citizens Bank, De Anza, Wells Fargo Bank, Bank of America, Security Pacific Bank, Bank of the W and United CA Bank.

HOSPITALS. Sunnyvale is located in the El Camino Hosp. District with the main hosp. in nearby Mt. View. Kaiser Hosp. maintains a clinic in Sunnyvale.

EDUCATION. Fourteen elementary, three intermediate, and six high schools serve Sunnyvale. Lib. facilities include the Sunnyvale Public Lib. and the Sunnyvale Patent Lib., one of only 23 in the US, and the only subject-classified patent collection in the US outside of WA, DC.

ENTERTAINMENT. Annual events include the Art Affair and the Sunnyvale Art and Wine Festival. The city is host to a number of major CA tennis tournaments. Sports and other entertainment can be found in the nearby San Francisco Bay area.

ACCOMMODATIONS. Hotels and motels in Sunnyvale include the Granada and Holiday inns, Royal Executive, Motel 6, Ambassador, Hilton, the Motel Orleans, Wittle, Der Ghan and Lawana.

FACILITIES. There are 13 parks in Sunnyvale, including WA, Serra, Ortega, Lakewood and Ponderosa. Jogging tracks are located at Freemont and Sunnyvale High and Mango Jr. High.

CULTURAL ACTIVITIES. Sunnyvale is served by the Sunnyvale Center Orchestra. The Performing Arts Center and the Creative Arts Center host numerous dramatic presentations and art exhibitions. Museums include the Engine House Museum. The Sunnyvale Historical Museum, located in Murphy Park, has exhibits on life in early Sunnyvale and other CA settlements.

LANDMARKS AND SIGHTSEEING SPOTS. The Villa Montalvo (estate of Senator Phelan, dating from 1912) is located in Saratoga. Additional sightseeing spots are available in the nearby San Francisco met. area.

Central Sunnyvale, California

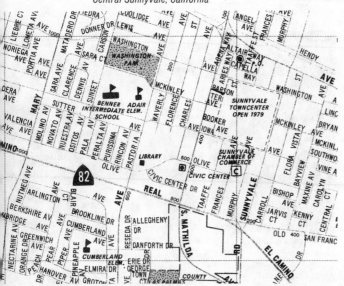

SYRACUSE
NEW YORK

CITY LOCATION-SIZE-EXTENT. Syracuse, the seat of Onondaga Co., encompasses 25.8 sq. mi. in upstate NY on the S bank of Onondaga Lake at 43°7' N lat. and 76°7' W long. Located at the geographical center of NY, the city's met. area extends into the neighboring counties of Oswego to the N, Madison to the E, Cortland to the S and Cayuga to the NE.

Central Syracuse, New York

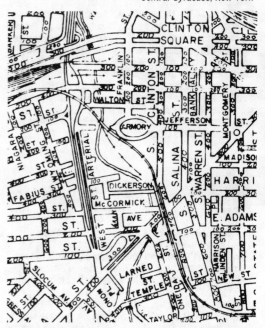

TOPOGRAPHY. The terrain of Syracuse, which is located in the Tug Hill plateau, is characterized by high plateaus and hills to the S rising to approx. 2,000' and the Erie-Ontario plain to the W. Its elev. ranges from 500' to 800'. Within the met. area are Otisco, Owasco, Skaneateles, Oneida and Onondaga lakes which empty into the Oneida River. The mean elev. is 400'.

CLIMATE. The climate of Syracuse is primarily continental and humid, modified by cold air masses moving through the Great Lakes region and down from the Hudson Bay area. The annual avg. rainfall of 35.63" is well distributed throughout the year. Most of the 112.3" avg. annual snowfall occurs from Dec. to Mar. Monthly mean temps. range from 24°F during Feb. to 71.2°F during July with an annual avg. of 47.7°F. The RH ranges from 51% to 87%. The avg. growing season is 171 days. Syracuse lies in the ESTZ and observes DST.

FLORA AND FAUNA. Animals native to Syracuse include the whitetail deer, opossum, otter, mink and raccoon. Common birds are the loon, thrush, warbler, broad-winged hawk and bluejay. Frogs, salamanders, turtles, lizards and snakes, including the venomous timber rattlesnake and copperhead, inhabit the area. Typical trees are the Norway maple, sugar maple, basswood and European buckthorn. Flowering plants include the rose, field daisy, bluet, honeysuckle, buttercup and jewelweed.

POPULATION. According to the US census, the pop. of Syracuse in 1970 was 197,297. In 1978, it was estimated that it had decreased to 182,543.

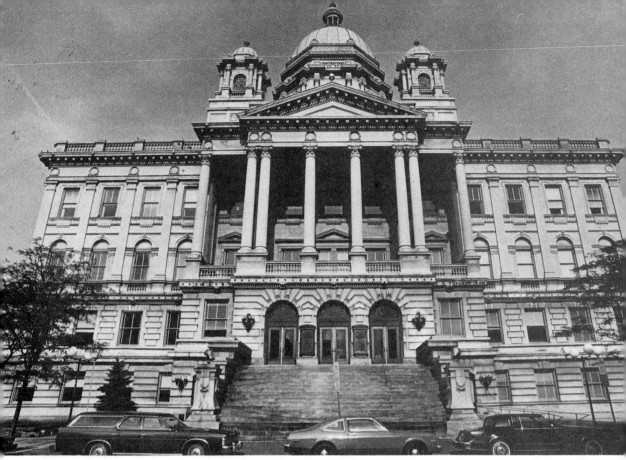

Onondaga County Courthouse, Syracuse, New York

ETHNIC GROUPS. In 1978, the ethnic distribution of Syracuse was approx. 83.5% Caucasian, 14% Black, 1% Hispanic and 1.5% other.

TRANSPORTATION. Interstate Hwys. 81 and 90, US hwy. 11 and state rtes. 5, 57 and 91 provide major motor access to Syracuse. The city is served by several *railroads*, including AMTRAK and ConRail. *Airlines* serving Syracuse-Hancock Intl. Airport are US Air, AA, EA, TW, NC and Empire. *Bus lines* include Greyhound, Onondaga Coach, Syracuse & Oswego, Central NY and the met. CENTRO. A barge canal connects the city to Lake Erie and the St. Lawrence Seaway.

COMMUNICATIONS. Communications, broadcasting and print media originating in Syracuse are: *AM radio stations* WSYR 570 (NBC, MOR); WHEN 620 (ABC, Adult Contemp.); WNDR 1260 (ABC/C, Top 40); WFBL 1390 (CBS, Top 40); WOLF 1490 (Indep., Top 40) and WYRD 1540 (Indep., Relig.); *FM radio stations* WAER 88.3 (Indep., Progsv.); WCNY 91.3 (NPR, Divers.); WNTQ 93.1 (ABC/FM, Btfl. Mus.); WSYR 94.5 (Indep., Btfl. Mus.) and WOND 107.9 (Indep., Clas.); *television stations* WSYR Ch. 3 (NBC); WTVH Ch. 5 (CBS); WNYS Ch. 9 (ABC) and WCNY Ch. 24 (PBS); *press:* two major newspapers are published in the city, the *Herald Journal*, issued evenings, and the *Post Standard*, issued mornings; other publications include the *Daily Orange, Adirondack Lift, Agway Cooperator, Catholic Sun, News for You, Record* and *Southside News.*

HISTORY. Up to the early 1600s, native American groups, including the Algonquins and Iroquois, lived in the area that is now Syracuse. Father Simon Le Moyne, a French Jesuit priest established, in 1654, Ft. St. Marie with the intention of converting the Indians. But the Dutch in New Amsterdam (NYC) opposed the French presence and the settlement was abandoned. Later the area passed into British hands, and by the 1780s was known as Webster's Landing, after the pioneer, Ephraim Webster. Among the factors that influenced the growth of towns in the Syracuse area were land grants made to Revolutionary War veterans, development of salt mining in "Devil Lake" and the completion of the Genesee and Peterboro Tpke. in 1800. In 1793, the first kettle designed to boil and refine salt was brought to Syracuse. James Geddes built the first salt works in 1804. Several villages grew up around the salt works, including Salina, later to be renamed Syracuse. The name change was inspired by a poem about the Sicilian village Syracuse, site of a lake where salt and fresh water mixed. In 1825 the village was incorporated. Syracuse developed quickly after the Erie Canal opened in 1820 and boosted the pop. from 250 in 1820 to over 15,000 in 1847. That year, the city received a charter. A wave of European immigrants settled in Syracuse after the 1840s. During the mid-1800s, the RRs also contributed to the city's growth. The salt industry peaked in 1862 and Syracuse was known as "Salt City" because it produced a lot of salt. By the time this industry declined in the late 1800s Syracuse's economy had shifted to manufacturing. The region was an important flour milling center by 1900. Syracuse continued to grow in the 1920s as rural residents migrated to the city. Today, Syracuse is an industrial center which also serves the surrounding agricultural area as a farming market.

GOVERNMENT. Syracuse has a mayor-council form of govt. The mayor, who is not a council member, serves a four-year term, while the council consists of five district representatives elected to two-year terms and four at large members who serve four-year terms and a council president who is elected to a four-year term.

ECONOMY AND INDUSTRY. The Syracuse met. area is NY's third largest manufacturing center. Electrical and non-electrical machinery industries currently employ the largest number of workers. Other major manufacturers are primary metals, food, transportation equipment, chemicals, pharmaceuticals, paper and paper products, printing, fabricated metals, glass, apparel, chinaware and candles. The city is the marketing center for a large farming comm. Avg. income per capita in 1977 was $5,207. The labor force in the met. area totaled 284,700 while unemployment was 7.1% in 1977.

BANKING. In 1978, total deposits at the five banks headquartered in Syracuse were approx. $2,572,526,000, while assets totaled $2,903,431,000. Among the banks serving the city are Onondaga Savings, Syracuse Savings, First Trust & Deposit, Lincoln First and Merchants Natl.

HOSPITALS. There are six hosps. in Syracuse. As the site of Upstate Medical Center in the state U of NY system, the city has become a natl. center for medical research and study. Other hosps. are Benjamin Rush Center, Comm. Gen., Crouse-Irving Memorial, St. Joseph's Health Center, Hutchings Psychiatric Center and the V.A. Medical Center.

EDUCATION. Syracuse U, a private institution, awards associate, bachelor, master and doctorate degrees. It was founded in 1870 by the Methodist Episcopal Church and moved to its present site in 1873. Enrollment was approx. 20,000 in 1978. State U of NY Upstate Medical Center established in 1950, functions as a medical school and research institution. Enrollment in 1978 was approx. 800. The Col. of Environmental Science and Forestry offers grad. and undergrad. degrees with more than

City Hall, Syracuse, New York

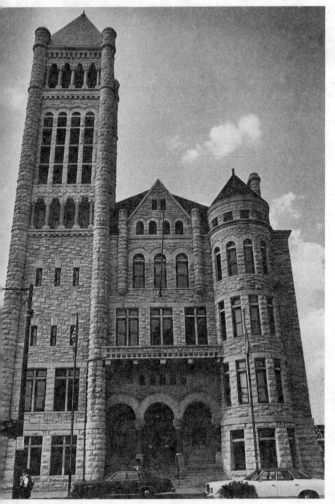

2,100 students enrolled in 1978. Other colleges and institutions in the area include Le Moyne Col., Onondaga Comm. Col., Central City Business Institute, Powelson Business Institute, and Maria Regina Col. The public school district has 25,000 students enrolled in 45 schools. Libs. include the Syracuse Public Lib., the Onondaga Lib. System and the Onondaga Free Lib.

ENTERTAINMENT. Annual festivals in Syracuse include the NY State Fair, held in Aug. which features displays of agricultural and industrial products and entertainment, including music and celebrity appearances. Professional sports entertainment is provided by the Syracuse Firebirds hockey team, the Centennials EBA basketball team and the Triple A Chiefs, a farm club of the Toronto Blue Jays. Collegiate sports are offered by the Syracuse U Orangemen and Le Moyne Col. The city is the hometown of two world champion boxers, Carmen Basilio and Billy Bachus.

ACCOMMODATIONS. There are numerous hotels and motels in Syracuse, including the Hotel Syracuse, Holiday, Dinkler Motor, Marriott, Hilton, Sheraton and Treadway inns and TraveLodge.

FACILITIES. The 2,300-acre Syracuse park system includes 173 parks, featuring a zoo, picnic sites, boating harbor, hiking and biking trails, jogging tracks, public golf courses, 48 tennis courts and ice skating rinks, among other facilities. Syracuse U is constructing a domed stadium to be completed in the fall of 1980. It will be one of the first domed stadiums in the E.

CULTURAL ACTIVITIES. The Syracuse Symphony Orchestra is noted as one of the 31 major symphony orchestras in the US. An annual concert series is presented by the Syracuse Friends of Chamber Music. During the year, Famous Artists and Civic Morning Musicals promote a variety of concerts while the Cultural Resources Council sponsors theatrical companies representing contemporary and ethnic dance forms. Theater organizations include Syracuse Stage, the Salt Lake City Playhouse and active comm. groups. Museums in the city include the Salt and Canal museums. The Everson Museum, founded in 1896, and formerly the Syracuse Museum of Fine Arts, features some of the first collections of American artwork in the country. Among its permanent collections are American paintings and ceramics, Chinese ceramics and English pottery and porcelain. Other art galleries are the Lowe Art Center at Syracuse U, which showcases student and faculty work, Folk Art Gallery and Hanover Gallery.

LANDMARKS AND SIGHTSEEING SPOTS. A replica of the 1656 French settlement, Ft. St. Marie, recalls the days of the Jesuit Priests and French colonists. Renovated buildings featuring distinctive architecture include the Syracuse Savings Bank, the Gridley, the Gere and the former US Post Office buildings. City Hall was constructed of Onondaga limestone in 1892. Listed on the Natl. Register of Historic Places, the Hall of Languages (1873) was the first building constructed at Syracuse U. The interior of the Co. Courthouse, built in 1907, is decorated with marble and ornate gilt. Located in historic Clinton/Hanover Sq. is the Soldiers and Sailors Monument. The main chapel of the Oakwood Cemetery was constructed in 1880. Kieffer's Cigar Store is a restored 19th-century business.

TACOMA
WASHINGTON

CITY LOCATION-SIZE-EXTENT. Tacoma, the third largest city in the state and the seat of Pierce Co., encompasses 47.8 sq. mi. on Commencement Bay of Puget Sound, 25 mi. S of Seattle, in W central WA at 47°14' N lat. and 122°26' W long. The greater met. area extends into King Co. to the NE and Thurston Co. to the SW.

TOPOGRAPHY. The terrain of Tacoma, which is situated in the Puget Sound lowlands, varies from rolling to hilly and slopes upward from the Bay. The Cascade Mts. lie to the E of the city, while the Olympic Mts. lie to the W. The mean elev. is 250'.

CLIMATE. The climate of Tacoma is coastal, characterized by warm, dry summers and wet, mild winters. The avg. annual temp of 50°F ranges from a Jan. mean of 37°F to a July mean of 63°F. There is an avg. of six days each summer with temps. exceeding 90°F. The annual avg. rainfall is 51.11" occurs mostly in winter, while summers are usually exceedingly dry. Nearly 50% of the avg. annual snowfall of 19" occurs during Jan. The RH ranges from 49% to 94%. The growing season avgs. approx. 166 days. Tacoma lies in the PSTZ and observes DST.

FLORA AND FAUNA. Animals native to Tacoma include the deer, black bear, chipmunk and weasel. Common birds include the woodpecker, chickadee, pipet and bluebird. Garter snakes, N alligator lizards and Pacific treefrogs, as well as the venomous Pacific rattlesnake, are also found in the area. The most common tree is the Douglas Fir. Smaller plants include the rhododendron, toothwort, jewelweed and spring beauty.

POPULATION. According to the US census, the pop. of Tacoma in 1970 was 154,407. In 1978, it was estimated that it had decreased to 151,267.

ETHNIC GROUPS. In 1978, the ethnic distribution of Tacoma was approx 91% Caucasian, 6.8% Black, 1.5% Hispanic and 0.7 other.

TRANSPORTATION. Interstate hwy. 5 and state hwy. Pacific. *Airlines* serving Seattle Tacoma Intl. Airport include AS, BN, CO, EA, FL, NW, PA, RW, UA, WA and WE. *Bus lines* serving the city include N and Union Greyhound, Trailways and the local Cascade System. Steamship lines furnish foreign, coastal, intercoastal and insular service through the Port of Tacoma.

COMMUNICATIONS. Communications, broadcasting and print media originating from Tacoma are: *AM radio stations* KTAC 850 (Indep., MOR); KMO 1360 (Indep., C&W) and KTNT 1400 (Indep., Contemp.); *FM radio stations* KPLU 88.5 (Indep., Btfl. Mus.); KPUS 90.1 (Univ., Educ.); KPEC 90.9 (Indep., MOR) and KTOY 91.7 (NPR, Top 40); KNBQ 97.3 (Indep. Var.); KBRD 103.9 (Indep., Btfl. Mus.) and KLAY 106.1 (Indep., Progsv.); *television stations* KTPS Ch. 62 (PBS); KSTW Ch. 11 (Indep.) and KCPQ Ch. 13 (PBS); *press:* one major daily serves the city, the evening *News-Tribune*; other publications include *Labor Advocate, Ft. Lewis Ranger, NW Airlifter, W Flyer* and *Tacoma Area Progress*

HISTORY. British explorer George Vancouver first explored the Tacoma area in 1792, but it was not until 1833 that the first ft. was constructed in the region. The Hudson Bay Co. constructed Ft. Nisqually, currently located in a Tacoma city park. In 1864, Civil War veteran Job Carr homesteaded the site of the original Tacoma, and part of his land was purchased in 1873 for the purpose of establishing the W terminal of the N Pacific RR. A sawmill was erected on the site and the resulting comm. was called "Commencement City". The name was changed, in 1869, to Tacoma. New Tacoma was founded in 1873, when the RR arrived at a site 1.5 mi. S of the earlier Tacoma and a post office was established at the new townsite. New Tacoma became the co. seat in 1880 and, in 1884, the older

Pantages Theater will be New Performing Arts Facility, Tacoma, Washington

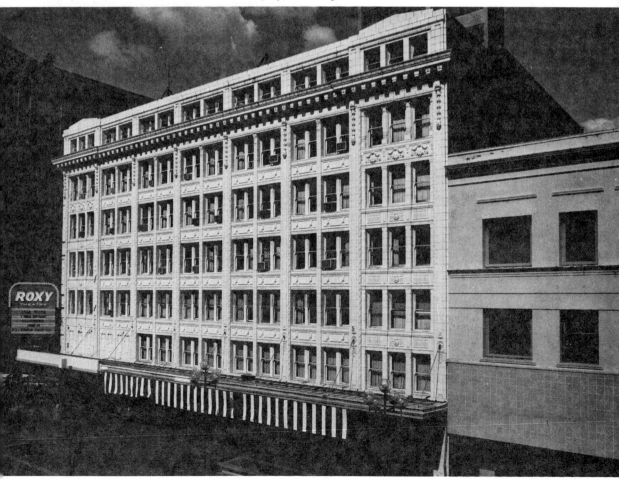

Tacoma and New Tacoma were consolidated into one city, called Tacoma. A transportation center, the city exported its first load of wheat in 1881. Annie Wright Seminary was established in the city in 1884 and the U of Puget Sound opened in 1886. In 1940, the city's suspension bridge earned the nickname "Galloping Gertie" when high winds caused it to bounce and fall apart. It has since been rebuilt. The city experienced rapid growth during WW II, due to the nearby military installations. Today, Tacoma, a distribution and industrial center, is the third largest city in WA.

GOVERNMENT. Tacoma has a council-mgr. form of govt. The nine council members, including the mayor as a voting member, are elected at large to four-year terms.

ECONOMY AND INDUSTRY. Govt. is the major employer in Tacoma, followed by trade, services, manufacturing and the military. Lumber and wood production is the primary manufacture industry, while the manufacture of furniture and chemicals, food processing and RR and machine repair are also important industries. Tacoma is a center of shipping and distribution. In June, 1979, the labor force for the Tacoma met. area was 173,600, while the rate of unemployment was 7.6%.

Central Tacoma, Washington

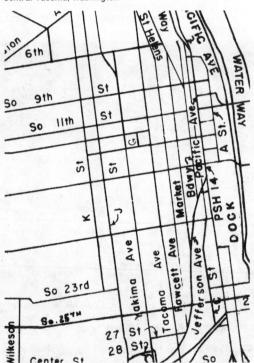

BANKING. There are 12 banking institutions in Tacoma. In 1978, total deposits for the six banks headquartered in the city were $943,161,000, while assets were $1,068,913,000. Banks include Puget Sound Natl., United Mutual Savings, State Mutual Savings, N Pacific, Tacoma and Union.

HOSPITALS. There are seven gen. care hosps. in Tacoma, Allenmore, Doctor's, Puget Sound, Tacoma Gen., St. Joseph's, Good Samaritan and Group Health. A children's hosp., the Mary Bridges, a V.A. Hosp., and a US Army medical facility are also located in the city.

EDUCATION. The U of Puget Sound, a privately-endowed liberal arts school under the auspices of the Methodist Church, is located in Tacoma. It awards bachelor and master degrees, and, in 1978, it enrolled approx. 4,000. Other institutions include the Pacific Lutheran U, Prometheus U, Ft.

Steilacoom Comm. Col., Tacoma Comm. Col., Faith Evangelical Seminary, Knapp Col. of Business, St. Joseph's Hosp., Tacoma Gen. Hosp., L. H. Bates Vocational-Technical Institute and Clover Park Vocational-Technical Education Center. Libs. include the Tacoma Public Lib. and the Pierce Co. Lib.

ENTERTAINMENT. Falstaf's Backstage Restaurant and Dinner Theater offers theater and dining entertainment in Tacoma. The W WA State Fair has been held in the city each Sept. since 1900, while the Payallup Valley Daffodil Festival is held each spring. The Tugs, a AAA farm team of the Cleveland Indians, offer Pacific League pro sports at Cheney Stadium, while the Loggers of the U of Puget Sound and the Raiders of Ft. Steilacoom Comm. Col. participate in intercollegiate sports.

ACCOMMODATIONS. There are several hotels and motels in Tacoma, including the Doric, TraveLodge and Holiday, Rodeway, Nendel's, Lakewood Motor and Sherwood inns.

FACILITIES. There are 1,432 acres of parks and playgrounds in the Tacoma city park system. The larger parks include Point Defiance, Swan Creek, Snakelake, Wapato, Titlow and Wright. The 640-acre Point Defiance Park contains woodland roads and trails, rose gardens, a Natural Habitat Aviary featuring birds from around the world, a deep sea aquarium, an otter display, Never Never Land (depicting storybook characters), a children's farm and animal zoo, Owen beach, boating and fishing facilities and a Japanese Garden. Wright Park contains a botanical conservatory with a large collection of orchids and tropical plants. Nearby is Mt. Rainer Natl. Park, providing 30 mi. of hiking and backpacking trails, numerous streams and lakes for fishing and nature walks. Also nearby is the NW Trek, a 548-acre wildlife park where visitors may observe animals native to the Pacific NW in their natural environment during walking tours or aboard enclosed trams. There are several public golf courses, including Spanaway, Meadow Park and Col. Tennis courts are provided at the Sprinker Recreation Center and throughout the city park system.

CULTURAL ACTIVITIES. Performing organizations in Tacoma include the Tacoma Symphony Orchestra, dance companies, U and col. theater groups, the Opera Society and the Little Theater. The WA State Historical Society Museum, one of the oldest on the W Coast, features collections devoted to the native Americans and the pioneers of the NW. Ft. Lewis Military Museum is dedicated to the preservation of the military history of the NW, while hand tools of the 1800s are on display at Old Ft. Nisqually. The Tacoma Art Museum provides art exhibits.

LANDMARKS AND SIGHTSEEING SPOTS. Job Carr Cabin, built in 1865, was the first house in Tacoma and is historically preserved. St. Peter's Church opened in 1873 and still stands today. Constructed in 1890, the Ezra Meeker Mansion was the home of a colorful pioneer who retraced the OR trail in a covered wagon when he was 78 years old. Old City Hall was constructed in 1893 and is now filled with shops. Tacoma has 32 buildings listed on the Natl. Register of Historic Places. One of the world's largest suspension bridges, Tacoma Narrows Bridge, is located in the city. It is 188' high and 2,800' long. The 150' tall Totem Pole, hand carved by Alaskan Indians, is the nation's tallest. Camp Six, also located in the city, is a replica of an early logging camp and is filled with photographs and tools used by early lumber jacks.

TAMPA
FLORIDA

CITY LOCATION-SIZE-EXTENT Tampa, the seat of Hillsborough Co. and the largest city on the W coast of the state, is located at the mouth of the Hillsborough River on Tampa Bay in W central FL and encompasses 84.5 sq. mi., a large portion of which is inland water, at 27°58' N lat. and 82°32' W long. The seat of Hillsborough Co, Tampa's greater met. area includes most of Hillsborough Co., approaches Pasco Co. to the N and extends into Pinellas Co. to the W, overlapping the met. area of St. Petersburg, which is located across Tampa Bay.

TOPOGRAPHY. The terrain of Tampa, which is situated in the coastal region of the Gulf on the FL peninsula on the E border of Tampa Bay, is very flat and laced with inland waters. Tampa Bay lies to the W of the city and Hillsborough Bay to the E and S. The city has a mean elev. of 19'.

CLIMATE. The climate of Tampa is humid sub tropical characterized by summer thundershowers, night ground fogs in winter (due to the flat terrain), and modified temps. thoughout the year due to the influence of the Gulf of Mexico and surrounding bays. The avg. annual mean temp. of 72.2°F ranges from monthly means of 61.1°F in Jan. to 82°F in Aug. Approx. 60% of the avg. annual rainfall of 48.62" occurs from June to Sept. RH ranges from 49% to 90%. Hurricanes are most likely to occur in June and Oct. Tampa lies in the ESTZ and observes DST.

FLORA AND FAUNA. Animals native to Tampa include the raccoon, opossum and whitetail deer. Common birds are the swallow, egret, heron, pelican, gull and blackbird. Frogs, salamanders, toads, fence lizards and kingsnakes as well as the venomous coral snake, water moccasin and rattlesnake, are found in the area. Typical trees are the oak, cypress, mango, mulberry and palm. Smaller plants include the palmetto, mangrove, bayberry, dayflower, honeysuckle and gladiolus.

POPULATION. According to the US census, the pop. of Tampa in 1970 was 277,714. In 1979, it was estimated that it had increased to 280,340.

ETHNIC GROUPS. In 1978, the ethnic distribution of Tampa was approx. 75% Caucasian, 19.7% Black and 14.5% Hispanic (a percentage of the Hispanic total is also included in the Caucasian total).

TRANSPORTATION. Interstate hwys. 4, 75 and 275, US hwys. 41, 92 and 301 and state Hwy. 60 provide major motor access to Tampa. *Railroad* service to the city is provided by the Seaboard Coast Line. *Airlines* serving Tampa Intl. Airport include BN, DL, EA, NA, NW, TW, US Air, Air FL and UA. The Peter O. Knight airport is available for private and corporate planes. *Bus lines* include Greyhound, Trailways and the local Tampa City. Tampa is a major US sea and fishing port.

COMMUNICATIONS. Communications, broadcasting and print media originating from Tampa are: *AM radio stations* WFLA 970 (NBC, MOR); WINQ 1010 (Indep., Relig.); WGBI 1050 (Indep., C&W); WTIS 1110 (Indep., C&W); WTMP 1150 (Mut. Blk.,); WDAE 1250 (ABC/I, Top 40) and WSLO 1300 (Indep., Relig., Span.) and WYOU 1500 (Indep., Span.); *FM radio stations* WUSF 89.7 (NPR, Clas. Educ.); WFLA 93.3 (Indep., Btfl. Mus.); WJYW 100.7 (Indep., Btfl. Mus.) and WRBQ 104.7 (Indep., Top 40); *television stations* WEDU Ch. 3 (PBS); WFLA Ch. 8 (NBC); WTSP Ch. 10 (ABC); WTVT Ch. 13 (CBS); WUSF Ch. 16 (PBS) WCLF Ch. 22 (Indep.) and WTOG Ch. 44 (Indep.); *press:* two major dailies serve the area, the *Tribune*, issued mornings, and the *Times*, issued evenings; other publications include the *Oracle, FL Sentinel-Bulletin, La Gaceta, FL Explorer, FL Trend, Lutz Party Line, MacDill Interbay Beacon, Citrus and Vegetables Magazine, The S Magazine, FL Builder* and *Family Pet.*

HISTORY. Native Americans of the Timucuan and Cahusa tribes originally inhabited the Tampa Bay area. In 1824, Robert J. Hackley of NY arrived in the region to build a plantation. Several months later, four companies of the US Army arrived to establish Ft. Brooke to protect the strategic harbor and supervise native Americans of the Seminole tribe, who had recently been placed in a reservation by the Army. The settlement that arose around the ft. became known as Tampa after the name bestowed on the area in 1601 by Antonio de Herrera, a Spanish cartographer. The first gen. store opened in 1828. In 1855, Tampa was incorporated. Although Union troops occupied Tampa during the Civil War, the city grew steadily in spite of the blockade. During the 1880s Henry B. Plant, a millionaire industrialist from Atlanta, laid the foundation for the

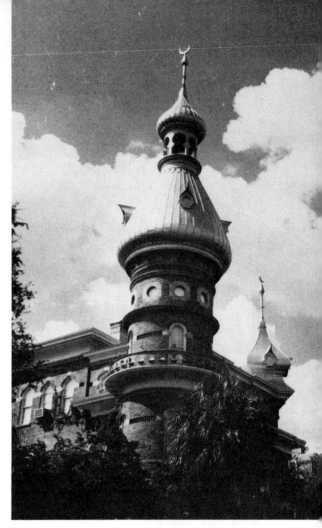

University of Tampa, Florida

city's tourist industry when he built a RR linking Tampa with the N. In 1886, Vincente M. Ybor established a cigar industry, and in 1888, phosphate mining began near the city. The Spanish American War (1898) added to Tampa's prosperity as the bay was used as an outfitting and embarkation port for American Troops. In the early 1900s, a real estate boom brought thousands of people to the city. Tourism increased and during WW II, Tampa became a shipbuilding center. Three AFB's were built, including MacDill. Industrial growth in the 1950s was remarkable. Today, Tampa is a major port for the phosphate and fishing industries.

GOVERNMENT. Tampa has a mayor-council form of govt. consisting of a council of seven members and a mayor. The council and mayor are elected at large to four-year terms.

ECONOMY AND INDUSTRY. Tampa is an important US seaport, handling approx. 48 million metric tons of cargo in 1978. It is the world's largest phosphate shipping port. Tampa is FL's second leading industrial city and has approx. 750 manufacturing plants, which employ approx. 15% of the city's workers. Major products include processed food and beverages. Tampa also produces chemicals, cigars, machinery and is the center of the world's largest citrus canning area. Tourism, the fishing industry and the MacDill AFB also make significant contributions to the economy. In June, 1979, the total labor force of the greater met. area, including St. Petersburg, was 590,500, while the rate of unemployment was 5.1%.

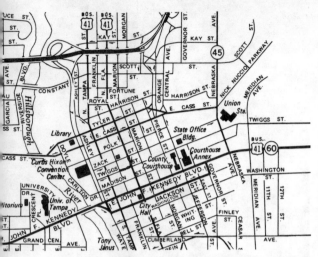

Central Tampa, Florida

BANKING. In 1978, total deposits for the 26 banks serving Tampa were $1,770,820,000, while assets were $2,182,647,000. Banks include First Natl. of FL, Exchange Natl., Met Bank & Trust Co., Flagship, Barnett, Landmark, Atlantic, Second Natl. and People's of Hillsborough City.

HOSPITALS. There are 16 gen., specialized and military hosps. in Tampa, including Memorial, Tampa Gen., Good Samaritan, Women's and St. Joseph's. A Veterans and a US Air Force Regional Hosp. are also located in the city.

EDUCATION. The U of Tampa, a private nonsectarian U founded in 1931, grants bachelor degrees and enrolled 2,274 in 1978. The U of S FL, a state U founded in 1960, offers bachelor, master and doctoral degrees and enrolled 23,091 in 1978. Other institutions include FL., Col., Hillsborough, Col., Tampa Gen. Hosp., Charon Williams Col., Butz Business Col. and Baptist Christian Col. The Tampa Hillsborough Co. Public Lib. serves the residents of the area.

ENTERTAINMENT. The Gaspariller Pirate Invasion, held annually each Feb., celebrates the historic invasion of Tampa Bay by the infamous pirate Jose Gaspar, and is FL's answer to the Mardi Gras. The State Fair in Mar. features FL agriculture, handicraft, arts and industry. Each Mar., Ybor City holds the Latin American Fiesta. Tampa is the home of the NFL-NFC Buccaneers football team and the NASL Rowdies pro soccer team. The U of S FL Golden Bulls participate in collegiate sports. Greyhound racing, horse racing and jai alai are available nearby.

Looking Across Hillsborough River, Tampa, Florida

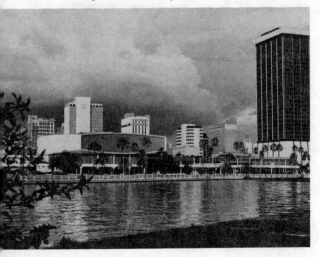

ACCOMMODATIONS. Hotels and motels in Tampa include the Downtown Hilton, Bay Harbor, Barclay Airport, Admiral Benbow, Causeway, Days, Hawaiian Village, several Holiday inns, the Host Intl. Hotel, the Tampa Airport Resort and Sheraton.

FACILITIES. Lowry Park houses a "Fairyland", featuring castles and characters from Mother Goose and other children's stories, as well as a small zoo, playground, miniature RR and amusement rides. Water sports are available at T. Davis Municipal Beach and other beaches. Public golf courses include Babe Zacharias, Loch Raven, Rocky Point and Rogers Park.

CULTURAL ACTIVITIES. Performing arts organizations serving Tampa include the FL Gulf Coast Symphony, the Tampa Concert Ballet, the San Carlo Opera Co. and the Tampa Ballet Theatre. The Henry B. Plant Museum features art objects and furnishings arranged according to period, while the Tampa Bay Art Center offers changing exhibits of paintings. The Museum of Science and Natural History is also located in Tampa.

LANDMARKS AND SIGHTSEEING SPOTS. Davis Islands are three man-made islands begun as a real estate venture and are now fine residential areas. Ybor City, virtually a self-contained city within itself, is home for most of the city's Cuban, Spanish and Italian pop. and contains the leading cigar factory in the US. Busch Gardens is a 300-acre park with more than 1,000 animals roaming the "African veldt". Trained animals and birds perform in separate theaters.

TOLEDO
OHIO

CITY LOCATION-SIZE-EXTENT. Toledo, the seat of Lucas Co.,encompasses 86 sq. mi. in NW OH at the W end of Lake Erie on both banks of the Maumee River, at 41°36' N lat. and 83°48' W long. The met. area includes the cities of Oregon to the E, Northwood to the E, Maumee to the S and Sylvania to the NW and extends S into Wood Co., E into Ottawa Co., W into Fulton Co. and N into Monroe Co., MI.

TOPOGRAPHY. Toledo lies in the Great Lakes Plains Region. The terrain is generally level with a slight slope towards the river and Lake Erie. The mean elev. is 587'.

CLIMATE. The climate of Toledo is continental and is modified by Lake Erie, which causes high humidity and excessive cloudiness. The avg. annual temp. of 49.7°F ranges from a Jan. mean of 25.7°F to a July mean of 73.2°F. The avg. annual rainfall of 31.59" is distributed evenly. Snowfall avgs. 39" annually, with most occurring during Dec. through Mar. The RH ranges from 52% to 90%. The avg. growing season is 160 days. Toledo lies in the ESTZ and observes DST.

FLORA AND FAUNA. Animals native to Toledo include the raccoon, opossum, whitetail deer, muskrat and squirrel. Common birds include the robin, blackbird, sparrow, cardinal (the state bird). and crow. Bullfrogs, garter snakes,salamanders, snapping turtles, toads and the venomous E massasauga rattlesnake are common to the area. Typical trees are the buckeye (the state tree), oak, maple, pine and elm. Smaller plants include the scarlet carnation (the state flower), honeysuckle, blackberry and rose.

POPULATION. According to the US census, the pop. of Toledo in 1970 was 383,818. In 1978, it was estimated that it had decreased to 356,100.

ETHNIC GROUPS. In 1978, the ethnic distribution of Toledo was approx. 83.8% Caucasian, 13.8% Black, 1.9% Hispanic, and 0.5% other races.

TRANSPORTATION. Interstate hwys. 75 and 80, US hwys. 20, 23 and 24 and state hwys. 2, 125 and 199 provide major motor access to Toledo. *Railroad* service is provided by AMTRAK, Chessie System, ConRail, Detroit & Toledo, Norfolk & W, Penn Central and Toledo, Angola & W. *Airlines* serving Toledo Express Airport are US Air, DL, EA, UA, Air FL, TW, Air WI and FL. *Bus lines* include Trailways, Greyhound, Shortway Charger Bus and the local Toledo Area Regional Transit Authority (TARTA). In 1978, the Port of Toledo handled 27,113,209 net tons of cargo.

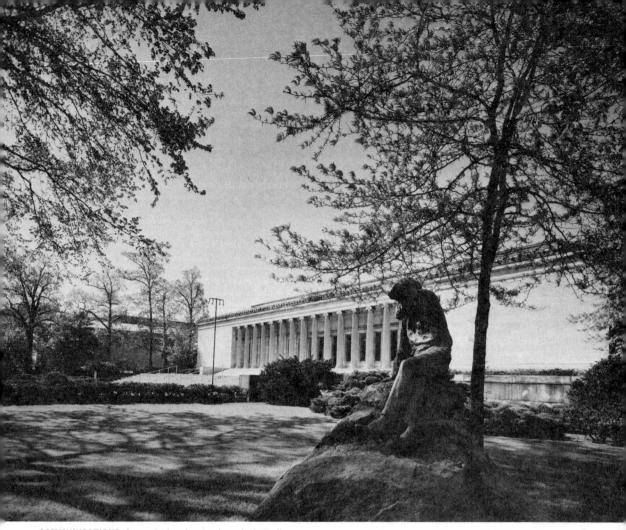

Museum of Art, Toledo, Ohio

COMMUNICATIONS. Communications, broadcasting and print media originating in Toledo are: *AM radio stations*: WCWA 1230 (ABC/E, Contemp., MOR); WSPD 1370 (NBC, MOR); WOHO 1470 (Indep., Top 40); WGOR 1520 (MBS, Relig.) and WTOD 1560 (ABC/I, C&W); *FM radio stations*: WAMP 88.3 (Indep., Soul, Contemp., News); WGTE 91.3 (NPR, Clas.); WWHE 92.5 (ABC/FM, Contemp., Rock); WKLR 99.9 (MBS/Blk.); WLQR 101.5 (Indep., Adult, MOR) and WIOT 104.7 (Indep., Progsv. Rock); *television stations*: WTOL Ch. 11 (CBS); Ch. 13 (NBC); WDHO Ch. 24 (ABC) and WGTE Ch. 30 (PBS); *press*: one major daily serves the area, the *Blade*, issued evenings; other publications include *Catholic Chronicle*, *The Collegian*, *Union Journal*, *American Flint*, *Jewish News* and *W Toledo Herald*.

HISTORY. The first inhabitants of the Toledo area were the native Americans of the Erie tribe. In 1794, after the Battle of Fallen Timbers, they ceded most of their lands remaining in the area at Ft. Industry. In 1817, the Port Lawrence settlement was established on the site of Ft. Industry. In 1833, this village merged with the village of Vistula to form Toledo. It is not clear why the name of Toledo was chosen, but according to local folklore, an interest in the author Washington Irving (then in Spain writing *Tales of Alhambra)*, led to the city's being named after Toledo, Spain. The 1835 solution of the "Toledo War", in which both OH and MI claimed Toledo, gave Toledo to OH and the upper peninsula to MI. The city was incorporated in 1837. Because of its strategic natural port location, Toledo immediately became a transportation center. The Erie & Kalamazoo RR, the first American RR W of the Alleghenies, completed in 1836, started in Toledo. During the 1840s, the Wabash and Erie, and Miami and Erie canals (each joining in Toledo), began operating in IN and OH. The intersecting transportation systems assured the city of its place as a major Great Lakes port. The discovery of oil and gas in the area encouraged the development of the glass industry. In 1888, the Libby Glass Co. was founded in the city by Edward Libby from MA, soon to be followed by Michael Owens, who began Owens Glass. After the turn of the century, the auto industry made its local emergence. An auto plant was opened in 1908. Auto parts manufacturing started on a major scale. Toledo soon became the largest oil and gas refining center between Chicago and the E Coast. Natural gas fuel provided impetus to make it the "glass capital of the world". During WW II, the jeep was developed in the city for the Army, and is still manufactured as a recreational vehicle. Today, Toledo ranks as one of the world's leading shippers of coal and the largest producer of auto parts.

GOVERNMENT. Toledo has a council-mgr. form of govt., consisting of a nine-member council, including the mayor, and a council-appointed mgr. All council members and the mayor are elected at large to two-year terms. The mayor is a voting member of the council.

ECONOMY AND INDUSTRY. Toledo has a diversified industrial base. Leading product areas are automotive, glass, petroleum, machinery and components, castings, coated fabrics, elevators, stampings, scales, electrical equipment, jet engines, food products, spray-

electrical equipment, jet engines, food products, spraying equipment, furnaces, metal working and plastics. It is an important transportation, warehousing and distribution center and is the regional center for the state's richest farm area. The Port of Toledo handled 27,113,209 net tons in 1978. The Toledo met. area labor force was 374,000 in June, 1979, while the unemployment rate was 6.8%. Spendable income per household in 1979 was approx. $18,000.

BANKING. In 1978, total deposits for the four banks headquartered in Toledo were $1,601,484,000, while assets were $1,985,496,000. Banks include Toledo Trust Co., First Natl., OH Citizens' Trust Co. and Huntington.

HOSPITALS. Nine gen. hosps. are located in Toledo, including Toledo, St. Vincent, Mercy, Riverside, Parkview, Medical Col., Flower, St. Luke's and St. Charles. The state psychiatric hospital is located here, as is a V.A. clinic.

EDUCATION. The U of Toledo, a state-supported U established in 1872, offers programs leading to degrees from bachelor to doctoral. In 1978, the U enrolled more than 17,400 students. The Medical Col. of OH, established in 1964, offers grad. training in 16 medical specialties. Offering both professional and grad. degrees, this institution enrolled more than 350 students in 1978. Michael J. Owens Technical Col., established in 1966, awards associate degrees. In 1978, the state-supported col. enrolled nearly 3,000 students. Other institutions located in the city include Toledo Bible Col., David Jr. Bus. Col., N Technical Institute, and Stautzenberger Col. of Bus. More than 82,000 students are enrolled in the city's public school system. Lib. facilities include the Toledo/Lucas Co. Public Lib. and the Toledo Bar Assn. Law Lib.

Central Toledo, Ohio

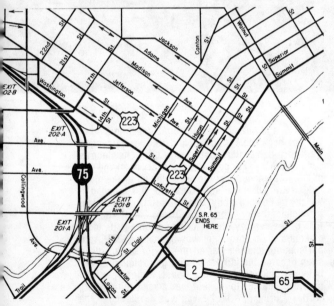

ENTERTAINMENT. The Westgate Dinner Theater provides dining entertainment in Toledo. Pro sports teams include the Goaldiggers (IHL, hockey), the Mudhens (IL, baseball) and the Troopers (women's football). Collegiate sports are offered by the U of Toledo Rockets.

ACCOMMODATIONS. Hotels and motels in Toledo include the Commodore Perry, Howard Johnson's and Holiday, Sheraton, Quality, Hillcrest, Ramada and Day's inns.

FACILITIES. Toledo offers more than 100 parks of varying sizes, comprising more than 2,000 acres and nine metroparks. Ottawa Park has a skating and hockey rink. Walbridge Park, on the river, has a boat launching ramp. Crosby Gardens Park offers trees, flowers and herb specimens. The city has 27 mi. of hiking trails, 20 mi. of horse trails, and 4.3 mi. of bicycle/fitness trails. The municipal zoo covers 33 acres and houses more

than 500 species of mammals, birds and reptiles and a large freshwater aquarium. Boating activity is concentrated in the many yacht clubs and marinas along the Maumee and Ottawa parks. There are 23 golf courses, including Collins Park, Ottawa and Detwiler. Public tennis courts are available through the city park system.

CULTURAL ACTIVITIES. There are three orchestras in Toledo—the Jack Runyon Orchestra, the Toledo Symphony Orchestra and the Johnny Knorr Orchestra. The Toledo Ballet Assn., the Opera Assn. and the Choral Society present regular performances. The U of Toledo and Bowling Green State U offer concerts and theatrical performances. Other theatrical groups include St. Hedwig's, the Village Players and the Toledo Repertoire. The Toledo Artists' Club offers regular exhibitions and the Arts Commission sponsors cultural activities. The Toledo Museum of Art has exhibits tracing art from ancient Egypt to the 20th century. The Blair Museum of Lithophanes and the Wolcott House Museum are also in the city.

LANDMARKS AND SIGHTSEEING SPOTS. Toledo's Old W End contains restored Victorian mansions. The Port Observation Deck and the Maumee Riverboat rides are also popular.

TOPEKA
KANSAS

CITY LOCATION-SIZE-EXTENT. Topeka, the capital of KS, is located on the KS River nearly 60 mi. above its junction with the MO River and encompasses 59.1 sq. mi. at 39°04' N lat. and 95°38' W long. Located in NE KS, it is near the geographical center of the US and is the seat of Shawnee Co. Its greater met. area includes most of Shawnee Co. and extends into the surrounding counties of Jefferson to the NE and Osage to the S.

TOPOGRAPHY. The terrain of Topeka is wide and flat along the KS River and is bordered on both sides by rolling prairie uplands. The city is close to the W edge of the prairie lands corn belt and the S edge of the glacial drift.

CLIMATE. The climate of Topeka is continental, characterized by large variations in year-to-year climatic conditions. The avg. yearly temp. of 54.7°F ranges from a Jan. mean 28.3°F to a July mean of 78.9°F. Most of the avg. annual rainfall of 33.38" occurs from May through Sept. Most of the snowfall occurs from Dec. through Mar. with an annual avg. of 21.4". RH ranges from 53% to 87%. The growing season avgs. 200 days. Disastrous storms in this area are possible, but infrequent. Topeka lies in the CSTZ and observes DST.

FLORA AND FAUNA. Animals native to Topeka include the raccoon, opossum, squirrel and deer. Common birds are the bluebird, cardinal, mockingbird and vulture. Bullfrogs, king snakes, toads, salamanders and collared lizards and snakes, including the venomous rattlesnake and copperhead inhabit the area. Typical trees are the oak, elm, willow and pine. Smaller plants include the sunflower, buckwheat, honeysuckle and ironweed.

POPULATION. According to the 1970 US census, the pop. of Topeka was 125,011. The projected 1980 census predicts an increase to 160,184.

ETHNIC GROUPS. In 1970, the ethnic distribution of Topeka was estimated to be 90.4% Caucasian, 8.3% Black and 1.4% foreign born.

TRANSPORTATION. Interstate hwys. 35 and 70 and US hwys. 24, 40, 59 and 75 and state Hwy. 4 provide major motor access to Topeka. *Railroads* serving the city include the Atchison, Topeka & Santa Fe, MO Pacific, Rock Island, Union Pacific and AMTRAK. *Airlines* serving Forbes Field include FL, while private facilities are available at the Topeka Billiard Airport. *Bus lines* serving the city include Intracity Transit Inc., Trailways and Greyhound.

COMMUNICATIONS. Communications, broadcasting and print media originating in Topeka are: *AM radio stations* WIBW 580 (CBS, News,

Talk); WREN 1250 (ABC/I, MOR); KEWI 1440 (Indep., Top 40) and KTOP 1490 (MBS, C&W); *FM radio stations* WIBW 97.3 (Indep., Top 40); KDUU 100.3 (MBS, Mod. Relig.); KTPK 106.9 (Indep., Mod. Ctry.) and KSWT 107.7 (Indep., Btfl. Mus.); *television stations* KTWU Ch. 11 (PBS); WIBW Ch. 13 (PBS); and KTSB Ch. 27 (NBC); *press:* three major dailies serve the city, the *Capital*, issued mornings, the *Journal*, issued evenings, and the *State Journal* (Sat. and Sun.); other publications include the *Daily Legal News*, *Capper's Weekly*, *KS Country Living*, *KS Farmer*, *KS Historical Quarterly*, *Journal of the KS Medical Society*, *KS Optometric Journal*, *KS Govt. Journal* and the *KS Stockman*.

HISTORY. Topeka was founded in 1854 by nine men who formed the Topeka Assn., a group of anti-slavery settlers mainly responsible for the establishment and early growth of KS. The city was incorporated in 1857. It was named the state capital after KS was admitted to the Union in 1861, following a decade of conflict between the abolitionists and the pro-slavery factions. During the conflict, the Free Soil Legislature had met in Topeka in 1856 and had been dispersed by fed. troops. Although slowed by the drought of 1860 and the Civil War, growth kept pace with the rebuilding and development efforts of the state after the war. Pop. in Topeka grew from 700 in 1862 to 5,000 in 1870. The RR started moving W from the city in 1869, and in 1878, the city became the headquarters and maintenance center for the Atchison, Topeka and Santa Fe RR. Today, the Santa Fe RR Co. repair shops are among the largest in the world.

GOVERNMENT. Topeka has a mayor-commission form of govt. under which the city is governed by a mayor and five commissioners, each of whom administers a dept. of the city: Mayor; Commissioner of Parks & Public Property; Commissioner of Streets and Public Improvements; Commissioner of Streets and Lighting and Commissioner of Finance and Revenue.

ECONOMY AND INDUSTRY. Products manufactured in Topeka include tires, freight cars and parts, yearbooks, paper, cellophane, pet food, food products and dairy products. In 1979, the total labor force of the greater met. area was approx. 100,200 while the rate of unemployment was 4.9%.

BANKING. There are 13 banks in Topeka. In 1978, total deposits for the 13 banks headquartered in the city were $770,136,000, while total assets were 916,012,000. Banks serving the city include First Natl. Bank, Merchant's Natl. Bank and Commerce Bank and Trust Co.

HOSPITALS. There are three gen. hosps. in Topeka; Memorial, St. Francis and Stormont-Vail. Specialized medical treatment is offered by the Menninger Foundation, which provides psychiatric and neurological treatment and research; the V.A.; Topeka State; KS Neurological and the Capper Foundation.

Central Topeka, Kansas

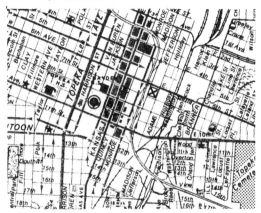

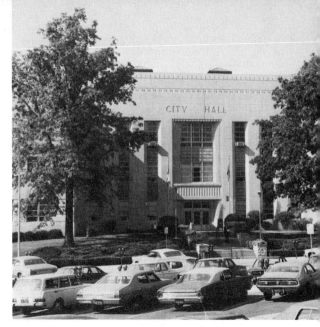

City Hall, Topeka, Kansas

EDUCATION. Washburn U, founded over a century ago as a Congregational school called Lincoln Col. enrolled 5,883 in 1978. Other colleges include the Clark School of Business and the Lattimore-Fink School of Medical Technology. There are over 16,000 students enrolled in the 69 public schools. Private schools include seven parochial elementary and high schools. The Topeka Public Lib. has over 26,000 volumes, two bookmobiles and a "book buggy" available to the residents.

ENTERTAINMENT: There are two dinner theaters in Topeka, the Showcase and Warehouse-on-the-Landing. Annual events include the Mexican Fiesta; Oktoberfest; and the Sunflower State Exposition, featuring entertainment, agricultural events and displays. Washburn U's Ichabods participate in intercollegiate sports.

ACCOMMODATIONS. There are several hotels and motels in Topeka, including the Ramada and Holiday inns, Howard Johnson's and Meadow Acres.

FACILITIES. Topeka's Gage Park covers 160 acres and features an Olympic size pool, picnic facilities, a miniature train for trips around the park, softball diamonds, the Reinisch Rose Garden, the Doran Rock Garden and the Topeka Zoological Park. Live plants and animals, habitat settings, climate conditions, cultural artifacts, visitor participation, interpretative graphics and audio visual learning experiences are incorporated and interrelated in the Zoo's Tropical Rain Forest tours. Golf courses are located at Forbes, Lake Shawnee, Sports Center, and the Topeka Public. Lake Shawnee offers camping and sailing facilities.

CULTURAL ACTIVITIES. The Topeka Civic Symphony Orchestra and the Comm. Concert Assn. sponsor concerts from Oct. to Apr. The Fine Arts Society presents chamber music at Washburn U White Concert Hall. Jazz and big band concerts are offered by the Topeka Jazz Workshop. Drama groups include the Washburn U Players and the Civic Theatre. Two ballet troupes, Ballet Mid-W and Topeka Ballet, are based in the city. A variety of concerts is presented at the Municipal Auditorium. The city maintains an Arts Council. There are more than 20 art galleries in Topeka. The Mulvane Art Museum on the campus of Washburn U contains collections of American painting and sculpture. The KS State Historical Society and Museum houses comprehensive exhibits of KS history including American and Indian galleries and agriculture and military halls.

LANDMARKS AND SIGHTSEEING SPOTS. The State House in Topeka contains John Stewart Curry and David Overmyer murals and other oil paintings as well as the "Pioneer Mother" and a bronze statue of Abraham Lincoln by Merrill Gage. Construction of the Ward-Meade Home and Botanical gardens overlooking the KS River Valley was begun in 1870. The gardens contain a variety of plants including many rare to the area. Potwin Place, an area dating back to 1887, contains stately homes and parks. Cedar Crest Gov.'s Mansion is a three-story Norman chateau built in 1928 which now serves as the gov.'s residence.

TORRANCE
CALIFORNIA

CITY LOCATION-SIZE-EXTENT. Torrance, a S CA ocean-side comm. in LA Co., is located 17 mi. SW of downtown LA and seven mi. NW of LA Harbor encompassing 21 sq. mi. at 33°49' N lat. and 118°18'5" W long. The W part of the city is bordered by the Pacific with a one and one-half mi. shore line. Part of the LA met. area, Torrance is the third largest city in LA Co. and is the 12th largest city in CA.

TOPOGRAPHY. Torrance lies in the relatively flat Pacific coastal plain with coastal mt. ranges to the N and E of the city. The mean elev. is 75'.

CLIMATE. The climate of Torrance is moderate, influenced by the nearby coastal mt. ranges, and is warmer and more humid than that of areas further inland. The avg. annual temp. of 62°F ranges from monthly means of 55°F during Jan. to 70°F during July. The annual rainfall of 12.22" occurs mostly during winter. RH ranges from 55% to 87%. Torrance is in the PSTZ and observes DST.

FLORA AND FAUNA. Animals native to Torrance include the opossum, gopher and skunk. Common birds are the house finch, scrubjay, starling, gull and egret. Pond turtles, tree frogs, lizards and toads as well as the venomous Pacific rattlesnake are also in the area. Typical trees are the oak, cork, fir, pine and willow. Smaller plants include the poppy, chaparral shrub, bunch grass, cinquefoil, tarweed and delphinium.

POPULATION. According to the US census, the population of Torrance in 1970 was 134,584. In 1978, it was estimated that it had decreased to approx. 128,593.

ETHNIC GROUPS. In 1978, the racial distribution of Torrance was approx. 85.99% Caucasian, .36% Black, 4.61% Hispanic, and 6.80% Asian (a percentage of the Hispanic total is also included in the Caucasian total).

TRANSPORTATION. Interstate Hwy. 405 and state hwys. 1, 91 and 107 provide major motor access to Torrance. *Railroads* serving the city are Santa Fe and Southern Pacific. All major *airlines* serve LA Intl. Airport, 11 mi. N of Torrance. The Torrance Municipal Airport offers general aviation facilities. *Bus lines* serving the city include Greyhound, the S CA Rapid Transit District and the local Torrance Transit System.

Central Torrance, California

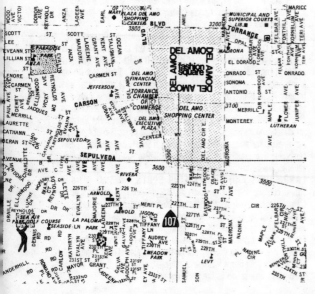

COMMUNICATIONS. Communications, broadcasting and print media originating from Torrance are: *FM radio station* KNHS 89.7 (Indep., Rock) and KFOX 93.7 (Indep.); no *AM radio stations* or *television stations* originate from the city, which receives broadcasting from nearby LA; *press*: one major daily serves the city, the *Daily Breeze*, issued evenings and Sundays; other publications include the weekly *News* and *Press-Herald*.

HISTORY. Torrance was founded in 1911 by Jared Sidney Torrance, a Pasadena real estate promoter who purchased portions of the Rancho San Pedro for a "garden-industrial" planned comm. It was incorporated in 1921. The Pacific Electric RR's Red Car trans. system, at the time the world's longest interurban electric railway, provided easy commuting for workers who moved to the city. In the early 1920s, the city expanded when the large Torrance oil field was discovered. Steady growth was maintained during the Great Depression due to Torrance's sound industrial foundation. In

1912 Gateway to Torrance, California

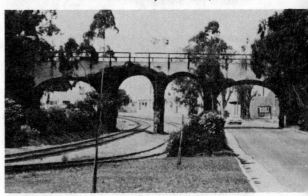

1936, construction began on the Civic Center, styled in "W.P.A. Moderne". During WW II, the city's economy boomed as it met defense requirements for the war effort. After the war, thousands of GI's took advantage of Torrance's mass-produced housing and moved to the city. Today, Torrance is the third largest city in LA Co.

GOVERNMENT. Torrance has a mayor-council mgr. form of govt. consisting of a seven-member council including the mayor, who is a voting member, and a council-appointed mgr. The mayor and council members are elected to four-year terms. The city clerk and the city treasurer in Torrance are also elected at large.

ECONOMY AND INDUSTRY. There are over 500 manufacturing plants in Torrance. Major products include steel, petroleum products, paints, aerospace equipment, plastic and electronics products. In 1978, the median household effective buying income was $20,664.

BANKING. There are 30 banks and 19 savings and loan assns. in Torrance. In 1978, total deposits for the one bank headquartered in the city were $27,668,000, while assets were $32,452,000. Banks include Torrance Natl., Union, United CA and CA First Natl.

HOSPITALS. There are three gen. care hosps. in Torrance, Harbor Gen., Little Company of Mary and Torrance Memorial. The Del Amo Hosp., an acute psychiatric unit, offers specialized medical treatment.

EDUCATION. El Camino Jr. Col., a publicly supported two-year institution, offers programs leading to the associate degree in transfer and terminal courses and enrolled 355 in 1978. The Unified School District is comprised of 21 elementary, seven middle, five high schools and one special education school. Total enrollment in 1978 was 24,586. The city is served by the Torrance Public Lib. and its five branches.

ENTERTAINMENT. Torrance annually hosts an Armed Forces Day

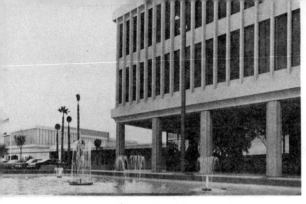

Civic Center, Torrance, California

celebration, a surf festival and an aqualade. El Camino Jr. Col.'s Warriors participate in area-wide intercollegiate sports.

ACOMMODATIONS. There are several hotels and motels in Torrance, including the El Rancho Motel, Holiday and Ramada inns.

FACILITIES. The Torrance met. park system includes 18 public parks and numerous playgrounds. Camping facilities are provided in El Nido Park, while El Retiro has lighted tennis courts and the new Delthorne features a jogging track.

CULTURAL ACTIVITIES. Dramatic productions are staged by the Children's Experimental Theatre and El Camino Col. in the Civic Center and Joslyn Center, the Torrance Music Festival is held each Oct.

LANDMARKS AND SIGHTSEEING SPOTS. The "Hollywood Riviera" section of Torrance contains many gracious homes, most of Italian-Mediterranean architecture. St. Joseph's Mission, constructed in 1919, originally served a comm. of Indians and Hispanics. Other buildings dating from the early 1900s include Torrance High School (1917), the Pacific Electric Depot (1912), the United CA Bank (1918) and El Roi Tan (1912), as well as private homes. The Alpine Village features Bavarian food, merchandise and entertainment. The original gateway to the city, the Bridge, was built by a RR company, and is still standing.

TRENTON
NEW JERSEY

CITY LOCATION-SIZE-EXTENT. Trenton, the state capital and seat of Mercer Co., encompasses 7.5 sq. mi. in W central NJ on the E bank of the Delaware River, 30 mi. from Philadelphia and 60 mi. from NYC, at 40°13' N lat. and 74°46' W long. The greater met. area extends across the river into Bucks Co., PA.

TOPOGRAPHY. The terrain of Trenton, situated in the Atlantic coastal plain, is characterized by compara-

tively flat land which slopes gently upward from near SL on the S to elevs. of approx. 500' to the N and NE. The Atlantic Ocean is approx. 40 mi. E of the city. The mean elev. is 50'.

CLIMATE. The climate of Trenton is continental, characterized by winds from the interior of the nation. The Appalachian Mts. to the W of the city moderate arctic air masses which frequently approach from the SE. The avg. annual temp. of 53.9°F ranges between monthly means of 32.2°F in Jan. and 75.7°F in July. The avg. annual rainfall of 43.85" is well distributed throughout the year. Coastal storms produce most of the 23.4" of avg. annual snowfall. The RH ranges from 46% to 79%. The sun shines an avg. of 60% of the daylight hours, with winter percentages only slightly lower than those of summer. The avg. growing season is 209 days. Trenton lies in the ESTZ and observes DST.

FLORA AND FAUNA. Animals native to Trenton include the opossum, whitetail deer, muskrat, mink, otter, raccoon and shrew. Common birds are the robin, bluebird, cardinal, bluejay and wren. Frogs, salamanders and turtles, as well as the venomous timber rattlesnake and copperhead, are found in the area. Typical trees are the red oak, maple, chestnut and ash. Smaller plants include the violet and cattail.

POPULATION. According to the US census, the pop. of Trenton in 1970 was 104,638. In 1980 it was estimated that it had decreased to 104,600.

ETHNIC GROUPS. In 1978, the ethnic distribution of Trenton was approx. 45% Caucasian, 51% Black, 3% Hispanic, 0.5% Asian and 0.5% other.

TRANSPORTATION. Interstate hwys. 95 and 295, US hwys. 1, 130 and 260 and state hwys. 29, 31 and 33 provide major motor access to Trenton. *Railroads* serving the area are AMTRAK, ConRail and IL Central Gulf. One *airline* serves Mercer Co. Airport—US Air. *Bus lines* include Suburban, Trailways and Greyhound and the local Mercer Metro.

COMMUNICATIONS. Communications, broadcasting and print media originating in Trenton are: *AM radio stations* WTTM 920 (MBS, Adult Contemp.); WBUD 1260 (Indep., All News) and WTNJ 1300 (Mut. Blk., Jazz); *FM radio stations* WTSR 91.3 (Col., Progsv., Educ.); WCHR 94.5 (Indep., Relig.); WPST 97.5 (Indep., Adult Rock) and WBJH 101.5 (NBC, Btfl. Mus.); *television station* WJNT Ch. 52 (PBS); *press:* two major dailies serve the area, the *Times,* issued evenings, and the *Trentonian,* issued mornings; other publications include *Mercer Co. Messenger, Hamilton Life, The Monitor, Times-Advertiser, NJ Business, NJ Municipalities, NJEA Review* and *Spotlight.*

HISTORY. Native Americans of the Delaware tribe inhabited the area of present-day Trenton when it was founded in 1679 by Quaker farmers led by Mahlon

World War I War Memorial, Trenton, New Jersey

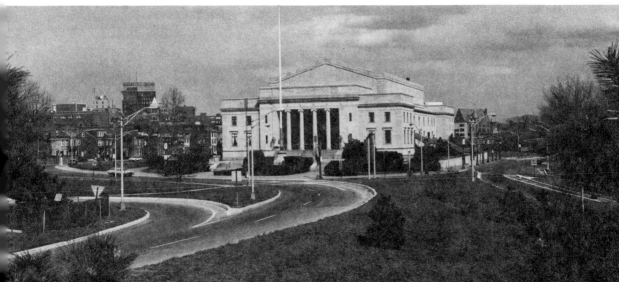

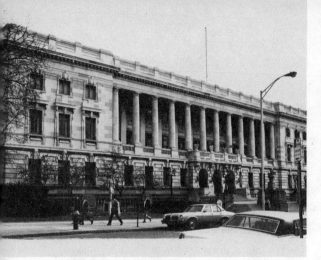

City Hall, Trenton, New Jersey

Stacy. The site, known as "The Falls" due to its location near the falls of the Delaware River, was sold by Mahlon Stacy, Jr. during the early 1700s to William Trent, Speaker of the House of Assembly. Renamed Trent's Town in 1719, the settlement later became Trenton. The comm. became a primary stopping point on the colonial stage line between NYC and Philadelphia. In 1776, Gen. George Washington led his army across the ice-clogged Delaware River near Trenton to surprise the Hessian garrison and take 1,000 prisoners. A week later, the Second Battle of Trenton was fought and Washington's army defeated the British troops under Gen. Charles Cornwallis. The city served as the nation's capital for two months in 1784, with Congress moving to NY the following year, and, in 1790, it became the NJ capital. It was incorporated in 1792. During the 1800s, Trenton developed into an industrial and trade center and a flow of factory workers into the city greatly increased its pop. After the turn of the 20th century, Trenton became the nation's leading producer of pottery and a major manufacturer of steel and rubber goods. A move to the suburbs, beginning in 1920, created a decline in Trenton's pop. Today, about 29% of the capital city's labor force are employed by state govt.

GOVERNMENT. Trenton has a mayor-council form of govt. The mayor and the seven council members are elected at large to four-year terms.

ECONOMY AND INDUSTRY. The largest employer in Trenton is govt., which employs approx. 29% of the labor force. Principal manufactured products are steel, electronics, processed foods, packed meats and apparel. In June, 1979, the met. area's labor force totaled 161,400, while the rate of unemployment was 5.5%. The avg. 1978 per capita income was $5,100.

Central Trenton, New Jersey

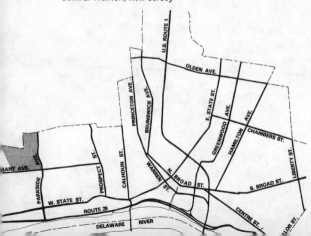

BANKING. In 1978, total deposits for the five banks headquartered in Trenton were $1,223,508,000, while total assets were $1,503,790,000. Banks include NJ Natl., Natl. State, Broad Street Natl. and Capitol State.

HOSPITALS. There are three hosps. in Trenton—Mercer Medical Center, St. Francis and Helene Fuld. The Trenton Psychiatric Hosp. is also located in the city.

EDUCATION. Trenton State Col., a liberal arts col. established in 1855 as the NJ State Normal and Model School, and upgraded in 1958 to state college status, awards the bachelor and master degrees. The 1978 enrollment was approx. 10,800. Rider Col., founded in 1865 as the Trenton Business Col., currently awards associate, bachelor and master degrees. In 1978 it enrolled approx. 870. Other institutions include Thomas A. Edison Col. and Mercer Co. Comm. Col. The city's 23 public schools enrolled approx. 17,000 in 1978. Lib. facilities include the Trenton Free Public Lib., the NJ State Lib. and the Mercer Co. Lib., with seven branches.

ENTERTAINMENT. Annual events in Trenton include St. Hedwig's Festival, Heritage Day and, in Sept., a Feast of Lights. The Trenton State Col. Lions and Mercer Co. Comm. Col. teams participate in intercollegiate sports. A soccer team participates in Italian-American Natl. Soccer Club competitions. The Champales offer pro softball.

ACCOMMODATIONS. There are many motels and hotels in Trenton, including Trenton Motor Lodge, the Inn of Trenton and Howard Johnson's.

FACILITIES. The Trenton park system includes Cadwalader, Stacy, Columbus, Mill Hill and N-25 Regional parks. Cadwalader Park contains a zoo and deer paddock. Nearby Washington Crossing State Park features a state forest nursery and the Pack Memorial Arboretum, containing native trees and shrubs. Public tennis courts can be found at Mercer Co. public indoor Tennis Center.

CULTURAL ACTIVITIES. The Greater Trenton Symphony Orchestra performs in the Trenton Soldiers' and Sailors' War Memorial Building, the city's concert hall. A Summer Festival of Performing Arts is held in the Open Air Theatre. Concerts and lectures are offered at the NJ State Museum, which houses art and science exhibits and a planetarium. Also available are the Trenton City Museum and The Contemporary Museum, which features Victorian restorations. The Flag Museum, which has an exhibit on the evolution of the American Flag, is located at Washington Crossing State Park.

LANDMARKS AND SIGHTSEEING SPOTS. The State House Historic District in Trenton has many historic homes and buildings displaying architectural styles which span the 18th, 19th and 20th centuries. Mill Hill Historic District, a residential section, was the location of the city's first industry, a grist mill. Old Barracks, one of the finest colonial barracks still standing in the country, were occupied at various times by British, Hessian and Continental troops and by Tory refugees. Trent House, the residence of Chief Justice William Trent and many other prominent men, is furnished in 1700s style and is famous for its curtains, which are copies of old fabrics. The Friends' Meeting House has housed the British Dragoons, American troops and a meeting of the convention of the NJ province. The old Masonic Lodge contains the gavel used by George Washington when he was a member of the Williamsburg Lodge. The Watson House, built in 1708 from stone and pegged timber, contains an underground, spring-fed vault. George Washington held a council of war on Jan. 2, 1777, in the Douglas Home. Other interesting locations include the Eagle Tavern, Berkeley Square and the Kelsey Building.

TUCSON
ARIZONA

CITY LOCATION-SIZE-EXTENT. Tucson, the seat of Pima Co., encompasses 91.6 sq. mi. on the Santa Cruz River at the foot of the Catalina Mts. in SE AZ, approx. 60 mi. N of the Mexico border, at 32°07' N lat. and 110°56' W long. The greater met. area extends N into Pinal Co.

TOPOGRAPHY. The terrain of Tucson, which is situated in the Basin and Range region of AZ, varies from flat to gently rolling, with many dry washes. Mts. to the N, E

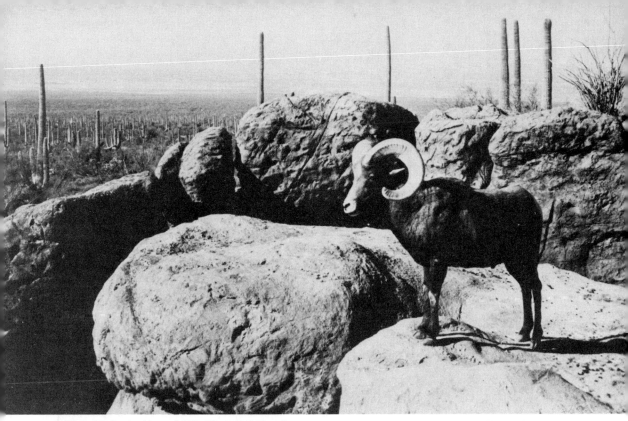

Bighorn sheep in desert setting, Tucson, Arizona

and S attain elevs. of over 5,000'. The mean elev. is 2,386'.

CLIMATE. The climate of Tucson is arid, characterized by a long hot season which begins in Apr. and ends in Oct. The avg. annual temp. of 67.4°F varies from monthly means of 50.3°F in Jan. and 86°F in July, while it is not uncommon for daytime temps. to reach 100°F during the summer. Approx. 50% of the avg. annual rainfall of 11.13" occurs during July through Sept. Occasional flash floods occur during the July through Sept. thunderstorms. The RH ranges from 16% to 65%. The annual snowfall avgs. 1.4". The growing season avgs. 250 days. Tucson lies in the MSTZ and does not observe DST.

FLORA AND FAUNA. Animals native to Tucson include the kangaroo rat, ringtail, javalina, bobcat, coyote, bat and jack rabbit. Typical birds include the roadrunner, hummingbird and pygmy owl. Horned lizards, leopard frogs, spadefoot toads and yellow mud turtles, as well as the venomous tiger rattlesnake, AZ coral snake and gila monster, may be found in the area. Typical trees include the pinyon and juniper. Smaller plants include the creosote bush, salt bush, prickly pear cactus, white bursage and paloverde.

POPULATION. One of the fastest growing cities of the 1970s, Tucson experienced a big increase in pop. between 1970 and 1977. According to the US census, the pop. of Tucson in 1970 was 262,933. In 1978, it was estimated that it had increased to 311,400.

ETHNIC GROUPS. In 1978, the ethnic distribution of Tucson was approx. 94.36% Caucasian, 3.72% Black, 22.8% Hispanic, 0.5% Asian and 1.4% other (a percentage of the Hispanic total is also included in the Caucasian total).

TRANSPORTATION. Interstate hwys. 10 and 19, US Hwy. 89 and state Hwy. 86 provide major motor access to Tucson. *Railroads* serving the city are AMTRAK, Pacific Fruit Express Co., Rock Island Lines and S Pacific. Ryan Field provides small craft facilities, while *airlines* serving Tucson Intl. Airport include Aero Mexico, Baja Cortez, Cochise Imperial, BN, CO, TW, FL, AA, RW and NC. *Bus lines* serving the city include Greyhound, Trailways and the local Sun Tran Transit System.

COMMUNICATION. Communications, broadcasting and print media originating from Tucson are: *AM radio stations* KIKX 580 (ABC/C, C&W); KEVT 690 (Indep., Span.); KCEE 790 (Indep., MOR); KMGX 940 (ABC/E, MOR); KTKT 990 (Indep., Top 40); KCUB 1290 (Indep., C&W); KHYT 1330 (MBS,

MOR); KTUC 1400 (ABC/I, MBS, News, Info., Sports); KOPO 1450 (CBS, MOR); KAIR 1490 (Indep., Btfl. Mus.); KUAT 1550 (Indep., Jazz, Talk) and KXEW 1600 (Indep., Span.); *FM radio stations* KUAT 90.5 (NPR, Clas.); KWFM 92.9 (ABC/FM, Rock, Progsv.); KRQQ 93.7 (Indep., Top 40); KAIR 94.9 (Indep., Btfl. Mus.); KCEE 96.1 (Indep., Btfl. Mus.); KFMM 99.5 (Indep., Relig.); *television stations* KVOA Ch. 4 (NBC); KUAT Ch. 6 (PBS); KGUN Ch. 9 (ABC); KZAZ Ch. 11 (Indep.) and KOLD Ch. 13 (CBS); *press*: two major dailies serve the area, the *Citizen*, issued evenings, and the *Star*, printed mornings; other publications include *AZ Daily Wildcat, AZ Catholic Lifetime, American Astrology* and *Tucson Magazine*.

HISTORY. A Hohokam Indian ranch existed on the site of present-day Tucson as early as 800 AD. In 1757, Father Bernard Middendorf, S.J., established a mission, but was forced by hostile Indians to abandon it later that year. Native Americans of the Sobaipuri tribe were transferred to the Tucson Indian Village in 1762 by an official of the Royal Spanish Army, who named the area San Jose. In 1775, Lt. Col. Don Hugo O'Connor, of the Royal Spanish Army, laid out the Presidio of San Augustin del Tucson on the site of the Stook-zone—"water at foot of black mt."—Indian Village. A comm. grew as Mexicans and Indians settled around the completed presidio. The first Tucson city council met in 1813, but disbanded the following year when King Ferdinand VII of Spain abolished the constitution. By 1820, the pop. of the village had grown to 181. Part of Mexico until the Gasden Purchase, Tucson came under US control in 1853. The first Butterfield Overland Mail coach reached Tucson in 1858. Two years later the village's pop. stood at 620. Tucson was occupied first by Confederate and later by Union troops during the Civil War. In 1864, Tucson was proclaimed a town by the govt., and fed. troops were removed over the protests of citizens who feared Apache attacks. The city served as the state capitol from 1867 through 1877. By 1870, more than 3,000 lived in Tucson, which was

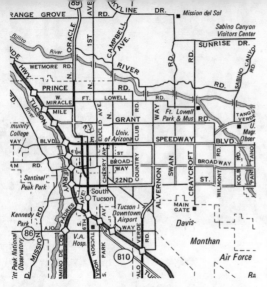

Tuscon, Arizona

incorporated as a village the following year. In 1877, Tucson was incorporated as a city. The city had a pop. of 7,007 when the S Pacific RR arrived in 1880. AZ U was founded in 1885. During the early 1900s, Tucson became a popular health and winter resort center due to its dry desert air. By 1969, the area had become the major copper mining region in the country. One of the oldest cities in the US, today Tucson is the home of Davis-Monthan AFB, Tactical Air Command.

GOVERNMENT. Tucson has a council-mgr. form of govt. The five council members, including the mayor as a voting member, are elected at large to two-year terms.

ECONOMY AND INDUSTRY. Major industries in Tucson are mining, construction, food products, stone, clay and glass products, printing, publishing, machinery and electronics. Tourism is an important industry, as the dry desert air and sunshine make the city a popular winter resort. The Davis-Monthan AFB is also a major employer. The 1979 labor force for the Tucson met. area was 185,100, while the rate of unemployment was 4.9%. The avg. per capita income in 1978 was $6,786.

BANKING. In 1978, total deposits for the five banks headquartered in Tucson were $99,108,000, while total assets were $112,800,000. Banks include Valley Natl., First Natl., AZ Bank, United and Great W.

HOSPITALS. There are seven gen. hosps. in Tucson, including El Dorado, Kino, St. Joseph, St. Mary's, Tucson Gen. and Tucson Medical Center. Several psychiatric facilities and a V.A. hosp. are also located in the city.

EDUCATION. The state-supported U of AZ, established in Tucson in 1891 as a land-grant col., awards grad., pro and undergrad. degrees. In 1978, it enrolled more than 28,000. The publicly-supported Pina Co. Comm. Col. awards associate degrees and, in 1978, it enrolled more than 21,000. The 99 schools in the Tucson public school system enrolled approx. 59,000 in 1978. Libs. include the Tucson Public Lib., the AZ Historical Society and the AZ State Museum Libs.

ENTERTAINMENT. Among the annual events in Tucson are the Square and Round Dance Festival and the Joe Garagiola Tucson Open. Rodeos include Fiesta De Los Vaqueros and the U of AZ Rodeo. Dinner theaters include the Play Box, Saguaro and Gas Light. The Gunners of WBA basketball, the Rangers of PCL baseball and the Rustlers of PHL hockey provide pro sports entertainment, while the U of AZ Wildcats participate in intercollegiate sports. The Cleveland Indians of AL baseball maintain winter training quarters in Tucson. Horse racing is held at Rillito Downs.

ACCOMMODATIONS. There are several hotels and motels in Tucson, including the Marriott, Doubletree, Granada Royale, Aztec, Santa Rita, Sheraton-Pueblo, Plaza Intl. and Hilton, Ramada and Holiday inns.

FACILITIES. There are 76 parks in the Tucson park system, including Palo Verde, Eastmoor, Himmel and Lakeside. Nearby is Tucson Mt. Park, encompassing 30,000 acres of the Tucson Mts. and embracing one of the largest areas of saguaro and natural desert growth in the SW. Also located

in the area are the Garden of Gethsemane, Sentinel Peak, Wish Shrine and the Tucson Botanical Gardens. Public golf courses are available at Arthur Park, Cliff Valley, El Rio and Randolf golf courses, while public tennis courts are provided at the Randolf Tennis Center.

CULTURAL ACTIVITIES. Tucson is served by the Tucson Symphony, Civic Orchestra, AZ Theater Co. and AZ Opera Co. The Tucson Museum of Art features crafts, textiles, furnishings and fine arts representing the area's Latin American heritage. Pioneer artifacts are housed at the AZ Historical Society, and the AZ State Museum emphasizes the archeology and ethnology of the state. Ft. Lowell Museum contains four rooms furnished as they were in 1885 and displays military equipment. The Mineral Museum is located on the U of AZ campus.

LANDMARKS AND SIGHTSEEING SPOTS. Many of the exhibits in the Grace H. Flandrau Planetarium, in Tucson, encourage visitor experimentation. The Dome Theater, located on the first floor, contains an atmospherium. The John C. Fremont House, built in 1858, is a restored Mexican-American casa occupied by Fremont during his term as territorial gov. Nearby Mission San Xavier de Bac is a well preserved example of early Spanish mission architecture.

TULSA
OKLAHOMA

CITY LOCATION-SIZE-EXTENT. Tulsa, the seat of Tulsa Co., encompasses 181.4 sq. mi. on both banks of the AR River in NE OK, approx. 105 mi. NE of OK City, at 36°12' N lat. and 95°54' W long. The greater met. area includes the cities of Turley to the N and Sapulpa to the SW and extends into the counties of Wagoner to the E, Okmulgee to the S, Creek to the W, Osage to the NW, Washington to the N and Rogers to the NE.

TOPOGRAPHY. The terrain of Tulsa, which is situated in the prairie plains, is gently rolling. There are many lakes in the area and the AR River runs through the city. The mean elev. is 617'.

CLIMATE. The climate of Tulsa is continental, while its intermediate position between the N and the S enables it to escape extremes in winter or summer temps. The avg. annual temp. of 60.0°F ranges from a Jan. mean of 37°F to a July mean of 82.6°F.Most of the avg. annual rainfall of 38" occurs during the late spring, summer and early fall, while most of the 9.3" avg. annual snowfall occurs during Jan. and Feb. The area is subject to violent windstorms and tornadoes throughout the year, although most occur during spring and early summer. The RH ranges from 49% to 86%. The growing season avgs. 216 days. Tulsa is in the CSTZ and observes DST.

FLORA AND FAUNA. Animals native to Tulsa include the raccoon, opossum, coyote and whitetail deer. Common birds are the mockingbird, bluebird, robin, catbird, scissor-tailed flycatcher and swallow. Snapping turtles, box turtles, bull frogs, toads and the venomous rattlesnake, cottonmouth and copperhead are found in the area. Common trees are the pine, oak, sycamore and sweet gum. Smaller plants include the honeysuckle, Indian paintbrush and black-eyed Susan.

POPULATION. According to the US census, the pop. of Tulsa in 1970 was 330,350. In 1978, it was estimated that it had increased to 360,000.

ETHNIC GROUPS. In 1978, the racial distribution of Tulsa was approx. 86.9% Caucasian, 10.7% Black, 1.4% Hispanic and 1.0% other.

TRANSPORTATION. The Glencoe and Muskogee turnpikes, interstate Hwy. 44, US hwys. 64, 66, 75 and 169 and state hwys. 11 and 51 provide major motor access to Tulsa. *Railroads* serving the city include Burlington N, ConRail, Frisco, IL Central Gulf, Katy, Santa Fe, S Pacific and Union Pacific. *Airlines* serving Tulsa Intl. Airport include AA, BN, CO, DL, FL, OZ and TW. *Bus lines* include K. G. Lines , Trailways, Greyhound and the local Met. Tulsa Transit Authority. The Port of Catoosa is part of the McClellan-Kerr AR River Navigation System.

COMMUNICATIONS. Communications, broadcasting and print media originating from Tulsa are: *AM radio stations* KRMG 740 (Indep., MOR); KAKC 970 (ABC/C, Contemp.); KFMJ 1050 (Indep., Relig.); KVOO 1170 (Indep., C&W); KXXO 1300 (CBS, All News) and KELI 1430 (Indep., Rock); *FM radio stations* KWGS 89.5 (Indep., Clas., Jazz); KBEZ 92.9 (Indep., Btfl. Mus.); KWEN 95.5 (Indep., Btfl. Mus.); KRAV 96.5 (Indep., Adult Contemp.); KMOD 97.5 (Indep., Progsv.); KCFO 98.5 (MBS, Relig.) and KKUL 103.3 (ABC/FM, Top 40); *television stations* KTEW Ch. 2 (NBC); KOTV Ch. 6 (CBS); KTUL Ch. 8 (ABC) and KOED Ch. 11 (PBS); *press:* two major dailies serve the area, the *Tribune,* issued evenings; and *World* issued mornings; other publications include *Star, Oil and Gas Journal, OK Eagle, Abundant Life, Tulsa Co. News, OK Business Magazine, Future-The Official Publication of the US Jaycees, OK Monthly* and *Military Collectors News.*

HISTORY. Native Americans of the Creek nation settled at the site of present-day Tulsa in the 1830s. They named their settlement Tallassee, after their old village in AL, and in time this name was shortened to Tulsa. In 1848, Lewis Perryman, himself a Creek, opened a trading post on his ranch near the AR River. For the next 30 years, Tulsa remained a small cattle town. A post office was opened on the ranch of Perryman's son, George, in 1879. Less than 1,000 people lived in the comm. in 1882, but construction of the RR that year brought more white settlers to the area and led to Tulsa's development as a cattle-shipping point. The town was incorporated in 1898, and by the turn of the century Tulsa's pop. stood at 1,390. The sleepy cattle town boomed in 1901 when oil was discovered at Red Fork. In 1905, oil was found in the immense Glenn Pool Field and Tulsa was established as a petroleum center. The town's pop. soared to 7,298 by 1907, and the following year, in 1908, Tulsa was chartered as a city. Between 1920 and 1930 the pop. nearly doubled—from 72,075 to 141,258. Following that surge, Tulsa's growth nearly halted for a decade, but was boosted during WW II by the influx of rural workers who arrived to work in the defense industries and the large bomber plant built by the govt. The plant is used today by private firms to manufacture commercial and industrial aircraft. In 1970, the long-awaited McClellan-Kerr AR River Navigation System made Tulsa a major inland port. Today, Tulsa is one of the fastest growing cities in the US and

Philbrook Art Museum, Tulsa, Oklahoma

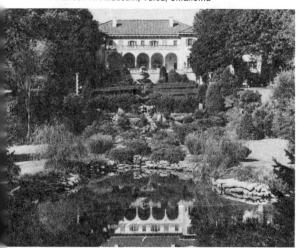

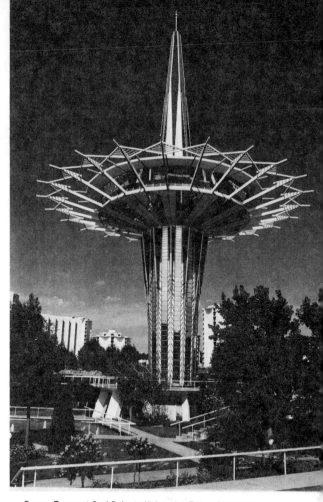

Prayer Tower at Oral Roberts University, Tulsa, Oklahoma

an important administrative center of the country's oil industry.

GOVERNMENT. Tulsa has a commission form of govt. The five commission members, including the mayor as a voting member, are elected at large to two-year terms. Each commissioner heads a city govt. department.

ECONOMY AND INDUSTRY. Once the "Oil Capital of the World", Tulsa currently has many administrative offices of oil-related companies, including the headquarters of more than 350 of these companies. Several large oil refineries are located in the city, including the state's largest. Transportation and aerospace are also important area industries. Major products manufactured in the approx. 1,000 firms located in the city include automotive equipment, tools, heating devices and food products. The Tulsa met. area had a labor force of 307,200 in June, 1979, while the rate of unemployment was 3.4%.

BANKING. In 1978, total deposits for the 28 banks headquartered in Tulsa were $3,036,726,000, while assets were $3,593,015,000. Banks include Bank of OK First Natl. Bank and Trust, Fourth Natl., Utica Natl. Bank and Trust, F & M Bank and Trust and Commerce and Trust Co.

HOSPITALS. There are four gen. hosps. in Tulsa, including St. Francis, Doctors, Hillcrest and St. John's. The Children's Medical Center, the OK Osteopathic Hosp. and several psychiatric facilities are also located in the city.

EDUCATION. The private U of Tulsa founded at Muskogee, Indian Territory, in 1894 and relocated in 1908, awards grad. and undergrad. degrees. In 1978, the U enrolled more than 6,000. Oral Roberts U, a privately-supported nonsectarian institution established in 1965 by the trustees of the Oral Roberts Evangelists Assn., awards bachelor and master degrees. The U enrolled more than 3,700 in 1978. The publicly-supported Tulsa Jr. Col., awarding associate degrees, enrolled more than 5,500 in 1978. Other institutions include OK Col. of Osteopathic Medicine and Surgery and OK School of Business, Accountancy, Law and Finance. The 95 elementary and 10 high schools in the public system enroll approx. 70,000. More than 3,000 attend 12 private schools. Libs. include the Tulsa City Co. Lib., the AMOCO Co. Lib. and the Cities Service Research Lib.

ENTERTAINMENT. Dining entertainment in Tulsa is offered by the Gaslight Dinner Theatre. Annual events include the Tulsa State Fair in late Sept. The Roughnecks of NASL soccer, the Rangers of TX League baseball and the Oilers of CHL hockey offer professional sports, while the Tulsa U Golden Hurricanes participate in intercollegiate sports. The International Finals of the Natl. Rodeo Competition are held in the city.

ACCOMMODATIONS. There are numerous hotels and motels in Tulsa, including the William Plaza Hotel, Skyline E and Airport, Sheraton Inns, Central and E Tradewinds, Howard Johnson's and LaQuinta Motor and Ramada inns.

FACILITIES. There are 90 parks, encompassing 4,000 acres, in Tulsa. The 2,817-acre Mohawk Park, the largest, contains a golf course and a zoo, and features more than 12,000 rose bushes. Tulsa is the home of the State Fairgrounds, which provides a livestock display barn, a show ring and an exposition center. Public golf courses are also located at LaFortuen and Mohawk parks. Public tennis courts are located at many city parks.

CULTURAL ACTIVITIES. Performances by the Tulsa Civic Ballet, Opera Co. and Philharmonic Orchestra are presented at the Performing Arts Center. "Oklahoma", the musical by Rogers and Hammerstein and "Dust on Her Petticoats", an outdoor drama about the role of pioneer women, are staged at the Discoveryland Amphitheatre. The Thomas Gilcrease Institute of American History and Art features an extensive collection of native American art and historical documents among its 5,000 works, and also houses the world's largest collection of works by American painters Thomas Moran, Frederic Remington and Charles M. Russell. The Philbrook Art Center displays Italian Renaissance paintings and native American art, Chinese jewelry, rooms in period decor and visiting exhibits. Articles from over 100 nations are exhibited in the World Museum Art Centre.

LANDMARKS AND SIGHTSEEING SPOTS. The oldest landmark in Tulsa is the Council Oak, a tree on Cheyenne Avenue under which, according to legend, Archie Yahola, a Creek elder, presided over tribal councils in 1836. Boston Avenue Methodist Church is an example of the application of modern skyscraper architecture to a large church. A 200-foot glass and steel prayer tower and a six-story, diamond-shaped lib. are part of the Oral Robert U, which conducts tours of its premises. Tours of the Sun Oil and Texaco refineries are also available.

Central Tulsa, Oklahoma

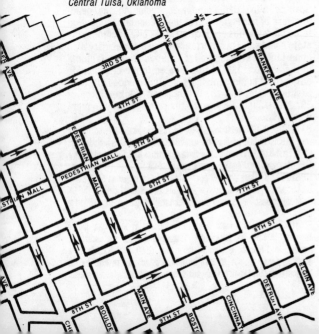

VIRGINIA BEACH
VIRGINIA

CITY LOCATION-SIZE-EXTENT. VA Beach, an independent Atlantic coastal city located in SE VA S of Cape Henry and N of NC, encompasses 310 sq. mi., including 38 mi. of beaches, at 36°50'8" N lat. and 75°58'5" W long. It ranks second among VA cities in pop. and third in land area. Its met. area extends into the city of Suffolk to the NW and Currituck Co. in NC, and encompasses the cities of Norfolk to the N, Portsmouth to the W and Chesapeake to the SW.

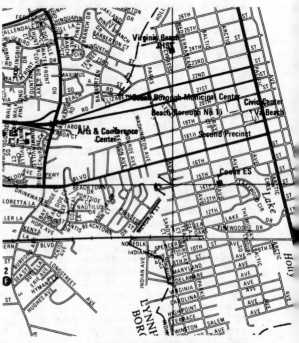

Ocean Front, Virginia Beach, Virginia

TOPOGRAPHY. VA Beach's level, low terrain is characteristic of the Tidewater Region. The Atlantic Ocean lies to the E and Chesapeake Bay lies to the N. The mean elev. is 16'.

CLIMATE. The climate of VA Beach is modified marine, influenced by the surrounding waters of the Atlantic Ocean and Chesapeake Bay. Winters are mild, summers warm and long, and spring and autumn usually pleasant. The avg. annual temp. of 60°F ranges from a Jan. mean of 41°F to a July mean of 79°F. Most of the 45" avg. annual rainfall occurs in March and June. The avg. annual snowfall of 7.2" occurs mostly during Jan. and Feb. The RH ranges from 50% to 87%. The avg. growing season is approx. 244 days. VA Beach lies in the ESTZ and observes DST.

FLORA AND FAUNA. Animals native to VA Beach include the opossum, rabbit and raccoon. Common birds are the shorebird, cardinal, mockingbird, bluejay and robin. Crab, oyster, bass and carp are present among area sealife. Many species of reptiles are found in the area, including the venomous copperhead, cottonmouth, coral snake and rattlesnake. Typical trees are the loblolly pine, magnolia, cypress and dogwood. Smaller plants include the water lily, azalea and cattail.

POPULATION. According to the US census, the pop. of VA Beach in 1970 was 172,106. In 1978, it was estimated that it had increased to 259,806.

ETHNIC GROUPS. In 1978, the ethnic distribution of VA Beach was approx. 91.1% Caucasian, 8.4% Black, 1% Asian and 4% other races (a percentage of the other races total is included in the Caucasian total).

TRANSPORTATION. Interstate Hwy. 64, US hwys. 13, 58 and 60 and state hwys. 149, 165, 166 and 190 provide major motor access to VA Beach. *Railroads* serving the city include VA & MD and S Railway. *Airlines* serving Norfolk Intl. Airport include US Air, NA, PD and UA. *Bus lines* serving the city include Greyhound, Trailways and the local Tidewater Regional Transit. The Port of Hampton Roads is the third largest container port on the Atlantic Ocean and handled more than 44 million tons of cargo in 1977.

COMMUNICATIONS. Communications, broadcasting and print media originating from VA Beach are: *AM radio stations* WVAB 1550 (MBS, Hits); no *FM radio stations* or *television stations* originate from the city, which receives broadcasting from nearby Norfolk; *press*: publications serving the city, are the daily and the weekly *Norfolk Ledger Star & Virginian Pilot, USMC Pictorial News* and the weekly *Sun.*

HISTORY. VA Beach was created in 1963 when the resort city VA Beach was merged with surrounding Princess Anne Co. Originally, the VA Beach site was settled in 1607 by English colonists who came ashore and eventually moved on to establish Jamestown. Princess Anne Co. was formed in 1691. During the Revolutionary War, Princess Anne was the location of a battle off Cape Henry, where a British defeat kept aid from reaching Cornwallis' troops at Yorktown. During the Civil War, the area was sympathetic toward the Confederacy, but remained under Union control. RR access and the infusion of Vanderbilt money, in the latter part of the 19th-century, converted VA Beach's rolling, empty sand dunes along the Atlantic into a premier resort center. VA Beach was incorporated as a town in 1906. During WW I, Germany torpedoed US merchant ships within view of the beach. VA Beach was booming by the 1920s. Its boardwalk was replaced with concrete and the city began annexing portions of Princess Anne Co. Following WW II, VA Beach had four military installations. Still growing as a resort, it also was becoming a suburb of Norfolk, but city leaders still sought a broader industrial base. In the 1960s, the area's continued expansion was aided by the completion of the Chesapeake Bay Bridge Tunnel and the opening of the VA Beach Expressway.

GOVERNMENT. VA Beach has a council-mgr. form of govt. The 11 council members, including the mayor as a voting member, are elected to four-year terms, seven by borough and four at large. The mayor, selected by the council from among its ranks, serves a two-year term.

ECONOMY AND INDUSTRY. The major industries in VA Beach are tourism, agriculture, commerce and construction. Govt. is also a major employer. There are 250 industrial companies in the city. Production of food, wood and paper products, fabrics, fiberglass boats, steel parts and furniture are significant to the city's economy. The city has more than 3,000 retail stores and trade engages 25% of its labor force. In April, 1979, the avg. per capita income was $6,578. In 1978, the total labor force of the greater met. area was 91,917, while the rate of unemployment was 5%.

BANKING. There are 11 banks with 54 branch offices and 20 savings and loan assns. in VA Beach. In 1978, total deposits for the two banks headquartered in the city were $22,739,000, while assets were $26,358,000. Banks include VA Beach and Commerce.

First colonists of Jamestown landed here in 1607, Virginia Beach, Virginia

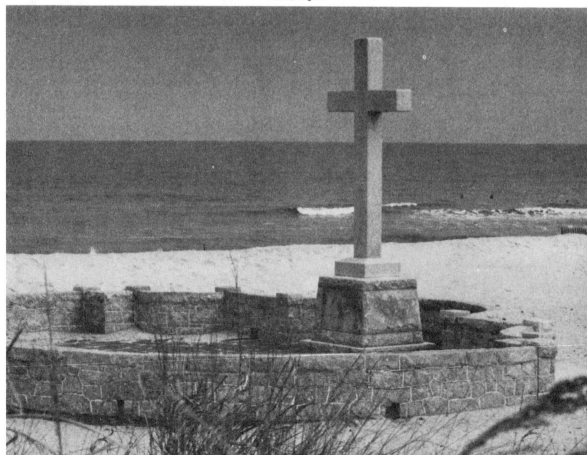

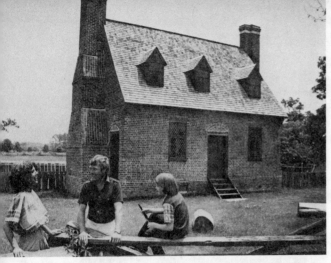

17th Century Lynnhaven House, Virginia Beach, Virginia

HOSPITALS. There are several hospitals in VA Beach, including the VA Beach and Bayside Memorial, which are presently being expanded. The health department has three facilities in the city and operates seven clinics at each location.

EDUCATION. The VA Beach Comm. Col., located in the Green Run area, offers courses leading to the associate degree. The public school system includes 42 elementary, eight jr. high and seven high schools and enrolls more than 55,000 students. The city's 18 private and parochial schools enroll an additional 3,600 students. Lib. facilities include the Public Lib., with five branches, and the Public Law Lib.

ENTERTAINMENT. Dining entertainment is offered by the Tidewater Dinner Theater. The ten-day Neptune Festival is held each fall in VA Beach. Other annual events include the Boardwalk Art Show, Music Festival, Folk Arts Festival and Shodeo.

ACCOMMODATIONS. There are many hotels and motels in VA Beach, including the Sheraton Beach, Hilton, Holiday, Cavalier Oceanfront, Princess Anne and Mariner Resort inns, as well as the Marjac, Seahawk and Triton Towers.

FACILITIES. The VA Beach park system includes 110 parks and school playground areas which feature several lakes, athletic field complexes, picnic areas, fishing and tennis facilities. Bayville Farms contains a specific area designed for use by the handicapped. Horse riding facilities are available at Princess Anne Park. Little Island Park is located along the ocean, while Red Wing Park is near the ocean front. Most of Seashore State Park's 2,770 acres are preserved as a natural area where rare forms of plant and animal life may be observed. Some 20 mi. of paved and natural-surfaced bike trails are featured at the VA Beach Bikeway. The Dept. of Parks and Recreation maintains a number of beaches throughout the city. A jogging track can be found on the Boardwalk. Public golf courses are located at Redwing and Bow Creek. There are also 13 marinas available in VA Beach.

CULTURAL ACTIVITIES. Musical performances are presented by the VA Beach Pops, the VA Beach Sunday Pops, orchestras, and the Comm. Chorus. The city is also served by a ballet company and Little Theater. The Civic Art Center houses the art gallery. Art exhibitions will also be held in the VA Beach Arts and Conference Center to be opened in 1980.

LANDMARKS AND SIGHTSEEING SPOTS. Owned by the Assn. for the Preservation of VA Antiquities in VA Beach, the Lynhaven House, built almost 300 years ago, is among the best preserved 17th-century dwellings in America. Other buildings of historical interest include the Adam Thoroughgood House (1836), the area's oldest brick house and the Francis Land House (1732). The Old Cape Henry Lighthouse, now a Natl. Historic Landmark, was authorized and funded by the country's first Congress. It was built in 1791 and guided mariners until 1881. The First Landing Cross on VA Beach marks the spot where America's first permanent settlers landed in 1607. Overlooking the sea is the Norwegian Lady, a nine-foot bronze figurehead commemorating the shipwreck (1891) of the Norwegian boat *Dictator*. A twin statue is located in Moss, Norway. The churchyard of The Old Dominion Church, which is a registered landmark, contains the graves of many past leaders in Princess Anne Co. The Little Creek Naval Amphibious Base has an "openhouse ship" on weekends. Restricted tours of the Oceana Naval Air Station are available to the public.

WARREN
MICHIGAN

CITY LOCATION-SIZE-EXTENT. Warren encompasses 34.2 sq. mi. in Macomb Co., adjacent to Detroit on the N, in SW MI at 42°30'5" N lat. and 83°01'6" W long. The greater met. area extends into Oakland Co. to the E and is part of the Detroit met. area.

TOPOGRAPHY. The topography of Warren, situated in the Great Lakes Plains, varies from slightly sloping terrain to rolling hills further to the W. Lake St. Clair is six mi. E of Warren and the Clinton River is three mi. to the N. The mean elev. is 800'.

CLIMATE. The continental climate in Warren is moderated by the effects of the Great Lakes on winds passing across them. The avg. annual temp. of 49°F ranges between monthly means of 24°F in Jan. and 72°F in July. The 32" of avg. annual rainfall is well distributed throughout the year. Most of the avg. annual snowfall of 36.1" occurs as individual snowstorms that avg. approx. 3" per storm. The RH ranges from 51% to 88%. The growing season avgs. 180 days. Warren lies in the ESTZ and observes DST.

FLORA AND FAUNA. Animals native to Warren include the fox, deer and muskrat. Typical birds are the blue jay, mockingbird, loon, and bittern. Bullfrogs, salamanders, snapping turtles, toads and lizards, as well as the venomous E massasauga (a pygmy rattler) are found in the area. Common trees are the maple, elm, oak and pine. Smaller plants include the honeysuckle, rose and blackberry.

POPULATION. According to the US census, the pop. of Warren in 1970 was 179,260. In 1978, it was estimated that it had decreased to approx. 170,000.

ETHNIC GROUPS. In 1978, the ethnic distribution of Warren was approx. 99.4% Caucasian, 0.1% Black, 0.1% Hispanic, 0.3% Asian and 0.1% other.

TRANSPORTATION. Interstate hwys. 75, 94, and 696 and state hwys. 53, 97 and 102 provide major motor access to Warren. *Railroads* serving the city include Grand Trunk W and ConRail. All major *airlines* serve Detroit Met. airport, 45 min. away. *Bus lines* serving the city include Greyhound and the local transit authority (SE MTA).

COMMUNICATIONS. Communications, broadcasting and print media originating in Warren include: no *AM radio stations* or *television stations* originate in Warren, which receives broadcasting from the Detroit met. area; *FM radio station* WPHS 91.5 (Indep., Btfl. Mus., Top 40); *press*: one daily serves the city, the *Macomb Daily*; weekly publications include the *Metro Shopping News*.

Central Warren, Michigan

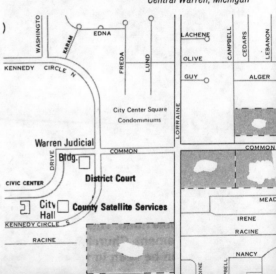

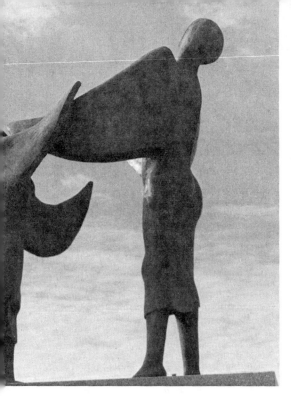

"Law and Justice" statue at Civic Center, Warren, Michigan

HISTORY. Warren was organized as a township in 1837 and became a village in 1893. It was incorporated as a city in 1957. The Detroit suburb is a center for auto research.

GOVERNMENT. Warren has a mayor-council form of govt. The three council members, including the mayor as a voting member, are elected at large to three-year terms.

ECONOMY AND INDUSTRY. Major industries in Warren include automotive, research, defense, electronics, chemicals, and steel. The total labor force in 1978 was 88,658, while the rate of unemployment was approx. 6.1%. The 1978 per capita income was approx. $6,000.

BANKING. In 1978, total deposits for the three banks headquartered in Warren were $283,401,000, while total assets were $318,311,000. Banks include Warren, Natl. Bank of Detroit, Bank of Commerce, and MI Natl. Bank of Macomb.

HOSPITALS. S Macomb, Bi-Co. Osteopathic, McNamara and Glen Edem hosps. are located in Warren. Msgr. Clement Kern offers specialized surgery facilities.

EDUCATION. Macomb Co. Commercial Col., a two-year public institution founded in Warren in 1954, awards associate degrees. Approx. 18,340 were enrolled in 1978. A branch, Center Campus, was also founded in 1954 to offer transfer and occupational programs. Granting the associate degree, this branch enrolled approx. 6,000 in 1978. The 84 schools in the Public School System enrolled approx. 49,000 in 1978. The Warren Public Lib. and its five branches provide library facilities in the city.

ENTERTAINMENT. Annual events include the Warren City Fair. The Macomb Co. Comm. Col.'s Monarchs participate in intercollegiate sports.

ACCOMMODATIONS. There are several hotels and motels in Warren, including the Flying Dutchman and the Executive and Holiday inns.

FACILITIES. Recreational facilities in Warren include Halmich Park, Stoney Creek Metro Park and Metro Beach. There are 20 public golf courses in one area.

CULTURAL ACTIVITIES. Musical performances are presented by the Warren Concert Band and the Warren Symphony. Nearby Detroit offers cultural activities also.

LANDMARKS AND SIGHTSEEING SPOTS. The General Motors Technical Center and the Army Tank Automotive Command are in Warren. Nearby Detroit offers many additional attractions.

WASHINGTON
DISTRICT OF COLUMBIA

CITY LOCATION-SIZE-EXTENT. Washington, the capital of the US, encompasses 70 sq. mi. in the District of Columbia (a municipal corporation and therefore not a part of any state) between VA and MD at the confluence of the Potomac and Anacostia rivers at 38°57' N lat. and 77°21' W long. The met. area extends into the MD counties of Charles to the S, Prince George to the E and Montgomery to the N, as well as the VA cos. of Arlington and Fairfax to the W, Loudon to the NW and Prince William to the SW and the independent cities of Alexandria, Fairfax and Fall Church.

TOPOGRAPHY. Washington lies in a broad flat area on the W edge of the middle Atlantic Coastal Plain, approx. 40 mi. E of the Blue Ridge Mts. and 35 mi. W of Chesapeake Bay. The city's mean elev. is 150'.

CLIMATE. The climate of Washington is continental. Summer thunderstorms often bring sudden and heavy rain showers, which may be attended by damaging winds, hail or lightning. Flooding in the area is usually caused by the effects of hurricanes, heavy rain in the Potomac Basin or a combination of melting snow and heavy rain. The avg. annual temp. of 55.5°F ranges from a Jan. mean of 33°F to a July mean of 76.9°F. The avg. annual rainfall is 40.49". The avg. annual snowfall of 19.4" occurs mainly during Dec. through Mar. The RH ranges from 45% to 91%. Washington lies in the ESTZ and observes DST.

FLORA AND FAUNA. Animals native to Washington include the fox, opossum, raccoon and squirrel. Common birds are the robin, thrasher, catbird, crow and vireo. Bullfrogs, salamanders, toads, king snakes, fence lizards and the venomous copperhead are common to the area. Typical trees are the oak, elm, sweetgum and ash. Smaller plants include the honeysuckle, holly, foxglove and bluets.

POPULATION. According to the US census, the pop. of Washington in 1970 was 756,668. In 1978, it was estimated that it had decreased to 676,000.

Jefferson Memorial, Washington, District of Columbia

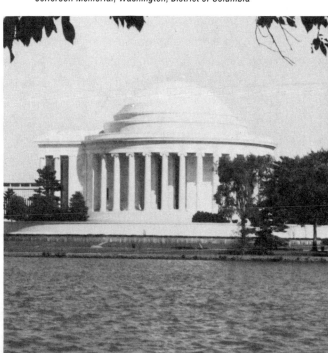

ETHNIC GROUPS. In 1978, the ethnic distribution of Washington was approx. 71.1% Black, 30.6% Caucasian and 2.1% Hispanic (a percentage of the Hispanic total is included in the Caucasian total).

TRANSPORTATION. Interstate hwys. 66, 95 and 270, US hwys. 1, 29 and 50 and state hwys. 4, 5, 27, 97 and 295 provide major motor access to Washington. *Railroad* service is provided by Auto-Train, the Metroliner, AMTRAK, Burlington N, Chessie System, CO & S, ConRail, Santa Fe and S Pacific and Union Pacific, among others. Intl. flight facilities are available at Dulles Intl. Airport, 25 mi., and Baltimore/Washington Intl. Airport, 20 mi. from downtown. *Airlines* serving Washington Natl. Airport, 3.5 mi. from downtown, with domestic flights are AA, US Air, BN, DL, EA, NA, NW, PD, TW and UA. *Bus lines* serving the city include Greyhound, Trailways and the local Metro System. The world's most modern rapid rail transit system, although still not completed, has three lines in operation.

COMMUNICATIONS. Communications, broadcasting and print media originating in Washington are: *AM radio stations* WGMS 570 (Indep., Clas.); WMAL 630 (ABC/I, MOR); WPIK 730 (MSB, C&W); WFAX 1220 (Indep., Relig.); WWDC 1260 (Indep., Rock); WEAM 1390 (Indep., Blk.); WTOP 1500 (CBS, All News) and WPGC 1580 (Indep., Contemp.); *FM radio stations* WAMU 88.5 (Amer., Divers.); WPFW 89.3 (Indep., A/MOR); WETA 90.9 (PBS, Spec. Prog.); WKYS 93.9 (NBC, Disco); WJMD 94.7 (Indep., Btfl. Mus.); WHUR 96.3 (Howard U, Spec. Prog.); WASH 97.1 (Metromedia, Contemp.); WMZQ 98.7 (Indep., Disco); WGAY 99.5 (Indep., Btfl. Mus.); WOOK 100.3 (ABC/FM, A/MOR); WWDC 101.1 (Indep., Contemp.); WGMS 103.5 (Indep., Divers.);

The Capital as seen from Pennsylvania Avenue, Washington, District of Columbia

WAVA 105.1 (Indep., Soft Rock) and WRQX 107.3 (ABC/I, Rock); *television stations* WRC Ch. 4 (NBC); WTTG Ch. 5 (Metromedia); WJLA Ch. 7 (ABC); WDVM Ch. 9 (CBS); WDCA Ch. 20 (Indep.); WETA Ch. 26 (PBS); WHMM Ch. 32 (Indep.) and cable; *press*: two major dailies serve the area, the *Post*, published mornings, and the *Star*, published mornings and evenings; other publications include *Co. News, The Hatchet, The New Observer, Smart Shopper, The Spotlight,* and *The Washingtonian,* the *Afro-American* and the *DC Gazette*.

HISTORY. In 1783, the US Congress decided to establish a permanent capital, but disagreement over the site of present-day Washington delayed the decision. In 1790, a compromise was achieved, and it was decided that the capital city be situated in the middle of the country (of that time period), so as to be equally accessible to both Northerners and Southerners. Pres. George Washington, who selected the site, chose a sparsely populated area on the Potomac bordered by MD and VA. In 1791, Andrew Elliott and Benjamin Banneker, a white surveyor and Black mathematician, respectively, worked together to delineate the boundaries of the DC. That same year, Pres. Washington appointed Pierre L'Enfant, a French engineer, to design the layout of the fed. city. The fed. govt. moved from Philadelphia to Washington in 1800. The city grew rather slowly. In 1802, Congress established a local govt. to help run the city. The city's growth was set back when, during the War of 1812,

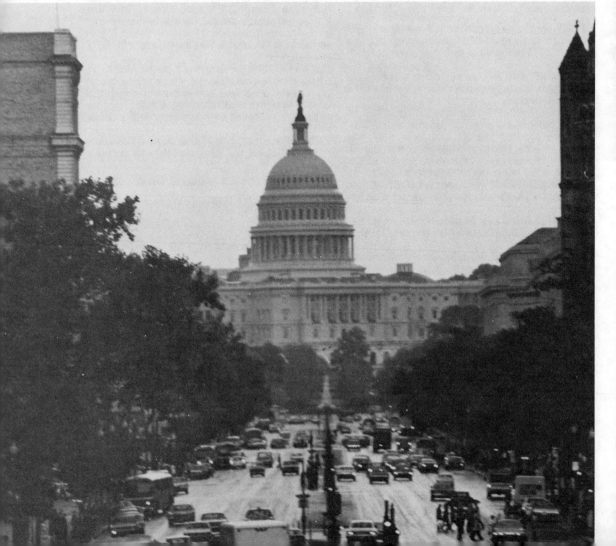

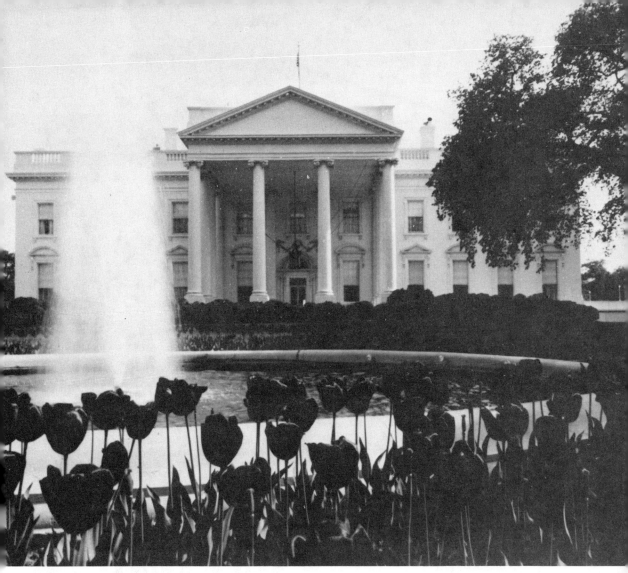

The White House, Washington, District of Columbia

British troops sacked and burned most of the govt. buildings, including the Capitol and White House. By 1819, the buildings had been restored. From an economic standpoint, Washington was a disappointment. It did not become the center of industry and commerce that had been envisioned. By the 1840s, there were about 50,000 residents and only a small part of the city was built up. As a result, Congress returned to VA the land that the state had donated to build Washington. The city was incorporated in 1846. During the Civil War, Washington expanded rapidly as thousands of Union soldiers were stationed there to guard the city from the Confed. After the War, Washington's growth continued. After 1865, tourism escalated when more than 100,000 people came to the capital city to witness the Grand Review of the Union Army. In 1871, a territorial govt. with a gov. was established; this was replaced in 1874 with a local govt. consisting of three commissioners appointed by the President. The Baltimore & Potomac RR station, constructed in 1874, became the city's first link to the RR system. In 1890, the 186-mi. Chesapeake & OH Canal connected Georgetown (a section of Washington) to Cumberland, MO. Washington's growth after the early 1900s always coincided with various natl. crises. In order to meet the demands of WW I, the civil service was enlarged, resulting in the relocation of many people to Washington. During the Great Depression of the 1930s, many people were attracted to Washington as the only city in which jobs were still available. The city's pop. peaked at 800,000 by 1950. While the actual city pop. is now slighly lower, the pop. of suburban areas close to Washington has increased. In 1964, a constitutional amendment gave Washingtonians the right to vote in pres. elections. This was followed by another amendment in 1973, which abolished the commission system of govt. in favor of an elected municipal council headed by a mayor. As the nation's capital, Washington today is a thriving center of govt. and tourism.

GOVERNMENT. Originally, Washington was a fed. district governed by Congress. As of 1973, the voters in the city elect their own officials to a mayor-council form of govt. consisting of 13 council members and a mayor. The mayor is elected at large to a four-year term. The 13 council members are elected to four-year terms, five at large and eight by district.

ECONOMY AND INDUSTRY. The fed. govt. is the major employer in Washington. The govt. employs approx. 25% of the area labor force. The leading private industry is tourism. The area is increasing in the number of R&D companies in electronics, physics and other sciences with applications to aircraft and space

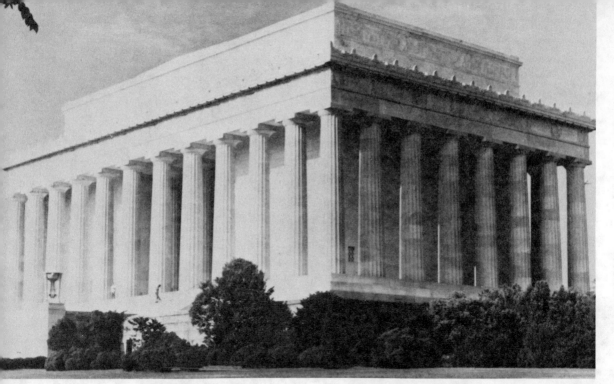

Lincoln Memorial, Washington, District of Columbia

vehicles. Manufacturing, primarily light industry, accounts for only 5% of the area's labor force. Printing and publishing firms are the major concerns. The Washington area had a labor force of 1,613,000 in Oct., 1979, and an unemployment rate of 6.4%.

BANKING. In 1978, total deposits for the 17 banks headquartered in Washington were $5,838,979,000, while assets were $7,086,581,000. Banks include Riggs Natl., American Security, Natl., Union First Natl. and Natl. Savings and Trust Co.

HOSPITALS. Washington has 20 gen. care hosps., several specialized and govt. facilities, and teaching hosps. These facilities include George Washington U. Capitol Hill, Doctors, Howard U. Georgetown U, WA Center, Children's, Columbia Hosp. for Women, Ft. Lincoln Family Medial Center, Greater SE Comm., Hadley Memorial Hosp. for Sick Children, Natl. Jewish, Providence, the Psychiatric Institute of Washington, Sibley Memorial and the V.A. Hosp. Several psychiatric facilities are also located in the city.

EDUCATION. Washington is noted for its educational institutions. Howard U, one of the nation's largest predominantly Black universities, was authorized by a charter of the 39th Congress in 1867. Offering grad. and undergrad. degrees, the U enrolled more than 9,800 students in 1978. Georgetown U, founded in 1789, was the nation's first private school to receive a U charter from the fed. govt. It offers 65 degree programs and includes a number of prominent public servants among its alumni. In 1978, it enrolled more than 11,700 students. George Washington U was established in 1821, and in 1978 it enrolled more than 23,100 students. It is a publicly-supported U offering degrees ranging from associate to doctoral. The U of DC, established in 1975, is a locally-controlled institution offering associate, bachelor and master degrees. In 1978, it enrolled more than 13,200 students. The American U is affiliated with the United Methodist Church. It was established in 1893 and in 1978 it enrolled more than 12,500 students. Other institutions include Campus-Free Col., the Catholic U of America, Dominican House of Studies, Gallaudet Col., Mt. Vernon Col., Oblate Col., SE U, Strayer Col., Trinity Col., Washington Intl. Col. and Wesley Theological Seminary. The public school system consists of over 170 schools, with 130,000 students in attendance. More than 75 private schools serve nearly 20,000 students. Lib. facilities include the Lib. of Congress, the

Downtown Washington, District of Columbia

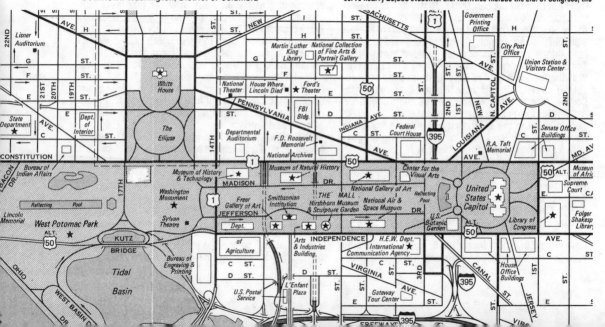

Martin Luther King Lib., Folger Shakespeare Lib., the Natl. Defense U Lib. and the lib. facilities of various organizations, including the Civil Service Commission, the Fed. Trade Comm., the Gen. Services Administration, the Natl. Geographic Society the Natl. Inst. of Education, the Natl. Science Foundation, the Organization of American States, the Smithsonian Inst., the House of Representatives, the Senate, the V.A. and the US depts. of Commerce, HEW, Justice, Labor, State, Air Force, Army, Interior, Navy and Transportation.

ENTERTAINMENT. Dinner theaters in Washington include Encore, Harlequin and Hayloft. The city hosts many annual events, including the Cherry Blossom Festival in late Mar. or early Apr., the Easter Egg Roll on Easter Monday, the President's Cup Regatta in June, a fireworks display at Washington Monument on July 4 and the Christmas Tree Lighting in mid-Dec. The inauguration of the Pres., occurring every four years on Jan. 20, is attended by many celebrations. Pro sports entertainment is offered by the Washington Redskins (NFL-NFC, football), the Diplomats (NASL, soccer), the Capitols (NHL, hockey) and the Bullets (NBA, Basketball). Collegiate sports are offered by the Georgetown U Hoyas, the Howard U Bisons, the Catholic U of America Cardinals and the George Washington U Colonials. Soccer, rugby and cricket are played by embassy teams in W Potomac Park.

ACCOMMODATIONS. Washington has many hotels and motels, including the Capitol Hilton, Dupont Plaza, Loew's L'Enfant, Madison, Embassy Room Hotel, Fairfax, Hotel Washington, Watergate, Washington Hilton, Bethesda Marriott, Sheraton, Arlington Hyatt and Stouffers. Various Howard Johnson's, TraveLodges and Ramada, Quality and Holiday inns are located throughout the vicinity.

FACILITIES. There are approx. 150 parks in the Washington system. Two of the largest parks are Dumbarton Oaks and Anacostia. Anacostia Park covers 750 acres and contains a bird sanctuary, tennis courts, a swimming pool, a skating rink and a recreation center. Sailing is available along the Potomac River. The Natl. Zoological Park houses more than 2,000 animals, including two panda bears given to the US by the Chinese govt. in 1972. The Natl. Arboretum contains 415 acres of flowering trees and shrubs. Public golf courses can be found at E Potomac Park and Rock Creek Park. Many public tennis courts are available.

CULTURAL ACTIVITIES. The John F. Kennedy Center for the Performing Arts serves as the permanent home of the American Ballet Theatre and the Natl. Symphony Orchestra in Washington. Touring dramatic, ballet and opera companies from all over the world perform at JFK. Within the JFK complex is the Eisenhower Theatre that is used for legitimate theater. Ford Theater, where Lincoln was shot, has been restored to its 1860s looks and provides mini-plays year round. The Smithsonian Institution operates a number of art galleries and museums around the city. Among the Smithsonian museums are the Natl. Museum of History & Technology and the Natl. Museum of Natural History. Smithsonian art galleries include the Natl. Portrait Gallery, the Hirshhorn Museum & Sculptor Garden and the Natl. Collection of Fine Arts. Besides the Smithsonian galleries, other galleries offer a wide range of art exhibits. The Museum of African Art emphasizes collections from Africa. Masterpieces of American painters can be viewed at the Corcoran Gallery. The Phillips Collection includes works from El Greco to the present.

LANDMARKS AND SIGHTSEEING SPOTS. As the nation's capital, Washington is full of sites and buildings closely identified with the nation's history and govt. Located on Capitol Hill are the US Capitol, which is the seat of the Legislative branch of govt. the US Supreme Court and the Lib. of Congress. To the W of Rock Creek Park is Georgetown, the oldest settlement in DC and the site of the C&O Canal and Georgetown U. Arlington Natl. Cemetery is the burial place of the nation's soldiers and heroes, including Pres. John F. Kennedy. The Washington story is also told in monuments. Some of the well-known monuments are the Washington, Jefferson, Lincoln and Theodore Roosevelt monuments. Buildings of interest connected with the day-to-day administration of the fed. govt. are: The White House (which houses the Executive Branch); and the Treasury, US Dept. of Agriculture and State Dept. buildings. Other buildings which have an historic or cultural significance are Blair House, which is the guest quarters for visiting dignitaries; the American Red Cross Building; Ford Theater, where Pres. Lincoln was shot; Petersen House, where Lincoln died; Anderson House,

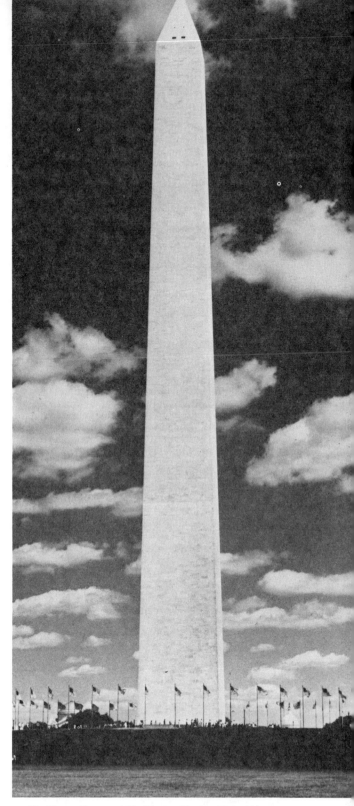

Washington Monument, Washington, District of Columbia

which serves as headquarters of the Society of Cincinnati (a military fraternity founded by Gen. George Washington in 1783); Washington Cathedral, a Gothic cathedral still under construction; The Islamic Center, the only US mosque for "orthodox" Muslims and Pierce Mill, an operating 19th-century flour mill.

WATERBURY
CONNECTICUT

CITY SIZE-LOCATION-EXTENT. Waterbury encompasses 28.2 sq. mi. along the Naugatuck River in New Haven Co., 18 mi. NW of New Haven, in W central CT at 73°2' W long. and 41°33' N lat. The greater met. area extends NW into Litchfield Co. and NE into Hartford Co.

TOPOGRAPHY. The terrain of Waterbury, which is situated in the W upland region of CT, varies from hilly, rugged areas to steep hills and ridges above the rivers. Hitchcock Lake lies to the E of the city, while Lake Quassapaug lies to the W. The mean elev. is 290'.

CLIMATE. The climate of Waterbury is continental marine, characterized by cold, dry winters and warm, maritime summers. The avg. annual temp. of 50°F ranges between monthly means of 25°F in Jan. and 70°F in July. The avg. annual rainfall of 44" is well distributed throughout the year. Snowfall avgs. 54" per year. The RH ranges from 43% to 87%. The growing season avgs. 174 days. Waterbury lies in the ESTZ and observes DST.

FLORA AND FAUNA. Animals native to Waterbury include the deer, squirrel and fox. Common birds include the cardinal, chickadee, goldfinch and blue jay. Salamanders, tree frogs, painted turtles, toads and milk snakes, as well as the venomous timber rattlesnake and copperhead, are also found in the area. Typical trees include the oak, birch, maple, dogwood, mountain laurel, hemlock and elm. Flowering plants include the rhododendron, rose, day lily and fireweed.

POPULATION. According to the US census, the pop. of Waterbury in 1970 was 108,333. In 1978, it was estimated that it had increased to 112,000.

ETHNIC GROUPS. In 1978, the ethnic distribution of Waterbury was approx. 81.1% Caucasian, 14.7% Black, 0.1% Asian and 4.1% other.

TRANSPORTATION. Interstate Hwy. 84 (Yankee Expressway) and state hwys. 8, 64, 66, 69 and 70 provide major motor access to Waterbury. *Railroad* service is provided by ConRail. A regional airport in nearby Oxford provides a helicopter shuttle service to NYC, Boston, Providence and Bradley Intl. Airport. *Airlines* serving Tweed-New Haven Airport, 25 mi. away, are EA, UA, US Air, AA and NA. *Bus lines* serving the city include Valley Transportation, Trailways and the local NE Transportation.

COMMUNICATIONS. Communications, broadcasting and print media originating from Waterbury are: *AM radio stations* WWCO 1240 (MBS, Contemp.); WATR 1320 (ABC/I, MOR) and WQQW 1590 (CBS, Adult Contemp.); *FM radio stations* WWYZ 92.5 (Indep., MOR) and WIOF

Waterbury, Connecticut

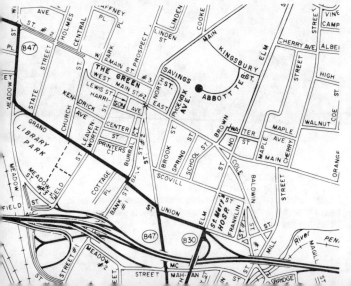

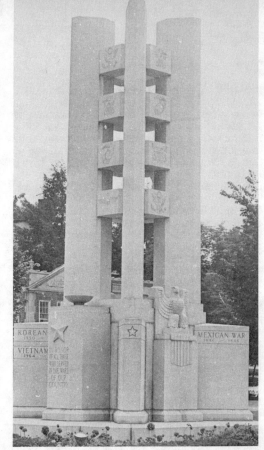

Veterans Memorial, Waterbury, Connecticut

104.1 (ABC/E, Contemp. Ctry.); *television station* WATR, Ch. 20 (NBC); *press* two major dailies serve the city, the *Republican*, issued mornings, and the *American*, issued evenings. Other publications include *Drycleaners News*, *NE Outdoors* and the weekly *Sunday Republican*.

HISTORY. In 1651, the present-day Waterbury area was settled by John Winthrop, Jr., who arrived from Pequot, CT, in search of iron and lead. Several mining families followed. The city was founded in 1674 when citizens from nearby Farmington purchased the site from native Americans, calling it the Plantation of Mattatuck. It was incorporated as a village and renamed Waterbury in 1686. Early attempts at farming failed due to the inadequacy of the soil and, by 1750, the citizens turned to manufacturing. The production of clocks began in the city in 1800 and, in 1802, the first waterwheel was built to drive simple machinery. The same year, the manufacture of brass buttons began, an industry which was to make Waterbury the "brass center of the world". The city was incorporated in 1853. During WW I, foreign and domestic laborers were attracted to the city by the new munitions industry. Between 1950 and 1960, industrial growth in Waterbury made it the only CT city to show an increase in pop. Today, Waterbury ranks among the top cities in the nation in the manufacture of brass and copper products.

GOVERNMENT. Waterbury has a mayor aldermanic form of govt. The 15 aldermen are elected at large to two-year terms. The mayor, elected at large to a two-year term, is not a member of council

ECONOMY AND INDUSTRY. There are approx. 400 manufacturing firms in the Waterbury area. The primary industry of brass and brass products is the basis for Waterbury's claim as "the Brass Center of the World". Other major industries include electronics, petrochemicals, chemicals, plastics, steel, research and clothing.

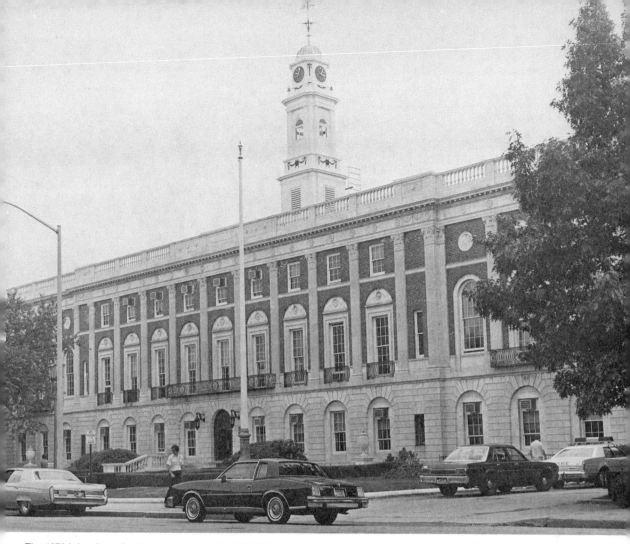

City Hall, Opened on January, 1916, Waterbury, Connecticut

The 1979 labor force for the met. area totaled 112,600, while the rate of unemployment was 5.6%.

BANKING. In 1978, total deposits for the three banks headquartered in the city were $1,455,390,000, while total assets were $1,737,685,000. Banks include First Fed. Savings and Loan, the Banking Center, Colonial Bank & Trust CT Natl, City Trust and Mattatuck Bank & Trust.

HOSPITALS. There are two gen. hosps. in Waterbury, St. Mary's and Waterbury.

EDUCATION. Post Col., established in Waterbury in 1890, is a private nonsectarian col. and business school. It awards associate degrees and, in 1978, it enrolled approx. 1,500. The publicly supported Mattatuck Comm. Col., founded in 1967, awards associate degrees. In 1978, it enrolled approx. 3,200. Other educational institutions include Waterbury State Technical Col. and the U of CT at Waterbury. There are 33 kindergartens, 21 elementary, three middle and three sr. high schools in the public system, which enrolls more than 16,000. The parochial system consists of 12 grammar, one middle and three high schools. The Silas Bronson Lib. and its two branches contain more than 163,000 volumes.

ENTERTAINMENT. Annual events in Waterbury include the Feast of Mt. Carmel, the Italian Festival and the Waterbury Annual Arts Festival. The El Giants of AA baseball provide pro sports, while the Mattatuck Comm. Col. Chiefs participate in intercollegiate sports.

ACCOMMODATIONS. There are several hotels and motels in Waterbury, including Johnson's and the Holiday, Red Bull and Waterbury Motor inns.

FACILITIES. There are 36 parks and 15 parklets in Waterbury, encompassing 892.52 acres. The major parks include Hamilton, Fulton, Washington Chase and Lakewood. The park system offers two 18-hole golf courses, an artificial skating rink, three outdoor swimming pools, 23 tennis courts, 28 ballfields, 14 basketball courts and one soccer field. Facilities for swimming, boating and fishing are provided at Lakewood and nearby Quassapaug and Hitchcock lakes.

CULTURAL ACTIVITIES. The Lincoln Center and Young Audiences, Inc., operate a performing arts program in Waterbury aimed at young people. It operates through the Arts Council and involves all school youth. Performing organizations include the 80-voice Waterbury Oratorio Society, the Civic Theatre, the Mattatuck Fife and Drum Corp. and the symphony orchestra. The Mattatuck Museum, founded in 1877, presents displays on the historical, industrial and cultural development of CT and features exhibitions by area artists. Library Park becomes an outdoor gallery during the summer Arts Festival, the state's oldest annual festival.

LANDMARKS AND SIGHTSEEING SPOTS. The Waterbury City Hall, designed by Cass Gilbert, opened Jan. 1, 1916. Also located in the city is the Republic and American Tower, dedicated in 1909 and modeled after the ancient Torre De Mangia in Siena, Tuscany, in Florence. It stands 240' tall and has 318 steps. The Father McGivney statue honors the founder of the Knights of Columbus. The Welton Drinking Fountain, a 2,500-lb. bronze horse erected on an 8.5' granite base, was dedicated in 1888 to resident Caroline J. Welton's favorite horse, "Knight". It was designed by Karl Gerhardt of Hartford, Ct. Charles H. Harrub bequeathed funds to the city for the building of two memorials. These statues are the Pilgrim Memorial, dedicated in 1930 to the founding fathers, and Veteran's Memorial, dedicated on Memorial Day, 1958, in honor of veterans of US wars. These monuments are contained in the Green, which is encircled by the mansions of the original settlers and includes the Italian Renaissance style Church of the Immaculate Conception.

WICHITA
KANSAS

CITY LOCATION-SIZE-EXTENT. Wichita, the seat of Sedgwick Co. and the largest city in the state, encompasses 99.57 sq. mi. in S central KS at 37°39' N lat. and 97°25' W long. The met area extends throughout most of Sedgwick Co. and E into Butler Co.

TOPOGRAPHY. Wichita lies on the confluence of the AR and Little AR rivers in the SE Plains Region. The terrain consists of generally flat farmlands. The mean elev. is 1,293'.

CLIMATE. The climate of Wichita is continental, characterized by hot summers and mild winters. Monthly mean temps. range from 31.4°F during Jan. to 80.3°F during July with an annual avg. of 56.6°F. From Apr. through Sept. 70% of the annual rainfall of 29.96" occurs. Thunderstorms occur about 56 days per year, some with hail. Snowfall occurs during Dec. through Mar. with an annual avg. of 15.6". The RH ranges from 50% to 83%. The windiest months are Mar. and Apr. with prevailing S winds. Occasional tornadoes have been observed in the area. The growing season lasts approx. 197 days. Wichita lies in the CSTZ and observes DST.

FLORA AND FAUNA. Animals native to Wichita include the opossum, coyote, raccoon and rabbit. Common birds are the cardinal, blue jay, crow, W meadowlark (state bird) and mockingbird. Characteristic to the area are bullsnakes, skinks, bullfrogs, toads and the venomous rattlesnake. Typical trees are the willow, oak, Siberian and American elm, cottonwood and mesquite. Smaller plants include the dandelion, petunia, clover, sunflower (state flower) and pasque flower.

POPULATION. According to the US census, the pop. of Wichita in 1970 was 276,554. In 1978, it was estimated that it had decreased to 261,862.

ETHNIC GROUPS. In 1978, the ethnic distribution of Wichita was approx. 87% Caucasian, 10% Black, 1.8% Hispanic, and 1.2% other.

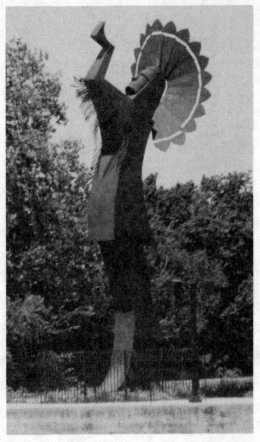

"Keeper of the Plains" Statue, Wichita, Kansas

Downtown, Wichita, Kansas

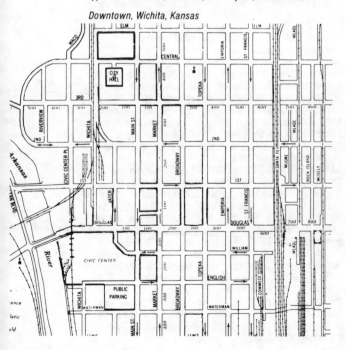

TRANSPORTATION. Interstate hwys. 35, 135 and 235, US hwys. 81 and 54 and state hwys. 2, 15, 42 and 96 provide major motor access to Wichita. The city is served by several *railroads* including Frisco, Rock Island, Missouri Pacific and Santa Fe. The *airlines* that serve Wichita MidContinental Airport are: CO, BN, TW, FL and SO. Airport service is also provided by McConnell AFB and several independent airports serve Wichita's large fleet of private aircrafts *Bus lines* to Wichita are provided by Trailways and the intracity Met. Transit Authority.

COMMUNICATIONS. Communications, broadcasting, and print media originating in Wichita are: *AM radio stations* KSGL 900 (Indep., Relig.); KFDI 1070 (Indep., C&W); KAKE 1240 (ABC/E, MOR); KFH 1330 (CBS, Adult Contemp.); KEYN 1410 (NBC, C&W) and KLEO 1480 (Indep., Top 40); *FM radio stations* KMUW (NPR, Var.); KDSA 91.1 (Indep., MOR, Ed.); KICT 95.1 (Indep., Mod, Ctry); KBRA 97.9 (Indep., Btfl. Mus.); KFDI 101.3 (Indep., Dups AM 45%); KEYN 103.7 (Indep., Top 40) and KARD 107.3 (Indep., Btfl. Mus.); *television stations* KARD Ch. 3 (NBC); KAKE Ch. 10 (ABC); KTVH Ch. 12 (CBS) and cable; press: there are two major dailies which serve the area *Wichita Beacon*, issued evenings and *Wichita Eagle*, issued mornings; other publications include *The Catholic Advocate; The Sunflower, Journal, Defender, Wichita, Times. The Wichitan* and *Wichita Light, All-Church Press*

HISTORY. Prior to white settlement, native Americans of the Wichita Tribe inhabited the site of present-day Wichita. The native Americans immigrated there to camp at the junction of two rivers during the Civil War, and whites followed in order to trade with them. Wichita was founded along the Chisholm cattle trail and incorporated in 1870. Two years later the Santa Fe

RR arrived and the city became an important cattle market. Wyatt Earp served as a lawman during 1875-1876 in Wichita, which was a noted frontier town in the 1880s. During the early 1900s oil was discovered near Wichita, stimulating additional development. In 1919, Wichita's history as an aviation center was initiated by the establishment of the town's first airplane factory. Economic stress during the Great Depression was alleviated in Wichita by the city's petroleum and aircraft industries. Aircraft production periodically boomed from WW II to the 1960s, but a slowdown in the nation's economy reduced the demand for small planes in the early 1970s and it was several years before the industry recovered. Today the city is the world's largest producer of small aircraft. A major manufacturing and agricultural marketing center, Wichita is the largest city in KS.

GOVERNMENT. Wichita has a council-mgr. form of govt. consisting of five members including the mayor. All members are elected at large to a four year term. The mayor is selected by and from the council and is a voting member of the council.

ECONOMY AND INDUSTRY. Major industries in Wichita are involved with exports, airplane parts, airplanes, petrochemicals, chemicals, meat packing, electronics and food processing. The average income per capita in 1977 was $7,418. In 1979, the labor force totaled 232,800 workers in the met. area with an unemployment rate of 2.2%.

BANKING. Wichita has more than 40 banking institutions serving the area. In 1978, total deposits for the 16 banks headquartered in the city were $1,578,420,000, while total assets were $1,933,378,000. Banks include Fourth Natl., First Natl., Central State, KS State, Union Natl., and SW Natl.

HOSPITALS. Wichita serves as the major medical center for the state, with a branch of the U of KS Medical School in the city and four major hospitals. These are Wesley Medical Center, St. Francis, St.Joseph's and Osteopathic. Of particular interest is the Institute of Logopedics, the world's largest speech and hearing residential rehabilitation center where research has made great strides in this field.

EDUCATION. Wichita State U (WSU), an institution within the Kansas state system of higher education, was founded in 1895 as Fairmount Col. Called the Mun. U of Wichita in 1926, WSU came into being in 1964 and is now the third largest col. in the state. The U is known for its Institute of Logopedics, the world's largest center for helping persons with speech and hearing handicaps. The U enrolled 15,723 stud. in 1978. Other institutions include the Electronic Computing Institution, Friends U, KS Newman Col., of U Medical School Branch, Wichita Automotive Institution, Wichita Bus. Col. and Wichita Technical Institution. Wichita's public school system includes about 100 elementary schools and 7 high schools. The city has also about 20 parochial and private schools. The Wichita Public Lib. system also provides a main center for educational assistance and nine branch libs.

ENTERTAINMENT. Each spring, a week-long celebration including a pageant, parades, dancing, carnivals, boat racing and hot-air balloon flying is held during the Wichita River Festival. Other events include the Annual Book and Art Fair, Okroberfest and a Square Dance Festival. Wichita has a pro baseball team in the AAA class known as the Aeros. The Wichita State U Shockers are the main collegiate sports interest. Friends U and KS Newman Col. participate in area collegiate sports.

ACCOMMODATIONS. Hotels and motels in Wichita include Broadview Hotel, Wichita Royale, Shepherd of the Hills, LaQuinta and English Village and Holiday, Ramada, Canterbury, Hilton, Diamond, Sheraton and Executive inns.

FACILITIES. Wichita maintains 69 parks with more than 2,808 acres of recreational space. The parks include Riverside, A. Price Woodward, O. J. Watson, Oak, Sim and Evergreen . There are eight public golf courses in the city. Tennis courts can be found at Wichita Racquet and Swim Club, Tennis West and Riverside Park Tennis Center. A ski lift can be found on Shocker Mt. The Sedgwick Co. Zoo is available to the public.

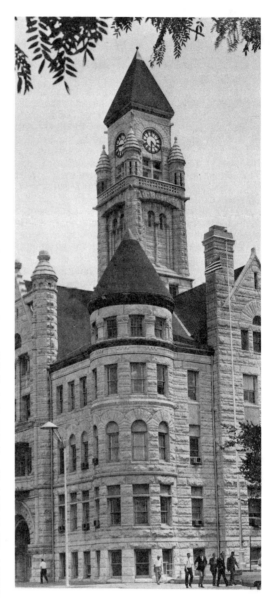

Wichita-Sedgwick County Historical Museum. Wichita, Kansas

CULTURAL ACTIVITIES. The Wichita Symphony Orchestra, the KS Chorale Society and the Wichita Jazz Festival give concerts. The Wichita Comm. Theater and the Wichita Art Assn. Children's Theater perform locally, as do the area's collegiate theater depts. Marple Theater provides a cabaret atmosphere and presents live music and stage entertainment. Lectures and films are presented by the Audubon Society. One of the largest collections of American art in the US, the Roland P. Murdock Collection, is displayed in the Wichita Art Museum. Other museums include the Wichita Art Assn., the Wichita Historical Museum, the Edwin A. Ulrich Museum of Art at Wichita State U Omnisphere Planetarium and the Mid-America All-Indian Center.

LANDMARKS AND SIGHTSEEING SPOTS. Historic Cowtown covers Wichita's history from 1868 to 1880 with 40 restored buildings, including the city's first permanent house and church and Wyatt Earp's jail. The Keeper of the Plains, a 44' sculpture of an Indian warrior, overlooks the confluence of the Big and Little AR rivers. Black Bears Great Plains Studio is another Wichita attraction.

362

WINSTON-SALEM
NORTH CAROLINA

CITY LOCATION-SIZE-EXTENT. Winston-Salem, located in central NC, approx. 70 mi. N of Charlotte and 30 mi. E of Greensboro, is the seat of Forsyth Co. and encompasses 58.2 sq. mi. at 36°6' N lat. and 80°14.7' W long. Its greater met. area includes most of Forsyth Co. and extends into the counties of Davie to the SW and Davidson to the SE.

TOPOGRAPHY. The terrain of Winston-Salem, located in the Piedmont area of NC, consists of gently rolling hills sloping upward towards the Blue Ridge Mts. to the W. The mean elev. is 884'.

CLIMATE. The climate of Winston-Salem is continental, characterized by moderate winters influenced by the nearby Appalachian Mts., which act as a barrier against cold N winter storms. The avg. annual temp. of 5°F ranges from monthly means of 39°F in Jan. to 77 °F in July. The annual rainfall of 42" is evenly distributed throughout the year. The avg. annual snowfall is 8.7". The RH ranges from 48% to 92%. The growing season is approx. 200 days. Winston-Salem lies in the ESTZ and observes DST.

FLORA AND FAUNA. Animals native to Winston-Salem include the opossum, raccoon and deer. Typical birds include the vireo, warbler, thrasher, robin and chuckwill's-widow. Dusky salamanders, frogs, tree frogs, Fowler's toads, ribbon snakes and the venomous rattlesnake and copperhead are found in the area. Typical trees are the oak, pine, elm and sweetgum. Smaller plants include the buckthorn, day lily, viburnum and wood sorrel.

POPULATION. According to the US census, the pop. of Winston-Salem in 1970 was 133,683. In 1978, it was estimated that it had increased to 145,000.

ETHNIC GROUPS. In 1978, the ethnic distribution of Winston-Salem was approx. 65.5% Caucasian, 34.1% Black and 0.5% Hispanic (a percentage of the Hispanic total is included in the Caucasian total).

TRANSPORTATION. Interstate hwy. 40, US hwys. 52, 158, 311 and 421 and state hwys. 67, 109 and 150 provide major motor access to Winston-Salem. *Railroads* serving the city include S, Winston-Salem Southbound and Norfolk & W. *Airlines* serving Smith Reynolds Airport include PI. *Bus lines* serving the city include Trailways, Greyhound and the local Winston-Salem Transit Authority.

Winston-Salem, North Carolina

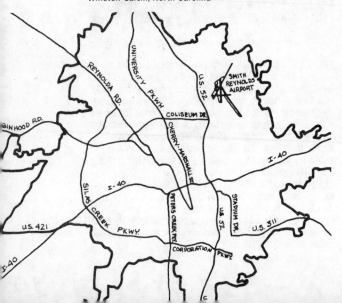

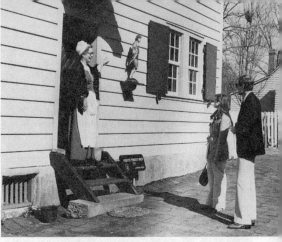

1771 Home in the 1766 Moravian Town of Old Salem, Winston-Salem, North Carolina

COMMUNICATIONS. Communications, broadcasting and print media originating in Winston-Salem are: *AM radio stations* WSJS 600 (NBC, MOR, Contemp.); WAAA 980 (Natl., Blk.); WAIR 1340 (Indep., Contemp., Top 40, Blk.); WTOB 1380 (Indep., Blk, Disco, Jazz); WSMK 1500 (ABC/I, C&W) and WPGD 1550 (Indep., Relig.); *FM radio stations* WFDD 88.5 (NPR, Clas., Educ.); WSEZ 93.1 (Indep., Easy Lis.); WTQR 104.1 (Indep., Ctry.) and WKZL 107.5 (Indep., Contemp., Top 40); *television stations* WFMY Ch. 2 (CBS); WGHP Ch. 8 (ABC); WXII Ch. 13 (NBC); WUNL Ch. 26 (Indep.); WGNN Ch. 45 (Indep.) and cable; *press*: two major dailies serve the city, the *Journal*, issued mornings and *Sentinel*, issued evenings; other publications include the *Chronicle* and *Suburbanite*.

HISTORY. In 1753, a group of Moravians (an early Protestant denomination) purchased 100,000 acres of land in the NC Piedmont. They named the region Wachovia, after the estate of an early European protector of the Moravian church. In 1766, the town of Salem, meaning "peace", was constructed nearby as the Moravian's permanent settlement. The comm. prospered and became a trading and crafts center. Cotton and wool industries contributed to the town's continued development. In 1849, Winston was founded by the NC Legislature and designated seat of the newly created co. of Forsyth. It was named for Revolutionary War hero Major Joseph Winston and located 1 mi. from Salem. Winston thrived along with its tobacco, furniture and textile industries. Since Winston and Salem shared the same interests and boundaries, the two towns were consolidated by a vote of their citizens in 1913. Today, Winston-Salem is a leading industrial center.

GOVERNMENT. Winston-Salem has a aldermanic-mgr. form of govt. The eight aldermen are elected by ward. The mayor, the political head of govt., presides at all Board of Aldermen meetings. All serve four-year terms.

ECONOMY AND INDUSTRY. A major tobacco manufacturing center, Winston-Salem is also one of the largest industrial centers of the S, producing textiles, furniture, electronic equipment, machinery and fabricated metal products. There are over 234 industries located in the city. In June, 1979, the labor force for the Greensboro-Winston-Salem-Highpoint met. area was 426,200, while the rate of unemployment was 4.5%. The avg. income per capita was $6,423 in 1977 and the avg. household income was $17,950.

BANKING. In 1978, total deposits for the six banks headquartered in Winston-Salem were $3,642,396,000, while assets were $4,561,498,000. Banks include Wachovia Bank and Trust Co., Forsyth Bank and Trust Co. and United Citizens.

HOSPITALS. There are four gen. hosps. in Winston-Salem, including Forsyth Memorial, NC Baptist, Mandala and Medical Park. Also located in the city is the Bowman Gray School of Medicine.

EDUCATION. Salem Col., a private liberal arts col. for women, was

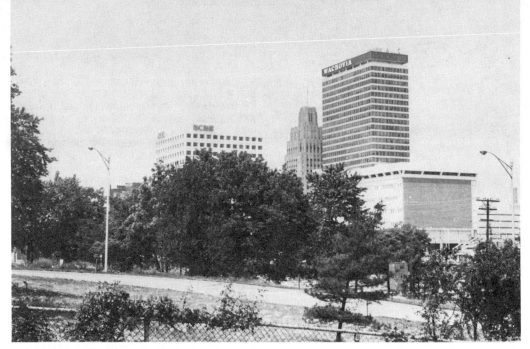

founded in 1772 by the Moravians, a Pre-Reformation Protestant denomination, and offers course work leading to bachelor degrees in music and teacher educ. Enrollment was 609 in 1978. Wake Forest U, a private institute founded in 1834 by the Baptist State Convention of NC, became coeducational in 1942. Awarding degrees from associate to doctorate, the U enrolled 4,630 students in 1978. Winston-Salem State U, a campus of the U of NC , is a public liberal arts and teachers col. founded in 1892 as the Slater Industrial Academy. It became a teachers col. in 1925 and was the nation's first black institution to grant degrees for teaching in the elementary grades. The U currently awards associate and bachelor degrees and enrolled 2,165 students in 1978. Other institutions include the NC Gov.'s School, a summer school program for the gifted; NC School of the Arts; NC Advancement School; Piedmont Bible Col.; Forsyth Technical Institution; NC School of the Arts (a campus of the U of NC); Piedmont Aerospace Institute and Winsalm Col. All of the public schools in the city and co. are under one administrative system. More than 24 private schools and 12 professional and trade schools serve the residents as well. Lib. facilities include the Winston-Salem Public Lib. and its branches.

ENTERTAINMENT. Professional sports entertainment is offered in Winston-Salem by the Red Sox (Central League, baseball). Wake Forest U's Demon Deacons participate in intercollegiate sports.

ACCOMMODATIONS. There are numerous hotels and motels in Winston-Salem, including the Winston-Salem Hyatt and the Sheraton Motor, Hilton, Holiday and Ramada inns.

FACILITIES. The Winston-Salem met. park system encompasses 50 parks, including Mineral Springs, Limberly and Tanglewood. Tanglewood Park, the largest, which occupies 1,117 acres and includes Mallard Lake, features golf, swimming, hiking, canoeing, picnicking and camping. It also provides paddle boats, an arboretum, horseback riding trails and stables. Fishing and boating facilities can be found at Salem Lake and Winston Lake. There are nine public golf courses, including Winston Lake, Hillcrest and Wilshire.

CULTURAL ACTIVITIES: Winston-Salem is served by several repertory companies and theaters, including the Piedmont Repertory Company and the Summit School Theatre. Comprised of art, music and dramatic groups, the Winston-Salem Arts Council is the oldest such organization in the country. Crafts are displayed for viewing and sale at the SE Center for Contemporary Art, an exhibition and education center for artists and the public. The city's numerous private art galleries also display SE crafts and antiques. The world's largest archives and manuscripts of early Moravian and American music is located in the Moravian Music Foundation. The Reynolds House, former home of R. J. Reynolds, is now a museum containing American paintings, furnishings and a ladies' costume collection spanning the first half of the 20th century. Anthropological, historical, and archeological exhibits are displayed in the Museum of Man. Other museums include the Museum of Early S Decorative Arts and the Winston-Salem Museum.

LANDMARKS AND SIGHTSEEING SPOTS. Old Salem, the restoration of the original Moravian town of Salem, is the site of many historic buildings erected between 1766 and 1850. Forty of the early structures, centered about a public square on approx. 20 city blocks, are still standing. Seven exhibit buildings are open—Single Brothers House (1769 and 1786); Miksch Tobacco Shop (1771); Winkler Bakery (1800); Boys School (1764); Salem Tavern (1784); John Vogler House (1819) and Market-Fire Museum (1803). Historic Bethabara, the first Moravian settlement in NC, includes a restored 1788 church, ft. and potter's house (1782). The Joseph Schlitz Brewing Co. offers tours of its plant.

WORCESTER
MASSACHUSETTS

CITY LOCATION-SIZE-EXTENT. Worcester, the seat of Worcester Co., encompasses 38.41 sq. mi. of land, at 42°16' N lat. and 71°52' W long., in central MA. Situated on the Blackstone River, it lies 39 mi. W of Boston.

TOPOGRAPHY. The terrain of Worcester, which is situated in the E N.E. upland, is a plateau-like area of low hills and valleys which rises from approx. 500' to 1,000' above sea level. Major bodies of water in the surrounding area include Lake Quinsigamond, Coes Reservoir, Indian Lake and Bell Pond. The mean elev. is 410'.

CLIMATE. The climate of Worcester is humid and continental and is largely influenced by the city's proximity to the Atlantic Ocean, Long Island Sound and the Berkshire Hills. Storms moving up the E coast bring NE and E winds with rain, fog or snow. Storms developing in TX-OK usually bring little rain, but do bring warm air into the region. The monthly mean temps. range from a Jan. mean of 23.6°F to a July mean of 69.9°F, with an avg. annual mean of 46.9°F. The avg. annual rainfall of 46.87" is evenly distributed throughout the year. Most of the 75" avg. annual snowfall

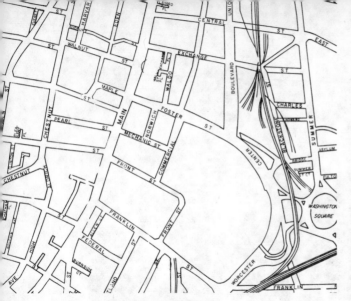

Downtown Worcester, Massachusetts

occurs between Dec. and Mar. The RH ranges from 48% to 83% and the growing season avgs. 149 days. Worcester is located in the ESTZ and observes DST.

FLORA AND FAUNA. Animals native to Worcester include the squirrel, rabbit, whitetail deer and raccoon. Common birds are the cardinal, mockingbird, thrush, bluebird and crow. Frogs, salamanders, a few species of turtles, snakes and lizards, as well as the venomous timber rattlesnake and the copperhead, inhabit the area. Typical trees include the white pine, oak and maple.

POPULATION. According to the US census, the pop. of Worcester in 1970 was 176,572. In 1980, it was estimated that it had decreased to 169,400.

ETHNIC GROUPS. In 1978, the ethnic distribution of Worcester was approx. 93.8% Caucasian, 1.9% Black, and 4.3% Hispanic.

TRANSPORTATION. Interstates 90, 190 and 290, US Hwy. 20 and state hwys. 9, 12 and 70 provide major motor access to Worcester. *Railroads* serving the city include ConRail, AMTRAK, Boston & ME and the Providence & Worcester. *Airlines* serving Worcester Municipal Airport include DL, and Precision. *Bus lines* serving the city include Greyhound, Trailways and the local Worcester Regional Transit Authority (WRTA).

COMMUNICATIONS. Communications, broadcasting and print media

Mechanics Hall, Worcester, Massachusetts

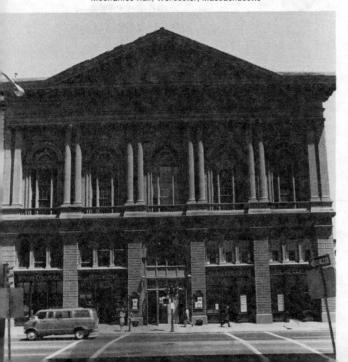

originating from Worcester are: *AM radio stations* WTAG 580 (NBC, MOR); WNEB 1230 (Indep., C&W); WORC 1310 (CBS Big Band); WFTQ 1440 (UPI, Contemp.); *FM radio stations* WCHC 89.1 (ABC/FM, Contemp.) WICN 90.5 (Indep., Divers.); WCUW 91.3 (Indep., Var. Span.) WSRS 96.1 (Indep., Btfl. Mus.); WAAF 107.3 (ABC/FM, AOR); *television stations* WSMW Ch. 27 (Indep.); *press*: two major daily publications serve the Worcester area, the *Telegram*, issued mornings, and the *Evening Gazette*, issued evenings.

HISTORY. The Nipmuck Indians inhabited the area of present-day Worcester when Ephraim Curtis settled there in 1670. Curtis and the settlers who followed were driven out of the settlement, called Quinsigamon Plantation, by Indians in 1675. A second settlement, established in the 1680s and named Worcester, after a British victory in Worcester, England, was also abandoned due to Indian attacks. The first permanent settlement was established in 1713 by Jonas Rice. It was incorporated as a town in 1722, and became the seat of Worcester Co. in 1731. The first N.E. reading of the Declaration of Independence took place in the city. A 1783 Worcester court ruling held that the MA Constitution did not permit slavery. During the early 1800s, the city became a transportation center, based in part on the comm.'s manufacturing output and the Blackstone Canal's linking of the city with Providence and the Atlantic Ocean in 1828. RRs were established in the city in 1839 and 1848. In 1848, Worcester was chartered as a city. During the post-Civil War period, Worcester's industrial base became more diversified, with expansion and the addition of wire manufacturing, a textile industry, a plant to make grinding wheels and a facility to produce the first practical envelope-folding machine. Immigration that started in the 1820s continued through the end of the century, with the arrival of many Italians, Swedes, E Europeans and blacks. Robert H. Goddard, the father of modern rocketry, conducted the first US rocket experiments in the city during the 1920s. In 1938 a hurricane caused extensive damage to the city. In 1966 the city established an inner-city renovation plan. Today Worcester is an industrial center with a rich cultural background.

GOVERNMENT. Worcester has a council-mgr. form of government consisting of nine members, including the mayor. The council members are elected at large to a two-year term. The mayor is the ceremonial head of the city, and is selected from and by the council; he serves a two-year term and is a council member with one vote. The city mgr. is chosen by the council and is the chief executive of the city.

ECONOMY AND INDUSTRY. Worcester is an important N.E. commercial and manufacturing center. About one-third of its total employment is concentrated in the manufacturing sector. Manufactured goods include primary metals, fabricated metals, non-electrical machinery, electrical equipment, textiles, apparel, leather goods, foods and printing. Retail trade, finance, real estate, insurance, and govt. are the chief non-manufacturing industries. Over 65% of employment opportunities in the city are in the non-manufacturing sector. More than half of the resident labor force is classified as professional, skilled worker or craftsman. In 1979, the total labor force of the met. area was 205,100, while the rate of unemployment was 4.2%.

BANKING. In 1978, total deposits for the eight banks headquartered in Worcester were $2,029,777,000, while total assets were $2,337,536,000. Among the banks serving the area are Worcester Co. Natl., Worcester Co. Institution for Savings, People's Savings Bank, Consumers Savings Bank, Guaranty Bank & Trust Co. and Mechanics Natl. Bank.

HOSPITALS. Among the hosps. serving the Worcester area are the

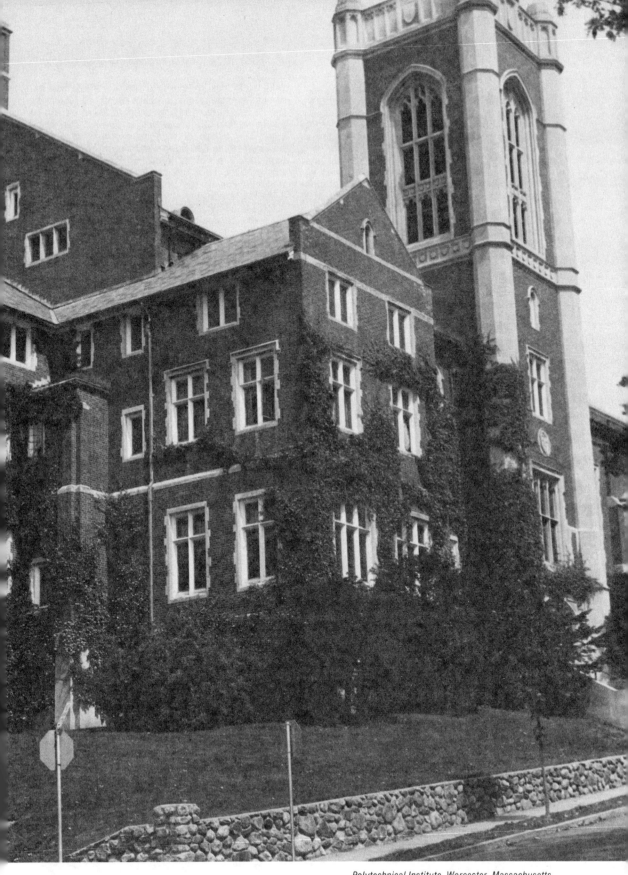

Polytechnical Institute, Worcester, Massachusetts

Memorial, St. Vincent and Worcester City (which serve as teaching hosps. for the prestigious U of MA Medical School) Fairlawn, Hahnemann, Doctors' and Worcester State. The world-famous Worcester Foundation for Experimental Biology is located in nearby Shrewsbury.

EDUCATION. Approximately 10 teaching and research institutions are located in Worcester. Prominent among them is Col. of the Holy Cross, a parochial, coed, liberal arts col. founded in 1843. N.E.'s oldest Roman Catholic col. enrolled 2,691 students in 1978. Worcester Polytechnical Inst., founded in 1865, had a 1978 enrollment of 3,192 and is a highly-regarded technical col. The presence of the U of MA Medical School greatly adds to Worcester's reputation as the medical center of central MA. Other schools in the area include Becker Jr. Col., Central N.E. Col. of Technology, N.E. School of Accounting, Quinsigamond Comm. Col., Assumption Col., Clark U, Salter Secretarial School, School of the Worcester Art Museum and Worcester Jr. Col. The comm. school concept in MA was pioneered by the City of Worcester. Six elementary and one high school house comm. school programs. These multi-purpose schools serve all ages and needs. There is a separate Vocational School Department which operates four schools to meet the needs of the vocationally-oriented student. Worcester's private schools include many Catholic schools, some Jewish schools and a number of private schools without religious affiliation. Most prominent among these are the col. preparatory schools. Libs. include Central MA Regional, Worcester Public and Worcester Co.

ENTERTAINMENT. For more than 120 years the city has hosted the Worcester Music Festival. The festival has attracted top performers from across the nation. Other annual events include the Greenhill Spectacular and the Lake Quinsigamond Rowing Regatta. Intercollegiate sports action is provided by the Holy Cross Col. Crusaders basketball and football teams and by the basketball teams of the Clark U Cougars and of Assumption Col.

ACCOMMODATIONS. Hotels and motels in the Worcester area include the Sheraton Lincoln, Howard Johnson's, Day's Lodge and the Holiday Inns.

City Hall, Worcester, Massachusetts

FACILITIES. There are 54 recreation sites totaling 1,251 acres in Worcester. Among the parks are Elm, Institute, Kendrick Field, Hadwen and Green Hill. Green Hill Park is the largest, covering 482.37 acres, and offers a barnyard zoo, Astro City, a space-age-styled playground, Story Book Village, winter sports such as skating, coasting and skiing and a new 1.2 mile jogging-exercise course. Activities available along the shores of Lake Quinsigamond, Lake Park and Regatta Point Park include swimming, picnicking, sailing, running, football and tennis. Golf courses are available at Green Hill Park, Worcester Country Club and Tatnuck Country Club. Hadwen Park has a ski lift.

CULTURAL ACTIVITIES. The City Mgr.'s Advisory Committee on the Arts sponsors programs and assists in the arts in Worcester. Musical organizations in the city include the Worcester Orchestra, Youth Orchestra, Worcester Chorus and Opera Worcester. Offering dramatic performances are the Foothills Theatre, the N.E. Repertory Company, Holy Cross Fenwick, the Entertainers' & Actors' Guild, Sock & Buskin, Children's Theatre and Worcester Co. Light Opera. Other performing organizations include the Ballet Society, the Poetry Assn. and the Worcester Comm. School for the Performing Arts. The Worcester Music Festival has been held for more than 120 years in the city and features nationally known performers in a series of events covering several weekends. Many of the area's performances are presented at Mechanics Hall and Worcester Auditorium. City museums include the Historical Museum and the Worcester Science Center, a 50-acre structure housing a zoo and a miniature train, in addition to its science displays. The Worcester Art Museum, founded in 1896, contains a collection of Japanese prints and houses an art school. The John Woodman Higgins Armory Museum features an extensive collection of medieval armor. The American Antiquarian Society maintains a collection of historical material dating from 1620 to 1820.

LANDMARKS AND SIGHTSEEING SPOTS. There are many historical structures and displays in Worcester. Mechanics Hall, with its impressive facade, is an example of the mid-19th century neo-Renaissance Italian style. It was designed by Eldridge Boyden and was dedicated in 1857.

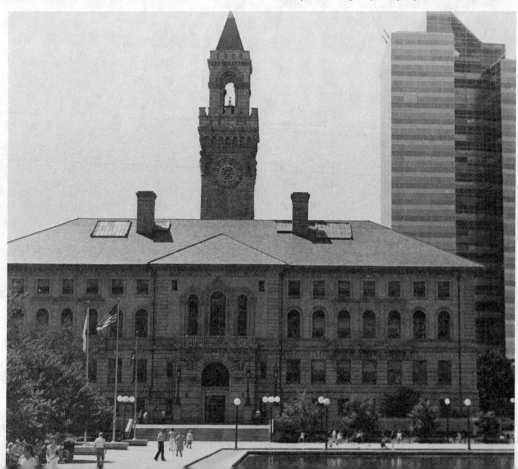

The many historical homes of interesting design include the American Antiquarian Society Home, G. A. R. Hall, Liberty Farm (an important link of the "Underground RR"), Salisbury Mansion, Whitcomb Mansion and Paine House. The Worcester Co. Horticultural Society offers exhibitions and summer shows. Relics of the early days of rockets and memorabilia of inventor Robert H. Goddard are housed in the Goddard Exhibition at Clark U.

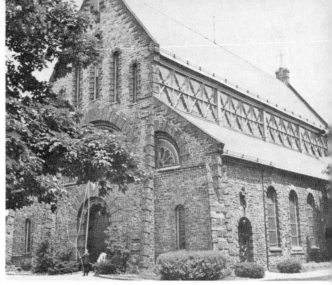

St. John's Episcopal, first church in Yonkers, New York

YONKERS
NEW YORK

CITY LOCATION-SIZE-EXTENT. Yonkers encompasses 21 sq. mi. in SE NY in Westchester Co., just N of the Bronx, at 40°57' N lat. and 73°53' W long. It is bounded on the W by the Hudson River, on the E by the Bronx River Parkway, on the N by the towns of Hastings-on-Hudson and Greenville and on the S by NYC and the met. area extends into that of NYC.

TOPOGRAPHY. The terrain of Yonkers, which is situated in the NE upland region, is characterized by hills and low mts. The mean elev. is 16'.

CLIMATE. The climate of Yonkers is continental, influenced by the W winds and sometimes moderated in summer by local sea breezes. The avg. annual temp. of 54°F ranges from a Jan. mean of 32°F to a July mean of 76°F. The avg. annual rainfall of 43" is well distributed. The avg. annual snowfall is 25". The RH ranges from 48% to 80%. The avg. growing season is approx. 200 days. Yonkers lies in the ESTZ and observes DST.

FLORA AND FAUNA. Animals native to Yonkers include the chipmunk, raccoon, opossum and skunk. Common birds are the cardinal, blue jay, starling and crow. Salamanders, leopard frogs, American toads, green snakes and box turtles, as well as the venomous timber rattlesnake and copperhead, are found in the area. Typical trees include the hemlock, oak, willow, spruce, maple and elm. Smaller plants include the rhododendron, azalea, tulip, rose, daffodil, meadowrue and petunia, the official flower of Yonkers.

POPULATION. According to the US census, the pop. of Yonkers in 1970 was 204,297. In 1978 it was estimated that it had decreased to 196,000.

ETHNIC GROUPS. In 1978 the racial distribution of Yonkers was approx. 75% Caucasian and 25% Black.

TRANSPORTATION. Interstate hwys. 9, 80, 87, 287, US hwy. 46 and state hwys. 4, 17 and 208 provide major motor access to Yonkers. *Railroads* serving the city include the Harlem, Hudson and Putnam branches of the ConRail system. The city has a 4.5 mi. waterfront providing shipping access and small boat docking. *Bus lines* operated by the Co. of Westchester provide transportation on 20 rtes. to all city areas and adjacent towns, with many going to NYC directly and seven connecting with NYC subways. *Airlines* serve Yonkers through Westchester Co. Airport, 20 min. N of the city. All major airlines serve the three major regional airports nearby: Newark, NJ and LaGuardia and Kennedy Intl. in NYC.

COMMUNICATIONS. Communications, broadcasting and print media serving Yonkers are: *AM radio stations* WVOX 1460 (MBS, Suburban Comm.); *FM radio station* WRTN 93.5 (MBS, Clas., MOR); no *television stations* originate from Yonkers which receives broadcasting from nearby NYC; *press*: one major newspaper is published in Yonkers, the evening *Herald Statesman*; other publications include the *Home News & Times*, *Tappan Ice Villager*, *Illustrated News*, *Westchester Co. Press*, *The Record of Yonkers* and *Yonkers Jewish Chronicle.*

HISTORY. The site of present-day Yonkers was inhabited by native Americans of the Algonquin and Iroquois tribes until purchased by the Dutch Republic in the early 1600s. Title was passed to the N.E. Company and then to Adrian van der Donck, who built a sawmill on the Nepperhan River. In Holland van der Donck was known as "Dejonkheer"—young nobleman—from which the city's name was subsequently derived. Towards the end of the 17th century, the area was acquired by the Philipse family. Frederick Philipse took over van der Donck's sawmill and built a grist mill. From here sloops transported flour down the Hudson to Philipse's warehouses in NYC. Philipse's Manor Hall was built in 1682 and later by a royal patent of 1693 the Philipse holdings (about one-third of modern Westchester Co., NY) were confirmed as the Philipse

Untermyer Park, Yonkers, New York

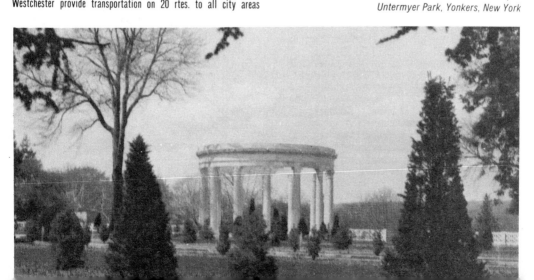

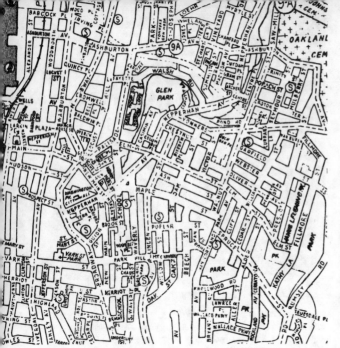

Central Yonkers, New York

Estate. The Philipses lost their holdings during the Revolutionary War when Colonel Frederick Philipse III was tried and found guilty of treason in absentia for siding with the British. The settlement grew slowly throughout the 18th century and during the first half of the 19th. In 1854, Elisha Otis started manufacturing elevators in Yonkers. In 1855, Yonkers was incorporated as a village. Yonkers received a city charter in 1872, when it had a pop. of 20,000. Yonkers today is a small, industrial and manufacturing center outside NYC and is included in the Port of NYC. The city's plans for growth in the coming years include the development of an industrial park and the Getty Sq. project which calls for the construction of an enclosed shopping mall downtown.

GOVERNMENT. Yonkers has a council-mgr. form of government consisting of 12 council members and the mayor. The mayor, who is a member of the council, is elected at large, while the council members are elected by ward, to two-year terms.

ECONOMY AND INDUSTRY. Major industries in Yonkers produce elevators, copper and cable wiring, electronic systems, graphic arts materials, syrups and sugars, spray valves, duplicating machines and ice cream. There are approx. 300 manufacuturing firms in the city. Manufacturing is the largest sector, followed by retail trade and government. It is estimated that the unemployment rate in June, 1978, was 8%. The city has the second highest median family income of cities with pop. over 200,000. In 1975, median per capita income in the city was $6,110.

BANKING. There are 20 banks in Yonkers. In 1978, total deposits for the one bank headquartered in the city were $39,496,000, while assets were $44,163,000. Banks include NY-Co. Trust Region, NY's first bank founded in 1784 by Alexander Hamilton; Hudson Valley Natl.; Chase Manhattan; the Manhattan Savings; Marine Midland and Natl. of Westchester.

HOSPITALS. There are four gen. care hosps. in Yonkers, including St. John's Riverside, St. Joseph's, Yonkers Gen. and Yonkers Professional.

EDUCATION. Elizabeth Seton Col., a jr. col. founded for women in 1960, grants associate degrees in arts and in applied science and enrolled approx. 1,200 students in 1978. St. Joseph's Seminary, a Roman Catholic institution under the sponsorship and control of the Archdiocese of NY for the preparation of candidates for the priesthood, awards professional degrees in theology and enrolled approx. 75 students in 1978. Other educational institutions within commuting distance include those located in NYC and its

environs. The Yonkers public school system maintains 30 elementary, seven jr. high and six sr. high schools, with a total enrollment of 25,370 students. There are 29 private and parochial schools with a 1977 enrollment of 7,660. Yonkers School for Adult Education maintains programs in ten centers throughout the city. The Yonkers Lib. system maintains five branches, one bookmobile and one minimobile.

ENTERTAINMENT. Yonkers hosts the annual Hudson Valley Speed Skating Championships at the Edward J. Murray Memorial Ice Skating Rink. Trotting is held at Yonkers Raceway on Central Avenue. Other spectator sports are available in nearby NYC.

ACCOMMODATIONS. There are several hotels and motels in Yonkers, including the City Line, Trade Winds Motor Court and the Tuckahoe Motor, Holiday and Yonkers Motor inns.

FACILITIES. There are 78 parks and playgrounds encompassing approx. 229.67 acres. There are a number of lakes in the area, including Tibbetts Brook, Sprain Ridge Co. and Untermeyer parks. Public golf courses are available at Dunwoodie and Sprain Lake. Yonkers Tennis Center offers both public and private courts. Other sporting facilities include 58 outdoor basketball courts, 44 ballfields, two pools and the Edward J. Murray Memorial Ice Skating Center. There are a number of lakes including Crestwood and Hill View Reservoir. Three picnic areas and pleasure boat facilities are also available.

CULTURAL ACTIVITIES. Dramatic productions are staged by the Yonkers Playhouse and the Greystone Actors Guild. The Hudson River Museum is the city's main cultural center, sponsoring concerts, musicals, dance, lectures and other performances by touring groups. Exhibits in the museum, which also houses the Andrus Space Transit Planetarium, range from historic artifacts and furnishings to modern art.

LANDMARKS AND SIGHTSEEING SPOTS. Philipse Manor Hall, built in 1682 and renovated in 1750 by Frederick Philipse III is now a NY state historical site. It also contains a museum. The Sherwood House, a Hudson Valley Colonial farmhouse built by Thomas Sherwood in 1740, is being restored and preserved by the Yonkers Historical Society.

YOUNGSTOWN
OHIO

CITY LOCATION-SIZE-EXTENT. Youngstown, seat of Mahoning Co., is on the Mahoning River in NE OH, just 10 mi. from the W border of PA and encompasses 33.6 sq. mi. at 41°16' N lat. and 80°40' W long. Its greater met. area extends into most of Mahoning Co. and Trumbull Co. to the N and overlaps the Warren met. area.

TOPOGRAPHY. Situated in the Appalachian Plateau re-

Youngstown, Ohio

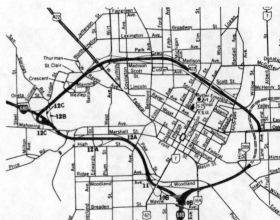

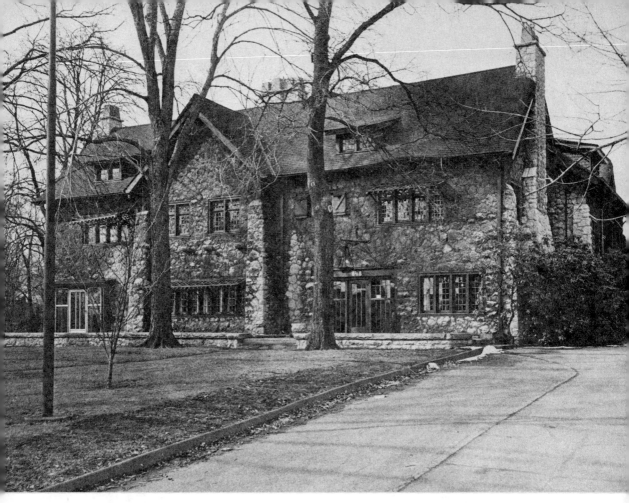

Arms Museum, Youngstown, Ohio

region, the terrain of Youngstown consists of rolling hills and valleys with numerous lakes in the area, both natural and man-made. The mean elev. of 840'.

CLIMATE. The climate of Youngstown is characterized by moderate temps., high humidity and cloudiness, and influenced by Lake Erie. The avg. annual temp. of 48.6°F ranges from a Jan. mean of 25°F to a July mean of 70°F. The 38" avg. annual rainfall is evenly distributed throughout the year. The avg. annual snowfall of 57.6" mainly occurs during snow flurries between Dec. and Mar. The RH ranges from 53% to 88%. The growing season avgs. 162 days. Youngstown is located in the ESTZ and observes DST.

FLORA AND FAUNA. Animals native to Youngstown include the raccoon, opossum and fox. Common birds are the cardinal (the state bird), robin, bluebird, swallow and sparrow. Box turtles, bullfrogs, salamanders, toads and milksnakes, as well as the venomous rattlesnake and copperhead, are found in the area. Typical trees are the elm, maple, oak and pine. Smaller plants include violets, roses and honeysuckle.

POPULATION. According to the US census, the pop. of Youngstown in 1970 was 140,909. In 1978, it was estimated that it had decreased to 120,000.

ETHNIC GROUPS. In 1978, the ethnic distribution of Youngstown was approx. 74.3% Caucasian, 25% Black and 2.6% Hispanic (a percentage of the Hispanic total is also included in the Caucasian total).

TRANSPORTATION. Interstate hwy. 680, US hwys. 62 and 422 and state hwys. 7, 164, 170, 193, 289, 616 and 625 provide major motor access to Youngstown. *Railroads* serving the city include the Chessie System, Chicago & NW, ConRail, Pittsburgh & Lake Erie, Youngstown & N, Youngstown and S Railway. *Airlines* serving Youngstown Municipal Airport are US Air and UA. *Bus lines* serving the city include Columbiana, Greyhound and Trailways.

COMMUNICATIONS. Communications, broadcasting and print media originating from Youngstown are: *AM radio stations* WKBN 570 (CBS, MOR, C&W); WBBW 1240 (ABC/I&E, Talk, News, Sports); WFMJ 1390 (Indep., Contemp.) and WGFT 1500 (ABC/C, ROck, Soul & Disco). *FM radio stations* WYSU 88.5 (NPR, Educ.); WQOD 93.3 (MBS, Divers.) WKBN 98.9 (Indep., Btfl. Mus.) and WSRD 101.1 (Indep., Prog.). *television stations* WFMJ Ch. 21 (NBC); WKBN Ch. 27 (CBS); WYTV Ch. 33 (ABC) and cable; *press*: one major daily serves the area, the *Vindicator*, issued evenings; other publications include the *Legal News* and *The Jambar.*

HISTORY. Youngstown was founded in 1797 by settlers from NY and named in honor of John Young, who purchased the site for the city. Development of the village was slow until construction of the first smelter in the area in 1802. In 1826, the first coal mine was opened in the Mahoning Valley. Youngstown was incorporated in 1848. Union Iron and Steel Co. opened the first steel plant in the city in 1892, further establishing the city's destiny as a great steel producer. Youngstown developed steadily as an industrial city during the 20th century, and today is fourth largest steel center in the US.

GOVERNMENT. Youngstown has a mayor-council form of govt. consisting of an eight-member council and a mayor. The council members are elected by district to a two-year term. The mayor, elected at large to a two year-term, is not a member and has no vote.

ECONOMY AND INDUSTRY. Youngstown ranks fourth in the nation in the production of pigiron and steel. Major products include a variety of steel products, communications systems, electronics, automotive parts, gloves

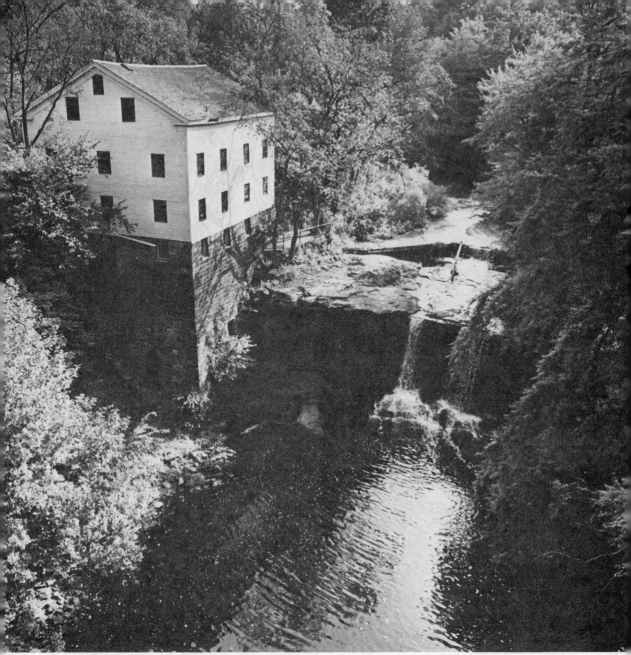

Old Mill, Lanternman Falls, Youngstown, Ohio

and aluminum products. In 1979, the total labor force of the greater met. area was approx. 237,500, while the rate of unemployment was 6.9%.

BANKING. In 1978, total deposits for the four banks headquartered in Youngstown were $1,001,415,000, while assets were $1,156,499,000. Banks include the Dollar Savings Bank and Trust Co. and Union Natl. Bank.

HOSPITALS. There are several hosps. in Youngstown, including Family Practice (Youngstown Hosp. Assn.), St. Elizabeth's, Woodside Revceiving and Youngstown Osteopathic. The N Columbiana Co. Comm. Hosp. and the Comm. Hosp. of Warren also serve the area.

EDUCATION. Youngstown State U was founded in 1908 by the YMCA and offers liberal arts, technical and professional courses. It also participates in the NE OH U Col. of Med. consortium and in a cooperative plan with Duke U in forestry. Grad. and undergrad. enrollment was 15,696 in 1978. Other teaching institutions include Penn-OH Col. and St. Elizabeth Hosp. The 99 schools in the public school system enrolled 56,000 in 1978. The Reuben McMillan Free Lib., with 18 branch libs., is available for the residents.

ENTERTAINMENT. The State U's Penguins participate in intercollegiate sports.

ACCOMMODATIONS. There are several hotels and motels in Youngstown, including the Knights, Day's and Holiday inns and Howard Johnson's.

FACILITIES. Youngstown has several parks, including Mill Creek Park, the largest, with more than 2,300 acres. Dogwood, Donnebrook, Hubbard, Lee Run, Meander and the municipal golf links are public golf courses in the area.

CULTURAL ACTIVITIES. Dramatic performances are presented at the Youngstown Playhouse. The Butler Institution of American Art contains paintings and etchings by American artists and miniatures of the American presidents. The Ford Nature Education Center includes a semiaquatic terrarium; aquariums with local fish, plants and crayfish, and displays of minerals and fauna.

LANDMARKS AND SIGHTSEEING SPOTS. The Arms Museum is housed in the restored home of one of the first families in the Youngstown area. The main floor remains as when they lived there, china, glassware and furniture are displayed with period household and farm items.

APPENDIXES

STATE CAPITALS

ALABAMA .... Montgomery
ALASKA .... Juneau
ARIZONA .... Phoenix
ARKANSAS .... Little Rock
CALIFORNIA .... Sacramento
COLORADO .... Denver
CONNECTICUT .... Hartford
DELAWARE .... Dover
FLORIDA .... Tallahassee
GEORGIA .... Atlanta
HAWAII .... Honolulu
IDAHO .... Boise
ILLINOIS .... Springfield
INDIANA .... Indianapolis
IOWA .... Des Moines
KANSAS .... Topeka
KENTUCKY .... Frankfort
LOUISIANA .... Baton Rouge
MAINE .... Augusta
MARYLAND .... Annapolis
MASSACHUSETTS .... Boston
MICHIGAN .... Lansing
MINNESOTA .... St. Paul
MISSISSIPPI .... Jackson
MISSOURI .... Jefferson City
MONTANA .... Helena
NEBRASKA .... Lincoln
NEVADA .... Carson City
NEW HAMPSHIRE .... Concord
NEW JERSEY .... Trenton
NEW MEXICO .... Santa Fe
NEW YORK .... Albany
NORTH CAROLINA .... Raleigh
NORTH DAKOTA .... Bismarck
OHIO .... Columbus
OKLAHOMA .... Oklahoma City
OREGON .... Salem
PENNSYLVANIA .... Harrisburg
RHODE ISLAND .... Providence
SOUTH CAROLINA .... Columbia
SOUTH DAKOTA .... Pierre
TENNESSEE .... Nashville
TEXAS .... Austin
UTAH .... Salt Lake City
VERMONT .... Montpelier
VIRGINIA .... Richmond
WASHINGTON .... Olympia
WEST VIRGINIA .... Charleston
WISCONSIN .... Madison
WYOMING .... Cheyenne

CITIES RANKED BY ESTIMATED POPULATION FIGURES

1. New York, City NY (1978) 7,414,800
2. Chicago, IL (1978) 2,940,000
3. Los Angeles, CA (1978) 2,795,000
4. Philadelphia, PA (1978) 1,765,000
5. Houston, TX (1978) 1,632,000
6. Detroit, MI (1978) 1,210,000
7. Dallas, TX (1979) 898,000
8. Baltimore, MD (1979) 830,000
9. San Diego, CA (1978) 830,000
10. San Antonio, TX (1978) 803,000
11. Phoenix, AZ (1979) 762,300
12. Indianapolis, IN (1978) 720,000
13. Honolulu, HI (1978) 720,000
14. Memphis, TN (1978) 680,000
15. Washington, DC (1978) 676,000
16. San Francisco, CA (1978) 657,000
17. Boston, MA (1978) 638,000
18. Milwaukee, WI (1978) 620,160
19. Cleveland, OH (1978) 580,000
20. San Jose, CA (1978) 578,600
21. New Orleans, LA (1978) 555,000
22. Jacksonville, FL (1978) 539,000
23. Columbus, OH (1978) 529,000
24. Denver, CO (1978) 516,000
25. St. Louis, MO (1978) 489,000
26. Kansas City, MO (1978) 485,007
27. Seattle, WA (1978) 470,000
28. Atlanta, GA (1978) 456,200
29. Nashville, TN (1978) 451,000
30. Pittsburgh, PA (1978) 421,000
31. Ft. Worth, TX (1979) 420,140
32. El Paso, TX (1979) 395,514
33. Cincinnati, OH (1978) 383,000
34. Oklahoma City, OK (1978) 379,800
35. Omaha, NE (1978) 375,400
36. Minneapolis, MN (1978) 375,000
37. Buffalo, NY (1978) 368,000
38. Portland, OR (1978) 368,000
39. Tulsa, OK (1978) 360,000
40. Toledo, OH (1978) 356,100
41. Miami, FL (1978) 354,000
42. Long Beach, CA (1978) 345,000
43. Oakland, CA (1978) 333,055
44. Austin, TX (1978) 331,577
45. Albuquerque, NM (1978) 330,000
46. Charlotte, NC (1978) 325,000
47. Newark, NJ (1978) 320,000
48. Louisville, KY (1979) 318,200
49. Tucson, AZ (1978) 311,400
50. Norfolk, VA (1978) 286,000
51. Tampa, FL (1979) 280,340
52. Birmingham, AL (1978) 278,000
53. St. Paul, MN (1978) 277,952
54. Rochester, NY (1978) 263,000
55. Wichita, KS (1978) 261,862
56. Sacramento, CA (1978) 260,000
57. Virginia Beach, VA (1978) 259,806
58. Akron, OH (1978) 245,000
59. Jersey City, NJ (1978) 244,200
60. St. Petersburg, FL (1978) 238,450
61. Colorado Springs, CO (1978) ... 230,000
62. Corpus Christi, TX (1978) 225,000
63. Shreveport, LA (1978) 220,000
64. Baton Rouge, LA (1978) 219,754
65. Richmond, VA (1978) 216,300
66. Jackson, MS (1978) 210,000
67. Anchorage, AK (1979) 204,809
68. Anaheim, CA (1978) 204,800
69. Mobile, AL (1978) 203,000
70. Fresno, CA (1978) 200,000
71. Dayton, OH (1978) 197,000
72. Yonkers, NY (1978) 196,000
73. Montgomery, AL (1978) 195,704
74. Lexington, KY (1978) 193,200
75. Grand Rapids, MI (1978) 190,000
76. Des Moines, IA (1978) 189,200
77. Knoxville, TN (1978) 187,000
78. Ft. Wayne, IN (1979) 185,500
79. Santa Ana, CA (1978) 183,900
80. Syracuse, NY (1978) 182,543
81. Salt Lake City, UT (1977) 180,000
82. Spokane, WA (1978) 176,700
83. Lubbock, TX (1978) 175,250
84. Madison, WI (1979) 173,051
85. Gary, IN (1978) 171,300
86. Kansas City, KS (1978) 170,708
87. Chattanooga, TN (1978) 170,046
88. Warren, MI (1978) 170,000
89. Columbus, GA (1978) 170,000
90. Worcester, MA (1980) 169,400
91. Lincoln, NE (1978) 168,800
92. Arlington, TX (1978) 168,000
93. Providence, RI (1978) 167,729
94. Springfield, MA (1978) 167,500
95. Newport News, VA (1978) 164,637
96. Huntington Beach, CA (1978) .. 164,500
97. Flint, MI (1977) 163,594
98. Las Vegas, NV (1978) 161,200
99. Riverside, CA (1978) 161,000
100. Topeka, KS (1980) 160,184

CITIES RANKED BY ESTIMATED POPULATION FIGURES (Continued)

101. Greensboro, NC (1979)	157,326	134. Youngstown, OH (1978)	120,000
102. Ft. Lauderdale, FL (1978)	156,400	135. Garden Grove, CA (1978)	118,454
103. Amarillo, TX (1979)	156,308	136. Pasadena, TX (1978)	118,000
104. Raleigh, NC (1978)	156,256	137. Alexandria, VA (1978)	116,900
105. Mesa, AZ (1979)	156,000	138. South Bend, IN (1978)	114,000
106. Little Rock, AR (1979)	155,000	139. Waterbury, CT (1978)	112,000
107. Paterson, NJ (1978)	154,256	140. Berkeley, CA (1978)	112,000
108. Tacoma, WA (1978)	151,267	141. Chesapeake, VA (1978)	111,896
109. Garland, TX (1978)	149,302	142. Livonia, MI (1978)	110,800
110. Bridgeport, CT (1978)	148,000	143. Pueblo, CO (1978)	110,668
111. Savannah, GA (1978)	148,000	144. Cedar Rapids, IA (1978)	110,400
112. Aurora, CO (1978)	146,000	145. Boise, ID (1978)	110,000
113. Winston-Salem, NC (1978)	145,000	146. Independence, MO (1978)	109,700
114. Huntsville, AL (1978)	143,500	147. Columbia, SC (1978)	109,600
115. Hialeah, FL (1978)	138,000	148. Portsmouth, VA (1978)	108,400
116. Peoria, IL (1978)	135,400	149. Irving, TX (1978)	107,000
117. Glendale, CA (1978)	134,300	150. Albany, NY (1978)	107,000
118. Springfield, MO (1978)	134,000	151. Durham, NC (1978)	107,000
119. New Haven, CT (1978)	133,000	152. San Bernardino, CA (1978)	107,000
120. Lakewood, CO (1978)	131,700	153. Ann Arbor, MI (1978)	107,000
121. Hampton, VA (1977)	131,300	154. Pasadena, CA (1978)	106,700
122. Stockton, CA (1978)	131,100	155. Sunnyvale, CA (1978)	106,050
123. Evansville, IN (1978)	130,100	156. Roanoke, VA (1978)	105,500
124. Beaumont, TX (1978)	129,990	157. Allentown, PA (1978)	105,069
125. Lansing, MI (1978)	129,000	158. Trenton, NJ (1980)	104,600
126. Torrance, CA (1978)	128,593	159. Elizabeth, NJ (1978)	104,000
127. Rockford, IL (1977)	128,101	160. Stamford, CT (1978)	103,300
128. Hollywood, FL (1978)	127,000	161. Hammond, IN (1978)	102,400
129. Erie, PA (1978)	125,800	162. Canton, OH (1978)	101,852
130. Fremont, CA (1978)	125,345	163. Davenport, IA (1978)	101,800
131. Hartford, CT (1978)	124,000	164. Cambridge, MA (1978)	101,300
132. Orlando, FL (1978)	122,090	165. Fall River, MA (1978)	100,430
133. Macon, GA (1978)	120,300	166. New Bedford, MA (1978)	100,075

CITIES RANKED BY SQUARE MILEAGE

1. Anchorage, AK	1,900.00	51. Lubbock, TX	83.80
2. Jacksonville, FL	840.00	52. Omaha, NE	83.00
3. Oklahoma City, OK	621.40	53. Amarillo, TX	80.06
4. Houston, TX	556.37	54. Cincinnati, OH	78.46
5. Nashville, TN	532.00	55. Knoxville, TN	77.10
6. Los Angeles, CA	463.90	56. Cleveland, OH	76.50
7. Indianapolis, IN	379.40	57. Lexington, KY	73.40
8. Dallas, TX	378.00	58. Beaumont, TX	71.70
9. Chesapeake, VA	353.00	59. Riverside, CA	71.30
10. Phoenix, AZ	325.20	60. Washington, DC	70.00
11. San Diego, CA	319.50	61. Salt Lake City, UT	69.50
12. Kansas City, MO	316.00	62. Newport News, VA	69.10
13. New York City, NY	314.00	63. Independence, MO	67.50
14. Virginia Beach, VA	310.00	64. Mesa, AZ	67.00
15. Memphis, TN	280.89	65. Louisville, KY	65.20
16. San Antonio, TX	263.50	66. Des Moines, IA	64.30
17. Ft. Worth, TX	244.00	67. Norfolk, VA	64.00
18. El Paso, TX	239.21	68. Springfield, MO	63.20
19. Chicago, IL	222.80	69. Davenport, IA	63.00
20. Columbus, GA	220.00	70. Irving, TX	63.00
21. New Orleans, LA	197.10	71. Richmond, VA	62.50
22. Tulsa, OK	181.40	72. St. Louis, MO	61.20
23. Columbus, OH	173.20	73. Savannah, GA	61.20
24. San Jose, CA	152.00	74. Greensboro, NC	60.60
25. Mobile, AL	141.90	75. Aurora, CO	60.00
26. Detroit, MI	139.60	76. Topeka, KS	60.00
27. Atlanta, GA	131.50	77. Minneapolis, MN	58.70
28. Philadelphia, PA	127.90	78. Lincoln, NE	58.66
29. Chattanooga, TN	126.90	79. Winston-Salem, NC	58.20
30. Denver, CO	115.08	80. Akron, OH	58.00
31. Huntsville, AL	113.00	81. Fresno, CA	58.00
32. Kansas City, KS	111.00	82. Little Rock, AR	56.90
33. Columbia, SC	108.60	83. St. Petersburg, FL	56.20
34. Austin, TX	106.00	84. Pittsburgh, PA	55.50
35. Jackson, MS	105.38	85. St. Paul, MN	55.44
36. Corpus Christi, TX	105.00	86. Ft. Wayne, IN	55.30
37. Wichita, KS	99.57	87. Pasadena, TX	55.00
38. Arlington, TX	99.00	88. Garland, TX	54.70
39. Fremont, CA	96.50	89. Hampton, VA	54.70
40. Milwaukee, WI	96.00	90. Las Vegas, NV	54.30
41. Sacramento, CA	93.90	91. Madison, WI	54.00
42. Portland, OR	93.50	92. Cedar Rapids, IA	53.61
43. Seattle, WA	91.60	93. Oakland, CA	53.40
44. Tucson, AZ	91.60	94. San Bernardino, CA	53.22
45. Shreveport, LA	90.00	95. Spokane, WA	52.42
46. Birmingham, AL	89.76	96. Long Beach, CA	50.10
47. Albuquerque, NM	87.70	97. Montgomery, AL	50.00
48. Toledo, OH	86.00	98. Macon, GA	49.50
49. Colorado Springs, CO	85.30	99. Pueblo, CO	49.46
50. Tampa, FL	84.50	100. Raleigh, NC	49.46

CITIES RANKED BY SQUARE MILEAGE (continued)

101. Boston, MA	49.40	134. Charlotte, NC	29.30
102. Dayton, OH	49.30	135. Glendale, CA	29.20
103. Baton Rouge, LA	48.70	136. Waterbury, CT	28.20
104. Tacoma, WA	47.80	137. Huntington Beach, CA	27.30
105. San Francisco, CA	46.60	138. Santa Ana, CA	27.20
106. Grand Rapids, MI	44.90	139. Hollywood, FL	26.90
107. Portsmouth, VA	43.00	140. Syracuse, NY	25.80
108. Roanoke, VA	43.00	141. Hammond, IN	24.10
109. Orlando, FL	42.87	142. Ann Arbor, MI	24.00
110. Gary, IN	42.70	143. Newark, NJ	24.00
111. Buffalo, NY	41.30	144. Sunnyvale, CA	22.95
112. Durham, NC	40.57	145. Hialeah, FL	22.00
113. Stockton, CA	40.12	146. Albany, NY	21.50
114. Anaheim, CA	40.00	147. Torrance, CA	21.00
115. Boise, ID	39.00	148. Yonkers, NY	21.00
116. Worcester, MA	38.41	149. Providence, RI	20.00
117. Peoria, IL	38.20	150. Canton, OH	18.99
118. Stamford, CT	38.10	151. New Bedford, MA	18.99
119. Evansville, IN	37.00	152. Erie, PA	18.90
120. Rochester, NY	36.70	153. Lakewood, CO	18.50
121. Livonia, MI	36.10	154. New Haven, CT	18.40
122. Rockford, IL	36.10	155. Baltimore, MD	18.30
123. Pasadena, CA	35.85	156. Allentown, PA	17.80
124. Lansing, MI	34.37	157. Bridgeport, CT	17.50
125. Miami, FL	34.30	158. Garden Grove, CA	17.40
126. Warren, MI	34.20	159. Hartford, CT	16.80
127. Youngstown, OH	33.60	160. Alexandria, VA	15.75
128. Pueblo, CO	33.50	161. Elizabeth, NJ	11.70
129. Fall River, MA	33.00	162. Jersey City, NJ	11.70
130. Flint, MI	32.90	163. Berkeley, CA	10.60
131. Springfield, MA	31.70	164. Paterson, NJ	8.40
132. Ft. Lauderdale, FL	31.00	165. Trenton, NJ	7.50
133. South Bend, IN	30.10	166. Cambridge, MA	6.25

CITY AREA CODES

City	Code	City	Code	City	Code
Akron, OH	216	Garland, TX	214	Pasadena, TX	713
Albany, NY	518	Gary, IN	219	Paterson, NJ	201
Albuquerque, NM	505	Glendale, CA	213	Peoria, IL	309
Alexandria, VA	703	Grand Rapids, MI	616	Philadelphia, PA	215
Allentown, PA	215	Greensboro, NC	919	Phoenix, AZ	602
Amarillo, TX	806	Hammond, IN	219	Pittsburgh, PA	412
Anaheim, CA	714	Hampton, VA	804	Portland, OR	503
Anchorage, AK	907	Hartford, CT	203	Portsmouth, VA	804
Ann Arbor, MI	313	Hialeah, FL	305	Providence, RI	401
Arlington, TX	817	Hollywood, FL	305	Pueblo, CO	303
Atlanta, GA	404	Honolulu, HI	808	Raleigh, NC	919
Aurora, CO	303	Houston, TX	713	Richmond, VA	804
Austin, TX	512	Huntington Beach, CA	714	Riverside, CA	714
Baltimore, MD	301	Huntsville, AL	205	Roanoke, VA	703
Baton Rouge, LA	504	Independence, MO	816	Rochester, NY	716
Beaumont, TX	713	Indianapolis, IN	317	Rockford, IL	815
Berkeley, CA	415	Irving, TX	214	Sacramento, CA	916
Birmingham, AL	205	Jackson, MS	601	St. Louis, MO	314
Boise, ID	208	Jacksonville, FL	904	St. Paul, MN	612
Boston, MA	617	Jersey City, NJ	201	St. Petersburg, FL	813
Bridgeport, CT	203	Kansas City, KS	913	Salt Lake City, UT	801
Buffalo, NY	716	Kansas City, MO	816	San Antonio, TX	512
Cambridge, MA	617	Knoxville, TN	615	San Bernardino, CA	714
Canton, OH	216	Lakewood, CO	303	San Diego, CA	714
Cedar Rapids, IA	319	Lansing, MI	517	San Francisco, CA	415
Charlotte, NC	704	Las Vegas, NV	702	San Jose, CA	408
Chattanooga, TN	615	Lexington, KY	606	Santa Ana, CA	714
Chesapeake, VA	804	Lincoln, NE	402	Savannah, GA	912
Chicago, IL	312	Little Rock, AR	501	Seattle, WA	206
Cincinnati, OH	513	Livonia, MI	313	Shreveport, LA	318
Cleveland, OH	216	Long Beach, CA	213	South Bend, IN	219
Colorado Springs, CO	303	Los Angeles, CA	213	Spokane, WA	509
Columbia, SC	803	Louisville, KY	502	Springfield, MA	413
Columbus, GA	404	Lubbock, TX	806	Springfield, MO	417
Columbus, OH	614	Macon, GA	912	Stamford, CT	203
Corpus Christi, TX	512	Madison, WI	608	Stockton, CA	209
Dallas, TX	214	Memphis, TN	901	Sunnyvale, CA	407
Davenport, IA	319	Mesa, AZ	602	Syracuse, NY	315
Dayton, OH	513	Miami, FL	305	Tacoma, WA	206
Denver, CO	303	Milwaukee, WI	414	Tampa, FL	813
Des Moines, IA	515	Minneapolis, MN	612	Toledo, OH	419
Detroit, MI	313	Mobile, AL	205	Topeka, KS	913
Durham, NC	919	Montgomery, AL	205	Torrance, CA	213
Elizabeth, NJ	201	Nashville, TN	615	Trenton, NJ	609
El Paso, TX	915	Newark, NJ	201	Tucson, AZ	602
Erie, PA	814	New Bedford, MA	617	Tulsa, OK	918
Evansville, IN	812	New Haven, CT	203	Virginia Beach, VA	804
Fall River, MA	617	New Orleans, LA	504	Warren, MI	313
Flint, MI	313	Newport News, VA	804	Washington, DC	202
Ft. Lauderdale, FL	305	New York City, NY	212	Waterbury, CT	203
Ft. Wayne, IN	219	Norfolk, VA	804	Wichita, KS	316
Ft. Worth, TX	817	Oakland, CA	415	Winston-Salem, NC	919
Fremont, CA	415	Oklahoma City, OK	405	Worcester, MA	617
Fresno, CA	209	Omaha, NE	406	Yonkers, NY	914
Garden Grove, CA	714	Orlando, FL	905	Youngstown, OH	216
		Pasadena, CA	213		

CITY ZIP CODES

Akron, OH 44300	Garland, TX* 75040	Pasadena, CA 91100
Albany, NY 12200	Gary, IN 46400	Pasadena, TX 77501
Albuquerque, NM 87100	Glendale, CA 91200	Paterson, NJ 07500
Alexandria, VA 22300	Grand Rapids, MI 49500	Peoria, IL 61600
Allentown, PA 18100	Greensboro, NC 27400	Philadelphia, PA 19100
Amarillo, TX 79100	Hammond, IN 46320	Phoenix, AZ 85000
Anaheim, CA 92800	Hampton, VA 23369	Pittsburgh, PA 15200
Anchorage, AK 99501	Hartford, CT 06100	Portland, OR 97200
Ann Arbor, MI 48108	Hialeah, FL 33010	Portsmouth, VA 23700
Arlington, TX* 76010	Hollywood, FL 33020	Providence, RI 02900
Atlanta, GA 30300	Honolulu, HI 96800	Pueblo, CO 81001
Aurora, CO* 80010	Houston, TX 77000	Raleigh, NC 27600
Austin, TX 78700	Huntington Beach, CA...92646	Richmond, VA 23200
Baltimore, MD 21200	Huntsville, AL 35800	Riverside, CA 92500
Baton Rouge, LA 70800	Independence, MO ... 64050	Roanoke, VA 24011
Beaumont, TX 77700	Indianapolis, IN 46200	Rochester, NY 14600
Berkeley, CA 94700	Irving, TX * 75060	Rockford, IL 61100
Birmingham, AL 35200	Jackson, MS 39200	Sacramento, CA 95800
Boise, ID 83700	Jacksonville, FL 33200	St. Louis, MO 63100
Boston, MA 02100	Jersey City, NJ 07300	St. Paul, MN 55100
Bridgeport, CT 06600	Kansas City, KS 66100	St. Petersburg, FL ... 33700
Buffalo, NY 14200	Kansas City, MO 64100	Salt Lake City, UT 84100
Cambridge, MA* 02138	Knoxville, TN 37900	San Antonio, TX 78200
Canton, OH 44700	Lakewood, CO * 80215	San Bernardino, CA ... 92400
Cedar Rapids, IA 52400	Lansing, MI 48900	San Diego, CA 92100
Charlotte, NC 28200	Las Vegas, NV 89100	San Francisco, CA 94100
Chattanooga, TN 37400	Lexington, KY 40500	San Jose, CA 95100
Chesapeake, VA 23320	Lincoln, NE 68500	Santa Ana, CA 92700
Chicago, IL 60600	Little Rock, AR 72200	Savannah, GA 31400
Cincinnati, OH 45200	Livonia, MI 48150	Seattle, WA 98100
Cleveland, OH 44100	Long Beach, CA 90800	Shreveport, LA 71100
Colorado Springs, CO .. 80900	Los Angeles, CA 90000	South Bend, IN 46600
Columbia, SC 29200	Louisville, KY 40200	Spokane, WA 99200
Columbus, GA 31900	Lubbock, TX 79400	Springfield, MA 01100
Columbus, OH 43200	Macon, GA 32100	Springfield, MO 65800
Corpus Christi, TX 78400	Madison, WI 53700	Stamford, CT 06900
Dallas, TX 75200	Memphis, TN 38100	Stockton, CA 95201
Davenport, IA 52800	Mesa, AZ* 85201	Sunnyvale, CA 94806
Dayton, OH 45400	Miami, FL 33100	Syracuse, NY 13200
Denver, CO 80200	Milwaukee, WI 53200	Tacoma, WA 98400
Des Moines, IA 50300	Minneapolis, MN 55400	Tampa, FL 33600
Detroit, MI 48200	Mobile, AL 36600	Toledo, OH 43600
Durham, NC 27700	Montgomery, AL 36100	Topeka, KS 66600
Elizabeth, NJ 07200	Nashville, TN 37200	Torrance, CA 90500
El Paso, TX 79900	Newark, NJ 07100	Trenton, NJ 08600
Erie, PA 16500	New Bedford, MA 02740	Tucson, AZ 85700
Evansville, IN 47700	New Haven, CT 06500	Tulsa, OK 74100
Fall River, MA 02720	New Orleans, LA 70100	Virginia Beach, VA 23451
Flint, MI 48500	Newport News, VA ... 23600	Warren, MI 48089
Ft. Lauderdale, FL 33300	New York City, NY 10000	Washington, DC 20000
Ft. Wayne, IN 46800	Norfolk, VA 23500	Waterbury, CT 06702
Ft. Worth, TX 76100	Oakland, CA 94600	Wichita, KS 67200
Fremont, CA 94536	Oklahoma City, OK ... 73100	Winston-Salem, NC .. 27100
Fresno, CA 93700	Omaha, NE 68100	Worcester, MA 01600
Garden Grove, CA 92640	Orlando, FL 32800	Yonkers, NY 10700

* Designates cities where one zip code covers the whole city. All others are multicoded (street address needed to determine full zip code).

Youngstown, OH 44500

UNITED STATES SENATORS OF THE 96TH CONGRESS

ALABAMA
Donald Stewart .... (D) Anniston
Howell Heflin .... (D) Tuscumbia

ALASKA
Mike Gravel .... (D) Anchorage
Ted Stevens .... (R) Anchorage

ARIZONA
Barry M. Goldwater .... (R) Scottsdale
Dennis DeConcini .... (D) Tucson

ARKANSAS
Dale Bumpers .... (D) Charleston
David Pryor .... (D) Little Rock

CALIFORNIA
Alan Cranston .... (D) Palm Springs
S. I. (Sam) Hayakawa .... (R) Mill Valley

COLORADO
Gary Hart .... (D) Denver
William L. Armstrong .... (R) Aurora

CONNECTICUT
Abraham A. Ribicoff .... (D) Hartford
Lowell P. Weicker Jr. .... (R) Greenwich

DELAWARE
William V. Roth Jr. .... (R) Wilmington
Joseph R. Biden Jr. .... (D) Wilmington

FLORIDA
Richard Stone .... (D) Tallahassee
Lawton Chiles .... (D) Lakeland

GEORGIA
Herman E. Talmadge .... (D) Lovejoy
Sam Nunn .... (D) Perry

HAWAII
Daniel K. Inouye .... (D) Honolulu
Spark M. Matsunaga .... (D) Honolulu

IDAHO
Frank Church .... (D) Boise
James A. McClure .... (R) Payette

ILLINOIS
Adlai E. Stevenson 3d .... (D) Chicago
Charles H. Percy .... (R) Wilmette

INDIANA
Birch Bayh .... (D) Indianapolis
Richard G. Lugar .... (R) Indianapolis

IOWA
John C. Culver .... (D) Cedar Rapids
Roger W. Jepsen .... (R) Davenport

KANSAS
Robert J. Dole .... (R) Russell
Nancy Landon Kassebaum ...... (R) Wichita

KENTUCKY
Wendell H. Ford .... (D) Owensboro
Walter D. Huddleston ..... (D) Elizabethtown

LOUISIANA
Russell B. Long .... (D) Baton Rouge
J. Bennett Johnston Jr. ...... (D) Shreveport

MAINE
Edmund S. Muskie .... (D) Waterville
William S. Cohen .... (R) Bangor

MARYLAND
Charles C. Mathias .... (R) Frederick
Paul S. Sarbanes .... (D) Baltimore

MASSACHUSETTS
Edward M. Kennedy .... (D) Boston
Paul E. Tsongas .... (D) Lowell

MICHIGAN
Donald W. Riegle Jr. .... (D) Flint
Carl Levin .... (D) Detroit

MINNESOTA
David Durenberger .... (R) Minneapolis
Rudolph E. Boschwitz .... (R) Wayzata

MISSISSIPPI
John C. Stennis .... (D) DeKalb
Thad Cochran .... (R) Jackson

MISSOURI
Thomas F. Eagleton .... (D) St. Louis
John C. Danforth .... (R) Jefferson City

MONTANA
John Melcher .... (D) Forsyth
Max Baucus .... (D) Missoula

NEBRASKA
Edward Zorinsky .... (D) Omaha
J. James Exon .... (D) Lincoln

NEVADA
Paul Laxalt .... (R) Carson City
Howard W. Cannon .... (D) Las Vegas

NEW HAMPSHIRE
John A. Durkin .... (D) Manchester
Gordon J. Humphrey .... (R) Swapee

NEW JERSEY
Harrison A. Williams Jr. ..... (D) Bedminster
Bill Bradley .... (D) Denville

NEW MEXICO
Harrison "Jack" Schmitt ...... (R) Silver City
Pete V. Domenici .... (R) Albuquerque

NEW YORK
Jacob K. Javits .... (R, L) New York
Daniel Patrick Moynihan ...... (D) New York

NORTH CAROLINA
Robert Morgan .... (D) Lillington
Jesse A. Helms .... (R) Raleigh

NORTH DAKOTA
Milton R. Young .... (R) LaMoure
Quentin N. Burdick .... (D) Fargo

UNITED STATES SENATORS OF THE 96TH CONGRESS (continued)

OHIO
John Glenn .... (D) Columbia
Howard M. Metzenbaum ... (D) Shaker Heights

OKLAHOMA
Henry Bellmon .... (R) Red Rock
David Lyle Boren .... (D) Oklahoma City

OREGON
Robert W. Packwood .... (R) Lake Oswego
Mark O. Hatfield .... (R) Salem

PENNSYLVANIA
Richard S. Schweiker .... (R) Worcester
H. John Heinz III .... (R) Pittsburgh

RHODE ISLAND
John H. Chafee .... (R) Warwick
Claiborne Pell .... (D) Newport

SOUTH CAROLINA
Ernest F. Hollings .... (D) Columbia
Strom Thurmond .... (R) Aiken

SOUTH DAKOTA
George McGovern .... (D) Mitchell
Larry Pressler .... (R) Humboldt

TENNESSEE
James R. Sasser .... (D) Nashville
Howard H. Baker Jr. .... (R) Huntsville

TEXAS
Lloyd Bentsen .... (D) Houston
John G. Tower .... (R) Wichita Falls

UTAH
Jake Garn .... (R) Salt Lake City
Orrin G. Hatch .... (R) Salt Lake City

VERMONT
Patrick J. Leahy .... (D) Burlington
Robert T. Stafford .... (R) Rutland

VIRGINIA
Harry F. Byrd Jr. .... (I) Winchester
John William Warner .... (R) Middleburg

WASHINGTON
Warren G. Magnuson .... (D) Seattle
Henry M. Jackson .... (D) Everett

WEST VIRGINIA
Robert C. Byrd .... (D) Sophia
Jennings Randolph .... (D) Charleston

WISCONSIN
Gaylord A. Nelson .... (D) Madison
William Proxmire .... (D) Madison

WYOMING
Malcolm Wallop .... (R) Big Horn
Alan K. Simpson .... (R) Cody

UNITED STATES REPRESENTATIVES OF THE 96TH CONGRESS

ALABAMA
Jack Edwards (1)* .... (R) Mobile
William L. "Bill" Dickinson (2) ...(R) Montgomery
Bill Nichols (3) .... (D) Sylacauga
Tom Bevill (4) .... (D) Jasper
Ronnie G. Flippo (5) .... (D) Florence
John H. Buchanan Jr. (6) .... (R) Birmingham
Richard C. Shelby (7) .... (D) Tuscaloosa

ALASKA
Don Young (At-large) .... (R) Anchorage

ARIZONA
John J. Rhodes (1) .... (R) Mesa
Morris K. Udall (2) .... (D) Tucson
Bob Stump (3) .... (D) Tolleson
Eldon Rudd (4) .... (R) Scottsdale

ARKANSAS
Bill Alexander (1) .... (D) Osceola
Edwin R. Bethune Jr. (2) .... (R) Searcy
John Paul Hammerschmidt (3) .. (R) Harrison
Beryl Anthony Jr. (4) .... (D) El Dorado

CALIFORNIA
Harold T. Johnson (1) .... (D) Roseville
Don H. Clausen (2) .... (R) Crescent City
Robert T. Matsui (3) .... (D) Sacramento
Vic Fazio (4) .... (D) Sacramento
John L. Burton (5) .... (D) San Francisco
Phillip Burton (6) .... (D) San Francisco
George Miller (7) .... (D) Martinez
Ronald V. Dellums (8) .... (D) Berkeley
Fortney H. Stark Jr. (9) .... (D) Oakland
Don Edwards (10) .... (D) San Jose
Leo J. Ryan (11) .... (D) Belmont
Paul N. McCloskey Jr. (12) ... (R) Menlo Park
Norman Y. Mineta (13) .... (D) San Jose
Norman D. Shumway (14) ...... (R) Stockton
Tony Coelho (15) .... (D) Merced
Leon E. Panetta (16) ...... (D) Carmel Valley
Charles Pashayan Jr. (17) .... (R) Fresno
William M. Thomas (18) ..... (R) Bakersfield
Robert J. Lagomarsino (19) ...... (R) Ventura
Barry M. Goldwater Jr. (20) ..... (R) Burbank
James C. Corman (21) ...... (D) Van Nuys
Carlos J. Moorhead (22) ...... (R) Glendale
Anthony C. Bellenson (23) ... (D) Los Angeles
Henry A. Waxman (24) ..... (D) Los Angeles
Edward R. Roybal (25) ...... (D) Los Angeles
John H. Rousselot (26) ...... (R) San Marino
Robert K. Dornan (27) .... (R) Redondo Beach
Julian C. Dixon (28) .... (D) Los Angeles
Augustus F. Hawkins (29) ... (D) Los Angeles
George E. Danielson (30) .. (D) Monterey Park
Charles H. Wilson (31) .... (D) Hawthorne
Glenn M. Anderson (32) ...... (D) Harbor City
Wayne Grisham (33) .... (R) La Mirada
Dan Lungren (34) .... (R) Long Beach
Jim Lloyd (35) .... (D) West Covina
George E. Brown Jr. (36) .... (D) Riverside
Jerry Lewis (37) .... (R) Highland
Jerry M. Patterson (38) ...... (D) Buena Park
William E. Dannemeyer (39) .... (R) Fullerton
Robert E. Badham (40) .... (R) Newport Beach
Bob Wilson (41) .... (R) San Diego
Lionel Van Deerlin (42) ...... (D) Chula Vista
Clair W. Burgener (43) .... (R) La Jolla

COLORADO
Pat Schroeder (1) .... (D) Denver
Tim Wirth (2) .... (D) Lakewood
Ray Kogovsek (3) .... (D) Pueblo
James P. (Jim) Johnson (4) ... (R) Fort Collins
Ken Kramer (5) .... (R) Colorado Springs

CONNECTICUT
William R. Cotter (1) .... (D) Hartford
Christopher J. Dodd (2) .... (D) Norwich
Robert N. Giaimo (3) .... (D) North Haven
Stewart B. McKinney (4) .... (R) Fairfield
William R. Ratchford (5) .... (D) Danbury
Anthony Toby Moffett (6) ..... (D) Unionville

DELAWARE
Thomas B. Evans Jr. (At-large) ...(R) Wilmington

FLORIDA
Earl Dewitt Hutto (1) .... (D) Panama City
Don Fuqua (2) .... (D) Altha
Charles E. Bennett (3) ...... (D) Jacksonville
Bill Chappell Jr. (4) .... (D) Ocala
Richard Kelly (5) .... (R) New Port Richey
C.W. Bill Young (6) .... (R) St. Petersburg
Sam M. Gibbons (7) .... (D) Tampa
Andy Ireland (8) .... (D) Winter Haven
Bill Nelson (9) .... (D) Melbourne
L.A. (Skip) Bafalis (10) ... (R) Fort Myers Beach
Dan Mica (11) .... (D) West Palm Beach
Edward J. Stack (12) .... (D) Hollywood
William Lehman (13) ..... (D) N. Miami Beach
Claude Pepper (14) .... (D) Miami
Dante B. Fascell (15) .... (D) Miami

GEORGIA
Bo Ginn (1) .... (D) Millen
Dawson Mathis (2) .... (D) Albany
Jack Brinkley (3) .... (D) Columbus
Elliott H. Levitas (4) .... (D) Atlanta
Wyche Fowler Jr. (5) .... (D) Atlanta
Newton Leroy Gingrich (6) .... (R) Carrollton
Larry P. McDonald (7) .... (D) Marietta
Billy Lee Evans (8) .... (D) Macon
Ed Jenkins (9) .... (D) Jasper
Doug Barnard (10) .... (D) Augusta

HAWAII
Cecil (Cec) Heftel (1) .... (D) Honolulu
Daniel K. Akaka (2) .... (D) Honolulu

UNITED STATES REPRESENTATIVES OF THE 96TH CONGRESS (continued)

IDAHO
Steven D. Symms (1) .... (R) Caldwell
George Hansen (2) .... (R) Pocatello

ILLINOIS
Bennett M. Stewart (1) .... (D) Chicago
Morgan F. Murphy (2) .... (D) Chicago
Martin A. Russo (3) .... (D) South Holland
Edward J. Derwinski (4) ...... (R) Flossmoor
John G. Fary (5) .... (D) Chicago
Henry J. Hyde (6) .... (R) Park Ridge
Cardiss Collins (7) .... (D) Chicago
Dan Rostenkowski (8) .... (D) Chicago
Sidney R. Yates (9) .... (D) Chicago
Abner J. Mikva (10) .... (D) Evanston
Frank Annunzio (11) .... (D) Chicago
Phillip M. Crane (12) ..... (R) Mount Prospect
Robert M. McClory (13) ...... (R) Lake Bluff
John N. Erlenborn (14) .... (R) Glen Ellyn
Tom Corcoran (15) .... (R) Ottawa
John B. Anderson (16) .... (R) Rockford
George M. O'Brien (17) .... (R) Joliet
Robert H. Michel (18) .... (R) Peoria
Tom Railsback (19) .... (R) Moline
Paul Findley (20) .... (R) Pittsfield
Edward R. Madigan (21) ...... (R) Lincoln
Daniel B. Crane (22) .... (R) Danville
Melvin Price (23) .... (D) East St. Louis
Paul Simon (24) .... (D) Carbondale

INDIANA
Adam Benjamin Jr. (1) .... (D) Hobart
Floyd J. Fithian (2) .... (D) Lafayette
John Brademas (3) .... (D) South Bend
Dan Quayle (4) .... (R) Fort Wayne
Elwood H. Hillis (5) .... (R) Kokomo
David W. Evans (6) .... (D) Indianapolis
John T. Myers (7) .... (R) Covington
H. Joel Deckard (8) .... (R) Evansville
Lee H. Hamilton (9) .... (D) Columbus
Phillip R. Sharp (10) .... (D) Muncie
Andrew Jacobs Jr. (11) ..... (D) Indianapolis

IOWA
Jim Leach (1) .... (R) Davenport
Thomas J. Tauke (2) .... (R) Dubuque
Charles E. Grassley (3) .... (R) New Hartford
Neal Smith (4) .... (D) Altoona
Tom Harkin (5) .... (D) Ames
Berkley Bedell (6) .... (D) Spirit Lake

KANSAS
Keith G. Sebellus (1) .... (R) Norton
James E. Jeffries (2) .... (R) Atchison
Larry Winn Jr. (3) .... (R) Overland Park
Dan Glickman (4) .... (D) Wichita
Robert "Bob" Whittaker (5) ...... (R) Augusta

KENTUCKY
Carroll Hubbard Jr. (1) .... (D) Mayfield
William Natcher (2) .... (D) Bowling Green
Romano L. Mazzoli (3) .... (D) Louisville
M. Gene Snyder (4) ... (R) Brownsboro Farms
Tim Lee Carter (5) .... (R) Tompkinsville
Larry J. Hopkins (6) .... (R) Lexington
Carl D. Perkins (7) .... (D) Hindman

LOUISIANA
Bob Livingston (1) .... (R) New Orleans
Lindy (Mrs. Hale) Boggs (2) ... (D) New Orleans
David C. Treen (3) .... (R) Metairie
Claude "Buddy" Leach (4) .... (D) Leesville
Jerry Huckaby (5) .... (D) Ringgold
W. Henson Moore (6) .... (R) Baton Rouge
John Breaux (7) .... (D) Crowley
Gillis W. Long (8) .... (D) Alexandria

MAINE
David F. Emery (1) .... (R) Rockland
Olympia J. Snowe (2) .... (R) Auburn

MARYLAND
Robert E. Bauman (1) .... (R) Easton
Clarence D. Long (2) .... (D) Ruxton
Barbara A. Mikulski (3) .... (D) Baltimore
Marjorie S. Holt (4) .... (R) Severna Park
Gladys Noon Spellman (5) .... (D) Laurel
Beverly B. Byron (6) .... (D) Frederick
Parren J. Mitchell (7) .... (D) Baltimore
Michael D. Barnes (8) .... (D) Kensington

MASSACHUSETTS
Silvio Conte (1) .... (R) Pittsfield
Edward P. Boland (2) .... (D) Springfield
Joseph D. Early (3) .... (D) Worcester
Robert F. Drinan (4) .... (D) Chestnut Hill
James M. Shannon (5) .... (D) Lawrence
Nicholas Mavroules (6) .... (D) Peabody
Edward J. Markey (7) .... (D) Malden
Thomas P. O'Neill Jr. (8) ...... (D) Cambridge
John J. Moakley (9) .... (D) Boston
Margaret Heckler (10) .... (R) Wellesley Hills
Brian J. Donnelly (11) .... (D) Dorchester
Gerry E. Studds (12) .... (D) Cohasset

MICHIGAN
John Conyers (1) .... (D) Detroit
Carl D. Pursell (2) .... (R) Plymouth
Howard Wolpe (3) .... (D) Lansing
Dave Stockman (4) .... (R) St. Joseph
Harold S. Sawyer (5) .... (R) Rockford
Bob Carr (6) .... (D) East Lansing
Dale E. Kildee (7) .... (D) Flint
Bob Traxler (8) .... (D) Bay City
Guy Vander Jagt (9) .... (R) Luther
Donald Joseph Albosta (10) .. (D) St. Charles
Robert W. Davis (11) .... (R) Gaylord

UNITED STATES REPRESENTATIVES OF THE 96TH CONGRESS (continued)

David E. Bonior (12) .... (D) Mt. Clemens
Charles C. Diggs Jr. (13) .... (D) Detroit
Lucien N. Nedzi (14) .... (D) Detroit
William D. Ford (15) .... (D) Taylor
John D. Dingell (16) .... (D) Trenton
William M. Brodhead (17) .... (D) Detroit
James J. Blanchard (18) .. (D) Pleasant Ridge
William S. Broomfield (19) .. (R) Birmingham

MINNESOTA
Arien Erdahl (1) .... (R) West St. Paul
Tom Hagedorn (2) .... (R) Truman
Bill Frenzel (3) .... (R) Golden Valley
Bruce F. Vento (4) .... (D) St. Paul
Martin Olav Sabo (5) .... (D) Minneapolis
Richard Nolan (6) .... (D) Waite Park
Arlan Stangeland (7) .... (R) Barnesville
James L. Oberstar (8) .... (D) Chisholm

MISSISSIPPI
Jamie L. Whitten (1) .... (D) Charleston
David Bowen (2) .... (D) Cleveland
G.V. (Sonny) Montgomery (3) ... (D) Meridian
Jon Clifton Hinson (4) .... (R) Tylertown
Trent Lott (5) .... (R) Gulfport

MISSOURI
William (Bill) Clay (1) .... (D) St. Louis
Robert A. Young (2) .... (D) St. Ann
Richard A. Gephardt (3) .... (D) St. Louis
Ike Skelton (4) .... (D) Lexington
Richard Bolling (5) .... (D) Kansas City
E. Thomas Coleman (6) ...... (R) Kansas City
Gene Taylor (7) .... (R) Sarcoxie
Richard H. Ichord (8) .... (D) Houston
Harold L. Volkmer (9) .... (D) Hannibal
Bill D. Burlison (10) ...... (D) Cape Girardeau

MONTANA
Pat Williams (1) .... (D) Helena
Ron Marlenee (2) .... (R) Scobey

NEBRASKA
Douglas K. Bereuter (1) .... (R) Utica
John J. Cavanaugh (2) .... (D) Omaha
Virginia Smith (3) .... (R) Chappell

NEVADA
Jim Santini (At-large) .... (D) Las Vegas

NEW HAMPSHIRE
Norman E. D'Amours (1) ..... (D) Manchester
James C. Cleveland (2) ..... (R) New London

NEW JERSEY
James J. Florio (1) .... (D) Camden
William J. Hughes (2) .... (D) Ocean City
James J. Howard (3) ... (D) Spring Lake Heights
Frank Thompson Jr. (4) .... (D) Trenton
Millicent H. Fenwick (5) ..... (R) Bernardsville
Edwin B. Forsythe (6) ...... (R) Moorestown

Andrew Maguire (7) .... (D) Ridgewood
Robert A. Roe (8) .... (D) Paterson
Harold C. Hollenbeck (9) ... (R) East Rutherford
Peter W. Rodino Jr. (10) .... (D) Newark
Joseph G. Minish (11) ..... (D) West Orange
Matthew J. Rinaldo (12) .... (R) Union
James A. Courter (13) ..... (R) Hackettstown
Frank J. Guarini (14) .... (D) Jersey City
Edward J. Patten (15) ..... (D) Perth Amboy

NEW MEXICO
Manuel Lujan Jr. (1) .... (R) Albuquerque
Harold Runnels (2) .... (D) Lovington

NEW YORK
William Carney (1) .... (R, C) Hauppauge
Thomas J. Downey (2) .... (D) West Islip
Jerome A. Ambro (3) ..... (D) East Northport
Norman F. Lent (4) .... (R, C) East Rockaway
John W. Wydler (5) .... (R, C) Garden City
Lester Wolff (6) .... (D, L) Great Neck
Joseph P. Addabbo (7) .. (D, R, L) Ozone Park
Benjamin S. Rosenthal (8) .... (D, L) Flushing
Geraldine A. Ferraro (9) ...... (D) Forest Hills
Mario Biaggi (10) .... (D, R, L) Bronx
James H. Scheuer (11) .... (D, L) Neponsit
Shirley Chisholm (12) .... (D, L) Brooklyn
Stephen J. Solarz (13) ...... (D, L) Brooklyn
Frederick W. Richmond (14) .. (D, L) Brooklyn
Leo C. Zefferetti (15) .... (D, C) Brooklyn
Elizabeth Holtzman (16) ..... (D, L) Brooklyn
John M. Murphy (17) .... (D) Staten Island
S. William Green (18) .... (R) New York
Charles B. Rangel (19) ...... (D, R) New York
Ted S. Weiss (20) .... (D, L) New York
Robert Garcia (21) .... (D, R, L) Bronx
Jonathan B. Bingham (22) ...... (D, L) Bronx
Peter A. Peyser (23) .... (D) Irvington
Richard L. Ottinger (24) ..... (D) Pleasantville
Hamilton Fish Jr. (25) ..... (R) Poughkeepsie
Benjamin A. Gilman (26) ..... (R) Middletown
Matthew F. McHugh (27) .... (D) Ithaca
Samuel S. Stratton (28) ...... (D) Amsterdam
Gerald B. H. Solomon (29) .. (R, C) Glens Falls
Robert C. McEwen (30) .... (R, C) Ogdensburg
Donald J. Mitchell (31) .... (R, C) Herkimer
James M. Hanley (32) .... (D) Syracuse
Gary A. Lee (33) .... (R) Ithaca
Frank Horton (34) .... (D, R) Rochester
Barber B. Conable (35) .... (R) Rochester
John J. La Falce (36) ...... (D, L) Tonawanda
Henry J. Nowak (37) .... (D, L) Buffalo
Jack Kemp (38) .... (R, C) Buffalo
Stanley N. Lundine (39) ...... (D) Jamestown

NORTH CAROLINA
Walter Jones (1) .... (D) Farmville
L. H. Fountain (2) .... (D) Tarboro

UNITED STATES REPRESENTATIVES OF THE 96TH CONGRESS (continued)

Charles Whitly (3) .... (D) Mt. Olive
Ike Andrews (4) .... (D) Siler City
Stephen L. Neal (5) ...... (D) Winston-Salem
Richardson Preyer (6) .... (D) Greensboro
Charles Rose (7) .... (D) Fayetteville
W. G. (Bill) Hefner (8) .... (D) Concord
James G. Martin (9) .... (R) Charlotte
James T. Broyhill (10) .... (R) Lenior
Lamar Gudger (11) .... (D) Asheville

NORTH DAKOTA
Mark Andrews (At-large) ...... (R) Mapleton

OHIO
Willis D. Gradison Jr. (1) ...... (R) Cincinnati
Thomas A. Luken (2) .... (D) Cincinnati
Tony P. Hall (3) .... (D) Dayton
Tennyson Guyer (4) .... (R) Findlay
Delbert Latta (5) .... (R) Bowling Green
William H. Harsha (6) .... (R) Portsmouth
Clarence J. Brown (7) .... (R) Urbana
Thomas N. Kindness (8) .... (R) Hamilton
Thomas Ludlow Ashley (9) ..... (D) Maumee
Clarence E. Miller (10) .... (R) Lancaster
J. William Stanton (11) ...... (R) Painesville
Samuel L. Devine (12) .... (R) Columbus
Donald J. Pease (13) .... (D) Oberlin
John F. Seiberling (14) .... (D) Akron
Chalmers P. Wylie (15) .... (R) Columbus
Ralph S. Regula (16) .... (R) Navarre
John M. Ashbrook (17) ...... (R) Johnstown
Douglas Applegate (18) ..... (D) Steubenville
Lyle Williams (19) .... (R) Niles
Mary Rose Oakar (20) .... (D) Cleveland
Louis Stokes (21) ... (D) Warrensville Heights
Charles A. Vanik (22) .... (D) Euclid
Ronald M. Mottl (23) .... (D) Parma

OKLAHOMA
James R. Jones (1) .... (D) Tulsa
Michael Lynn Synar (2) .... (D) Muskogee
Wesley Wade Watkins (3) .... (D) Ada
Tom Steed (4) .... (D) Shawnee
Mickey Edwards (5) ...... (R) Oklahoma City
Glenn English (6) .... (D) Cordell

OREGON
Les AuCoin (1) .... (D) Portland
Al Ullman (2) .... (D) Baker
Robert B. Duncan (3) .... (D) Portland
James Weaver (4) .... (D) Eugene

PENNSYLVANIA
Michael Myers (1) .... (D) Philadelphia
William H. Gray III (2) ...... (D) Philadelphia
Raymond F. Lederer (3) ..... (D) Philadelphia
Charles F. Dougherty (4) .... (R) Philadelphia
Richard T. Schulze (5) ...... (R) West Chester
Gus Yatron (6) .... (D) Reading

Robert W. Edgar (7) .... (D) Broomall
Peter H. Kostmayer (8) ...... (D) New Hope
Bud Shuster (9) .... (R) Everett
Joseph M. McDade (10) ... (R) Clarks Summit
Daniel J. Flood (11) .... (D) Wilkes-Barre
John P. Murtha (12) .... (D) Johnstown
R. Lawrence Coughlin (13) ... (R) Norristown
William S. Moorhead (14) .... (D) Pittsburgh
Donald Lawrence Ritter (15) ... (R) Coopersburg
Robert S. Walker (16) .... (R) East Petersburg
Allen E. Ertel (17) .... (D) Montoursville
Doug Walgren (18) .... (D) Pittsburgh
William F. Goodling (19) .... (R) York
Joseph M. Gaydos (20) ..... (D) McKeesport
Donald A. Bailey (21) .... (D) Greensburg
Austin J. Murphy (22) ..... (D) Monongahela
William F. Clinger Jr. (23) ...... (R) Warren
Marc L. Marks (24) .... (R) Sharon
Eugene V. Atkinson (25) ...... (D) Aliquippa

RHODE ISLAND
Fernard St. Germain (1) ..... (D) Woonsocket
Edward P. Beard (2) .... (D) Cranston

SOUTH CAROLINA
Mendel J. Davis (1) .... (D) Charleston
Floyd D. Spence (2) .... (R) Lexington
Butler Derrick (3) .... (D) Edgefield
Carroll A. Campbell Jr. (4) ... (R) Fountain Inn
Ken Holland (5) .... (D) Rock Hill
John W. Jenrette Jr. (6) ... (D) North Myrtle Beach

SOUTH DAKOTA
Thomas A. Daschle (1) .... (D) Aberdeen
James Abdnor (2) .... (R) Mitchell

TENNESSEE
James Quillen (1) .... (R) Kingsport
John J. Duncan (2) .... (R) Knoxville
Marilyn Lloyd (3) .... (D) Chattanooga
Albert Gore Jr. (4) .... (D) Carthage
William Hill Boner (5) .... (D) Nashville
Robin Beard (6) .... (R) Memphis
Ed Jones (7) .... (D) Yorkville
Harold E. Ford (8) .... (D) Memphis

TEXAS
Sam B. Hall (1) .... (D) Marshall
Charles Wilson (2) .... (D) Lufkin
James M. Collins (3) .... (R) Dallas
Ray Roberts (4) .... (D) McKinney
Jim Mattox (5) .... (D) Dallas
Wm. Philip Gramm (6) .... (D) College Station
Bill Archer (7) .... (R) Houston
Robert Eckhardt (8) .... (D) Houston
Jack Brooks (9) .... (D) Beaumont
James J. Pickle (10) .... (D) Austin
Marvin Leath (11) .... (D) Marlin
Jim Wright (12) .... (D) Ft. Worth

UNITED STATES REPRESENTATIVES OF THE 96TH CONGRESS (continued)

Jack Hightower (13) .... (D) Vernon
Joe Wyatt Jr. (14) .... (D) Victoria
E. de la Garza (15) .... (D) Mission
Richard C. White (16) .... (D) Bethesda
Charles W. Stenholm (17) ...... (D) Stamford
G. T. (Mickey) Leland (18) .... (D) Houston
Kent Hance (19) .... (D) Lubbock
Henry B. Gonzalez (20) ..... (D) San Antonio
Thomas G. Loeffler (21) .... (R) Hunt
Ronald E. Paul (22) .... (R) Lake Jackson
Abraham Kazen Jr. (23) .... (D) Laredo
Martin Frost (24) .... (D) Dallas

UTAH
Gunn McKay (1) .... (D) Salt Lake City
Dan Marriott (2) .... (R) Salt Lake City

VERMONT
James M. Jeffords (At-large) .... (R) Rutland

VIRGINIA
Paul S. Trible Jr. (1) ...... (R) Tappahannock
G. Wm. Whitehurst (2) ..... (R) Virginia Beach
David E. Satterfield (3) .... (D) Richmond
Robert W. Daniel Jr. (4) ..... (R) Spring Grove
Dan Daniel (5) .... (D) Danville
M. Caldwell Butler (6) .... (R) Roanoke
J. Kenneth Robinson (7) ..... (R) Winchester
Herbert E. Harris II (8) .... (D) Alexandria
William C. Wampler (9) .... (R) Bristol
Joseph L. Fisher (10) .... (D) Arlington

*Numbers indicate district represented

WASHINGTON
Joel Pritchard (1) .... (R) Seattle
Allan Byron Swift (2) .... (D) Bellingham
Don Bonker (3) .... (D) Olympia
Mike McCormack (4) .... (D) Richland
Thomas S. Foley (5) .... (D) Spokane
Norman N. Dicks (6) .... (D) Bremerton
Michael E. Lowry (7) ...... (D) Mercer Island

WEST VIRGINIA
Robert H. Mollohan (1) .... (D) Fairmont
Harley O. Staggers (2) .... (D) Keyser
John M. Slack (3) .... (D) Charleston
Nick J. Rahall II (4) .... (D) Beckley

WISCONSIN
Les Aspin (1) .... (D) East Troy
Robert W. Kastenmeier (2) ... (D) Sun Prairie
Alvin Baldus (3) .... (D) Menomonie
Clement J. Zablocki (4) .... (D) Milwaukee
Henry S. Reuss (5) .... (D) Milwaukee
William A. Steiger (6) .... (R) Oshkosh
David R. Obey (7) .... (D) Wausau
Toby Roth (8) .... (R) Appleton
F. James Sensenbrenner Jr. (9)...(R) Shorewood

WYOMING
Richard Bruce Cheney (At-large) ... (R) Casper

NON-VOTING DELEGATES

WASHINGTON, D.C.
Walter E. Fauntroy .... (D) D.C.
GUAM
Antonio Borja Won Pat .... (D) Agana
VIRGIN ISLANDS
Melvin Evans .... (R) St. Croix
PUERTO RICO
Jaime Benitez .... (Pop., D) Cayey

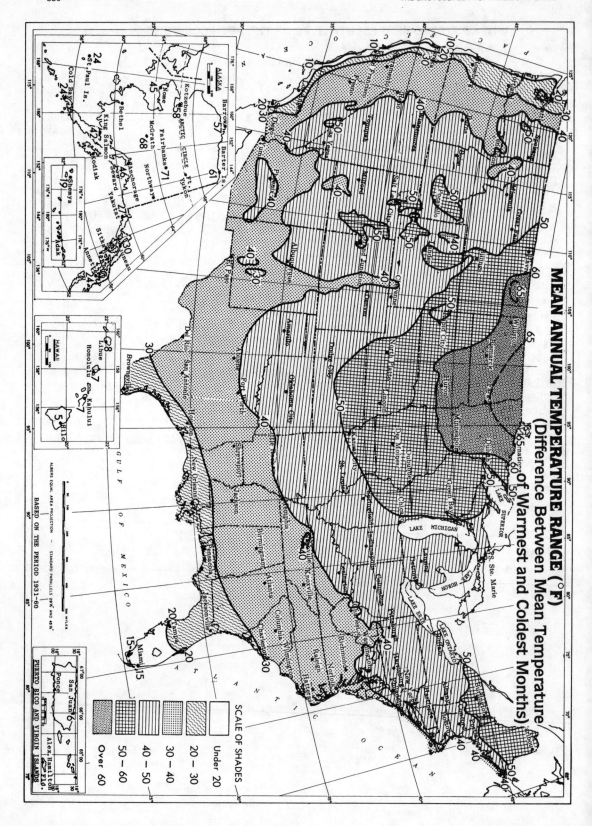

MEAN ANNUAL TEMPERATURE RANGE (°F)
(Difference Between Mean Temperature of Warmest and Coldest Months)

SCALE OF SHADES

Under 20
20 — 30
30 — 40
40 — 50
50 — 60
Over 60

ALBERS EQUAL AREA PROJECTION — STANDARD PARALLELS 29½° AND 45½°
BASED ON THE PERIOD 1931-60

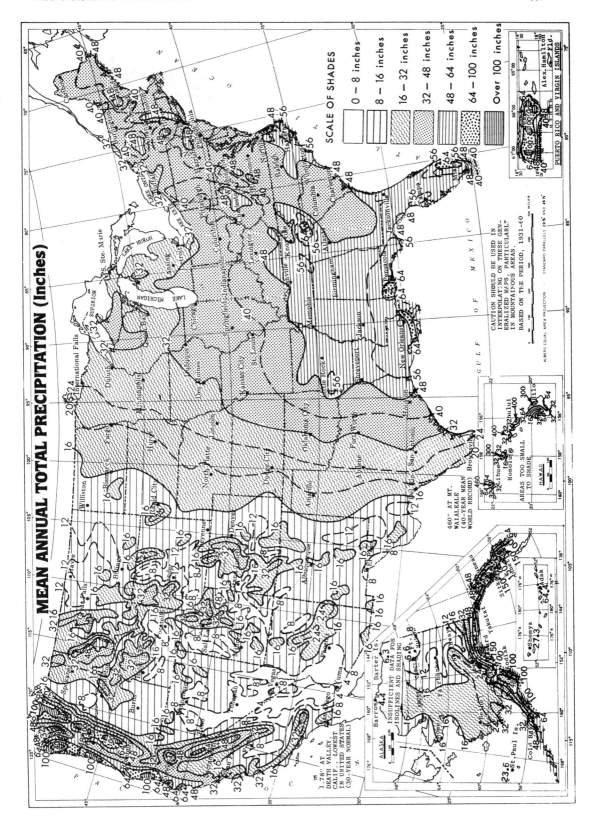

MEAN ANNUAL TOTAL PRECIPITATION (Inches)

SCALE OF SHADES

0 – 8 inches
8 – 16 inches
16 – 32 inches
32 – 48 inches
48 – 64 inches
64 – 100 inches
Over 100 inches

CAUTION SHOULD BE USED IN
INTERPOLATING ON THESE GEN-
ERALIZED MAPS, PARTICULARLY
IN MOUNTAINOUS AREAS.
BASED ON THE PERIOD, 1931–60

ALBERS EQUAL AREA PROJECTION — STANDARD PARALLELS 29½° AND 45½°

PUERTO RICO AND VIRGIN ISLANDS

HAWAII

460" AT MT.
WAIALEALE
(40-YEAR MEAN)
WORLD RECORD)

1.78" AT
DEATH VALLEY,
CALIF.: LOWEST
IN UNITED STATES
(30-YEAR NORMAL)

ALASKA

INSUFFICIENT DATA FOR
ISOLINES AND SHADING

AREAS TOO SMALL
TO SHADE

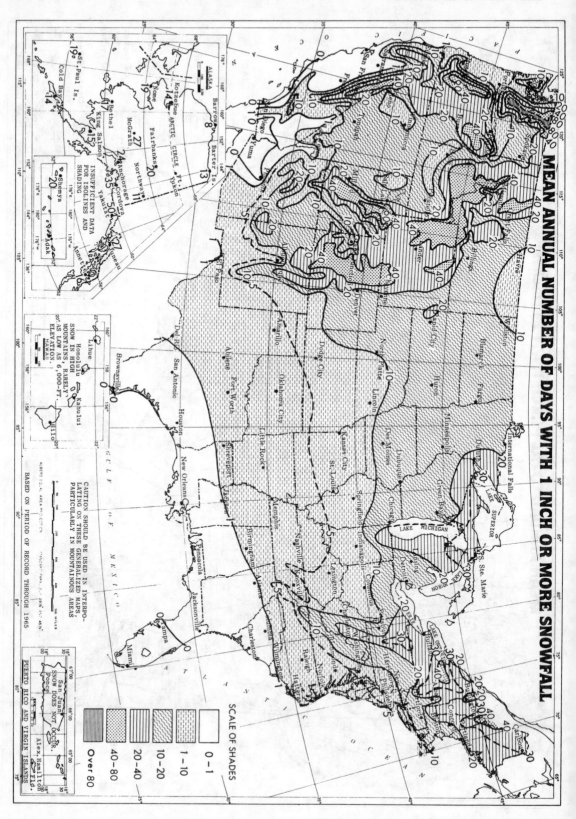

MEAN ANNUAL NUMBER OF DAYS WITH 1 INCH OR MORE SNOWFALL

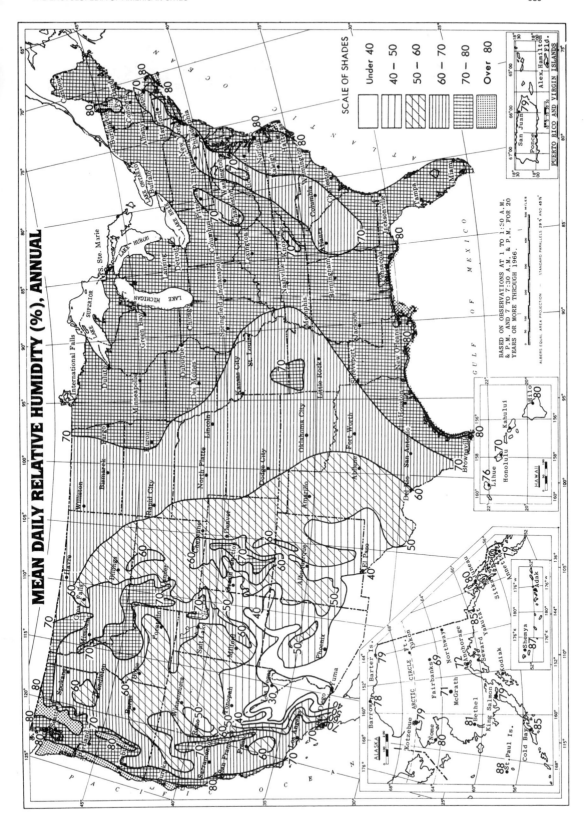

MEAN DAILY RELATIVE HUMIDITY (%), ANNUAL

SCALE OF SHADES

Under 40
40 – 50
50 – 60
60 – 70
70 – 80
Over 80

BASED ON OBSERVATIONS AT 1 TO 1:30 A.M.
& P.M. AND 7 TO 7:30 A.M. & P.M. FOR 20
YEARS OR MORE THROUGH 1966.

ALBERS EQUAL AREA PROJECTION — STANDARD PARALLELS 29½° AND 45½°

PUERTO RICO AND VIRGIN ISLANDS

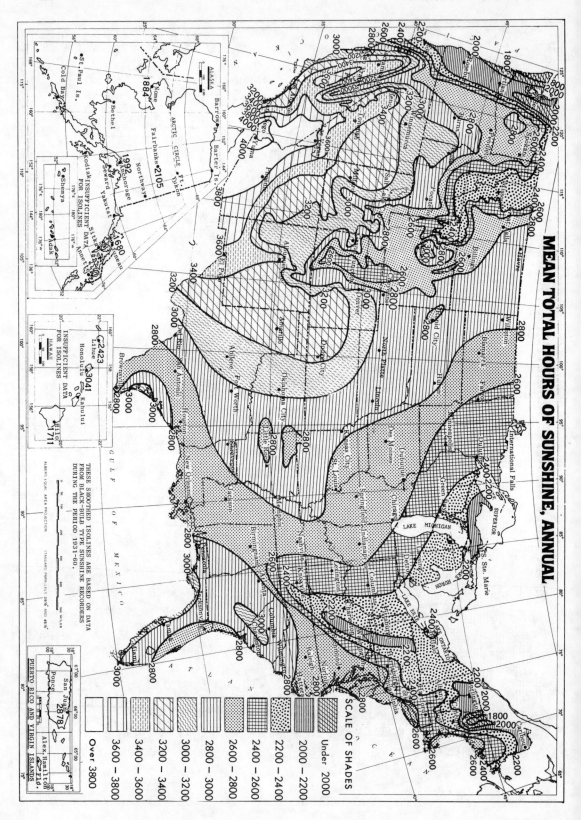

MEAN TOTAL HOURS OF SUNSHINE, ANNUAL

ABBREVIATIONS

& .... and	EA .... Eastern Air Lines, Inc.
° .... degree, degrees	EDT .... Eastern Daylight Time
' .... foot, feet; minute, minutes	EL .... Eastern League
" .... inch, inches; second, seconds	elev., elevs. .... elevation, elevations
% .... percent	EST .... Eastern Standard Time
AA .... American Airlines, Inc.; American	F .... Fahrenheit
Association	Feb. .... February
AAA .... American Automobile Association	fed., Fed. .... federal, Federal
A and M .... Agricultural and Mechanical	ff. .... following
ABC .... American Broadcasting Company	FL .... Florida; Frontier Airlines, Inc.
AD .... anno Domini	FM .... frequency modulation
Adm. .... Admiral	Fr. .... Father
AFB .... Air Force Base	Fri. .... Friday
AFC .... American Football Conference	frwy., Frwy., frwys. ... freeway, Freeway, freeways
AHL .... American Hockey League	FSL .... Florida State League
AK .... Alaska	Ft. .... Fort
AL .... Alabama; American League	FT .... Flying Tiger Line, Inc., The
a.m. .... ante meridiem	FW .... Wright Air Lines, Inc.
AM .... amplitude modulation	GA .... Georgia
AOR .... Album Oriented Rock	gen., Gen. .... general, General
approx. .... approximate, approximately	gov., Gov., govs. ..... governor, Governor, governors
Apr. .... April	govt., govts. .... government, governments
AR .... Arkansas	grad., grads. .... graduate, graduates
AS .... Alaska Airlines, Inc.	Grk. .... Greek
assn., Assn. assns. ..... association, Association,	HA .... Hawaiian Airlines, Inc.
associations	HI .... Hawaii
asst. .... assistant	hosp., Hosp., hosps. .... hospital, Hospital, hospitals
atty., Atty. .... attorney, Attorney	hwy., Hwy., hwys. .... highway, Highway, highways
Aug. .... August	I .... Independent
Ave., aves. .... Avenue, avenues	IA .... Iowa
avg., avgs. .... average, averages	ID .... Idaho
AZ .... Arizona	IHL .... International Hockey League
BA .... bachelor of arts	IL .... Illinois; International League
BC .... before Christ	IN .... Indiana
Blk. .... Black	Inc. .... Incorporated
blvd., Blvd. .... boulevard, Boulevard	Indep. .... Independent
BN .... Braniff Airways, Inc.	intl., Intl. .... international, International
brig., Brig. .... brigadier, Brigadier	Jan. .... January
BS .... bachelor of science	jr., Jr. .... junior, Junior
Btfl. .... Beautiful	KC .... Kansas City
c. .... circa	kHz .... kilohertz
CA .... California	KO .... Kodiak Western Alaska Airlines, Inc.
Capt. .... Captain	KS .... Kansas
CBS .... Columbia Broadcasting System	KY .... Kentucky
Ch., ... Channel	LA .... Los Angeles; Louisiana
CHL .... Central Hockey League	lat. .... latitude
CL .... California League	LI .... Long Island
Clas. .... Classical	lib., Lib. libs. .... library, Library, libraries
Co. .... Company, County,	long. .... longitude
CO .... Colorado; Continental Air Lines, Inc.	lt., Lt. .... lieutenant, Lieutenant
col., Col., cols. .... college, College, colleges;	MA .... Massachusetts; master of arts
colonel, Colonel	Mar. .... March
Comm. .... Commodore; Community	MBA .... master of business administration
Conf. .... Conference	MBS .... Mutual Broadcasting System
Confed. .... Confederate	MD .... doctor of medicine; Maryland
Contemp. .... Contemporary	ME .... Maine
Corp. .... Corporation	met. .... metropolitan
CrL .... Carolina League	mgr. .... manager
CSA .... Confederate States of America	mHz .... megahertz
CST .... Central Standard Time	mi. .... mile, miles
CT .... Connecticut	MI .... Michigan
C&W .... Country and Western	MISL .... Major Indoor Soccer League
DC .... District of Columbia	MN .... Minnesota
Dec. .... December	MO .... Missouri
dept., Dept., depts. ..... department, Department,	Mon. .... Monday
departments	MOR .... Middle of the Road
Dir. .... Director	Mr. .... Mister
Divers. .... Diversified	Mrs. .... Mistress
DL .... Delaware; Delta Air Lines, Inc.	MS .... master of science; Mississippi
Dr. .... Doctor	MST .... Mountain Standard Time
DST .... Daylight Saving Time	mt., Mt., mts., Mts. .... mount, Mount, mountain,
E .... east, eastern	Mountain, mountains, Mountains

ABBREVIATIONS (continued)

MT	Montana
Mus.	Music
Mut.	Mutual
MVA	Mississippi Valley Airlines
MWL	Midwest League
N	north, northern
NA	National Airlines, Inc.
NASL	North American Soccer League
natl., Natl.	national, National
NBA	National Basketball Association
NBC	National Broadcasting Company
NC	North Carolina; North Central Airlines, Inc.
ND	North Dakota
NE	Air New England, Inc.; Nebraska; northeast, northeastern
N.E.	New England
NEHL	Northeast Hockey League
NET	National Educational Television
NFC	National Football Conference
NH	New Hampshire
NHL	National Hockey League
NJ	New Jersey
NL	National League
NM	New Mexico
Nov.	November
NPR	National Public Radio
NV	Nevada
NW	northwest, northwestern; Northwest Airlines, Inc.
NWL	Northwest League
NY	New York; New York Airways, Inc.
NYC	New York City
NYPL	New York-Pennsylvania League
NYPMHL	New York-Pennsylvania Minor Hockey League
Oct.	October
OH	Ohio
OK	Oklahoma
OR	Oregon
OZ	Ozark Air Lines, Inc.
p.	page
PA	Pan American World Airways, Inc.; Pennsylvania
PBS	Public Broadcasting System
PCL	Pacific Coast League
PG	postgraduate
PhD	doctor of philosophy
PHL	Pacific Hockey League
PI	Piedmont Aviation, Inc.
pkwy., Pkwy., pkwys.	parkway, Parkway, parkways
p.m.	post meridiem
pop.	population
pp.	pages
PR	Puerto Rico
precip.	precipitation
pres., Pres.	president, President
Prog.	Programming
Progsv.	Progressive
PST	Pacific Standard Time
PX	Aspen Airways, Inc.
R&B	Rhythm and Blues
R&D	research and development
Rd.	Road
RD	Airlift International, Inc.
Relig.	Religious
Rev.	Reverend
RH	relative humidity
RI	Rhode Island
RP	Republic Airlines, Inc.

RR, RRs	railroad, Railroad, railroads, Railroads
Rte., rtes.	Route, routes
RV	Reeve Aleutian Airways, Inc.
RW	Hughes Air Corp., dba Hughes Airwest
S	south, southern
Sat.	Saturday
SB	Seaboard World Airlines, Inc.
SC	South Carolina
SD	South Dakota
SE	southeast, southeastern
Sen.	Senator
Sept.	September
SL	Southern League
S&L, S&Ls	Savings and Loan Association; savings and loan associations
SO	Southern Airways, Inc.
Span.	Spanish
Spec.	Special
sq.	square
sr., Sr.	senior, Senior
St.	Street; Saint
Sun.	Sunday
SW	southwest, southwestern
temp., temps.	temperature, temperatures
Thurs.	Thursday
TI	Texas International Airlines, Inc.
TN	Tennessee
Tnpk., tnpks	Turnpike, turnpikes
topog.	topography
TS	Aloha Airlines, Inc.
Tues.	Tuesday
TV	television
TW	Trans World Airlines, Inc.
TX	Texas
TxL	Texas League
U	University
UA	United Air Lines, Inc.
UN	United Nations
undergrad.	undergraduate
US	United States
USA	United States of America
USAF	United States Air Force
US Air	US Airlines, Inc. (formerly Allegheny Airlines, Inc.)
USCG	United States Coast Guard
USMC	United States Marine Corps
USN	United States Navy
USS	United States Ship
UT	Utah
VA	Virginia
V.A.	Veterans Administration
Var.	Variety
vol., vols.	volume, volumes
v.p., VP	vice-president, Vice-President
vs.	versus
VT	Vermont
W	west, western
WA	Washington; Western Air Lines, Inc.
WE	Wien Air Alaska, Inc.
Wed.	Wednesday
WHA	World Hockey Association
WHL	World Hockey League
WI	Wisconsin
WV	West Virginia
WY	Wyoming
XY	Munz Northern Airlines, Inc.
YMCA	Young Men's Christian Association
YWCA	Young Women's Christian Association
Z	Zone
ZV	Air Midwest

ACKNOWLEDGEMENTS

In the course of our effort to research and assemble the material for the ENCYCLOPEDIA, we have had the help and cooperation of individuals and organizations, to whom we owe a debt of gratitude. We would like to take this opportunity to extend our thanks and appreciation to each and all for their help and concern and our apologies to those whom we have repeatedly bothered with requests and demands in the name of thoroughness and perfection. Special thanks are extended to the American Automobile Association and Ms. K. E. Simmons, Manager of Production Services in the Natl. Travel Dept. for their kind permission to make use of their maps and extensive services. We are also grateful for the cooperation of the following contributors: Louise A. Morris, Librarian, Dept. of Planning and Urban Renewal, Akron, OH; Mary Catherine Norviel, Administrative Asst. of Visitor's Division, Convention and Visitor's Center, and Sandra Brown, Asst. to the Mayor, Albuquerque, NM; John Q. Ward, Administrative Analyst, City Manager's Office, Amarillo, TX; James L. Wilson, Associate Planner, and Jim Wilson, Photographer, Planning and Comm. Development, Alexandria, VA; James A. Kelly, Director, Bureau of Planning, Allentown, PA; Linda R. Bell, Director, Visitor Promotions and Services, Anchorage, AK; Janice Williams, Administrative Intern, Ann Arbor, MI; Jeff Wolfskill, Arlington, TX; Jocelyn Ross, Director of Research, City Hall, Dorthy Carr, Deputy Director, Mayor's Office of Communications, and Jaci Morris, Chamber of Commerce, Atlanta, GA; Jan Hilton, Administrative Asst., City Manager's Office, Austin, TX; Mayor Fred H. Hood, Aurora, CO; Susan Wright, Mayor's office, Baltimore, MD; Myrtle Corgey, City Clerk, and Jim Wright, Manager of Communications, Chamber of Commerce, Baton Rouge, LA; Forrest A. Craven, Acting City Manager, Berkeley, CA; Benita E. Hagen, Manager of Information Services, Chamber of Commerce, Birmingham, AL; Historical Collections, Bridgeport Public Library, Bridgeport, CT; Mayor Richard R. Eardly, and Leon M. Grisham, Administrative Asst., Boise, ID; Mayor Kevin H. White, and Martha G. King, Special Asst. to the Mayor, Boston, MA; Mayor James D. Griffin, and Beth Abbott, Dept. of Comm. Development, Buffalo, NY; John Roger Boothe, Head of Urban Design, Cambridge, MA; Earl V. Gholston, Comm. Planner, Dept. of Planning and Zoning, Canton, OH; Candace Marshall, Administrative Asst., City Manager's Office, Charlotte, NC; Mayor Charles A. Rose, and the Convention and Visitor's Bureau, Chattanooga, TN; James N. Bradshaw, Information Planner, Chesapeake, VA; Mayor Jane Byrne, and Owen J. Doughterty, Press Aide to the Mayor, Chicago, IL; Paul L. Wertheimer, Public Information Officer, City Hall, and William Donaldson, City Manager, Cincinnati, OH; Andrew M. Juniewicz, Press Secretary, Cleveland, OH; Sterling M. Campbell, Public Affairs Administrator, Colorado Springs, CO; Mayor Harry C. Jackson, and Merne H. Posey, Information and Research Specialist, Columbus, GA; Pamela R. Johnston, Dept. of Development, and Patty Miller, Mayor's office, Columbus, OH; Archie Walker, Asst. City Manager, and Jennifer L. Durham, Dept. Head, Information Services, City Hall, Corpus Christi, TX; Pamela G. Bonnell, Librarian, Research Library, and Robin T. Mercer, Administrative Asst., City Hall, Dallas, TX; Jayne Rolphes, Communications Specialist, City Manager's Office, Dayton, OH; Mayor W. H. McNichols, Jr., Denver, CO; Mayor Richard E. Olson, and Anne L. Slatterly, Chamber of Commerce, Des Moines, IA; Mayor Coleman A. Young, and James L. Graham, Press Secretary to the Mayor, Detroit, MI; Margarette Rollins, City Clerk, and Dawn H. Hall, Administrative Asst., Durham, NC; Dennis W. Hudacsko, Coordinator, Comm. Projects, Dept. of Comm. Development, Elizabeth, NJ; Mayor Thomas D. Westfall, Mayor Ray Salazar, Margie Ranc, Public Information Officer, Leon Metz, Executive Asst. to the Mayor, and Glenda Miles, Research and Records Manager, El Paso, TX; Mayor Louis S. Tullio, and Gene H. Eckerson, Communications Officer, Erie, PA; Mayor Russell G. Lloyd, Joan Marchand, Photographer, and Meribeth Richardt, Evansville, IN; Mayor Carleton Viveiros, and Denise Rankin, Mayor's Press Aide, Fall River, MA; Constance W. Hoffman, Asst. City Manager, Ft. Lauderdale, FL; Ladona Huntly, Public Affairs Officer, and Larry Wardlaw, Asst. Public Affairs Officer, Ft. Wayne, IN; Vernell Sturns, Asst. City Manager, and Nat O'Day, Planning Dept., Fort Worth, TX; Keith Johnson, Administrative Asst., Fremont, CA; Mayor Daniel K. Whitehurst, and Rose Fisher, Chamber of Commerce, Fresno, CA; Gwen Wiesner, Administrative Services Director, Garden Grove, CA; P. A. Williams, Director, Economic Development and Public Information, Garland, TX; Leland T. Jones, Executive Secretary, Gary, IN; Len Tehrrien, Glendale, CA; James H. Knack, Planning Director, Emaline Peck, Mayor's Office, and Gary L. Carey, Planner I, Grand Rapids, MI; Chris Huff, Land Use Planner, and Stephen E. McIlwain, City Attorney, Hammond, IN; Diane Hughes, Hampton, VA; Theodore A. Brindamour, Division Engineer, Dept. of Public Works, Wendy Rambach Moore, Director of Communications, Convention and Visitor's Bureau, and Charles Norwood, Public Information Supervisor, CT Dept. of Commerce, Hartford, CT; James Chandler, City Manager, Hollywood, FL; Robert Mumby, Research Analyst, Office of Information and Complaints, V. G. "Jerry" Panzo, Director of Information Services, Abe Poepoe, Chief of Information, Mayor's Office, and Hawaii Visitor's Bureau, Honolulu, HI; Mayor Ronald R. Pattinson, and William G. Reed, Public Information Officer, Office of Public Information, Huntington Beach, CA; Mayor Jim McConn, and Jim Young, Asst. Director, Communications Division, Houston, TX; Tom Dozier, Director, City Planning Commission, and Mayor Joe W. Davis, Huntsville, AL; Donna Ullrich-Eaton, Information Specialist, and Carolyn Mainey, Independence, MO; Donna J. Marsham, Comm. Information Dept., Chambor of Commerce, Indianapolis, IN; the City News Bureau, Jacksonville, FL; Jerome M. Hiller, Planning Director, Division of Planning, and Lena Consonni, Jersey City, NJ; Mayor John Reardon, Dean Katerndahl, Director, Dept. of Economic Development, and Jan Hart, Kansas City, KS; Richard Lovett, Director, Dept. of Public Information, Kansas City, MO; Dr. Patricia G. Ball, Director, Public Affairs, Knoxville, TN; Regina M. March, Secretary to the City Administrator, Lakewood, CO; Steven E. Dougan, Administrative Asst., Mayor's Office, Don Hanna, Planning Director, and the Michigan Travel Commission, Lansing, MI; Donn Blake, Special Projects Coordinator, Las Vegas, NV; Carolyn H. Saylor, Asst. Director, Convention Bureau, Lexington, KY; Mayor Helen G. Boosalis, and Connie Guilliaume, Secretary, Mayor's Office, Lincoln, NE; Mayor Webb Hubbell, Vicki Bufford, Information Service Dept., Chamber of Commerce, and Sherry Bain, Little Rock, AR; John J. Nagy, Planning Director, and Sharon E. Falk, Mayor's Office, Livonia, MI; John E. Dever, City Manager, and Robert C. Creighton,

Asst. City Manager, Long Beach, CA; Mayor William Stansbury, James E. Reed, Asst. Director of Public Affairs, Mayor's Office, Michael H. Starks, News Bureau Director, and Madonna Douglas, Louisville, KY; Grey Lewis, Asst. Manager, Chamber of Commerce, and Mayor Dirk West, Lubbock, TX; Glenda Ferrell, Director of Better Business and Research, Chamber of Commerce, Macon, GA; Mayor Paul R. Soglin, and Ann Waidelich, Librarian, Municipal Reference Service, Madison, WI; Michael C. Ritz, Director, Planning and Development, and Randa Lipman, Sales Asst./Public Information Specialist, Convention and Visitor's Bureau, Memphis, TN; Tanya Collins, Public Information Coordinator, Mesa, AZ; Joseph Grassie, City Manager, and Miami-Metro Dept. of Commerce, Miami, FL; Patricia Stawicki, Mayor's Office, and Michael J. Kremar, Research Analyst-Legislative Reference Bureau, Milwaukee, WI; Mayor Albert J. Hofstede, Oliver Byrum, Planning Director, and Jennifer Deakyne, Public Information Office, Minneapolis, MN; Mayor Lambert C. Mims, Mobile, AL; Mayor Emory Folmar, and Rhonda L. Zbinden, Director, Convention and Visitor's Services, Montgomery, AL; Mayor Richard Fulton, Nashville, TN; Carmen A. Baise, Deputy Mayor, Newark, NJ; Mayor John A. Markey, New Bedford, MA; Elaine Noe, Director, Visitor's and Convention Bureau, New Haven, CT; J. Handelman, Information Director, and Tana M. Adde, Public Information Office, New Orleans, LA; Hal H. Holker, Director, Dept. of Development, Newport News, VA; Mrs. Kline, Mayor's Action Office, NY State Office of General Services, Promotion and Public Affairs, and Convention and Visitor's Bureau, New York City, NY; Susan Gallagher, Public Communications Coordinator, Dept. of Conventions and Marketing, Norfolk, VA; Mayor Lionel J. Wilson, Oakland, CA; James J. Cook, City Manager, Oklahoma City, OK; Mayor Al Veys, and Mr. Douglas, Omaha, NE; Grace A. Chewning, City Clerk, and Phyllis D. Freedman, Librarian, Municipal Reference Library, Orlando, FL; Peter Apanel, Pasadena, CA; Bettie Fife, Director, Comm. Affairs, Pasadena, TX; Norma Harrison, Public Information Officer, Mayor's Office, Paterson, NJ; Mrs. Woods, Peoria, IL; John Moore, Information Officer, Philadelphia, PA; Julie Birch, Management Asst., City Manager's Office, Phoenix, AZ; Mayor Richard S. Caliguiri, Pittsburgh, PA; Mayor Neil Goldschmidt, and Dan Churchill, Administrative Asst., Mayor's office, Portland, OR; Robert P. Creecy, Management Analyst, Portsmouth, VA; Joseph A. Chrostowski, City Historian, Archives, and Patrick J. Conley, Administrative Asst. to the Mayor, Providence, RI; Jaycee P. Maret, Director, Research and Public Information Office, Raleigh, NC; William J. Leidinger, City Manager, Frank J. McNally, Asst. to the Mayor, and Met. Richmond Chamber of Commerce, Richmond, VA; Fritz Zimmer, Administrative Intern, City Manager's Office, Riverside, CA; Dr. Noel C. Taylor, Mayor, and Elizabeth A. Stahl, Economic Developer/Public Information Officer, City Manager's Office, Roanoke, VA; Constance B. James, Director, Public Information, City Manager's Office, Rochester, NY; Judy Porter, Director of Tourism, and the Convention and Visitor's Bureau, Sacramento, CA; Mayor James F. Conway, St. Louis, MO; Mayor George Latimer, and Peg O'Keefe, Director of Public Information, St. Paul, MN; Jennifer Fogle, Director, Information Services, Chamber of Commerce, St. Petersburg, FL; Mayor Ted L. Wilson, and John D. Hushey, Administrative Asst. to the Mayor, Salt Lake City, UT; Mayor Lila Cockrell, and Nancy Brennan, Public Information Officer, Convention and Visitor's Bureau, San Antonio, TX; Marshall W. Julian, City Administrator, and Thelma Press, Executive Director, Mayor's Council for Intl. Friendship and Goodwill, San Bernardino, CA; Lauren Schlau, Research Projects Manager, Convention and Visitor's Bureau, and George Story, Director, Citizen's Assistance and Information Dept., San Diego, CA; S. Dale Hess, Asst. General Manager, and Nancy L. Henry, Director, Visitor Services, Convention and Visitor's Bureau, San Francisco, CA; Stanley Z. Twardus, Director, Economic Development, San Jose, CA; Bruce Spragg, City Manager, and Janice Guy, City Council Clerk, Santa Ana, CA; Mike Vaquer, Public Information Officer, Met. Planning Commission, Savannah, GA; Shelly Yapp, Acting Director, Allen Loverud and Al Crosetti, Planning Analysts, Executive Dept., Office of Policy Planning, Seattle, WA; Mayor W.T. Hanna Jr., and Miss Cooper, Mayor's Secretary, Shreveport, LA; James G. Masters, Asst. City Attorney, Michael J. Danch, Landscape Architect, St. Joseph Co. Area Plan Commission, Hildy L. Kingma, Research Associate, Comm. Development Program, City Hall, and Steve Queior, Research Director, Chamber of Commerce, South Bend, IN; Vaughn P. Call, Manager, City Plan Commission, and Michael Carlson, Mayor's Asst., Spokane, WA; Donald H. Kelly, City Clerk, and Sheryl L. Hymer, Administrative Clerk, City Clerk's Office, Springfield, MO; Barbara Foreman, Mayor's Executive Aide, Stamford, CT; Mayor Arnold I. Rue, Stockton, CA; Judy V. Bulk, Administrative Asst., Comm. Relations, Sunnyvale, CA; John E. Cerio, Mayor's Executive Asst., Syracuse, NY; Patricia A. Sias, Historic Preservation Officer, Comm. Development Dept., Tacoma, WA; Roger Wehling, City Planner, and Frances Henriquez, City Clerk's Office, Tampa, FL; Walter Kane, City Manager, and Ted Reeves, Public Information Director, Toledo, OH; Sherry Nelson, City Clerk, and Claire Gall, Secretary to the Mayor, Torrance, CA; Judith M. Granat, A.I.C.P., Senior Planner, Dept. of Planning and Development, Trenton, NJ; James K. Koshmider, Administrative Asst. to the Mayor, Tuscon, AZ; Mrs. Roach, Mayor's Secretary, Tulsa, OK; Pamela M. Lingle, Asst. Public Information Officer, Municipal Center, Virginia Beach, VA; Mrs. Boewe, Mayor's Secretary, Warren, MI; Florence Tate, Press Secretary to the Mayor, Dwight S. Gropp, Executive Secretary, Executive Office, and James O. Gibson, Asst. City Administrator, Planning and Development, Washington, D.C.; Mayor Edward Bergin, Waterbury, CT; David Furnas, Public Affairs Director, City Hall, William Clark Ellington, Jr., City Historian, and the Wichita Police Dept., Wichita, KS; Gary Smith, Manager, Convention and Visitor's Bureau, Chamber of Commerce, Winston-Salem, NC; Francis J. McGrath, City Manager, Worcester, MA; John Zakiasl, Mayor's Asst., Yonkers, NY; Jean Landers, Mayor's Secretary, Youngstown, OH; Ed Demoney, and Theodore E. Allison, Secretary, Board of Governors of the Federal Reserve Board; the U.S. Dept. of Labor, Bureau of Labor Statistics; the Federal Communications Commission; the Natl. Oceanic and Atmospheric Administration; and the Natl. Center for Education Statistics.

                                                                                                                                                                     The Editors

INDEX